Dedication

This volume is dedicated to the heart health of women
for generations to come, as personified by the granddaughters of Dr Nanette Wenger
Abigail Jane Beaird and Molly Charlotte Beaird
Katherine Grace Wiatrak and Juliette Faye Wiatrak

and of the current generation, as personified by the mother of Dr Peter Collins
Alice Collins

WOMEN & HEART DISEASE
Second edition

Edited by

Nanette Kass Wenger
Professor of Medicine (Cardiology)
Emory University School of Medicine
Chief of Cardiology
Grady Memorial Hospital
Consultant
Emory Heart and Vascular Center
Atlanta, Georgia, USA

and

Peter Collins
Professor of Clinical Cardiology
Department of Cardiac Medicine
National Heart and Lung Institute
Faculty of Medicine
Imperial College of Science, Technology and Medicine
London, UK

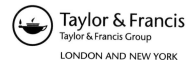
Taylor & Francis
Taylor & Francis Group

LONDON AND NEW YORK

© 2005 Taylor & Francis, an imprint of the Taylor & Francis Group

First published in the United Kingdom in 2005
by Taylor & Francis,
an imprint of the Taylor & Francis Group,
2 Park Square, Milton Park
Abingdon, Oxon OX14 4RN, UK

Tel.:   +44 (0) 20 7017 6000
Fax.:   +44 (0) 20 7017 6699
Email: info.medicine@tandf.co.uk
Website: http://www.tandf.co.uk/medicine

British Library Cataloguing in Publication Data

Data available on application

Library of Congress Cataloging-in-Publication Data

Data available on application

ISBN 1-84184-288-5

Distributed in North and South America by

Taylor & Francis
2000 NW Corporate Blvd
Boca Raton, FL 33431, USA

Within Continental USA
Tel.: 800 272 7737; Fax.: 800 374 3401
Outside Continental USA
Tel.: 561 994 0555; Fax.: 561 361 6018
E-mail: orders@crcpress.com

Distributed in the rest of the world by
Thomson Publishing Services
Cheriton House
North Way
Andover, Hampshire SP10 5BE, UK
Tel.: +44 (0) 1264 332424
E-mail: salesorder.tandf@thomsonpublishingservices.co.uk

Composition by Scribe Design Ltd, Ashford, Kent, UK
Printed and bound by Antony Rowe Ltd., Chippenham, Wiltshire, UK

Contents

List of contributors

T.F.L. Adams RN BSN
Mayo Clinic
200 First Street SW
Rochester, MN 55905
USA

D.E. Anderson PhD
Laboratory of Cardiovascular Science
National Institute on Aging
5600 Nathan Shock Blvd
Baltimore, MD 21224
USA

M.A.F. Apacible RN BSN
School of Nursing
School of Medicine
University of California San Francisco
2 Koret Way, N631
San Francisco, CA 94143
USA

C.M. Apovian MD
Director, Center for Nutrition and Weight
   Management
Boston Medical Center
Associate Professor of Medicine
Boston University School of Medicine
Boston Medical Center
Robinson Building
88 E. Newton Street
Boston, MA 02118
USA

C.N. Bairey Merz MD
Medical Director
Division of Cardiology
Cedars-Sinai Research Institute
Cedars-Sinai Medical Center
UCLA School of Medicine
444 S. San Vicente Blvd
Los Angeles, CA 90048
USA

E. Barrett-Connor MD
Professor and Chief, Division of Epidemiology
Department of Family and Preventive Medicine
School of Medicine
University of California San Diego
9500 Gilman Drive
La Jolla, CA 92093
USA

S.S. Bassuk ScD
Division of Preventive Medicine
Brigham & Women's Hospital
900 Commonwealth Avenue East
Boston, MA 02215
USA

D.G. Beevers MD
University Department of Medicine
City Hospital
Birmingham B18 7QH
UK

V.A. Bittner MD MSPH
Professor of Medicine
Division of Cardiovascular Disease
University of Alabama at Birmingham
703 19th Street South
Birmingham, AL 35294
USA

J. Bogousslavsky MD
Chief, Department of Neurology
Centre Hospitalier Universitaire Vaudois
CH-1011 Lausanne
Switzerland

D. Bott-Kitslaar RN MSN
Mayo Clinic
200 First Street SW
Rochester, MN 55905
USA

C.S. Broberg MD
Fellow, Adult Congenital Heart Disease Unit
Royal Brompton Hospital
Sydney Street
London SW3 6NP
UK

J. Chambers MD
Cardiothoracic Unit
Guy's and St Thomas' Hospital
Lambeth Palace Road
London SE1 7EH
UK

M.A. Chesney PhD
Deputy Director
National Center for Complementary and
    Alternative Medicine
National Institutes of Health
31 Center Drive
Bethesda, MD 20892
USA

K. Chinnaiyan MD
Beaumont Health Center
Preventive Cardiology
4949 Coolidge Highway
Royal Oak, MI 48073
USA

P. Collins MA MD (Cantab)
Professor of Clinical Cardiology
Department of Cardiac Medicine
National Heart and Lung Institute
Faculty of Medicine
Imperial College of Science, Technology and
    Medicine
Dovehouse Street
London SW3 6LY
UK

R. Costa MD
Cardiovascular Research Foundation
55 E. 59th Street
New York, NY 10022
USA

E. Critea MD
Cardiovascular Research Foundation
55 E. 59th Street
New York, NY 10022
USA

M. Cushman MD MSc
Associate Professor of Medicine and Pathology
University of Vermont/Fletcher Allen Health Care
208 South Park Drive
Colchester, VT 05446
USA

S. Daoud MD
University of Wisconsin
Madison, WI 53792
USA

D. Détaint MD
Division of Cardiovascular Disease and Internal
    Medicine
Mayo Clinic
200 1st Street SW
Rochester, MN 55905
USA

F.H. Edwards MD
Professor of Surgery
Chief, Division of Cardiothoracic Surgery
University of Florida/Shands Jacksonville
655 W. 8th Street
Jacksonville, FL 32209
USA

M. Enriquez-Sarano MD
Division of Cardiovascular Disease and Internal
  Medicine
Mayo Clinic
200 1st Street SW
Rochester, MN 55905
USA

W. Foster MD
University Department of Medicine
City Hospital
Birmingham B18 7QH
UK

A. Fowler BS
Beaumont Health Center
Preventive Cardiology
4949 Coolidge Highway
Royal Oak, MI 48073
USA

B.A. Franklin PhD
Director, Cardiac Rehabilitation and Exercise
  Laboratories
Beaumont Health Center
Preventive Cardiology
4949 Coolidge Highway
Royal Oak, MI 48073
USA

E.S.S. Froelicher RN MA PhD
Professor of Physiological Nursing
School of Nursing
Department of Epidemiology and Biostatistics
School of Medicine
University of California San Francisco
2 Koret Way, N631
San Francisco, CA 94143
USA

M.A. Gatzoulis MD PhD
Director, Adult Congenital Heart Disease Unit
Royal Brompton Hospital
Sydney Street
London SW3 6NP
UK

J.K. Ghali MD
Professor of Medicine
Section of Cardiology
Department of Internal Medicine
Louisiana State University Health Sciences Center
Shreveport, LA 71130
USA

R.J. Gibbons MD
Professor of Medicine
Mayo Clinic College of Medicine
200 First Street SW
Rochester, MN 55905
USA

P. Hardiman MBBS MD
Senior Lecturer
Department of Obstetrics and Gynaecology
Royal Free and University College Medical School
Rowland Hill Street
London NW3 2PF
UK

D. Hasdai MD
Associate Professor of Cardiology
Sackler Faculty of Medicine
Tel Aviv University
Director, Coronary Care Unit
Rabin Medical Center
Beilinson Campus
Petah Tikva 49100
Israel

S.N. Hayes MD
Director, Mayo Clinic Women's Health Clinic
200 First Street SW
Rochester, MN 55905
USA

D.M. Herrington MD MHS
Wake Forest University School of Medicine
Medical Center Blvd
Winston-Salem, NC 27157
USA

R.H. Hongo MD
Cardiac Electrophysiology Section
University of California San Francisco
500 Parnassus Avenue
San Francisco, CA 94121
USA

S.A. Hunt MD
Professor of Cardiovascular Medicine
Stanford University Medical Center
300 Pasteur Drive
Palo Alto, CA 94305
USA

G. Jackson MD
Consultant Cardiologist
Cardiac Department
Guy's and St. Thomas' Hospitals
Lambeth Palace Road
London SE1 7EH
UK

P.R. James MD BSc
Consultant Cardiologist
Cardiac Unit
Royal Sussex County Hospital
Eastern Road
Brighton BN2 5BE
UK

A. John MD PhD
Cardiovascular Magnetic Resonance Unit
Royal Brompton Hospital
Sydney Street
London SW3 6NP
UK

A.M. Kanaya MD
Assistant Professor of Medicine
Division of General Internal Medicine
Women's Health Clinical Research Center
University of California
San Francisco, CA 94143
USA

J.C. Kaski MD DSc
Professor of Cardiovascular Science
Coronary Artery Disease Research Unit
Department of Cardiological Sciences
St George's Hospital Medical School
Cranmer Terrace
London SW17 0RE
UK

K.-T. Khaw MBBChir
Professor of Clinical Gerontology
University of Cambridge School of Clinical
    Medicine
Box 251, Addenbrooke's Hospital
Cambridge CB2 2QQ
UK

D.W. Kitzman MD
Professor of Medicine – Cardiology and Geriatrics
Director of Echocardiography
Section of Cardiology
Wake Forest University School of Medicine
Medical Center Blvd
Winston-Salem, NC 27157
USA

K. Lakhani MSc
Research Fellow
Department of Obstetrics and Gynaecology
Royal Free and University College Medical School
Rowland Hill Street
London NW3 2PF
UK

M.J. Landzberg MD
Director, Boston Adult Congenital Heart and
    Pulmonary Hypertension Group
Department of Cardiology
Children's Hospital and Brigham and Women's
    Hospital
300 Longwood Avenue
Boston, MA 02115
USA

A.J. Lansky MD
Cardiovascular Research Foundation
55 E. 59th Street
New York, NY 10022
USA

G.Y.H. Lip MD
Consultant Cardiologist and Professor of
    Cardiovascular Medicine
Director, Haemostasis, Thrombosis and Vascular
    Biology Unit
University Department of Medicine
City Hospital
Birmingham B18 7QH
UK

A. Mahnke MD PhD
Cardiovascular Magnetic Resonance Unit
Royal Brompton Hospital
Sydney Street
London SW3 6NP
UK

J.E. Manson MD
Division of Preventive Medicine
Brigham & Women's Hospital
900 Commonwealth Avenue East
Boston, MA 02215
USA

K. Martin RN MS
Los Medanos College
2700 E. Leland Road
Pittsburg, CA 94565
USA

B.P. McClain MS
Wake Forest University School of Medicine
Medical Center Blvd
Winston-Salem, NC 27157
USA

M.E. McDonnell MD
Section of Endocrinology
Boston Medical Center
Evans Building 201
88 E. Newton Street
Boston, MA 02118
USA

L. Mehta MD
Beaumont Health Center
Preventive Cardiology
4949 Coolidge Highway
Royal Oak, MI 48073
USA

M.A. Mendelson MD
Director, Heart Disease and Pregnancy Program
Division of Cardiology
Northwestern Medical Faculty Foundation
201 E. Huron Street
Chicago, IL 60611
USA

A.P. Miller MD
Chief Fellow in Cardiology
Vascular Biology and Hypertension Program
Division of Cardiovascular Disease
University of Alabama at Birmingham
703 19th Street South
Birmingham, AL 35294
USA

T.D. Miller MD
Professor of Medicine
Mayo Clinic College of Medicine
200 First Street SW
Rochester, MN 55905
USA

D.C. Morris MD
Director
Emory Heart Center
1365 Clifton Rd NE
Atlanta, GA 30322
USA

C.M. Oakley MD
Professor (Emeritus) of Clinical Cardiology
Imperial College School of Medicine
Hammersmith Hospital
London W12 0HS
UK

S. Oparil MD
Professor of Medicine, Physiology and Biophysics
Director, Vascular Biology and Hypertension
  Program
University of Alabama at Birmingham
703 19th Street South
Birmingham, AL 35294
USA

K. Orth-Gomér MD PhD
Karolinska Institute
Department of Public Health Sciences
Division of Psychosocial Factors and Health
SE-171 77 Stockholm
Sweden

B. Piechowski-Jóźwiak MD
Assistant, Department of Neurology
The Medical University of Warsaw, Poland
Fellow, Department of Neurology
Centre Hospitalier Universitaire Vaudois
CH-1011 Lausanne
Switzerland

I.L. Piña MD
Professor of Medicine
Cardiology Division and Section of Heart Failure
  and Transplantation
Case Western Reserve University
11100 Euclid Avenue
Cleveland, OH 44106
USA

J.T. Powell MD PhD
Consultant Vascular Surgeon
Department of Vascular Surgery
Imperial College
St Dunstan's Road
London W6 8RP
UK

S. Prasad BSc MD
Consultant Cardiologist
Cardiovascular Magnetic Resonance Unit
Royal Brompton Hospital
Sydney Street
London SW3 6NP
UK

P. Raggi MD
Professor of Cardiology
Tulane University School of Medicine
1430 Tulane Avenue
New Orleans, LA 70112
USA

T. Ribbons MBChB
Department of Vascular Surgery
Imperial College
St Dunstan's Road
London W6 8RP
UK

A. Rosengren MD
Sahlgrenska University/Ostra
SE-416 85 Göteborg
Sweden

M.M. Scheinman MD
University of California San Francisco
500 Parnassus Avenue
San Francisco, CA 94121
USA

J.B. Schwartz MD
Director of Research
Jewish Home of San Francisco
Clinical Professor of Medicine, Cardiology and
  Clinical Pharmacology
University of California San Francisco
302 Silver Avenue
San Francisco, CA 94112
USA

S.B. Shah MD
Assistant Professor of Medicine and Radiology
Cardiology Unit
University of Rochester
Rochester, NY 14642
USA

L.J. Shaw PhD
Director of Outcomes Research
Atlanta Cardiovascular Research Institute
5665 Peachtree Dunwoody Road NE
Atlanta, GA 30342
USA

P.J. Steer BSc MBBS MD
Professor of Obstetrics
Head, High-risk Obstetrics Unit
Chelsea and Westminster Hospital
369 Fulham Road
London SW10 9NH
UK

J.C. Stevenson MB BS
Imperial College London
Royal Brompton Hospital
Sydney Street
London SW3 6NP
UK

A.J. Tajik MD
Division of Cardiovascular Disease and Internal
    Medicine
Mayo Clinic
200 1st Street SW
Rochester, MN 55905
USA

V. Vaccarino MD PhD
Department of Medicine
Division of Cardiology
Emory Center for Outcomes Research
Emory University School of Medicine
1256 Briarcliff Road
Atlanta, GA 30322
USA

D.S. Wald MA MD
Clinical Research Fellow and Specialist Registrar in
    Cardiology
Wolfson Institute of Preventive Medicine
University of London
Charterhouse Square
London EC1M 6BQ
UK

Patricia Ward MA
Cardiovascular Research Foundation
55 E. 59th Street
New York, NY 10022
USA

N.J. Weissman MD
Associate Professor of Medicine
Georgetown University Director
Cardiac Ultrasound and Ultrasound Care Labs
Washington Hospital Center
110 Irving Street NW
Washington, DC 20010
USA

N.K. Wenger MD
Professor of Medicine (Cardiology)
Emory University School of Medicine
Chief of Cardiology
Grady Memorial Hospital
Consultant, Emory Heart and Vascular Center
Faculty Office Building
49 Jesse Hill Jr. Drive SE
Atlanta, GA 30303
USA

P.W.F. Wilson MD
Program Director GCRC
Department of Endocrinology, Diabetes, and
    Medical Genetics
Medical University of South Carolina
96 Jonathan Lucas St
Charleston, SC 29425
USA

S.M. Yentis BSc MBBS MD
Consultant Anaesthetist
Magill Department of Anaesthesia, Intensive Care
    and Pain Management
Chelsea and Westminster Hospital
369 Fulham Road
London SW10 9NH
UK

Introduction

Women and heart disease

'You've Come a Long Way, Baby'[*][1]

Information about coronary heart disease (CHD) and cardiovascular disease in women is rapidly escalating, likely as a component of the concept of sex-specific medicine during the past decade. Unequivocally, the landmark 2001 Institute of Medicine report *Exploring the Biological Contributions to Human Health: Does Sex Matter?*[2] has been the beacon for better understanding of the differences in human diseases between the sexes and translation of these differences into clinical practice. We are beginning to see the reversal of the traditional under-representation of women in clinical research studies, and specifically, in research studies on the diagnosis and treatment of CHD.[3,4] Many of the newer therapies and procedures for CHD, albeit with continuing under-representation of women, have increasingly reported sex-specific clinical trial data. New requirements by regulatory agencies both in the US and overseas promise to provide sex-specific data on pharmacologic therapy for women.

Public information and education about women and heart disease has also escalated. This appears exceedingly important as most women report receiving health information from magazines and other media outlets.[5] In April 2003, the cover story for *TIME* magazine highlighted the issue of women and heart disease, a major reversal in the focus of cardiovascular reporting. The year 2004 saw major advances in the US, beginning with the National Heart, Lung, and Blood Institute's Heart Truth Campaign, a national effort to highlight that the female heart is vulnerable to heart disease. Concomitantly, the American Heart Association's Red Dress Campaign, a public education venture being replicated in many nations throughout the world, aims to reverse the erroneous perception that heart disease is predominantly a male problem. The importance of such education is that unless women consider coronary disease to be part of their illness experience, they are unlikely to heed preventive messages across the lifespan or to respond appropriately to the chest pain symptoms of CHD.

The last several years has witnessed the publication of clinical trials demonstrating that menopausal hormone therapy fails to provide cardiac protection for women, and conversely has been associated with specific risk. Those data have refocused attention on lifestyle and pharmacologic interventions documented to be effective for the prevention of cardiovascular and coronary heart disease in women. The American Heart Association in 2004 released *Evidence-based Guidelines for Cardiovascular Disease Prevention in Women*.[6] This provides the woman the ability, in cooperation with her treating physician, to define her personal cardiovascular risk and undertake appropriate interventions. It also offers the opportunity to refocus patterns of clinical practice to optimize the heart health of women.

In this second edition of *Women and Heart Disease*, we present contributions from international leaders in women's heart health and disease, offering a concise and well-referenced resource to the practicing physician that incorporates the latest available information. It is this emerging new information about

---

*'You've Come a Long Way, Baby' is a registered trademark of Philip Morris, Inc.

cardiovascular disease in women, and its application in daily clinical practice, that is likely to improve clinical cardiovascular outcomes for women.

The editors acknowledge with gratitude the spectacular chapter authors for their scholarly comprehensive reviews and timely submission of the relevant information. Appreciation as well to Alan Burgess, Senior Publisher; Margaret Smart, Senior Administrative Assistant; Giovanna Ceroni, former Production Editor; and Pam Lancaster, Production Editor from the publishing office of Taylor & Francis Medical Books, for their enthusiasm, encouragement, and superb organizational skills in the development of this volume. Special commendation to Julia C. Wright, Administrative Assistant to Dr

Wenger, for her painstaking and meticulous incorporation of the editorial changes and for facilitating correspondence with the chapter authors. We acknowledge as well the wonderful women worldwide who were participants in the registries, case series, and clinical trials that enabled delineation of the characteristics of heart disease specific to women. As noted by the Society for Women's Health Research, there are 'Some Things Only a Woman Can Do™'[7] and such participation by women in clinical research studies is a pivotal contribution.

Nanette Kass Wenger MD
Peter Collins MD

References

1. Wenger MD. You've Come a Long Way, Baby. Cardiovascular health and disease in women: problems and prospects. *Circulation* 2004; **109**:558–60.
2. Wizemann TM, Pardue M-L (eds). *Exploring the Biological Contributions to Human Health. Does Sex Matter?* Committee on Understanding the Biology of Sex and Gender Differences. Board on Health Sciences Policy, Institute of Medicine. Washington, DC: National Academy Press, 2001.
3. Agency for Healthcare Research and Quality. *Results of Systematic Review of Research on Diagnosis and Treatment of Coronary Heart Disease in Women.* Evidence Report/Technology Assessment No. 80. AHRQ Pub. No. 03-E034. Rockville, MD: US Department of Health and Human Services, Public Health Services, May 2003.
4. Agency for Healthcare Research and Quality. *Diagnosis and Treatment of Coronary Heart Disease in Women: Systematic Reviews of Evidence on Selected Topics.* Evidence Report/Technology Assessment No. 81. AHRQ Pub. No. 03-E036. Rockville, MD: US Department of Health and Human Services, Public Health Services, May 2003.
5. Mosca L, Ferris A, Fabunmi R, Robertson RM. Tracking women's awareness of heart disease. An American Heart Association National Study. *Circulation* 2004; **109**:573–9.
6. Mosca L, Appel LJ, Benjamin EJ, et al. American Heart Association. Evidence-based guidelines for cardiovascular disease prevention in women. Expert Panel/Writing Group. *Circulation* 2004; **109**:672–92.
7. www.womancando.org [accessed September 1, 2004].

Part 1
Coronary Heart Disease

1

Epidemiology of coronary heart disease in women

Kay-Tee Khaw

Introduction

Coronary heart disease (CHD) is the leading cause of death and a major cause of disability in industrialized countries; it is rapidly also becoming the leading cause of death in nonindustrialized countries worldwide. While the male excess in CHD is well recognized, CHD is also the leading cause of death in women in most industrialized countries.

Definitions

The World Health Organization (WHO) defines CHD, or ischemic heart disease, as 'the cardiac disability, acute or chronic, arising from reduction or arrest of blood supply to the myocardium in association with disease processes in the coronary arterial system'. These processes include atherosclerosis of the coronary arteries and related phenomena such as atheromatous plaque rupture and thrombosis. CHD is manifest clinically as angina pectoris (reversible chest pain on effort), myocardial infarction (chest pain, serial electrocardiographic changes, and raised serum cardiac muscle enzyme levels), cardiac failure, arrhythmias and/or sudden death, usually related to acute arrhythmias.[1]

Most comparisons using routinely collected vital statistics rely on mortality rates for CHD. These have some disadvantages including issues of diagnostic reliability. While morbidity and disability due to CHD are also of major concern, few other routine sources are likely to provide satisfactory data. A large proportion of persons sustaining a myocardial infarction either die suddenly before reaching hospital or are cared for at home; hospital admission or discharge statistics depend on admission policies and accessibility, which vary enormously from country to country and over time. Where community myocardial infarction registers have been specially set up, as with the WHO MONICA (Monitoring Trends and Determinants in Cardiovascular Disease) studies,[2] these have shown that mortality statistics are closely correlated with incidence.

Case fatality

There has been much debate about whether case fatality from acute myocardial infarction differs in women compared with men. Hospital-based data have been inconclusive, but some analyses have indicated that women have a worse prognosis following acute myocardial infarction compared with men. However, only about 20% of coronary deaths occur in hospital and there is no convincing evidence for worse outcome in women from population-based data. The WHO community-based MONICA studies from 38 populations have reported average 28-day case fatality for acute myocardial infarction of about 50%, broadly similar in women and men.[1,2] Of those dying within 28 days, only between 30 and 40% were ever hospitalized. Men were more likely to die suddenly, both within 1 hour and within 24 hours of

Table 1.1   Coronary heart disease (CHD) as a percentage of all deaths in women and men at different ages in England and Wales and the US[3,4]

	Total number of CHD deaths, all ages	All	Percentage of deaths in age group (years)			
			45–55	55–64	65–74	75+
England and Wales 2002						
Women	46 129	16	7	11	17	18
Men	56 704	22	22	25	22	22
US 1999						
Women	262 391	22	10	15	18	26
Men	267 268	22	20	24	24	26

onset, compared with women. On average, 37% of deaths in men occurred within 1 hour compared with 30% of deaths in women. It is possible that the higher case fatality reported in women hospitalized for acute myocardial infarction compared with men in some studies may to some extent reflect women surviving long enough to be admitted to hospital before dying.

Mortality by age and sex

Table 1.1 shows the percentage of all deaths in women and men at different ages in England and Wales and the US.[3,4] Approximately a fifth of all deaths are due to CHD; the proportion is substantially greater in men compared with women between ages 45 and 74 years. Table 1.2 shows the percentages of all deaths in women due to CHD at all ages, and

compares this to the percentages for breast cancer and other reproductive cancers in England and Wales and the US. CHD deaths constitute the major proportion of all deaths.

Figure 1.1 shows mortality rates for CHD by age and sex in the UK and in the US and also the ratio in women compared with men. Rates rise sharply with increasing age in both sexes. One of the most striking features is the male excess for CHD. The sex difference is apparent throughout life, but most marked at younger ages, with the male:female ratio decreasing from about 3.5:1 in the US and 4.5:1 in the UK to 1.2:1 in the US and 1.5:1 in the UK at ages 75+. However, while the relative difference declines, the absolute difference in CHD rates between women and men actually increases with increasing age, particularly in the UK, since CHD rates increase with increasing age. There is no evidence of a differential sharp upturn at the time of menopause in women compared with men.

Table 1.2 Deaths among women in England and Wales 2002 and the US 1999[3,4]

	England and Wales 2002		US 1999	
	n	%	n	%
All causes	280 383	100	1 215 939	100
Coronary heart disease	59 560	21	262 391	22
Breast cancer	13 019	5	41 144	3
Uterine cancer	1358	<1	6468	<1
Cervical cancer	995	<1	4205	<1

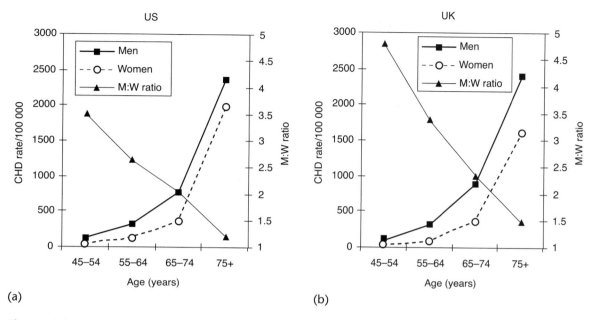

Figure 1.1
Coronary heart disease (CHD) mortality rates by sex and age group and ratio of CHD mortality in men compared with women in the US (a) and UK (b) 1999.[4]

International comparisons

Figure 1.2 shows age-standardized CHD mortality rates by sex for selected countries between 1999 and 2000.[4,5] The highest documented rates are now seen in countries in Eastern Europe. Additionally, many developing countries, of which Mauritius is shown as an example, now have rates higher than those of more industrialized countries such as those in Western Europe or the US. There is enormous international variation, with women in the highest rate countries having over tenfold the rates of women in Japan. While men show a consistent relative excess of CHD, there is a strong international correlation between rates in women and men; countries where men have high rates are also countries where women have high rates and women in the high rate countries have about sixfold the rate in Japanese men. Age-specific rates for an illustrative selection of countries shown in Fig. 1.3 indicate that the age-standardized comparisons reflect consistent differences over all age groups.

Time trends

Figure 1.4 shows time trends for selected countries from 1969 to 2001[4,5] and illustrates different patterns in these countries. The US and UK had the highest rates in 1968 and both have shown striking declines in three decades. Rates in Japan, low to start with, have continued to decline until 1996. In contrast, CHD rates in Mauritius, a developing country, have been increasing since the 1970s, with a continuing rise in women compared with men. The Russian Federation has shown the most striking patterns, with major sharp fluctuations in the 1990s, on a base of very high rates.

Figure 1.5 showing percentage changes for selected countries between 1989 and 1999[4,5] indicates the marked and divergent time trends for CHD in different countries even within a 10-year time period. While most Western European countries have shown marked declines in CHD mortality over the 10-year period, East European countries in contrast show marked rises. The profound temporal trends also indicate that the major determinants of mortality

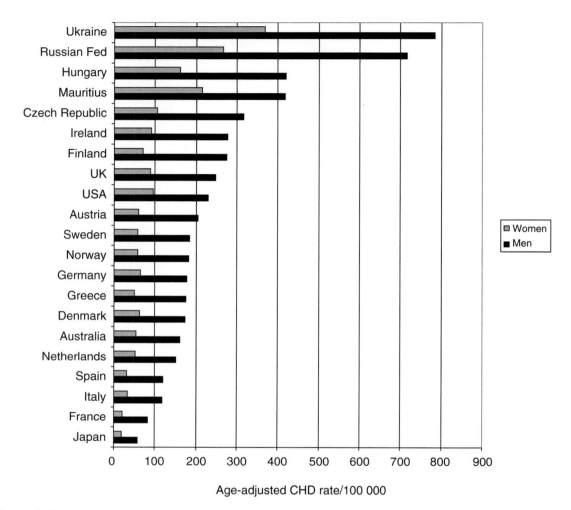

Figure 1.2
Age-adjusted coronary heart disease (CHD) rates for women and men aged 35–74 years in selected countries, 1999–2000.[4,5]

rates are likely to be potentially modifiable environmental factors rather than genetic susceptibility. Further evidence for this is apparent from migrant studies. Japanese women living in the US have twice the CHD rates of Japanese women in Japan. There has been much discussion about the decline in CHD mortality in countries such as the US and how far this may be due to improved case fatality (possibly due to improved medical therapy and/or changing severity of disease) or to decline in incidence. The WHO MONICA studies are designed to study the impact of

recent therapies on case fatality and the impact of coronary risk factors on event rates; the evidence to date indicates that changes in mortality reflect to a large extent changes in incidence.

In marked contrast to previous decades, both in the UK and US, the percentage decline for women has been greater than that for men. Nevertheless, changes in rates in women and men are correlated over the different countries, suggesting that whatever the factors are determining mortality, they affect women and men in different countries at more or

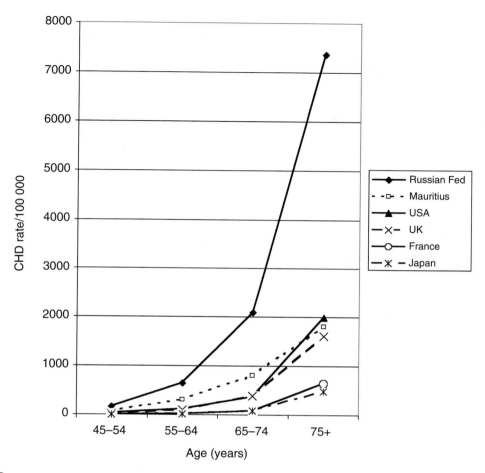

Figure 1.3
Coronary heart disease (CHD) mortality rates by age in women in selected countries, 1999–2000.[4,5]

less the same time and in the same direction. When these changes have been examined in more detail, there is little evidence of a cohort pattern, indicating that these factors appear to act on the whole population and have a relatively immediate effect.

Regional and social class differences

Even within any one country, there are marked differences in CHD rates by geographic region and by social class.[5,6] Age-standardized CHD mortality rates vary by over twofold between different regions in

Great Britain. Table 1.3 shows standardized mortality ratios for CHD for women and men by social class in three time periods in Great Britain. The social class differential is greater for women than for men. These social class differentials have not decreased over time and have actually increased in men.

Preventive strategies

The societal response to the problem of CHD may be twofold: to improve treatment, care, and rehabilitation of those with CHD, and to prevent the occurrence of CHD. Later chapters in this book will focus

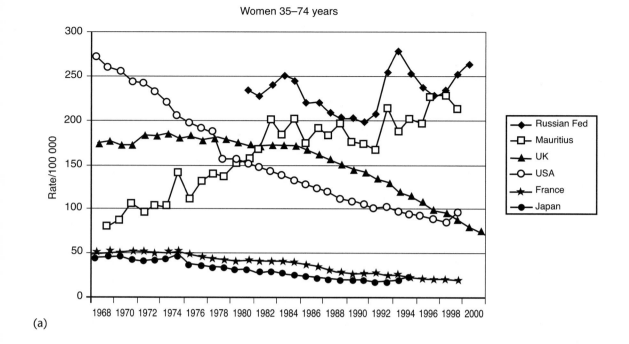

(a)

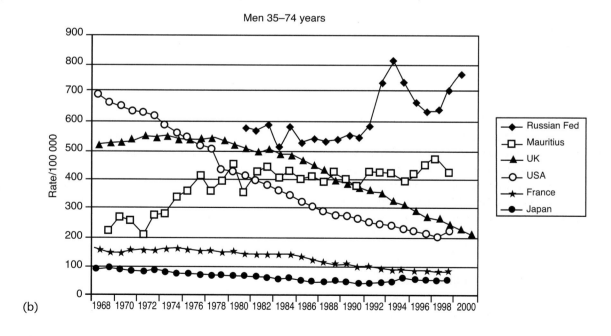

(b)

Figure 1.4
Trends in age-adjusted coronary heart disease mortality rates 1968–2001 for women (a) and men (b)
aged 35–74 years in selected countries.[4,5]

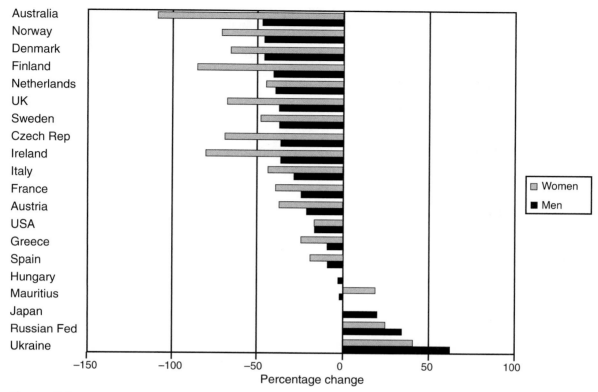

Figure 1.5
Percentage change in mortality rates from coronary heart disease in women and men aged 35–74 years from 1989 to 1999 in selected countries.[4,5]

on the clinical care of women with CHD; general preventive approaches will be considered here. The striking geographic variations, temporal trends, and migrant studies indicate that a large proportion of CHD is potentially preventable. There is a wealth of evidence implicating many biological and environmental factors in the etiology of CHD.[7] Of these, the role of the classical risk factors – blood cholesterol levels, blood pressure, and cigarette smoking – have been the best documented. Strategies aimed at preventing CHD may be individual-based or population-based.[8] The individual-based strategy aims to identify specific high-risk individuals for individual-based targeted intervention (such as reduction of high cholesterol levels using pharmacologic or behavioral changes), whereas the population-based strategy aims to change risk factor levels in the population as a whole (such as by changing dietary patterns or reducing smoking in the whole community). The major factors determining differences in CHD risk between individuals in any one population may not be the same as those factors determining differences in rates between populations. This has implications when considering preventive strategies for both women and men.

Risk factors (see also Chapter 2)

Numerous risk factors have been implicated in CHD. There is increasing evidence to show that many of the risk factors first documented in men apply similarly to women. It is reasonable to postulate that most risk

Table 1.3 Age-standardized death rates per 100 000 population from coronary heart disease (CHD) for women and men aged 35–64 years by sex and social class in England and Wales 1976/81–1986/92[5,6]

Social class	Age-standardized CHD death rates/100 000		
	1976/81	*1981/85*	*1986/92*
Women			
I/II Professional/intermediate	39	45	29
IIIN Skilled non-manual	56	57	39
IIIM Skilled manual	85	67	59
IV/V Partly skilled/unskilled	105	76	68
Ratio manual:non-manual	2.23	1.49	2.18
Men			
I/II Professional/intermediate	246	186	160
IIIN Skilled non-manual	382	267	162
IIIM Skilled manual	309	269	231
IV/V Partly skilled/unskilled	363	293	266
Ratio manual:non-manual	1.19	1.34	1.58

factors are likely to have similar qualitative or biologic effects in women; the exceptions might be the sex-specific factors such as sex hormones.

Table 1.4 shows cross-sectional data for distributions of the classical risk factors in women and men in England in 2002;[9] patterns are similar in most developed countries. In general risk factor levels increase with age, although they level off at older ages. At younger ages, women tend to have lower levels of the risk factors systolic blood pressure and serum cholesterol compared with men; this pattern reverses at older ages. Unlike other risk factors, the prevalence of cigarette smoking habit declines with age in both women and men. These cross-sectional patterns reflect not only the influence of age on risk factors, but may also be affected by selective survival (men with high levels of risk factors are more likely to die at younger ages) and birth cohort effects.

The evidence for the major importance of raised blood cholesterol for CHD in both women and men is now overwhelming. Raised blood pressure, fibrinogen levels, cigarette smoking habit, diabetes, and obesity – particularly central obesity – are also well documented risk factors in women. Of these risk factors, reduction of blood pressure and cholesterol have been demonstrated to be of cardiovascular benefit in randomized trials which have included women, although a recent meta-analysis suggested that current evidence was insufficient to determine conclusively whether drug treatment of hyperlipidemia may reduce CHD events in women without known cardiovascular disease.[10] Several other risk factors such as plasma homocysteine levels and inflammatory markers which have been demonstrated to be of importance in men also influence risk in women, although as yet trial data demonstrating benefit of reduction of these risk factors in women are not available.

The magnitude of the relative risk of subsequent CHD associated with the major risk factors is similar in women and men, which is consistent with similar qualitative biological effects. However, the absolute risk of CHD is higher in men compared with women. For example, several prospective studies have shown that while increasing cholesterol or blood pressure level is associated with a similar relative increase in risk of CHD in both women and men, for any given level of cholesterol or blood pressure, men still have approximately twofold the absolute rate of CHD compared with women, after adjusting for age and other risk factors.[11,12] This has implications for individual-based preventive therapies. Assuming a 20% reduction in CHD with treatment of hypercholesterolemia in all age and sex groups, the estimated number of women needing to be treated to prevent one coronary event within 5 years is greater than for men the same age.[13] The estimated benefits are also

Table 1.4 Distribution of selected risk factors by age and sex in England 2002[9]

	25–34	35–44	45–54	55–64	65–74	75+
			Age (years)			
Systolic BP (mmHg)			Mean levels			
Women	120	123	131	138	145	152
Men	129	130	133	140	143	146
			% with high blood pressure†			
Women	6	13	33	63	70	79
Men	17	24	37	53	62	71
Cholesterol (mmol/l)			Mean levels			
Women	4.9	5.2	5.7	6.1	6.5	6.3
Men	5.1	5.5	5.8	5.8	5.8	5.5
			% ≥5.0 mmol/l			
Women	44	59	74	89	91	89
Men	50	70	78	82	78	72
Body mass index (kg/m^2)			Mean levels			
Women	26.0	26.9	27.2	27.8	27.7	27.0
Men	26.6	27.3	27.9	27.9	28.1	27.1
			% >30 kg/m^2			
Women	21	23	26	29	28	22
Men	18	24	28	28	26	19
Smoking			% current			
Women	32	32	26	23	17	8
Men	37	31	26	23	14	10

†Systolic blood pressure (BP) ≥140 mmHg or diastolic BP ≥90 mmHg or taking medication prescribed for blood pressure.

greater at older ages where CHD rates are higher. Thus, the risk–benefit balance is more sensitive in women to any potential adverse effects of therapy.

Lifestyle risk factors (see also Chapter 2)

There are also a plethora of lifestyle factors implicated in CHD which can be broadly classified as dietary, physical activity, and psychosocial. Some of these may have effects through influencing levels of known physiological risk factors such as lipid levels, blood pressure, and fibrinogen, but others may have effects through other mechanisms involved in atherosclerosis and thrombosis. As with the physiological risk factors, it is important to note that much of the evidence is based on men only, although it may seem

reasonable to assume here too that many of the biological effects may be similar in women and men. There are virtually no randomized trials of primary prevention of CHD using lifestyle measures in women. Some secondary prevention trials have included women, although these have all had insufficient numbers and inadequate power to examine results in women separately.

Sex hormones (see also Chapters 25 and 26)

Women and men obviously differ in endogenous sex hormone levels and a general assumption has been that women have less CHD than men because either high estrogen levels are protective or high testosterone levels are adverse for CHD.

There is surprisingly little evidence from studies of endogenous hormone levels to support such a hypothesis. Such work is limited by the problems in characterizing sex hormone levels in individuals and prospective studies have only been able to examine sex hormone levels in middle or later life. While increased CHD risk in women who have an early menopause has been reported,[14] prospective studies have found no relationship between measured endogenous estrogen or testosterone and CHD in women.[15] Conversely, studies examining endogenous testosterone levels in men have found no consistent significant relationships with CHD or risk factors; if anything, the associations with endogenous testosterone levels appear to be in a beneficial direction.[16] Additionally, endogenous estrogen or testosterone levels are unlikely to explain the differences in CHD rates in women in different populations. The lowest endogenous estrogen levels are in fact found in women who have low CHD rates, such as Japanese and Chinese women, whereas high endogenous estrogen levels are seen in US women who have higher CHD rates.[17] Again, these hormone differences are unlikely to be genetic, as Japanese and Chinese women in the US have higher endogenous estrogen levels.

In terms of exogenous hormone use, despite early observational studies suggesting a protective effect of menopausal estrogen use, the Women's Health Initiative and other randomized trials have now indicated that menopausal hormone therapy with estrogen or with estrogen and progestin combinations has no benefit for CHD.[18–20]

The evidence to date therefore provides no good support for the hypothesis that differences in estrogen or testosterone levels per se measured in later life may explain the male excess in CHD and that any explanation involving sex hormones must lie in more complex areas such as receptor sensitivity or exposures earlier in life.

Conclusions

Women have consistently lower CHD rates than men. The classical risk factors – blood pressure, raised blood cholesterol, and cigarette smoking –

appear to confer the same relative increase in CHD risk in women, and some of the sex difference in CHD can be explained by lower levels of risk factors in women, at least at younger ages. In particular, cigarette smoking habit has been substantially lower in the past in women compared with men, but trends appear to be reversing in younger cohorts. Some of the apparent protection that women seem to have from CHD may diminish as prevalence of cigarette smoking in women increases and even exceeds that in men.

However, the absolute risk of CHD at any age, even after adjusting for risk factors, is about two to three times greater in men. This has implications for individual-based preventive interventions such as pharmacologic treatment of hypertension and hypercholesterolemia. Even if these confer similar relative benefits for CHD in women and men, the absolute benefit is likely to be lower in women. Thus, the risk–benefit balance may be different and more finely balanced in women compared with men when individual preventive treatments are considered.

Nevertheless, CHD is the leading cause of death in women in industrialized countries and preventive interventions need to be targeted at women as well as men. The huge international variation in mortality and incidence rates in women, together with time trends and findings from migrant studies, indicate that a substantial proportion of CHD in women can be prevented. While there has been some debate as to whether the same lifestyle preventive advice given to men should apply to women, the rates in women closely correlate with rates in men, thus indicating that the environmental and lifestyle factors that lead to high CHD rates in men also lead to high rates in women. Thus, population-based approaches which aim to modify lifestyle factors such as diet, smoking, and physical activity are likely to benefit both women and men. The observation that women in countries with high CHD rates have over sixfold the rates in men living in countries with low CHD rates indicates that the role of environmental influences far outweighs the impact of any biologic differences between women and men in CHD susceptibility. A major priority for research is to elucidate further the major environmental etiologic factors that determine high CHD incidence and mortality in populations. In the interim, there is abundant evidence to support measures that lead to reduction in overall levels of CHD risk factors in both women and men in the population through dietary changes such as increasing fruit and vegetable intake, reduction of saturated fat intake, increased physical activity and, most notably, stopping cigarette smoking.

References

1. Tunstall-Pedoe H (ed). Prepared by Tunstall-Pedoe H, Kuulasmaa K, Tolonen H, Davidson M, Mendis S, with 64 other contributors for the WHO MONICA Project. *MONICA Monograph and Multimedia Sourcebook*. Geneva: World Health Organization, 2003 [http://www4.ktl.fi/monica/public/monograph.html].

2. Hammar N, Alfredsson L, Rosen M, Spetz CL, Kahan T, Ysberg AS. A national record linkage to study acute myocardial infarction incidence and case fatality in Sweden. *Int J Epidemiol* 2001; 30 (Suppl 1):S30–34.

3. Office for National Statistics. *Mortality Statistics*. DHI Series No. 34 2001 and Series DH2 No. 29. London: Office for National Statistics London, 2002 [http://www.statistics.gov.uk/downloads/theme_health/].

4. World Health Organization. Statistical information (WHOSIS), 2004 [http://www3.who.int/whosis/menu.cfm].

5. Petersen S, Peto V, Rayner M. *Coronary Heart Disease Statistics 2004*. London: British Heart Foundation, 2004 [http://www.heartstats.org/].

6. Office for National Statistics. *Health Inequalities*. London: The Stationery Office, 1997.

7. Marmot M, Elliott P (eds). *Coronary Heart Disease Epidemiology*. Oxford: Oxford University Press, 1997.

8. Rose G. *The Strategy of Preventive Medicine*. Oxford: Oxford University Press, 1992.

9. Health Survey for England 2002 [http://www.publications.doh.gov.uk/stats/trends1.htm].

10. Walsh JM, Pignone M. Drug treatment of hyperlipidemia in women. *JAMA* 2004; 291:2243–52.

11. Isles CG, Hole DJ, Hawthorne VM, Lever AF. Relation between coronary risk and coronary mortality in women of the Renfrew and Paisley survey: comparison with men. *Lancet* 1992; 339:702–6.

12. Verschuren WMM, Kromhout D. Total cholesterol and mortality at a relatively young age: do women and men differ? *BMJ* 1995; 311:779–83.

13. Khaw KT, Rose G. Cholesterol screening programmes: how much benefit? *BMJ* 1989; 299:606–7.

14. Stampfer MJ, Colditz GA, Willett WC. Menopause and heart disease: a review. *Ann N Y Acad Sci* 1990; 592:192–203.

15. Barrett-Connor E, Goodman-Gruen D. Prospective study of endogenous sex hormones and fatal cardiovascular disease in post-menopausal women. *BMJ* 1995; 311:1193–6.

16. Wu FC, von Eckardstein A. Androgens and coronary artery disease. *Endocr Rev* 2003; 24:183–217.

17. Rossouw JE, Anderson GL, Prentice RL, et al. Writing Group for the Women's Health Initiative Investigators. Risks and benefits of estrogen plus progestin in healthy postmenopausal women: principal results from the Women's Health Initiative randomized controlled trial. *JAMA* 2002; 288: 321–33.

18. Anderson GL, Limacher M, Assaf AR, et al. Women's Health Initiative Steering Committee. Effects of conjugated equine estrogen in postmenopausal women with hysterectomy: the Women's Health Initiative randomized controlled trial. *JAMA* 2004; 291:1701–12.

19. Samsioe G. HRT and cardiovascular disease. *Ann N Y Acad Sci* 2003; 997:358–72.

20. Goldin BR, Adlercreutz H, Gorbach SL, et al. The relationship between estrogen levels and diets of Caucasian American and Oriental immigrant women. *Am J Clin Nutr* 1986; 33:945–63.

2

Cardiovascular disease risk factors in women

Peter W.F. Wilson

Introduction

Atherosclerotic disease is a source of great morbidity and mortality in North America, Europe, and developing regions of the world. Coronary heart disease (CHD), cardiovascular disease (CVD), and cerebrovascular disease are largely attributable to atherosclerosis. This chapter will focus on risk factors for atherosclerotic outcomes in women. The mortality burden of CVD appears to be similar in men and women and CVD accounts for approximately 40% of deaths in men and 41% in women.[1] Rates for CHD mortality used to be higher, peaked in the US during the 1970s, and have declined more than 30% since that time. Multiple factors related to prevention and care of patients appear to account for the decline.[2,3] The decrease in CHD death has been more consistent over the past decade in men than for women.

Atherosclerotic disease risk factors

Risk factors can be grouped into several categories and definitely modifiable, potentially modifiable, and fixed risk factors is a common method of classification (Table 2.1). Cholesterol, blood pressure, cigarette smoking, lifestyle, and behavioral factors are on the definitely modifiable list. The potentially modifiable risk factors usually include newer measurements that are being actively investigated as contributors to greater risk of atherosclerotic disease.

The scientific information for these factors is generally less certain than for the definitely modifiable factors. The fixed risk factors for CHD include age, sex, and family history. Genetics may contribute to each of these groupings and alter CHD risk. For example, the genetic disorder familial hypercholesterolemia is now considered a definitely modifiable condition, and modern lipid-lowering therapy can reduce CHD risk in these individuals. Variations in lipoproteins and other metabolic factors may have a genetic basis and can augment risk of atherosclerotic disease, especially when specific environmental or dietary conditions are present. Myocardial infarction rates in Americans are consistently greater in men than in women at all ages for adults aged 35–85 in the Framingham Heart Study (Fig. 2.1).[1]

Table 2.1 Coronary risk factors for initial coronary heart disease

Definitely modifiable	Potentially modifiable	Fixed
Cholesterol	Lp(a)	Age
HDL cholesterol	Oxidized lipids	Sex
Triglycerides	Hematologic	Family
Blood pressure	Glucose intolerance	history
Cigarette smoking	LVH/LV mass	
Diabetes		
Obesity		
Sedentary lifestyle		
Alcohol		

HDL, high-density lipoprotein; Lp(a), lipoprotein (a); LVH, left ventricular hypertrophy; LV, left ventricular.

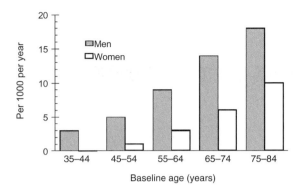

Figure 2.1
Myocardial infarction incidence in the Framingham cohort follow-up 1948–84. Data from reference 1.

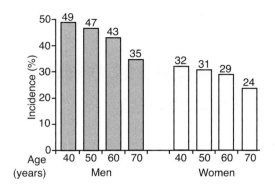

Figure 2.2
Lifetime risk of coronary heart disease: Framingham men and women. Modified from reference 4.

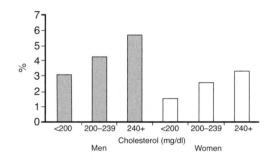

Figure 2.3
Cumulative lifetime risk of coronary heart disease by cholesterol level: Framingham men and women, baseline age 40–49 years. Modified from reference 5.

The lifetime risk of CHD is highly related to age and sex. At age 40 years the Framingham men experienced a 49% risk of developing CHD (angina pectoris, myocardial infarction, or CHD death) prior to death. The lifetime incidence was lower for older persons who had never experienced CHD, and at age 70 years the lifetime risk for CHD in men was 35% (Fig. 2.2). The lifetime risks for CHD in women were lower at each age in comparison with the men. Overall, the lifetime risk for CHD was approximately 40% in men and 30% in women.[4] In contrast, the lifetime risk for developing breast cancer in women is approximately 10%, a rate that is much lower than a woman's lifetime risk for CHD. A follow-up report showed that lifetime risks were also related to total cholesterol level in both sexes and higher cholesterol levels at age 40–49 led to greater risk of CHD in a stepwise fashion (Fig. 2.3).[5]

CHD may manifest itself in several different ways. Angina pectoris is the most common first CHD event in women,[6] followed by myocardial infarction, and CHD death; sudden cardiac death is extremely uncommon in women. Different patterns of first CHD events have been observed for men, with myocardial infarction the most common first CHD event, followed by angina pectoris and coronary death.[6] The frequency of sudden cardiac death has diminished considerably in recent years, as identification of susceptible patients and appropriate medical care has improved greatly.[7–12] Importantly,

after age 40 years, sudden cardiac death is most likely to be related to atherosclerotic disease.

Age

CHD in women tends to occur after menopause, and rates are significantly higher than for other common diseases of aging, including fractures, cerebrovascular disease, breast cancer, and uterine cancer. Decreased estrogen production after menopause has been thought to be an important determinant of

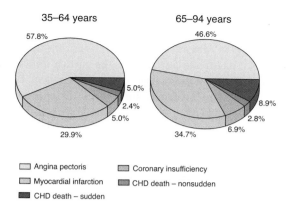

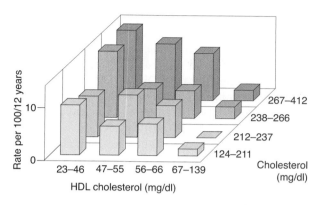

Figure 2.4
Percent of first coronary heart disease (CHD) types in women by age groups. Modified from reference 6 with permission.

Figure 2.5
12-year incidence of myocardial infarction in Framingham cohort women. HDL, high-density lipoprotein. Modified from reference 14.

increased risk for CHD in older women. In Framingham women the first CHD event was angina pectoris in more than half of the cases, and myocardial infarction was the second most common initial CHD. At older age the proportion who presented with angina declined and the proportion with myocardial infarction increased (Fig. 2.4).[6]

Lipids (see also Chapter 4)

Higher levels of cholesterol are related to the development of CHD. In women the greater CHD risk is typically not observed prior to menopause, even if cholesterol levels are quite elevated. Using a cholesterol level of 200 mg/dl as the comparison, a level of 250 mg/dl has typically led to a twofold risk of CHD death and a level of 300 mg/dl led to a threefold risk of CHD death, and these relative risk effects are relatively similar in men and women.[13]

High-density lipoprotein (HDL) cholesterol is a major fraction of cholesterol in the plasma and is an important determinant of risk for CHD and myocardial infarction even when the total cholesterol level is known. The 12-year incidence of myocardial infarction was positively related to cholesterol level and inversely related to HDL cholesterol level in Framingham women (Fig. 2.5).[14] At a total cholesterol level <211 mg/dl the HDL cholesterol levels

were inversely related to risk of developing myocardial infarction in these women. The total/HDL cholesterol ratio is another way to represent the relation between these simple lipid measures and CHD risk, which is highly related to this ratio. Total cholesterol and low-density lipoprotein (LDL) cholesterol had similar predictive capabilities in the prediction of CHD in women in multivariable models that also included age and HDL cholesterol, suggesting that total cholesterol is adequate for screening purposes at a population level (Fig. 2.6).[15]

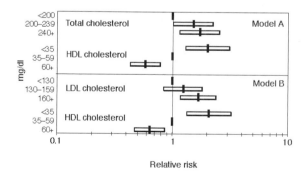

Figure 2.6
12-year coronary heart disease incidence in women according to lipid categories. HDL, high-density lipoprotein; LDL, low-density lipoprotein. Modified from reference 15.

A large variety of lipoprotein particles have been identified, and several techniques are available to assess their density, diameter, electrophoretic characteristics, and nuclear magnetic resonance properties. Initially the LDL particles received the most attention, as apolipoprotein B is present in the LDL fraction. Research interest has spread to investigate the role of all particle groups, as newer methods have allowed rapid assessment of the numbers and concentrations of lipoprotein particles.[16–19] There are complex inter-relations between the number of particles and some of the commonly measured lipids. For example, with increasing concentrations of triglycerides the percentage of smaller, denser LDL particles increases and the frequency of large, buoyant LDL particles decreases.[16] The smaller, denser LDL particles may be associated with greater risk in men and women, but the added usefulness of these measurements for the assessment of CVD risk in prospective studies is not assured at this time.[20,21]

Lipoprotein (a) (Lp(a)) is an accepted determinant of CHD risk, and this particle includes an LDL moiety that is linked to a protein chain that bears homology to plasminogen. The length of the apoprotein (a) varies and is heritable. A variety of methods have been undertaken to assay Lp(a),[22] and standard-ization has been difficult because the particles vary in composition from person to person.[22] Levels of Lp(a) are higher in Africans and African Americans than in whites.[23] In African populations the particle concentrations follow a normal statistical distribution, but Lp(a) levels are lower and the distribution is skewed in whites. Lp(a) has generally been shown to be a CHD risk factor in men and women, especially at the higher concentrations (>30 mg/dl) in whites.[24] Routine screening for Lp(a) levels has been recommended for persons with premature CHD that is not explained by conventional risk factor levels.[25,26]

The advent of 3-hydroxy-3-methylglutaryl coenzyme A reductase inhibitors in the late 1980s led to an improved ability to reduce LDL cholesterol. A large number of diet and lipid therapy trials ensued and favorable treatment effects on subclinical and clinical disease were observed for the coronary and carotid arteries, initial CHD events, recurrent CHD events, and stroke.[27–36] In general, more cholesterol-lowering has led to a greater reduction in risk of initial and recurrent CHD in these studies. The efficacy of cholesterol therapy in these trials has largely been premised upon the intention to treat and not on the degree of blood cholesterol-lowering achieved or the ability to reach predefined target levels of cholesterol or LDL cholesterol.

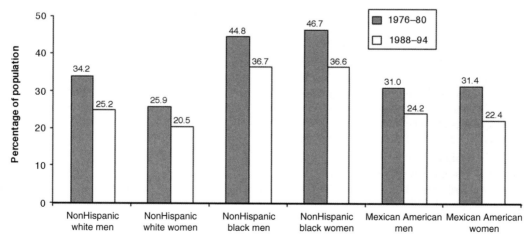

Figure 2.7
Age-adjusted prevalence trends for high blood pressure at age 20–74 by race/ethnicity and sex, from surveys in the US during 1976–80 and 1988–94. (Source: National Health and Nutrition Examination Survey (NHANES) II (1976–80) and NHANES III (1988–94). Data are based on multiple measurements of blood pressure. From reference 1.

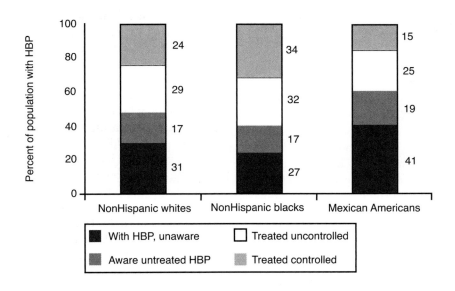

Figure 2.8
Extent of awareness, treatment and control of blood pressure by race/ethnicity: US 1988–94. HBP, high blood pressure. Modified from reference 37 with permission.

Blood pressure (see also Chapter 31)

The age-adjusted prevalence of high blood pressure has decreased from the late 1970s to the 1990s for several ethnic groups in the US. Throughout the interval the nonHispanic blacks have had higher rates of hypertension (>140/90 mmHg) than whites or Hispanics; in all ethnic groups the prevalence of hypertension is lower in women than in men (Fig. 2.7). In these surveys many persons in the US were unaware that they had high blood pressure or were inadequately treated for the condition. As seen in Fig. 2.8, approximately 50% of persons with high blood pressure were treated and only 15–24% were under control. A sizable fraction, ranging from 27–41% of persons with high blood pressure, were unaware that they were affected.[37]

Risk of CHD is highly related to blood pressure level and levels of systolic pressure are typically more highly associated with the development of clinical disease than levels of diastolic blood pressure. Systolic and diastolic hypertension generally confer a relative risk of 1.6 for CHD; for combined systolic and diastolic hypertension the relative risk is 2.0.[38,39] Pulse pressure is also related to CVD outcomes, especially in older men and women, as diastolic pressures typically are lower in the elderly than those observed in middle age.[40]

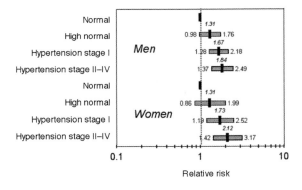

Figure 2.9
12-year incidence of coronary heart disease according to blood pressure category. Modified from reference 15.

Blood pressure levels that do not meet the criteria for hypertension increase the risk for a first major CHD event, and long-term comparisons have shown that the risk of CHD is increased in persons with high normal blood pressure (systolic pressure 130–139 mmHg with diastolic 85–89 mmHg) (Fig. 2.9).[15] As high normal pressure level is a common condition, this level of blood pressure accounts for a sizable fraction of CHD events and on a population basis is nearly as important as hypertension itself.[41]

The overall effect of blood pressure on CVD death has been summarized in a review analysis of 61 prospective observational studies of blood pressure and mortality.[42] At age 40–69 years a difference of 20 mmHg in systolic pressure or 10 mmHg in diastolic pressure was related to approximately a twofold difference in death rate from CHD.

A large number of clinical trials have been undertaken to lower blood pressure and have demonstrated that CHD risk is reduced when diastolic and systolic blood pressure levels are lowered with diet or a variety of drugs, although safety with some treatments has been an issue.[43–45] Research has recently concentrated on treatment in special groups, especially older persons and those with elevated systolic pressure. These trials have demonstrated efficacy in reducing vascular disease risk in the Systolic Hypertension and the Elderly Program (SHEP), the Systolic Treatment in Europe Trial (Syst-Eur), and the Systolic Treatment in China trial (Syst-China).[46–48] Women were often under-represented in the earlier clinical trials that tested the use of newer hypertensive medications and strategies.

The Antihypertensive and Lipid-Lowering treatment to prevent Heart Attack Trial (ALLHAT), a study with more than 40 000 US participants, tested the efficacy of several treatment modalities for elevated blood pressure in older Americans. This study found that thiazide diuretics were as effective as calcium channel blockers and angiotensin-converting enzyme (ACE) inhibitors as initial therapy in the prevention of CHD risk.[49] The addition of a statin provided no further benefit, but the difference in cholesterol levels between placebo users and those randomized to the active agent used was approximately 10% during the trial.[49,50] Different results were obtained in the combined blood pressure and lipid treatment arms from the Anglo-Scandinavian Cardiac Outcomes Trial (ASCOT), which used blood pressure medications and more potent statin therapy that effected a difference in cholesterol levels that exceed 40 mg/dl. In the ASCOT trial lower CVD risk was related to both the lipid and the blood pressure treatments.[34] In each of these studies the results in women generally paralleled those observed for men.

Obesity, nutrition and heart disease (see also Chapter 6)

Excess adiposity has been defined by the World Health Organization using body mass index (BMI =

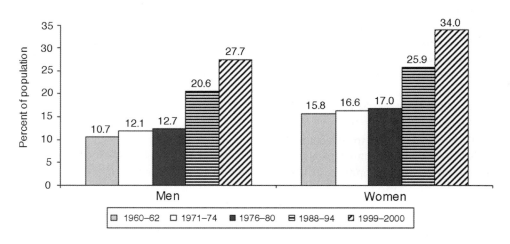

Figure 2.10
Age-adjusted prevalence of obesity in the US: 1960–62, 1971–74, 1976–80, 1988–94, and 1999–2000. Obesity is defined as a body mass index ≥30 kg/m². Source: respective health examination surveys, Centers for Disease Control and Prevention/National Center for Health Statistics. Modified from reference 1.

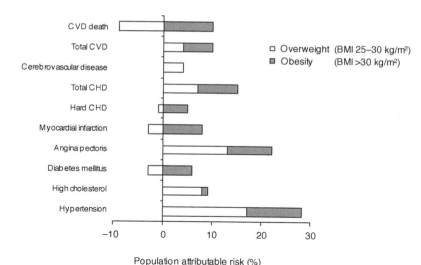

Figure 2.11
Population attributable risk percent effects for overweight and obesity on cardiovascular disease (CVD) risk factors and events in women. CHD, coronary heart disease; BMI, body mass index. Modified from reference 54.

body weight in kilograms divided by the square of height in meters) and abdominal girth (greatest circumference of the abdomen when a subject is standing).[51] Using these measures, overweight is present for a BMI 25–29.9 kg/m[2] and obesity for a BMI >30 kg/m[2]. Increased abdominal adiposity is defined as >90 cm (35.4 inches) for women and >100 cm (39.4 inches) for men.

The prevalence of obesity has increased dramatically over the course of the past 30 years in the US.[52] Data from US surveys have shown that the prevalence of obesity has risen from 10% to 27% in men and from 16% to 34% in women from the year 1960 to 2000 (Fig. 2.10). Correspondingly, the prevalence of overweight has also increased, and it is now estimated that >50% of US adults are either overweight or obese.[1,51]

Obesity contributes to the development of several CHD risk factors, especially hypertension, diabetes mellitus, low HDL cholesterol, elevated triglycerides, and elevated levels of inflammatory markers. Weight gain during adult years is highly related to developing a greater risk factor burden, and this phenomenon has been observed with relatively modest weight increases in prospective studies such as the Framingham offspring investigation.[53] Using population attributable risk estimation procedures, obesity accounts for approximately 15% of CHD, 15% of angina pectoris, and 15% of hypertension in long-term analyses of Framingham women, and

similar effects were observed for the overweight category as well (Fig. 2.11).[54] These data suggest that being overweight is more than sufficient to increase risk for CHD. Excess adiposity underlies the risk factors that appear to directly increase risk for CHD and other adverse chronic disease outcomes.

Cholesterol levels have diminished modestly in the US population over the past two decades and the average cholesterol in adults is approximately 204 mg/dl.[55] Lower consumption of fat is largely responsible for the change in blood cholesterol over time,[56] and switching from the usual US diet that includes 35–41% of calories as fat to an American Heart Association Step I diet with <30% calories as fat would be expected to change cholesterol levels by 15% from baseline.[57] Dietary cholesterol guidelines promulgated by expert committees now recommend consumption of a variety of foods, including fruits, vegetables, and grains; and that a healthy body weight, desirable cholesterol level in the blood, and desirable blood pressure levels are all important.[58] Adult blood cholesterol levels <200 mg/dl are becoming the target and approximately half of the population is not at goal with these criteria. An aggressive goal of an LDL cholesterol <100 mg/dl has been set for persons with known CVD and it has been estimated that only 18% of the candidates are at goal.[59]

Increased oxidation has been proposed as an important contributor to atherosclerosis and interest has emerged in nutrients that have antioxidant properties.[60] Vitamins B, C, and E have been studied the most and several observational studies suggested that greater intake of these vitamins in regular food or as supplements had favorable effects on cardiovascular risk;[61,62] controlled clinical trials, recently in the setting of a 2 × 2 factorial trial with other anti-atherosclerotic regimens, have generally not demonstrated reductions in risk.[28,63,64]

Greater alcohol intake has consistently been related to a reduced risk of CHD, and an intake in the range of more than two drinks a day in men and more than one drink a day in women appears to confer this benefit.[65–68] Favorable effects on HDL cholesterol levels are thought to be important in exerting this effect, as well as anti-inflammatory and anti-platelet effects. Greater alcohol intake is not without hazards and greater risk of gastrointestinal bleeding, hemorrhagic stroke, accidents, suicide, and cirrhosis may occur with increased intake.[69,70]

Smoking (see also Chapter 5)

The prevalence of cigarette smoking has declined in the US since the 1960s. Data from the National Health and Nutrition Examination Survey from 1988–1994 (NHANES III) showed that cigarette smoking rates were lowest among individuals with more than 12 years of education for white, black, and Mexican American participants, but approximately 20% of US adults smoked cigarettes regularly (Fig. 2.12). Higher smoking rates were present for those with less education, especially whites with less than 12 years of education.[71]

Cigarette smoking generally doubles the risk of CHD outcomes. Both regular and filter cigarettes have similar adverse effects on CHD risk.[72] Low-tar and low-nicotine cigarettes have shown no reduction in CHD risk in comparisons with products that are higher in tar and nicotine.[73] Cessation of cigarette smoking was associated with half the risk for CVD death in 1–2 years after quitting in men screened as part of the Multiple Risk Factor Intervention Trial (MRFIT) study,[74] and the effects for smoking cessation on the clinical course of CHD risk in women were similar.[75]

Passive smoking has been related to an increased risk of CHD that is approximately 30% greater than the risk for non-smokers,[76] and it has also been reported that persons exposed to environmental smoke have increased intima medial thickness of their carotid arteries, an indication of subclinical arteriosclerosis, in comparison with nonsmokers.[77]

Physical activity and fitness (see also Chapter 7)

Persons with a more active lifestyle generally experience lower risk for CHD. Early studies investigated

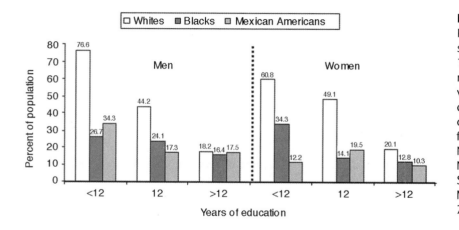

Figure 2.12
Prevalence of current smoking in adults aged 18–24 by education and race/ethnicity. Ethnic variation in cardiovascular disease risk factors among children and young adults: findings from the Third National Health and Nutrition Examination Survey (1988–94). Modified from reference 71 with permission.

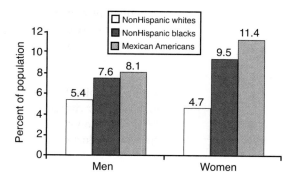

Figure 2.13
Age-adjusted prevalence of physician-diagnosed diabetes mellitus in Americans aged 20 and older by sex and race/ethnicity in the US 1988–94. Findings from the third National Health and Nutrition Examination Survey (1988–94). Modified from reference 86.

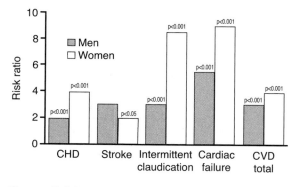

Figure 2.14
Diabetes and cardiovascular disease (CVD) risk in the Framingham cohort aged 35–64 years: 30-year follow-up. CHD, coronary heart disease. Modified from reference 87.

occupations and risk for CHD, but more recent research has concentrated on leisure time physical activity. A key report for men from the Harvard Alumni Study showed that greater exercise was inversely related to risk of fatal and nonfatal myocardial infarction over an 8-year interval.[78] This result and others showed that physical activity reported in middle-aged adults was important in reducing CHD risk.[79] There is an increased risk for sudden cardiac death during or following exercise in persons who generally perform little exercise, but adverse events are uncommon.[80,81] Current recommendations call for physical activity 30 minutes a day at least five times a week.[82–84]

Greater fitness that has been documented by longer exercise treadmill times has been related to reduced risk for CHD in men and women.[85] Persons in the lowest quintile of fitness experienced the highest CHD event rates and even modest degrees of fitness were related to lower risk of CHD. Greater activity and fitness have favorable effects on several CHD risk factors. Higher HDL cholesterol levels, less cigarette smoking, less adiposity, and better nutritional habits are frequent accompaniments and may help to explain the lower CHD risk for active men and women.

Diabetes mellitus and the metabolic syndrome (see also Chapter 3)

An increased prevalence of type 2 diabetes mellitus is following on the heels of the obesity epidemic in the United States. The prevalence of type 2 diabetes mellitus rises with age in both sexes and at age 50 years approximately 4% of the population is affected. The lowest prevalence of type 2 diabetes mellitus is commonly observed in nonHispanic whites, higher levels are seen in nonHispanic blacks, and the highest levels have been reported for Mexican Americans and Native Americans (Fig. 2.13).[86]

Risk of CHD is increased twofold among younger men with type 2 diabetes mellitus, and risk varies according to type of vascular complication. In Framingham, as well as several other studies, a three-fold risk for CHD has been observed for younger women with type 2 diabetes mellitus (Fig. 2.14).[87] Data from Finland have suggested that the risk for a heart attack in a person with diabetes is very similar to the risk for a person who has had a heart attack and is at risk for subsequent heart attack. This result led to the concept of type 2 diabetes mellitus as a

Table 2.2 National Cholesterol Education Program Adult Treatment Panel III: the metabolic syndrome[89]

Risk factor	Definition
1. Waist circumference	>102 cm (>40 in) men
	>88 cm (>35 in) women
2. Triglycerides	≥150 mg/dl
3. HDL cholesterol	<40 mg/dl men
	<50 mg/dl women
4. Blood pressure	≥130/≥85 mmHg
5. Fasting glucose	>110 mg/dl

HDL, high-density lipoprotein.

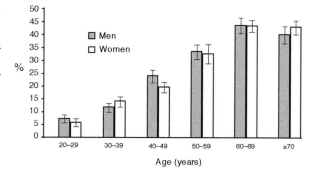

Figure 2.15
Age-specific prevalence of the metabolic syndrome in the third National Health and Nutrition Examination Survey. Data are presented as percentages (standard error). Modified from reference 96.

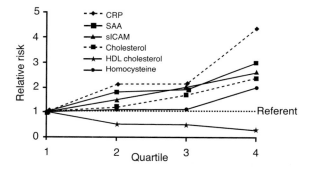

Figure 2.16
Inflammation markers and cardiovascular disease in Women's Health Study. CRP, high-sensitivity C-reactive protein; SAA, serum amyloid A; sICAM, soluble intercellular adhesion molecule 1; HDL, high-density lipoprotein. Modified from reference 101.

CHD risk equivalent, and emphasizes the need for aggressive treatment of risk factors in persons with type 2 diabetes mellitus to prevent CHD events.[88]

Cardiovascular risk reduction efforts have only recently targeted persons with type 2 diabetes mellitus and lower thresholds for LDL cholesterol and blood pressure for persons with type 2 diabetes mellitus are now recommended.[89,90] The basis for these aggressive approaches came from subgroup analyses of treatment effects for blood pressure and lipid-lowering in type 2 diabetic persons in randomized clinical trials.

The efficacy of this approach has been published in a Danish trial of men and women with aggressive therapy for hyperglycemia, hypertension, dyslipidemia, and microalbuminuria in persons with type 2 diabetes mellitus.[91]

Data to support concerted glucose control as a CHD prevention strategy has obtained support from observational studies, and glucose and HbA$_{1C}$ (glycosylated hemoglobin) data from clinical trials have been impressive for the prevention of microvascular eye and kidney complications, but little added benefit has been shown for tight glucose control with current regimens for CVD prevention.[91–95] This issue is now being addressed with large-scale multifactorial intervention trials in patients with type 2 diabetes mellitus.

Several CVD risk factors occur at a frequency greater than expected and insulin resistance is thought to account for clustering of these traits, especially higher blood pressure, impaired fasting glucose, increased triglycerides, decreased HDL cholesterol, and greater abdominal adiposity. The presence of three or more of these five abnormalities has been named the metabolic syndrome, and some of the criteria are sex-specific (Table 2.2).[89]

The metabolic syndrome is present in approximately 24% of US men and women according to US survey data from the early 1990s, and the prevalence is highly related to age, ranging from 7% in persons at 20–29 years to 43% in persons 60–69 years (Fig. 2.15).[96] The presence of the metabolic syndrome in adults has been shown to confer an increased risk of diabetes mellitus, CHD, and CVD death.[97–99]

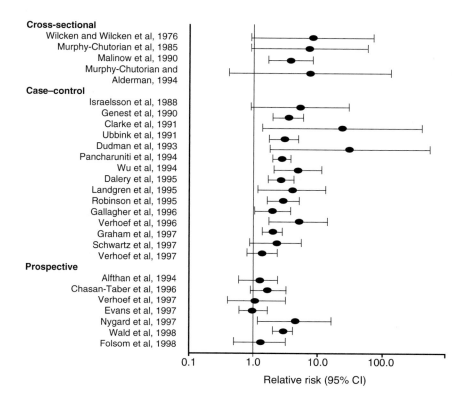

Cross-sectional
Wilcken and Wilcken et al, 1976
Murphy-Chutorian et al, 1985
Malinow et al, 1990
Murphy-Chutorian and
Alderman, 1994
Case–control
Israelsson et al, 1988
Genest et al, 1990
Clarke et al, 1991
Ubbink et al, 1991
Dudman et al, 1993
Pancharuniti et al, 1994
Wu et al, 1994
Dalery et al, 1995
Landgren et al, 1995
Robinson et al, 1995
Gallagher et al, 1996
Verhoef et al, 1996
Graham et al, 1997
Schwartz et al, 1997
Verhoef et al, 1997
Prospective
Alfthan et al, 1994
Chasan-Taber et al, 1996
Verhoef et al, 1997
Evans et al, 1997
Nygard et al, 1997
Wald et al, 1998
Folsom et al, 1998

0.1   1.0   10.0   100.0

Relative risk (95% CI)

Figure 2.17
Coronary heart disease and elevated homocysteine levels. CI, confidence interval. Modified from reference 108 with permission.

Inflammation (see also Chapter 9)

A variety of factors related to hematologic, endothelial, or inflammatory processes have been studied for their relation to CVD. Early studies investigated leukocyte count and these were followed by fibrinogen determinations. In a meta-analysis, the top third of fibrinogen levels led to a doubling of risk for initial and recurrent CVD events.[100] Several markers of inflammation are highly related to CHD risk and quartile analyses for adhesion molecules, hs-CRP (C-reactive protein), and fibrinogen have generally been positive. Each of these markers was highly related to greater risk of subsequent CHD in categorical analyses that used quintiles of each factor (Fig. 2.16).[101] Subsequent research in a large number of studies has shown that CRP is highly related to increased risk of atherosclerotic events, including initial and recurrent CVD, as well as stroke.[102–105] Measurement of inflammatory markers, specifically CRP, is now considered a reasonable adjunct to the major risk factors to

further assess absolute risk for coronary disease primary prevention.[106]

Blood levels of the amino acid homocysteine have been studied for their relation to CVD risk in both sexes. Investigations in the early 1990s showed that lower intake of B vitamins (folate, vitamin B_6, vitamin B_{12}) was related to greater concentrations of homocysteine.[107] Persons with higher homocysteine levels experienced greater risk for CVD, and the results were stronger in the earlier reports than in more recent investigations (Fig. 2.17).[108,109] Folate fortification of cereals and grains was undertaken in the United States during the late 1990s and has appeared to reduce the frequency of elevated homocysteine levels in the free-living population.[110] Additional folate intake from supplementary vitamins and multivitamins may be contributing to a reduced importance for homocysteine as a CVD risk factor.

Homocysteine may be a more important contributor to greater CHD risk in specific situations. Extremely high homocysteine levels, despite folate supplementation, are commonly observed in persons with impaired kidney function, and may contribute to the accelerated atherosclerosis observed with this condition.[111] Clinical trials are underway to test the utility of folate supplementation to reduce atherosclerosis in men and women with reduced kidney function.[112]

Genetics

Genetic abnormalities and variants in common genes contribute to risk of atherosclerotic disease and research is very active in this field.[113,114] Diseases such as familial hypercholesterolemia have been shown to have several potential causes and taken together they probably account for approximately 5% of the case burden of persons with myocardial infarction.[115] In both sexes the alleles of the apolipoprotein E have been related to cholesterol and triglyceride levels in young adults, risk of CVD in middle age, and dementia in older age.[116–118] The apolipoprotein E4 allele is present in approximately 24% of the population, confers a relative risk for CHD of 1.5, and has led to the realization that this gene variant accounts for approximately 10–15% of CHD.[117,119] Furthermore, the different alleles of the apolipoprotein E gene may affect responses to diet and lipid-altering medications.[120,121] Variants of the several other genes, including those encoding ACE,[122] Lp(a),[123] cholesterol ester transfer protein,[124] hepatic lipase,[125] and methylene tetrahydrofolate reductase (MTHFR) (related to folate and homocysteine metabolism),[126] are examples of candidate genes that have been studied for their relation to metabolic factors and CVD risk and the risk of candidates is growing rapidly. Gene–environment effects appear to be operative in the case of apolipoprotein E and MTHFR. Several observational studies have undertaken large-scale genome efforts to screen for relations between genetic markers and the presence of a variety of cardiovascular phenotypes in men and women, considering abnormal cholesterol levels, hypertension, and other risk factors.[127] This research typically involves the use of anonymous markers every 5–10 centimorgans along the human chromosome and includes 300 or more genetic tests for each individual. Positive results are then used to perform fine mapping and further genetic testing in an effort to identify genes that are responsible for the different phenotypes.

Subclinical cardiovascular disease

Atherosclerosis develops and progresses at different rates in the vasculature. The aorta is the region that is most likely to develop early atherosclerosis and fatty streaks are common during adolescence, as noted in earlier studies of war victims and recent investigations from the Premature Development of Atherosclerosis in Youth (PDAY) study.[128,129] Early adulthood often leads to fibrous plaque formation and calcification of the aorta, especially in the arch and distally near the bifurcation into the iliac arteries. This calcification is equally common in men and women at age 50 and the severity of the calcification on radiograms has been shown to predict the occurrence of CVD events over and above traditional risk factors.[130]

Modern techniques can provide assessment of subclinical vascular disease in smaller arteries. The carotid arteries have been studied with B mode ultrasound and more recently with magnetic resonance imaging. Greater carotid stenosis in older persons has correlated with the burden of smoking, blood pressure, and cholesterol across the adult years,[131] and increased intima medial thickening of the carotid arteries in the elderly has been shown to be predictive of subsequently developing CVD.[132] The usefulness of this testing is limited by the need for accurate measurements and trained sonographers.

Computerized scanning of the coronary arteries for the presence of calcification has been proposed as a useful strategy to identify persons at high risk for the development of clinical CVD.[133,134] Data are limited at present, but large investigations such as the Multi-Ethnic Study of Atherosclerosis should help to provide a critical assessment of the added usefulness of these newer screening modalities in nonselected population cohorts.[135]

Renal disease

Proteinuria was noted in the 1980s to be related to an increased risk of CHD[136] and more recent research has focused on microalbuminuria (>30 mg/g urinary creatinine) as a marker of renal impairment in persons with hypertension or diabetes mellitus. Modest decrements in estimated glomerular filtration rate and presence of microalbuminuria have been shown to be important predictors of decline in renal function and in the development of CVD in both sexes.[137,138] Assessment of albumin excretion is now recommended at regular intervals for persons with diabetes mellitus or hypertension.

Long-term treatment of hypertension and type 2 diabetes mellitus has led to extension of life, but chronic kidney failure may occur. These two diseases are now the most common diagnoses for persons who have to start chronic dialysis.[139] Once kidney failure has developed the prognosis is quite poor, as heart disease appears to enter an acclerated phase, resulting in cardiac failure or cardiac death in a significant number of those affected. New guidelines for aggressive treatment of blood pressure and lipids have been developed for these patients and an American Heart Association group of experts has recommended that chronic kidney failure itself be considered a heart disease risk factor.[140]

Multivariable coronary heart disease risk estimation

Risk for CVD events can be estimated with multivariable prediction equations using a score sheet, pocket calculator, or computer. The variables age, systolic blood pressure, smoking, cholesterol, HDL cholesterol, and diabetes mellitus are commonly used to estimate risk for initial CHD events, employing separate equations for men and women. This approach has been validated in the United States across several observational studies for both sexes.[15,141] Estimation of CHD risk is generally valid for middle-class, white populations in North America and Europe where risk factors and heart disease rates approximate the experience of studies such as Framingham that provided the estimates. Overestimates of CHD risk may be obtained in other locales, especially where CHD risk is low, such as in Spain or Hawaii.[141,142]

An example of CHD risk prediction based on the experience of Framingham women is shown in Fig. 2.18. The vertical bar on the left side of the figure

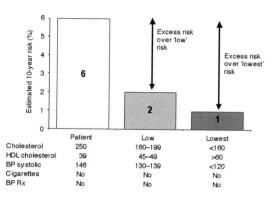

	Patient	Low	Lowest
Cholesterol	250	160–199	<160
HDL cholesterol	39	45–49	>60
BP systolic	146	130–139	<120
Cigarettes	No	No	No
BP Rx	No	No	No

Figure 2.18
Estimated 10-year hard coronary heart disease risk in a 55-year-old woman according to levels of various factors. Lipids are denoted in mg/dl and blood pressure in mmHg. HDL, high-density lipoprotein; BP, blood pressure; Rx, prescription. Modified from reference 141.

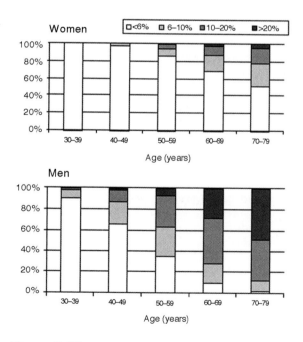

Figure 2.19
Estimated 10-year hard coronary heart disease risk in Framingham offspring and cohort. Modified from reference 143.

represents the estimated absolute risk for CHD over 10 years for a representative 55-year-old woman with a cholesterol of 250 mg/dl, HDL cholesterol of 39 mg/dl, systolic blood pressure of 146 mmHg, and no cigarette smoking or blood pressure therapy. Comparisons for a woman the same age with 'low' risk factor levels and with the 'lowest' risk factor levels are shown in the other vertical bars. The excess risk is the difference between the estimated risk for the patient and the individual comparisons, and the relative risk is the ratio of the estimated risk for the patients and the individual comparisons.

The distribution of the 10-year estimated risks for CHD in Framingham men and women are shown in Fig. 2.19 with the frequencies for women at the top of the figure and the information for men at the bottom. It can be seen that low risks for CHD (<6% over 10 years) predominate in women up to age 70 years and that for every age group considered the men tend to have much higher risks for CHD events.[143]

Using a slightly different set of variables, equations that estimate CHD risk have been developed in Germany to predict initial CHD events in men.[144] European investigators from several countries have

also developed algorithms to estimate risk of CHD mortality.[145] For persons with type 2 diabetes mellitus, British investigators have developed a CHD risk estimating equation, and this approach includes factoring in levels of glycosylated hemoglobin and duration of diabetes mellitus.[146]

Estimating CHD risk can help clinicians to match the estimated risk of CHD with aggressiveness of risk factor management. Separate risk estimating equations have been developed for the prediction of stroke, intermittent claudication, and the individual components of CHD.[147–149]

Estimation of CHD risk with multivariable equations is a dynamic process and new information is constantly being evaluated as it may change the approach. An important ingredient to assess is whether it improves the overall prediction of CHD within a population.[141,150] Accuracy and precision of the new measurement, standardization of the technique, low correlation with existing predictive variables, validation in other observational studies, and biological relevance are examples of features that have to be considered prior to the inclusion of newer variables into risk estimating approaches.[145,150–152]

References

1. American Heart Association. *Heart Disease and Stroke Statistics – 2003 Update*. Dallas, TX: American Heart Association, 2002.
2. Guidry UC, Evans JC, Larson MG, Wilson PW, Murabito JM, Levy D. Temporal trends in event rates after Q-wave myocardial infarction: the Framingham Heart Study. *Circulation* 1999; **100**:2054–9.
3. McGovern PG, Pankow JS, Shahar E, et al. Recent trends in acute coronary heart disease – mortality, morbidity, medical care, and risk factors. The Minnesota Heart Survey Investigators. *N Engl J Med* 1996; **334**:884–90.
4. Lloyd-Jones DM, Larson MG, Beiser A, Levy D. Lifetime risk of developing coronary heart disease. *Lancet* 1999; **353**:89–92.
5. Lloyd-Jones DM, Wilson PW, Larson MG, et al. Lifetime risk of coronary heart disease by cholesterol levels at selected ages. *Arch Intern Med* 2003; **163**:1966–72.
6. Lerner DJ, Kannel WB. Patterns of coronary heart disease morbidity and mortality in the sexes: a 26-year follow-up of the Framingham population. *Am Heart J* 1986; **111**:383–90.
7. Folsom AR, Chambless LE, Duncan BB, Gilbert AC, Pankow JS. Prediction of coronary heart disease in middle-aged adults with diabetes. *Diabetes Care* 2003; **26**:2777–84.
8. Maron BJ. Sudden death in young athletes. *N Engl J Med* 2003; **349**:1064–75.
9. Maron BJ. Contemporary considerations for risk stratification, sudden death and prevention in hypertrophic cardiomyopathy. *Heart* 2003; **89**:977–8.
10. Priori SG, Aliot E, Blomstrom-Lundqvist C, et al. Update of the guidelines on sudden cardiac death of the European Society of Cardiology. *Eur Heart J* 2003; **24**:13–15.
11. Maron BJ, Shirani J, Poliac LC, Mathenge R, Roberts WC, Mueller FO. Sudden death in young competitive athletes: clinical, demographic, and pathological profiles. *JAMA* 1996; **276**:199–204.

12. Maron BJ. Hypertrophic cardiomyopathy: a systematic review. *JAMA* 2002; **287**:1308–20.

13. Gotto AM Jr, LaRosa JC, Hunninghake D, et al. The cholesterol facts: a summary of the evidence relating dietary fats, serum cholesterol, and coronary heart disease: a joint statement by the American Heart Association and the National, Heart, Lung, and Blood Institute. *Circulation* 1990; **81**:1721–33.

14. Abbott RD, Wilson PW, Kannel WB, Castelli WP. High density lipoprotein cholesterol, total cholesterol screening, and myocardial infarction. The Framingham Study. *Arteriosclerosis* 1988; **8**:207–11.

15. Wilson PW, D'Agostino RB, Levy D, Belanger AM, Silbershatz H, Kannel WB. Prediction of coronary heart disease using risk factor categories. *Circulation* 1998; **97**:1837–47.

16. Austin MA, King MC, Vranizan KM, Krauss RM. Atherogenic lipoprotein phenotype. A proposed genetic marker for coronary heart disease risk. *Circulation* 1990; **82**:495–506.

17. Otvos JD, Jeyarajah EJ, Bennett DW, Krauss RM. Development of a proton nuclear magnetic resonance spectroscopic method for determining plasma lipoprotein concentrations and subspecies distributions from a single, rapid measurement. *Clin Chem* 1992; **38**:1632–8.

18. Reaven GM, Abbasi F, Bernhart S, et al. Insulin resistance, dietary cholesterol, and cholesterol concentration in postmenopausal women. *Metabolism* 2001; **50**:594–7.

19. Campos H, McNamara JR, Wilson PWF, Ordovas JM, Schaefer EJ. Differences in low density lipoprotein subfractions and apolipoproteins in premenopausal and postmenopausal women. *J Clin Endocrinol Metab* 1988; **67**:30–5.

20. Gardner CD, Fortmann SP, Krauss RM. Association of small low-density lipoprotein particles with the incidence of coronary artery disease in men and women. *JAMA* 1996; **276**:875–81.

21. Lamarche B, St Pierre AC, Ruel IL, Cantin B, Dagenais GR, Despres JP. A prospective, population-based study of low density lipoprotein particle size as a risk factor for ischemic heart disease in men. *Can J Cardiol* 2001; **17**:859–65.

22. Marcovina SM, Albers JJ, Scanu AM, et al. Use of a reference material proposed by the International Federation of Clinical Chemistry and Laboratory Medicine to evaluate analytical methods for the determination of plasma lipoprotein(a). *Clin Chem* 2000; **46**:1956–67.

23. Gidding SS, Liu K, Bild DE, et al. Prevalence and identification of abnormal lipoprotein levels in a biracial population aged 23 to 35 years (the CARDIA Study). The Coronary Artery Risk Development in Young Adults Study. *Am J Cardiol* 1996; **78**:304–8.

24. Schaefer EJ, Lamon-Fava S, Jenner JL, et al. Lipoprotein(a) levels and risk of coronary heart disease in men: the Lipid Research Clinics Coronary Primary Prevention Trial. *JAMA* 1994; **271**:999–1003.

25. Scanu AM. Lp(a) lipoprotein – coping with heterogeneity. *N Engl J Med* 2003; **349**:2089–90.

26. Scanu AM. Lipoprotein(a) and the atherothrombotic process: mechanistic insights and clinical implications. *Curr Atheroscler Rep* 2003; **5**:106–13.

27. Blankenhorn DH, Nessim SA, Johnson RL, Sanmarco ME, Azen SP, Cashin-Hemphill L. Beneficial effects of combined colestipol–niacin therapy on coronary atherosclerosis and coronary venous bypass grafts. *JAMA* 1987; **257**:3233–40.

28. Brown BG, Zhao XQ, Chait A, et al. Simvastatin and niacin, antioxidant vitamins, or the combination for the prevention of coronary disease. *N Engl J Med* 2001; **345**:1583–92.

29. Shepherd J, Cobbe SM, Ford I, et al. Prevention of coronary heart disease with pravastatin in men with hypercholesterolemia. West of Scotland Coronary Prevention Study Group. *N Engl J Med* 1995; **333**:1301–7.

30. Frick MH, Elo O, Haapa K, et al. Helsinki Heart Study: primary-prevention trial with gemfibrozil in middle-aged men with dyslipidemia. Safety of treatment, changes in risk factors, and incidence of coronary heart disease. *N Engl J Med* 1987; **317**:1237–45.

31. The 4S Group. Randomised trial of cholesterol lowering in 4444 patients with coronary heart disease: the Scandinavian Simvastatin Survival Study (4S). *Lancet* 1994; **344**:1383–9.

32. Kreger BE, Kannel WB, Cupples LA. Electrocardiographic precursors of sudden unexpected death: the Framingham Study. *Circulation* 1987; **75** (Suppl 2):22–4.

33. Rubins HB, Robins SJ, Collins D, et al. Gemfibrozil for the secondary prevention of coronary heart disease in men with low levels of high-density lipoprotein cholesterol. Veterans Affairs High-Density Lipoprotein Cholesterol Intervention Trial Study Group. *N Engl J Med* 1999; **341**:410–18.

34. Sever PS, Dahlof B, Poulter NR, et al. Prevention of coronary and stroke events with atorvastatin in hypertensive patients who have average or lower-than-average cholesterol concentrations, in the Anglo-Scandinavian Cardiac Outcomes Trial–Lipid Lowering Arm (ASCOT-LLA): a multicentre

randomised controlled trial. *Lancet* 2003; **361**: 1149–58.

35. Heart Protection Study Collaborative Group. MRC/BHF Heart Protection Study of cholesterol lowering with simvastatin in 20,536 high-risk individuals: a randomised placebo-controlled trial. *Lancet* 2002; **360**:7–22.

36. Shepherd J, Blauw GJ, Murphy MB, et al. Pravastatin in elderly individuals at risk of vascular disease (PROSPER): a randomised controlled trial. *Lancet* 2002; **360**:1623–30.

37. Hyman DJ, Pavlik VN. Characteristics of patients with uncontrolled hypertension in the United States. *N Engl J Med* 2001; **345**:479–86.

38. Basile JN. The importance of systolic blood pressure control and cardiovascular disease prevention. *Curr Treat Options Cardiovasc Med* 2003; **5**:271–7.

39. Kannel WB. Elevated systolic blood pressure as a cardiovascular risk factor. *Am J Cardiol* 2000; **85**:251–5.

40. Franklin SS, Larson MG, Khan SA, et al. Does the relation of blood pressure to coronary heart disease risk change with aging? The Framingham Heart Study. *Circulation* 2001; **103**:1245–9.

41. Vasan RS, Larson MG, Leip EP, et al. Impact of high-normal blood pressure on the risk of cardiovascular disease. *N Engl J Med* 2001; **345**:1291–7.

42. Lewington S, Clarke R, Qizilbash N, Peto R, Collins R. Age-specific relevance of usual blood pressure to vascular mortality: a meta-analysis of individual data for one million adults in 61 prospective studies. *Lancet* 2002; **360**:1903–13.

43. Pahor M, Psaty BM, Alderman MH, Applegate WB, Williamson JD, Furberg CD. Therapeutic benefits of ACE inhibitors and other antihypertensive drugs in patients with type 2 diabetes. *Diabetes Care* 2000; **23**:888–92.

44. Sacks FM, Svetkey LP, Vollmer WM, et al. Effects on blood pressure of reduced dietary sodium and the Dietary Approaches to Stop Hypertension (DASH) diet. DASH-Sodium Collaborative Research Group. *N Engl J Med* 2001; **344**:3–10.

45. Furberg CD, Psaty BM, Meyer JV. Nifedipine. Dose-related increase in mortality in patients with coronary heart disease. *Circulation* 1995; **92**:1326–31.

46. Systolic Hypertension in the Elderly Program Cooperative Research Group. Prevention of stroke by antihypertensive drug treatment in older persons with isolated systolic hypertension: final results of the Systolic Hypertension in the Elderly Program (SHEP). *JAMA* 1991; **265**:3255–64.

47. Staessen JA, Fagard R, Thijs L, et al. Randomised double-blind comparison of placebo and active treatment for older patients with isolated systolic hypertension. The Systolic Hypertension in Europe (Syst-Eur) Trial Investigators. *Lancet* 1997; **350**:757–64.

48. Wang JG, Staessen JA, Gong L, Liu L. Chinese trial on isolated systolic hypertension in the elderly. Systolic Hypertension in China (Syst-China) Collaborative Group. *Arch Intern Med* 2000; **160**:211–20.

49. ALLHAT Officers and Coordinators for the ALLHAT Collaborative Research Group. Major outcomes in high-risk hypertensive patients randomized to angiotensin-converting enzyme inhibitor or calcium channel blocker vs diuretic: The Antihypertensive and Lipid-Lowering Treatment to Prevent Heart Attack Trial (ALLHAT). *JAMA* 2002; **288**:2981–97.

50. ALLHAT Officers and Coordinators for the ALLHAT Collaborative Research Group. Major cardiovascular events in hypertensive patients randomized to doxazosin vs chlorthalidone: the antihypertensive and lipid-lowering treatment to prevent heart attack trial (ALLHAT). *JAMA* 2000; **283**:1967–75.

51. Expert Panel. *Clinical Guidelines on the Identification, Evaluation, and Treatment of Overweight and Obesity in Adults. [1].* Bethesda, MD: Public Health Service, NIH, NHLBI, 1998.

52. Mokdad AH, Serdula MK, Dietz WH, Bowman BA, Marks JS, Koplan JP. The spread of the obesity epidemic in the United States, 1991–1998. *JAMA* 1999; **282**:1519–22.

53. Wilson PW, Kannel WB, Silbershatz H, D'Agostino RB. Clustering of metabolic factors and coronary heart disease. *Arch Intern Med* 1999; **159**:1104–9.

54. Wilson PW, D'Agostino RB, Sullivan L, Parise H, Kannel WB. Overweight and obesity as determinants of cardiovascular risk: the Framingham experience. *Arch Intern Med* 2002; **162**:1867–72.

55. Lichtenstein AH, Kennedy E, Barrier P, et al. Dietary fat consumption and health. *Nutr Rev* 1998; **56**:S3–19.

56. Inskeep PB, Davis KM, Reed AE. Pharmacokinetics of the acyl coenzyme A:cholesterol acyl transferase inhibitor CP-105,191 in dogs – the effect of food and sesame oil on systemic exposure following oral dosing. *J Pharm Sci* 1995; **84**:131–3.

57. Schaefer EJ, Lamon-Fava S, Ausman LM, et al. Individual variability in lipoprotein cholesterol response to National Cholesterol Education Program Step 2 diets. *Am J Clin Nutr* 1997; **65**:823–30.

58. Krauss RM, Eckel RH, Howard B, et al. AHA Dietary Guidelines: revision 2000: A statement for healthcare professionals from the Nutrition Committee of the American Heart Association. *Circulation* 2000; **102**:2284–99.

59. Pearson TA, Laurora I, Chu H, Kafonek S. The lipid treatment assessment project (L-TAP): a multicenter survey to evaluate the percentages of dyslipidemic patients receiving lipid-lowering therapy and achieving low-density lipoprotein cholesterol goals. *Arch Intern Med* 2000; **160**:459–67.

60. Steinberg D, Parthasarathy S, Carew TE, Khoo JC, Witztum JL. Beyond cholesterol: modifications of low-density lipoproteins that increase its atherogenicity. *N Engl J Med* 1989; **320**:915–24.

61. Rimm EB, Stampfer MJ, Ascherio A, Giovannucci E, Colditz GA, Willett WC. Vitamin E consumption and the risk of coronary heart disease in men. *N Engl J Med* 1993; **328**:1450–6.

62. Stampfer MJ, Hennekens CH, Manson JE, et al. Vitamin E consumption and risk of coronary heart disease in women. *N Engl J Med* 1993; **328**:1444–9.

63. Yusuf S, Dagenais G, Pogue J, Bosch J, Sleight P. Vitamin E supplementation and cardiovascular events in high-risk patients. The Heart Outcomes Prevention Evaluation Study Investigators. *N Engl J Med* 2000; **342**:154–60.

64. Heart Protection Study Collaborative Group. MRC/BHF Heart Protection Study of antioxidant vitamin supplementation in 20,536 high-risk individuals: a randomised placebo-controlled trial. *Lancet* 2002; **360**:23–33.

65. Kannel WB, Ellison RC. Alcohol and coronary heart disease: the evidence for a protective effect. *Clin Chim Acta* 1996; **246**:59–76.

66. Klatsky AL. Alcohol, coronary disease, and hypertension. *Annu Rev Med* 1996; **47**:149–60.

67. Shaper AG. Alcohol and coronary heart disease. *Eur Heart J* 1995; **16**:1760–4.

68. Rimm EB, Willett WC, Hu FB, et al. Folate and vitamin B6 from diet and supplements in relation to risk of coronary heart disease among women. *JAMA* 1998; **279**:359–64.

69. Ellison RC. Cheers! *Epidemiology* 1990; **1**:337–9.

70. Boffetta P, Garfinkel L. Alcohol drinking and mortality among men enrolled in an American Cancer Society Prospective Study. *Epidemiology* 1990; **1**:342–8.

71. Winkleby MA, Robinson TN, Sundquist J, Kraemer HC. Ethnic variation in cardiovascular disease risk factors among children and young adults: findings from the Third National Health and Nutrition Examination Survey, 1988–1994. *JAMA* 1999; **281**:1006–13.

72. Castelli WP, Garrison RJ, Dawber TR, McNamara PM, Feinleib M, Kannel WB. The filter cigarette and coronary heart disease: the Framingham Study. *Lancet* 1981; **2**:109–13.

73. Palmer JR, Rosenberg L, Shapiro S. 'Low yield' cigarettes and the risk of nonfatal myocardial infarction in women. *N Engl J Med* 1989; **320**:1569–73.

74. Ockene JK, Kuller LH, Svendsen KH, Meilahn E. The relationship of smoking cessation to coronary heart disease and lung cancer in the Multiple Risk Factor Intervention Trial (MRFIT). *Am J Public Health* 1990; **80**:954–8.

75. Bolego C, Poli A, Paoletti R. Smoking and gender. *Cardiovasc Res* 2002; **53**:568–76.

76. Steenland K. Passive smoking and the risk of heart disease. *JAMA* 1992; **267**:94–9.

77. Howard G, Burke GL, Szklo M, et al. Active and passive smoking are associated with increased carotid wall thickness. The Atherosclerosis Risk in Communities Study. *Arch Intern Med* 1994; **154**: 1277–82.

78. Paffenbarger RS Jr, Hyde RT, Wing AL, Hsieh C-C. Physical activity, all-cause mortality, and longevity of college alumni. *N Engl J Med* 1986; **314**:605–13.

79. Paffenbarger RS Jr, Hyde RT, Wing AL, Lee IM, Jung DL, Kampert JB. The association of changes in physical-activity level and other lifestyle characteristics with mortality among men. *N Engl J Med* 1993; **328**:538–45.

80. Mittleman MA, Maclure M, Tofler GH, Sherwood JB, Goldberg RJ, Muller JE. Triggering of acute myocardial infarction by heavy physical exertion. Protection against triggering by regular exertion. Determinants of Myocardial Infarction Onset Study Investigators. *N Engl J Med* 1993; **329**:1677–83.

81. Mittleman MA, Siscovick DS. Physical exertion as a trigger of myocardial infarction and sudden cardiac death. *Cardiol Clin* 1996; **14**:263–70.

82. Thompson PD, Buchner D, Pina IL, et al. Exercise and physical activity in the prevention and treatment of atherosclerotic cardiovascular disease: a statement from the Council on Clinical Cardiology (Subcommittee on Exercise, Rehabilitation, and Prevention) and the Council on Nutrition, Physical Activity, and Metabolism (Subcommittee on Physical Activity). *Arterioscler Thromb Vasc Biol* 2003; **23**:E42–9.

83. Thompson PD, Lim V. Physical activity in the prevention of atherosclerotic coronary heart disease. *Curr Treat Options Cardiovasc Med* 2003; **5**:279–85.

84. Thompson PD. Exercise and physical activity in the prevention and treatment of atherosclerotic cardiovascular disease. *Arterioscler Thromb Vasc Biol* 2003; **23**:1319–21.

85. Blair SN, Kampert JB, Kohl HW 3rd, et al. Influences of cardiorespiratory fitness and other precursors on

cardiovascular disease and all-cause mortality in men and women. *JAMA* 1996; **276**:205–10.

86. Harris MI, Flegal KM, Cowie CC, et al. Prevalence of diabetes, impaired fasting glucose, and impaired glucose tolerance in U.S. adults. The Third National Health and Nutrition Examination Survey, 1988–1994. *Diabetes Care* 1998; **21**:518–24.

87. Wilson PW. Diabetes mellitus and coronary heart disease. *Am J Kidney Dis* 1998; **32** (Suppl 3):S89–100.

88. Haffner SM, Lehto S, Ronnemaa T, Pyorala K, Laakso M. Mortality from coronary heart disease in subjects with type 2 diabetes and in nondiabetic subjects with and without prior myocardial infarction. *N Engl J Med* 1998; **339**:229–34.

89. Executive Summary of the Third Report of the National Cholesterol Education Program (NCEP) Expert Panel on Detection, Evaluation, and Treatment of High Blood Cholesterol in Adults (Adult Treatment Panel III). *JAMA* 2001; **285**: 2486–97.

90. Sowers JR, Epstein M, Frohlich ED. Diabetes, hypertension, and cardiovascular disease: an update. *Hypertension* 2001; **37**:1053–9.

91. Gaede P, Vedel P, Larsen N, Jensen GV, Parving HH, Pedersen O. Multifactorial intervention and cardiovascular disease in patients with type 2 diabetes. *N Engl J Med* 2003; **348**:383–93.

92. Singer DE, Nathan DM, Anderson KM, Wilson PWF, Evans JC. Association of HbA1c with prevalent cardiovascular disease in the original cohort of the Framingham Heart Study. *Diabetes* 1992; **41**:202–8.

93. Kuusisto J, Mykkanen L, Pyorala K, Laakso M. NIDDM and its metabolic control predict coronary heart disease in elderly subjects. *Diabetes* 1994; **43**:960–7.

94. Turner RC. The U.K. Prospective Diabetes Study. A review. *Diabetes Care* 1998; **21** (Suppl 3):C35–8.

95. Turner RC, Cull CA, Frighi V, Holman RR. Glycemic control with diet, sulfonylurea, metformin, or insulin in patients with type 2 diabetes mellitus: progressive requirement for multiple therapies (UKPDS 49). UK Prospective Diabetes Study (UKPDS) Group. *JAMA* 1999; **281**:2005–12.

96. Ford ES, Giles WH, Dietz WH. Prevalence of the metabolic syndrome among US adults: findings from the third National Health and Nutrition Examination Survey. *JAMA* 2002; **287**:356–9.

97. Isomaa B, Almgren P, Tuomi T, et al. Cardiovascular morbidity and mortality associated with the metabolic syndrome. *Diabetes Care* 2001; **24**:683–9.

98. Lakka HM, Laaksonen DE, Lakka TA, et al. The metabolic syndrome and total and cardiovascular disease mortality in middle-aged men. *JAMA* 2002; **288**:2709–16.

99. Sattar N, Gaw A, Scherbakova O, et al. Metabolic syndrome with and without C-reactive protein as a predictor of coronary heart disease and diabetes in the West of Scotland Coronary Prevention Study. *Circulation* 2003; **108**:414–19.

100. Danesh J, Collins R, Appleby P, Peto R. Association of fibrinogen, C-reactive protein, albumin, or leukocyte count with coronary heart disease: meta-analyses of prospective studies. *JAMA* 1998; **279**:1477–82.

101. Ridker PM, Hennekens CH, Buring JE, Rifai N. C-reactive protein and other markers of inflammation in the prediction of cardiovascular disease in women. *N Engl J Med* 2000; **342**:836–43.

102. Ridker PM, Cushman M, Stampfer MJ, Tracy RP, Hennekens CH. Plasma concentration of C-reactive protein and risk of developing peripheral vascular disease. *Circulation* 1998; **97**:425–8.

103. Ridker PM, Glynn RJ, Hennekens CH. C-reactive protein adds to the predictive value of total and HDL cholesterol in determining risk of first myocardial infarction. *Circulation* 1998; **97**:2007–11.

104. Ridker PM, Rifai N, Rose L, Buring JE, Cook NR. Comparison of C-reactive protein and low-density lipoprotein cholesterol levels in the prediction of first cardiovascular events. *N Engl J Med* 2002; **347**:1557–65.

105. Rost NS, Wolf PA, Kase CS, et al. Plasma concentration of C-reactive protein and risk of ischemic stroke and transient ischemic attack: The Framingham Study. *Stroke* 2001; **32**:2575–9.

106. Pearson TA, Mensah GA, Alexander RW, et al. Markers of inflammation and cardiovascular disease: application to clinical and public health practice: a statement for healthcare professionals from the Centers for Disease Control and Prevention and the American Heart Association. *Circulation* 2003; **107**:499–511.

107. Selhub J, Jacques PF, Wilson PWF, Rush D, Rosenberg IH. Vitamin status and intake as primary determinants of homocysteinemia in the elderly. *JAMA* 1993; **270**:2693–8.

108. Christen WG, Ajani UA, Glynn RJ, Hennekens CH. Blood levels of homocysteine and increased risks of cardiovascular disease: causal or casual? *Arch Intern Med* 2000; **160**:422–34.

109. Homocysteine and risk of ischemic heart disease and stroke: a meta-analysis. *JAMA* 2002; **288**:2015–22.

110. Jacques PF, Selhub J, Bostom AG, Wilson PW, Rosenberg IH. The effect of folic acid fortification on plasma folate and total homocysteine concentrations. *N Engl J Med* 1999; **340**:1449–54.

111. Bostom AG, Gohh RY, Liaugaudas G, et al. Prevalence of mild fasting hyperhomocysteinemia in renal transplant versus coronary artery disease patients after fortification of cereal grain flour with folic acid. *Atherosclerosis* 1999; **145**:221–4.

112. Bostom AG, Selhub J, Jacques PF, Rosenberg IH. Power shortage: clinical trials testing the 'homocysteine hypothesis' against a background of folic acid-fortified cereal grain flour. *Ann Intern Med* 2001; **135**:133–7.

113. Nabel EG. Cardiovascular disease. *N Engl J Med* 2003; **349**:60–72.

114. Breslow JL. Genetic markers for coronary heart disease. *Clin Cardiol* 2001; **24**(7 Suppl):II-7.

115. Goldstein JL, Hazzard WR, Schrott HG, Bierman EL, Motulsky AB. Hyperlipidemia in coronary heart disease I. Lipid levels in 500 survivors of myocardial infarction. *J Clin Invest* 1973; **52**:1533–43.

116. Dallongeville J, Lussier-Cacan S, Davignon J. Modulation of plasma triglyceride levels by apoE phenotype: a meta-analysis. *J Lipid Res* 1992; **33**:447–54.

117. Wilson PW, Myers RH, Larson MG, Ordovas JM, Wolf PA, Schaefer EJ. Apolipoprotein E alleles, dyslipidemia, and coronary heart disease. The Framingham Offspring Study. *JAMA* 1994; **272**:1666–71.

118. Corder EH, Saunders AM, Strittmatter WJ, et al. Gene dose of apolipoprotein E type 4 allele and the risk of Alzheimer's disease in late onset families. *Science* 1993; **261**:921–3.

119. Luc G, Bard J-M, Arveiler D, et al. Impact of apolipoprotein E polymorphism on lipoproteins and risk of myocardial infarction: The ECTIM Study. *Arterioscler Thromb* 1994; **14**:1412–19.

120. Lopez-Miranda J, Ordovas JM, Mata P, et al. Effect of apolipoprotein E phenotype on diet-induced lowering of plasma low density lipoprotein cholesterol. *J Lipid Res* 1994; **35**:1965–75.

121. Mooser V, Helbecque N, Miklossy J, Marcovina SM, Nicod P, Amouyel P. Interactions between apolipoprotein E and apolipoprotein(a) in patients with late-onset Alzheimer disease. *Ann Intern Med* 2000; **132**:533–7.

122. Cambien F, Poirier O, Lecer L, et al. Deletion polymorphism in the gene for angiotensin-converting enzyme is a potent risk factor for myocardial infarction. *Nature* 1993; **359**:641–4.

123. Marcovina SM, Hegele RA, Koschinsky ML. Lipoprotein(a) and coronary heart disease risk. *Curr Cardiol Rep* 1999; **1**:105–11.

124. Zhong S, Sharp DS, Grove JS, et al. Increased coronary heart disease in Japanese-American men with mutation in the cholesteryl ester transfer protein gene despite increased HDL levels. *J Clin Invest* 1996; **97**:2917–23.

125. Despres JP, Couillard C, Gagnon J, et al. Race, visceral adipose tissue, plasma lipids, and lipoprotein lipase activity in men and women: the Health, Risk Factors, Exercise Training, and Genetics (HERITAGE) family study. *Arterioscler Thromb Vasc Biol* 2000; **20**:1932–8.

126. Klerk M, Verhoef P, Clarke R, et al. MTHFR 677C→T polymorphism and risk of coronary heart disease: a meta-analysis. *JAMA* 2002; **288**:2023–31.

127. Shearman AM, Ordovas JM, Cupples LA, et al. Evidence for a gene influencing the TG/HDL-C ratio on chromosome 7q32.3–qter: a genome-wide scan in the Framingham Study. *Hum Mol Genet* 2000; **9**:1315–20.

128. Relationship of atherosclerosis in young men to serum lipoprotein cholesterol concentrations and smoking. A preliminary report from the Pathobiological Determinants of Atherosclerosis in Youth (PDAY) Research Group. *JAMA* 1990; **264**:3018–24.

129. McGill HC, McMahan CA, Herderick EE, et al. Effects of coronary heart disease risk factors on atherosclerosis of selected regions of the aorta and right coronary artery. PDAY Research Group. Pathobiological Determinants of Atherosclerosis in Youth. *Arterioscler Thromb Vasc Biol* 2000; **20**:836–45.

130. Wilson PW, Kauppila LI, O'Donnell CJ, et al. Abdominal aortic calcific deposits are an important predictor of vascular morbidity and mortality. *Circulation* 2001; **103**:1529–34.

131. Wilson PWF, Hoeg JM, D'Agostino RB, et al. Cumulative effects of high cholesterol levels, high blood pressure, and cigarette smoking on carotid stenosis. *N Engl J Med* 1997; **337**:516–22.

132. O'Leary DH, Polak JF, Kronmal RA, Manolio TA, Burke GL, Wolfson SKJ. Carotid-artery intima and media thickness as a risk factor for myocardial infarction and stroke in older adults. Cardiovascular Health Study Collaborative Research Group. *N Engl J Med* 1999; **340**:14–22.

133. Raggi P, Callister TQ, Cooil B, et al. Identification of patients at increased risk of first unheralded acute myocardial infarction by electron-beam computed tomography. *Circulation* 2000; **101**:850–5.

134. Raggi P, Cooil B, Callister TQ. Use of electron beam tomography data to develop models for prediction of hard coronary events. *Am Heart J* 2001; **141**:375–82.

135. Bild DE, Bluemke DA, Burke GL, et al. Multi-ethnic study of atherosclerosis: objectives and design. *Am J Epidemiol* 2002; **156**:871–81.

136. Kannel WB, Stampfer MJ, Castelli WP, Verter J. The prognostic significance of proteinuria: The Framingham Study. *Am Heart J* 1984; **108**:1347–52.

137. Culleton BF, Larson MG, Wilson PW, Evans JC, Parfrey PS, Levy D. Cardiovascular disease and mortality in a community-based cohort with mild renal insufficiency. *Kidney Int* 1999; **56**:2214–19.

138. Tight blood pressure control and risk of macrovascular and microvascular complications in type 2 diabetes: UKPDS 38. UK Prospective Diabetes Study Group. *BMJ* 1998; **317**:703–13.

139. Levey AS, Beto JA, Coronado BE, et al. Controlling the epidemic of cardiovascular disease in chronic renal disease: what do we know? What do we need to learn? Where do we go from here? *Am J Kidney Dis* 1998; **32**:853–906.

140. Sarnak MJ, Levey AS, Schoolwerth AC, et al. Kidney disease as a risk factor for development of cardiovascular disease: a statement from the American Heart Association Councils on Kidney in Cardiovascular Disease, High Blood Pressure Research, Clinical Cardiology, and Epidemiology and Prevention. *Circulation* 2003; **108**:2154–69.

141. D'Agostino RB Sr, Grundy S, Sullivan LM, Wilson P. Validation of the Framingham Coronary Heart Disease Prediction Scores: results of a multiple ethnic groups investigation. *JAMA* 2001; **286**:180–7.

142. Marrugat J, Solanas P, D'Agostino R, et al. Coronary risk estimation in Spain using a calibrated Framingham function. *Rev Esp Cardiol* 2003; **56**:253–61.

143. Pasternak RC, Abrams J, Greenland P, Smaha LA, Wilson PW, Houston-Miller N. 34th Bethesda Conference: Task force #1 – Identification of coronary heart disease risk: is there a detection gap? *J Am Coll Cardiol* 2003; **41**:1863–74.

144. Assmann G, Cullen P, Schulte H. Simple scoring scheme for calculating the risk of acute coronary events based on the 10-year follow-up of the prospective cardiovascular Munster (PROCAM) study. *Circulation* 2002; **105**:310–15.

145. Conroy RM, Pyorala K, Fitzgerald AP, et al. Estimation of ten-year risk of fatal cardiovascular disease in Europe: the SCORE project. *Eur Heart J* 2003; **24**:987–1003.

146. Stevens RJ, Kothari V, Adler AI, Stratton IM. The UKPDS risk engine: a model for the risk of coronary heart disease in Type II diabetes (UKPDS 56). *Clin Sci (Lond)* 2001; **101**:671–9.

147. Wolf PA, D'Agostino RB, Belanger AJ, Kannel WB. Probability of stroke: a risk profile from the Framingham Study. *Stroke* 1991; **3**:312–18.

148. Murabito JM, D'Agostino RB, Silbershatz H, Wilson PWF. Intermittent claudication: a risk profile from the Framingham Heart Study. *Circulation* 1997; **96**:44–9.

149. Anderson KM, Odell PM, Wilson PWF, Kannel WB. Cardiovascular disease risk profiles. *Am Heart J* 1991; **121**:293–8.

150. Wilson PW, Smith SC Jr, Blumenthal RS, Burke GL, Wong ND. 34th Bethesda Conference: Task force #4 – How do we select patients for atherosclerosis imaging? *J Am Coll Cardiol* 2003; **41**:1898–906.

151. Wilson PW. Metabolic risk factors for coronary heart disease: current and future prospects. *Curr Opin Cardiol* 1999; **14**:176–85.

152. Mosca L. C-reactive protein – to screen or not to screen? *N Engl J Med* 2002; **347**:1615–17.

3

The A, B, C, D, and E of diabetes and heart disease in women

Alka M. Kanaya and Elizabeth Barrett-Connor

Introduction

In the United States, diabetes is equally common in women and men,[1] although rates may be higher in ethnic minority women in whom diabetes is more common, reflecting common sex differences in obesity in these groups.[2] Diabetes increases the risk of coronary heart disease (CHD) in both sexes,[3] one- to twofold in men and two- to fourfold in women.[4] In this chapter we review the epidemiologic evidence for sex differences in the association between diabetes and heart disease, and consider the evidence for sex differences among diabetic patients in response to interventions. The interventions reviewed are limited to data from clinical trials modifying HbA$_{1c}$, **B**lood pressure, **C**holesterol, **D**iet, and **E**xercise (the A, B, C, D, and E of clinical trial results). Trial results provide evidence for (or against) causality and inform recommendations for prevention therapies in patients with or at high risk of type 2 diabetes.

Epidemiology

Until recently, nearly all prospective studies of heart disease risk factors that included standard tests of glycemia, and that tested for an independent effect of diabetes or hyperglycemia on cardiovascular outcomes, were conducted in men. The largest study, the Multiple Risk Factor Intervention Trial (MRFIT),

enrolled 347 978 middle-aged adults, all men, in the 1970s.[5] After 12 years there was a threefold increased risk of cardiovascular disease mortality in men who had diabetes compared with those who did not.[5] This risk was independent of smoking, cholesterol, and hypertension, but, as shown in Fig. 3.1, each risk factor added to the excess risk of cardiovascular death associated with diabetes.[5]

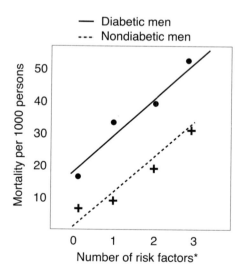

Figure 3.1
Impact of diabetes on cardiovascular mortality.
*Risk factors analyzed were smoking, dyslipidemia, and hypertension. Modified from reference 5 with permission.

In a 1985 review, Epstein[6] reported a significant positive association of glucose levels with incident heart disease independent of major heart disease risk factors in five of 19 prospective studies; only four of the 19 studies included women. In a 1999 meta-analysis, Coutinho et al.[7] found 20 prospective studies that included a total of 95 783 adults; only 6% were women. Those with impaired fasting glucose (IFG) between 6.1 and 6.9 mmol/l (110–125 mg/dl) had a relative risk (RR) of 1.33 (95% confidence interval (CI), 1.06–1.67) for cardiovascular events; those with impaired glucose tolerance (IGT) with a 2-hour post-challenge glucose between 7.8 and 11.0 mmol/l (140–199 mg/dl) had RR of 1.58 (95% CI 1.10–2.10).[7] There is unequal overlap between IFG and IGT[8] suggesting that these groups represent different proportions of the glucose spectrum.[9] In the large DECODE (Diabetes Epidemiology: Collaborative analysis Of Diagnostic criteria in Europe) prospective study of European adults, neither women nor men with IFG alone were at increased risk of death, while those with IGT alone were at significantly increased risk, similar in both sexes (hazard ratio (HR) 1.56, 95% CI 1.33–1.83 in men and HR 1.66, 95% CI 1.24–2.23 in women).[10]

In every country men have more fatal heart disease than women between the ages of 45 and 64.[11] The reason for this sex difference is unknown, but women with diabetes appear to have a two- to four-fold increased risk of CHD mortality compared with nondiabetic women, while men with diabetes have about a one- to twofold increased risk compared with nondiabetic men. It is unknown how diabetes equalizes or reduces the usual sex difference in risk of CHD. A few meta-analyses attempted to assess the sex-specific risk of fatal and nonfatal CHD events associated with diabetes,[3,12,13] and reached somewhat different conclusions. A recent meta-analysis by Kanaya and colleagues found that the sex difference was largely obliterated in studies that controlled for other common heart disease risk factors.[3] A recent review from the Agency for Healthcare Research and Quality reported that the increased risk of diabetes for CHD death in women was similar to that in men after adjusting for classical heart disease risk factors such as age, cholesterol, hypertension, and smoking.[14] These results suggest that the reduced sex difference in CHD rates in the presence of diabetes is caused by sex differences in the cluster of diabetes-associated risk factors.

In 1970, Bierman et al. recognized the clustering of heart disease risk factors, noting that persons with diabetes had more of these risk factors.[15] In 1983, Wingard and colleagues[16] reported that diabetic women from three different cohorts had more clustered risk factors than diabetic men. At about the same time, it became clear that the main lipid abnormality in persons with diabetes was not total or low-density lipoprotein (LDL) cholesterol, but was a low high-density lipoprotein (HDL) cholesterol level in the presence of a high triglyceride level, with larger differences in women with diabetes compared with women without than seen in similar comparisons of men with and without diabetes[17] (Fig. 3.2). This dyslipidemia, called pattern B dyslipidemia, is a marker for small dense LDL, a particularly atherogenic LDL. In 1988, Reaven[18] named the cluster syndrome X and proposed that it included pattern B dyslipidemia, hyperglycemia, and hypertension, and was caused by insulin resistance. This definition of syndrome X did not include obesity or central adiposity, and did not consider sex differences.

Increasing attention has focused on the role of this cluster as a heart disease risk factor. In 2001 the National Cholesterol Education Program and the third Adult Treatment Panel report recommended that individuals with three or more of these risk factors be classified as having the metabolic syndrome.[19] These features included elevated waist circumference (>102 cm in men and >88 cm in women) and low HDL cholesterol (<40 mg/dl in men and <50 mg/dl in women), reflecting the sex differences in these factors. Other components of the metabolic syndrome were not sex-specific and included triglycerides ≥150 mg/dl, high blood pressure (≥130/≥85 mmHg), and elevated fasting glucose (≥110 mg/dl). These criteria were based primarily on studies of Caucasians of northern European ancestry; the panel report recommended a lower cut-off point of waist circumference in those genetically predisposed to the metabolic syndrome. Using data from the third National Health and Nutrition Examination Survey, it was estimated that 22% of the adult US population has the metabolic syndrome,[20] almost three times the prevalence of diabetes in the same population.[1]

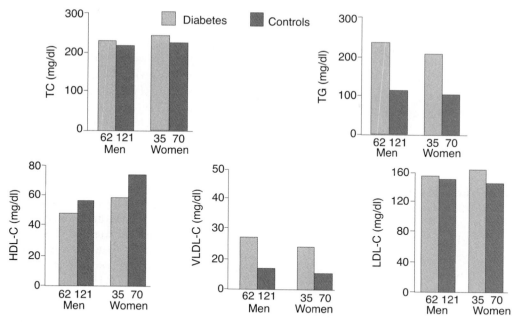

Figure 3.2
Rancho Bemardo study: lipids and lipoproteins by diabetes status. TC, total cholesterol; TG, triglycerides; HDL-C, high-density lipoprotein cholesterol; VLDL-C, very-low-density lipoprotein cholesterol; LDL-C, low-density lipoprotein cholesterol. Modified from reference 17 with permission of Oxford University Press.

The metabolic syndrome has been associated with increased risk of cardiovascular death. In the Kuopio Ischaemic Heart Disease Risk Factor Study of 1209 healthy Finnish middle-aged men, those with the metabolic syndrome were almost three times more likely to die of cardiovascular disease or CHD than those without the syndrome after adjustment for conventional cardiovascular risk factors.[21] No similar study has been published for women.

Because of the very high risk of heart disease in persons with diabetes, diabetes has been proposed (and widely accepted) to be considered a heart disease equivalent.[19] Haffner and colleagues[22] examined the 7-year incidence of myocardial infarction (MI) among a large number of diabetic (1059) and nondiabetic (1373) men in a Finnish study. In this study, the 7-year incidence of MI among nondiabetic men with a history of CHD was similar to the MI incidence among diabetic men without a history of CHD, as shown in Fig. 3.3. In a pooled analysis from the Organization to Assess Strategies for Ischemic Syndromes study, diabetic women and

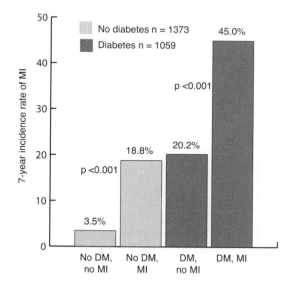

Figure 3.3
Type 2 diabetes (DM) and coronary heart disease: 7-year incidence of fatal/nonfatal myocardial infarction (MI) from the East West Study. Modified from reference 22 with permission.

men who were hospitalized with unstable angina or non-Q-wave MI in six countries and followed for 2 years had similar cardiovascular mortality rates to men and women with a past history of cardiovascular disease.[23] However, in a 22-year follow-up of

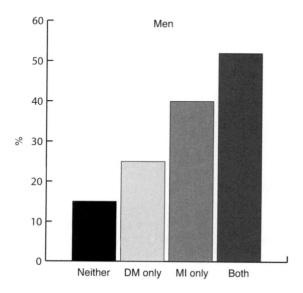

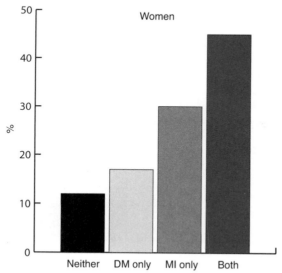

Figure 3.4
Age-adjusted coronary heart disease mortality rates – Rancho Bernardo study: 22-year follow-up by type 2 diabetes (DM) and myocardial infarction (MI) status.

community-dwelling older adults from California, women and men with known CHD and no diabetes had almost double the rates of CHD death (37.5% in men and 25.9% in women) than women and men with diabetes with no known CHD (17% in men and 11.2% in women) (Fig. 3.4) (Barrett-Connor, unpublished data).

While most long-term complications of diabetes occur at a similar frequency for both women and men, one notable exception may be heart failure. An early report from the Framingham Heart Study found that twice as many men with diabetes and five times as many women with diabetes compared with their nondiabetic counterparts had echocardiographic criteria for congestive heart failure.[24] Additionally, diabetic women had a 10% greater left ventricular mass compared with nondiabetic women in the Framingham study.[25] However, a more recent report from the Framingham Heart Study found that the overall lifetime risk of developing heart failure is similar (approximately 20%) in both women and men.[26] Heart failure in the presence of diabetes is not entirely explained by known coronary artery disease, and is thought by some to be a unique entity characterized by diastolic dysfunction.[27] Some studies have found that poor glycemic control is related to the increased risk of heart failure,[28] and others have reported that left ventricular hypertrophy is related to the clustering of risk factors in the metabolic syndrome.[29]

A: HbA$_{1c}$

HbA$_{1c}$ is a measure of glycemic control over the past 3–4 months. The recommended goal for A$_{1c}$ for diabetic patients is currently less than 7%.[30] The American Diabetes Association recommendation was based on randomized controlled trials showing that lowering of A$_{1c}$ reduced the microvascular and neuropathic complications of diabetes.[31] The few large trials that evaluated the effects of intensive glucose control on macrovascular outcomes such as CHD did not show statistically significant benefit and did not present sex-specific results.[32–34]

The first large multicenter placebo-controlled clinical trial of any medication to prevent heart disease was the University Group Diabetes Program (UGDP), begun in 1961.[32] A total of 823 patients with mild hyperglycemia were enrolled in this 10-year trial. Despite a 7–8 mmol/l decrease in the achieved glucose levels among those assigned to a variable dose of insulin versus placebo, there was no significant difference in the incidence of cardiovascular or coronary heart disease. More recently the United Kingdom Prospective Diabetes Study (UKPDS)[34,35] examined the effect of improved glycemic control on vascular disease outcomes in 3867 adults (39% women) with newly diagnosed type 2 diabetes. The main intervention compared the effect of one of two sulfonylureas or insulin with conventional diet management. At the end of the trial, the intensive management group achieved a HbA$_{1c}$ of 7.0% (6.2–8.2) versus 7.9% (6.9–8.8) in the conventional management group. Compared with the conventional group, the risk in the intensive group was 12% lower for all diabetes-related endpoints (p = 0.03), with most of the risk reduction attributable to a 25% risk reduction in microvascular outcomes. There was a trend towards decreased risk of MI in the intensive group (RR 0.84, 95% CI 0.71–1.00, p = 0.052).[34] No sex-specific data were published.

The weak effect on coronary risk in the UKPDS compared with the impressive benefit against microvascular disease suggests either that factors other than glucose are major contributors to heart disease etiology or that the achieved level of glucose control is inadequate for the prevention of heart disease. A subset analysis of the main UKPDS study supports the latter thesis, showing a significant 14% reduction in MI risk for every 1% decrement of A$_{1c}$.[36]

A supplementary UKPDS study that examined the effect of metformin versus diet control among 753 overweight persons with newly diagnosed type 2 diabetes found a significant risk reduction in the metformin group for MI (RR 0.61, 95% CI 0.41–0.89) and for all-cause mortality (RR 0.64, 95% CI 0.45–0.91).[35] This effect cannot be directly attributed to glucose control, because metformin has other beneficial effects and, unlike insulin or the sulfonylureas, does not cause weight gain.

Results from the Diabetes Control and Complications Trial (DCCT), a clinical trial conducted in patients with type 1 diabetes, also showed that intensive insulin therapy significantly reduced the risk of microvascular complications compared with conventional insulin therapy, but the 40% reduced risk of CHD was not statistically significant.[37] The DCCT had little power to show a reduction in CHD – subjects were young and events were rare.

A trial that implemented a multifactorial intervention in patients with type 2 diabetes, including dietary modification, increased physical activity, intensive glycemic control, hypertension control, and lipid control versus conventional therapy, found that the intensive multifactorial intervention significantly reduced cardiovascular disease (HR 0.47, 95% CI 0.24–0.73).[38] Given the nature of the intervention it is not clear which of the many interventions, or combination of interventions, was most predictive of this benefit. Additionally, although 41 women (26% of the study population) were included in this trial, sex-specific results were not presented.

B: Blood pressure (see also Chapter 31)

The currently recommended blood pressure goal for persons with diabetes is <130/85 mmHg.[31,39] Several trials have examined blood pressure goals and optimal pharmacologic agents for the treatment of hypertension in type 2 diabetes. A recent systematic review of randomized trials found that a target diastolic blood pressure of <80 mmHg is optimal based on trial evidence, while the systolic blood pressure target has not been rigorously evaluated.[40]

Most large hypertension trials that compared the effects of blood pressure control with cardiovascular outcomes included a good proportion of women and diabetic participants. However, none of the subgroup analyses for diabetic subjects have included sex-specific results (Table 3.1).[41–47] The Systolic Hypertension in the Elderly Program (SHEP), a diuretic-based intervention, and the Systolic Hypertension in Europe (Syst-Eur), a calcium channel blocker-based intervention, were placebo-controlled trials conducted in older adults.[41,42] The active treatments reduced systolic blood pressure and total cardiovascular events, with a similar risk reduction (number needed to treat (NNT) = 12) in both

Table 3.1 Results of hypertension control trials in diabetic persons

Study acronym*, reference	Follow-up (years)	No. (with DM)	No. (women with DM)	Intervention	Cardiovascular events		Total mortality	
					RRR	ARR	RRR	ARR
SHEP[41]	5	583	NR	Thiazide vs usual care	34%	8% (1–14%)	36%	2% (–4% to 8%)
Syst-Eur[42]	2	492	NR	CCB vs placebo	62%	8% (3–13%)	41%	5% (–1% to 9%)
HOPE[45]	5	3577	NR	Ramipril vs placebo	25%	5% (2–7%)	24%	3% (1–5%)
RENAAL[46]	3.4	1513	557	Losartan vs placebo	10% (NS)	2% (–3% to 7%)	2% increase (NS)	–1% (–5% to 3%)
HOT[43]	3.8	1503	NR	Target DBP <80 or <90; felodipine, ACEI or βB	48%	5% (2–8%)	44%	3% (0–5%)
UKPDS[44]	8.4	1148	NR	Target <180/105 vs <150/85; captopril or atenolol	34%	NR	16%	4% (–1% to 9%)
ABCD[47]	5.3	470	153	Target DBP 75 vs 80–89; nisoldipine or enalapril	NR	NR	49%	5% (0–10%)

DM, diabetes mellitus; RRR, relative risk reduction; ARR, absolute risk reduction; NR, not reported; CCB, calcium channel blocker; NS, not significant; DBP, diastolic blood pressure; ACEI, angiotensin-converting enzyme inhibitor; βB, beta-blocker.
*See reference for explanation.

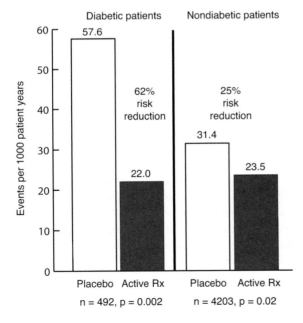

Figure 3.5
Syst-Eur trial on hypertension control: effect of systolic blood pressure control (Rx, prescription) on all cardiovascular events at 2 years. Modified from reference 42 with permission.

studies. In these trials, the effect of intensive blood pressure control on risk reduction was greater among persons with diabetes than among those without diabetes in both studies (Fig. 3.5).[42]

Diastolic blood pressure goals were evaluated in the Hypertension Optimal Treatment (HOT) study, which included 1501 diabetic patients.[43] Among the subgroup with diabetes, there was a 48% risk reduction of cardiovascular events in those randomized to the most intensive diastolic pressure control (80 mmHg) versus those in the least intensive control group (90 mmHg) (NNT = 20). In contrast, there was no significant benefit of intensive control among trial participants overall.

The UKPDS included a separate treatment group of 1148 (44% were women) newly diagnosed diabetic subjects with hypertension. They were randomly assigned to a 'tight control' target of 150/85 mmHg using either atenolol or captopril or a 'less tight' target blood pressure of 180/105 mmHg avoiding angiotensin-converting enzyme (ACE) inhibitors and beta-blockers.[44] Results were not specified for men and women separately. Overall participants assigned to tight control achieved a mean blood pressure of 144/82 mmHg versus 150/85 in the less

Subgroups	Relative risk	Favors lisinopril	Favors chlorthalidone
Nonfatal MI + CHD death	1.00 (0.87–1.14)		
All-cause mortality	1.02 (0.91–1.13)		
Stroke	1.07 (0.90–1.28)		
Combined CHD	1.03 (0.93–1.14)		
Combined CVD	1.08 (1.00–1.17)		
Heart failure	1.22 (1.05–1.42)		

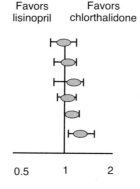

0.5   1   2

Figure 3.6
Antihypertensive and Lipid-Lowering treatment to prevent Heart Attack Trial (ALLHAT) diabetes patients: lisinopril/chlorthalidone comparisons. MI, myocardial infarction; CHD, coronary heart disease; CVD, cardiovascular disease. Modified from reference 49 with permission.

Subgroups	Relative risk	Favors amlodipine	Favors chlorthalidone
Nonfatal MI + CHD death	0.99 (0.87–1.13)		
All-cause mortality	0.96 (0.87–1.07)		
Stroke	0.90 (0.75–1.08)		
Combined CHD	1.04 (0.94–1.14)		
Combined CVD	1.06 (0.98–1.15)		
Heart failure	1.42 (1.23–1.52)		

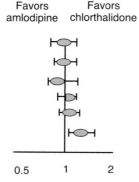

0.5   1   2

Figure 3.7
Antihypertensive and Lipid-Lowering treatment to prevent Heart Attack Trial (ALLHAT) diabetes patients: amlodipine/chlorthalidone comparisons. MI, myocardial infarction; CHD, coronary heart disease; CVD, cardiovascular disease. Modified from reference 49 with permission.

tight control group, and had a relative risk reduction of 34% (p = 0.019). The benefit of intensive hypertension control in the UKPDS greatly outweighed the benefit of intensive glycemic control on all of the published outcomes.[40]

Although the benefit of blood pressure control in diabetes is irrefutable, the effects of different drug classes in the treatment of hypertension among individuals with and without diabetes has been the subject of intense debate.[48] This debate is further complicated by the fact that most persons with or without diabetes eventually require more than one blood pressure agent to maintain treatment goals. One of the few head-to-head comparisons was the Antihypertensive and Lipid-Lowering treatment to prevent Heart Attack Trial (ALLHAT), which compared ACE inhibitors, calcium channel blockers, and thiazide diuretics.[49] In a prespecified analysis of the 12 063 ALLHAT participants with diabetes, there were no significant differences by treatment among

the groups in the combined outcome of nonfatal MI and CHD death or in all-cause mortality (Figs 3.6 and 3.7).[49] The risk of heart failure was lowest in the diuretic group (ACE inhibitor vs diuretic: RR 1.22, 95% CI 1.04–1.42; amlodipine vs diuretic: RR 1.42, 95% CI 1.23–1.52), and the ACE inhibitor group had a borderline elevated risk for cardiovascular disease compared with the diuretic group.[49] Based on this study and prior trial evidence that included renal disease outcomes, the currently recommended treatment for hypertension in persons with diabetes includes thiazide diuretics, beta-blockers, ACE inhibitors, angiotensin receptor blockers, and calcium channel blockers.

The use of beta-blockers in diabetes has been debated in the literature, with concerns about decreased insulin release from the pancreas, worsening of lipid and glycemic control, prolongation and masking of hypoglycemic symptoms, fatigue, and erectile dysfunction. Long-term data from 18

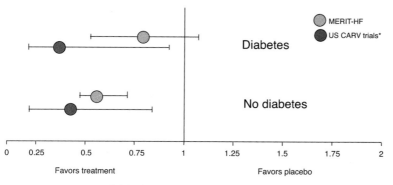

	Metoprolol CR/XL/placebo	Carvedilol/placebo
Diabetes	495/1990 (25%)	195/696 (28%)
No diabetes	489/2001 (24%)	112/398 (28%)

Figure 3.8
Effect of beta-blockade in mild-moderate congestive heart failure: all-cause mortality. *Not a planned endpoint. Modified from Metoprolol CR/XL Randomized Intervention Trial in Congestive Heart Failure (MERIT-HF) Study Group and the US carvedilol trials in heart failure (US CARV trials), references 51 and 52.

randomized trials of beta-blockers for hypertension involving 18 883 persons (mostly without diabetes) found convincing evidence that beta-blockers decreased the risk of stroke (29%) and congestive heart failure (42%), but not CHD (7%, not significant).[50]

The use of beta-blockers in patients with mild or moderate congestive heart failure has been studied in randomized controlled trials, with somewhat inconsistent results. The Metoprolol CR/XL Randomized Intervention Trial in Congestive Heart Failure (MERIT-HF) study enrolled 3991 patients with ejection fraction less than 40%, 25% with diabetes,

and found a 34% risk reduction for all-cause mortality.[51] The 984 participants in the MERIT-HF diabetic subgroup, however, had a less impressive benefit from beta-blockade that was not statistically significant. In contrast, a stratified analysis of the US carvedilol trials in heart failure showed a similar favorable risk reduction in persons with and without diabetes (Fig. 3.8).[51,52] At present, the weight of the evidence supports long-term benefit of beta-blocker use in patients with diabetes, with or without heart failure. Although few of these investigators showed sex-specific data, most commented that there was no difference in the outcomes between sexes.

	No. of participants	No. of events Placebo	No. of events Statin	Risk reduction
Women				
4S	827	91	60	
CARE	576	39	23	
AFCAPS/TexCAPS	997	13	7	
LIPID	1516	104	90	
Overall	3916	247	180	29% (13–42)
Men				
4S	3617	531	371	
WOSCOPS	6595	248	174	
CARE	3583	235	189	
AFCAPS/TexCAPS	5608	170	109	
LIPID	7498	611	467	
Overall	26 901	1795	1310	31% (26–36)

Relative odds and 95fi CIs

Figure 3.9
Effect of gender in major statin trials (4S, Scandinavian Simvastatin Survival Study; CARE, Cholesterol And Recurrent Events trial; AFCAPS/TexCAPS, Air Force/Texas Coronary Atherosclerosis Prevention Study; LIPID, Long-term Intervention with Pravastatin in Ischemic Disease trial; WOSCOPS, West of Scotland Coronary Prevention Study). CI, confidence interval. Modified from reference 54 with permission.

Table 3.2 Results of cholesterol-lowering trials among individuals with type 2 diabetes

Study acronym*, reference	Follow-up (years)	No. (with DM)	No. (women with DM)	Baseline lipid (mg/dl)	% change	Therapy	Outcome	RRR
Statin studies:								
WOSCOPS[57]	4.9	76	None	LDL 193	−26% LDL	Pravastatin	CHD death	NR
AFCAPS/TexCAPS[58]	5.2	155	None	LDL 150	−25% LDL	Lovastatin	CHD death, NFMI, angina	37%
4S[59]	5.5	202	NR	LDL 186	−34% LDL	Simvastatin	CHD death, NFMI	55%
CARE[60]	4.9	586	115	LDL 135	−27% LDL	Pravastatin	CHD death, NFMI	13%
LIPID[61]	6.1	782	NR	LDL 147	−25% LDL	Pravastatin	CHD death, NFMI	19% (NS)
Post-CABG[62]	4.3	116	17	LDL 151	−38% LDL	Lovastatin	CV death, MI, CVA, revasc.	47%
ALLHAT[63]	4.8	3638	NR	LDL 146	−28% LDL	Pravastatin	CHD	11% (NS)
HPS[55]	4.8	2912	NR	LDL 131	−29% LDL	Simvastatin	Vascular event	33%
ASCOT[56]	3.3	2532	NR	LDL 133	−32% LDL	Atorvastatin	CHD death, NFMI	17% (NS)
Fibrate studies:								
Helsinki Heart Study[64]	5	135	None	LDL 201	−10% LDL −26% TG +6% HDL	Gemfibrozil	CHD death, NFMI	68%
BIP[65]	6.2	309	NR	TG 145 HDL 35 LDL 149	−21% TG +18% HDL −6% LDL	Bezafibrate	MI or sudden death	NR (9% overall)
DAIS[66]	3.3	418	113	TG 222 HDL 40 LDL 131	−28% TG +6% HDL −5% LDL	Fenofibrate	Progression in angiographic CAD	40%
VA-HIT[67]	5.1	627	None	TG 156 HDL 32 LDL 104	−31% TG +6% HDL 0% LDL	Gemfibrozil	CHD death, NFMI, CVA	24%

DM, diabetes mellitus; RRR, relative risk reduction; NR, not reported; LDL, low-density lipoprotein cholesterol; TG, triglycerides; HDL, high-density lipoprotein cholesterol; CHD, coronary heart disease; NFMI, nonfatal myocardial infarction; MI, myocardial infarction; CVA, cerebrovascular accident; CAD, coronary artery disease; NS, not significant.
*See reference for explanation.

C: Cholesterol (see also Chapter 4)

The current recommended goal for LDL cholesterol for persons with diabetes is <100 mg/dl.[31] As noted above, elevated LDL is not a major lipid abnormality in diabetes, but LDL is the cholesterol fraction that has been most implicated in cardiovascular complications in persons with diabetes. In an analysis from the UKPDS study, a 1.0 mmol/l (or 39 mg/dl) increase in LDL was associated with a 57% increased risk in CHD, whereas a 0.1 mmol/l (or 3.9 mg/dl) increase in HDL cholesterol was associated with a net 15% reduction of CHD risk.[53]

The treatment of hypercholesterolemia has been transformed by the introduction of the 3-hydroxy-3-methylglutaryl coenzyme A reductase inhibitors, commonly known as statins. In a meta-analysis of four major statin trials that included both sexes, women had the same overall relative risk reduction as men (relative risk reduction 29% in women and 31% in men), although the results in three of the four individual studies of women were not statistically significant due to the smaller number of women in each study[48] (Fig. 3.9).[54] Table 3.2[55-67] shows results for several randomized controlled trials that evaluated the effect of various cholesterol-lowering agents in persons with or without established CHD and analyzed subgroups with diabetes separately. Most placebo-controlled trials of cardiovascular disease with cholesterol-lowering agents found significant

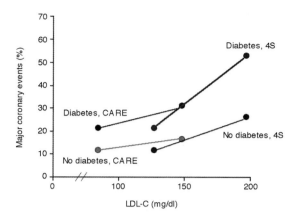

Figure 3.10
Lowering of low-density lipoprotein cholesterol (LDL-C) in patients with diabetes: Scandinavian Simvastatin Survival Study (4S) and Cholesterol and Recurrent Events trial (CARE). Modified from reference 68 with permission from Excerpta Medica Inc.

risk reduction in those randomized to the active treatment, and the magnitude of the risk reduction for the diabetic subgroup was usually equal to or greater than the reduction in risk among the participants without diabetes[68] (Fig. 3.10).

The Heart Protection Study (HPS) is the largest trial to date of primary and secondary prevention of cardiovascular disease using lipid-lowering therapy.[55,69] Of the 20 536 UK adults who were randomized in this study, 5963 (29%) had diabetes.[55] Overall, there was a 24% relative risk reduction in major vascular events at 5 years among those randomized to 40 mg/day of simvastatin compared with placebo. Among the 3051 diabetic participants without cardiovascular disease at baseline, there was a 31% reduction in the relative risk of a major vascular event – similar in both sexes and independent of duration of diabetes or glucose control[56] (Fig. 3.11).

A recent trial of statin therapy designed specifically for patients with diabetes, the Collaborative AtoRvastatin Diabetes Study (CARDS), was terminated prematurely when interim analysis demonstrated efficacy of low-dose atorvastatin vs placebo in the prevention of major cardiovascular events.[70,71]

In addition to demonstrated ability to reduce first or recurrent cardiovascular events among persons with diabetes, initiation of statin therapy as soon as possible after an acute coronary syndrome reduced recurrent ischemic events in the Myocardial Ischemia Reduction with Aggressive Cholesterol Lowering (MIRACL) study, which included 715 (23%) diabetic subjects.[72] Although results were not

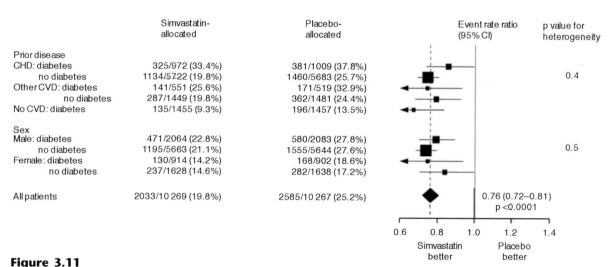

Figure 3.11
Effect of simvastatin on first cardiovascular event in select subgroups: the Heart Protection Study. CI, confidence interval; CHD, coronary heart disease; CVD, cardiovascular disease. Modified from reference 55 with permission from Elsevier.

Table 3.3 Interventions and main results from studies of lifestyle intervention for the prevention of diabetes

Study acronym*, reference	Mean follow-up (years)	Intervention group (n)	Control group (n)	Mean weight change* (kg)	RRR (95% CI)	NNT†
Da Qing Study[75]	6	130 diet only, 141 exercise, 126 diet + exercise	133	NR	31% diet, 46% exercise, 42% diet + exercise	17 for 6 years; 14 for 6 years; 16 for 6 years
Finnish DPS[76]	3.2	265	257	−4.2, −0.8	58%	22 for 1 year, or 5 for 5 years
DPP[77]‡	2.8	1079	1082	−5.6, −0.1	58% (48–66%)	7 for 3 years

RRR, relative risk reduction for incidence of diabetes; CI, confidence interval; NNT, number needed to treat; NR, not reported.
*See reference for explanation.
†Mean weight loss (−) or gain (+) for the intervention group, then the control group.
‡Results presented for intensive lifestyle intervention vs standard lifestyle intervention only.

presented separately by sex, subjects with or without diabetes had similar outcomes, with a 16% relative risk reduction in the combined endpoint of readmission, recurrent ischemia, infarction or death.

D: Diet

The American Diabetes Association recommends improved nutrition to attain optimal blood glucose levels, lipid profile, and blood pressure levels.[73] Most clinical trials of diet and diabetes have been small and of short duration, designed to study these intermediate metabolic outcomes. An ongoing clinical trial, the LOOK AHEAD study, is evaluating the effect of weight loss on cardiovascular outcomes among overweight adults with type 2 diabetes.[74] The intensive lifestyle intervention group is designed to achieve and maintain weight loss through decreased caloric intake and increased physical activity; the control group receives diabetes support and education.

Three published randomized controlled trials that studied volunteers at high risk for diabetes each found that improvement in diet and physical activity could reduce or delay the onset of type 2 diabetes (Table 3.3).[75–77] The Diabetes Prevention Program (DPP), the largest and most recent trial, randomized a total of 3234 adults to one of three groups: intensive lifestyle intervention, metformin therapy with standard lifestyle advice, and a control group with

standard lifestyle advice plus a placebo.[77] DPP participants were at least 25 years old, had a body mass index of 24 kg/m² or higher (or 22 kg/m² for Asians), and had IGT plus a fasting plasma glucose of 95–125 mg/dl (5.3–6.9 mmol/l); 67% of the DPP participants were women. The goals in the intensive lifestyle intervention were (1) weight loss of 7%, and (2) moderate physical activity for at least 150 minutes per week. During the first 6 months, the intensive lifestyle intervention group were offered 16 individual sessions with a case manager who covered topics on diet, exercise, and behavior modification, followed by regular monthly sessions that included group classes on exercise and weight loss every 3 months and two supervised exercise sessions weekly.

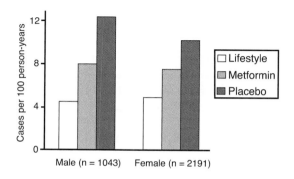

Figure 3.12
Diabetes Prevention Program: diabetes incidence rates by sex.

The DPP trial was ended 1 year early, after 2.9 years, when the incidence of diabetes was 58% lower in the lifestyle intervention group, and 31% lower in the metformin group, than in the placebo group. The results were the same in both sexes (Fig. 3.12). The incidence of diabetes was 4.8 per 100 person-years for the lifestyle intervention group, 7.8 for the metformin group, and 11.0 for the placebo group. About seven persons needed lifestyle intervention for 3 years to prevent or delay one case of diabetes.

At 6 months, about half of the participants in the DPP intensive lifestyle intervention group achieved the weight loss goal and about three-quarters achieved the exercise goal. After 2.9 years, the average weight loss in the DPP was 12 lbs for the lifestyle group, 5 lbs for the metformin group, and less than 0.5 lb for the placebo group. Although the investigators concluded that the weight loss explained more of the benefit than the exercise intervention,[78] weight change is much easier to quantify than changes in physical activity.

There is no clinical trial proof that diet and exercise prevent heart disease in persons with or without diabetes. The DPP was not powered to look at cardiovascular outcomes, but the prevention or delay of diabetes is expected to reduce the risk of cardiovascular disease. In support of a potential cardiovascular benefit, intensive lifestyle intervention in DPP significantly reduced several cardiovascular risk factors including measures of inflammation.[78]

E: Exercise (see also Chapter 7)

Current national guidelines recommend 30 minutes or more of moderate physical activity on most days of the week or 150 minutes/week.[79,80] As with diet therapy, the effect of physical activity has been studied in mostly short clinical trials with intermediate metabolic endpoints, and there are no reported controlled exercise trials with cardiovascular events as outcomes.

Most experts believe that physical activity helps with weight loss and weight maintenance, and has other cardiovascular benefits as well, but controversy remains about the optimal amount of time and level of physical activity. In a trial of 201 sedentary and overweight women without diabetes who were randomized to either high or low intensity exercise for either high or moderate duration for 1 year, investigators found that there was similar weight loss with either vigorous or moderate intensity of exercise, but a longer duration of exercise was associated with greater overall weight loss.[81]

In short-term trials, exercise has been associated with favorable changes in both lipids and blood pressure. In a systematic review of 52 trials that lasted for 12 weeks or longer and included approximately 4700 subjects overall, exercise was associated with a mean 5.0% reduction of LDL cholesterol, 3.7% reduction of triglycerides, and a 4.6% increase in HDL.[82] The most commonly observed lipid change was a significant increase in HDL, which was observed in both men and women of all ages in approximately half of the studies reviewed. In another review of 44 trials, exercise intervention was associated with an average 3.4 mmHg decrease in systolic blood pressure and 2.4 mmHg decrease in diastolic blood pressure.[83] Those with hypertension had a more marked benefit in blood pressure reductions than those without hypertension (−7.4 mmHg systolic and −5.8 mmHg diastolic for hypertensive subjects vs −2.6 mmHg systolic and −1.8 mmHg diastolic for nonhypertensive subjects). Sex-specific results were not discussed in this review.

The best evidence for benefit of exercise among persons with diabetes comes from a review of nine clinical trials that examined the acute effect of exercise training on HbA_{1c} in 337 individuals with type 2 diabetes (21% women), which showed an average reduction of A_{1c} of 0.5–1.0%.[84,85] Although these trials included women, sex-specific results are not shown.

Conclusion

Diabetes increases the risk of cardiovascular disease in both sexes, more in women than in men, possibly attributable to their greater differences in traditional cardiovascular risk factors. Review of the trial data finds good evidence that aggressive blood pressure and lipid control decreases cardiovascular outcomes among diabetic patients. The evidence for glucose control is weak, possibly reflecting either the multifactorial etiology of heart disease or the inadequate glucose control. There are no trials reporting the effect of diet or exercise on cardiovascular disease endpoints in patients with or without diabetes. For each of these subtopics, presented from A through E, most trials included some women, but few reported sex-specific results. Although it is likely that interventions will yield similar benefits (and risks) in women and men, it would be nice to be certain, and we encourage the presentation of sex-specific data in the future.

References

1. Harris MI, Hadden WC, Knowler WC, Bennett PH. Prevalence of diabetes and impaired glucose tolerance and plasma glucose levels in U.S. population aged 20–74 yr. *Diabetes* 1987; **36**:523–34.

2. Hazuda HP, Mitchell BD, Haffner SM, Stern MP. Obesity in Mexican American subgroups: findings from the San Antonio Heart Study. *Am J Clin Nutr* 1991; **53**:1529S-34S.

3. Kanaya AM, Grady D, Barrett-Connor E. Explaining the sex difference in coronary heart disease mortality among patients with type 2 diabetes mellitus: a meta-analysis. *Arch Intern Med* 2002; **162**:1737–45.

4. Pyorala K, Laakso M, Uusitupa M. Diabetes and atherosclerosis: an epidemiologic view. *Diabetes Metab Rev* 1987; **3**:463–524.

5. Stamler J, Vaccaro O, Neaton JD, Wentworth D. Diabetes, other risk factors, and 12-yr cardiovascular mortality for men screened in the Multiple Risk Factor Intervention Trial. *Diabetes Care* 1993; **16**:434–44.

6. Epstein FH. [Coronary heart disease: epidemiologic–genetic aspects.] *Soz Praventivmed* 1985; **30**:33–6 [in German].

7. Coutinho M, Gerstein HC, Wang Y, Yusuf S. The relationship between glucose and incident cardiovascular events. A metaregression analysis of published data from 20 studies of 95,783 individuals followed for 12.4 years. *Diabetes Care* 1999; **22**:233–40.

8. Harris MI, Eastman RC, Cowie CC, Flegal KM, Eberhardt MS. Comparison of diabetes diagnostic categories in the U.S. population according to the 1997 American Diabetes Association and 1980–1985 World Health Organization diagnostic criteria. *Diabetes Care* 1997; **20**:1859–62.

9. Gabir MM, Hanson RL, Dabelea D, et al. The 1997 American Diabetes Association and 1999 World Health Organization criteria for hyperglycemia in the diagnosis and prediction of diabetes. *Diabetes Care* 2000; **23**:1108–12.

10. Glucose tolerance and mortality: comparison of WHO and American Diabetes Association diagnostic criteria. The DECODE study group. European Diabetes Epidemiology Group. Diabetes Epidemiology: collaborative analysis of diagnostic criteria in Europe. *Lancet* 1999; **354**:617–21.

11. Kalin MF, Zumoff B. Sex hormones and coronary disease: a review of the clinical studies. *Steroids* 1990; **55**:330–52.

12. Orchard TJ. The impact of gender and general risk factors on the occurrence of atherosclerotic vascular disease in non-insulin-dependent diabetes mellitus. *Ann Med* 1996; **28**:323–33.

13. Lee WL, Cheung AM, Cape D, Zinman B. Impact of diabetes on coronary artery disease in women and men: a meta-analysis of prospective studies. *Diabetes Care* 2000; **23**:962–8.

14. Diagnosis and treatment of coronary heart disease in women: systematic reviews of evidence on selected topics, 2003 [http://www.ahrq.gov/clinic/epcindex.htm#cardiovascular].

15. Bierman EL, Porte D Jr, Bagdade JD. Hypertriglyceridemia and glucose intolerance in man. *Horm Metab Res* 1970; **2** (Suppl 2):209–12.

16. Wingard DL, Barrett-Connor E, Criqui MH, Suarez L. Clustering of heart disease risk factors in diabetic compared with nondiabetic adults. *Am J Epidemiol* 1983; **117**:19–26.

17. Barrett-Connor E, Grundy SM, Holdbrook MJ. Plasma lipids and diabetes mellitus in an adult community. *Am J Epidemiol* 1982; **115**:657–63.

18. Reaven GM. Banting lecture 1988. Role of insulin resistance in human disease. *Diabetes* 1988; **37**:1595–607.

19. Executive Summary of the Third Report of the National Cholesterol Education Program (NCEP) Expert Panel on Detection, Evaluation, and Treatment of High Blood Cholesterol in Adults (Adult Treatment Panel III). *JAMA* 2001; **285**:2486–97.

20. Ford ES, Giles WH, Dietz WH. Prevalence of the metabolic syndrome among US adults: findings from the third National Health and Nutrition Examination Survey. *JAMA* 2002; **287**:356–9.

21. Lakka HM, Laaksonen DE, Lakka TA, et al. The metabolic syndrome and total and cardiovascular disease mortality in middle-aged men. *JAMA* 2002; **288**:2709–16.

22. Haffner SM, Lehto S, Ronnemaa T, Pyorala K, Laakso M. Mortality from coronary heart disease in subjects with type 2 diabetes and in nondiabetic subjects with and without prior myocardial infarction [see comments]. *N Engl J Med* 1998; **339**:229–34.

23. Malmberg K, Yusuf S, Gerstein HC, et al. Impact of diabetes on long-term prognosis in patients with unstable angina and non-Q-wave myocardial infarction: results of the OASIS (Organization to Assess Strategies for Ischemic Syndromes) Registry. *Circulation* 2000; **102**:1014–19.

24. Kannel WB, McGee DL. Diabetes and cardiovascular disease. The Framingham study. *JAMA* 1979; **241**:2035–8.

25. Galderisi M, Anderson KM, Wilson PW, Levy D. Echocardiographic evidence for the existence of a distinct diabetic cardiomyopathy (the Framingham Heart Study). *Am J Cardiol* 1991; **68**:85–9.

26. Lloyd-Jones DM, Larson MG, Leip EP, et al. Lifetime risk for developing congestive heart failure: the Framingham Heart Study. *Circulation* 2002; **106**:3068–72.

27. Bell DS. Diabetic cardiomyopathy. A unique entity or a complication of coronary artery disease? *Diabetes Care* 1995; **18**:708–14.

28. Devereux RB, Roman MJ, Paranicas M, et al. Impact of diabetes on cardiac structure and function: the strong heart study. *Circulation* 2000; **101**:2271–6.

29. Phillips RA, Krakoff LR, Dunaif A, Finegood DT, Gorlin R, Shimabukuro S. Relation among left ventricular mass, insulin resistance, and blood pressure in nonobese subjects. *J Clin Endocrinol Metab* 1998; **83**:4284–8.

30. Mosca L, Appel LJ, Benjamin EJ, et al. Evidence-based guidelines for cardiovascular disease prevention in women. *Circulation* 2004; **109**:672–93.

31. Standards of medical care for patients with diabetes mellitus. *Diabetes Care* 2003; **26** (Suppl 1): S33–50.

32. A study of the effects of hypoglycemic agents on vascular complications in patients with adult-onset diabetes. II. Mortality results. *Diabetes* 1970; **19**:789–815.

33. Abraira C, Colwell J, Nuttall F, et al. Cardiovascular events and correlates in the Veterans Affairs Diabetes Feasibility Trial. Veterans Affairs Cooperative Study on Glycemic Control and Complications in Type II Diabetes. *Arch Intern Med* 1997; **157**:181–8.

34. Intensive blood-glucose control with sulphonylureas or insulin compared with conventional treatment and risk of complications in patients with type 2 diabetes (UKPDS 33). UK Prospective Diabetes Study (UKPDS) Group [published erratum appears in *Lancet* 1999; **354**:602] [see comments]. *Lancet* 1998; **352**:837–53.

35. Effect of intensive blood-glucose control with metformin on complications in overweight patients with type 2 diabetes (UKPDS 34). UK Prospective Diabetes Study (UKPDS) Group [see comments] [published erratum appears in *Lancet* 1998; **352**:1557]. *Lancet* 1998; **352**:854–65.

36. Stratton IM, Adler AI, Neil HA, et al. Association of glycaemia with macrovascular and microvascular complications of type 2 diabetes (UKPDS 35): prospective observational study. *BMJ* 2000; **321**:405–12.

37. The effect of intensive treatment of diabetes on the development and progression of long-term complications in insulin-dependent diabetes mellitus. The Diabetes Control and Complications Trial Research Group. *N Engl J Med* 1993; **329**:977–86.

38. Gaede P, Vedel P, Larsen N, Jensen GV, Parving HH, Pedersen O. Multifactorial intervention and cardiovascular disease in patients with type 2 diabetes. *N Engl J Med* 2003; **348**:383–93.

39. Chobanian AV, Bakris GL, Black HR, et al. The Seventh Report of the Joint National Committee on Prevention, Detection, Evaluation, and Treatment of High Blood Pressure: the JNC 7 report. *JAMA* 2003; **289**:2560–72.

40. Vijan S, Hayward RA. Treatment of hypertension in type 2 diabetes mellitus: blood pressure goals, choice of agents, and setting priorities in diabetes care. *Ann Intern Med* 2003; **138**:593–602.

41. Curb JD, Pressel SL, Cutler JA, et al. Effect of diuretic-based antihypertensive treatment on cardiovascular disease risk in older diabetic patients with isolated systolic hypertension. Systolic Hypertension in the Elderly Program Cooperative Research Group. *JAMA* 1996; **276**:1886–92.

42. Tuomilehto J, Rastenyte D, Birkenhager WH, et al. Effects of calcium-channel blockade in older patients with diabetes and systolic hypertension. Systolic Hypertension in Europe Trial Investigators. *N Engl J Med* 1999; **340**:677–84.

43. Hansson L, Zanchetti A, Carruthers SG, et al. Effects of intensive blood-pressure lowering and low-dose aspirin in patients with hypertension: principal results of the Hypertension Optimal Treatment (HOT) randomised trial. HOT Study Group. *Lancet* 1998; **351**:1755–62.

44. Tight blood pressure control and risk of macrovascular and microvascular complications in type 2 diabetes: UKPDS 38. UK Prospective Diabetes Study Group [see comments] [published erratum appears in *BMJ* 1999; **318**:29]. *BMJ* 1998; **317**:703–13.

45. Effects of ramipril on cardiovascular and microvascular outcomes in people with diabetes mellitus: results of the HOPE study and MICRO-HOPE substudy. Heart Outcomes Prevention Evaluation Study Investigators. *Lancet* 2000; **355**:253–9.

46. Brenner BM, Cooper ME, de Zeeuw D, et al. Effects of losartan on renal and cardiovascular outcomes in patients with type 2 diabetes and nephropathy. *N Engl J Med* 2001; **345**:861–9.

47. Estacio RO, Jeffers BW, Gifford N, Schrier RW. Effect of blood pressure control on diabetic microvascular complications in patients with hypertension and type 2 diabetes. *Diabetes Care* 2000; **23** (Suppl 2):B54–64.

48. Neal B, MacMahon S, Chapman N. Effects of ACE inhibitors, calcium antagonists, and other blood-pressure-lowering drugs: results of prospectively designed overviews of randomised trials. Blood Pressure Lowering Treatment Trialists' Collaboration. *Lancet* 2000; **356**:1955–64.

49. Major outcomes in high-risk hypertensive patients randomized to angiotensin-converting enzyme inhibitor or calcium channel blocker vs diuretic: the Antihypertensive and Lipid-Lowering Treatment to Prevent Heart Attack Trial (ALLHAT). *JAMA* 2002; **288**:2981–97.

50. Psaty BM, Smith NL, Siscovick DS, et al. Health outcomes associated with antihypertensive therapies used as first-line agents. A systematic review and meta-analysis. *JAMA* 1997; **277**:739–45.

51. Effect of metoprolol CR/XL in chronic heart failure: Metoprolol CR/XL Randomised Intervention Trial in Congestive Heart Failure (MERIT-HF). *Lancet* 1999; **353**:2001–7.

52. Wedel H, Demets D, Deedwania P, et al. Challenges of subgroup analyses in multinational clinical trials: experiences from the MERIT-HF trial. *Am Heart J* 2001; **142**:502–11.

53. Turner RC, Millns H, Neil HA, et al. Risk factors for coronary artery disease in non-insulin dependent diabetes mellitus: United Kingdom Prospective Diabetes Study (UKPDS: 23) [see comments]. *BMJ* 1998; **316**:823–8.

54. LaRosa JC, He J, Vupputuri S. Effect of statins on risk of coronary disease: a meta-analysis of randomized controlled trials. *JAMA* 1999; **282**:2340–6.

55. Collins R, Armitage J, Parish S, Sleigh P, Peto R. MRC/BHF Heart Protection Study of cholesterol-lowering with simvastatin in 5963 people with diabetes: a randomised placebo-controlled trial. *Lancet* 2003; **361**:2005–16.

56. Sever PS, Dahlof B, Poulter NR, et al. Prevention of coronary and stroke events with atorvastatin in hypertensive patients who have average or lower-than-average cholesterol concentrations, in the Anglo-Scandinavian Cardiac Outcomes Trial – Lipid Lowering Arm (ASCOT-LLA): a multicentre randomised controlled trial. *Lancet* 2003; **361**:1149–58.

57. Shepherd J, Cobbe SM, Ford I, et al. Prevention of coronary heart disease with pravastatin in men with hypercholesterolemia. West of Scotland Coronary Prevention Study Group. *N Engl J Med* 1995; **333**:1301–7.

58. Downs JR, Clearfield M, Weis S, et al. Primary prevention of acute coronary events with lovastatin in men and women with average cholesterol levels: results of AFCAPS/TexCAPS. Air Force/Texas Coronary Atherosclerosis Prevention Study. *JAMA* 1998; **279**:1615–22.

59. Pyorala K, Pedersen TR, Kjekshus J, Faergeman O, Olsson AG, Thorgeirsson G. Cholesterol lowering with simvastatin improves prognosis of diabetic patients with coronary heart disease. A subgroup analysis of the Scandinavian Simvastatin Survival Study (4S). *Diabetes Care* 1997; **20**:614–20.

60. Goldberg RB, Mellies MJ, Sacks FM, et al. Cardiovascular events and their reduction with pravastatin in diabetic and glucose-intolerant myocardial infarction survivors with average cholesterol levels: subgroup analyses in the cholesterol and recurrent events (CARE) trial. The Care Investigators. *Circulation* 1998; **98**:2513–19.

61. Prevention of cardiovascular events and death with pravastatin in patients with coronary heart disease and a broad range of initial cholesterol levels. The Long-Term Intervention with Pravastatin in Ischaemic Disease (LIPID) Study Group. *N Engl J Med* 1998; **339**:1349–57.

62. Hoogwerf BJ, Waness A, Cressman M, et al. Effects of aggressive cholesterol lowering and low-dose anticoagulation on clinical and angiographic outcomes in patients with diabetes: the Post Coronary Artery Bypass Graft Trial. *Diabetes* 1999; **48**:1289–94.

63. Major outcomes in moderately hypercholesterolemic, hypertensive patients randomized to pravastatin vs usual care: the Antihypertensive and Lipid-Lowering Treatment to Prevent Heart Attack Trial (ALLHAT-LLT). *JAMA* 2002; **288**: 2998–3007.

64. Koskinen P, Manttari M, Manninen V, Huttunen JK, Heinonen OP, Frick MH. Coronary heart disease incidence in NIDDM patients in the Helsinki Heart Study. *Diabetes Care* 1992; **15**:820–5.

65. Secondary prevention by raising HDL cholesterol and reducing triglycerides in patients with coronary artery disease: the Bezafibrate Infarction Prevention (BIP) study. *Circulation* 2000; **102**:21–7.

66. Effect of fenofibrate on progression of coronary-artery disease in type 2 diabetes: the Diabetes Atherosclerosis Intervention Study, a randomised study. *Lancet* 2001; **357**:905–10.

67. Rubins HB, Robins SJ, Collins D, et al. Diabetes, plasma insulin, and cardiovascular disease: subgroup analysis from the Department of Veterans Affairs high-density lipoprotein intervention trial (VA-HIT). *Arch Intern Med* 2002; **162**:2597–604.

68. Kreisberg RA. Diabetic dyslipidemia. *Am J Cardiol* 1998; **82**:67U–73U; discussion 85U–6U.

69. MRC/BHF Heart Protection Study of cholesterol lowering with simvastatin in 20,536 high-risk individuals: a randomised placebo-controlled trial. *Lancet* 2002; **360**:7–22.

70. Colhoun HM, Thomason MJ, Mackness MI, et al. Design of the Collaborative AtoRvastatin Diabetes Study (CARDS) in patients with type 2 diabetes. *Diabetic Med* 2002; **19**:201–11.

71. Scheen AJ. Premature interruption of ASCOT and CARDS clinical trials of cardiovascular prevention with atorvastatin in patients with arterial hypertension or diabetes mellitus: compromise between ethics and statistics in evidence-based medicine. *Rev Med Liege* 2003; **58**:585–90 [in French].

72. Schwartz GG, Olsson AG, Ezekowitz MD, et al. Effects of atorvastatin on early recurrent ischemic events in acute coronary syndromes: the MIRACL study: a randomized controlled trial. *JAMA* 2001; **285**:1711–18.

73. Franz MJ, Bantle JP, Beebe CA, et al. Evidence-based nutrition principles and recommendations for the treatment and prevention of diabetes and related complications. *Diabetes Care* 2003; **26** (Suppl 1):S51–61.

74. Ryan DH, Espeland MA, Foster GD, et al. Look AHEAD (Action for Health in Diabetes): design and methods for a clinical trial of weight loss for the prevention of cardiovascular disease in type 2 diabetes. *Control Clin Trials* 2003; **24**:610–28.

75. Pan XR, Li GW, Hu YH, et al. Effects of diet and exercise in preventing NIDDM in people with impaired glucose tolerance. The Da Qing IGT and Diabetes Study. *Diabetes Care* 1997; **20**:537–44.

76. Tuomilehto J, Lindstrom J, Eriksson JG, et al. Prevention of type 2 diabetes mellitus by changes in lifestyle among subjects with impaired glucose tolerance. *N Engl J Med* 2001; **344**:1343–50.

77. Knowler WC, Barrett-Connor E, Fowler SE, et al. Reduction in the incidence of type 2 diabetes with lifestyle intervention or metformin. *N Engl J Med* 2002; **346**:393–403.

78. Haffner SM. Diabetes Prevention Program update: lifestyle changes superior to drugs in cutting CVD risk in pre-diabetics. *Endocrinologist* 2003; **13**:S14 (abstract).

79. Pate RR, Pratt M, Blair SN, et al. Physical activity and public health. A recommendation from the Centers for Disease Control and Prevention and the American College of Sports Medicine. *JAMA* 1995; **273**:402–7.

80. Albright A, Franz M, Hornsby G, et al. American College of Sports Medicine position stand. Exercise and type 2 diabetes. *Med Sci Sports Exerc* 2000; **32**:1345–60.

81. Jakicic JM, Marcus BH, Gallagher KI, Napolitano M, Lang W. Effect of exercise duration and intensity on weight loss in overweight, sedentary women: a randomized trial. *JAMA* 2003; **290**:1323–30.

82. Leon AS, Sanchez OA. Response of blood lipids to exercise training alone or combined with dietary intervention. *Med Sci Sports Exerc* 2001; **33**:S502–15; discussion S528–9.

83. Fagard RH. Exercise characteristics and the blood pressure response to dynamic physical training. *Med Sci Sports Exerc* 2001; **33**:S484–92; discussion S493–4.

84. Thompson PD, Crouse SF, Goodpaster B, Kelley D, Moyna N, Pescatello L. The acute versus the chronic response to exercise. *Med Sci Sports Exerc* 2001; **33**:S438–45; discussion S452–3.

85. Thompson PD, Buchner D, Pina IL, et al. Exercise and physical activity in the prevention and treatment of atherosclerotic cardiovascular disease: a statement from the Council on Clinical Cardiology (Subcommittee on Exercise, Rehabilitation, and Prevention) and the Council on Nutrition, Physical Activity, and Metabolism (Subcommittee on Physical Activity). *Circulation* 2003; **107**:3109–16.

4

Lipid abnormalities: recognition and management

Nanette K. Wenger

Introduction

Coronary heart disease (CHD) is a prevalent and lethal problem for adult women in the US and most industrialized nations. Risk reduction interventions therefore assume utmost importance. The identification that four of five US women and one of three of their primary care providers were unaware of CHD as the leading cause of mortality for women likely contributes to the under-recognition and under-treatment of lipid abnormalities, as well as other coronary risk factors, in women.

Lipids and coronary risk

Most data relating hypercholesterolemia to an increase in coronary events and in coronary mortality derive from studies conducted in men. The available studies in women show a less powerful relationship; this may be explained in part by most survey data not including women older than 69 years of age (in whom CHD prevalence is greater) and not addressing levels of high-density lipoprotein (HDL) cholesterol (HDL-C), which are typically higher in women. Although increased total cholesterol, low-density lipoprotein (LDL) cholesterol (LDL-C), and triglyceride (TG) levels are associated with an increased cardiovascular risk for women, these

relationships appear diminished in older women. Low HDL-C and increased TG predict risk for both younger and older women.[1] Low HDL-C and an increased total cholesterol/HDL-C ratio better predicted cardiovascular mortality in Framingham women than did LDL-C.[2,3] Data from the Lipid Research Clinics Followup Study further confirm that an HDL-C level below 50 mg/dl better predicts cardiovascular risk for women than does total cholesterol or LDL-C.[4] Elevated TG levels, particularly in association with low HDL-C levels, may be an independent risk factor for coronary mortality in women.[4,5]

Potential plaque-stabilizing effects of cholesterol-lowering[6] include a decrease in the number of macrophages, increase in smooth muscle cell maturation, increased interstitial collagen content, decreased expression of matrix metalloproteinases (MMP-1, MMP-2, MMP-3, MMP-9), decreased tissue factor expression, decreased CD40 ligand/ CD40 suggesting decreased plaque thrombogenicity, decreased expression of adhesion molecules (vascular cell adhesion molecule-1, monocyte chemoattractant protein-1), and lessening of oxidative stress.

Studies of LDL-lowering with statins identify an important anti-inflammatory mechanism. Aggressive lowering of LDL-C more rapidly decreased the concentration of C-reactive protein,[7] with the potential for greater plaque stabilization.

A recent systematic review of research related to CHD in women found that overall evidence was inconclusive regarding the association of abnormal lipoprotein levels and CHD risk.[8] Twelve-year follow-up of the Finnmark Study suggested that the pattern of risk associated with hyperlipidemia in middle-aged women was similar to that for middle-aged men,[9] i.e. increased CHD mortality rates with higher levels of total cholesterol, LDL-C and TG, and lower levels of HDL-C. Serum TG and HDL-C were strongly inversely intercorrelated. Smoking reduced HDL-C more in women than in men. However, the pattern of risk among older women appears to be different than for men, with increased mortality risk associated only with lower HDL-C and higher TG levels. Potential pharmacologic intervention to increase HDL-C, as with cholesteryl ester transfer protein (CETP) inhibition, is a promising area of investigation.[10]

Sex disparities in lipid screening and management

Sex-specific data on the treatment of hypercholesterolemia from the National Health and Nutrition Examination Survey (NHANES) 1990–2000[11] identified that women more frequently had their cholesterol levels checked than men (72.3% vs 66.9%), but that equal numbers of women and men were aware of hypercholesterolemia, about 35%. Nonetheless, 14% of men were treated, in contrast to 10.2% of women, and 7.5% of the men had a cholesterol concentration of <200 mg/dl in contrast to 3.7% of women. In general, most studies of patients with established cardiovascular disease suggest that men have their cholesterol measured more often and treated more aggressively, with resultant lower LDL-C levels, than women.

The majority of women with CHD on lipid-lowering therapy do not attain LDL-C treatment goals. For example, 63% of the women with established CHD enrolled in the Heart and Estrogen/progestin Study (HERS) trial (1993) did not meet the National Cholesterol Education Program (NCEP) Adult Treatment Panel (ATP) I (1988) LDL-C goal of <130 mg/dl, with 91% of women not meeting the NCEP ATP II (1993) LDL-C goal of <100 mg/dl.[12] The mean baseline LDL-C level in HERS women was 145 mg/dl, although 47% of these women were taking a lipid-lowering medication.[13]

In the PREVENT (Prospective Randomized Evaluation of the Vascular Effects of Norvasc Trial) study that included 20% of women as participants, there was continued evidence for the underutilization of lipid-lowering therapy in women at academic medical centers in the US and Canada. At the onset of the trial in 1994, 17% of the men were at a target LDL-C of <100 mg/dl as compared with 6% of the women. At the end of the trial in 1997, 31% of the men achieved the target LDL-C in contrast to 12% of the women.[14]

The Women's Atorvastatin Trial on CHolesterol (WATCH)[15] documented that the NCEP ATP III target goals are attainable in women; 87% of the women without cardiovascular disease and 80% of the women with established cardiovascular disease achieved the LDL-C target levels with drug titration.

A review of the limited evidence and explanations for suboptimal screening and treatment of dyslipidemia in women[16] suggests lower rates among women than men. However, the majority of studies that examined screening and treatment for dyslipidemia failed to report analyses by sex or to describe the degree of disparity between women and men. Warranting further study are the contributions of the patient, the clinician, and the health system factors to these disparities.

Clinical trial evidence for the benefit of lipid management in women (Table 4.1)[17–25]

In early studies of lipid-lowering treatments, exclusion of women or their under-representation in clinical trials limited the development of evidence-based guidelines for lipid management in healthy women and in those with established CHD.

A systematic review of lipid-lowering treatment to reduce the risk of CHD in women,[26] identified that although 20 clinical trials of the effects of lipid-lowering therapy included women, only nine of these published results stratified by sex. Data for women in two additional trials was obtained from the study investigators. Thus, the analysis reflected the results from 11 trials that included 15 917 women. Based on these data, lipid-lowering therapy reduced the risk of CHD mortality by 26%, nonfatal myocardial infarc-

Table 4.1 Major lipid-lowering trials using statin therapy for prevention of coronary heart disease (CHD)

Study acronym*, reference	No. of patients	No. of women (%)	Prevention category	Risk reduction – major CHD events in women
4S[17]	4444	827 (19)	Secondary	35%
CARE[18]	4159	576 (14)	Secondary	46%
LIPID[19]	9014	1516 (17)	Secondary	11%
AFCAPS/TexCAPS[20]	6605	997 (15)	Primary	46%
PROSPER[21]	5804	3000 (52)	Both	NS benefit for women
HPS[22]	20 536	5082 (25)	Primary	19%
ALLHAT-LLT[23]	10 355	5051 (49)	Primary (14% CHD)	Sex-specific data not reported – NS in total cohort
GREACE[24]	1600	344 (21)	Secondary	54%
ASCOT-LLA[25]	10 305	1942 (19)	Primary	NS benefit for women

NS, not significant.
*See reference for explanation.

tion (MI) by 36%, and major CHD events by 21% in women with known CHD. There was insufficient evidence that lipid-lowering therapy reduced rates of revascularization procedures and no evidence of a reduction of risk for total mortality. This review cited insufficient evidence in women without established CHD to determine whether lipid-lowering therapy reduced the risk for any clinical outcome. However, the small number of outcome events in women may have provided inadequate power to detect differences. Nonetheless, lipid management appears prudent for women at increased coronary risk, given their adverse outcomes with manifest CHD.

Therapeutic lifestyle changes

Diet and exercise were beneficial in preventing the increase in LDL-C and weight gain during perimenopause to menopause in the Women's Healthy Lifestyle Project clinical trial;[27] benefit occurred both in hormone users and nonusers.

Clofibrate, colestipol, niacin

Although women were included as participants in the secondary prevention randomized controlled trials of clofibrate, subgroup analyses of clinical endpoints in women were not reported.[28,29] Neither were sex-specific outcomes reported in a comparison of

aggressive versus moderate lipid-lowering in patients following coronary artery bypass graft surgery, the Post Coronary Artery Bypass Graft Trial.[30] There was no significant clinical endpoint difference save for a decrease in revascularization procedures with aggressive lipid-lowering with lovastatin and, if needed, cholestyramine in the total cohort.

Sex-specific endpoints for mortality were reported in a randomized controlled trial of colestipol versus placebo in 2278 patients, including both primary and secondary prevention populations, with 1184 women participants.[31] Cardiovascular mortality was improved for men but not for women.

Sex-specific data were not reported for the secondary prevention study comparing nicotinic acid and clofibrate versus placebo; 113 of the 555 participants in this Stockholm Ischemic Heart Disease study were women.[32]

Partial ileal bypass surgery

In the comparison of partial ileal bypass surgery with usual care for lipid-lowering Program On the Surgical Control of Hyperlipidemias (POSCH), 78 of the 838 participants were women. No significant improvement in the composite outcome of coronary death or nonfatal MI was present for women, although there was significant improvement for the total cohort; this may reflect the small number of women participants.[33]

Statin drugs (Table 4.1)[17-25]

There were no sex-specific clinical endpoints reported in the ASymptomatic Carotid Artery Progression Study (ASCAPS) primary prevention trial examining the effect of lovastatin on early carotid atherosclerosis and cardiovascular events,[34] although 473 of the 919 participants with moderately elevated LDL-C levels randomized to lovastatin versus placebo were women.

The Scandinavian Simvastatin Survival Study (4S) randomized 4444 coronary patients with angina or following MI, whose total cholesterol was 213–309 mg/dl and TG was <200 mg/dl, to 20–40 mg of simvastatin versus placebo. Nineteen percent of the participants were women; they were more likely to have had angina without MI than men. During a 5.4-year median follow-up, the relative risk of clinical events in treated women was 1.16 for all-cause mortality, 0.86 for CHD mortality, 0.66 for major coronary events, and 0.51 for myocardial revascularization procedures. Thus there was a 34% decrease in the risk of major coronary events, although too few female deaths occurred in this population to assess a mortality benefit. Estrogen use in 4S women was <4%, such that the effect of this therapy could not be ascertained.[17]

The Cholesterol And Recurrent Events (CARE) trial compared 4159 patients following MI randomized to pravastatin 40 mg daily versus placebo; 14% of the participants were women. Similar improvement in lipid levels occurred in the women and men. All had average cholesterol levels at baseline: total cholesterol <240 mg/dl, LDL-C 115–174 mg/dl, TG <354 mg/dl. At a mean follow-up of 5 years, pravastatin-treated women had a 43% reduction in the primary endpoint of coronary death or nonfatal MI; 46% decrease in combined coronary events; 48% decrease in percutaneous transluminal coronary angioplasty; a nonsignificant 40% decrease in coronary artery bypass grafting surgery; and 56% decrease in stroke rate.[18]

In the Long-term Intervention with Pravastatin in Ischemic Disease (LIPID) trial, which evaluated 9014 patients with MI or unstable angina, 17% of the study population were women.[19] The baseline total cholesterol level was 155–271 mg/dl and TG level <445 mg/dl. At 6 years, 40 mg of pravastatin daily compared with placebo decreased major coronary events in women by 11%, but this failed to achieve statistical significance consequent to small numbers of coronary events in women.

The effect of 20–40 mg of lovastatin versus placebo added to dietary therapy was examined in 6605 participants in the primary prevention Air Force/Texas Coronary Atherosclerosis Prevention Study (AFCAPS/ TexCAPS); 15% of the participants were women. For enrollment men were required to have an HDL-C <45 mg/dl and women <47 mg/dl. There was a 46% decrease in first major coronary events in treated women.[20] Again this did not reach statistical significance because of the low overall event rate in women.

The Medical Research Council/British Heart Foundation Heart Protection Study (HPS) enrolled patients aged 40–80 years with a total cholesterol level in excess of 135 mg/dl at increased risk of coronary death due to MI or coronary disease, occlusive disease of noncoronary arteries, or diabetes mellitus or treated hypertension. Statin therapy was not considered clearly indicated or contraindicated by the patient's primary physician. Of the 20 536 participants, 25% (5082 individuals) were women.[22] There was a clear benefit of therapy with 40 mg of simvastatin daily, with a reduction of about 24% in major vascular events, equally seen in women and men, younger and older participants, and diabetic and nondiabetic participants. Importantly, comparable benefit was obtained with baseline LDL-C levels above and below the current NCEP ATP III optimal target level of <100 mg/dl.

In the Myocardial Ischemia Reduction with Aggressive Cholesterol Lowering (MIRACL) trial, intensive statin therapy with 80 mg of atorvastatin daily in patients with acute coronary syndromes reduced death, nonfatal MI, resuscitated cardiac arrest or recurrent ischemia requiring hospitalization by 15% and nonfatal and overall stroke rate by 50% at 16 weeks.[35,36] In all, 1074 of the 3086 participants were women, but sex-specific data were not reported. The major benefit was on recurrent symptomatic ischemia requiring rehospitalization. The mean baseline LDL-C level was 124 mg/dl.

There was no difference in all-cause mortality or in coronary death and nonfatal MI in the 40 mg pravastatin compared with usual care therapy in the Antihypertensive and Lipid Lowering Treatment to Prevent Heart Attack Trial, Lipid Lowering Trial, (ALLHAT-LLT);[23] 5051 of the 10 355 participants were women. LDL-C was 120–189 mg/dl at entry without known CHD; 100–129 mg/dl with known CHD. Sex-specific clinical endpoints were not reported. However, the degree of lipid-lowering in ALLHAT-LLT was far less than that encountered in other major statin trials that showed coronary risk reduction.

The PROSPER (a PROspective Study of Pravastatin in the Elderly at Risk) trial involved 5804 subjects, 3000 of them women, aged 70–82 years with a total cholesterol of 155–350 mg/dl. They were randomized to pravastatin 40 mg daily versus placebo and followed for an average of 3.2 years. In all, 50% had vascular disease and 50% were at high risk of such disease.[21] There was a reduction in the combined primary endpoint of coronary death, nonfatal MI, and fatal or nonfatal stroke, and also of CHD death or nonfatal MI. However, there was no reduction in the stroke endpoints (possibly due to inadequate statistical power or to the short duration of trial) and there was an increase in total cancers. Although there was significant reduction in coronary death, no significant treatment effect was evident on vascular or nonvascular death. Significant benefit occurred only in the male subjects.

In the GREek Atorvastatin and Coronary-heart disease Evaluation (GREACE) study, comparison was made of atorvastatin 10–80 mg daily with a target LDL-C of <100 mg/dl to usual care; 344 of the 1600 participants were women. The only subgroup analysis reported for women was for all clinical events, with a relative risk of 0.46 in the treatment group. Significant improvement in MI, stroke, revascularization procedures, mortality and heart failure was reported for the entire cohort.[24]

ASCOT-LLA (Anglo-Scandinavian Cardiac Outcomes Trial, Lipid Lowering Arm) assessed the effect on nonfatal MI and fatal CHD of atorvastatin 10 mg compared with placebo in patients with total cholesterol levels that were average or lower than average.[25] A total of 1942 women was included among the 10 305 hypertensive patients in this primary prevention study. The trial was terminated prematurely for a 36% reduction in the primary endpoint of coronary death or nonfatal MI in the overall cohort at a median follow-up of 3.3 years, but there was no significant improvement for women.

A recent randomized statin trial, REVERSAL (Reversal of Atherosclerosis with Aggressive Lipid Lowering) compared the 18-month change in

atheroma volume measured by intravascular ultrasound (IVUS) of 80 mg of atorvastatin versus 40 mg of pravastatin. One hundred and forty of the 502 evaluable patients were women; participants had at least a 20% angiographic coronary stenosis and an LDL-C of 125–250 mg/dl.[37] Both women and men had decreased atheroma volume with aggressive lipid-lowering with atorvastatin, in contrast to an increase in volume with moderate lipid-lowering with pravastatin. Whether this reflected greater LDL-C lowering (−47% vs −26%) or decreased C-reactive protein ($\downarrow$ 36.4% vs $\downarrow$ 5.2%) or both with atorvastatin versus pravastatin is unknown, but the data provide further evidence for benefit of lower levels of LDL-C.

PROVE IT-TIMI 22 (Pravastatin and Atorvastatin Evaluation and Infection Therapy-Thrombolysis in Myocardial Infarction 22) compared the clinical outcomes of 4162 patients (22% women) with an acute coronary syndrome within the preceding 10 days randomized to atorvastatin 80 mg versus pravastatin 40 mg to ascertain the effect of intensive versus standard lipid lowering on early recurrent coronary events.[38] LDL-C reduction of 42% with atorvastatin versus 10% with pravastatin was associated with a 16% reduction in the composite endpoint of all-cause mortality, MI, hospitalization for unstable angina, coronary revascularization and stroke with intensive lipid lowering, 22.4% for atorvastatin versus 26.3% for pravastatin. Mean LDL-C was 62 mg/dl for atorvastatin versus 95 mg/dl for pravastatin. Clinical event curves separated within 30 days, showing an early and consistent benefit of intensive lipid lowering throughout the study. Benefit was present for both women and men.

Sex-specific recommendations for lipid management (see also Chapter 39)

National Cholesterol Education Program 2001

Although the LDL-C goal levels are not sex-specific in NCEP ATP III,[39] premature CHD in a first-degree relative has a sex-based age differential, being defined as younger than age 55 for men as compared with age

65 for women. A low HDL-C is defined as <40 mg/dl for both sexes. However, in the definition of the metabolic syndrome, the desirable waist circumference is <40 inches for men and <35 inches for women; and the desirable HDL-C is <40 mg/dl for men and 50 mg/dl for women. Calculation of the 10-year risk also confers points differentially for women and men with the same age range and same total cholesterol levels.

NCEP ATP III recommends statin therapy for women 45–70 years of age, in that at the time these recommendations were published (2001) no data were available to support recommendations for women older than age 75. Benefit was subsequently demonstrated for elderly women in HPS but not in PROSPER.

Updated NCEP ATP III guidelines,[40] based on data from five major recent clinical trials, offer new options for lower LDL-C goals and lower thresholds for pharmacotherapy for very high-risk patients. For such patients an optimal LDL-C goal of <70 mg/dl is provided, with initiation of therapeutic lifestyle changes at an LDL-C ≥100 mg/dl and consideration of drug therapy if the LDL-C is <100 mg/dl. Combining a fibrate or nicotinic acid with an LDL-lowering drug can be considered for such patients with high TG or low HDL-C levels. For moderately high-risk patients an LDL-C goal <100 mg/dl is an optimal goal and drug therapy may be initiated with a baseline LDL-C of 100–124 mg/dl.

American Heart Association 2004

In February of 2004 the American Heart Association (AHA) presented the first evidence-based guidelines for cardiovascular disease prevention in women.[41] The recommendations relative to lipid management are as follows:

- Heart healthy diet. Consistently encourage an overall healthy eating pattern that includes an intake of a variety of fruits, vegetables, grains, low-fat or nonfat dairy products, fish, legumes, sources of protein low in saturated fat (e.g. poultry, lean meats, plant sources). Limit saturated fat intake to <10% of calories, limit cholesterol intake to <300 mg/day, and limit intake of transfatty acids (class I, level B).

- Lipid, lipoproteins. Optimal levels of lipids and lipoproteins in women are LDL-C <100 mg/dl, HDL-C >50 mg/dl, TG <150 mg/dl and non-HDL-C <130 mg/dl and should be encouraged through lifestyle approaches (class I, level B).

- Lipids – diet therapy. In high-risk women or when LDL-C is elevated, saturated fat intake should be reduced to <7% of calories, cholesterol to <200 mg/day and transfatty acid intake should be reduced (class I, level B).

- Lipid pharmacotherapy in high-risk women. Initiate LDL-C-lowering therapy (preferably a statin) simultaneously with lifestyle therapy in high-risk women with LDL-C ≥100 mg/dl unless contraindicated (class I, level A) and initiate statin therapy in high-risk women with an LDL-C <100 mg/dl (class I, level B). Initiate niacin or fibrate therapy when HDL-C is low, or nonHDL-C is elevated in high-risk women (class I, level B).

- Lipid pharmacotherapy in intermediate-risk women. Initiate LDL-C-lowering therapy (preferably a statin) if LDL-C level is ≥130 mg/dl on lifestyle therapy (class I, level A) or niacin or fibrate therapy when HDL-C is low or nonHDL-C is elevated after LDL-C goal is reached (class I, level B).

- Lipid pharmacotherapy in low-risk women. Consider LDL-C-lowering therapy in low-risk women with 0 or 1 risk factor when LDL-C level is ≥190 mg/dl or if multiple risk factors are present when LDL-C is ≥160 mg/dl (class IIA, level B) or niacin or fibrate therapy when HDL-C is low or nonHDL-C elevated after LDL-C goal is reached (class IIA, level B)

The AHA further indicates that combined estrogen plus progestin hormone therapy should not be initiated (class III, level A) or continued (class III, level C) to prevent CVD in postmenopausal women. Other forms of menopausal hormone therapy (e.g. unopposed estrogen) should not be initiated or continued to prevent CVD in postmenopausal women pending the results of ongoing trials (class III, level C). Results of the Women's Health Initiative (WHI) estrogen-only arm, published shortly after the AHA Guidelines elevated this quality of evidence to level A.[42]

Challenges relative to recent clinical trial data for menopausal hormone therapy
(see also Chapter 26)

Because the occurrence of CHD escalates in women at older age, particularly in the menopausal years, attention was directed to the role of menopausal hormone therapy in reducing cardiovascular risk.

The US NCEP ATP II (1993) recommended consideration of menopausal hormone use as the initial lipid-lowering therapy for women. Subsequent data from major randomized controlled trials of menopausal hormone therapy have indicated no evidence-based rationale for the use of such therapy for primary or secondary coronary prevention. Thus hormone therapy is not recommended in NCEP ATP III.[39]

Despite favorable effects of estrogen plus progestin on HDL-C and LDL-C levels (albeit with an unfavorable increase in TG concentration) in the Heart and Estrogen/progestin Replacement Study follow-up (HERS-II), this regimen did not reduce the risk of cardiovascular events including revascularization, unstable angina, heart failure, stroke, transient ischemic attack, peripheral arterial disease, etc., in women with established CHD. Thus the recommendations are that this regimen of 0.625 mg of conjugated equine estrogen plus 2.5 mg of medroxyprogesterone acetate daily should not be used to decrease the risk of cardiovascular events in women with CHD.[43] In HERS, changes in lipid levels with hormone therapy did not predict CHD outcomes.[44] Despite improvement in lipid profiles, other randomized trials of menopausal hormone therapy have failed to identify improved coronary outcomes for women with CHD.

Similarly, in the WHI estrogen/progestin study, a randomized controlled trial in 16 608 healthy women aged 50–79 years assigned to 0.625 mg conjugated equine estrogen plus 2.5 mg medroxyprogesterone acetate daily versus placebo, the trial was terminated prematurely after an average of 5.2 years of follow-up because of an unfavorable global risk score and an increased risk of invasive breast cancer.[45] In WHI, the overall health risks exceeded the benefits, with a 26% increased risk of invasive breast cancer, a 29% increased risk of coronary events, a 41% increased risk of stroke, and doubled risk for venous throm-

boembolism. These contrasted with benefits of a 37% decrease in colorectal cancer, a 33% decrease in hip fracture, and a 24% decrease in total fracture. The conclusion of the investigators was that because of the excess coronary and stroke risks and no benefit from this hormone regimen it should not be initiated or continued for the primary prevention of CHD.[45]

Subsequently, the parallel WHI estrogen study, which randomized 10 739 women after hysterectomy to 0.625 mg conjugated equine estrogen versus placebo was terminated prematurely after nearly 7 years of average follow-up because of lack of improvement in the global risk score and an increase in stroke risk.[42] Heart disease risk was not affected, there was a decreased risk for hip fracture, a nonsignificant decrease in breast cancer risk and no decrease in risk for colon cancer.

Thus menopausal hormone therapy fails to confer coronary benefit and may increase the early risk of adverse cardiovascular events. Recommendations from the US Food and Drug Administration are that women consult their physicians regarding established approaches to lowering coronary risk.[46]

Absence of sex-specific data regarding other lipid interventions

In the Lyon Diet Heart Study, a dietary lipid-lowering trial, data were not reported separately by sex, nor was there an indication of the number of women enrolled. The entire cohort had improved cumulative survival independent of the lipid effect.[47]

Randomized trial information is not available for women regarding dietary supplements designed to lower LDL-C levels such as soluble fiber, soy protein, and plant sterol or stanol esters.

Further, randomized trial data are unavailable for women for niacin interventions – with niacin effective in lowering TG and lipoprotein (a) levels and raising HDL-C; nor for fibrate (excellent TG-lowering drugs) or bile acid sequestrant therapy.

Ezetimibe, added to a statin, comparably lowers LDL-C levels in women and men;[48] clinical outcome data are lacking.

Summary

Impressive clinical trial data have unequivocally established the benefit of statin therapy in the prevention of cardiovascular events in women. A good quality meta-analysis found that both women and men with hyperlipidemia, treated with statins, had favorable modification of their lipid profile and a 30% reduction in the risk of major CHD events.[49] Although men experienced a 20% reduction in total mortality, this was not evident in women, likely due to the small numbers of women included in the trials. In a more recent randomized trial among patients with CHD or at high risk for its occurrence, treatment with simvastatin 40 mg daily reduced the risk of major vascular events by about 25% in both women and men, regardless of pretreatment cholesterol level, age, or diabetic status.[21] Despite their higher prevalence of co-morbidities, women in several large randomized controlled trials of lipid-lowering with statins had comparable reduction in clinical events to their male counterparts. A recent systematic review of lipid-lowering therapy in women that included data from large multinational statin studies[50] concluded that treatment of hyperlipidemia in women with known cardiovascular disease reduced coronary events: CHD mortality, nonfatal MI and revascularization, but did not affect total mortality. Limited enrollment of women, small numbers of fatal events, and relatively young age of women participants may be explanatory. Lipid lowering did not affect total or CHD mortality in women without cardiovascular disease; although lipid lowering may reduce CHD events, current evidence is inclusive. Statins have an impressive safety profile for both women and men.

Widespread intensive application of 3-hydroxy-3-methylglutaryl coenzyme A reductase inhibitor (statin) lipid-lowering therapies for women, currently underutilized, warrants high priority. Whether LDL-C lowering below the current NCEP ATP III target of below 100 mg/dl or below 70 mg/dl for high-risk patients will provide added benefit should be ascertained from ongoing clinical trials. Recent trials[37,38] add support to the benefit of lower levels of LDL-C.

The expertise of Karl Woodworth in the literature search is acknowledged with appreciation.

References

1. Manolio TA, Pearson TA, Wenger NK, Barrett-Connor E, Payne GH, Harlan WR. Cholesterol and heart disease in older persons and women. Review of an NHLBI workshop. *Ann Epidemiol* 1992; **2**:161–76.
2. Kannel WB. Metabolic risk factors for coronary heart disease in women: perspective from the Framingham Study. *Am Heart J* 1987; **114**:413–19.
3. Kannel WB, Wilson PWF. Risk factors that attenuate the female coronary disease advantage. *Arch Intern Med* 1995; **155**:57–61.
4. Bass KM, Newschaffer CJ, Klag MJ, Bush TL. Plasma lipoprotein levels as predictors of cardiovascular death in women. *Arch Intern Med* 1993; **153**:2209–16.
5. LaRosa JC. TGs and coronary risk in women and the elderly. *Arch Intern Med* 1997; **157**:961–8.
6. Libby P, Aikawa M. Mechanisms of plaque stabilization with statins. *Am J Cardiol* 2003; **91**:4B-8B.
7. Kinlay S, Timms T, Clark M, et al., for the Vascular Basis Study Group. Comparison of effect of intensive lipid lowering with atorvastatin to less intensive lowering with lovastatin on C-reactive protein in patients with stable angina pectoris and inducible myocardial ischemia. *Am J Cardiol* 2002; **89**:1205–7.
8. Grady D, Chaput L, Kristof M. *Results of Systematic Review of Research on Diagnosis and Treatment of Coronary Heart Disease in Women.* Evidence Report/Technology Assessment No. 80. (Prepared by the University of California, San Francisco-Stanford Evidence-based Practice Center under Contract No. 290-97-0013.) AHRQ Publication No. 03–0035. Rockville, MD: Agency for Healthcare Research and Quality, May 2003.
9. Njølstad I, Arnesen E, Lund-Larsen PG. Smoking, serum lipids, blood pressure, and sex differences in myocardial infarction. A 12–year follow-up of the Finnmark Study. *Circulation* 1996; **93**:450–6.
10. Doggrell SA. Raising high-density lipoprotein cholesterol with inhibitors of cholesteryl ester transfer

protein – a new approach to coronary artery disease. *Expert Opin Invest Drugs* 2004; **13**:1365–8.

11. Ford ES, Mokdad AH, Giles WH, Mensah GA. Serum total cholesterol concentrations and awareness, treatment, and control of hypercholesterolemia among US adults. Findings from the National Health and Nutrition Examination Survey, 1999 to 2000. *Circulation* 2003; **107**:2185–9.

12. The Expert Panel. Summary of the second report of the National Cholesterol Education Program (NCEP) Expert Panel on Detection, Evaluation, and Treatment of High Blood Cholesterol in Adults (Adult Treatment Panel II). *JAMA* 1993; **269**:3015–23.

13. Schrott HG, Bittner V, Vittinghoff E, Herrington DM, Hulley S, for the HERS Research Group. Adherence to National Cholesterol Education Program treatment goals in postmenopausal women with heart disease. The Heart and Estrogen/progestin Replacement Study (HERS). *JAMA* 1997; **277**:1281–6.

14. Miller M, Byington R, Hunninghake D, Pitt B, Furberg CD, for the Prospective Randomized Evaluation of the Vascular Effects of Norvasc Trial (PREVENT) Investigators. Sex bias and underutilization of lipid-lowering therapy in patients with coronary artery disease at academic medical centers in the United States and Canada. *Arch Intern Med* 2000; **160**:343–7.

15. McPherson R, Angus C, Murray P, Genest J Jr, for the WATCH Investigators. Efficacy of atorvastatin in achieving National Cholesterol Education Program low-density lipoprotein targets in women with severe dyslipidemia and cardiovascular disease or risk factors for cardiovascular disease: The Women's Atorvastatin Trial on Cholesterol (WATCH). *Am Heart J* 2001; **141**:949–56.

16. Kim C, Hofer TP, Kerr EA. Review of evidence and explanations for suboptimal screening and treatment of dyslipidemia in women. A conceptual model. *J Gen Intern Med* 2003; **18**:854–63.

17. Miettinen TA, Pyörälä K, Olsson AG, et al., for the Scandinavian Simvastatin Study Group. Cholesterol-lowering therapy in women and elderly patients with myocardial infarction or angina pectoris. Findings from the Scandinavian Simvastatin Survival Study (4S). *Circulation* 1997; **96**:4211–18.

18. Lewis SJ, Sacks FM, Mitchell JS, et al., for the CARE Investigators. Effect of pravastatin on cardiovascular events in women after myocardial infarction: the Cholesterol and Recurrent Events (CARE) Trial. *J Am Coll Cardiol* 1998; **32**:140–6.

19. The Long-Term Intervention with Pravastatin in Ischaemic Disease (LIPID) Study Group. Prevention of cardiovascular events and death with pravastatin in patients with coronary heart disease and broad range of initial cholesterol levels. *N Engl J Med* 1998; **339**:1349–57.

20. Downs JR, Clearfield M, Weis S, et al., for the AFCAPS/TexCAPS Research Group. Primary prevention of acute coronary events with lovastatin in men and women with average cholesterol levels. *JAMA* 1998; **279**:1615–22.

21. Shepherd J, Blauw GJ, Murphy MB, et al., on behalf of the PROSPER study group. Pravastatin in elderly individuals at risk of vascular disease (PROSPER): a randomised controlled trial. *Lancet* 2002; **360**:1623–30.

22. Heart Protection Study Collaborative Group. MRC/BHF Heart Protection Study of cholesterol lowering with simvastatin in 20 536 high-risk individuals: a randomised placebo-controlled trial. *Lancet* 2002; **360**:7–22.

23. The ALLHAT Officers and Coordinators for the ALLHAT Collaborative Research Group. Major outcomes in moderately hypercholesterolemic, hypertensive patients randomized to pravastatin vs usual care. The Antihypertensive and Lipid-Lowering Treatment to Prevent Heart Attack Trial (ALLHAT-LLT). *JAMA* 2002; **288**:2998–3007.

24. Athyros VG, Papageorgiou AA, Mercouris BR, et al. Treatment with atorvastatin to the National Cholesterol Education Program goal versus 'usual' care in secondary coronary heart disease prevention. The GREek Atorvastatin and Coronary-heart-disease Evaluation (GREACE) study. *Curr Med Res Opin* 2002; **18**:220–8.

25. Sever PS, Dahlöf B, Poulter NR, et al., for the ASCOT investigators. Prevention of coronary and stroke events with atorvastatin in hypertensive patients who have average or lower-than-average cholesterol concentrations, in the Anglo-Scandinavian Cardiac Outcomes Trial – Lipid Lowering Arm (ASCOT-LLA): a multicentre randomised controlled trial. *Lancet* 2003; **361**:1149–58.

26. Grady D, Chaput L, Kristof M. *Diagnosis and Treatment of Coronary Heart Disease in Women: Systematic Reviews of Evidence on Selected Topics.* Evidence Report/Technology Assessment No. 81. (Prepared by the University of California, San Francisco-Stanford Evidence-based Practice Center under Contract No. 290-97-0013.) AHRQ Publication No. 03-0037. Rockville, MD: Agency for Healthcare Research and Quality, May 2003.

27. Kuller LH, Simkin-Silverman LR, Wing RR, Meilahn

EN, Ives DG. Women's Healthy Lifestyle Project: a randomized clinical trial. Results at 54 months. *Circulation* 2001; **103**:32–7.

28. Anonymous. Ischaemic heart disease: a secondary prevention trial using clofibrate. Report by a research committee of the Scottish Society of Physicians. *BMJ* 1971; **4**:775–84.

29. Anonymous. Trial of clofibrate in the treatment of ischaemic heart disease. Five-year study by a group of physicians of the Newcastle upon Tyne region. *BMJ* 1971; **4**:767–75.

30. Anonymous. The effect of aggressive lowering of low-density lipoprotein cholesterol levels and low-dose anticoagulation on obstructive changes in saphenous-vein coronary-artery bypass grafts. The Post Coronary Artery Bypass Graft Trial Investigators [erratum appears in *N Engl J Med* 1997; **337**:1859]. *N Engl J Med* 1997; **336**:153–62.

31. Dorr AE, Gundersen K. Schneider JC Jr, Spencer TW, Martin WB. Colestipol hydrochloride in hypercholesterolemic patients – effect on serum cholesterol and mortality. *J Chronic Dis* 1978; **31**:5–14.

32. Rosenhamer G, Carlson LA. Effect of combined clofibrate–nicotinic acid treatment in ischemic heart disease. *Atherosclerosis* 1980; **37**:129–42.

33. Buchwald H, Varco RL, Matts JP, et al. Effect of partial ileal bypass surgery on mortality and morbidity from coronary heart diease in patients with hypercholesterolemia. Report of the Program on the Surgical Control of the Hyperlipidemias (POSCH). *N Engl J Med* 1990; **323**:946–55.

34. Furberg CD, Adams HP Jr, Applegate WB, et al. Effect of lovastatin on early carotid atherosclerosis and cardiovascular events. Asymptomatic Carotid Artery Progression Study (ACAPS) Research Group. *Circulation* 1994; **90**:1679–87.

35. Schwartz GG, Olsson AG, Ezekowitz MD, Ganz P, Oliver MF, Waters D, for the Myocardial Ischemia Reduction with Aggressive Cholesterol Lowering (MIRACL) Study Investigators. Effects of atorvastatin on early recurrent ischemic events in acute coronary syndromes: The MIRACL Study: a randomized controlled trial. *JAMA* 2001; **285**:1711–18.

36. Waters DD, Schwartz GG, Olsson AG, et al., for the MIRACL Study Investigators. Effects of atorvastatin on stroke in patients with unstable angina or non-Q-wave myocardial infarction. A Myocardial Ischemia Reduction with Aggressive Cholesterol Lowering (MIRACL) Substudy. *Circulation* 2002; **106**:1690–5.

37. Nissen SE, Tuzcu EM, Schoenhagen P, et al., for the REVERSAL Investigators. Effect of intensive compared with moderate lipid-lowering therapy on progression of coronary atherosclerosis: a randomized controlled trial. *JAMA* 2004; **291**:1071–80.

38. Cannon CP, Braunwald E, McCabe CH, et al., for the Pravastatin or Atorvastatin Evaluation and Infection Therapy-Thrombolysis in Myocardial Infarction 22 Investigators. Intensive versus moderate lipid lowering with statins after acute coronary syndromes. *N Engl J Med* 2004; **350**:1495–504.

39. Expert Panel on Detection, Evaluation, and Treatment of High Blood Cholesterol in Adults. Executive Summary of the Third Report of the National Cholesterol Education Program (NCEP) Expert Panel on Detection, Evaluation, and Treatment of High Blood Cholesterol in Adults (Adult Treatment Panel III). *JAMA* 2001; **285**:2486–97.

40. Grundy SM, Cleeman JI, Merz CNB, et al., for the Coordinating Committee of the National Cholesterol Education Program. Implications of recent clinical trials for the National Cholesterol Education Program Adult Treatment Panel III Guidelines. *Circulation* 2004; **110**:227–39.

41. Mosca L, Appel LJ, Benjamin EJ, et al. American Heart Association. Evidence-based guidelines for cardiovascular disease prevention in women. Expert Panel/Writing Group. *Circulation* 2004; **109**:672–92.

42. The Women's Health Initiative Steering Committee. Effects of conjugated equine estrogen in postmenopausal women with hysterectomy: the Women's Health Initiative randomized controlled trial. *JAMA* 2004; **291**:1701–12.

43. Grady D, Herrington D, Bittner V, et al., for the HERS Research Group. Cardiovascular disease outcomes during 6.8 years of hormone therapy. Heart and Estrogen/progestin Replacement Study Follow-up (HERS II). *JAMA* 2002; **288**:49–57.

44. Shlipak MG, Chaput LA, Vittinghoff E, et al., for the Heart and Estrogen/progestin Replacement Study (HERS) Investigators. Lipid changes on hormone therapy and coronary heart disease events in the Heart and Estrogen/progestin Replacement Study (HERS). *Am Heart J* 2003; **146**:870–5.

45. Writing Group for the Women's Health Initiative Investigators. Risks and benefits of estrogen plus progestin in healthy postmenopausal women. Principal results from the Women's Health Initiative randomized controlled trial. *JAMA* 2002; **288**:321–33.

46. http://www.fda.gov/bbs/topics/NEWS/2003/NEW00 863.html [accessed July 26, 2003].

47. de Lorgeril M, Salen P, Martin J-L, Monjaud I, Delaye J, Mamelle N. Mediterranean diet, traditional risk

factors, and the rate of cardiovascular complications after myocardial infarction. Final report of the Lyon Diet Heart Study. *Circulation* 1999; **99**:779–85.

48. Goldberg AC, Sapre A, Liu J, Capece R, Mitchel YB for the Ezetimibe Study Group. Efficacy and safety of ezetimibe coadministered with simvastatin in patients with primary hypercholesterolemia: a randomized, double-blind, placebo-controlled trial. *Mayo Clin Proc* 2004; **79**:620–9.

49. LaRosa JC, He J, Vupputuri S. Effect of statins on risk of coronary disease: a meta-analysis of randomized controlled trials. *JAMA* 1999; **282**:2340–6.

50. Walsh JME, Pignone M. Drug treatment of hyperlipidemia in women. *JAMA* 2004; **291**:2243–52.

5

Other risk interventions: smoking

Maria Amada F. Apacible, Kirsten Martin and
Erika S. Sivarajan Froelicher

Introduction

Smoking is closely linked to cardiovascular disease and cancer, which are the leading causes of death for women in developed countries.[1] Yet, there are few studies that focus specifically on the concerns unique to women. There are several explanations for this gap in the literature: (1) the delay in peak levels of smoking in women, (2) the research focus on men as the primary population perceived to be at risk for smoking-related illnesses, and (3) the associated emphasis on studies for smoking cessation interventions for men.[2] However, the evidence is clear that the ill health consequences of smoking are equally, if not more devastating, in women than in men.[3] Therefore, until research is able to provide specific guidance for smoking cessation interventions addressing the particular needs of women, it is reasonable to follow current guidelines outlined by the Agency for Healthcare Research and Quality.[4] The purpose of this chapter is to explain current recommendations for smoking cessation interventions in adult women.

Clinical practice guidelines

The current guidelines were developed by a panel of national experts who critically reviewed and analyzed available scientific research, from which they identified effective smoking cessation treatments validated through experimental research studies. The resulting evidence-based guidelines are summarized in the document, *Treating Tobacco Use and Dependence: Clinical Practice Guideline*, henceforth referred to as the Guideline.[4]

The Guideline established five major intervention steps referred to as the '5As.' These are: (1) **A**sk about tobacco use and document status for every patient visit; (2) **A**dvise the patient to quit in a clear personalized manner; (3) **A**ssess willingness to make a quit attempt; (4) **A**ssist patient to make a quit attempt; and (5) **A**rrange for follow-up.[4] These steps are useful for clinicians regardless of the practice setting.

Step One: ASK – screen for tobacco use status

The goal of this intervention is to identify every smoker every time she is seen by a clinician. In order to accomplish this, a systematic screening tool should be in place (Fig. 5.1).[4,5] It may be done in simple a manner, by adding assessment of smoking status to the routine vital signs at each visit. If a woman is identified as a smoker, further assessment of level of nicotine dependence can be used to guide treatment and care. The Fagerstrom Questionnaire for Nicotine Dependence (FTND) is a widely used instrument to assess severity of nicotine dependence, based on scores from zero to ten.[6,7] The FTND may be self-administered by women. Clinicians with limited time for assessing level of nicotine addiction may consider using only two of the Fagerstrom questions: (1) how soon after you wake up do you smoke your first cigarette, and (2) do you have a hard time refraining from smoking in places where it is

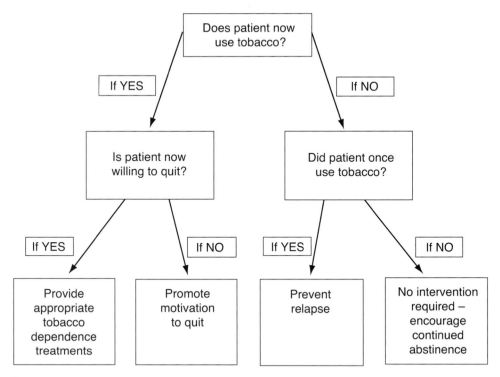

Figure 5.1
Treating tobacco use and dependence: clinical practice guideline.[4] Screen for tobacco use status.

prohibited? Responses to these questions are useful in assessing level of nicotine addiction.

Step Two: ADVISE – strongly urge all smokers to quit

The next intervention is strong, clear, and personalized advice to stop smoking. The advice should be delivered in a direct and sensitive manner, but should clearly inform the woman of the impact of smoking on her health. For example, 'As your health provider, I need you to understand that quitting smoking is the most important thing you can do to protect your health now and in the future. I think that it is absolutely vital that you stop smoking now and I will help you.' The message should be fitted to that particular individual's concerns, and address family history, age, gender, social situation, past health behaviors, and personal health status. For

example, if a woman has high blood pressure or has had a myocardial infarction (MI), that woman needs to understand the direct connection between smoking and her current condition. It is also important to explain that continued smoking will place her at increased risk for a subsequent MI. Smoking after angioplasty places her at increased risk for restenosis.

Step Three: ASSESS – determine willingness to make a quit attempt

After counseling the woman to stop smoking, it is important to determine if she is willing to quit at this time. Willingness to stop smoking may be assessed using a simple yes/no question, such as, 'Are you willing to stop smoking now?' Willingness may also be assessed using an intention question, such as, 'Are you willing to stop smoking in the next month?' It is also possible to use a willingness scale, such as a zero to ten scale, with zero signifying no intention to quit smoking and ten indicating maximum willingness to quit smoking. If the woman is willing to quit, have her set a quit day and provide an individualized intervention, whether brief or intensive, that is appropriate for her level of nicotine dependence and coincides with her preferences.

Smokers who are unwilling to quit

If the woman states an unwillingness to quit at this time, then it is appropriate to provide a motivational intervention. In order to provide an effective intervention, it is important to determine the source of her reluctance to stop smoking. Regardless of the barrier, providing pertinent information that directly addresses the issues or anticipatory guidance for potential problems may encourage the woman to move further along toward quitting. If she becomes willing to quit, it is then appropriate to provide interventions that assist her in her efforts. However, if the patient continues to state that she is unwilling to quit, the Guideline[4] provides for a motivational intervention called the '5Rs'. The 5Rs consist of: (1) **R**elevance, (2) **R**isks, (3) **R**ewards, (4) **R**oadblocks, and (5) **R**epetition. Smokers may be unwilling to quit because of misinformation, concerns about the effects of quitting, or because of low levels of self-efficacy or feelings of failure related to previously unsuccessful quit attempts.

Relevance. Encourage the woman to identify factors that are personally relevant to her smoking behaviors and how those impact her present and future health. Motivational information has the greatest impact when it is directly related to a woman's disease risk or status, family, social situation, co-morbid health conditions, age, or other personal experiences. A woman who has been admitted to the hospital for a smoking-related illness should be counseled about the connection between her smoking and her current health status. Women who are unwilling to quit because of previously unsuccessful attempts should be counseled that it is common to make several quit attempts before successful quitting is achieved. Women should also understand that with appropriate assistance and support their likelihood of success is much greater.

Risks. The clinician should ask the woman to identify the potential negative health consequences of smoking, and emphasize those that are pertinent to her. It should be made clear to the woman that smoking low-tar/low-nicotine cigarettes and other forms of tobacco such as cigars, pipes or smokeless tobacco do not eliminate these risks. Examples of acute risks are: shortness of breath and related activity intolerance, asthma exacerbations, impotence, and infertility.[4] Long-term risks include heart attack, stroke, emphysema, lung and other cancers; the potential for long-term disability, extended care, and early death.[4] There is further risk of heart disease and lung cancer in partners of smokers from environmental exposure; as well as increased rates of smoking, asthma, middle ear disease, sudden infant death syndrome, and respiratory infections in children exposed to environmental smoke.[4]

Rewards. The clinician should encourage the woman to identify potential benefits of smoking cessation. It may be useful to highlight those benefits that are most personally relevant for the woman. Examples of rewards include: improved health; better ability to taste food; improved sense of smell; monetary savings; better self-esteem; better smelling clothes, home and car; improved performance at physical activities; a better feeling of physical well-being; no worries about exposing others to smoke; having healthier babies and children; setting a healthy example for children; reduced wrinkling and aging of skin.[4]

Roadblocks. The clinician should help the woman identify barriers or impediments to smoking cessation with special attention to those that are amenable to intervention (pharmacologic treatment or problem-solving). Encourage the woman to see her impediments as surmountable with assistance and treatment. Typical barriers might include: withdrawal symptoms, fear of failure, depression, stress, lack of support, fear of weight gain, and enjoyment of tobacco.

Repetition. The motivational intervention should be repeated every time an unmotivated, smoking woman is seen in a clinical setting. Reviewing the individual smoker's relevance, risks, rewards, and roadblocks at each visit may help her move towards readiness to start a smoking cessation intervention. It also emphasizes the importance of smoking cessation to health and makes the patient aware of the clinician's level of concern regarding smoking.

Step Four: ASSIST – aid the patient to quit smoking

For the woman who is ready to quit smoking, the first step toward smoking cessation is developing a quit plan. The components of a plan include: (1) setting a quit date, ideally within 2 weeks of the time when they are seen and state their willingness to stop smoking; (2) telling family, friends, and co-workers about quitting and requesting understanding and support; (3) anticipate challenges to planned quit attempt, particularly within the first few weeks when risk of relapse is highest; (4) remove all tobacco products from the environment including ashtrays, matches, and cigarettes.[4] Prior to quitting smokers should avoid smoking in places where much time will be spent after the quit date, such as in the car or house. If a woman is identified in the hospital, a quit date is not necessary because of the smoking ban inside the hospital. However, this woman should be offered counseling and pharmacologic support as part of her smoking cessation intervention and a plan should be made to continue treatment following discharge. Signing a behavioral contract to stop smoking has proved an effective technique in aiding patients to remain abstinent from smoking, regardless of whether initiated in the hospital or in the clinic. This process helps to formalize the woman's commitment to quit and is an effective tool for counseling. Also, it extends support from the clinician to the patient through the process of its development. The contract should be simple and explicit, specifying the support provided by the clinician, the rewards of successful adherence, and the consequences of not adhering to expected behavior including the harmful health consequences of continued smoking. The contract must be written, reviewed, and signed, so that both the woman and the clinician agree with the stated terms.

The Guideline[4] recommends that five major components be part of any brief intervention for smoking cessation. These components include: (1)

providing practical counseling for abstinence, stress management, relapse prevention, problem-solving, and skills training; (2) providing intra-treatment social support directly from the clinician to the woman; (3) assisting the woman in obtaining other social support outside the clinical setting (extratreatment social support); (4) recommending the use of approved pharmacotherapy when appropriate; and (5) providing supplementary materials to assist with smoking cessation efforts. All five components should be part of any intervention offered to smokers regardless of whether they request referral for more intensive therapy.

Provide practical counseling

Practical counseling includes assisting women to identify and anticipate situations that increase the risk of relapse. This should incorporate a review of past quit attempts and factors that contributed to previous relapses. It is critical to anticipate triggers or challenges that may arise and discuss strategies of how the woman may overcome or avoid them. Common triggers of relapse include social situations such as living with another smoker, drinking alcohol, increased life stress; or internal states such as negative affect. Successful coping strategies to emphasize include anticipatory planning, avoidance, stress reduction, and the development of alternative health behaviors. It is vital that women understand the addictive nature of smoking and the potential withdrawal symptoms that they may experience while attempting to quit. Smokers should be counseled that withdrawal symptoms will peak at 24–48 hours after smoking their last cigarette, gradually declining over the following 1–2 weeks. It is imperative to emphasize the importance of total abstinence, women should understand that smoking even one puff after the quit date increases the likelihood of complete relapse.

Provide intra-treatment social support

Intra-treatment social support is simply providing the woman with encouragement, support, and information that demonstrates a sincere concern about her health. It includes creating a supportive clinical environment that encourages the patient to stop smoking. In practical terms, it means structuring clinical time to give the patient opportunities to talk about her quit attempt including concerns, fears, and successes.

Assist the patient to obtain extra-treatment social support

The provision of extra-treatment social support is critical in sustaining the smoking cessation effort. Extra-treatment social support includes all social support obtained outside of the treatment environment. It includes encouraging family members, friends, and significant others to support the patient in the quit attempt by actions such as not smoking around the person attempting to quit and not offering them cigarettes. If appropriate, the provider may need to provide simultaneous smoking cessation interventions to several household members who smoke, or encourage them to be present at counseling and appointments for the individual making the quit attempt. This is particularly important for women living with another smoker because living with another smoker is a strong predictor of relapse in women.[8] It may require role-playing and helping the woman to plan how she will ask for the support that is needed, identifying community resources such as telephone support lines, websites, support group meetings, or helping the woman find a another smoker who is also attempting to quit with whom she can partner for support.

Recommend the use of approved pharmacotherapy when appropriate

Provision of appropriate pharmacotherapies is strongly recommended and has proven effective in increasing the success of smoking cessation efforts. Women should understand how these medications work to increase smoking cessation success and reduce withdrawal symptoms. They should also be counseled about how to use medications as prescribed and understand the potential side effects. The first-line pharmacotherapy agents include: bupropion SR, nicotine replacement therapy in the forms of patch, gum, inhaler, and nasal spray. The

clinical guidelines for prescribing pharmacotherapy in smoking cessation are summarized in Table 5.1.[4]

Provide supplementary materials

When the woman leaves the health-care setting, it is strongly recommended that she be provided with supplementary materials that are racially, culturally, educationally, and age appropriate. It is common for women to choose individual methods of smoking cessation and decline more intensive therapies; providing self-help materials is a low-cost method of intervention for a woman with this preference. The clinician should be aware of the many federal agencies, nonprofit organizations, and local and state health departments that offer resources in order to have a wide variety of materials to suit the diverse needs of patients. A wide selection of materials should be available in the health-care setting to provide appropriate help for patients who require any type of smoking cessation intervention.

Step Five: ARRANGE for follow-up

Women need a specific plan for follow-up either in the clinic or by phone. Periodic assessment of smoking cessation status and supportive interventions are associated with increased success in smoking cessation.[4] Also, increased numbers of contact hours between the woman and the provider are predictive of successful smoking cessation.[4] Finally, follow-up allows for modifications or revisions to be made to the overall smoking cessation plan in light of the patient's changing smoking status and current situation.

Although most patients choose to stop smoking on their own or with the assistance of brief interventions, there are women who may prefer and benefit from more intensive therapy. There is evidence that intensive interventions are more effective than brief interventions and should be used whenever possible, depending on the resources available and patient preference. Therefore, clinicians have an obligation to know which resources are available in their communities, and be willing to make appropriate referrals. Clinicians should also be able to provide women with information regarding the types, costs,

Table 5.1 First-line pharmacotherapies for smoking cessation (approved for use for smoking cessation by the US Food and Drug Administration)[4]

Pharmacotherapy	Precautions/ contraindications	Side effects	Dosage	Duration	Availability	Cost per day
Bupropion SR	History of seizure History of eating disorders	Insomnia Dry mouth	150 mg every morning for 3 days then 150 mg twice daily (begin treatment 1–2 weeks pre-quit)	7–12 weeks maintenance, up to 6 months	Zyban (prescription only)	$3.50
Nicotine gum	–	Mouth soreness Dyspepsia	1–24 cigs/day – 2 mg gum (up to 24 pieces/day) 25+ cigs/day – 4 mg gum (up to 24 pieces/day)	Up to 12 weeks	Nicorette, Nicorette Mint, Nicorette Orange (OTC only)	Brand name: $4.54 for 10 2-mg pieces, $5.00 for 10 4-mg pieces Store brand: $3.00 for 10 2-mg pieces, $3.70 for 10 4-mg pieces
Nicotine inhaler	–	Local irritation of mouth and throat	6–16 cartridges/day	Up to 6 months	Nicotrol inhaler (prescription only)	$10.95 for 10 cartridges
Nicotine nasal spray	–	Nasal irritation	8–40 doses/day	3–6 months	Nicotrol NS (prescription only)	$5.64 for 12 doses
Nicotine patch	–	Local skin reaction Insomnia	21 mg/24 hours 14 mg/24 hours 7 mg/24 hours 15 mg/16 hours	4 weeks, then 2 weeks, then 2 weeks 8 weeks	Nicoderm CQ, (OTC only), generic patches (prescription and OTC) Nicotrol (OTC only)	Brand name: $3.50 Store brand: $2.11

OTC, over the counter.

methods, and contacts of the available community programs, encouraging the woman to choose the program that best suits her needs.

Relapse prevention

Because of the chronic nature of nicotine dependence, relapse prevention is a major component of any smoking cessation intervention. All former smokers should be assessed for smoking relapse at every visit. Although most relapses occur early in the days to weeks following the quit date, some people remain more vulnerable and may relapse after months or even years of smoking abstinence. Relapse prevention interventions take the form of either brief (minimal) or more intensive, pharmacologic treatments. However, every former smoker should receive a minimum of a brief smoking relapse intervention, which includes congratulations on any successes and strong encouragement to remain abstinent. Particular attention needs to be paid to women who have recently stopped smoking and are at increased risk for relapse. The clinician needs to engage the patient in active discussion about: (1) the benefits derived from smoking cessation, (2) any successes the patient has had in quitting including duration of abstinence and reduction in withdrawal, and (3) any problems encountered or anticipated threats to maintaining abstinence. The use of open-ended questions and the woman's active engagement in problem-solving are important to supporting continued abstinence.

If significant threats to abstinence are identified during the brief relapse prevention evaluation, the woman may require more intensive or prescriptive intervention. One commonly reported problem is lack of support for cessation, for which the clinician may need to schedule follow-up visits or phone calls with the woman. It may also be appropriate to assist the patient in identifying sources of support within her own environment, or to refer the patient to an organization that offers cessation counseling or support. Another commonly reported problem is negative mood or depression, which may require counseling, medication, or referral for mental health services. Strong or prolonged withdrawal symptoms are also a frequent complaint in the period following smoking cessation. If the woman reports craving, anxiety or other withdrawal symptoms, appropriate treatment may include extending the use of approved pharmacotherapy or combining medications to reduce symptoms. The fourth threat to continuing abstinence is weight gain. Recommend starting or increasing physical activity, but discourage strict dieting that may exacerbate cravings.[9] Emphasize the importance of a healthy diet. Reassure the patient that some weight gain after quitting is normal and self-limiting.[10] Maintain the woman on pharmacotherapy known to attenuate or delay weight gain until the critical relapse period has passed. If necessary, refer the woman to a specialist or program for treatment. The final common indication for intensive therapy is flagging motivation or feelings of deprivation. Reassure the woman that such feelings are common and recommend engaging in rewarding activities. Assess her for periodic

tobacco use, and emphasize that beginning to smoke (even a single puff) will increase urges and make cessation more difficult.

Special considerations in smoking cessation intervention for women

The failure of many smoking cessation intervention studies to report results by gender, and the lack of studies focused on the concerns unique to women, do not allow for the drawing of firm conclusions about smoking cessation interventions for women. However, information regarding women and smoking cessation has accumulated since the current guidelines were developed and may influence their implementation. Observations and clinical experience gained in more recent studies indicate that there may be gender differences in the way women are impacted by and experience smoking. These differences may also extend to intervention responses and experiences during the relapse period.

Physiological and psychosocial aspects of smoking in women

Women's sensitivity, tolerance, and dependence on the effects of smoking appear to have physical, behavioral, and psychosocial factors. In terms of physiological vulnerability, women have an apparent increased sensitivity to the physical consequences of smoking. When controlling for age, amount, and number of years smoking, women reported increased incidence of respiratory symptoms, decreased lung function, and decreased global health ratings.[3] Women have also reported greater severity of withdrawal symptoms on quitting.[9] Even when women and men smoked the same number of cigarettes, women had lower plasma levels of nicotine and decreased tolerance for the negative effects of nicotine (such as nausea).[11] Researchers have extrapolated that women have increased sensitivity to nicotine and do not need as high a blood level to achieve desired effects. Consequently it is hypothesized that women have lower levels of physical dependence on nicotine and smoke less for its stimulant effects, but rather for a complex combination of reasons. There are data that women are more likely to smoke to alleviate stress, moderate negative affect, and control weight. This may help explain lower quit rates for women compared with men in programs designed primarily around single interventions including monotherapy nicotine replacement.[2] Although pharmacologic therapy is first-line therapy for all smokers in combination with cognitive-behavioral therapy, this combination may be more critical in the smoking cessation efforts of women.

Stress (see also Chapter 40)

Stress is a common trigger for smoking initiation, maintenance, and relapse in both women and men. However, women may have greater vulnerability in response to stress and stressful life events. Women appear more likely to identify smoking as a means of coping with stress and relieving anxiety than men. Study results have indicated that women's cessation rates tend to decrease as stress levels increase.[12] Women also appear to be more likely to relapse and less likely to quit in the presence of stressful life events, particularly stress related to health and financial issues.[13] If confirmed by further studies, these results would be consistent with findings from other drug dependence studies where women identified physical health, finances, and interpersonal losses as major triggers for relapse and challenges to initiating smoking cessation.[14] Therefore, it may be prudent to consider counseling women about stress as a potential trigger for relapse and providing appropriate stress reduction therapies during smoking cessation interventions.

Depression (see also Chapter 41)

A third area of vulnerability for women in smoking cessation appears to be depression. Despite conflicting data, a recent meta-analysis of 15 studies has brought some insight into key issues for women.[15] It appears that a single episode of depression in the past does not affect success in a smoking cessation program. However, women who have a history of recurrent depression are at an apparent increased risk for relapse, while men with a history of recurrent depression do not seem to share the same risk.[16] Overall, women who smoke have higher rates of depression at 22% as compared with a rate of 18% among men.[17] Depressed women also appear to have decreased rates of self-efficacy, which may affect their motivation and ability to stop smoking. Screening for depression may be helpful prior to initiating smoking cessation intervention. Also, smokers with a history of recurrent depression appeared to have higher abstinence rates with mood managed therapies than those who received other types of cessation therapies. Thus it would be reasonable to consider such therapies in the development of an individualized smoking cessation intervention.[15]

Weight concerns (see also Chapter 6)

The fourth and most frequently cited issue of concern for women with smoking cessation is weight control.[10] Women appear more likely to be concerned about weight gain, and may report higher levels of reluctance to stop smoking as a result.[10,18] In a recent study, as weight gain increased during the early stages of smoking cessation, relapse rates also appeared to increase, but whether this effect was causative or correlational is as yet undetermined.[19] Regardless, it would be appropriate to screen and counsel women about the likelihood of weight gain and offer interventions that directly address this concern. Although the focus of this paper is adult women smokers, it is important to note for future clinical and public health considerations that currently the group that is most resistant to smoking cessation interventions comprises adolescent, young women. The apparent reason for this high level of treatment resistance is concern regarding weight gain.[2]

Social support and cohabitation with another smoker

Women who smoke tend to report lower levels of general social support and have fewer social contacts than women who do not. In the National Health and

Nutrition Examination Survey and the Lung Health Study, lack of social support and living alone were key predictors of smoking relapse.[20,21] Adult women who smoke appear to have a greater than 50% chance of either living alone or living with a partner who smokes, both of which may be predictive of smoking cessation failure.[20,21] In the Women's Initiative for Nonsmoking study, the greatest predictor of relapse was cohabitation with a smoker. Although counter-intuitive, women who lived with another smoker reported decreased levels of social support when they were attempting to stop smoking.[8,22] Therefore, when assessing a woman smoker's resources for a quit attempt, it may be prudent to more carefully assess levels of social support with particular attention to living situation and smoking status of other people who may live in the same household. If levels of social support are in question, it may be necessary for the clinician to consider counseling other members in the household regarding smoking cessation or providing the woman patient with additional sources of social support through referral or more frequent follow-up care.

Other predictors of relapse

Among women, lower levels of education and living at or beneath the poverty level have been associated with increased smoking rates and decreased cessation rates. Women who have less than 12 years of education and lower income levels smoke at a rate of approximately 30%, whereas women who have more than 12 years of education and live above the poverty level smoke at rates of about 11%.[20] There may be several explanations for these differences, but they remain largely understudied. However, when designing smoking cessation interventions it is important to know that women with more education seem more likely to perceive the benefits of smoking cessation, and are more likely to quit than women of

lower socioeconomic status with less educa-tion.[20,22–31] Therefore, the clinician may need to be prepared to see more women with less education and lower socioeconomic status who are smokers and be able to provide appropriate resources for these women. To provide comprehensive health promo-tion and risk reduction for women, it is important that in addition to smoking cessation counseling, all women are able to benefit from the preventive Guideline recommendations.

Directions for future study

Clearly, smoking cessation intervention for women is an area in need of much research. However, several questions may provide more useful direction in clini-cal practice. These questions include: (1) how do smoking cessation support groups for women impact cessation rates, (2) what is the optimal pharmacologic therapy for the prevention of relapse in women, and (3) what types of smoking cessation therapies are most effective in depressed or weight concerned women?

Conclusions

Because of its enormous impact on health and society, smoking is one of the most studied health-related behaviors, yet it is one of the most under-treated risk factors in women's health care. Thousands of studies exist documenting its health consequences, but there are still substantial questions about women and smoking that remain unanswered and understudied, particularly for smoking cessation interventions. Because the need for intervention is compelling, it is critical that clini-cians implement evidence-based recommendations as they currently exist until research is able to provide more specific interventions for women.[32]

References

1. World Health Organization. *Women and the Tobacco Epidemic: Challenges for the 21st Century*. Canada: Institute for Global Tobacco Control, 2001.
2. United States Department of Health and Human Services. *Women and Smoking: A Report of the Surgeon General*. Atlanta, GA: Centers for Disease Control and Prevention, 2001.
3. Langhammer A, Johnsen R, Gulsvik A, Holmen TL, Bjermer L. Sex differences in lung vulnerability to tobacco smoking. *Eur Respir J* 2003; **21**:1017–23.
4. Fiore MC, Bailey WC, Cohen SJ, et al. *Treating Tobacco Use and Dependence. Quick Reference Guide for Clinicians*. Rockville, MD: US Department of Health and Human Services, Public Health Service, 2000.
5. Rigotti N, MacKool K, Shiffman S. Predictors of smoking cessation after coronary bypass surgery: results of a randomized trial with five year follow-up. *Ann Intern Med* 1994; **120**:287–93.
6. Fagerstrom KO. Measuring degree of physical dependence to tobacco smoking with reference to individualization of treatment. *Addict Behav* 1978; **3**:234–41.
7. Fagerstrom KO, Schneider NG. Measuring nicotine dependence: a review of the Fagerstrom Tolerance Questionnaire. *J Behav Med* 1989; **12**:159–82.
8. Froelicher ES, Christopherson DJ, Miller NH, Martin K. Women's initiative for nonsmoking (WINS) IV: description of 277 smokers hospitalized with cardiovascular disease. *Heart Lung* 2002; **31**:3–14.
9. Pinto BM, Borrelli B, King TK, et al. Weight control smoking among sedentary women. *Addict Behav* 1999; **24**:75–86.
10. Meyers AW, Klesges RC, Winders SE, Ward KD, Peterson BA, Eck LH. Are weight concerns predictive of smoking cessation? A prospective analysis. *J Consult Clin Psychol* 1997; **65**:448–52.
11. Zeman MV, Hiraki L, Sellers EM. Gender differences in tobacco smoking: Higher relative exposure to smoke than nicotine in women. *J Womens Health Gend Based Med* 2002; **11**:147–53.
12. Wetter DW, Kenford SL, Smith SS, Fiore MC, Jorenby DE, Baker TB. Gender differences in smoking cessation. *J Consult Clin Psychol* 1999; **67**:555–62.
13. McKee SA, Maciejewski PK, Falba T, Mazure CM. Sex differences in the effects of stressful life events on changes in smoking status. *Addiction* 2003; **98**:847–55.
14. Weaver GD, Turner NH, O'Dell KJ. Depressive symptoms, stress and coping among women recovering from addiction. *J Subst Abuse Treat* 2000; **18**:161–7.
15. Hitsman B, Borrelli B, McChargue DE, Spring B, Niaura R. History of depression and smoking cessation outcome: a meta-analysis. *J Consult Clin Psychol* 2003; **71**:657–63.
16. Covey LS, Glassman AH, Stetner F. Naltrexone effects on short-term memory and long-term cessation. *J Addict Dis* 1999; **18**:31–40.
17. Killen JD, Fortmann SP, Schatzberg A, Hayward C, Varady A. Onset of major depression during treatment for nicotine dependence. *Addict Behav* 2003; **28**:461–70.
18. Borrelli B, Spring B, Niaura R, Hitsman B, Papandonatos G. Influences of gender and weight gain on short-term relapse to smoking cessation trial. *J Consult Clin Psychol* 2001; **69**:511–15.
19. Perkins KA. Smoking cessation in women. *CNS Drugs* 2001; **15**:391–411.
20. Ford ES, Ahluwalia IB, Galuska DA. Social relationships and cardiovascular disease risk factors: findings from the third national health and nutrition examination survey. *Prev Med* 2000; **30**:83–92.
21. Nides MA, Rakos RF, Gonzales D, et al. Predictors of initial smoking cessation and relapse through the lung health study. *J Consult Clin Psychol* 1995; **62**:60–9.
22. Froelicher ES, Miller NH, Li W, Maher-Imhof R, Sohn M, Bacchetti P. Predictors of smoking cessation in women with cardiovascular disease: the Women's Health Initiative for Nonsmoking (WINS). *Circulation* 2002; **106**:II-666.
23. Froelicher ES, Miller NH, Christopherson DJ, et al. High rates of sustained smoking cessation in women hospitalized with cardiovascular disease: the Women's Initiative for Nonsmoking (WINS). *Circulation* 2004; **109**:587–93.
24. Sivarajan Froelicher E, Christopherson DJ. Women's Initiative for Nonsmoking (WINS) I: design and methods. *Heart Lung* 2000; **29**:429–37.
25. Martin K, Sivarajan Froelicher E, Houston Miller N. Women's Initiative for Nonsmoking (WINS) II: the intervention. *Heart Lung* 2000; **29**:438–45.
26. Sivarajan Froelicher E, Kozuki Y. Theoretical application of smoking cessation interventions to individuals with medical conditions: Women's Initiative for Nonsmoking (WINS): Part III. *Int J Nurs Stud* 2002; **39**:1–15.

27. Mahrer-Imhof R, Froelicher E, Li W. Women's Initiative for Nonsmoking (WINS V): under-use of nicotine replacement therapy. *Heart Lung* 2002; **31**:368–73.

28. Sohn M, Hartley C, Sivarajan Froelicher E, Benowitz NL. Tobacco use and dependence. *Semin Oncol Nurs* 2003; **19**:250–60.

29. Hutchinson KH, Sivarajan Froelicher E. Populations at risk for tobacco-related diseases. *Semin Oncol Nurs* 2003; **19**:276–83.

30. Sivarajan Froelicher E, Sohn M, Max W, Bacchetti P. Women's Initiative for Nonsmoking (WINS) VII: evaluation of health service utilization and costs among women smokers with cardiovascular disease. *J Cardiopulm Rehabil* 2004; **24**:218–28.

31. Sivarajan Froelicher E, Li WW, Mahrer-Imhof R, Christopherson R, Stewart AL. Women's Initiative for Nonsmoking (WINS) VI: reliability and validity of health and psychosocial measures in women smokers with cardiovascular disease. *Heart Lung* 2004; **33**:162–75.

32. Expert Panel/Writing Group: Mosca L, Appel LJ, Benjamin EJ, Berra K, et al. Evidence-based guidelines for cardiovascular disease prevention in women. *Circulation* 2004; **109**:672–93.

6

Other risk interventions: obesity

Marie E. McDonnell and Caroline M. Apovian

Introduction

Obesity and *overweight* are common conditions that greatly increase the risk of cardiovascular disease (CVD) in women and men, both directly and through associated conditions.[1,2] During the second half of the twentieth century, the prevalence of obesity grew to epidemic proportions in several industrialized nations. Of major concern is that women appear to be at particular risk, with postmenopausal women, Mexican-American and nonHispanic black women having the highest rates of obesity in the United States. Moreover, epidemiologic data show that increased adiposity has a greater relative impact on cardiovascular risk in women than it has in men.[3]

This chapter addresses the problem of obesity as a risk factor for CVD, specifically in women. While both women and men share much of the same biology, it is clear that there are factors unique to a woman's life cycle that have significant impact on her weight and body fat composition. This concept is important in the study of the epidemiology, pathophysiology and treatment of obesity. For example, neurobiologic research has identified peptides that regulate patterns of appetite and eating behavior, and therefore have therapeutic potential. Some of these peptides, such as leptin, have also been linked to fertility.[4] This suggests that just as the biological models of female and male fertility differ, so there may be subtle gender differences in body fat regulation. Such links in biological function not only reveal the complexity of obesity, but also suggest that gender lends insight into etiologies, global health impact, and the efficacy of specific therapies.

Definition and measurement

Conditions of excess weight are well defined by the World Health Organization using the body mass index (BMI) as a simple measurement tool. The BMI is calculated by dividing weight in kilograms by the square of height in meters, and correlates strongly with total body fat content in most adults. Normal weight in Western countries corresponds to a BMI between 18 kg/m^2 and 24.9 kg/m^2. Obesity is defined as a BMI of 30 kg/m^2 or above, and is then further delineated into subgroups based on risk (see Table 6.1).[5] On either side of the obesity epidemic is a population that is pre-obese, or overweight (BMI

Table 6.1 Obesity class and disease risk

Body mass index (kg/m^2)	Classification	Disease risk* (Waist circumference) Men ≤40 in Women ≤35 in	>40 in >35 in
<25.0–29.9	Overweight	Increased	High
30.0–34.9	Obesity I	High	Very high
35.0–39.9	Obesity II	Very high	Very high
>40	Obesity III	Extremely high	Extremely high

*For type 2 diabetes mellitus, hypertension, and cardiovascular disease.
Adapted from reference 5.

25–29.9 kg/m²) and one that is extremely obese (BMI ≥40 kg/m²).

There are three cautions to consider in using the BMI definitions. First, fat distribution may predict risk in patients who have a normal BMI. Increased waist circumference, a surrogate marker for abdominal adiposity, independently predicts the development of insulin resistance, diabetes mellitus, hypertension, hyperlipidemia, and polycystic ovarian syndrome (PCOS) in women. A waist circumference of ≥35 inches (88 cm) in women or ≥40 inches (102 cm) in men defines central obesity. The ratio of the waist circumference to hip circumference, albeit more cumbersome, is another tool that has been shown to independently predict CVD. A ratio of ≥0.96 in men and ≥0.81 in women is associated with increased risk for CVD. Second, in some cultures with varying body types, the normal range for BMI may underestimate, or potentially overestimate, the population at risk. For example, in Asian nations, a BMI of 23 is considered overweight, since at the same BMI, Asians on average have a higher percent body fat and a greater waist circumference than Caucasians.[6] Third, the definitions include individuals who have an overweight or obese BMI but who do not have excess adipose tissue, but rather a larger proportion of lean mass. This is rarely an important consideration in women, however, since women generally have a higher percentage body fat than men.

Epidemiology of obesity

The National Health and Nutrition Examination Survey (NHANES) showed that in the year 1999–2000, the age-adjusted prevalence of obesity in the US adult population was 30.5 %.[7] This represents an increase of nearly 8% from the previous survey of the period between 1988 and 1994, and a doubling since 1980. Extreme obesity has risen in prevalence from 3% to nearly 5% during the 1990s. With another 33% of the US population being pre-obese, or overweight, and with the majority of adults continuing to gain weight throughout life, the prevalence of obesity is not likely to decrease soon. Moreover, judging from the increased prevalence of overweight in children and adolescents internation-

ally, the problem will become even more challenging in the near future.

Obesity is more prevalent among women in Western cultures, although *overweight* is more common in men. In the US, 34% of women versus 27.7% of men are obese; yet, 27.9% of women versus 39.5% of men are overweight. In Europe, obesity rates are lower, but the same pattern exists: 19% of women and 13% of men are obese versus 35% of women and 50% of men are overweight.[8] Postmenopausal women appear to bear the brunt of the epidemic. Among US women between the ages of 60 and 69, 64% are either overweight or obese. This is twice the prevalence of overweight and obesity in women between the ages of 20 and 29.

North Americans gain on average 1 lb per year during their adult life, although women in their postmenopausal years may gain up to 5 lbs per year in the absence of formal attention to weight.[9] According to current statistics, if a 50-year-old woman with a height of 63 inches and weight of 134 lbs (BMI = 24 kg/m²) at the onset of menopause gains 5 lbs per year, she could become obese by age 57 (BMI = 30 kg/m²) and in that short time *double* her risk of CVD.[3]

Obesity and cardiovascular disease

The risk of having a myocardial infarction (MI) increases proportionately to BMI. Mortality rates clearly rise in proportion to degree of obesity,[10] explained in large part by the multiple co-morbid conditions which are associated with CVD: hypertension, dyslipidemia, type 2 diabetes, coronary artery disease, stroke, sleep apnea, and congestive heart failure. Hypertension (see also Chapter 31), for example, is three times more common in obese subjects than in normal weight individuals,[11] and weight loss lowers blood pressure. Insulin resistance (see also Chapter 3), which includes a disease spectrum ranging from impaired glucose tolerance and the metabolic syndrome to overt type 2 diabetes mellitus, appears to be even more common among the obese than hypertension.[3] The increased prevalence of obesity in the US during the last decade of

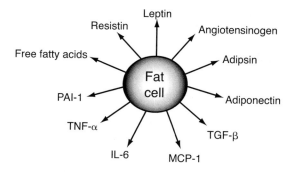

Figure 6.1
Adipocytes release cytokines that mediate inflammation, metabolism, and other physiologic pathways: interleukin-6 (IL-6), tumor necrosis factor-α (TNF-α), plasminogen activator inhibitor-1 (PAI-1), monocyte chemoattractant protein-1 (MCP-1), transforming growth factor-β (TGF-β).

the 1990s was accompanied by a 25% increase in the prevalence of type 2 diabetes. In a large epidemiologic study of female nurses in the US, an increase in BMI from 23 kg/m² to 25 kg/m² was associated with a fourfold risk of developing type 2 diabetes compared with women whose BMI was <22 kg/m². Not surprisingly, a weight loss of at least 5 kg led to a 50% reduction in the incidence of type 2 diabetes.[12]

Obesity is also considered an *independent* risk factor for CVD;[13,14] there is increasing evidence that excess fat tissue has a direct effect on the development of atherosclerosis through the production of bioactive molecules, termed adipocytokines (Fig. 6.1). Several of these substances are associated with inflammation.

Adipose tissue produces hormones that directly affect the cardiovascular system

Adipose tissue is a highly active endocrine organ, composed of fat cells that metabolize and store fat, and preadipocytes, which reside in the vascular/stromal compartment. There are two types of adipose – brown adipose tissue (BAT) and white adipose tissue (WAT). While the physiologic role of BAT in humans may involve thermogenesis, it is not yet established. However, the physiology of WAT has become increasingly clear. The function of WAT is not simply limited to passive fat storage, but rather to produce several bioactive adipocytokines. These include leptin, tumor necrosis factor-α (TNF-α), interleukin-6 (IL-6), transforming growth factor-β (TGF-β), plasminogen activator inhibitor-1 (PAI-1), angiotensinogen, adipsin, acylation-stimulating protein, and metallothionein.

Many of the proteins secreted by adipose tissue have specific roles in the development of obesity-associated complications, such as insulin resistance, endothelial dysfunction, arterial hypertension, and atherosclerosis. *TNF-α* is a cytokine produced by WAT that is markedly upregulated in obesity and interferes with insulin receptor signaling, therefore contributing to insulin resistance.[14] TNF-α also acts to suppress the release of *adiponectin*, an adipocytokine that promotes insulin sensitivity. *Resistin* is a protein expressed in adipose tissue that may be elevated in individuals with type 2 diabetes.[15] It has been implicated in mechanisms of insulin resistance and oxidative stress, which have relevance to the pathophysiology of vascular dysfunction. *IL-6* is an established serum marker of vascular inflammation and is elevated in obese subjects along with C-reactive protein. Both of these markers fall after weight loss as modest as 10%.[16,17] *PAI-1* is an inhibitor of fibrinolysis and is elevated in the serum of obese patients. Increased PAI-1 contributes to a prothrombotic state, which may promote atherogenesis and increase CVD risk.

Angiotensinogen is the substrate for a two-step enzyme cleavage that eventually yields the potent vasoconstrictor angiotensin II. Angiotensin II causes contraction of vascular smooth muscle and stimulates aldosterone release from the adrenal glands, with an end effect of increased blood pressure. Until recently, angiotensinogen was thought to be produced only in the liver. The knowledge that adipocytes produce the precursor to the active product of the renin–angiotensin system has linked obesity more directly to hypertension, and potentially to congestive heart failure (CHF). Morbid obesity has been a known risk factor for CHF for some time, but recent data show that lesser degrees of obesity portend independent risk for CHF as well.[18]

Fat cells located in the abdomen, such as omental fat, are metabolically unique, which may explain why the 'apple' body shape is associated with a higher CVD risk than the 'pear.' Intra-abdominal adipocytes are more lipolytically active than those from other fat depots, and the larger the fat cell, the more unregulated the lipolysis. The elevation in free fatty acids, often measured in obese subjects, leads to lipid deposition in liver and muscle cells, leading ultimately to impaired insulin sensitivity.[19] In addition, the adipocytokine adiponectin is decreased in centrally obese subjects. Adiponectin may therefore be a protective hormone that is suppressed in obesity by an unknown mechanism.

Obesity produces an inflammatory state

Several adipocytokines are known to initiate a vascular inflammatory response and also to affect vessel functions such as smooth muscle cell proliferation and apoptosis. These effects appear to have clinical significance. For example, TNF-α is released by fat cells and is an independent predictor of cardiovascular events in older persons.[20]

Obesity is associated with impaired endothelial function that worsens as the BMI increases,[21] related to both inflammation and insulin resistance. Loss of vasodilator, anti-inflammatory, and anti-thrombotic actions of the endothelium in obesity contributes to the pathophysiology of clinical atherothrombotic events. Obese individuals exhibit endothelial vasomotor dysfunction in the coronary and peripheral circulations, suggesting reduced bioavailability of vascular endothelium-derived nitric oxide.[22] Since the severity of impaired vasomotor function relates to the future risk of adverse outcomes in patients with atherosclerosis, such impairment could partially explain the increased number of cardiovascular events in the obese. Fasting levels in humans of the soluble adhesion molecules intercellular cell adhesion molecule-1 and vascular cell adhesion molecule-1, known markers of endothelial dysfunction, increase according to BMI and the degree of insulin resistance.[23] Other studies have since shown that weight loss is not only correlated with decreased levels of such markers, but also with improved endothelial function, as measured by flow-mediated dilation of the brachial artery.[24,25]

Etiology of obesity

It is generally understood that the body's failure to maintain normal body fat stores results from a complex interaction between genetic and environmental influences. The inherited component of fat excess most likely operates through susceptibility genes, with increased risk for developing obesity in a favorable environment. Supporting this theory are migration studies, which show a marked increase in weight when a specific population changes environmental conditions.[26] Cultural factors have great impact on environment – affecting food availability, the composition of the diet, and degree of physical activity. In industrialized societies, obesity is more common among poor women, whereas in underdeveloped countries, wealthier women are more often obese. In both children and women, obesity correlates with the amount of time spent watching television.[27,28]

Energy homeostasis – what makes us fat versus lean?

Energy homeostasis is the physiologic regulatory system whereby energy availability of an organism tends to remain balanced and stable. It follows, then, that the problem of excess adiposity must lie in one or more defects in this system. Finding such defects is challenging, in light of substantial evidence that human energy homeostasis is regulated by both endocrine and neural components that affect both *energy intake* and *expenditure*. A complex and pliable system is necessary, since in comparison to the internal physiologic environment, the external human environment is highly variable. Body weight, or fat stores, reflect the energy available to an organism, which is crucial to its survival, yet can change drastically due to external factors. For example, a small change of 0.5% in negative energy balance over 30 years would result in a 15-kg weight loss. The body has a fuel-sensing mechanism, or 'fuel gage,' however, and such alterations in stable weight by food deprivation, or in the opposite direction with overfeeding, induce physiologic changes that resist perturbations and maintain homeostasis. When the fuel gage senses a decrease, the appetite increases and

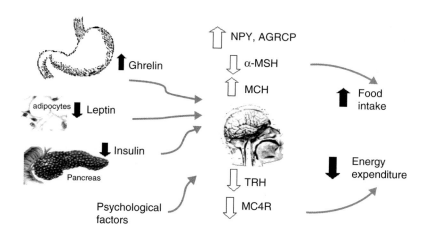

Figure 6.2
The complex control of appetite, as shown by some of the major components known to regulate food intake. Some of the mechanisms which increase appetite are linked to a decreased energy expenditure, promoting fat storage. NPY, neuropeptide Y; AGRP, Agouti-related peptide; α-MSH, melanocyte-stimulating hormone; MCH, melanin-concentrating hormone; TRH, thyrotropin-releasing hormone; MC4R, type 4 receptor for MSH.

energy expenditure decreases, and with excess fuel, the opposite occurs. Of the two compensatory mechanisms, however, the former is stronger and the latter frequently fails. Since survival is more acutely threatened by starvation than obesity, it is logical for the human body to be set up to store fat. This is the basis for the 'thrifty genotype' hypothesis, which holds that evolution has promoted inherited mutations over thousands of years that create a defective fuel-sensing mechanism, thus permitting obesity to develop in an environment where food is abundant and physical activity is low.[29,30]

Data from controlled human feeding studies indicate that becoming obese induces a 'set-point' change for weight maintenance. Metabolism shifts such that subjects who were once obese but lost weight must take in fewer calories to maintain the same weight as a subject who has been weight-stable.[31] Such metabolic changes have been attributed to the thrifty genotype being 'turned on.' It is during the period when the obese individual is actively losing weight that intervention – whether behavioral, biochemical or hormonal – is likely to be most effective.

Metabolism is therefore remarkably complex, and requires constant management by the central nervous system. The brain maintains energy balance largely by linking fuel-sensing to food-seeking behavior. The resulting behavior is stimulated by *appetite, pleasure,* and *reward.* Appetite is influenced by many signals that are integrated by the brain,

mostly within the hypothalamus (Fig. 6.2). These signals in turn are integrated with pathways associated with pleasure and reward, namely serotonergic, catecholaminergic, and opioid signaling pathways. Undoubtedly, sensory inputs such as taste and smell are also powerful mediators of pleasure pathways. The reader is directed to a detailed review of the neurohormonal control of appetite and feeding.[32]

Energy expenditure is one target of neurohormonal regulation of fat stores. Humans expend energy through physical activity, resting metabolic rate, and the thermic effect of food. A significant component of daily energy consumption is therefore fixed: basal metabolic rate accounts for about 70% of daily energy expenditure, while physical activity contributes only 5–10%. Although several lines of evidence suggest that obesity in humans may be in part determined by reduced energy expenditure, insights from research on the possible pathways have lagged behind those related to altered appetite.

Obesity results from both genes and environment

While we understand that in a modern industrialized human society, a state of excess energy storage in the form of fat is counterproductive for survival, it is still unclear exactly why we are becoming fatter. Genetic predisposition plays a role, although its importance is not clear. For example, obesity prevalence in the

US and Europe exists on a bell-shaped curve, with a small percentage of the population at the extremes of BMI. This phenomenon could either be due to genetic variation *or* to a normal distribution of environments across several regions. It *is* clear, however, that the rising prevalence of obesity worldwide is occurring too rapidly to be explained by a change in the gene pool.

Nevertheless, not all individuals living in convenient, food-abundant societies are obese. The variable susceptibility to obesity in response to environment must be modulated by specific genes. It has been estimated that 30–50% of variability in total body fat stores may be genetically determined. Familial obesity strongly supports this, where several members of the same family are obese. Likewise, identical twins have very similar BMIs whether reared together or apart, and their BMIs are much more strongly correlated than those of dizygotic twins. Inheritance is not Mendelian, however, and varies depending on factors such as family history of type 2 diabetes and central adiposity.

A growing body of evidence suggests that both the 'fuel gage' and resting metabolic rates are inherited. Markers of a defective fuel-sensing mechanism which permits obesity include central obesity and type 2 diabetes. The complex phenotype of type 2 diabetes, often seen across multiple generations in one family, probably includes a decreased resting energy expenditure and defective lipid oxidation, placing future progeny at risk for obesity as long as food is abundant.[33] Additional evidence for genetic variation in metabolism comes from data showing that African American women have a lower resting metabolic rate for a given body weight and lean body mass when compared with Caucasian women matched for age and BMI.[34]

The concept of purely genetic mutations leading to obesity followed the discovery of the adipocytokine leptin. Described in 1994, leptin plays a role in signaling the state of fat reserves to the brain, which then affects food intake and energy expenditure. Leptin rises in the fed state, and falls when the body is starving. Leptin deficiency, then, drives hunger, suppresses energy expenditure, and inhibits reproductive competence – all advantageous adaptations in the context of starvation. Although replacement of leptin promoted an impressive weight loss in leptin-

Table 6.2 Some obesity genes in humans

Mutated gene	Normal gene product	Mechanism of obesity
Lep (ob)	Leptin	Brain perceives starvation in absence of leptin
LepR (db)	Leptin receptor	Brain perceives starvation in absence of leptin
POMC	Pro-opiomelanocortin, a hypothalamic hormone	Reduced or absent production of the satiety signal melanocyte-stimulating hormone (MSH)
MC4R	Type 4 receptor for MSH	Satiety signal from MSH is not received in the brain
PC-1	Prohormone convertase-1, a processing enzyme	Defective production of a neuropeptide important for satiety
PPARγ	Peroxisome proliferator activated receptor	Unknown

deficient mice, leptin deficiency was found to be the cause of obesity in only a few human cases. The majority of obese persons, in fact, demonstrate high circulating leptin levels, and do not respond well to therapeutic recombinant leptin.[35,36] This defines a state of leptin resistance in common obesity, probably caused by alterations of the leptin receptor in combination with neurohormonal influences.

Genes may play a greater role in certain individuals with obesity. The identified genetic defects and syndromes in humans make up <1% of all obesity (Table 6.2).

Common obesity results from increased energy intake, decreased energy expenditure, or a combination of the two

When the environment promotes this combination, individuals with genetic susceptibility become obese. Declining physical activity, ingestion of foods high in fat and calories, and oversized food portions are driving the international trend of obesity. Apart from rare syndromes involving leptin, its receptor and the melanocortin system, the defects in the complex appetite control network that account for common obesity are not well understood. If a patient falls far from the average path for weight gain in their family or environment (see *Epidemiology of obesity* above), it is appropriate to consider treatable secondary causes, including endocrine disease.

Endocrine diseases are atypical causes of obesity

Hypothyroidism is a common condition, particularly among women, that is an uncommon cause of obesity. Hashimoto's thyroiditis is the most prevalent etiology. Decreased circulating thyroxine leads to decreased metabolic rate, and therefore may cause excess fat storage. An elevated screening plasma TSH (thyroid-stimulating hormone) level measured during the initial evaluation of the obese patient indicates a possible role of hypothyroidism, and requires treatment with levothyroxine.

Excess corticosteroid exposure, whether endogenous (Cushing's syndrome) or exogenous (therapeutic glucocorticoid use), often leads to excess adiposity, typically with a central distribution. Cushing's disease is the most common cause of Cushing's syndrome, and is caused by excess ACTH (adrenocorticotropic hormone) production by a pituitary corticotroph adenoma. True Cushing's syndrome is exceedingly rare, and clinical suspicion should only arise when a patient has a constellation of symptoms and signs, including obesity, hypertension, hirsutism, easy bruising, wide purple striae on the abdomen, and osteoporosis. Obesity itself can make the laboratory evaluation difficult, and referral to an endocrinologist for diagnosis is usually warranted.

Acromegaly is a rare and insidious condition that results from excess growth hormone secretion by a tumor, usually in the pituitary gland. The symptoms and signs relate to the growth of many tissues, such as skin, connective tissue, cartilage, bone, viscera, and many epithelial tissues. Patients with acromegaly are obese by BMI measurement, but generally have more lean body mass relative to fat mass. However, patients still become insulin-resistant and commonly develop hypertension, dyslipidemia and heart failure – all likely mediated in part by direct growth hormone effects. An elevated IGF-1 (insulin-like growth factor-1; somatomedin C) level in a patient with clinical excess growth hormone suggests acromegaly. The primary treatment is surgical resection.

Hypothalamic damage, caused by a tumor, trauma or inflammation, is associated with polyphagia and rapid weight gain. Dysfunction of the hypothalamus can lead to altered satiety, hunger, and energy expenditure – leading to varying degrees of obesity. Other evidence of hypothalamic damage, including diabetes insipidus, hypoadrenalism and/or hypogonadism, usually suggests the diagnosis, thus prompting magnetic resonance imaging of the brain.

Obesity across the female life cycle

The average woman gains body fat at predictable times during her life, with the most common time being near and after the menopause. During menopause, a woman's risk of CVD approaches that of men. Epidemiologic evidence suggests that the rise in CVD prevalence in postmenopausal women is related to weight gain, and possibly fat redistribution, that a large subset of women experience after menses cease. Weight gain is predictable during specific periods throughout a woman's lifetime. When obesity develops early, other health risks accrue, often making subsequent weight loss increasingly difficult. We have chosen to chronologically highlight some of the major conditions related to obesity that manifest during the female lifecycle.

Fetal undernourishment

The relation between fetal growth and obesity in later life is a complicated one. Several studies have shown that people who were heavy at birth or at 1 year of age tended to be slightly more obese as adults. Other studies indicate that small babies tend to have more abdominal fat as adults. More evidence is emerging, however, that undernourishment *in utero* predisposes to obesity later in life. Several studies have examined birth records of infant survivors of the Dutch Famine, which occurred in western Netherlands at the end of World War II. By age 50 years, the female survivors who had been exposed to famine in *early* gestation had a significantly higher BMI (7.4%) than nonexposed women.[37] This adds to evidence that hunger and low protein intake during pregnancy place offspring at risk for developing obesity in an environment where calorically dense foods are readily available. Such a phenomenon suggests *in utero* programming of the genotype, resulting in an energy-storing phenotype.

Pubescent weight gain

Obesity in adolescent girls is associated with earlier menarche.[38] Several studies have shown that girls who undergo menarche at a relatively young age tend to be more obese as adults, which reflects the common persistence of childhood obesity into adulthood.[39] Premature adrenarche, defined in girls as the appearance of pubic or axillary hair before age 8, usually occurs in overweight adolescents and may be a marker for future co-morbidity. These adolescents appear to be at higher risk for developing obesity, metabolic syndrome, and PCOS.

Polycystic ovarian syndrome (see also Chapter 27)

PCOS, also known as Stein–Leventhal syndrome, is a common syndrome, affecting 5–10% of women of reproductive age. Women with PCOS usually come to medical attention with either irregular menses, infertility or symptoms of hyperandrogenism, such as hirsutism. Approximately 50–60% of women with PCOS are obese, and most have insulin resistance.[40] While defects have been identified at many levels in the reproductive endocrine axis (hypothalamic, pituitary, gonad, adipocyte), many theories to explain the etiology of PCOS involve a role of hyperinsulinemia leading to overproduction or overaromatization of sex hormones in the ovary. This theory follows well with the clinical observation that both weight loss and insulin-sensitizing medications

reduce serum insulin levels and restore fertility in women with PCOS. Moreover, medications used to treat PCOS, including metformin and the thiazolidinediones, simultaneously improve insulin resistance and normalize ovulatory cycles. Weight loss as modest as 5–7% can decrease androgen levels and restore spontaneous ovulation in most patients with PCOS.

Metabolic syndrome

The metabolic syndrome, also known as syndrome X, is composed of several features, including abdominal adiposity, insulin resistance, hypertension, and dyslipidemia. The risk of CVD attributed to the metabolic syndrome appears to be especially high in women, and it is estimated that half of all cardiovascular events in women are related to the metabolic syndrome.[41] Although it affects approximately 20–30% of the middle-aged population, many features probably develop in the third decade. Increased BMI increases the risk of the metabolic syndrome markedly, as does physical inactivity.

Infertility

A woman's BMI at age 18 predicts menstrual irregularity. An 18-year-old woman with a BMI of 30 kg/m^2 is 2.5 times as likely to have primary ovulatory infertility than an 18-year-old woman with a BMI of 20 kg/m^2.[41] Furthermore, obesity in earlier fertile years, age 20–22, predicts a substantial incidence of obesity by the age of 35–37 years.[43] Neuropeptides likely play a role in obesity-related infertility. Leptin, for example, appears to act as a permissive factor during puberty, both centrally at the hypothalamus and peripherally at the ovary.[44] Resistance to leptin, a feature of common obesity, may therefore contribute to infertility.

Pregnancy

Pregnancy has been associated with excess weight gain and development of overweight.[45] Maternal obesity is a significant risk factor for developing gesta-

Table 6.3 Institute of Medicine (IOM) recommendations for weight gain during pregnancy

Pre-pregnancy BMI (kg/m²)	Recommended total gain (kg)
Low (BMI <19.8)*	12.5–18
Normal (BMI 19.8–26)	11.5–16
High (BMI >26–29)†	7–11.5

*The body mass index (BMI) ranges delineated by the IOM differ from the World Health Organization and National Institutes of Health guidelines.
†The recommended target gain for obese women (BMI >29 kg/m²) is at least 6.8 kg.
Adapted from reference 47.

tional diabetes mellitus, pre-eclampsia, eclampsia, puerperal infections, and thromboembolic complications. Obese women who become pregnant have higher maternal and fetal complications, including macrosomia, birth trauma, neural tube defects, antepartum stillbirth, cesarean delivery, and large-for-gestational-age infants.[46] Importantly, maternal obesity is an excellent predictor of childhood obesity.

Women who gain more than 16 kg during pregnancy are more likely to retain at least 6 kg postpartum. Excess weight gain above the recommended range (see Table 6.3)[47] and failure to lose weight after pregnancy are predictors of long-term obesity. Breast-feeding and aerobic exercise postpartum may be helpful to control long-term weight.[48]

Menopause

Most women gain weight during the menopause (see *Epidemiology of obesity*, above), while the risk for cardiovascular events rises. There is no evidence, however, that the estrogen withdrawal characteristic of menopause *directly* leads to weight gain. On the contrary, estrogen therapy during menopause does not prevent weight gain, and may even exacerbate it. It becomes important, then, to consider other *indirect* factors that may contribute to obesity during menopause. For example, secondary effects of decreased estrogen in menopause, such as depression, may lead to weight gain. Another example is smoking cessation, which is strongly encouraged to reduce CVD risk, and is associated with weight gain if not specifically addressed.[49,50] Of note, women tend to

gain more weight than men after smoking cessation.[51]

In a synergistic fashion with obesity, other distinct effects of estrogen withdrawal may lead to increased risk of CVD. Estrogen withdrawal may limit lipid oxidation, for example, which could lead to preferential deposition of fat in the abdomen, regardless of age and overall adiposity.[52] Moreover, central adiposity is one of several features of the metabolic syndrome commonly seen in the transition from pre- to post-menopause, including a shift toward a more atherogenic lipid profile and increased glucose and insulin levels.[53]

Weight gain in the elderly

As women age, they engage in less physical activity and their resting metabolic rate decreases due to the decrease in lean body mass from relative inactivity. In the past, women in developed countries gained weight steadily until age 60, when body weight began to decline; however, recent trends show that weight gain continues into the 70s. Intra-abdominal fat proportion also increases. Conditions associated with aging, including urinary incontinence and osteoarthritis, both predispose to and exacerbate weight gain. Urinary incontinence, for example, disproportionately affects women and may reduce their inclination to exercise. Furthermore, obesity can exacerbate urine leakage, further reducing motivation. Obesity doubles a woman's risk of osteoarthritis.[3] The inevitable limitation in physical mobility has clearly been shown to increase BMI. In addition, elderly women at higher BMIs are less likely to score well on a standardized physical performance test.[54] This creates a vicious circle, thus posing a substantial challenge to the treatment of obesity in the elderly.

Studies on the ramifications of weight loss in the elderly are inconclusive. However, weight loss in obese elderly women appears to reduce cardiovascular risk as well as improve well-being and independence, and should be advised. Of note, weight loss in this group is associated with a decrease in bone mineral density, and clinicians should be diligent in advising bone-protective strategies to all elderly women, with particular attention to those who want to lose weight.[55]

Treatment of obesity

Given the predictability of weight gain during a woman's lifetime, prevention of excess weight is clearly the best way to 'treat' the obesity epidemic. Effective strategies must simultaneously address the population as a whole as well as the individual. Public health plans span the realms of childhood education policy, the food industry, and access to health care. In regard to the individual, there is good evidence that careful lifestyle modification in Western society prevents weight gain, as shown in healthy, premenopausal women who control caloric intake.[9]

The evaluation and assessment of patients with overweight and obesity is thorough and appropriately time-consuming. There are several aspects of the patient's condition that are routinely covered at the initial visit (see Box 6.1). Patients are encouraged to bring family and friends, since some subpopulations seem to adopt different strategies for weight management, and maladaptive strategies can be 'passed down' from family members.[56] Goal-setting is an important feature of the initial and subsequent visits, since patients typically have inappropriate expectations for weight loss. The goal of treatment is a weight loss of 5–10% of initial body weight in 6 months at a rate of approximately 1–2 lbs per week. Further weight loss can be considered after a period of weight maintenance.

Obesity is a chronic disease. The high rate of recidivism has brought experts to the conclusion that obesity requires lifelong therapy.[57] A range of different treatment approaches exists to help the individual make major lifestyle changes, from basic nutrition education to behavioral modification and cognitive therapy. A typical multidisciplinary program provides at least 16 weekly group lifestyle/behavior modification sessions, followed by visits at regular intervals. The group sessions are usually conducted by a dietitian or psychologist.

The cornerstone of therapy is a diet where caloric intake is below energy expended. A balanced calorie deficit diet (BCDD) provides 1000–1200 kcal/day for women and 1200–1500 kcal/day for men. Although there is no evidence that a particular diet composition has an advantage over another in regard to weight loss, the authors have had positive results from prescribing a diet with the majority of calories from lean proteins and vegetables, with a balanced amount of complex carbohydrates in the form of fresh fruits and whole grains, and minimal simple sugars and fat.

Very low calorie diets (VLCD) provide approximately 250–800 kcal/day and can be used in certain circumstances for rapid improvement of sleep apnea, hyperglycemia, hypertension, and preoperative risk. This approach requires intensive medical monitoring as well as vitamin and mineral supplementation to meet recommended daily allowances. Many medically supervised weight management programs also use liquid meal replacements as well as the protein modified fast to provide VLCDs to their patients.[58] Patients on these diets should be monitored weekly by a team of physicians, dietitians and/or physician assistants. Nonetheless, patients should be informed that while VLCDs may promote greater weight loss than BCDDs initially, studies have shown that weight loss after 1 year is not significantly greater.[59]

Exercise is a crucial element of any weight reduction program. Not only does it promote weight loss by increasing energy expenditure, but it also improves mood and quality of life and decreases the size of visceral fat depots independent of weight loss. Overweight and obese men who achieve cardiorespiratory fitness have a lower all-cause and CVD mortality risk than normal weight sedentary men. This may extend to women as well. Metabolic parameters such as insulin, glucose, and lipid levels also improve with exercise alone. Exercise should be initiated slowly and increased gradually to a goal of moderate intensity exercise for at least 200 or more

---

Box 6.1 Initial assessment of obesity

- Body mass index and risk category
- Waist circumference
- Co-morbid medical illness
- Co-morbid psychiatric illness
- Contributing medications (e.g. steroids, insulin)
- Previous dieting history
- Readiness, motivation, ability to change
- Reason for seeking treatment
- Emotional support
- Financial considerations

Table 6.4 Anti-obesity medication actions

Drug	Mechanism
FDA-approved for short-term use	
Benzphetamine, phendimetrazine, phentermine, diethylpropion	↑ NE and DA release
Mazindol	↓ NE reuptake
FDA-approved for long-term use	
Sibutramine	↓ NE, 5-HT reuptake
Orlistat	Blocks intestinal lipases (not systemically absorbed)
Investigational agents*	
Bupropion	Enhances NE activity
Topiramate	Enhances GABA, blocks glutamate receptors
Zonisamide	Enhanced 5-HT, dopamine activity
Rimonabant	Blocks cannabinoid receptor

FDA, US Food and Drug Administration; NE, noradrenaline; DA, dopamine; 5-HT, serotonin; GABA, γ-aminobutyric acid.
*Not FDA-approved for the treatment of obesity as of April, 2004.

minutes/week, which has been shown to prevent weight regain in women.[60]

Patients with a BMI ≥30, or 27 kg/m^2 with significant co-morbidities (e.g. type 2 diabetes) should be considered for pharmacotherapy as an adjuvant to lifestyle modification. There are several available medications that have been shown to reduce weight (Table 6.4), and the authors have extensive experience with their use within a multidisciplinary weight loss program. They are classified as either anorectic agents or malabsorptive agents. Pharmacotherapeutic agents are discontinued if patients do not lose an accepted amount of weight, usually at least 4 lbs

per month. Future directions in obesity pharmacology include, among others, a cannabinoid antagonist, PYY (peptide YY) agonists, antagonists of gut peptides, and drugs that target leptin resistance.

Herbal and dietary supplements that claim to promote weight loss such as chitosan, chromium picolonate, conjugated linoleic acid, ephedra (prohibited by the Food and Drug Administration in 2003) and *Garcinia cambogia* are relatively unregulated with minimal proof of efficacy. Well-designed studies of efficacy and safety are warranted to investigate herbal supplements for weight loss, which would benefit both patients and providers.

Surgical treatment for obesity, or bariatric surgery, is an option for morbidly obese individuals who have failed medical therapies for weight loss. The time allotted for an individual to be deemed a medical treatment failure varies according to the presence of life-threatening co-morbidities, e.g. obstructive sleep apnea or uncontrolled hypertension. The National Institutes of Health has set forth guidelines for the selection of appropriate patients for surgery (Table 6.5).[5] There are several types of bariatric procedures, but the two approved by the NIH are the Roux-en-Y gastric bypass (RYGB) and the vertical-banded gastroplasty (VBG). In experienced institutions, the operative mortality risk for both procedures is <1%. Weight reduction has been quantified as percent of preoperative body weight in excess of ideal body weight (%EBW) that is lost after surgery. Surgical success is considered loss of 60% of EBW, or approximately 30% of preoperative weight.

The RYGB is both a 'restrictive' and 'malabsorptive' procedure. The upper stomach is completely closed off, thereby excluding more than 95% of the stomach, all of the duodenum, and 15–20 cm of the proximal jejunum from digestive continuity. Mean excess weight loss in RYGB patients typically ranges

Table 6.5 National Institutes of Health guide for selecting treatment based on body mass index (BMI)

			BMI (kg/m^2)		
	25–26.9	27–29.9	30–34.9	35–39.9	>40
Diet, physical activity and behavior therapy	✔	✔	✔	✔	✔
Pharmacotherapy		✔*	✔	✔	✔
Surgery				✔*	✔

*With co-morbidities.
Adapted from reference 5.

from 65% to 75%, with a small rate of recidivism 3–5 years after the procedure. Insulin resistance typically improves early on; up to 83% of patients with type 2 diabetes are normoglycemic within 2 years post-operatively.[61] The VBG achieves weight loss by restricting caloric intake. The stomach is partitioned close to the gastro-esophageal junction, creating a small-capacity upper gastric pouch with a small outlet. Large meals become impossible, or induce vomiting. Gastroplasty is not nearly as effective as RYGB, due in part to pouch expansion, and has a 15–20% rate of reoperation for either stomal outlet stenosis or severe gastro-esophageal reflux.

Although bariatric surgery is the most effective therapy for morbid obesity, there are many areas open for investigation. For example, preliminary investigations suggest that there is likely a hormonal component to weight loss induced by altering the route by which nutrients pass through the gut. However, it is unknown whether changes in certain peptides and appetite mediators are major determinants of postoperative weight loss, and whether physicians could use these markers to predict an individual's success after bariatric surgery. We therefore look forward to prospective data from the NIH program Longitudinal Assessment of Bariatric Surgery (LABS). Major efforts in the areas of epidemiology, basic and clinical research will hopefully reach the following goals: (1) better define the risks and benefits of bariatric surgery, including gender-specific outcomes, (2) form evidence-based recommendations for patient selection and management, and (3) elucidate the mechanisms by which surgery affects obesity-related co-morbid conditions, energy expenditure, nutrient partitioning, appetitive behaviors, and psychosocial factors.

Conclusion

While obesity is an epidemic in most industrialized nations in the twenty-first century, it is a powerful modifiable risk factor for CVD, particularly for women. Failure to halt the epidemic results from a combination of three factors: physiologic mechanisms which promote positive energy balance, the inherent challenge of behavior-dependent preventive strategies, and the lack of easily accessed and effective long-term therapy for obesity. An examination of the female life cycle reveals that weight gain during specific time periods is predictable and, importantly, obesity becomes more life-threatening as a woman ages. While it remains unclear whether estrogen withdrawal independently increases a woman's risk for cardiovascular events, obesity is one of several known factors, including dyslipidemia and central adiposity, which likely contribute to the postmenopausal increase in cardiovascular risk. While investigations into treatments of obesity continue, preventive measures should be instituted at any and all stages of a woman's lifetime.

References

1. Hubert HB. The importance of obesity in the development of coronary risk factors and disease: the epidemiological evidence. *Annu Rev Public Health* 1986; **7**:493–502.
2. Manson JE, Colditz GA, Sampfer MJ, et al. A prospective study of obesity and risk of coronary heart disease in women. *N Engl J Med* 1990; **322**:882–9.
3. Must A, Spadano J, Coakley EH. The disease burden associated with overweight and obesity. *JAMA* 1999; **282**:1523–9.
4. Farooqi IS, Matarese G, Lord GM, et al. Beneficial effects of leptin on obesity, T-cell hyporesponsiveness, and neuroendocrine/metabolic dysfunction of human congenital leptin deficiency. *J Clin Invest* 2002; **100**:1093–103.
5. NHLBI Obesity Education Initiative Expert Panel. The NHLBI Practical Guide to Identification, Evaluation and Treatment of Overweight and Obesity in Adults. NIH Pub. No. 00-4084, October, 2000.
6. Wang J, Thornton J, Russell M, Burastero S, Heymsfield S, Pierson R. Asians have lower body mass index but higher percent body fat than do whites: comparisons of anthropometric measurements. *Am J Clin Nutr* 1994; **60**:23–8.

7. Flegal KM, Carroll MD, Ogden CL, et al. Prevalence and trends in obesity among US adults, 1999–2000. *JAMA* 2002; **288**:1723–7.

8. Bergstrom A, Pisani P, Tenet V, et al. Overweight as an avoidable cause of cancer in Europe. *Int J Cancer* 2001; **91**:421–30.

9. Simkin-Silverman L, Wing RR, Boraz MA, et al. Maintenance of cardiovascular risk factor changes among middle-aged women in a lifestyle intervention trial. *Woman's Health* 1998; **4**:255–71.

10. Allison DB, Fontaine KR, Manson JE. Annual deaths attributable to obesity in the Unites States. *JAMA* 1999; **282**:1530–8.

11. Van Itallie TB. Health implications of overweight and obesity in the United States. *Ann Intern Med* 1985; **103**:983–8.

12. Colditz GA, Willett WC, Rotnitzky A, Manson JE. Weight gain as a risk factor for clinical diabetes mellitus. *Ann Intern Med* 1995; **122**:481–6.

13. Grundy SM. Obesity, metabolic syndrome and coronary atherosclerosis. *Circulation* 2002; **5**:2696–8.

14. Eckel RH, Krauss RM, for the AHA Nutrition Committee. American Heart Association call to action: obesity as a major risk factor for coronary heart disease. *Circulation* 1998; **97**:2099–100.

15. Youn B-S, Yu K-Y, Park HJ, et al. Plasma resistin concentrations measured by enzyme-linked immunosorbent assay using a newly developed monoclonal antibody are elevated in individuals with type 2 diabetes mellitus. *J Clin Endocrinol Metab* 2004; **89**:150–6.

16. Esposito K, Pontillo A, Di Palo C, et al. Effect of weight loss and lifestyle changes on vascular inflammatory markers in obese women. A randomized trial. *JAMA* 2003; **289**:1799–804.

17. Monzillo LU, Hamdy O, Horton E, et al. Effect of lifestyle modification on adipokine levels in obese subjects with insulin resistance. *Obes Res* 2003; **11**: 1048–54.

18. Kenchaiah S, Evans JC, Levy D, et al. Obesity and the risk of heart failure. *N Engl J Med* 2002; **347**:305–13.

19. Boden G, Lebed B, Schatz M, et al. Effects of acute changes of plasma free fatty acids on intramyocellular fat content and insulin resistance in healthy subjects. *Diabetes* 2001; **50**:1612–17.

20. Cesari M, Penninx BW, Newman AB, et al. Inflammatory markers and onset of cardiovascular events: results from the Health ABC study. *Circulation* 2003; **108**:2317–22.

21. Al Suwaidi J, Higano ST, Holmes DR Jr, et al. Obesity is independently associated with coronary endothelial dysfunction in patients with normal or mildly diseased coronary arteries. *J Am Coll Cardiol* 2001; **37**:1523–8.

22. Steinberg HO, Chaker H, Learning R, Johnson A, Brechtel G, Baron AD. Obesity/insulin resistance is associated with endothelial dysfunction: implications for the syndrome of insulin resistance. *J Clin Invest* 1996; **97**:2601–10.

23. Leinonen E, Hurt-Camejo E, Wiklund O, Hulten LM, Hiukka A, Taskinen MR. Insulin resistance and adiposity correlate with acute-phase reaction and soluble cell adhesion molecules in type 2 diabetes. *Atherosclerosis* 2003; **166**:387–94.

24. Hambdy O, Ledbury S, Mullooly C, et al. Lifestyle modification improves endothelial dysfunction in obese subjects with the insulin resistance syndrome. *Diabetes Care* 2003; **26**:2119–25.

25. Gokce N, Vita JA, McDonnell M, et al. Effect of medical and surgical weight loss on endothelial vasomotor function in obese patients. *Am J Cardiol* 2005; **95**:266–8.

26. WHO. Monica Project: genographical variation in the major risk factors of coronary heart disease in men and women aged 34–64 years. *World Health Stat Q* 1998; **41**:115–40.

27. Gortmaker SL, Must A, Sobol AM, et al. Television viewing as a cause of increasing obesity among children in the United States. *Arch Pediatr Adolesc Med* 1996; **150**:356–62.

28. Hu FB, Li T, Colditz G, Willett W, Manson J. Television watching and other sedentary behaviors in relation to risk of obesity and type 2 diabetes mellitus in women. *JAMA* 2003; **289**:1785–91.

29. Hales CN, Barker DJ. Type 2 (non-insulin-dependent) diabetes mellitus: the thrifty phenotype hypothesis. *Diabetologia* 1992; **35**:595–601.

30. Neel JV. The 'thrifty genotype' in 1998. *Nutr Rev* 1999; **57**:S2–9.

31. Hirsch J, Hudgins LC, Leibel RL, Rosenbaum M. Diet composition and energy balance in humans. *Am J Clin Nutr* 1998; **67** (3 Suppl):551S–5S.

32. Flier JS. Obesity wars: molecular progress confronts an expanding epidemic. *Cell* 2004; **116**:337–50.

33. De Pergola G, Pannacciulli N, Minenna A, Cannito F, Giorgino R. Fuel metabolism in adult individuals with a wide range of body mass index: effect of a family history of type 2 diabetes. *Diabetes Nutr Metab* 2003; **16**:41–7.

34. St Onge MP, Jones A, Heymsfield S, Albu J. Body weight and fat-free mass do not explain resting metabolic rate differences between African-American and Caucasian women. *Obes Res* 2003; **11**(Suppl): A63.

35. Considine RV, Sinha MK, Heiman ML, et al. Serum immunoreactive-leptin concentraion in normal weight and obese humans. *N Engl J Med* 1996; **334**:292–5.

36. Heymsfield SB, Greenberg AS, Fujioka K, et al. Recombinant leptin for weight loss in obese and lean adults: a randomized, controlled, dose-escalation trial. *JAMA* 1999; **282**:1568–75.

37. Ravelli ACJ, van Der Meulen JH, Osmond C, Barker DJP, Bleker OP. Obesity at the age of 50y in men and women exposed to famine prenatally. *Am J Clin Nutr* 1999; **70**:811–16.

38. Wattingney WA, Srimvasan SR, Chen W, et al. Secular trend of earlier onset of menarch with increasing obesity in black and white girls. The Bogalusa Heart Study. *Ethn Dis* 1999; **9**:181–9.

39. Freedman DS, Khan LK, Serdula MK, Dietz WH, Srinivasan SR, Berenson GS. The relation of menarcheal age to obesity in childhood and adulthood: the Bogalusa heart study. *BMC Pediatr* 2003; **3**:3.

40. Hoeger K. Obesity and weight loss in polycystic ovary syndrome. *Obstet Gynecol Clin North Am* 2001; **28**:85–97.

41. Rich-Edwards JW, Goldman MB, Willett WC, et al. Adolescent body mass index and infertility caused by ovulatory disorder. *Am J Obstet Gynecol* 1994; **17**:171–7.

42. McTigue KM, Garret JM, Popkin BM. The natural history of the development of obesity in a cohort of young US adults between 1981 and 1998. *Ann Intern Med* 2002; **136**:201–9.

43. Mijailovic M, Mijailovic V, Micic D. Childhood onset of obesity: does an obese child become an obese adult? *J Pediatr Endocrinol Metab* 2001; **14**(Suppl 5):1335-8.

44. Wilson PW, Kannel WB, Silbershatz H, D'Agostino RB. Clustering of metabolic factors and coronary heart disease. *Arch Intern Med* 1999; **159**:1104–9.

45. Gunderson EP, Murtaugh MA, Lewis CE, Quesenberry CP, West DS, Sidney S. Excess gains in weight and waist circumference associated with childbearing: the coronary artery risk development in young adults study (CARDIA). *Int J Obes Relat Metab Disord* 2004; **28**:525–35.

46. Cedergren MI. Maternal morbid obesity and the risk of adverse pregnancy outcome. *Obestet Gynecol* 2004; **103**:219–24.

47. Institute of Medicine Subcommittee on Nutritional Status and Weight Gain During Pregnancy. *Nutrition During Pregnancy: Part I: Weight Gain, Part II: Nutrient Supplements.* Washington, DC: National Academy Press, 1990: 70–2.

48. Rooney BL, Schauberger CW. Excess pregnancy weight gain and long-term obesity: one decade later. *Obstet Gynecol* 2002; **100**:245–52.

49. Flegal KM, Troiano RP, Pamuk ER, Kuczmarski RJ, Campbell SM. The influence of smoking cessation on the prevalence of overweight in the United States. *N Engl J Med* 1995; **333**:1165–70.

50. Janzon F, Hedblad B, Bergland G, Engstrom G. Changes in blood pressure and body weight following smoking cessation in women. *J Intern Med* 2004; **255**:266–72.

51. Fiore MC, Novotny TE, Pierce JP, Hatziandreu EJ, Patel KM, Davis RM. Trends in cigarette smoking in the United States: the changing influence of gender and race. *JAMA* 1989; **261**:49–55.

52. Lwin R, Oster R, Darnell B, Foster J, Azziz R, Gower B. The effect of oral estrogen on postprandial lipid oxidation, fat mass and lean body mass in postmenopausal women. *Obes Res* 2003; **11** (Suppl):A50.

53. Poehlman ET, Toth MJ, Gardner AW. Changes in energy balance and body composition at menopause: a controlled longitudinal study. *Ann Intern Med* 1995; **123**:673–5.

54. Apovian CM, Frey CM, Wood GC, Rogers JZ, Still CD, Jensen GL. Body mass index and physical function in older women. *Obes Res* 2002; **10**:740–7.

55. Knoke JD, Barrett-Connor E. Weight loss: a determinant of hip-bone loss in older men and women: the Rancho Bernardo study. *Am J Epidemiol* 2003; **158**:1132–8.

56. Breitkopf CR, Berenson AB. Correlates of weight loss behaviors among low-income African American, Caucasian, and Latina women. *Obstet Gynecol* 2004; **103**:231–9.

57. Crawford D. Population strategies to prevent obesity. *BMJ* 2002; **325**:728–9.

58. Palgi A, Read JL, Greenberg I, Hoefer MA, Bistrian BR, Blackburn GL. Multidisciplinary treatment of obesity with a protein-sparing modified fast: results in 668 outpatients. *Am J Public Health* 1985; **75**:1190–4.

59. Saris WHM. Very-low-calorie-diets and sustained weight loss. *Obes Res* 2001; **9** (Suppl):295S-301S.

60. Jakicic JM, Winters C, Lang W, Wing RR. Effects of intermittent exercise and use of home exercise equipment on adherence of weight loss and fitness in overweight women: a randomized trial. *JAMA* 1999; **282**:1554–60.

61. Pories WJ, Swanson MS, MacDonald KG, et al. Who would have thought it? An operation proves to be the most effective therapy for adult-onset diabetes mellitus. *Ann Surg* 1995; **222**:339–50.

7

Other risk interventions: exercise

Shari S. Bassuk and JoAnn E. Manson

Introduction

Researchers generally agree that physical activity provides cardiovascular benefits, although the amount or 'dose' (a function of intensity, frequency, and duration) of activity required for optimal health continues to be debated. A 1990 meta-analysis of 27 cohort studies in mostly male populations concluded that physically active individuals have about half the coronary heart disease (CHD) risk of those who are sedentary,[1] and studies conducted within the last decade also indicate that physically active women experience lower CHD rates than their inactive counterparts. Physical activity may slow the initiation and progression of atherosclerotic disease via favorable effects on body weight, blood pressure, insulin sensitivity and glycemic control, lipid profile, fibrinolysis, endothelial function, and inflammatory defense systems. This chapter reviews recent observational and clinical trial data on the role of physical activity in the prevention of overt and subclinical vascular disease. Dose–response issues and implications for public health practice are considered.

The long-standing belief that physical activity must be vigorous in order to be salutary has been overturned in the last decade by epidemiologic studies showing otherwise. Earlier guidelines advocating vigorous exercise for at least 20 minutes three times per week have been supplemented by a well-publicized 1995 recommendation by the Centers for Disease Control (CDC) and the American College of Sports Medicine (ACSM) that adults engage in 30 minutes of moderate-intensity physical activity on most, and preferably all, days of the week.[2] This has also been the standard endorsed by the US Surgeon General since 1996.[3] In 2002, the Institute of

Medicine (IOM) concurred that moderately intense activity is beneficial, but it doubled the daily goal from 30 to 60 minutes, concluding that one half-hour is not sufficient to maintain a healthy weight nor to achieve maximal health benefits.[4] The IOM guideline was issued in a report focused on setting forth diet and nutrition goals for the US public.

Although the IOM has received praise for highlighting physical activity as an essential part of a healthy lifestyle, its recommendation has also been criticized for failing to balance the issue of efficacy with that of feasibility, both of which are essential to achieve a public health goal. Data from the National Health Interview Survey indicate that 73% of US women and 66% of men fail to meet the 30-minute

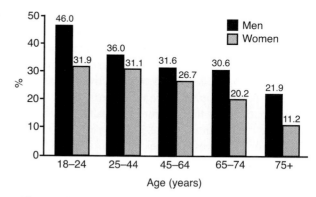

Figure 7.1
Percent of US adults engaging in regular leisure-time physical activity, by gender and age. (Regular activity = light-to-moderate activity five times or more per week for 30 minutes each time, or vigorous activity three times or more per week for 20 minutes or more each time.) Data from reference 5.

guideline; and 41% of women and 35% of men engage in no leisure-time physical activity at all (Fig. 7.1).[5] Setting 'the bar' even higher, to 60 minutes, may erode motivation that the American public, already largely unable to fulfill less stringent goals, might muster to boost its activity level. Based on this fact and on our review of available scientific data, we, along with many researchers and policy-makers, believe that the public health message should continue to be that moderately intense exercise for one half-hour per day confers significant and measurable cardiovascular benefits. Indeed, physical activity guidelines issued in 2003 by the American Heart Association (AHA) and endorsed by the ACSM reaffirm the 30-minute goal for the prevention of cardiovascular disease (CVD),[6] as do the AHA's 2004 CVD prevention guidelines specifically targeted toward women.[7] This is not to deny, however, that a dose–response relationship between physical activity and cardiovascular outcomes exists; in populations with low baseline activity levels, another half-hour of exercise per day would, on average, be expected to confer additional protection against CVD beyond that of the initial 30 minutes.[8]

Clinical cardiovascular disease

Coronary heart disease

Observational epidemiologic studies provide strong empirical support for the prescription of 30 minutes per day of moderate-intensity activity. Among 73 743 postmenopausal women aged 50–79 years participating in the Women's Health Initiative, walking briskly for at least 2.5 hours per week (i.e. a half-hour five times per week) was associated with a 30% reduction in cardiovascular events over 3.2 years of follow-up.[9] After adjustment for total exercise energy expenditure, brisk walking and more vigorous exercise were associated with similar risk reductions in cardiovascular events, and the results did not vary substantially according to race, age, or baseline body mass index (BMI) (Fig. 7.2).

The cardiovascular benefits of walking, the most common leisure activity among US adults, have also been demonstrated in other studies of middle-aged

and older women. In the Nurses' Health Study, an 8-year follow-up of 72 488 healthy female nurses aged 40–65 years, 3 hours of brisk walking per week had the same protective effect as 1.5 hours of vigorous exercise per week.[10] Women engaging in either form of exercise had a 30–40% lower rate of myocardial infarction than sedentary women. In the Women's Health Study, which followed 39 372 healthy middle-aged female health professionals for 7 years, walking at least 1 hour per week was associated with a 50% reduction in CHD risk in individuals reporting no vigorous physical activity.[11] Among 1564 middle-aged University of Pennsylvania alumni followed for 30 years, walking ten or more blocks per day as compared with walking less than four blocks per day was associated with a 33% reduction in CVD incidence.[12] In the Study of Osteoporotic Fractures, a 10-year follow-up of 9704 community-dwelling white women aged 65 years or older, participants with weekly walking energy expenditures averaging 300 kilocalories (kcal) or more (i.e. about ≥1 hour of walking per week) experienced an approximate 34% reduction in CVD mortality as compared with those with weekly walking energy expenditures below 70 kcal.[13] Among 1645 women and men aged 65 and older in a large health maintenance organization, walking more than 4 hours per week, as compared with walking less than 1 hour per week, significantly reduced the risk of hospitalization for cardiovascular reasons.[14]

Cardiovascular benefits of walking have been observed in male populations as well, albeit somewhat less strongly, perhaps due to generally higher physical activity levels for men as compared with women. Nevertheless, in the Health Professionals Follow-up Study, a 12-year follow-up of 44 452 male health professionals aged 40–75 years, a half-hour per day or more of brisk walking was associated with an 18% reduction in CHD incidence.[15] In the Honolulu Heart Program, men aged 71–93 years who walked 1.5 miles per day experienced half the risk of CHD of those who walked less than 0.25 mile per day.[16] In the Zutphen Elderly Study, men aged 64–84 years who walked or cycled at least three times per week for 20 minutes experienced a 31% reduction in CHD mortality over a 10-year follow-up period, compared with their counterparts who did not meet this physical activity

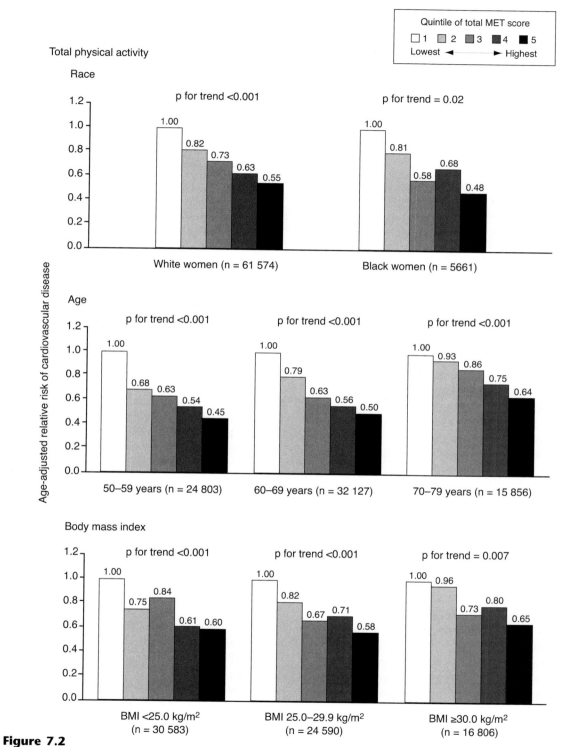

Figure 7.2
Age-adjusted relative risks of cardiovascular disease according to quintile of total metabolic equivalent (MET) score in subgroups defined by race, age, and body mass index (BMI). The reference category is the lowest quintile of MET score. Reproduced from reference 9 with permission. Copyright © 2002, Massachusetts Medical Society.

criterion.[17] Studies in men suggest that vigorous exercise is associated with even greater reductions in the risk of CVD than is moderate-intensity exercise.[15,17–19]

Although these studies did not examine physical activity patterns across the lifespan, other investigations suggest that adopting a physically active lifestyle even in late adulthood can lower cardiovascular risk. For example, the British Regional Heart Study, which examined changes in physical activity over 14 years among 5934 men aged 40–59 years at baseline, found that men who took up even light activity in later life experienced a 34% reduction in cardiovascular mortality over the subsequent 4 years as compared with those who remained inactive.[20] Similarly, the Study of Osteoporotic Fractures, which assessed physical activity changes over 6 years among 7553 women aged 65 years and older at baseline, reported that women who increased their physical activity level were 36% less likely to die of cardiovascular causes during the subsequent 7 years than were women who stayed sedentary.[13] Nevertheless, both studies also indicate that exercise must be current and habitual to confer cardiovascular protection; men and women who became inactive in later life had a similar risk of cardiovascular death to those who had remained inactive over the course of follow-up.

Bouts of activity lasting as little as 10 minutes have been shown to improve the cardiovascular risk profile of otherwise sedentary individuals.[21,22] Only one prospective study has examined the relationship between short bouts of exercise and CVD itself. In a 5-year follow-up of 7307 middle-aged and elderly male Harvard alumni, exercise sessions lasting 15 minutes, 30 minutes, or 45 minutes all offered equal protection against CVD after adjustment for total energy expenditure.[23] To date, there are no comparable studies of this issue in female populations. However, it is not unreasonable to speculate that comparable findings would be observed among similarly aged women. From a public health perspective, this knowledge may help motivate busy individuals to view exercise as a manageable part of their daily routine rather than as a time-consuming activity to be reserved for rare occasions.

Although many epidemiologic studies of physical activity have focused on aerobic exercise, resistance exercise may also be important in reducing CHD

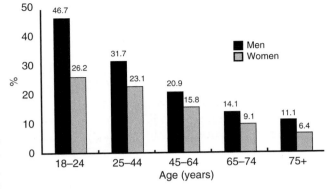

Figure 7.3
Percent of US adults engaging in any strengthening activities, by gender and age. (Strengthening activities = leisure-time physical activities specifically designed to strengthen muscles.) Data from reference 5.

incidence. In the Health Professionals Follow-up Study, men who trained with weights for at least 30 minutes per week were 23% less likely to develop CHD over an 8-year follow-up period than men who did not train with weights.[15] Aerobic and resistance exercise also confer noncardiovascular benefits, most notably improved bone density and the preservation of musculoskeletal function,[3] which may be particularly important for women, who are more susceptible to osteoporotic fractures than are men. For these reasons, it is of concern that only 16% of US women aged 45–64 and <10% of women aged 65 or older report ever engaging in strengthening activities (Fig. 7.3).[5]

The above studies, which relied on self-reported physical activity patterns as the predictor variable, offer direct support for current public health guidelines for CVD prevention, which target physical activity, a behavior, rather than physical fitness, an attained physiologic state. However, cardiorespiratory fitness as assessed by maximal treadmill exercise test has also been shown to correlate inversely with cardiovascular mortality in women[24] and men[25–27] without symptoms of CHD. In a 20-year follow-up of 2994 women aged 30–80 years in the Lipid Research Clinics Study, the risk of cardiovascular mortality and of all-cause mortality decreased by 17% and 11%, respectively, for every metabolic equivalent (MET) increment in exercise capacity, after adjustment for multiple cardiovascular risk factors.[24] In an 8-year follow-up of 5721 women aged 35 and older (the St James Women Take Heart Study), all-cause mortality declined by 17% for each 1-MET increase in exercise capacity, after adjustment for coronary risk profile;[28] cardiovascular endpoints were not reported, however.

Although regular aerobic physical activity is known to improve physical fitness, the degree to which being inactive and being unfit represent distinct cardiovascular risk factors remains uncertain.[29] The amount and intensity of exercise needed to reduce one's risk of developing CHD likely depends on one's age and fitness level. This observation may account for inconsistencies in epidemiologic findings regarding the level of exercise intensity necessary for coronary risk reduction. In general, studies that have shown that moderate-intensity activity decreases CHD incidence or mortality have been conducted in women or older men, who tend to be less fit, whereas studies that have reported that vigorous activity is required to reduce cardiovascular risk have been conducted in young or middle-aged men, who tend to be more fit.[18,19]

On a related note, distinguishing between absolute versus relative intensity of exercise may be important when assessing dose–response relationships between physical activity and CHD and formulating activity guidelines. Among older men in the Harvard Alumni Study, there was a strong inverse relation between relative intensity of activity – i.e. an individual's perceived level of exertion – and risk of CHD, regardless of whether participants exercised enough to meet current activity guidelines.[30] While physical activity guidelines are most often framed in terms of absolute intensities (e.g. moderate-intensity activities are defined as those requiring 3 to <6 METs, and vigorous activities as those requiring ≥6 METs), there is a growing recognition that such guidelines should take into account perceived intensity of exercise as well.[6,31]

Stroke

Evidence from prospective studies indicates that physical activity is associated with a reduced risk of stroke, although data are less extensive and less consistent than for CHD. A meta-analysis of 18 cohort studies with follow-up periods ranging from 2 to 32 years found that moderately active and highly active persons were 17% and 25% less likely, respectively, to have a stroke or die of stroke-related causes than were persons with low activity.[32] On the basis of six ischemic and three hemorrhagic stroke studies in the meta-analysis, physical activity appears to offer protection against both types of stroke. Compared with low-activity individuals, moderately active persons had a 9% and 15% lower risk of incident ischemic stroke and hemorrhagic stroke, respectively; the corresponding figures for highly active persons were 21% and 34%.[32] Unfortunately, variation in the measurement and classification of physical activity in the original studies precluded a clear definition for the 'high', 'moderate', and 'low' activity categories. Moreover, the meta-analysis did not provide gender-specific results, although eight of the 18 studies included a substantial number of women. In the Nurses' Health Study, which followed 72 488 middle-aged women for 8 years, there was a strong inverse gradient of risk with volume of physical activity;[33] this was primarily due to the relation with ischemic stroke as opposed to hemorrhagic stroke, with women in the highest activity category experiencing only half the risk of ischemic stroke as the least active respondents after adjustment for BMI and other vascular risk factors. On the other hand, in the Physicians' Health Study, an 11-year follow-up of 21 823 men aged 40–84 years, a linear dose–response effect was observed for hemorrhagic but not ischemic stroke incidence.[34] However, the Aerobics Center Longitudinal Study, which followed 16 878 men aged 40–87 for 10 years, found a strong association between cardiorespiratory fitness level and total stroke mortality, which persisted after adjustment for conventional risk factors. Compared with men in the bottom quintile of fitness, individuals in the top two quintiles of fitness and those in the middle two quintiles experienced similar reductions in stroke mortality – 68% and 63%, respectively.[35] Data on stroke subtypes were not collected. A report published after completion of the meta-analysis showed a strong inverse relationship between cardiorespiratory fitness and the incidence of total stroke and ischemic stroke among 2011 men aged 42–60 followed for 11 years in the Kuopio Ischemic Heart Disease Risk Factor Study.[36]

Coronary and peripheral artery atherosclerosis

There is some epidemiologic evidence to suggest that physical activity can also slow the progression of asymptomatic coronary and peripheral artery disease. Relationships between regular physical activity and measures of coronary and peripheral arteriosclerosis have been observed in population-based cross-sectional studies, albeit inconsistently. In a sample of 2274 men and women aged 65 years and older participating in the Cardiovascular Health Study,[37] investigators examined the association between exercise intensity and indicators of subclinical cardiovascular disease, including ankle-brachial blood pressure index (ABI) and B-mode ultrasound carotid intima-media thickness (IMT). Low ABI is a marker of leg atherosclerosis, and high IMT indicates carotid atherosclerosis. Exercise intensity, classified as high, moderate, or low according to the most vigorous of 15 leisure-time activities performed during the prior 2 weeks, exhibited a dose–response relationship in the expected direction with ABI but not with IMT. After adjustment for total leisure-time energy expenditure, an inverse relationship between exercise intensity and >50% carotid stenosis also emerged, but only in women. Among respondents reporting moderate-intensity exercise, energy expenditure was unrelated to either ABI or carotid IMT. Work-related physical activity was not examined in this cohort of elderly individuals, most of whom were retired. However, in a companion study of 14 430 men and women aged 45–64 years (the Atherosclerosis Risk In Communities (ARIC) study), work-related physical activity was associated with lower IMT in both genders even though leisure-time activity was not.[38] Nevertheless, a study of 630 male and female US Army personnel aged 39–45 years failed to find a relationship between work-related, sports-related, or leisure-time physical activity and the extent of calcified coronary atherosclerosis measured by electron-beam computed tomography.[39]

There are limited prospective data on the relationship between physical activity and asymptomatic peripheral artery disease or coronary atherosclerosis in general populations. However, four population-based cohort studies – three in Scandinavia and one in the United States – support the hypothesis that physical activity retards the initiation or progression of atherosclerosis.

In the Tromso Study, a 15-year follow-up of 3128 middle-aged Norwegians, leisure-time physical activity was classified as a three-level ordinal variable, with levels roughly corresponding to no activity, moderate-intensity activity for at least 4 hours per week, and vigorous activity for at least 2 hours per week.[40] Intensity of physical activity was inversely related to carotid IMT in men but not women. The investigators offered several plausible explanations for the apparent effect modification by gender. First, the activity level among women, who as a group were more sedentary than the men, may have been too low to show a benefit. Second, because women may have been more likely than men to engage in housekeeping or caregiving activities requiring physical exertion, leisure-time activity may be less indicative of overall activity in women than in men. Lastly, the benefit of exercise may occur via improvements in physiologic parameters in which women have a comparative advantage over men, such as blood pressure or high-density lipoprotein (HDL) cholesterol level.

Using a physical activity classification scheme similar to that of the Tromso investigators, Swedish researchers examined whether intensity of activity was associated with asymptomatic leg atherosclerosis in a cohort of 363 male residents of Malmo who were followed for 13 years (the 'Men Born in 1914 Study').[41] After adjustment for potential confounders, intensity of physical activity at age 55 and increases in activity intensity between age 55 and 68 were predictive of higher ABI at age 68, suggesting that exercise may prevent atherosclerotic lesions even in those who become active relatively late in life.

Among 854 middle-aged Finnish men in the Kuopio Ischemic Heart Disease Risk Factor Study, a high level of cardiorespiratory fitness was predictive of a significant slowing in the progression of early atherosclerosis.[42] Maximal oxygen uptake during baseline exercise testing exhibited strong, inverse, and graded associations with 4-year increases in maximal IMT, mean IMT, plaque height, and surface roughness. No association between self-reported physical activity (total energy expenditure, duration, frequency, or mean intensity level) and 4-year changes in these carotid parameters was detected, however.

The Los Angeles Atherosclerosis Study examined the relationship between leisure-time physical activity and early atherosclerotic progression in 500 middle-aged male and female employees of a utility company.[43] Physical activity, an ordinal three-level variable based both on intensity of activity and number of times per week the activity was performed, was strongly and inversely related to changes in mean carotid IMT over a 3-year period. The magnitude of the association was similar for both genders.

When interpreting the inverse associations between physical activity and clinical or subclinical atherosclerotic disease reported in observational studies, both the possibility that unmeasured or unknown factors may influence the selection and participation of study participants (selection bias) and the possibility that unmeasured or unknown third factors account for the association (confounding) must be considered. However, the consistency of the results across studies supports a causal association, as does the biologic plausibility due to the known salutary effects of increased physical activity on the coronary risk factor profile.

Cardioprotective mechanisms

Experimental as well as observational data indicate that habitual physical activity has beneficial effects on both atherosclerotic and thrombotic risk factors. These effects include reducing adiposity, blood pressure, diabetes, dyslipidemia, and inflammation, and enhancing insulin sensitivity, glycemic control, fibrinolysis, and endothelial function. Whether physical activity confers cardioprotection primarily via anti-atherosclerotic or anti-thrombotic pathways is not known.

Body weight (see also Chapter 6)

The primary basis for the IOM's aforementioned recommendation of 1 hour of moderate-intensity physical activity per day is that lesser amounts of activity have not been consistently shown to ensure weight maintenance within the healthy BMI range of

$18.5–25.0 \ kg/m^2$ or to promote weight loss in the absence of curtailing food intake. Exercising for weight control may be particularly salient for women, as data from the National Health and Nutrition Examination Surveys (NHANES) indicate that, during the past three decades, caloric intakes of US women increased by a much higher percentage than did those of men. From 1971 to 2000, the daily caloric intake of the average woman rose 22%, from 1542 to 1877 kcal, while the average man increased his intake by 7%, from 2450 to 2618 kcal.[44] During this period, the prevalence of obesity soared. In the NHANES survey of 1960–62, an estimated 31.6% of adults were overweight (BMI $25–29.9 \ kg/m^2$) and 13.4% were obese (BMI $\geq30 \ kg/m^2$). By the NHANES survey of 1999–2000, the proportion of overweight adults had increased only slightly, to 34.0%, while the proportion of obese adults more than doubled, to 30.5%.[45,46] An estimated 33.4% of US women and 27.5% of men are obese.

Several lines of evidence suggest that an hour of activity per day may indeed be necessary to control weight without also practicing dietary restraint. In an IOM-compiled database of 407 healthy stable-weight adults whose energy expenditures had been estimated with the doubly-labeled water method, considered the gold standard of energy expenditure measurement, persons with a BMI between 18.5 and $25.0 \ kg/m^2$ expended a daily energy equivalent of at least 1 hour of moderate activity – or, as the IOM phrased it, walking at least 4.4 miles per day at the rate of 2–4 miles per hour.[4] Moreover, descriptive studies of formerly obese individuals suggest that 80 minutes per day of moderately intense activity or 35 minutes per day of vigorous activity is required for long-term weight loss maintenance.[47–49] In the National Weight Control Registry, a sample of 629 women and 155 men who lost an average of 30 kg and maintained a minimum weight loss of 13.6 kg for 5 years, the self-reported median weekly energy expenditure was 11 830 kJ (404 kcal/day), a level that corresponds to 1.5 hours per day of brisk walking for a 65-kg woman.[48]

On the other hand, recent findings from randomized trials of exercise in overweight, sedentary individuals who were asked to adhere to their usual diet indicate that lesser amounts of physical activity can also have a beneficial effect on weight control.

For example, a trial that randomly assigned 173 postmenopausal women with a mean age of 61 years and mean BMI of 30.5 kg/m² to a year-long program of nonsupervised moderate-intensity exercise for 45 minutes per day on 5 days per week or to a stretching control group found significant reductions in adiposity even among participants whose exercise amounts fell short of the prescribed intervention.[50] Women assigned to the intervention group, who reported exercising a mean of 3.5 days for 176 minutes per week, experienced a mean BMI reduction of 0.3 kg/m², whereas control subjects' BMI increased by 0.3 kg/m². Moreover, women who were highly active (exercised >195 minutes/week) or moderately active (135–195 minutes/week) lost significantly more total body fat and intra-abdominal fat than did control-group women. Mean total body fat loss was 4.2% in highly active women, 2.4% in moderately active women, and 0.4% in controls. Mean intra-abdominal fat loss was 6.9% in highly active women and 5.9% in moderately active women; controls gained 0.1%.

Similarly, an 8-month intervention in which sedentary women and men with a mean age of 53 years and mean BMI of 30 kg/m² were randomly assigned to one of three exercise regimens – total exercise energy expenditures were roughly equivalent to (a) jogging 17–18 miles per week, (b) jogging 11 miles per week, or (c) walking 11 miles per week – or to a nonexercising control group found a mean weight decrease of 2.9 kg, 0.6 kg, and 0.9 kg in the three exercise groups and a mean weight increase of 1 kg in the control group.[51] An extrapolation of these results by the investigators suggests that 6–7 miles of brisk walking per week – which can easily be accomplished by exercising 30 minutes (or less) per day on most days of the week – without concurrent dietary change would suffice to prevent weight gain for the majority of middle-aged individuals.

A trial among sedentary young adults with a mean age of 23 years and mean BMI of 29 kg/m² found that 16 months of supervised moderate-intensity exercise (primarily walking) for 45 minutes per day on 5 days per week while keeping total energy intake constant prevented weight gain in women and produced weight loss in men.[52] Women assigned to the exercise group maintained their baseline weight, BMI, and fat mass, while women in the nonexercising control group experienced significant increases in these parameters – 2.9 kg, 1.1 kg/m², and 2.1 kg, respectively. Men assigned to the exercise group had significant decreases in weight (5.2 kg), BMI (1.6 kg/m²), and fat mass (4.9 kg), as compared with men in the nonexercising control group, who had negligible changes in these variables. Although lesser amounts of activity were not tested in this trial, calculations using nationally representative data suggest that a mere 100 kcal/day change in energy balance could prevent weight gain in the majority of US adults aged 20–40 years, and that modest increases in physical activity, such as 15 minutes of walking per day, or reductions in caloric intake, such as eating fewer bites at each meal, would produce the desired change.[53]

While the exact shape of the dose–response curve between physical activity and body weight remains controversial, it is unlikely that all of the cardiovascular benefits derived from physical activity are a function of weight regulation. For example, walking is associated with a reduced incidence of CVD even after adjustment for changes in BMI over time,[10] and clinical trials show that dieters who exercise develop a more favorable lipid profile than dieters who do not exercise, even when weight loss is equivalent between the two groups.[54] Therefore, focusing on excess weight – as powerful a CVD risk factor as it is – as the primary guidepost yields an incomplete picture when assessing exercise's impact on cardiovascular health.

Blood pressure (see also Chapter 31)

Prospective observational studies in men indicate that increased physical activity or cardiorespiratory fitness may protect against the development of hypertension.[55–57] Three cohort studies – the ARIC study in the United States[58] and two studies in Finland[59,60] – have conducted gender-specific analyses of the association between physical activity and incident hypertension. The ARIC investigators, who followed 7459 men and women aged 45–64 for 6 years, and Haapenen and colleagues,[59] who followed 1340 men and 1500 women aged 35–63 for 10 years, each reported an inverse association between physical activity and incident hypertension in men but not women. However, the largest of the three studies, a

10-year follow-up of 8302 Finnish men and 9139 women aged 25–64 years, found that increased physical activity, a composite of amount and intensity of recreational, occupational, and commuting-related activity, significantly predicted a lower risk of hypertension in both genders.[60] After adjustment for baseline systolic blood pressure, BMI, and other potential confounders, the relative risks of hypertension associated with light, moderate, and high physical activity were 1.00, 0.60, and 0.59 (p for trend <0.001), respectively, in men, and 1.0, 0.80, and 0.72 (p for trend = 0.006), respectively, in women.

Among men in the ARIC study, nonsport leisure activities such as walking or cycling were more predictive of reduced hypertension risk than were sport and exercise activities typically performed at high intensity levels.[58] When the leisure and sport indices were included in the same predictive model, the association between the leisure index and incident hypertension persisted, whereas the association for the sports index did not. Similarly, in the study by Haapanen and colleagues, vigorous physical activity was not an important predictor of hypertension risk in men after adjustment for total physical activity.[59] Data from randomized clinical trials also indicate that regular moderate-intensity exercise lowers blood pressure as or more effectively than does high-intensity exercise; such effects occur in both normotensive and hypertensive subjects and are independent of weight change. In a recent meta-analysis of 54 randomized trials (2419 participants), aerobic exercise was associated with a reduction in mean blood pressure of 3.9/2.6 mmHg across all initial blood pressure levels, with a mean reduction of 4.9/3.7 mmHg in hypertensive patients; the degree of blood pressure reduction did not differ by frequency or intensity of exercise.[61] Another meta-analysis of 47 aerobic exercise trials (2543 participants) reported mean blood pressure decreases of 2/1 mmHg (2%/1%) in normotensive persons and decreases of 6/5 mmHg (4%/5%) in hypertensive persons.[62] In a meta-analysis of 16 trials (650 participants) that employed walking as the sole activity intervention, decreases of 3/2 mmHg were observed in both normotensive and hypertensive individuals after an average of 25 weeks of treatment.[63] All of these meta-analyses included trials with a large percentage of female participants and found that the effectiveness

of the intervention did not vary by gender. Resistance exercise may also reduce hypertension.[64]

Insulin sensitivity and glycemic control (see also Chapter 3)

Observational and clinical trial data suggest that regular physical activity, either alone or combined with dietary therapy, improves insulin sensitivity, glycemic control, and the metabolic profile among both nondiabetic and diabetic populations.[65] Moderate- and high-intensity exercise may be equally efficacious. The Insulin Resistance Atherosclerosis Study found significant cross-sectional relationships of similar magnitude between both moderate- and vigorous-intensity physical activity and insulin sensitivity among middle-aged women and men with and without type 2 diabetes.[66] The Cross-Cultural Activity Participation Study reported that 30-minute increases in 'moderate/vigorous' and 'moderate' physical activity per day were cross-sectionally associated with 3.4% and 5.2% lower fasting insulin levels, respectively, among women aged 40–83 years unselected for diabetes status.[67] A meta-analysis of 14 trials (11 of which were randomized; 504 participants) of physical activity interventions lasting 8 weeks or more found that exercise training produced modest but clinically important reductions in glycosylated hemoglobin (HbA_{1c}) levels among middle-aged diabetics.[68] Aerobic exercise interventions – which, on average, consisted of three 53-minute sessions per week of walking or cycling over an 18-week period – were associated with a mean 0.67% reduction in HbA_{1c} level; resistance training – two to three sets ranging from 10 to 20 repetitions at 50% of respondents' repetition maximum – yielded a comparable reduction of 0.64%.

Several prospective observational studies have found that walking is predictive of a reduced CVD incidence or CVD mortality among women and men with type 2 diabetes.[69–72] Among Nurses' Health Study participants with diabetes who reported no vigorous exercise, for example, the 14-year relative risks for incident cardiovascular events across increasing quartiles of walking energy expenditure were 1.0, 0.85, 0.63, and 0.56 (p for trend = 0.03), after adjustment for BMI and other confounders.[69]

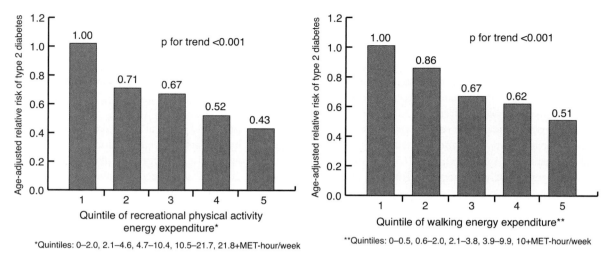

Figure 7.4
Age-adjusted relative risks of type 2 diabetes according to quintile of total recreational physical activity energy expenditure, whole sample (left panel) and quintile of walking energy expenditure, among women who did not perform vigorous activities (right panel). Nurses' Health Study. Data from reference 74.

In an 8-year follow-up of 2449 adults with diabetes in the National Health Interview Survey, walking 2 or more hours per week was associated with a 41% reduction in CVD mortality as compared with walking no hours per week.[71] An ongoing large-scale clinical trial, the Look AHEAD (Action For Health in Diabetes) study funded by the National Institute of Diabetes and Digestive and Kidney Diseases, should provide valuable randomized data about the long-term (≥10 years) effects of sustained weight loss through exercise and decreased caloric intake on the risk of CVD in obese persons with diabetes.[73]

Diabetes (see also Chapter 3)

Prospective observational studies have also consistently shown a marked reduction in the incidence of type 2 diabetes among physically active individuals as compared with their sedentary peers (Fig. 7.4). In the Nurses' Health Study, moderate-intensity activity (e.g. brisk walking) and more vigorous activity resulted in comparable reductions in diabetes incidence over an 8-year follow-up, after adjustment for total exercise energy expenditure and BMI.[74] A 6-year follow-up of 1728 Pima Indians in Arizona – a community with one of the world's highest incidences of type 2 diabetes and a high prevalence of obesity – found that recreational physical activity at levels meeting the 30-minute, moderate-intensity public health guideline was associated with a 26% reduction in diabetes incidence in women (p = 0.03) and a 12% reduction in men (p = 0.06), after controlling for age and BMI.[75]

Intervention studies in high-risk populations also suggest that physical activity lowers the risk of diabetes. In the Da Qing Impaired Glucose Tolerance and Diabetes Study, 577 middle-aged Chinese women and men with impaired glucose tolerance were randomized to one of three treatment groups – diet only, exercise only, or diet plus exercise – or to a control group.[76] Over 6 years, the three interventions were associated with statistically significant reductions of 31%, 46%, and 42% in diabetes risk, respectively. Similar reductions in diabetes incidence were observed in both lean and overweight individuals. In the Finnish Diabetes Prevention Study, 522 middle-aged, overweight women and men with impaired glucose tolerance were randomly assigned to an intensive lifestyle intervention designed to promote healthy eating and exercise patterns or to a control group.[77] Members of the diet and exercise intervention group lost significantly more weight than did the control group (3.5 vs 0.8 kg) and reduced their risk of developing diabetes by 58% over a 3-year interval. The US Diabetes Prevention Program, a 3-year follow-up of 3234 American women and men aged 25–85 years with impaired glucose tolerance and BMI of 24 kg/m^2 or more, also reported a 58% reduction in diabetes risk among the intervention group, whose members, on average, performed moderate-intensity exercise for 30 minutes per day and lost 5–7% of their body weight during the trial.[78] This study oversampled older individuals, as well as individuals of ethnic groups that suffer disproportionately from diabetes (i.e. African, Hispanic, and Asian Americans; Pacific Islanders; and American Indians), and found that the lifestyle intervention was effective in reducing diabetes risk in all age and ethnic groups. Indeed, among people aged 60 years and older – a group with a diabetes prevalence of nearly 20% – the intervention was associated with a 71% reduction in diabetes risk.

Dyslipidemia (see also Chapter 4)

In contrast to the findings for hypertension and glycemic control, strong dose–response associations between exercise intensity and blood lipids – specifically, HDL cholesterol and triglyceride levels – have been reported in observational studies.[79] A recent 8-month trial that randomly assigned overweight, dyslipidemic women and men aged 40–65 years to various exercise regimens or to a nonexercising control group found that although exercise did not affect plasma levels of total and low-density lipoprotein (LDL) cholesterol, it did yield significant improvements in various LDL subfraction parameters in addition to the expected favorable changes in HDL cholesterol and triglycerides.[80] (Only participants who complied with their assigned exercise program – 84 of 159 individuals – were included in the main analyses.) These effects were far more striking among the 'high-amount/high-intensity' exercise group, who expended the caloric equivalent of jogging 17–18 miles per week,

than among the 'low-amount/high-intensity' and 'low-amount/moderate-intensity' groups, who expended the equivalent of jogging or walking 11 miles per week, respectively. A comparison of the latter two exercise groups showed that they experienced similar improvements in lipoprotein profile to each other. On the basis of these results, the investigators suggest that lipoprotein profiles are more strongly related to amount, rather than intensity, of physical activity. However, because a 'high-amount/moderate-intensity' exercise group was not studied, this conclusion may not be warranted. Favorable effects of aerobic exercise (walking at 70% heart rate reserve for three 50-minute sessions per week) and resistance training on plasma lipoprotein levels were also found in a 10-week randomized trial of women aged 70–87 years, further evidence that exercise can ameliorate cardiovascular risk even in elderly persons.[81] In both trials, the beneficial effects of exercise occurred without concurrent changes in diet.

Hemostasis

The cardioprotective effect of physical activity may partly result from its favorable influence on hemostatic factors. Among 1507 women and men aged 25–64 years in the Northern Sweden MONICA Study (Monitoring of Trends and Determinants in Cardiovascular Disease), tissue plasminogen activator (tPA) activity increased linearly with greater leisure-time physical activity, while plasminogen activator inhibitor-1 activity decreased.[82] In the British Regional Heart Study, a 20-year follow-up of 3810 men aged 40–59 years, habitual leisure-time physical activity showed significant and inverse dose–response relationships with fibrinogen, plasma and blood viscosity, platelet count, coagulation factors VIII and IX, von Willebrand factor, fibrin D-dimer, and tPA antigen, even after adjustment for multiple potential confounders.[83] Initially sedentary men who became active in later life had a similar hemostatic profile to men with a consistent history of high activity, whereas men who became inactive in later life had a profile similar to those who had been inactive for the duration of follow-up; these findings suggest that exercise must be current to produce favorable changes in hemostasis. Randomized intervention studies have consistently found that regular moderate-intensity exercise produces significant improvements in fibrinolytic capacity in formerly sedentary individuals.[84,85] However, sparse and inconsistent data from trials testing the effect of regular physical activity performed at varying intensities on blood coagulation and platelet reactivity preclude definite conclusions regarding these two pathways.[84,86]

Inflammation (see also Chapter 9)

Regular physical activity may favorably modulate immune system function and inflammatory responses, critical processes in the pathogenesis of CVD.[87] Elevated levels of the acute-phase reactant C-reactive protein (CRP) powerfully predict cardiovascular events in prospective studies,[88] and high-sensitivity CRP testing has recently been endorsed by the AHA as a useful screening tool in persons considered to be at moderate cardiovascular risk by conventional measures.[89]

In the nationally representative NHANES III survey, the multivariate-adjusted relative risks for elevated CRP (defined as ≥85th percentile of the sex-specific distribution) were 0.98, 0.85, and 0.53 for respondents who engaged in light, moderate, and vigorous leisure-time activity, respectively, during the previous month compared with those engaging in no leisure-time activity during that time.[90] In an analysis limited to healthy respondents without CHD, diabetes, or other chronic conditions, frequency of physical activity was also associated in a dose-dependent manner with CRP level.[91] Compared with those engaging in leisure-time physical activity three or fewer times per month, persons engaging in such activity 4–21 times per month and persons engaging in such activity 22 or more times per month were 23% and 37% less likely, respectively, to have an elevated CRP level (p for trend = 0.02). Recreational or household-related physical activity was also associated in a dose-dependent manner with several inflammatory markers, including CRP, interleukin-6, and white blood cell count, in three large cohorts of elderly persons unselected for CVD – the Cardiovascular Health Study,[92] the British Regional Heart Study,[83] and the MacArthur Studies of Successful Aging.[93] Cardiorespiratory fitness as assessed by maximal treadmill exercise test has also been shown to correlate strongly and inversely with CRP levels in women[94] and men[95] without a history of CVD. In the Aerobics Center Longitudinal Study, for example, the relative risks of having an elevated CRP were 1.00, 0.43, 0.33, 0.23, and 0.17 for individuals in the lowest (least fit) to the highest (most fit) quintile, respectively.[95]

Limited data from intervention studies also suggest a beneficial effect of regular exercise on inflammation. In a nonrandomized trial, 9 months of distance running led to a 31% decrease in CRP levels among 12 subjects training for a marathon, while CRP levels remained stable in ten sedentary controls.[96] In a 'before–after' trial of a 6-month individualized exercise intervention in which 43 participants exercised for a mean of 2.5 hours per week, mononuclear cell production of atherogenic cytokines fell by 58% (p <0.001), whereas the production of atheroprotective cytokines rose by 36% (p <0.001).[97] A 35% decrease in CRP level was also noted (p = 0.12).

Whether or not the inverse association between physical activity and CRP is independent of the former's effect on adiposity is controversial. Although all of the observational studies above found significant relationships between physical activity and CRP even after adjustment for BMI, physical activity–CRP associations were attenuated after control for BMI and leptin (a surrogate marker for fat mass) among healthy men and women participating in the Health Professionals Follow-up Study and the Nurses' Health Study II, respectively.[98] Physical activity was also unrelated to CRP after adjustment for BMI among healthy men in the Physicians' Health Study.[99] Similarly, in several smaller observational studies,[100,101] correlations between exercise and CRP could be accounted for by a lower degree of body fat of the more active participants.

Endothelial function

There are few epidemiologic data on the association between regular physical activity and endothelial function in apparently healthy individuals. Small intervention studies in men at usual risk of CVD have not consistently demonstrated salutary effects of exercise on endothelial parameters.[102] However, in trials of male patients with hypertension, hypercholesterolemia, diabetes, coronary artery disease, or heart failure, aerobic exercise training has been shown to increase nitric oxide and prostacyclin availability and to improve endothelial-dependent vasodilatation.[102–106] Comparable studies in women are lacking. Because the vascular endothelium is also involved in other aspects of cardiovascular health, such as mediating the balance between fibrinolytic and prothrombotic processes and controlling inflammatory responses, it likely represents an important pathway by which exercise exerts multiple cardioprotective effects.

Summary and recommendations

Observational epidemiologic data suggest that as little as 30 minutes per day of moderate-intensity physical activity, including brisk walking, can reduce the incidence of clinical cardiovascular events. Regular physical activity also appears to slow the initiation or progression of asymptomatic coronary and peripheral artery atherosclerosis. Cardioprotective mechanisms of physical activity include the reduction of adiposity, blood pressure, insulin resistance, diabetes incidence, dyslipidemia, and inflammation, and the enhancement of insulin sensitivity, glucose tolerance, and fibrinolytic and endothelial function. Clinical trials find favorable changes in many of these physiologic parameters following moderate-intensity exercise interventions.

In a sedentary society such as the United States, the identification of strategies for facilitating sustained exercise at a level sufficient to result in measurable improvements to public health should be a top priority. The challenge to clinicians and policymakers is determining how best to promote appropriate levels of regular physical activity to their patients and the general public, respectively. Based on our review of available scientific data, as well as a balancing of efficacy and feasibility concerns, we concur with the AHA and ACSM that the clinical and public health message regarding exercise should remain '30 minutes per day of moderate activity is beneficial; and more is better, to a reasonable extent.'

Although more than two in three adults do not exercise enough to meet the 30-minute guideline, only one in three persons who saw a physician in the prior year were counseled about physical activity at their last visit, according to data from the National Health Interview Survey.[107] Low rates of clinician counseling are generally attributed to lack of time and training,[108] yet counseling about physical activity need not be time-intensive or intricate. Data from the multicenter Activity Counseling Trial suggest that clinicians can easily learn to incorporate 3–4 minutes of physical activity advice into the routine office visits of sedentary patients,[109] and that these brief counseling interventions can help patients to become more active.[110] Unfortunately, the ACT trial is one of very few methodologically rigorous studies on this topic. Because of a dearth of such research, the US Preventive Services Task Force, while endorsing high-intensity behavioral counseling, has been unable to evaluate fully the effectiveness of moderate- to low-intensity counseling by primary care clinicians in promoting increased physical activity.[111] Additional studies are urgently needed not only of this issue but also, more broadly, of the characteristics of other individual- and community-based interventions, initiatives, and policies that may be useful in fostering healthful exercise behaviors.[112] While awaiting such studies, however, health-care professionals seeking guidance on how to help patients increase their physical activity level may wish to consult recent AHA guidelines for prescribing aerobic and resistance exercise for persons with and without CVD.[113,114] A recent commentary also offers a simple blueprint for physicians who are perplexed about how to incorporate brief counseling about physical activity into their daily practices.[115] Given the high prevalence of sedentary behavior, a widespread effort to help patients achieve even modest increases in regular physical activity will likely have a favorable impact on cardiovascular morbidity and mortality. As the eminent British epidemiologist Geoffrey Rose has observed,[116] the overall disease burden in a given population generally undergoes a more dramatic reduction when a large segment of the population adopts small improvements in health behaviors than when a small segment of the population adopts large improvements.

References

1. Berlin JA, Colditz GA. A meta-analysis of physical activity in the prevention of coronary heart disease. *Am J Epidemiol* 1990; **132**:612–28.
2. Pate RR, Pratt M, Blair SN, et al. Physical activity and public health. A recommendation from the Centers for Disease Control and Prevention and the American College of Sports Medicine. *JAMA* 1995; **273**:402–7.
3. US Department of Health and Human Services. *Physical Activity and Health: A Report of the Surgeon General*. Atlanta, GA: US Department of Health and Human Services, Centers for Disease Control and Prevention, National Center for Chronic Disease Prevention and Health Promotion, 1996.
4. Institute of Medicine. *Dietary Reference Intakes for Energy, Carbohydrates, Fiber, Fat, Protein, and Amino Acids*. Washington, DC: National Academies Press, 2002.
5. Schoenborn CA, Barnes PM. *Leisure-time Physical Activity among Adults: United States, 1997–98*. Advance Data from Vital and Health Statistics No. 325. Hyattsville, MD: National Center for Health Statistics, 2002.
6. Thompson PD, Buchner D, Pina IL, et al. Exercise and physical activity in the prevention and treatment of atherosclerotic cardiovascular disease: a statement from the Council on Clinical Cardiology (Subcommittee on Exercise, Rehabilitation, and Prevention) and the Council on Nutrition, Physical Activity, and Metabolism (Subcommittee on Physical Activity). *Circulation* 2003; **107**:3109–16.
7. Mosca L, Appel LJ, Benjamin EJ, et al. Evidence-based guidelines for cardiovascular disease prevention in women. *Circulation* 2004; **109**:672–93.
8. Kohl HW III. Physical activity and cardiovascular disease: evidence for a dose-response. *Med Sci Sports Exerc* 2001; **33** (6 Suppl):S472–83.
9. Manson JE, Greenland P, LaCroix AZ, et al. Walking compared with vigorous exercise for the prevention of cardiovascular events in women. *N Engl J Med* 2002; **347**:716–25.
10. Manson JE, Hu FB, Rich-Edwards JW, et al. A prospective study of walking as compared with vigorous exercise in the prevention of coronary heart disease in women. *N Engl J Med* 1999; **341**:650–8.
11. Lee IM, Rexrode KM, Cook NR, Manson JE, Buring JE. Physical activity and coronary heart disease in women: is 'no pain, no gain' passe? *JAMA* 2001; **285**:1447–54.
12. Sesso HD, Paffenbarger RS, Ha T, Lee IM. Physical activity and cardiovascular disease risk in middle-aged and older women. *Am J Epidemiol* 1999; **150**:408–16.
13. Gregg EW, Cauley JA, Stone K, et al. Relationship of changes in physical activity and mortality among older women. *JAMA* 2003; **289**:2379–86.
14. LaCroix AZ, Leveille SG, Hecht JA, Grothaus LC, Wagner EH. Does walking decrease the risk of cardiovascular disease hospitalizations and death in older adults? *J Am Geriatr Soc* 1996; **44**:113–20.
15. Tanasescu M, Leitzmann MF, Rimm EB, Willett WC, Stampfer MJ, Hu FB. Exercise type and intensity in relation to coronary heart disease in men. *JAMA* 2002; **288**:1994–2000.
16. Hakim AA, Curb JD, Petrovitch H, et al. Effects of walking on coronary heart disease in elderly men: the Honolulu Heart Program. *Circulation* 1999; **100**:9–13.
17. Bijnen FC, Caspersen CJ, Feskens EJ, Saris WH, Mosterd WL, Kromhout D. Physical activity and 10-year mortality from cardiovascular diseases and all causes: the Zutphen Elderly Study. *Arch Intern Med* 1998; **158**:1499–505.
18. Yu S, Yarnell JW, Sweetnam PM, Murray L. What level of physical activity protects against premature cardiovascular death? The Caerphilly study. *Heart* 2003; **89**:502–6.
19. Lee IM. No pain, no gain? Thoughts on the Caerphilly study. *Br J Sports Med* 2004; **38**:4–5.
20. Wannamethee SG, Shaper AG, Walker M. Changes in physical activity, mortality, and incidence of coronary heart disease in older men. *Lancet* 1998; **351**:1603–8.
21. Jakicic JM, Wing RR, Butler BA, Robertson RJ. Prescribing exercise in multiple short bouts versus one continuous bout: effects on adherence, cardiorespiratory fitness, and weight loss in overweight women. *Int J Obes Relat Metab Disord* 1995; **19**:893–901.
22. Murphy M, Nevill A, Neville C, Biddle S, Hardman A. Accumulating brisk walking for fitness, cardiovascular risk, and psychological health. *Med Sci Sports Exerc* 2002; **34**:1468–74.
23. Lee IM, Sesso HD, Paffenbarger RS Jr. Physical activity and coronary heart disease risk in men: does the duration of exercise episodes predict risk? *Circulation* 2000; **102**:981–6.
24. Mora S, Redberg RF, Cui Y, et al. Ability of exercise

testing to predict cardiovascular and all-cause death in asymptomatic women: a 20-year follow-up of the Lipid Research Clinics Prevalence Study. *JAMA* 2003; **290**:1600–7.

25. Gibbons LW, Mitchell TL, Wei M, Blair SN, Cooper KH. Maximal exercise test as a predictor of risk for mortality from coronary heart disease in asymptomatic men. *Am J Cardiol* 2000; **86**:53–8.

26. Blair SN, Kohl HW 3rd, Barlow CE, Paffenbarger RS Jr, Gibbons LW, Macera CA. Changes in physical fitness and all-cause mortality. A prospective study of healthy and unhealthy men. *JAMA* 1995; **273**:1093–8.

27. Ekelund LG, Haskell WL, Johnson JL, Whaley FS, Criqui MH, Sheps DS. Physical fitness as a predictor of cardiovascular mortality in asymptomatic North American men. The Lipid Research Clinics Mortality Follow-up Study. *N Engl J Med* 1988; **319**:1379–84.

28. Gulati M, Pandey DK, Arnsdorf MF, et al. Exercise capacity and the risk of death in women: the St James Women Take Heart Project. *Circulation* 2003; **108**:1554–9.

29. Williams PT. Physical fitness and activity as separate heart disease risk factors: a meta-analysis. *Med Sci Sports Exerc* 2001; **33**:754–61.

30. Lee IM, Sesso HD, Oguma Y, Paffenbarger RS. Relative intensity of physical activity and risk of coronary heart disease. *Circulation* 2003; **107**: 1110–16.

31. American College of Sports Medicine Position Stand. The recommended quantity and quality of exercise for developing and maintaining cardiorespiratory and muscular fitness, and flexibility in healthy adults. *Med Sci Sports Exerc* 1998; **30**:975–91.

32. Lee CD, Folsom AR, Blair SN. Physical activity and stroke risk: a meta-analysis. *Stroke* 2003; **34**:2475–81.

33. Hu FB, Stampfer MJ, Colditz GA, et al. Physical activity and risk of stroke in women. *JAMA* 2000; **283**:2961–7.

34. Lee IM, Hennekens CH, Berger K, Buring JE, Manson JE. Exercise and risk of stroke in male physicians. *Stroke* 1999; **30**:1–6.

35. Lee CD, Blair SN. Cardiorespiratory fitness and stroke mortality in men. *Med Sci Sports Exerc* 2002; **34**:592–5.

36. Kurl S, Laukkanen JA, Rauramaa R, Lakka TA, Sivenius J, Salonen JT. Cardiorespiratory fitness and the risk for stroke in men. *Arch Intern Med* 2003; **163**:1682–8.

37. Siscovick DS, Fried L, Mittelmark M, Rutan G, Bild D, O'Leary DH. Exercise intensity and subclinical cardiovascular disease in the elderly: the Cardiovascular Health Study. *Am J Epidemiol* 1997; **145**:977–86.

38. Folsom AR, Eckfeldt JH, Weitzman S, et al. Relation of carotid artery wall thickness to diabetes mellitus, fasting glucose and insulin, body size, and physical activity. Atherosclerosis Risk in Communities (ARIC) Study Investigators. *Stroke* 1994; **25**:66–73.

39. Taylor AJ, Watkins T, Bell D, et al. Physical activity and the presence and extent of calcified coronary atherosclerosis. *Med Sci Sports Exerc* 2002; **34**: 228–33.

40. Stensland-Bugge E, Bonaa KH, Joakimsen O, Njolstad I. Sex differences in the relationship of risk factors to subclinical carotid atherosclerosis measured 15 years later: the Tromso Study. *Stroke* 2000; **31**:574–81.

41. Engstrom G, Ogren M, Hedblad B, Wollmer P, Janzon L. Asymptomatic leg atherosclerosis is reduced by regular physical activity. Longitudinal results from the cohort 'Men Born in 1914'. *Eur J Vasc Endovasc Surg* 2001; **21**:502–7.

42. Lakka TA, Laukkanen JA, Rauramaa R, et al. Cardiorespiratory fitness and the progression of carotid atherosclerosis in middle-aged men. *Ann Intern Med* 2001; **134**:12–20.

43. Nordstrom CK, Dwyer KM, Merz CN, Shircore A, Dwyer JH. Leisure time physical activity and early atherosclerosis: the Los Angeles Atherosclerosis Study. *Am J Med* 2003; **115**:19–25.

44. Centers for Disease Control and Prevention. Trends in intake of energy and macronutrients – United States, 1971–2000. *MMWR* 2004; **53**:80–2.

45. Flegal KM, Carroll MD, Kuczmarski RJ, Johnson CL. Overweight and obesity in the United States: prevalence and trends, 1960–1994. *Int J Obes Relat Metab Disord* 1998; **22**:39–47.

46. Flegal KM, Carroll MD, Ogden CL, Johnson CL. Prevalence and trends in obesity among US adults, 1999–2000. *JAMA* 2002; **288**:1723–7.

47. Schoeller DA, Shay K, Kushner RF. How much physical activity is needed to minimize weight gain in previously obese women? *Am J Clin Nutr* 1997; **66**:551–6.

48. Klem ML, Wing RR, McGuire MT, Seagle HM, Hill JO. A descriptive study of individuals successful at long-term maintenance of substantial weight loss. *Am J Clin Nutr* 1997; **66**:239–46.

49. Wing RR. Physical activity in the treatment of the adult overweight and obesity: current evidence and research issues. *Med Sci Sports Exerc* 1999; **31** (11 Suppl):S547–52.

50. Irwin ML, Yasui Y, Ulrich CM, et al. Effect of exercise on total and intra-abdominal body fat in postmenopasual women: a randomized trial. *JAMA* 2003; **289**:323–30.

51. Slentz CA, Duscha BD, Johnson JL, et al. Effects of the amount of exercise on body weight, body composition, and measures of central obesity: STRRIDE – a randomized controlled study. *Arch Intern Med* 2004; **164**:31–9.

52. Donnelly JE, Hill JO, Jacobsen DJ, et al. Effects of a 16-month randomized controlled exercise trial on body weight and composition in young, overweight men and women: the Midwest Exercise Trial. *Arch Intern Med* 2003; **163**:1343–50.

53. Hill JO, Wyatt HR, Reed GW, Peters JC. Obesity and the environment: where do we go from here? *Science* 2003; **299**:853–5.

54. Stefanick ML, Mackey S, Sheehan M, Ellsworth N, Haskell WL, Wood PD. Effects of diet and exercise in men and postmenopausal women with low levels of HDL cholesterol and high levels of LDL cholesterol. *N Engl J Med* 1998; **339**:12–20.

55. Paffenbarger RS Jr, Wing AL, Hyde RT, Jung DL. Physical activity and incidence of hypertension in college alumni. *Am J Epidemiol* 1983; **117**:245–57.

56. Blair SN, Goodyear NN, Gibbons LW, Cooper KH. Physical fitness and incidence of hypertension in healthy normotensive men and women. *JAMA* 1984; **252**:487–90.

57. Hayashi T, Tsumura K, Suematsu C, Okada K, Fujii S, Endo G. Walking to work and the risk for hypertension in men: the Osaka Health Survey. *Ann Intern Med* 1999; **131**:21–6.

58. Pereira MA, Folsom AR, McGovern PG, et al. Physical activity and incident hypertension in black and white adults: the Atherosclerosis Risk in Communities Study. *Prev Med* 1999; **28**:304–12.

59. Haapanen N, Miilunpalo S, Vuori I, Oja P, Pasanen M. Association of leisure time physical activity with the risk of coronary heart disease, hypertension and diabetes in middle-aged men and women. *Int J Epidemiol* 1997; **26**:739–47.

60. Hu G, Barengo NC, Tuomilehto J, Lakka TA, Nissinen A, Jousilahti P. Relationship of physical activity and body mass index to the risk of hypertension: a prospective study in Finland. *Hypertension* 2004; **43**:25–30.

61. Whelton SP, Chin A, Xin X, He J. Effect of aerobic exercise on blood pressure: a meta-analysis of randomized, controlled trials. *Ann Intern Med* 2002; **136**:493–503.

62. Kelley GA, Kelley KA, Tran ZV. Aerobic exercise and resting blood pressure: a meta-analytic review of randomized, controlled trials. *Prev Cardiol* 2001; **4**:73–80.

63. Kelley GA, Kelley KS, Tran ZV. Walking and resting blood pressure in adults: a meta-analysis. *Prev Med* 2001; **33**:120–7.

64. Hurley BF, Roth SM. Strength training in the elderly: effects on risk factors for age-related diseases. *Sports Med* 2000; **30**:249–68.

65. Skerrett PJ, Manson JE. Reduction in risk of coronary heart disease and diabetes. In: Ruderman N, Devlin JT, Schneider SH, Kriska A (eds). *Handbook of Exercise in Diabetes*. Alexandria, VA: American Diabetes Association, 2002:155–81.

66. Mayer-Davis EJ, D'Agostino R Jr, Karter AJ, et al. Intensity and amount of physical activity in relation to insulin sensitivity: the Insulin Resistance Atherosclerosis Study. *JAMA* 1998; **279**:669–74.

67. Irwin ML, Mayer-Davis EJ, Addy CL, et al. Moderate-intensity physical activity and fasting insulin levels in women: the Cross-Cultural Activity Participation Study. *Diabetes Care* 2000; **23**:449–54.

68. Boule NG, Haddad E, Kenny GP, Wells GA, Sigal RJ. Effects of exercise on glycemic control and body mass in type 2 diabetes mellitus: a meta-analysis of controlled clinical trials. *JAMA* 2001; **286**:1218–27.

69. Hu FB, Stampfer MJ, Solomon C, et al. Physical activity and risk for cardiovascular events in diabetic women. *Ann Intern Med* 2001; **134**:96–105.

70. Batty GD, Shipley MJ, Marmot M, Smith GD. Physical activity and cause-specific mortality in men with Type 2 diabetes/impaired glucose tolerance: evidence from the Whitehall study. *Diabet Med* 2002; **19**:580–8.

71. Gregg EW, Gerzoff RB, Caspersen CJ, Williamson DF, Narayan KM. Relationship of walking to mortality among US adults with diabetes. *Arch Intern Med* 2003; **163**:1440–7.

72. Tanasescu M, Leitzmann MF, Rimm EB, Hu FB. Physical activity in relation to cardiovascular disease and total mortality among men with type 2 diabetes. *Circulation* 2003; **107**:2435–9.

73. Ryan DH, Espeland MA, Foster GD, et al. Look AHEAD (Action for Health in Diabetes): design and methods for a clinical trial of weight loss for the prevention of cardiovascular disease in type 2 diabetes. *Control Clin Trials* 2003; **24**:610–28.

74. Hu FB, Sigal RJ, Rich-Edwards JW, et al. Walking compared with vigorous physical activity and risk of type 2 diabetes in women: a prospective study. *JAMA* 1999; **282**:1433–9.

75. Kriska AM, Saremi A, Hanson RL, et al. Physical activity, obesity, and the incidence of type 2 diabetes in a high-risk population. *Am J Epidemiol* 2003; **158**:669–75.

76. Pan XR, Li GW, Hu YH, et al. Effects of diet and

exercise in preventing NIDDM in people with impaired glucose tolerance. The DaQing IGT and Diabetes Study. *Diabetes Care* 1997; **20**:537–44.

77. Tuomilehto J, Lindstrom J, Eriksson JG, et al. Prevention of type 2 diabetes mellitus by changes in lifestyle among subjects with impaired glucose tolerance. *N Engl J Med* 2001; **344**:1343–50.

78. Knowler WC, Barrett-Connor E, Fowler SE, et al. Reduction in the incidence of type 2 diabetes with lifestyle intervention or metformin. *N Engl J Med* 2002; **346**:393–403.

79. Leon AS, Sanchez OA. Response of blood lipids to exercise training alone or combined with dietary intervention. *Med Sci Sports Exerc* 2001; **33** (6 Suppl):S502–15.

80. Kraus WE, Houmard JA, Duscha BD, et al. Effects of the amount and intensity of exercise on plasma lipoproteins. *N Engl J Med* 2002; **347**:1483–92.

81. Fahlman MM, Boardley D, Lambert CP, Flynn MG. Effects of endurance training and resistance training on plasma lipoprotein profiles in elderly women. *J Gerontol A Biol Sci Med Sci* 2002; **57**:B54–60.

82. Eliasson M, Asplund K, Evrin PE. Regular leisure time physical activity predicts high activity of tissue plasminogen activator: the Northern Sweden MONICA Study. *Int J Epidemiol* 1996; **25**:1182–8.

83. Wannamethee SG, Lowe GD, Whincup PH, Rumley A, Walker M, Lennon L. Physical activity and hemostatic and inflammatory variables in elderly men. *Circulation* 2002; **105**:1785–90.

84. Lee KW, Lip GY. Effects of lifestyle on hemostasis, fibrinolysis, and platelet reactivity: a systematic review. *Arch Intern Med* 2003; **163**:2368–92.

85. Smith DT, Hoetzer GL, Greiner JJ, Stauffer BL, DeSouza CA. Effects of ageing and regular aerobic exercise on endothelial fibrinolytic capacity in humans. *J Physiol* 2003; **546**:289–98.

86. Rauramaa R, Li G, Vaisanen SB. Dose–response and coagulation and hemostatic factors. *Med Sci Sports Exerc* 2001; **33** (6 Suppl):S516–20.

87. Libby P, Ridker PM, Maseri A. Inflammation and atherosclerosis. *Circulation* 2002; **105**:1135–43.

88. Ridker PM. Clinical application of C-reactive protein for cardiovascular disease detection and prevention. *Circulation* 2003; **107**:363–9.

89. Pearson T, Mensah GA, Alexander RW, et al. Markers of inflammation and cardiovascular disease: application to clinical and public health practice. *Circulation* 2003; **107**:499–511.

90. Ford ES. Does exercise reduce inflammation? Physical activity and C-reactive protein among US adults. *Epidemiology* 2002; **13**:561–8.

91. Abramson JL, Vaccarino V. Relationship between physical activity and inflammation among apparently healthy middle-aged and older US adults. *Arch Intern Med* 2002; **162**:1286–92.

92. Geffken DF, Cushman M, Burke GL, Polak JF, Sakkinen PA, Tracy RP. Association between physical activity and markers of inflammation in a healthy elderly population. *Am J Epidemiol* 2001; **153**:242–50.

93. Reuben DB, Judd-Hamilton L, Harris TB, Seeman TE. The associations between physical activity and inflammatory markers in high-functioning older persons: MacArthur Studies of Successful Aging. *J Am Geriatr Soc* 2003; **51**:1125–30.

94. LaMonte MJ, Durstine JL, Yanowitz FG, et al. Cardiorespiratory fitness and C-reactive protein among a tri-ethnic sample of women. *Circulation* 2002; **106**:403–6.

95. Church TS, Barlow CE, Earnest CP, Kampert JB, Priest EL, Blair SN. Associations between cardiorespiratory fitness and C-reactive protein in men. *Arterioscler Thromb Vasc Biol* 2002; **22**:1869–76.

96. Mattusch F, Dufaux B, Heine O, Mertens I, Rost R. Reduction of the plasma concentration of C-reactive protein following nine months of endurance training. *Int J Sports Med* 2000; **21**:21–4.

97. Smith JK, Dykes R, Douglas JE, Krishnaswamy G, Berk S. Long-term exercise and atherogenic activity of blood mononuclear cells in persons at risk of developing ischemic heart disease. *JAMA* 1999; **281**:1722–7.

98. Pischon T, Hankinson SE, Hotamisligil GS, Rifai N, Rimm EB. Leisure-time physical activity and reduced plasma levels of obesity-related inflammatory markers. *Obes Res* 2003; **11**:1055–64.

99. Rohde LE, Hennekens CH, Ridker PM. Survey of C-reactive protein and cardiovascular risk factors in apparently healthy men. *Am J Cardiol* 1999; **84**:1018–22.

100. Rawson ES, Freedson PS, Osganian SK, Matthews CE, Reed G, Ockene IS. Body mass index, but not physical activity, is associated with C-reactive protein. *Med Sci Sports Exerc* 2003; **35**:1160–6.

101. Manns PJ, Williams DP, Snow CM, Wander RC. Physical activity, body fat, and serum C-reactive protein in postmenopausal women with and without hormone replacement. *Am J Human Biol* 2003; **15**:91–100.

102. Moyna NM, Thompson PD. The effect of physical activity on endothelial function in man. *Acta Physiol Scand* 2004; **180**:113–23.

103. Hambrecht R, Wolf A, Gielen S, et al. Effect of exercise on coronary endothelial function in patients with coronary artery disease. *N Engl J Med* 2000; **342**:454–60.

104. Roberts CK, Vaziri ND, Barnard J. Effect of diet and exercise intervention on blood pressure, insulin, oxidative stress, and nitric oxide availability. *Circulation* 2002; **106**:2530–2.

105. Hambrecht R, Adams V, Erbs S, et al. Regular physical activity improves endothelial function in patients with coronary artery disease by increasing phosphorylation of endothelial nitric oxide synthase. *Circulation* 2003; **107**:3152–8.

106. Walsh JH, Yong G, Cheetham C, et al. Effects of exercise training on conduit and resistance vessel function in treated and untreated hypercholesterolaemic subjects. *Eur Heart J* 2003; **24**:1681–9.

107. Wee CC, McCarthy EP, Davis RB, Phillips RS. Physician counseling about exercise. *JAMA* 1999; **282**:1583–8.

108. Kottke TE, Brekke ML, Solberg LI. Making 'time' for preventive services. *Mayo Clin Proc* 1993; **68**:785–91.

109. Albright CL, Cohen S, Gibbons L, et al. Incorporating physical activity advice into primary care: physician-delivered advice within the Activity Counseling Trial. *Am J Prev Med* 2000; **18**:225–34.

110. Writing Group for the Activity Counseling Trial Research Group. Effects of physical activity counseling in primary care: the Activity Counseling Trial: a randomized controlled trial. *JAMA* 2001; **286**:677–87.

111. US Preventive Services Task Force. Behavioral counseling in primary care to promote physical activity: recommendation and rationale. *Ann Intern Med* 2002; **137**:205–7.

112. Task Force on Community Preventive Services. Recommendations to increase physical activity in communities. *Am J Prev Med* 2002; **22**(4 Suppl):67–72.

113. Fletcher GF, Balady GJ, Amsterdam EA, et al. Exercise standards for testing and training: a statement for healthcare professionals from the American Heart Association. *Circulation* 2001; **104**:1694–740.

114. Pollock ML, Franklin BA, Balady GJ, et al. AHA Science Advisory. Resistance exercise in individuals with and without cardiovascular disease: benefits, rationale, safety, and prescription: an advisory from the Committee on Exercise, Rehabilitation, and Prevention, Council on Clinical Cardiology, American Heart Association. *Circulation* 2000; **101**:828–33.

115. Manson JE, Skerrett PJ, Greenland P, VanItallie TB. The escalating pandemics of obesity and sedentary lifestyle: a call to action for clinicians. *Arch Intern Med* 2004; **164**:249–58.

116. Rose G. *The Strategy of Preventive Medicine*. New York: Oxford University Press, 1992.

8

Serum homocysteine and coronary heart disease*

David S. Wald

Introduction

The clinical observation linking serum homocysteine with cardiovascular disease (CVD) was made over 35 years ago[1] and since then much evidence has accumulated on the subject. However, opinion on whether homocysteine causes CVD remains divided.[2] Resolving the uncertainty is important as serum homocysteine levels can be lowered by taking additional folic acid, raising the prospect of a simple means of prevention.[3] This chapter examines the evidence for a causal relation between homocysteine

and coronary heart disease (CHD) and considers the implications for prevention.

Homocysteine metabolism

Homocysteine is an amino acid formed during the metabolism of the essential amino acid methionine, the major methyl group donor in mammals necessary for DNA synthesis. Homocysteine is metabolized in two ways (Fig. 8.1). It is remethylated to methionine,

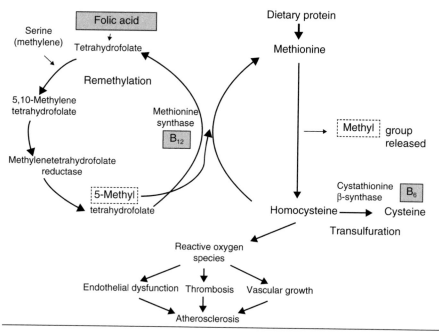

Figure 8.1
Summary of the major pathways of homocysteine metabolism and atherosclerosis.

with 5-methyl tetrahydrofolate acting as the methyl group donor, a process dependent on vitamin B_{12}, the enzyme methionine synthase, and tetrahydrofolate (derived from natural folate or from the B vitamin folic acid). Tetrahydrofolate is then remethylated to replenish 5-methyl tetrahydrofolate, a process dependent on the enzyme methylenetetrahydrofolate reductase (MTHFR) and the amino acid serine. Homocysteine is also metabolized by transulfuration to cystathionine, a process dependent on vitamin B_6 and the enzyme cystathionine β-synthase. Impairment of either of these two processes can increase serum homocysteine concentrations.

The blood level of homocysteine is ordinarily tightly controlled in most individuals with an average level in Western populations of about 12 µmol/l. The level in women is about 1 µmol/l lower than in men.[4] This may be related to the larger muscle mass of men, since about 75% of homocysteine is formed in conjunction with creatine synthesis[5] or it may be due to a homocysteine-lowering effect of estrogens.[6]

Lowering homocysteine with B vitamins

Homocysteine can be lowered by increasing the intake of the B vitamins, folic acid, vitamin B_{12} or vitamin B_6. The Homocysteine Lowering Trialists Collaboration showed that folic acid was the most effective of the B vitamins in lowering serum homocysteine.[3] A dose of 1 mg per day lowered serum homocysteine by 25% (or about 3 µmol/l from the population average level of 12 µmol/l); doses above 1 mg per day produced no additional benefit. Vitamin B_{12} (0.5 mg per day) produced only an additional 7% reduction and B_6 had no further detectable effect. Subsequent trials have shown that the full homocysteine-lowering effect of folic acid is achieved with about 0.8 mg folic acid per day, and most of the effect by 0.4 mg.[7,8] Folic acid lowers serum homocysteine from all pre-treatment levels in Western populations, although the reduction is greater from higher levels.[7] Folic acid supplementation is more effective than dietary change; an unrealistically large amount of folate-containing foods would need to be eaten each day to reach the equivalent homocysteine-lowering effect of a daily 0.8 mg folic acid supplement. This is because the folate concentration of foods is relatively low and the bioavailability of natural folate is about half that of folic acid.

The link between homocysteine and coronary heart disease: homocystinuria

The association between homocysteine and CHD was identified in 1969 by McCully who described premature atherosclerotic disease at autopsy in two children who died with the rare autosomal recessive condition, homocystinuria.[1] Homocystinuria is a deficiency of one of three enzymes involved in homocysteine metabolism (Fig. 8.1), leading to three distinct disorders: cystathionine β-synthase deficiency, MTHFR deficiency, and the B_{12} metabolic defects that result in impaired methionine synthase activity. Heterozygotes for these three disorders have about three times the population average serum homocysteine concentration and a high risk of CVD. Homozygotes have serum homocysteine levels 10–50 times the population average and a very high risk of premature CVD; about 50% of them experience an arterial or venous disease event by the age of 30.[9] A high homocysteine level is the only biochemical change common to all three disorders; no other substance is consistently high or low. It follows therefore that the high homocysteine causes the increased risk of CVD in people with homocystinuria. Two studies among homozygotes with homocystinuria treated with vitamins B_6, B_{12}, and folic acid indicate that risk can be reduced. Treatment with these vitamins led to only two vascular events when 30 would have been expected (from previous observation in untreated patients) in one study,[10] and no events when 29 would have been expected in the other.[11] While these were not randomized trials, selection bias could not reasonably explain so large a difference with two events observed versus 59 expected.

Pathogenic mechanisms

Other than providing a reservoir for regenerating methionine and thereby maintaining the methylation process throughout the body, homocysteine serves no useful biological function and high levels are thought to promote atherosclerosis. Three interlinked mechanisms have been postulated: endothelial dysfunction, thrombosis, and vascular growth (Fig. 8.1).

Endothelial effects

In vitro experimental evidence suggests that homocysteine causes endothelial injury through auto-oxidation to reactive oxygen radicals[12,13] (the superoxide anion, hydroxyl radical, and hydrogen peroxide) which expose the underlying endothelial matrix, leading to smooth muscle cell proliferation and platelet activation.[14] Homocysteine also oxidizes low-density lipoprotein (LDL), and may therefore promote cellular uptake of LDL, an important step in the atherosclerotic process.[15] Homocysteine is known to impair normal endothelial function and repair mechanisms by reducing the formation of endothelial-derived nitric oxide.[16] Ordinarily, nitric oxide detoxifies homocysteine by forming S-nitroso-homocysteine, a potent platelet inhibitor and vasodilator, but exposure to high homocysteine levels impairs this protective effect.[16] Homocysteine impaired endothelium-dependent vasodilation has been demonstrated in vitro,[16] in primates,[17] and in humans with homocystinuria.[18]

Thrombosis

Homocysteine has been shown to increase the production of procoagulant factors and inactivate anticoagulant factors. In vitro, high concentrations of homocysteine induce endothelial cell tissue factor expression and activity which may initiate coagulation.[19] Homocysteine alters the natural antithrombotic mechanisms by enhancing the activity of factors XII and V and depressing the activation of protein C and thrombomodulin.[20,21] Homocysteine also stimulates platelet generation of thromboxane A_2, a potent vasoconstrictor and proaggregant.[22]

Vascular growth

Homocysteine stimulates the signal transduction pathways in vascular smooth muscle cells and collagen expression and may promote smooth muscle proliferation at sites of injured endothelium.[23,24] In a rat carotid endarterectomy model, experimental elevation of plasma homocysteine increased initimal hyperplasia fourfold[25] and in humans, patients with homocystinuria have been shown to have marked carotid wall hypertrophy.[26]

Although there is still uncertainty over the precise mechanisms involved, a role for homocysteine either in the long-term development of atherosclerotic lesions or the later onset thrombosis on damaged endothelial surfaces (or both) is biologically plausible.

Retrospective and prospective epidemiologic studies

Retrospective and prospective studies provide evidence of the dose–response relationship across the range of serum homocysteine in the population. Approximately one-quarter of the data in these studies were collected from women and since the effects of homocysteine on CHD are similar in men and women, the data are summarized together. Overall, there is about a twofold risk gradient from the highest to the lowest fifth of serum homocysteine values.

In retrospective studies homocysteine was measured after the diagnosis of CHD in cases (generally with nonfatal myocardial infarction, MI) and in unaffected controls. Over 30 such studies have been published and all show a positive association between CHD and serum homocysteine. Figure 8.2 shows the results of a meta-analysis of 12 published retrospective studies (combining data from 1517 cases of MI) that reported the proportional difference in risk for a specified serum homocysteine difference adjusted for age and in some studies other cardiovascular risk factors (or reported data from which this could be calculated).[27–38] Six of the 12 studies included data on women and one, with a risk estimate close to the median of all studies, examined data from women alone.[35] The risk of a CHD event (odds ratio) for a 3 µmol/l decrease in serum homocysteine (achievable by taking 0.8 mg folic acid) is shown for each study, together with the summary estimate for all studies combined. The summary odds ratio was 0.78 (95% confidence interval (CI) 0.72–0.85) for a 3 µmol/l decrease in

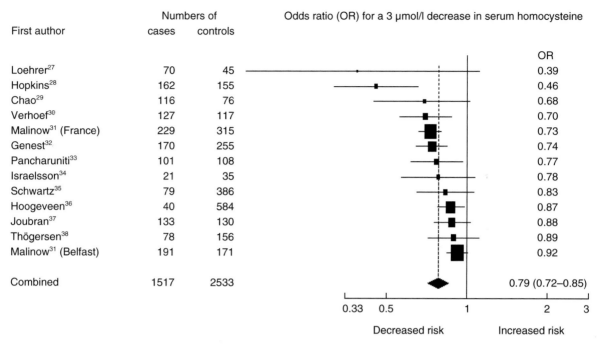

Figure 8.2
Results of 12 retrospective studies of serum homocysteine and coronary heart disease events:[27–38] values are odds ratios (95% confidence intervals) for a 3 μmol/l decrease in serum homocysteine. Results are adjusted for age and sex and in some studies other cardiovascular risk factors, but not for regression dilution bias.

homocysteine, or 0.75 (0.68–0.82) adjusted for regression dilution bias (p = 0.001).[39] This result is likely to over-estimate the true effect as some of the studies did not adjust for confounding by other cardiovascular risk factors (such as smoking, serum cholesterol, and blood pressure) and possibly because atherosclerotic disease may increase homocysteine, due to reduced renal function.[40]

Prospective studies by their design reduce any effect of disease on homocysteine. In these studies blood was taken from healthy subjects who were then followed up for several years. Samples from those who later developed CHD events and from matched controls were then tested (a so-called nested case–control design). Figure 8.3 shows the results of a meta-analysis of 16 published prospective studies (including data from women in eight studies) of serum homocysteine and CHD events (death or

nonfatal MI, n = 3144).[41] The odds ratios shown were adjusted for age, sex, smoking habits, blood pressure, and serum cholesterol in all the studies except one which was adjusted for age and sex alone. The summary odds ratio was 0.89 (0.85–0.92) for a 3 μmol/l decrease in serum homocysteine or 0.85 (0.80–0.90) adjusted for regression dilution bias. These results are similar to those published from another recent meta-analysis of 11 prospective studies.[42]

The retrospective and prospective studies show a positive association between serum homocysteine and CHD. These studies on their own are insufficient to determine whether the association is one of cause and effect because they may be subject to confounding by unknown cardiovascular risk factors or by imprecision in measuring known ones. However, there is an additional source of evidence – the genetic

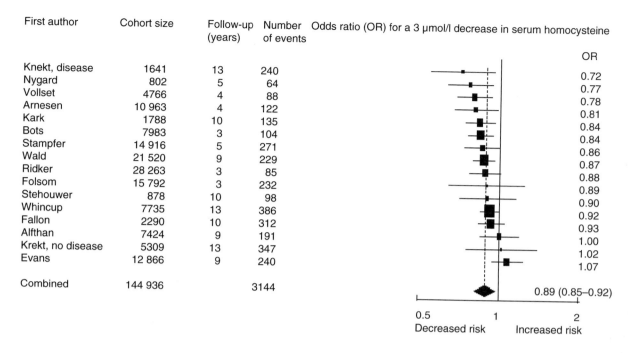

First author	Cohort size	Follow-up (years)	Number of events	Odds ratio (OR) for a 3 µmol/l decrease in serum homocysteine	OR
Knekt, disease	1641	13	240		0.72
Nygard	802	5	64		0.77
Vollset	4766	4	88		0.78
Arnesen	10 963	4	122		0.81
Kark	1788	10	135		0.84
Bots	7983	3	104		0.84
Stampfer	14 916	5	271		0.86
Wald	21 520	9	229		0.87
Ridker	28 263	3	85		0.88
Folsom	15 792	3	232		0.89
Stehouwer	878	10	98		0.90
Whincup	7735	13	386		0.92
Fallon	2290	10	312		0.93
Alfthan	7424	9	191		1.00
Krekt, no disease	5309	13	347		1.02
Evans	12 866	9	240		1.07
Combined	144 936		3144		0.89 (0.85–0.92)

0.5   1   2
Decreased risk   Increased risk

Figure 8.3

Results of prospective studies of serum homocysteine and coronary heart disease events: values are odds ratios (95% confidence intervals) for a 3 µmol/l decrease in serum homocysteine, adjusted for age, sex, smoking, serum cholesterol, and blood pressure (age and sex alone in one study) but not for regression dilution bias. Reproduced from reference 41 with permission from the BMJ Publishing Group.

epidemiological studies of the thermolabile C677T *MTHFR* polymorphism – and these help resolve the uncertainty.

Genetic epidemiology: studies on the *MTHFR* gene

Moderately raised serum homocysteine levels (about 25% above average levels) occur as a result of a single mutation in the *MTHFR* gene (cytosine to thymidine (C→T) at base pair position 677) that renders the enzyme thermolabile with reduced activity.[43] The presence of this polymorphism in the population provides a natural experiment capable of testing whether moderately raised homocysteine levels cause CHD. The C→T mutation is common (about 10% of

individuals are homozygous (TT) and about 47% are heterozygous (CT)) such that it has been possible to conduct studies of the risk of CHD in persons with and without the mutation, and many are now available.

The difference in homocysteine levels between persons homozygous for the abnormal allele (TT) and persons homozygous for the normal allele (CC), from a meta-analysis of 33 studies, is about 2.7 µmol/l.[41] The effect of the TT genotype on serum homocysteine levels varies between individuals and communities because it is subject to environmental influence, in particular serum folate.[44] The variable increase in serum homocysteine means that heterogeneity between studies is to be expected (and has been observed). The heterogeneity and the relatively small difference in homocysteine between TT and CC mean that large numbers are needed to show a statistically

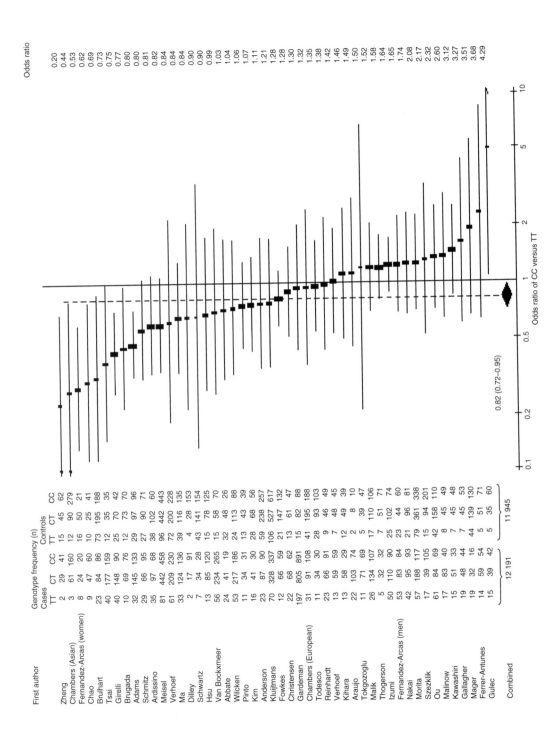

Figure 8.4

Results of published studies of the association between mutation of the *MTHFR* gene and coronary heart disease events: values are odds ratios (95% confidence intervals) for homozygotes for the mutant allele (TT) versus wild type (CC). Reproduced from reference 41 with permission from the BMJ Publishing Group.

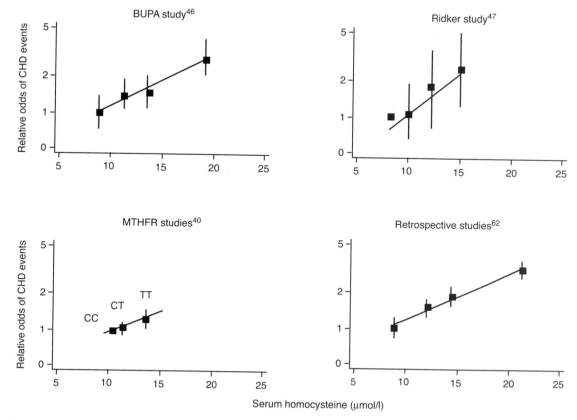

Figure 8.5
Dose–response plots of the incidence of coronary heart disease (CHD) events against serum homocysteine from two prospective studies,[46,47] a meta-analysis of 46 studies on *MTHFR*,[40] and a meta-analysis of seven retrospective studies.[62]

significant association with CHD. It is only recently that sufficient data have become available (through the publication of over 40 studies) to permit a meta-analysis with sufficient statistical power.

Figure 8.4 shows the odds ratios of CHD (95% CI) for CC homozygotes relative to TT homozygotes in order of increasing effect, from a meta-analysis of 46 studies combining data from 12 193 cases and 11 945 controls. Nine of these studies collected data from men alone, two from women alone and 35 from populations consisting of both men and women. The overall summary odds ratio is 0.83 (95% CI 0.72–0.94; p = 0.01), indicating that the risk of CHD is, on average, 17% lower in CC homozygotes than in TT homozygotes.[41] Another meta-analysis yielded a similar result (0.86 (0.78–0.95)).[45] The odds ratio of

0.83 for the average homocysteine difference of 2.7 μmol/l is equivalent to an odds ratio of 0.81 (0.69–0.88) for the 3 μmol/l decrease in homocysteine produced by folic acid (calculated by raising 0.83 to the power of 3/2.7). This is similar to the summary estimate from the prospective studies for the same decrease in serum homocysteine (odds ratio 0.85 (0.80–0.90)).

Interpretation of the evidence on causality

The results from the prospective and the MTHFR studies can be interpreted in two ways – a direct (or

Table 8.1 Summary results (95% confidence intervals) from the *MTHFR* gene studies and the prospective studies on coronary heart disease, deep vein thrombosis, and stroke*

Study type	No. of studies	No. of cases	Odds ratio for 3 µmol/l homocysteine decrease		Odds ratio expressed as risk reduction
Coronary heart disease					
MTHFR	46	12 193	0.81 (0.69–0.88)	0.84 (0.80–0.89)	16% (11–20%)
Prospective†	16	3144	0.85 (0.80–0.90)		
Deep vein thrombosis					
MTHFR	26	3439	0.75 (0.62–0.92)		25% (8–38%)
Stroke					
MTHFR	7	1217	0.74 (0.43–1.28)	0.76 (0.67–0.85)	24% (15–33%)
Prospective†	8	676	0.76 (0.67–0.86)		

*Results taken from reference 41.
†Prospective studies adjusted for regression dilution bias, and for age, sex, blood pressure, and serum cholesterol in all studies, except age and sex only in one.

causal) explanation or an indirect (or noncausal) explanation. An indirect (noncausal) explanation would depend on the prospective and MTHFR studies both showing associations with homocysteine through confounding. In the MTHFR studies the homocysteine difference arises from a single gene mutation effectively allocated at random throughout the population through the random segregation of alleles during gametogenesis and conception – known as Mendelian randomization. There is, therefore, no basis for expecting that persons with and without the mutant gene would systematically differ in other cardiovascular risk factors. The data from these studies confirm this; there were no statistically significant differences in serum cholesterol levels, blood pressure, or smoking habits between persons with the TT and CC genotypes.[41] The confounding would therefore have to involve some unknown cardiovascular risk factor, controlled by a gene linked to the *MTHFR* gene (i.e. at a neighboring chromosomal locus). Importantly, the proposed genetic linkage could not account for confounding in the prospective studies because it would be too weak to do so, accounting for only one-quarter of the twofold increase in risk observed from the 10th to 90th centiles in the prospective studies. The indirect interpretation relies on two separate explanations for the effects in the prospective and genetic epidemiologic studies that produce nearly identical results for a given difference in

serum homocysteine even though any confounding would differ across the two types of study. This is so complex and improbable that it can be reasonably rejected, leaving the direct (causal) explanation as the simpler and more plausible interpretation of the results.

Dose–response relationship between homocysteine and coronary heart disease

Figure 8.5 shows dose–response plots of the incidence of CHD events against serum homocysteine. Two are shown based on data from prospective studies (one from a study in men[46] and the other from a study in women[47]), with summary estimates of risk close to the median for all prospective studies, one from a meta-analysis of retrospective studies (seven that published individual data on serum homocysteine in cases and controls – so permitting a plot of the combined results)[30–33,36–38] and one from a meta-analysis of the MTHFR studies (plots of relative risk over a narrower range of homocysteine in persons with the CC, CT and TT genotypes).[41]

With disease incidence on the vertical axis (using a proportional or logarithmic scale), the plots yield reasonably straight lines, indicating a constant proportional reduction in risk from any starting point

Table 8.2 Randomized trials of homocysteine reduction with folic acid, vitamin B$_6$ and vitamin B$_{12}$ with vascular disease endpoints[53]

Study	Population	Start	Primary outcome	Intervention	Size
Cambridge Heart Antioxidant Study, UK	MI/angina	1998	MI	Folic acid, 5 mg/day vs placebo	4000
Oxford Study of the Effectiveness of Additional Reductions in Cholesterol and Homocysteine, UK	MI	1998	MI	Folic acid 2 mg/day and vit B$_{12}$ 1 mg/day vs placebo; (SEARCH) study	12 000
Norwegian Study of Homocysteine Lowering with B Vitamins in Myocardial Infarction (NORVIT) Study, Norway	MI	1998	MI	Folic acid 5 mg/day for 2 weeks, then 0.8 mg vs placebo; vit B$_6$, 40 mg/day vs placebo	3000
Bergan Vitamin study, Norway	Stroke/TIA	1997	Stroke	Folic acid 5 mg/day for 2 weeks, then 0.8 mg vs placebo; vit B$_6$, 40 mg/day vs placebo	2000
Prevention with a Combined Inhibitor and Folate in Coronary Heart Disease (PACIFIC) study, Australia	MI/angina and risk factors	1998	Peripheral vascular disease	Folic acid 0.2 or 2 mg/day, vs placebo	10 000
Vitamins To Prevent Stroke (VITATOPS) study, Australia	Stroke/TIA	1999	Stroke	Folic acid 2 mg/day, vit B$_6$, 25 mg/day and vit B$_{12}$, 0.4 mg/day, vs placebo	5000
Vitamins in Stroke Prevention (VISP) study, USA	Stroke/TIA	1998	Stroke	Folic acid 2.5 mg/day, vit B$_6$, 25 mg/day and vit B$_{12}$, 0.4 mg/day vs folic acid 0.02 mg/day and vit B$_{12}$, 0.06 mg/day	3600
Womens Antioxidant and Cardiovascular Disease Study, USA	Vascular disease and risk factors	1998	Vascular disease	Folic acid 2.5 mg/day, vit B$_6$, 50 mg/day and vit B$_{12}$, 1 mg/day vs placebo	8000
Heart Outcomes Prevention Evaluation Study (HOPE-2), Canada	Vascular disease	1999	Peripheral vascular disease	Folic acid 2.5 mg/day, vit B$_6$, 50 mg/day and vit B$_{12}$, 1 mg/day	5000
Vitamin and Thrombosis Trial, Netherlands	DVT/PE	2000	Venous thrombosis	Folic acid 5 mg/day, vit B$_{12}$ 0.4 mg/day, vit B$_6$ 50 mg/day	600

MI, myocardial infarction; TIA, transient ischemic attack; DVT, deep vein thrombosis; PE, pulmonary embolism.

of serum homocysteine. The 95% confidence intervals about the risk estimates exclude a threshold within the population range of values. It follows from the continuous dose–response plots in Fig. 8.5 that, as with the other cardiovascular risk factors, intervention to lower serum homocysteine should not be limited to people with a high serum homocysteine, but should be offered to everyone at high risk whatever the reason for the high risk. The small average homocysteine difference (1 μmol/l) between women and men is therefore of no practical importance as both can expect the same proportionate reduction in risk for a given reduction in serum homocysteine.

Implications for prevention

The summary results from the MTHFR and prospective studies are combined in Table 8.1.[41] The effects on deep vein thrombosis and stroke are also shown to demonstrate the general cardiovascular effect. The overall (weighted average) odds ratio for CHD is 0.84 (0.80–0.89) – an expected reduction in risk of 16% (11% to 20%). This risk reduction is relatively modest compared with the effect of treatments that lower serum cholesterol or blood pressure. Nonetheless, the public health impact would be large because CHD is so common (about 120 000 deaths in the UK and about 400 000 deaths in the US each year).

The ongoing randomized trials of homocysteine reduction

It is generally felt that clinical practice should not change until there are randomized trials that show the effect of treatment on disease events. This, however, is too simplistic. For example, there is no randomized trial evidence of the effect of giving up smoking on the risk of CHD but causality is accepted. It is argued that we have previously been misled by associations in epidemiologic studies (for example, the antioxidant vitamin E and CHD as shown in the US Nurses Study and the US male Health Professionals study[48,49]), since randomized trials failed to demonstrate an effect.[50,51] This is

however not the case because in these examples there was no basis to exclude confounding as the reason for the association. This was always acknowledged and is why randomized trials were needed.[48,49] There was also genuine uncertainty over whether hormone replacement therapy reduced cardiovascular risk, which is why randomized trials were carried out.[52] In the case of homocysteine and CHD the position is different. Unlike vitamin E and hormone replacement therapy there is the genetic evidence from the MTHFR and from the homocystinuria studies, which taken together with the evidence from the prospective studies, leave no reasonable doubt over causality. Randomized trials are not necessary to show that high homocysteine levels cause CVD, but, if sufficiently large and of sufficient duration, may provide evidence of risk reversal and an indication of the time required to realize the full potential 16% reduction in CHD risk.

Table 8.2 lists the ongoing large randomized trials of folic acid, vitamin B_6, and vitamin B_{12} in relation to CVD events.[53] Because the expected effect of homocysteine reduction on CHD prevention is modest, the trials need to be extremely large to have sufficient statistical power to show it. A trial of recurrent CHD events (a secondary prevention trial) would require about 15 000 participants followed for 5 years to demonstrate the expected 16% reduction in CHD events. None of the ongoing trials are this large. The introduction of folic acid fortification of flour (to prevent neural tube defects) in the US and other countries has, furthermore, reduced the statistical power by reducing the already small homocysteine difference between treated and control groups (since the control as well as the treated individuals are now receiving some folic acid through their diet).

Five randomized trials have so far been published. There has been a tendency for these to be interpreted as either positive or negative when, in fact, they lack the statistical power to be informative;[54–58] their confidence intervals are consistent with no effect and with the expected modest effect. Furthermore, their average follow-up period of 2 years may be too short to show the expected effect on CVD events. With serum cholesterol reduction, for example, it takes over 2 years to show the expected risk reduction in CHD events[59] and a similar period might be needed with serum homocysteine reduction.

Over the next few years evidence from other randomized trials will emerge and it will be important to avoid interpreting nonsignificant results as negative – to avoid concluding that no evidence of an effect is evidence of no effect.[60] The focus should be on whether the confidence intervals for the effect on CHD events include the expected relative risk of 0.84 for a 3 μmol/l homocysteine reduction. Only if they include 1.0 but exclude 0.84 is there reason to question this expectation.

Conclusion

Five observations arise from the evidence on homocysteine and CHD summarized in this chapter. (1) The genetic (MTHFR) studies show a moderate increase in risk for a moderate increase in serum homocysteine. (2) The prospective studies show an association between serum homocysteine and CVD after allowance for confounding. (3) These two types of study are susceptible to different sources of error but show quantitatively similar associations, a result that is unlikely to have occurred through different potential sources of confounding acting independently. (4) Evidence from in vitro and in vivo experimental studies show that increases in blood homocysteine increase vascular damage through plausible pathologic mechanisms. (5) The homocystinurias cause high serum homocysteine levels and high risks of premature CVD, and lowering serum homocysteine reduces this high risk. These observations provide a strong case for a cause and effect relationship between homocysteine and CHD and therefore a protective role for folic acid in CHD prevention.

Pre-conception folic acid is already of proven benefit to women in the prevention of neural tube defect births and over half the countries in the world have taken action to fortify the diet with up to 0.4 mg folic acid per day for this purpose.[61] In the light of the evidence on homocysteine and CHD, consideration should now be given to increasing the fortification level to 0.8 mg per day to achieve the full potential impact on CHD prevention.

References

1. McCully KS. Vascular pathology of homocyteinemia: implications for the pathogenesis of arteriosclerosis. *Am J Pathol* 1969; **56**:111–28.
2. Hankey GJ, Eikelboom JW. Homocysteine and vascular disease. *Lancet* 1999; **354**:407–13.
3. Homocysteine Lowering Trialists Collaboration. Lowering blood homocysteine with folic acid based supplements: meta-analysis of randomised trials. *BMJ* 1998; **316**:894–8.
4. Selhub J, Jacques PF, Wilson PWF, Rush D, Rosenberg IH. Vitamin status and intake as primary determinants of homocysteinemia in an elderly population. *JAMA* 1993; **270**:2693–8.
5. Mudd SH, Pool JR. Labile methyl balance for normal humans on various dietary regimens. *Metabolism* 1975; **24**:721–3.
6. Kamg SS, Wong PWK, Zhou J, Cook HY. Total homocysteine in plasma and amniotic fluid of pregnant women. *Metabolism* 1986; **35**:889–91.
7. Wald DS, Bishop L, Wald NJ, et al. Randomised trial of folic acid supplementation on serum homocysteine levels. *Arch Intern Med* 2001; **161**:695–700.
8. van Oort FVA, Melse-Boonstra A, Brouwer IA, et al. Folic acid and reduction of plasma homocysteine concentrations in older adults: a dose–response study. *Am J Clin Nutr* 2003; **77**:1318–23.
9. Mudd SH, Skovby F, Levy HL, et al. The natural history of homocystinuria due to cystathionine beta-synthase deficiency. *Am J Hum Genet* 1985; **37**:1–31.
10. Kluijtmans LAJ, Boers GHD, Kraus JP, et al. The molecular basis of cystathionine-synthase deficiency in Dutch patients with homocystinuria: effect of CBS genotype on biochemical and clinical phenotype and on response to treatment. *Am J Hum Genet* 1999; **65**:59–67.
11. Yap S, Naughten E. Homocysteinemia due to cystathionine beta synthase deficiency in Ireland: 25 years experience of a newborn screened and treated population with reference to a clinical outcome and biochemical control. *J Inherit Metab Dis* 1998; **21**:738–47.

12. Wall RT, Harlan JM, Harker LA, Striker GE. Homocysteine-induced endothelial cell injury in vitro: a model for the study of vascular injury. *Thromb Res* 1980; **18**:405–10.

13. Misra HP. Generation of superoxide free radical during the auto-oxidation of thiols. *J Biol Chem* 1974; **249**:2151–5.

14. Harker LA, Slichter SJ, Scott CR, Ross R. Homocysteinaemia: vascular injury and arterial thrombosis. *N Engl J Med* 1974; **291**:537–43.

15. Heinecke JW, Rosen H, Suzuki LA, Chait A. The role of sulphur containing amino acids in superoxide production and modification of low density lipoprotein by arterial smooth muscle cells. *J Biol Chem* 1987; **262**:10098–103.

16. Stamler JS, Osborne JA, Jaraki O, et al. Adverse vascular effects of homocysteine are modulated by endothelium-derived relaxing factor and related oxides of nitrogen. *J Clin Invest* 1993; **91**:308–18.

17. Lentz SR, Sobey CG, Piegors DJ, et al. Vascular dysfunction in monkeys with diet-induced hyperhomocysteinaemia. *J Clin Invest* 1996; **98**:24–9.

18. Celermajer DS, Sorensen K, Ryalls M, et al. Impaired endothelial function occurs in the systemic arteries of children with homozygous homocystinuria but not in their heterozygous parents. *J Am Coll Cardiol* 1993; **22**:854–8.

19. Fryer RH, Wilson BD, Gubler DB, et al. Homocysteine, a risk factor for premature vascular disease and thrombosis, induces tissue factor activity in endothelial cells. *Arterioscler Thromb* 1993; **13**: 1327–33.

20. Rodgers GM, Kane WH. Activation of endogenous factor V by a homocysteine-induced vascular endothelial cell activator. *J Clin Invest* 1986; **77**: 1909–16.

21. Lentz SR, Sadler JE. Inhibition of thrombomodulin surface expression and protein C activation by the thrombogenic agent homocysteine. *J Clin Invest* 1991; **88**:1906–14.

22. Graeber JE, Slott JH, Ulane RE, et al. Effect of homocysteine and homocystine on platelet and vascular arachidonic acid metabolism. *Pediatr Res* 1982; **16**:490–3.

23. Brown JC, Rosenquist TH, Monaghan DT. ERK2 activation by homocysteine in vascular smooth muscle cells. *Biochem Biophys Res Commun* 1998; **251**:669–76.

24. Majors A, Ehrhart LA, Pezacka EH. Homocysteine as a risk factor for vascular disease. Enhanced collagen production and accumulation by smooth muscle cells. *Arterioscler Thromb Vasc Biol* 1997; **17**:2074–81.

25. Southern FN, Cruz N, Fink LK, et al. Hyperhomocysteinaemia increases intimal hyperplasia in a rat carotid endarterectomy model. *J Vasc Surg* 1998; **28**:909–18.

26. Megnien JL, Gariepy J, Saudubray JM, et al. Evidence of carotid artery wall hypertrophy in homozygous homocystinuria. *Circulation* 1995; **91**:1161–74.

27. Loehrer FM, Angst CP, Haefeli WE, Jordon PP, Ritz R, Fowler B. Low whole-blood S-adenosylmethionine and correlation between 5-methylenetetrahydrofolate and homocysteine in coronary artery disease. *Arterioscler Thromb Vasc Biol* 1996; **18**:727–33.

28. Hopkins PN, Wu LL, Hunt SC, James BC, Vincent GM, Williams RR. Higher plasma homocysteine and increased susceptibility to adverse effects of low folate in early familial coronary artery disease. *Arterioscler Thromb Vasc Biol* 1995; **15**:1314–20.

29. Chao CL, Tsai HH, Lee CM, et al. The graded effect of hyperhomocysteinemia on the severity and extent of coronary atherosclerosis. *Atherosclerosis* 1999; **147**:379–86.

30. Verhoef P, Stampfer MJ, Buring JE, et al. Homocysteine metabolism and risk of myocardial infarction: relation with vitamins B6, B12 and folate. *Am J Epidemiol* 1996; **143**:845–59.

31. Malinow MR, Ducimetiere P, Luc G, et al. Plasma homocysteine levels and graded risk for myocardial infarction: findings in two populations at contrasting risk for coronary disease. *Atherosclerosis* 1996; **126**:27–34.

32. Genest JJ, McNamara JR, Salem DN, Wilson PWF, Schaefer EJ, Malinow MR. Plasma homocysteine levels in men with premature coronary artery disease. *J Am Coll Cardiol* 1990; **16**:1114–19.

33. Pancharuniti N, Lewis CA, Sauberlich HE, et al. Plasma homocyst(e)ine, folate, and vitamin B12 concentrations and risk for early onset coronary artery disease. *Am J Clin Nutr* 1994; **59**:940–8.

34. Israelsson B, Brattstrom LE, Hultberg BL. Homocysteine and myocardial infarction. *Atherosclerosis* 1988; **71**:227–33.

35. Schwartz SM, Siscovick DS, Malinow MR, et al. Myocardial infarction in young women in relation to plasma total homocysteine, folate, and a common variant in the methylenetetrahydrofolate reductase gene. *Circulation* 1997; **96**:412–17.

36. Hoogeveen EK, Kostense PJ, Beks PJ, et al. Hyperhomocysteinemia is associated with an increased risk of cardiovascular disease, especially in non-insulin-dependent diabetes mellitus. *Arterioscler Thromb Vasc Biol* 1998; **18**:133–8.

37. Joubran R, Asmi M, Busjahn A, Vergopoulos A, Luft

FC, Jouma M. Homocysteine levels and coronary heart disease in Syria. *J Cardiovasc Risk* 1998; **5**:257–61.

38. Thögersen AM, Nilsson TK, Dahlen G, et al. Homozygosity for the mutation C[677T] of 5,10-methylenetetrahydrofolate reductase and total plasma homocysteine are not associated with greater than normal risk of a first myocardial infarction in northern Sweden. *Coron Artery Dis* 2001; **12**:85–90.

39. Clarke R, Lewington S, Donald A, et al. Underestimation of the importance of homocysteine as a risk factor for cardiovascular disease in epidemiological studies. *J Cardiovasc Risk* 2001; **8**:363–9.

40. Wald DS, Law ML, Morris J. Serum homocysteine and the severity of coronary artery disease. *Thromb Res* 2003; **111**:55–7.

41. Wald DS, Law M, Morris J. Homocysteine and cardiovascular disease: evidence on causality from a meta-analysis. *BMJ* 2002; **325**:1202–6.

42. Homocysteine Studies Collaboration. Homocysteine and risk of ischaemic heart disease and stroke. *JAMA* 2002; **288**:2015–22.

43. Frosst P, Blom HJ, Milos R. A candidate genetic risk factor for vascular disease: a common mutation in methylenetetrahydrofolate reductase. *Nat Genet* 1995; **10**:111–13.

44. Kluijtmans LAJ, Kastelein JJP, Lindemans J, et al. Thermolabile methylenetetrahydrofolate reductase in coronary artery disease. *Circulation* 1997; **96**:2573–7.

45. Klerk M, Verhoef P, Clarke R, Blom H, Kok FJ, Schoutten EG. MTHFR 677C to T polymorphism and risk of coronary heart disease. *JAMA* 2002; **288**:2023–31.

46. Wald NJ, Watt HC, Law MR, Weir DG, McPartlin J, Scott JM. Homocysteine and ischaemic heart disease: results of a prospective study with implications regarding prevention. *Arch Intern Med* 1998; **158**:862–7.

47. Ridker PM, Manson JE, Buring JE, Shih J, Matias M, Hennekens CH. Homocysteine and risk of cardiovascular disease among postmenopausal women. *JAMA* 1999; **281**:1817–21.

48. Stampfer MJ, Hennekens CH, Manson JE, Colditz GA, Rosner B, Willett WC. Vitamin E consumption and the risk of coronary disease in women. *N Engl J Med* 1993; **328**:1444–9.

49. Rimm EB, Stampfer MJ, Ascherio A, Giovannucci E, Colditz GA, Willett WC. Vitamin E consumption and the risk of coronary heart disease in men. *N Engl J Med* 1993; **328**:1450–6.

50. The Heart Outcomes Evaluation Study Investigators. Vitamin E supplementation and cardiovascular events in high-risk patients. *N Engl J Med* 2000; **342**:154–60.

51. Heart Protection Study Collaborative Group. MRC/BHF Heart Protection Study of antioxidant vitamin supplementation in 20 536 high-risk individuals: a randomised placebo-controlled study. *Lancet* 2002; **360**:23–33.

52. Grady D, Herrington D, Bittner V, et al. Cardiovascular disease outcomes during 6.8 years of hormone therapy: Heart and Estrogen/progestin Replacement Study follow-up (HERS II). *JAMA* 2002; **288**:49–57.

53. Clarke R, Collins R. Can dietary supplements with folic acid or vitamin B6 reduce cardiovascular risk? Design of clinical trials to test the homocysteine hypothesis of vascular disease. *J Cardiovasc Risk* 1998; **5**:249–55.

54. Schnyder G, Roffi M, Pin R. Decreased rate of coronary restenosis after lowering of plasma homocysteine levels. *N Engl J Med* 2001; **345**:1593–600.

55. Baker F, Picton D, Blackwood S, et al. Blinded comparison of folic acid and placebo in patients with ischaemic heart disease: an outcome trial (abstract). *Circulation* 2002; **106** (Suppl II):2-741.

56. Liem A, Reynierse-Buitenwerf GH, Zwinderman AH, et al. Secondary prevention with folic acid: effects on clinical outcomes. *J Am Coll Cardiol* 2003; **41**:2105–13.

57. Toole JF, Malinow MR, Chambless LE, et al. Lowering homocysteine in patients with ischemic stroke to prevent recurrent stroke, myocardial infarction, and death. The Vitamin Intervention for Stroke Prevention (VISP) Randomized Trial. *JAMA* 2004; **291**:565–75.

58. Lange H, Suryapranata H, De Luca G, et al. Folate therapy and in-stent restenosis after coronary stenting. *N Engl J Med* 2004; **350**:2673–81.

59. Law M, Wald NJ, Thompson SG. By how much and how quickly does reduction in serum cholesterol concentration lower risk of ischaemic heart disease? *BMJ* 1994; **308**:367–72.

60. Altman DG, Bland JM. Absence of evidence is not evidence of absence. *BMJ* 1995; **311**:485.

61. Wald NJ, Sneddon J, Densem J, Frost C, Stone R. Prevention of neural tube defects: results of the MRC vitamin study. *Lancet* 1991; **338**:132–7.

62. Wald DS, Law M, Morris JK. The dose–response relation between serum homocysteine and cardiovascular disease: implications for treatment and screening. *Eur J Cardiovasc Prev Rehabil* 2004; **11**:250–3.

9

Novel risk factors: C-reactive protein

Mary Cushman

Introduction

Intense interest has recently focused on determining the clinical applications of novel risk factor assessment for coronary heart disease (CHD). In this regard, several domains of risk that can be assessed by measurement of circulating factors have been considered. These domains include coagulation, fibrinolysis, inflammation, and endothelial function, with research related to plaque stability, sex hormones, and oxidative stress on the horizon. Elevated homocysteine as a risk factor is reviewed in Chapter 8.

There are two major purposes of research on novel risk factors: (1) to assess risk factors that will improve identification of individuals at high risk of CHD, so they can be considered for risk-reducing treatments they might not otherwise receive, and (2) to generate hypotheses on new mechanisms of atherogenesis that can be studied in basic research settings. The latter purpose holds much promise in that success may ultimately lead to new therapeutic strategies. As for public health applications, it appears that the use of novel risk factors might be most appropriate for further risk assessment among asymptomatic patients at intermediate global risk based on risk assessment tools such as the Framingham Risk Score.[1] This is because persons at high risk already require aggressive preventive therapy, while persons at low risk would be less likely to benefit from preventive treatments given their low risk status. For those at intermediate risk, presence of a novel risk factor might indicate earlier or more aggressive risk

factor intervention. This chapter will focus on the role of inflammation factors in the primary prevention of CHD, focusing on the most promising clinical measure to date, C-reactive protein (CRP).

Inflammation is central to atherogenesis.[2] The earliest stage of plaque formation, the fatty streak, is primarily an inflammatory lesion, with upregulation of endothelial surface adhesion molecules, leukocyte adhesion and migration into the subendothelium, foam cell formation, and T lymphocyte activation. At later stages in plaque progression, inflammation plays a crucial role in plaque rupture. The coagulation system is also an important component, with thrombus formation on a ruptured or eroded atherosclerotic plaque as the pathological basis of acute myocardial infarction (MI). Inflammation and coagulation balance are closely interconnected, with activation of one leading to activation of the other, and vice versa.[3] There are statistical correlations among circulating levels of inflammation and coagulation factors. For example, fibrinogen and CRP are correlated owing to fibrinogen's role as both an inflammation-sensitive protein and a coagulation factor. CRP also may activate coagulation, as indicated by its ability to indirectly stimulate monocytes to release tissue factor.[4,5]

Since the early 1990s, with the development of highly sensitive assays for detection of CRP, over 20 studies have confirmed that higher CRP is associated with increased risk of future MI or stroke in both healthy persons and in those with existing vascular disease.[6] It is important to draw a distinction

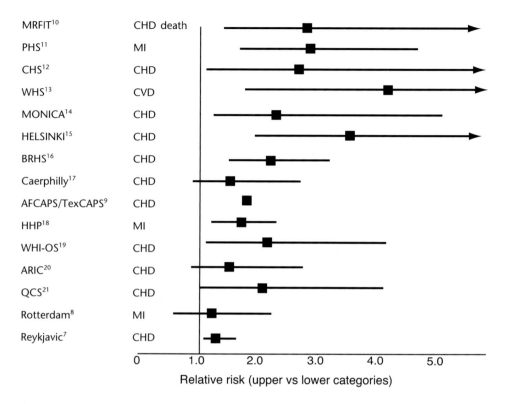

Figure 9.1
Relative risk (95% confidence interval) of future myocardial infarction (MI) or coronary heart disease (CHD) with higher C-reactive protein in prospective studies of participants without cardiovascular disease at baseline. Data are from references 7–21.

between the highly sensitive CRP assays (so-called 'hs-CRP') and traditional less sensitive assays that are used to monitor chronic infections. The latter may not be used in vascular risk assessment, even though values may be reported with this assay within the range of the high sensitivity assay.

Epidemiology of C-reactive protein

Findings of many observational studies of CRP and risk of future vascular events conducted among those healthy at baseline are depicted in Fig. 9.1.[7–21] In these studies, asymptomatic participants underwent baseline risk factor screening and were followed for

variable durations of time. Baseline levels of CRP were then related to the risk of future vascular outcomes. Although some heterogeneity of findings is observed, a consistent association of higher CRP with future vascular events is apparent. These findings have also been extended to prediction of peripheral artery disease,[22] but not venous thrombosis,[23] a different manifestation of vascular disease.

In evaluation of the epidemiologic data, there is less information available from studies specifically analyzing the association of CRP with coronary disease risk among women. In a 2004 meta-analysis, the association of CRP with risk of coronary events was similar in women and men, based on studies involving 1325 cases in women and over 4000 men.[7] The two largest studies of women were the Women's Health Study, an ongoing prevention trial including

28 345 female health professionals, and the Women's Health Initiative (WHI) Observational Study, a study of 75 343 women who were ineligible or unwilling to participate in the WHI hormone and dietary modification trials. Both studies consisted of primarily middle-aged women with follow-up of 8 and 2.9 years, respectively, after CRP and other risk factors were assessed. In the Women's Health Study, CRP provided better risk prediction of MI than low-density lipoprotein (LDL) cholesterol.[24] CRP measurement also added to information gained from determination of global risk with the Framingham Risk Score.[25] Another report from a large study included 18 569 residents of Reykjavik, Iceland, who were followed for nearly 20 years. Over 2400 cases of coronary outcomes were analyzed, but sex-specific incidences were not reported.[7]

Role of C-reactive protein screening

In considering carefully the role for CRP screening for middle-aged women, it is necessary to understand the absolute risk of events with higher CRP. Few studies have measured CRP in all study participants and then followed them over time to allow calculation of absolute incidences. Most studies have not been designed to do this, as they have only measured CRP using a nested case–control study design (measurement on a subset). In the Women's Health Study, CRP was measured in most of the 28 345 participants, and the coronary event rate with elevated CRP was low at about 3.5% over 8 years of follow-up, despite a high relative risk of over 4 for higher CRP. Even women with high CRP and high LDL cholesterol (>130 mg/dl) in this study only had an 8-year rate of MI of 4%, while women with high CRP and lower LDL had an 8-year rate of about 2% (Fig. 9.2).[24,26] This raises the question of whether CRP screening in middle-aged women would be cost-effective or efficient.[27]

It is possible that CRP screening for consideration of prevention of a first MI or stroke would be more useful in older than younger subjects, as they have a much higher incidence of cardiovascular events. However, little information on elderly women is

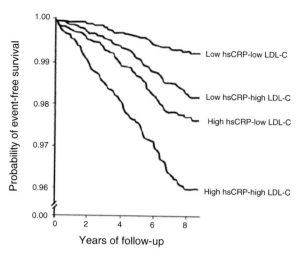

Figure 9.2
Incidence of a first coronary event among women by baseline categories of high-sensitivity C-reactive protein (hsCRP) and low-density lipoprotein (LDL) cholesterol. Data are from the Women's Health Study. Reprinted from reference 26 with permission.

available. After accounting for other cardiovascular risk factors, there was no association of higher CRP with risk of MI in the 7983 older participants of the Rotterdam Study (age 55+ years), although this analysis included only 157 cases and 500 controls and sex-specific analysis was not presented.[8] In the Health, Aging and Body Composition study, which included 2225 men and women aged 70–79 years, with 3.6 years of follow-up, CRP was weakly associated with future CHD events (n = 188), and more closely associated with future stroke (n = 60) or congestive heart failure (n = 92).[28] Separate analyses by sex were not undertaken, and further follow-up is needed to achieve adequately powered analysis. More data focusing on the elderly population are needed, as the public health impact of CRP evaluation in this group might be highest.

As an assay contemplated for clinical use, CRP meets many desired criteria, including good assay reproducibility, a simple laboratory method, low within-person variability, low cost, consistent epidemiologic findings, and additivity to information gained from standard risk assessment.

The clinical use of CRP testing was addressed by a consensus conference in 2003.[29] It was recommended

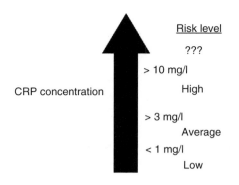

Figure 9.3
Proposed values of C-reactive protein (CRP) indicating increased vascular risk. Adapted from reference 29.

that CRP screening be considered for cardiovascular risk assessment among persons at intermediate vascular risk, based on global risk assessment using a tool such as the Framingham Risk Score. In addition, a cut-off point of >3 mg/l was suggested as a level indicating increased cardiovascular risk (Fig. 9.3).[29] This concentration of CRP would appear to classify approximately one-third of middle- and older-aged adults as having increased risk on the basis of inflammation. The consensus statement also noted that a CRP value above 10 mg/l might indicate clinical inflammation and an underlying cause should be considered. Since that report, it has become apparent that CRP values above 10 mg/l in women may be associated with an even higher risk of CHD than lower values, so this recommendation might require reconsideration.[25] Further, for patients with a value >10 mg/l it is not known what the appropriate work-up should be to determine the presence of an inflammatory disease. In one study of 4517 men and women aged 65 and older without vascular disease, 6% of subjects had CRP >10 mg/l (Cushman, unpublished data). CRP values in this range might be observed with a variety of obvious and occult medical conditions, including cancer. When considering the costs and effectiveness of CRP screening, consideration of the extent of medical evaluation required, and the costs of evaluation of very high levels, is needed.

Pharmacological considerations for C-reactive protein (see also Chapters 4, 25, 26 and 42)

Several drugs are known to influence CRP concentrations. Of relevance to women, statins and menopausal hormone therapy are most relevant. All the statin drugs are known to lower CRP concentrations by about 15%, despite weak associations of CRP with lipid levels. In the CARE (Cholesterol and Recurrent Events) secondary prevention trial and in AFCAPS/TexCAPS (Air Force/Texas Coronary Atherosclerosis Prevention Study), baseline CRP concentration helped identify subgroups who received benefit from statins, even though their lipid levels were not elevated (Fig. 9.4).[9] Specifically, in AFCAPS/TexCAPS, a trial assessing prevention of first MI, 5 years of treatment with lovastatin was similarly effective in MI prevention among those with LDL cholesterol below the median value and CRP above the median value as compared with the overall treated population.[9] These findings raise the possibility that CRP- or inflammation-lowering is an additional mechanism of action of statins in vascular

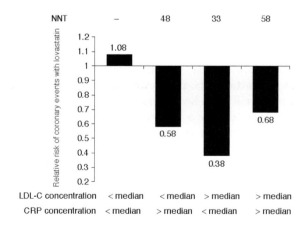

Figure 9.4
Relative risk reduction of coronary events with lovastatin versus placebo in categories of C-reactive protein (CRP) and low-density lipoprotein cholesterol (LDL-C). NNT, number needed to treat. Data are from reference 9.

risk reduction. Indeed, statin therapy appears to have anti-inflammatory mechanisms in addition to lipid-lowering.

In a randomized trial of standard versus high-dose statin therapy among 3745 patients with acute coronary syndromes, those with CRP <2 mg/l after 30 days on treatment had a lower risk of recurrent CHD than other patients, irrespective of the statin dose and achieved LDL cholesterol.[30] In another study, CRP-lowering with statins was correlated with regression of angiographic coronary disease.[31] Whether these data indicate that CRP assessment should be used to guide lipid therapy is uncertain.

To address these questions further, a large trial is ongoing assessing a statin compared with placebo in prevention of first MI among those with normal LDL cholesterol and higher CRP concentrations.[26] This and other studies will help to shape the clinical role of CRP testing for risk assessment and aggressive lipid intervention. Prior to this, CRP screening to prescribe statin therapy in primary prevention settings would be premature.

In 1998 the Heart and Estrogen/progestin Replacement Study (HERS) results indicated no vascular benefit of randomized treatment with conjugated equine estrogen plus medroxyproges-terone acetate compared with placebo among women with established CHD.[32] In a secondary analysis, it appeared that there was an increased early vascular risk and possible later benefit of hormone therapy. Shortly following this, reports appeared documenting a near-doubling of CRP concentration with most commonly used forms of menopausal estrogen therapy, with or without a progestin.[33] It was previously known that hormone therapy was also associated with coagulation activation. Similar effects on CRP were not observed for selective estrogen receptor modulators such as raloxifene and tamoxifen, the latter even lowering CRP.[34,35] Notably, these agents either protect or have no effect on risk of MI. The CRP findings were perplexing, as hormone therapy has anti-inflammatory effects in vitro and in animal models, and simultaneously lowers other acute phase reactants including adhesion molecules, while raising CRP.[33] A lack of effect of transdermal estrogen on CRP[36] suggests that the CRP-raising effect of oral estrogen is related to a first-pass liver effect. Whether this large effect of hormones on CRP

leads to adverse coronary outcomes is currently unknown. Newer data suggest that lower doses of oral estrogen therapy do not alter, or may even reduce CRP concentration,[37,38] leading to interesting hypotheses about the potential utility of low-dose formulations of estrogen for menopausal symptoms or vascular disease prevention.[39]

In 2002, the WHI trial of estrogen plus progestin was stopped early due to an increased risk of adverse health outcomes with estrogen plus progestin[40] (see Chapters 26 and 42). There was a 30% increased risk of MI with estrogen plus progestin over 5.6 years in this study. In an analysis of cases and controls partic-ipating in this study who either did or did not develop MI or stroke, higher baseline CRP concentration did not identify a group of women at higher risk of devel-oping MI or stroke.[41,42] However, these analyses were based on a relatively small number of cases, and it is not known whether the increase in CRP with hormones translates to increased vascular risk. If this were documented, given the other anti-inflammatory effects of hormones, the finding would support a hypothesis of a causal role for CRP in atherogenesis.

Biology of C-reactive protein and atherosclerosis

The associations of circulating inflammation factors with CHD risk probably reflect both the detection of atherosclerosis, and factors related to the progression of atherosclerosis. Imaging techniques, primarily used in clinical research settings since the 1990s, allow quantitative assessment of the atherosclerosis burden across the lifespan, and have facilitated detailed assessment of the inter-relation of novel risk factors and atherosclerosis. Higher CRP levels are associated with impaired endothelial function, and even with increased carotid intima-media thickness in healthy children.[42] Although associations are not always large, in most studies CRP was also higher in healthy adults with, compared with without, sub-clinical atherosclerosis detected with noninvasive tests.[44] In at least one study, higher CRP was associ-ated with greater progression of carotid atherosclero-sis over ~3 years among Japanese patients with hypertension.[45] Among those with angina scheduled

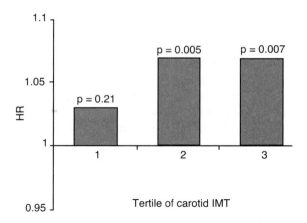

Figure 9.5
Relative risk of stroke by baseline C-reactive protein (CRP) and carotid intima-media thickness (IMT) in the elderly. The relative risk of stroke per 2.38 mg/l higher CRP is shown by thirds of the distribution of carotid IMT. The significance level of an interaction term between CRP and carotid IMT to predict stroke was p = 0.003. Analyses were adjusted for age, sex, ethnic group, diabetes, smoking status, hypertension, systolic blood pressure, and total cholesterol. Data are from reference 47.

for coronary bypass surgery, elevated CRP was associated with presence of unstable carotid artery plaques, visualized by ultrasound.[46]

It may be that inflammation is more important in the presence of subclinical disease than in its absence. This was well illustrated in a study that assessed stroke risk. Among nearly 5400 elderly subjects followed for 10 years, CRP was a better predictor of first-time stroke among those with more subclinical atherosclerosis, suggesting an inter-relation of inflammation and atherosclerosis as an important determinant of clinical events (Fig. 9.5).[47] In a smaller study, the risk of MI was also higher among those with higher coronary artery calcium scores if CRP was also elevated.[48] In an autopsy study of subjects with sudden cardiac death, CRP levels were associated with plaque pathology. CRP was highest in those with acute plaque rupture, followed by those with plaque erosion, then stable plaque, and with the lowest levels in controls who died of noninflammatory conditions.[49] CRP concentrations were also higher in those with greater staining intensity for CRP in macrophages and in the lipid core of plaques, as well as in those with a larger number of thin cap atheroma. Given the findings to date, it is likely that

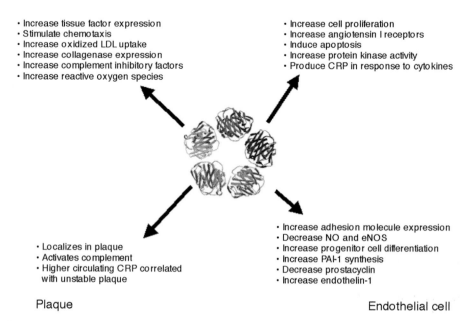

Figure 9.6
Possible roles of C-reactive protein (CRP) in atherosclerosis. LDL, low-density lipoprotein. NO, nitric oxide; eNOS, endothelial nitric oxide synthase; PAI-1, plasminogen activator inhibitor-1. Modified from reference 26.

underlying subclinical atherosclerosis, the precursor to clinical events,[50] causes inflammation, yet inflammation that can be detected through measurement of circulating factors also contributes to the progression of the disease.[51]

Whether or not CRP represents a causal and modifiable risk factor for CHD is a topic of current debate and ongoing study. As for a causal association with CHD, there is little argument that inflammation plays a role in atherogenesis. However, as reviewed by Hirschfield and Pepys in 2003, many studies document possible biological roles for CRP itself, suggesting that CRP is an integral component of the inflammatory processes involved in atherogenesis, and not simply a marker of other inflammation-related mechanisms.[52] Many of these effects of CRP are depicted in Fig. 9.6.[26] Research into drug effects on inflammation and novel drug development

targeting CRP or inflammation will help disentangle these questions. Newer findings, such as the need for depolymerization of the CRP pentamer in order to effect endothelial activation,[53] may provide potential targets for drug development.

At this time it may be appropriate to screen intermediate-risk healthy patients using CRP testing. However, a major obstacle to this is the lack of well-documented interventions once elevated CRP is detected. In addition, the risks to the patient in terms of costs of evaluation and emotional distress require study. This is particularly important given that no specific treatment for elevated CRP can be recommended. Any differing role of CRP in risk prediction in different ethnic groups has not been addressed. The results of ongoing trials, including drug development efforts, will better elucidate the role of this blood test in the future.

References

1. Greenland P, Smith SC Jr, Grundy SM. Improving coronary heart disease risk assessment in asymptomatic people: role of traditional risk factors and noninvasive cardiovascular tests. *Circulation* 2001; **104**:1863–7.

2. Ross R. Atherosclerosis – an inflammatory disease. *N Engl J Med* 1999; **340**:115–26.

3. Levi M, van der Poll T, Buller HR. Bidirectional relation between inflammation and coagulation. *Circulation* 2004; **109**:2698–704.

4. Cermak J, Key N, Bach R, Balla J, Jacob H, Vercellotti G. C-reactive protein induces human peripheral blood monocytes to synthesize tissue factor. *Blood* 1993; **82**:513–20.

5. Paffen E, Vos HL, Bertina RM. C-reactive protein does not directly induce tissue factor in human monocytes. *Arterioscler Thromb Vasc Biol* 2004; **24**:975–81.

6. Libby P, Ridker PM. Inflammation and atherosclerosis: role of C-reactive protein in risk assessment. *Am J Med* 2004; **116** (Suppl 6A):9S-16S.

7. Danesh J, Wheeler JG, Hirschfield GM, et al. C-reactive protein and other circulating markers of inflammation in the prediction of coronary heart disease. *N Engl J Med* 2004; **350**:1387–97.

8. van der Meer IM, de Maat MP, Kiliaan AJ, van der Kuip DA, Hofman A, Witteman JC. The value of C-reactive protein in cardiovascular risk prediction: the Rotterdam Study. *Arch Intern Med* 2003; **163**:1323–8.

9. Ridker PM, Rifai N, Clearfield M, et al. Measurement of C-reactive protein for the targeting of statin therapy in the primary prevention of acute coronary events. *N Engl J Med* 2001; **344**:1959–65.

10. Kuller LH, Tracy RP, Shaten J, Meilahn EN. Relation of C-reactive protein and coronary heart disease in the MRFIT nested case–control study. *Am J Epidemiol* 1996; **144**:537–47.

11. Ridker PM, Cushman M, Stampfer MJ, Tracy RP, Hennekens CH. Inflammation, aspirin, and the risk of cardiovascular disease in apparently healthy men. *N Engl J Med* 1997; **336**:973–9.

12. Tracy RP, Lemaitre RN, Psaty BM, et al. Relationship of C-reactive protein to risk of cardiovascular disease in the elderly: results from the Cardiovascular Health Study and the Rural Health Promotion Project. *Arterioscler Thromb Vasc Biol* 1997; **17**:1121–7.

13. Ridker PM, Buring JE, Shih J, Matias M, Hennekens CH. A prospective study of C-reactive protein and risk of future cardiovascular events among apparently healthy women. *Circulation* 1998; **98**:731–3.

14. Koenig W, Sund M, Frolich M, et al. C-reactive protein, a sensitive marker of inflammation, predicts future risk of coronary heart disease in initially

healthy middle-aged men: results from the MONICA (Monitoring Trends and Determinants in Cardiovascular Disease) Augsburg cohort study, 1984 to 1992. *Circulation* 1999; **99**:237–42.

15. Roivainen M, Viik-Kajander M, Palosuo T, et al. Infections, inflammation and the risk of coronary heart disease. *Circulation* 2000; **101**:252–7.

16. Danesh J, Whincup P, Walker M, et al. Low grade inflammation and coronary heart disease: prospective study and updated meta-analyses. *BMJ* 2000; **321**:199–204.

17. Mendall MA, Strachan DP, Butland BK, et al. C-reactive protein: relation to total mortality, cardiovascular mortality and cardiovascular risk factors in men. *Eur Heart J* 2000; **21**:1584–90.

18. Sakkinen P, Abbott RD, Curb JD, Rodriguez BL, Yano K, Tracy RP. C-reactive protein and myocardial infarction. *J Clin Epidemiol* 2002; **55**:445–51.

19. Pradhan AD, Manson JE, Rossouw JE, et al. Inflammatory biomarkers, hormone replacement therapy, and incident coronary heart disease: prospective analysis from the Women's Health Initiative observational study. *JAMA* 2002; **288**:980–7.

20. Folsom AR, Aleksic N, Catellier D, Juneja HS, Wu KK. C-reactive protein and incident coronary heart disease in the Atherosclerosis Risk In Communities (ARIC) study. *Am Heart J* 2002; **144**:233–8.

21. St. Pierre AC, Bergeron J, Pirro M, et al. Effect of plasma C-reactive protein levels in modulating the risk of coronary heart disease associated with small, dense, low-density lipoproteins in men (The Quebec Cardiovascular Study). *Am J Cardiol* 2003; **91**:555–8.

22. Ridker PM, Cushman M, Stampfer MJ, Tracy RP, Hennekens CH. Plasma concentration of C-reactive protein and risk of developing peripheral vascular disease. *Circulation* 1998; **97**:425–8.

23. Tsai AW, Cushman M, Rosamond WD, et al. Coagulation factors, inflammation markers, and venous thromboembolism: the longitudinal investigation of thromboembolism etiology (LITE). *Am J Med* 2002; **113**:636–42.

24. Ridker PM, Rifai N, Rose L, Buring JE, Cook NR. Comparison of C-reactive protein and low-density lipoprotein cholesterol levels in the prediction of first cardiovascular events. *N Engl J Med* 2002; **347**:1557–65.

25. Ridker PM, Cook N. Clinical usefulness of very high and very low levels of C-reactive protein across the full range of Framingham Risk Scores. *Circulation* 2004; **109**:1955–9.

26. Ridker PM. Rosuvastatin in the primary prevention of cardiovascular disease among patients with low levels of low-density lipoprotein cholesterol and elevated high-sensitivity C-reactive protein: rationale and design of the JUPITER trial. *Circulation* 2003; **108**:2292–7.

27. Blake GJ, Ridker PM, Kuntz KM. Potential cost-effectiveness of C-reactive protein screening followed by targeted statin therapy for the primary prevention of cardiovascular disease among patients without overt hyperlipidemia. *Am J Med* 2003; **114**:485–94.

28. Cesari M, Penninx BW, Newman AB, et al. Inflammatory markers and onset of cardiovascular events: results from the Health ABC study. *Circulation* 2003; **108**:2317–22.

29. Pearson TA, Mensah GA, Alexander RW, et al. Markers of inflammation and cardiovascular disease: application to clinical and public health practice: a statement for healthcare professionals from the Centers for Disease Control and Prevention and the American Heart Association. *Circulation* 2003; **107**:499–511.

30. Ridker PM, Cannon CP, Morrow D, et al. C-reactive protein levels and outcomes after statin therapy. *N Engl J Med* 2005; **352**:20–8.

31. Nissen SE, Tuzcu EM, Schoenhagen P, et al. Statin therapy, LDL cholesterol, C-reactive protein and coronary artery disease. *N Engl J Med* 2005; **352**:29-38.

32. Hulley S, Grady D, Bush T, et al. Randomized trial of estrogen plus progestin for secondary prevention of coronary heart disease in postmenopausal women. *JAMA* 1998; **280**:605–13.

33. Cushman M, Legault C, Barrett-Connor E, et al. Effect of postmenopausal hormones on inflammation-sensitive proteins: the Postmenopausal Estrogen/Progestin Interventions (PEPI) study. *Circulation* 1999; **100**:717–22.

34. Walsh BW, Paul S, Wild RA, et al. The effects of raloxifene compared with hormone replacement therapy on homocysteine and C-reactive protein in healthy postmenopausal women: a randomized controlled trial. *J Clin Endocrinol Metab* 2000; **85**:214–18.

35. Cushman M, Costantino JP, Tracy RP, et al. Tamoxifen and cardiac risk factors in healthy women: suggestion of an anti-inflammatory effect. *Arterioscler Thromb Vasc Biol* 2001; **2**:255–61.

36. Sattar N, Perera M, Small M, Lumsden MA. Hormone replacement therapy and sensitive C-reactive protein concentration in women with type-2 diabetes. *Lancet* 1999; **354**:487–8.

37. Prestwood KM, Unson C, Kulldorff M, Cushman M.

The effect of different doses of micronized 17beta-estradiol on C-reactive protein, interleukin-6, and lipids in older women. *J Gerontol A Biol Sci Med Sci* 2004; **59**:827–32.

38. Wakatsuki A, Ikenoue N, Shinohara K, Watanabe K, Fukaya T. Effect of lower dosage of oral conjugated equine estrogen on inflammatory markers and endothelial function in healthy postmenopausal women. *Arterioscler Thromb Vasc Biol* 2004; **24**:571–6.

39. Ferrara A, Quesenberry CP, Karter AJ, Njoroge CW, Jacobson AS, Selby JV. Current use of unopposed estrogen and estrogen plus progestin and the risk of acute myocardial infarction among women with diabetes: the Northern California Kaiser Permanente Diabetes Registry, 1995–1998. *Circulation* 2003; **107**:43–8.

40. Rossouw JE, Anderson GL, Prentice RL, et al. Risks and benefits of estrogen plus progestin in healthy postmenopausal women: principal results from the Women's Health Initiative randomized controlled trial. *JAMA* 2002; **288**:321–33.

41. Manson JE, Hsia J, Johnson KC, et al. Estrogen plus progestin and the risk of coronary heart disease. *N Engl J Med* 2003; **349**:523–34.

42. Wassertheil-Smoller S, Hendrix SL, Limacher M, et al. Effect of estrogen plus progestin on stroke in postmenopausal women: the Women's Health Initiative: a randomized trial. *JAMA* 2003; **289**:2673–84.

43. Jarvisalo MJ, Harmoinen A, Hakanen M, et al. Elevated serum C-reactive protein levels and early arterial changes in healthy children. *Arterioscler Thromb Vasc Biol* 2002; **22**:1323–8.

44. Tracy RP, Psaty BM, Macy E, et al. Lifetime smoking exposure affects the association of C-reactive protein with cardiovascular disease risk factors and subclini-cal disease in healthy elderly subjects. *Arterioscler Thromb Vasc Biol* 1997; **17**:2167–76.

45. Hashimoto H, Kitagawa K, Hougaku H, Etani H, Hori M. Relationship between C-reactive protein and progression of early carotid atherosclerosis in hypertensive subjects. *Stroke* 2004; **35**:1625–30.

46. Lombardo A, Biasucci LM, Lanza GA, et al. Inflammation as a possible link between coronary and carotid plaque instability. *Circulation* 2004; **109**:3158–63.

47. Cao JJ, Thach C, Manolio TA, et al. C-reactive protein, carotid intima-media thickness, and incidence of ischemic stroke in the elderly. The Cardiovascular Health Study. *Circulation* 2003; **108**:166–70.

48. Park R, Detrano R, Xiang M, et al. Combined use of computed tomography coronary calcium scores and C-reactive protein levels in predicting cardiovascular events in nondiabetic individuals. *Circulation* 2002; **106**:2073–7.

49. Burke AP, Tracy RP, Kolodgie F, et al. Elevated C-reactive protein values and atherosclerosis in sudden coronary death: association with different pathologies. *Circulation* 2002; **105**:2019–23.

50. Kuller LH, Shemanski L, Psaty BM, et al. Subclinical disease as an independent risk factor for cardiovascular disease. *Circulation* 1995; **92**:720–6.

51. Tracy RP. Inflammation in cardiovascular disease: cart, horse, or both? *Circulation* 1998; **97**:2000–2.

52. Hirschfield GM, Pepys MB. C-reactive protein and cardiovascular disease: new insights from an old molecule. *Q J Med* 2003; **96**:793–807.

53. Khreiss T, Jozsef L, Potempa LA, Filep JG. Conformational rearrangement in C-reactive protein is required for proinflammatory actions on human endothelial cells. *Circulation* 2004; **109**:2016–22.

10

Diagnostic procedures: exercise testing/exercise and pharmacologic radionuclide procedures

Todd D. Miller and Raymond J. Gibbons

Introduction

Stress testing remains the cornerstone of noninvasive evaluation of coronary heart disease (CHD). The most commonly used forms of stress testing in the United States are standard exercise treadmill testing and stress imaging. The most frequently utilized stress imaging procedures include single-photon emission computed tomography (SPECT) and echocardiography. The stress modalities employed with these imaging technologies include treadmill exercise or intravenous infusion of a pharmacologic agent (most commonly the vasodilators adenosine or dipyridamole with SPECT and the synthetic sympathomimetic dobutamine with echocardiography). This chapter will focus on standard exercise treadmill testing and stress SPECT in women. Stress echocardiography and nuclear imaging procedures other than stress SPECT are addressed elsewhere (see Chapter 11).

Women were under-represented in early studies of stress testing. In a meta-analysis of 147 studies published between 1967 and 1986 comparing exercise-induced ST segment depression with coronary angiography, only 10% of 24 074 patients studied were women.[1] There is now a larger literature examining the use of exercise treadmill testing and stress SPECT in women. In many recent studies 30% or more of the population have been female. Some studies have examined only women, and many studies have compared accuracy of these techniques between women and men.[2]

Certain principles apply to all stress testing modalities. Stress testing is most commonly performed for diagnostic and prognostic purposes.[3] The gold standard for establishing the presence or absence of coronary artery disease (CAD) remains coronary angiography. Studies that examine the diagnostic accuracy of stress testing compare the stress test results to coronary angiography. Stress test results are characterized as true positive (TP), false positive (FP), true negative (TN), or false negative (FN). Test performance is described in terms of sensitivity (TP/TP + FN), specificity (TN/TN + FP), positive predictive value (TP/TP + FP), negative predictive value (TN/TN + FN), and accuracy (TP + TN/all tests). Since TP and TN rates are <100% and FP and FN rates are >0% for all stress test modalities, the results of a stress test are not truly 'diagnostic' of CAD but only increase or decrease the likelihood that CAD is present or absent after clinical assessment has been performed (Bayes' theorem). Studies that assess prognosis (also commonly referred to as risk stratification) use one of two endpoints: angiographically defined severe (left main and/or 3-vessel) CAD or actual patient outcome. An advantage of using this latter endpoint is the ability to examine the entire study population which undergoes stress testing rather than just the smaller subset of patients referred for coronary angiography. Commonly accepted cut-off points to define low-, intermediate-, and high-risk patients are annual cardiac mortality rates <1%, 1%–3%, and >3%, respectively.[4]

Although this separation of test indication by diagnostic and prognostic purposes is somewhat artificial since testing is commonly done for both reasons in individual patients, test performance is commonly assessed according to either diagnostic or prognostic accuracy.

Prevalence of disease and verification bias

Two issues that markedly impact the apparent accuracy of a stress test relate to the prevalence of CAD in the population being studied and the selection of patients for coronary angiography, a concept known as verification bias (or post-test referral bias). Both of these issues affect the apparent accuracy of all types of stress tests.

Tests generally are less accurate in populations where the prevalence of CAD is low. It is well established that there is a 10–20-year lag in the incidence of CHD in women versus men. As a result the prevalence of CHD is lower in age-matched women versus men, although this gender gap narrows as age increases[5] (Fig. 10.1). The likelihood that a patient with obstructive CAD will have a positive stress test is related to the severity of CAD (positive tests are more common in patients with 3-vessel versus 1-vessel CAD). Since populations with a low prevalence of CAD also have a low prevalence of severe (left main and/or 3-vessel) disease, true positive tests are uncommon, which lowers sensitivity (TP/TP + FN). Additionally, since positive test results occur in patients for reasons other than obstructive CAD, many of the positive tests in low prevalence populations will be 'false positives', thereby lowering specificity (TN/TN + FP). Since premenopausal women have a low prevalence of CHD, the accuracy of stress testing in this population is more limited than in older women.

Parameters that measure test accuracy such as sensitivity and specificity are derived from the highly selected subset of the population referred for coronary angiography. The design of most clinical studies that examine stress test accuracy involves first performing stress testing on a large group of patients and then measuring sensitivity and specificity on the

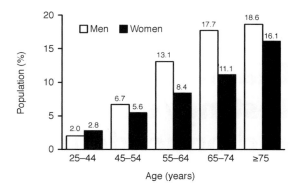

Figure 10.1
Prevalence of coronary heart disease by age and sex according to National Health and Nutrition Examination Survey III, 1988–1994. Reproduced from reference 5.

minority of patients who undergo coronary angiography. Test accuracy on the much larger group of patients not referred for coronary angiography is not determined with this type of study design. Since clinicians who order the stress tests are much more likely to refer to angiography patients with a positive versus a negative test result, the number of positive tests (both TP and FP) is considerably greater than the number of negative tests (both TN and FN) in the angiographic cohort. The net effect of verification bias is to artificially increase sensitivity (TP/TP + FN) and to artificially decrease specificity (TN/TN + FP). One method to overcome the effect of verification bias is to catheterize the entire study population referred for stress testing regardless of the test result. Unfortunately this approach requires an expensive study design in a research setting and has been applied in only a few studies.[6,7] Another approach is to develop a statistical model based on the study cohort referred to coronary angiography to identify the characteristics of this cohort that were associated with referral to coronary angiography. This model is then applied to the entire study population who underwent stress testing to derive estimates of sensitivity and specificity based on the entire study population. This methodology has limitations but arrives at estimates of sensitivity and specificity that are likely more accurate than the apparent sensitivity and specificity derived from the highly selected minority of patients referred to angiography. Only a few studies have utilized this approach.[8–15] *Since most published studies do not adjust for verification bias, their estimates of sensitivity and specificity (which follow throughout this chapter) should be interpreted with great caution.*

Standard treadmill exercise testing

General use

Standard treadmill exercise testing remains a widely utilized form of stress testing. Its advantages over stress imaging procedures include greater availability, simplicity, and lower cost. The hallmark of an abnormal test for diagnostic purposes is ST segment depression. Several meta-analyses examining the diagnostic accuracy of the exercise electrocardiogram (ECG) have been published.[1,3,16] These meta-analyses noted a wide range of values for sensitivity and specificity in individual studies. Average values in the meta-analyses for sensitivity were 67–72% and for specificity 69–84%.[1,3,16] Values for sensitivity and specificity varied modestly depending upon whether patients with prior myocardial infarction (MI), digoxin use, ST depression on the resting ECG, or left ventricular hypertrophy were included or excluded from the analyses. A more recent meta-analysis of the exercise ECG in studies published between 1990 and 1997 of patients who also underwent either exercise SPECT or exercise echocardiography reported a lower average value for sensitivity of 52% but a similar average value for specificity of 71%.[17]

The standard exercise test has also been validated for prognostic purposes. The single most important variable is exercise capacity,[3] usually expressed as minutes on the treadmill or as metabolic equivalents (METs). Variables that reflect exercise-induced ischemia also have prognostic value. These variables are more accurate prognostic indicators when considered together rather than individually. A number of prognostic scores have been developed. The most widely used score is the Duke treadmill score:[18,19]

Score = exercise time (minutes Bruce protocol)
− 5 × ST segment deviation (mm)
− 4 × angina index (0 = none, 1 = non-limiting angina, 2 = angina reason for test termination)

Risk categories based on this score are low (score ≥+5, annual cardiovascular mortality 0.25%), intermediate (score +4 to −10, mortality 1.25%), and high (score <−10, mortality 5%). More recently a number of additional variables have been shown to have prognostic value, including chronotropic incompetence,[20] delayed heart rate recovery after exercise,[21] and ventricular ectopy during and after exercise.[22]

Diagnostic studies in women

Kwok et al.[23] published a comprehensive meta-analysis of studies performed over a 30-year period (1966–1995) examining the accuracy of the exercise ECG in women. They identified 19 studies[24–42] involving 3721 women that met selection criteria (published manuscript, English language, separate reporting of results in women if men also included, and ≥50 women with exercise ECG and coronary angiography). Results are listed in Table 10.1. Weighted mean values were sensitivity 61% (95% confidence intervals 54–68%), specificity 70% (64–75%), positive likelihood ratio 2.25 (1.84–2.66), and negative likelihood ratio 0.55 (0.47–0.62).

Inspection of Table 10.1 reveals a wide range of values among the individual studies for both sensitivity (27–91%) and specificity (46–86%). Methodology was markedly different among studies. The number of women enrolled ranged from 56 to 660. Seven of the studies contained fewer than 100 women. Fourteen of the studies used exercise ECG alone and five also used imaging (the results of which influence referral to coronary angiography). The prevalence of CAD varied from 18% to 67%. Overall, mean age was 56 years with a range of mean age in the individual studies from 49 to 63 years. These numbers suggest that many of the women included in these studies were pre- or peri-menopausal. Other methodologic differences among studies were the inclusion or exclusion of patients with prior MI, digoxin use, and baseline ECG abnormalities. The studies were approximately equally divided between the definition

Table 10.1 Meta-analysis of 19 studies of exercise electrocardiogram 1966–1995 (adapted from reference 23 – not corrected for referral bias)

First author	Tests studied	No. of women (%)*	Mean age (years)	Prevalence of CAD (%)	Baseline ECG abnormalities excluded†	Participants taking digoxin excluded	Upsloping ST‡ positive	Sensitivity of exercise ECG	Specificity of exercise ECG	Likelihood ratio (+)	Likelihood ratio (−)
Barolsky[24]	ECG	92 (52)	50	33	Yes	No	Yes	0.60	0.68	1.86	0.59
Chae[25]	ECG Tl-201	243 (100)	62	67	No	No	Yes	0.27	0.79	1.27	0.93
Chikamori[26]	ECG	132 (36)	63	46	Yes	Yes	Yes	0.82	0.54	1.76	0.34
Ellestad[27]	ECG	188 (34)	59	41	Yes	No	Yes	0.65	0.71	2.25	0.49
Friedman[28]	ECG Tl-201	60 (100)	53	47	No	No	Yes	0.32	0.75	1.29	0.9
Guiteras[40]	ECG	112 (100)	49	38	Yes	No	No	0.71	0.73	2.63	0.39
Hlatky[29]	ECG	613 (27)	53	32	Yes	No	No	0.57	0.86	4.06	0.5
Hung[30]	ECG Tl-201	92 (100)	51	30	Yes	Yes	No	0.75	0.59	1.85	0.42
Marwick[31]	ECG echo	161 (100)	60	37	Yes	No	No	0.77	0.56	1.74	0.41
Masini[32]	ECG	83 (100)	55	47	Yes	Yes	Yes	0.72	0.52	1.5	0.54
Morise[33]	ECG Tl-201	552 (40)	56	37	No	No	Yes	0.51	0.76	2.1	0.65
Pratt[34]	ECG	200 (100)	51	40	Yes	No	No	0.69	0.56	1.56	0.56
Richardson[35]	ECG	62 (100)	53	18	Yes	Yes	Yes	0.91	0.51	1.85	0.18
Robert[36]	ECG	250 (100)	55	44	Yes	–	–	0.61	0.59	1.47	0.67
Sawada[37]	ECG echo	57 (100)	57	49	No	No	No	0.29	0.83	1.66	0.86
Severi[38]	ECG	122 (28)	55	34	Yes	No	No	0.71	0.46	1.3	0.64
Sketch[39]	ECG	56 (22)	50	20	No	No	No	0.45	0.78	2.04	0.7
Weiner[41]	ECG	109 (33)	52	34	Yes	Yes	Yes	0.59	0.81	3.06	0.5
Weiner[42]	ECG	580 (28)	NA	28	No	No	No	0.76	0.64	2.14	0.37
Weighted means								0.61	0.7	2.25	0.55
(95% CI)								(0.54–0.68)	(0.64–0.75)	(1.84–2.66)	(0.47–0.62)

CAD, coronary artery disease; ECG, electrocardiogram; NA, not available; CI, confidence interval.

*Percentage of total subjects who were women.

†These studies excluded participants with bundle branch block, Q waves, and left ventricular hypertrophy on the resting ECG.

‡Upsloping ST segment depression considered a positive exercise electrocardiographic test.

of angiographic CAD as a 50% or 70% stenosis and the definition of an ischemic exercise ECG to include or exclude upsloping ST segment depression. *It is important to emphasize that the values for sensitivity and specificity for the individual studies listed in Table 10.1 have not been corrected for post-test referral bias.* Additionally, other studies have noted that the accuracy of standard treadmill testing in women can be increased by considering other exercise test variables (including exercise capacity and duration of ST segment depression) rather than ST segment depression alone when interpreting the test results,[43] by using heart rate adjusted ST segment depression criteria,[44] and by considering estrogen status.[45]

Ten of the studies in Table 10.1 reported results in both women and men. In men sensitivity was 70% and specificity was 77%. Given the many differences in methodology, these data should not be over-interpreted but suggest that the exercise ECG is modestly less accurate in women than men. *However, these gender differences in test performance are probably less than commonly believed.*

Potential explanations for lower diagnostic accuracy of the exercise ECG in women

Lower accuracy of the exercise ECG in women has been attributed to a number of factors. The main reason for reduced sensitivity is likely due to lower prevalence of both overall CAD and severe (left main/3-vessel) CAD as discussed above. Average prevalences of overall and severe CAD in women in the angiographic studies have been approximately 40% and 15%, respectively.[23,46] Lower sensitivity may also be related to poorer exercise performance in woman. Exercise performance is usually judged by exercise duration or by myocardial oxygen demand, which can be indirectly estimated by peak exercise heart rate or the product of exercise heart rate times systolic blood pressure (rate–pressure product). Exercise duration and myocardial oxygen demand are often but not always correlated. Some entities (poor motivation, orthopedic conditions) may limit both parameters, but there are other entities (deconditioning, use of beta-blockers) that have a differential effect on these variables. A consistent finding in the litera-

ture has been lower exercise duration in women versus men,[3,47] but recent large series have reported similar peak heart rates and only slightly lower peak blood pressures in women compared with men.[48,49]

Part of the explanation for reduced specificity of the exercise ECG in women is also related to lower prevalence of CAD. The effects of post-test referral bias have been discussed earlier. A practice pattern based on referral of most patients with positive tests and very few patients with negative tests to coronary angiography results in exposing a high number of false-positive tests to a comparatively low number of true-negative tests, resulting in a low value for specificity. However, even after correcting for referral bias, one report suggests that test accuracy still appears to be lower in women than men.[50]

Potential biological reasons for women to develop ST segment depression in the absence of obstructive CAD include the effects of female hormones and differences in coronary artery tone and microvascular function. Estrogen has been noted to have a chemical structure similar to digoxin[39] and has been implicated as a cause of ST segment depression.[45,51,52] This effect of estrogen can be offset by concomitant use of progesterone[52] (Fig. 10.2). Limited evidence

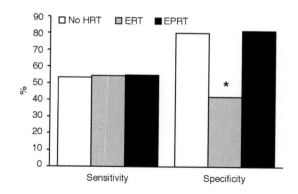

Figure 10.2
Sensitivity and specificity for the stress electrocardiogram compared with gated single-photon emission computed tomography for women on no hormone replacement therapy (no HRT), estrogen replacement therapy (ERT), and estrogen plus progesterone replacement therapy (EPRT). *p <0.01 compared with other groups. Reproduced from reference 52 with permission from American College of Cardiology Foundation.

suggests that estrogen replacement therapy but not naturally occurring estrogen accounts for the increased occurrence of false-positive ST segment depression in women.[53] The majority of patients with cardiac syndrome X (typical angina, positive stress test, normal coronary arteries) are women. Earlier studies examining the pathophysiology of this condition reported conflicting results concerning myocardial ischemia, but recent studies using magnetic resonance imaging (MRI) indicate that myocardial ischemia occurs in some of these patients. Buchthal et al.[54] reported that 20% of female syndrome X patients have decreases in the phosphocreatine:ATP ratio during handgrip exercise. In another MRI study of 20 syndrome X patients (16 women), Panting et al.[55] found that subendocardial hypoperfusion occurs during adenosine infusion.

Prognostic studies in women

There are fewer prognostic compared with diagnostic studies of treadmill exercise testing in women. The Duke treadmill score was originally developed in a population which was 70% male.[18] In a subsequent study the Duke authors compared the prognostic value of the Duke treadmill score in 2249 men and 976 women who underwent both treadmill testing and cardiac catheterization.[56] The authors reported gender differences for women versus men including lower mean treadmill score (−0.3 vs 1.6), lower prevalence of CAD (32% vs 72%) and lower 2-year mortality (1.9% vs 4.9%). The Duke treadmill score provided similar relative prognostic value in both women and men (Fig. 10.3).[56] In a study using the Coronary Artery Surgery Study registry database, Weiner et al.[57] examined the prognostic value of exercise testing in 3086 men and 747 women. Among 28 clinical and exercise test variables, exercise duration was the strongest predictor of outcome. In a subset of 2291 men and 242 women with follow-up for up to 16 years, an exercise test risk classification scheme (based on exercise duration and ST depression) was effective for risk stratification in both women and men (Fig. 10.4).[57] Morise et al.[58] developed a scoring system based on clinical and exercise variables (which included ST segment depression, exercise heart rate, and Duke angina index but not

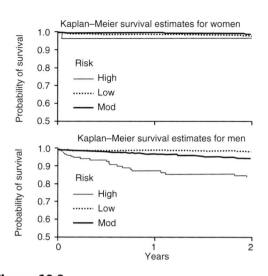

Figure 10.3
Kaplan–Meier curves for 2-year survival for women and men with low-, moderate-, and high-risk Duke treadmill scores. The Duke treadmill score was an independent predictor of survival in both genders. Reproduced from reference 56 with permission from American College of Cardiology Foundation.

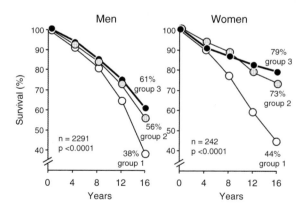

Figure 10.4
Cumulative survival for men and women in the Coronary Artery Surgery Study registry based on the results of exercise testing: group 1 (high-risk) >1 mm ST depression and final stage Bruce protocol <1; group 2 (intermediate risk) >1 mm ST depression and final stage >1 or no ST depression and final stage <2; group 3 (low-risk) no ST depression and final stage >3. Reproduced from reference 57 with permission from Excerpta Medica.

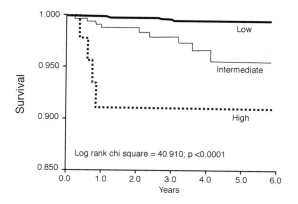

Figure 10.5
Kaplan–Meier survival curves for three exercise test score probability groups. Reproduced from reference 58 with permission from Elsevier.

exercise duration) in a group of 442 women who underwent exercise treadmill testing and coronary angiography and then validated this score in a separate angiographic cohort of 256 women. The prognostic value of this score was then tested in a larger population of 1678 patients. Although only 16 deaths occurred over a mean follow-up of 2.6 years, the score could effectively risk stratify the population (Fig. 10.5).[58] Roger et al.[59] examined the prognostic value of treadmill exercise testing in a community-based population of 1452 men and 741 women and reported similar results for each gender. Workload, positive ECG, and exercise-induced angina were significantly associated by univariate analysis with time to a cardiac event in both women and men. In the multivariate analysis, the only exercise test variable associated with outcome was exercise duration. Although duration was greater in men (10.9 METs) than women (8.5 METs), the predictive power of this variable was similar in women (risk ratio 0.77; 95% CI 0.67–0.89) and men (0.83; 0.77–0.89). These studies in primarily symptomatic populations have been extended to asymptomatic female populations. Three studies, from the Cooper Clinic (3120 women),[60] the St James Women Take Heart Project (5721 women),[61] and the Lipid Research Clinics Prevalence Study (2994 women),[62] have reported that exercise capacity predicts mortal-

ity in asymptomatic women. One of these studies[62] also reported that low heart rate recovery also predicts outcome.

Radionuclide procedures

General use

Nuclear cardiology procedures can be applied to measure left ventricular function and myocardial perfusion. Historically, measurement of left ventricular function (radionuclide angiography) was performed using the radioisotope technetium (Tc)-99m pertechnetate administered either as a bolus (the first-pass technique) or by labeling the patient's red blood cells (the gated-equilibrium technique). The prototype myocardial perfusion agent for several years was thallium (Tl)-201. In the early 1990s Tc-99m-based perfusion agents (sestamibi and tetrofosmin) were approved by the Food and Drug Administration for clinical use. Advantages of these agents over Tl-201 include a higher primary peak energy window (140 vs 80 keV) and minimal myocardial redistribution following injection. Another technical advance was the replacement of the planar imaging method by the tomographic imaging technique. These advances permit gating of the myocardial perfusion images for measurement of left ventricular function. Most laboratories now perform stress SPECT with one of these Tc-99m-based radioisotopes to measure both left ventricular function and myocardial perfusion with the same study.

Stress SPECT has many advantages over standard treadmill testing, including: (1) higher sensitivity for diagnostic testing; (2) incremental prognostic information in selected patients; (3) ancillary information, such as measurement of left ventricular ejection fraction and localization of ischemia; (4) use in patients with an uninterpretable resting ECG, including left bundle branch block, paced ventricular rhythm, and Wolff–Parkinson–White pattern or significant (>1 mm) resting ST segment depression; and (5) use in patients undergoing pharmacologic stress. The major disadvantage of stress SPECT compared with standard treadmill testing is higher cost. In the Medicare population, charges for stress

SPECT are approximately five times those of standard treadmill testing.[4] Stress SPECT should therefore be thoughtfully applied to selected patients in whom the higher cost can be justified by the advantages of stress SPECT over standard treadmill testing.

Several meta-analyses examining the diagnostic accuracy of stress SPECT have been published. The average values for exercise SPECT for sensitivity are 87% and for specificity 64–73%.[17,63] Values for vasodilator SPECT are similar with sensitivity 89% and specificity 75%.[63] As is the case for standard treadmill testing, many of the individual studies included small, highly selected patient populations, and *the values derived for sensitivity and specificity have not been corrected for the effect of referral bias.* In an attempt to overcome the effects of referral bias on specificity, a number of studies have examined 'normalcy rate'. Normalcy rate addresses the concept of specificity (the percentage of patients free of disease who have a normal test) but does not compare true negatives and false positives in the cohort of patients referred to coronary angiography. Instead, normalcy rate is calculated as the percentage of normal tests in the larger population of all patients undergoing stress testing who are at a low likelihood (usually defined as pre-test probability <5%) of CHD on the basis of Bayesian analysis. Average normalcy rate is 91%.[63]

There is an extensive literature that totals more than 30 000 patients examining the prognostic value of stress SPECT.[63] Men account for the majority of patients in most studies. The annual risk of cardiac death or nonfatal infarction in patients with a normal scan is generally <1%, although this risk may be higher in selected patient subsets. The annual risk of a hard event in patients with an abnormal study is generally 2–7%, with higher risk associated with a more severely abnormal scan. Most prognostic studies currently use summed perfusion scores, which are calculated as the summation of perfusion grades assigned to each individual segment in a multisegment myocardial model. These scores include the summed stress score (from the stress images), the summed rest score (from the rest images), and the summed difference or reversibility score (the difference between the summed stress and rest scores). In most studies the variable that has been the strongest prognostic indicator is the summed stress score, which reflects the extent and severity of combined infarction and ischemia. Other prognostic indicators available from stress SPECT include left ventricular ejection fraction, quantitated infarct size, transient left ventricular cavity dilation, and, in studies using Tl-201, increased lung uptake.

Assessment of left ventricular function in women

Women have smaller left ventricular volumes, even after correction for body surface area, and in most studies modestly higher ejection fraction than men.[64–67] Gated SPECT LVEF (left ventricular ejection fraction) may overestimate ejection fraction in women due to smaller chamber size and greater inaccuracy with measuring end-systolic volume. In one study mean gated SPECT LVEF was 51% ± 10% in men and 61% ± 11% in women.[67] Lower limits of normal for ejection fraction by gated SPECT were 43% for men and 50% for women in one study[65] and 41% for men and 49% for women in another study.[66] Although exercise radionuclide angiography is no longer commonly performed, studies using this technique did provide interesting insight into gender differences of the left ventricular response to exercise.[64,68,69] Compared with men, normal responses in women included more left ventricular dilatation and a smaller increase in ejection fraction (and sometimes even a decrease) in response to exercise.

Diagnostic myocardial perfusion results in women

In a meta-analysis of 56 studies published between 1977 and 1986 that examined the accuracy of exercise Tl-201 imaging primarily by the planar imaging technique (tomographic imaging was used in only five of the studies), Detrano et al.[70] reported that the only two variables independently associated with test sensitivity were inclusion of patients with prior MI and the percentage of men in the study group. The percentage of men was not significantly associated with specificity. In older studies using planar imaging that focused specifically on women,[71–73] wide ranges of sensitivity (54–75%) and specificity (59–97%) were reported. In a study that used a combination of

Table 10.2 Diagnostic stress single-photon emission computed tomography studies in women (not corrected for referral bias)

First author	No. of women	Mean age (years)	Prevalence of CAD (%)	Stress type	Exercise radioisotope	Sensitivity	Specificity	Normalcy
Miller[15]	272	63*	62*	TMET	Mibi/Tl-201	0.95	0.21	–
Santana-Boado[14]	63	60	32	Ergo (+Dip 35%)	Mibi	0.85	0.91	–
Iskandrian[74]	266	–	78*	TMET	Tl-201	0.72	0.69	–
	117*	–	–	TMET	Tl-201	–	–	0.93
Taillefer[75]	48	58	67 (50% stenosis)	TMET	Tl-201/Mibi	0.75 Tl-201/ 0.72 Mibi	0.50 Tl-201/ 0.81 Mibi	–
	–	–	58 (70% stenosis)	TMET	Tl-201/Mibi	0.79 Tl-201/ 0.75 Mibi	0.50 Tl-201/ 0.85 Mibi	–
	30	45	–	TMET	Tl-201/Mibi	–	–	0.77 Tl-201/ 0.87 Mibi
Chae[76]	243	62	–	TMET	Tl-201	0.71	0.65	–
VanTrain[77]	52	–	71	TMET	Tl-201	0.95	0.62	–
	20	–	–	TMET	Tl-201	–	–	0.75
Pharmacologic								
Miller[15]	205	63*	62*	Adeno–Dip	Mibi/Tl-201	0.99	0.17	–
Travin[78]	58	68	72	Dip	Mibi	1.00	0.19	–
Ho[79]	44	62	57	Dip–Dob	Tl-201	0.79	0.75	–
Elhendy[80]	70	58	64	Dob	Mibi	0.64	0.72	–
Iskandrian[74]	233	–	78*	Adeno	Tl-201	0.84	0.85	–
	117*	–	–	Adeno	Tl-201	–	–	0.95
Taillefer[75]	37	63	86 (50% stenosis) 62 (70% stenosis)	Dip	Tl-201/Mibi	0.75 Tl-201/ 0.72 Mibi / 0.91 Tl-201/ 0.87 Mibi	1.00 Tl-201/ 1.00 Mibi / 0.71 Tl-201/ 0.79 Mibi	–
Amanullah[81]	130	72	72	Adeno	Mibi	0.93	0.78	–
	71	56	–	Adeno	Mibi	–	–	0.93
Kong[82]	43	63	72	Dip	Tl-201	0.87	0.58	–
Iskandrian[83]	63	63	83	Dip	Tl-201	0.87	–	–

CAD, coronary artery disease; TMET, treadmill exercise test; Ergo, ergonometer; Adeno, adenosine; Dob, dobutamine; Mibi, technetium-99m sestamibi; Tl-201, thallium-201; Dip, dipyridamole.
*Refers to total number of women (both exercise and pharmacologic stress) in the study.

planar and SPECT imaging, Morise et al.[33] found that Tl-201 imaging added incremental information to clinical and exercise ECG variables for detection of CAD presence and extent in both women and men. For disease detection the area under the receiver operating characteristic (ROC) curve showed a similar increase with the addition of Tl-201 imaging variables from 0.77 ± 0.02 to 0.83 ± 0.02 in men and from 0.76 ± 0.02 to 0.81 ± 0.02 in women.

A summary of diagnostic studies[14,15,74-83] using stress SPECT in woman separated by exercise and pharmacologic stress is shown in Table 10.2. This table illustrates the relatively small number of published studies of this technique and the small sample sizes in many of the studies. The wide range of values for sensitivity (exercise 71–95%, pharmacologic 64–100%) and even wider range for specificity (exercise 21–91%, pharmacologic 17–100%) in the individual studies reflects differences in methodologies and patients selected for coronary angiography. (*Note that none of the values shown in Table 10.2 have been corrected for verification bias.*) In the study by Miller et al.,[15] adjustment for referral bias (by the Diamond method) changed apparent sensitivity (for both exercise and pharmacologic stress combined) from 97% to 58% and apparent specificity from 20% to 84%. Roger et al.[13] performed a similar study examining exercise echocardiography in women and reported changes in sensitivity from 79% to 28% and specificity from 37% to 85% after adjustment for referral bias. These studies illustrate that referral bias has a major impact on the apparent accuracy of all stress testing modalities. Attempts to judge accuracy of these techniques using coronary angiography as an endpoint can be misleading without adjustment for referral bias.

A small number of studies directly compared accuracy of stress SPECT in women versus men. Two studies[14,74] reported lower sensitivity, whereas three others reported no difference.[77,78,82] All five studies reported no difference in specificity.[14,74,77,78,82]

Potential explanations for lower diagnostic accuracy of stress SPECT in women versus men

Although the gender differences in the test performance of stress SPECT are not well established, there

are a number of factors that could affect test accuracy in women. Analogous to the previous discussion of exercise ECG in women, the main issue affecting sensitivity is prevalence of CAD and severe (left main/3-vessel) CAD in the population. Santana-Boado et al.[14] reported lower sensitivity (85% women vs 93% men) and lower prevalence of CAD (32% women vs 80% men), and Iskandrian et al.[74] reported similar findings (sensitivity for exercise 72% and for pharmacologic 84% in women, for exercise 92% and for pharmacologic 94% in men; prevalence of CAD 78% women, 89% men).

Two gender-related issues that may lower accuracy of SPECT imaging in women are smaller left ventricular chamber size and breast attenuation. Sensitivity may be lower in patients with small hearts because perfusion defects are more difficult to detect in small hearts. Hansen et al.[84] reported that diagnostic accuracy of SPECT Tl-201 was lower in women than men but that this difference disappeared when patients were stratified by left ventricular chamber size. They postulated that the lower accuracy in small hearts was due to the effects of visual blurring. In a subsequent study,[85] however, these authors were unable to demonstrate that diagnostic accuracy in women improved by using either a size- and gender-based normal database or a filtering system that compensated for blurring. Taillefer et al.[86] used a different approach to try to eliminate the effects of blurring on small hearts by applying gating and studying the end-diastolic images only compared with the conventionally acquired summed images. In 53 women who underwent Tc-99m sestamibi SPECT, significantly more ischemic defects were detected by the end-diastolic versus conventional summed technique (173 vs 106, $p<0.001$) with an insignificant trend towards higher sensitivity (84% vs 74%).

The major effect of breast attenuation is to lower specificity. Attenuation artifacts can be fixed or reversible (due to variable attenuation resulting from shifting position of the breasts between the rest and stress studies). In a study using planar Tl-201 imaging, Goodgold et al.[87] reported a significant improvement in specificity for women from 18% to 92% simply by changing the definition of abnormal scan from any perfusion abnormality to only reversible defects or a 'significant' fixed defect. From

Horizontal axis

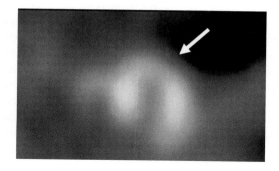

Short axis

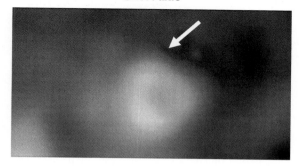

Figure 10.6
A typical example of breast artifact in single-photon emission computed tomography images demonstrating attenuation of technetium-99m sestamibi uptake (arrow) in the apical portion of the left ventricle in the horizontal long-axis view (above) and the anterior and lateral aspects of the left ventricle in the short-axis view at the apical level of the left ventricle (below).

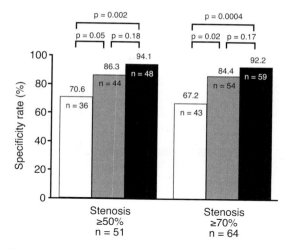

Figure 10.7
Specificity of thallium-201 (open bars), technetium-99m sestamibi (gray bars), and technetium-99m sestamibi with gated single-photon emission computed tomography (solid bars) for patients without coronary artery disease combined with the group of normal volunteers based on stenosis severity ≥50% (left) and stenosis severity ≥70% (right). Reproduced from reference 75 with permission from American College of Cardiology Foundation.

a practical standpoint the large majority of mild fixed defects in the anterior and/or anterolateral segments at the apical and mid levels of the left ventricle in women are due to breast attenuation and generally are not considered abnormal (Fig. 10.6). Other attempts to overcome the effects of breast attenuation and improve specificity include gating for analysis of wall motion[75,88,89] and the use of the higher energy technetium-based isotopes in place of Tl-201.[75] By combining the results of 34 women with a normal coronary angiogram with 30 normal female volunteers, Taillefer et al.[75] reported that 'specificity' increased from 67% for Tl-201 ungated SPECT to 92% for Tc-99m sestamibi gated SPECT (p = 0.0004)

(Fig. 10.7). None of these approaches, however, addresses the problem of reversible defects due to variable breast attenuation. Attenuation-correction techniques have the potential to address this issue but require more extensive testing to demonstrate their superiority.[90]

Prognostic SPECT studies in women

There are pooled data in the literature on over 7500 women with normal stress SPECT and over 5000 women with abnormal stress SPECT,[48,91–114] although results separated by gender were not included in all studies. The annual rate of cardiac death or MI in women with a normal study is <1%. This finding is important because 70–80% of women referred for stress SPECT have normal images.[107,114,115] The event rate in women with an abnormal study is substantially higher and is proportional to the degree of abnormality on the SPECT images. In an early study

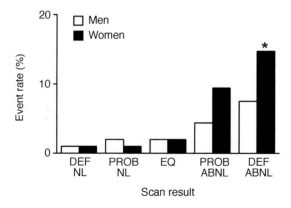

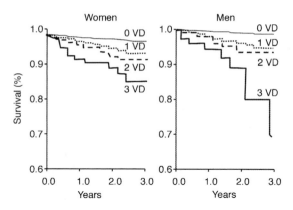

Figure 10.8
Event rates (cardiac deaths and nonfatal myocardial infarctions) in men (open bars) and women (solid bars) as a function of scan result (definitely normal, DEF NL; probably normal, PROB NL; equivocal, EQ; probably abnormal, PROB ABNL; definitely abnormal, DEF ABNL). The event rate in women with definitely abnormal scan results was significantly greater than that in men (*p <0.001). Reproduced from reference 98 with permission from American College of Cardiology Foundation.

Figure 10.9
Kaplan–Meier curves for cardiac survival in women and men as a function of extent of reversible single-photon emission computed tomography perfusion defects, expressed as involvement of 0–3 coronary vessels diseased (VD). Reproduced from reference 107 with permission from Excerpta Medica.

of 243 women who underwent exercise Tl-201 SPECT and coronary angiography, Chae et al.[25] found that multivessel Tl-201 abnormality and exercise heart rate were the only independent predictors of left main/3-vessel CAD. Hachamovitch et al.[98] reported on 2742 men and 1394 women who underwent resting Tl-201/exercise Tc-99m sestamibi SPECT and were followed up for a mean of 20 months. In both sexes the event rate increased according to worsening summed stress score. SPECT imaging variables added incremental prognostic value to clinical and exercise variables but added only 17% more information in men versus 37% more information in women (p <0.0001). Risk stratification was more effective in women because event rates were similarly low in both sexes with normal scans but were considerably higher in women than men with abnormal scans (Fig. 10.8).[98] Data from the Economics of Noninvasive Diagnosis (END) study involving 8411 patients demonstrated that the extent

of ischemia by stress (exercise 7486, pharmacologic 925) SPECT predicted cardiac mortality with equal accuracy in 3402 women and 4500 men[107] (Fig. 10.9). A series of studies from Cedars Sinai have demonstrated the prognostic value of adenosine SPECT in women. In the first study of 130 women who underwent rest Tl-201/adenosine Tc-99m sestamibi SPECT and coronary angiography, the only independent predictors of severe or extensive CAD were the pre-scan likelihood of CAD (p <0.05) and the summed stress score (p <0.0001).[116] In a subsequent study of 923 women who underwent adenosine SPECT and were followed up for a mean of 26 months, these investigators reported that the summed stress score added significant incremental prognostic information to clinical and physiologic variables and could effectively risk stratify the population.[106] In the most recent study, the prognostic value of rest Tl-201/adenosine Tc-99m sestamibi SPECT was compared in 2656 women and 2677 men who were followed up for a mean of 27 months.[114] The summed stress score added significant incremental prognostic information to pre-scan variables in both sexes (Fig. 10.10). The summed stress score was equally effective for stratifying cardiac mortality

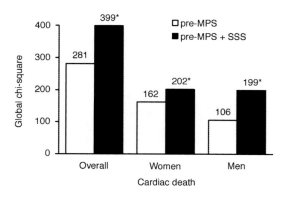

Figure 10.10
Chi-square values from the Cox proportional hazards models for prediction of cardiac death for the overall study cohort, for women, and for men. Increases in chi-square values were significant in all groups (*p <0.00001) comparing pre-myocardial perfusion score (pre-MPS) to pre-myocardial perfusion score plus summed stress score (pre-MPS + SSS). Reproduced from reference 114 with permission from American College of Cardiology Foundation.

risk (ROC area women = 0.78 ± 0.02, men = 0.83 ± 0.02, p = NS).

Summary and recommendations

There is an extensive published literature demonstrating that standard treadmill testing and exercise and pharmacologic SPECT are useful for diagnostic and prognostic purposes in women. The true diagnostic accuracy of these techniques is difficult to determine due to issues related to verification bias. Early studies of exercise ECG included many premenopausal women, in whom the prevalence of CHD is very low, leading to low values for sensitivity and specificity. These results created a perception that standard treadmill testing is of little to no value in women. More recent studies suggest that sensitivity and specificity may be lower in women than men, but gender differences appear to be modest. Comparison of the diagnostic accuracy of stress

SPECT between women and men is especially difficult because of the wide range of values for sensitivity and specificity reported for this technique. Some studies suggest that there are pathophysiologic gender differences (hormones, endothelial function, microvascular function, exercise capacity, left ventricular chamber size, breast attenuation) that may contribute to lower test accuracy of standard treadmill testing and stress SPECT in women. Despite these potential limitations risk stratification appears to be equally accurate in women and men when the same technique (either standard treadmill testing or stress SPECT) is applied.

Some investigators have suggested that stress imaging or even coronary angiography be performed as the initial procedure for evaluation of chest pain in women.[117–119] No study has been performed that prospectively randomizes women presenting for evaluation of chest pain to different testing strategies and proves the cost-effectiveness of a selected strategy over others. Many women have a normal or near-normal resting ECG and can adequately exercise and can be effectively risk stratified using the standard exercise treadmill test.[56] Consider the following example. A 45-year-old premenopausal woman has been experiencing brief episodes of substernal, stabbing chest pain not related to exertion or emotion for the past 3–4 weeks. Her risk factor profile for CHD reveals the following: lifetime nonsmoker, no family history of premature CHD; blood pressure 110/70 mmHg; fasting blood glucose 86 mg/dl; low-density lipoprotein cholesterol 152 mg/dl. Her physical examination and resting ECG are normal. Does this patient need a stress imaging study or will a standard treadmill test suffice? Her pre-test probability of CHD is 10%. Assume she performs a standard treadmill test and completes 10 minutes of the Bruce protocol, with normal heart rate and blood pressure response and without chest pain or ischemic ECG changes. Her post-test probability of CHD is 5%. Her Duke treadmill score is 10, consistent with a 4-year probability of survival of 99%.[19] These values are generally considered to be in a high enough accuracy range to permit clinical decision-making without additional testing.[4]

Nonetheless, some authorities still might raise the following issues. (1) In the example the exercise ECG

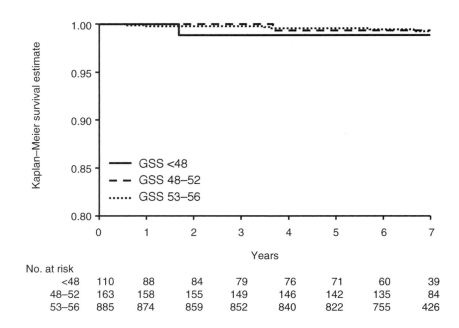

Figure 10.11
Kaplan–Meier survival estimate to cardiac death in the patient cohort with low clinical risk according to the global stress score (GSS): low risk, 53–56; intermediate risk, 48–52; high risk, <48. These patients had excellent survival regardless of the GSS. Reproduced from reference 120 with permission from American College of Cardiology Foundation.

was stated to be negative, but isn't this patient likely to have a false-positive ECG? Couldn't performing a stress imaging study as the initial strategy obviate the need for two tests (standard treadmill followed by stress imaging) caused by a false-positive ECG? Miller et al.[49] examined concordance rates between the exercise ECG and myocardial perfusion imaging in 3213 women and 5458 men with an interpretable exercise ECG and without known CAD. More women (14%) than men (10%) had a positive ECG with normal images (presumed false-positive ECG). The difference between the sexes was statistically significant (p <0.001), but the percentage of false-positive tests was low (<15%) in both sexes, and the absolute difference between the sexes was modest. These results suggest that standard treadmill testing should be the first test performed for evaluation of CHD in both sexes, and exercise imaging could be performed as a sequential testing strategy in the small percentage of patients where the suspicion of a false-positive ECG is high. (2) Even though this patient's post-test probability of CHD with a negative exercise ECG is 5%, couldn't the standard treadmill test still miss severe CHD in a small percentage of patients? Poornima et al.[120] examined the utility of myocardial

perfusion imaging in 1461 symptomatic patients with low-risk Duke treadmill scores to determine if imaging could detect high-risk patients that the standard treadmill test was failing to detect. The value of imaging depended on a patient's clinical risk. In 21% of the patients identified as high clinical risk, imaging (based on the summed stress score) could risk stratify the population further, identifying low-risk (annual cardiac mortality <1%) and high-risk individuals (annual cardiac mortality approaching 3%). However, in the larger (79%) subset of the population with low clinical risk, imaging could not provide further risk stratification. Outcome was excellent (annual cardiac mortality ≈0.25%) in all groups regardless of the results of imaging (Fig. 10.11). In other words, in our patient example with low clinical risk and a low-risk treadmill score, outcome would be predicted to be excellent even if the perfusion images demonstrated a severe abnormality. Stress imaging does not appear to be justified in such patients. At the present time there are insufficient data to recommend routine stress imaging as the initial test for evaluating CHD in women.[3,4] Selected women with baseline resting ECG abnormalities (Wolff–Parkinson–White pattern, left bundle branch block, ventricular pacing, or >1 mm ST segment depression), prior coronary revascularization, or inability to adequately exercise are candidates for an initial stress imaging study.[3,4] A large body of evidence has validated stress SPECT imaging for risk stratification in women.

References

1. Gianrossi R, Detrano R, Mulvihill D, et al. Exercise-induced ST depression in the diagnosis of coronary artery disease: a meta-analysis. *Circulation* 1989; **80**:87–98.

2. Mieres JH, Shaw LJ, Arai A, et al. Cardiac Imaging Committee, Council on Clinical Cardiology, Cardiovascular Imaging and Intervention Committee, Council on Cardiovascular Radiology and Intervention. The role of noninvasive testing in the clinical evaluation of women with suspected coronary artery disease. *Circulation* 2005 (in press).

3. Gibbons RJ, Balady GJ, Bricker JT, et al. ACC/AHA 2002 guideline update for exercise testing: a report of the American College of Cardiology/American Heart Association Task Force on Practice Guidelines (Committee on Exercise Testing) 2002 [http:// www. acc.org/clinical/guidelines/exercise/dirIndex.htm].

4. Gibbons RJ, Abrams J, Chatterjee K, et al. ACC/AHA 2002 guideline update for the management of patients with chronic stable angina: a report of the American College of Cardiology/American Heart Association Task Force on Practice Guidelines (Committee to Update the 1999 Guidelines for the Management of Patients with Chronic Stable Angina) 2002 [http:// www.acc.org/clinical/guidelines/stable/stable.pdf].

5. American Heart Association. Heart disease and stroke statistics – 2004 update. American Heart Association web site [www.aha.org].

6. Froelicher VF, Lehmann KG, Thomas R, et al. The electrocardiographic exercise test in a population with reduced workup bias: diagnostic performance, computerized interpretation, and multi-variable prediction. *Ann Intern Med* 1998; **128**:965–74.

7. Lewis JF, Lin L, McGorray S, et al. Dobutamine stress echocardiography in women with chest pain. Pilot phase data from the National Heart, Lung and Blood Institute Women's Ischemia Syndrome Evaluation (WISE). *J Am Coll Cardiol* 1999; **33**:1462–8.

8. Diamond GA. Reverend Bayes' silent majority: an alternative factor affecting sensitivity and specificity of exercise electrocardiography. *Am J Cardiol* 1986; **5**:1175–80.

9. Diamond GA. How accurate is SPECT thallium scintigraphy? *J Am Coll Cardiol* 1990; **16**:1017–21.

10. Schwartz RS, Jackson WG, Celio PV, Richardson LA, Hickman JR Jr. Accuracy of exercise 201-Tl myocardial scintigraphy in asymptomatic young men. *Circulation* 1993; **87**:165–72.

11. Morise AP, Diamond GA. Comparison of the sensitivity and specificity of exercise electrocardiography in biased and unbiased population of men and women. *Am Heart J* 1995; **130**:741–7.

12. Cecil MP, Kosinski AS, Jones MT, et al. The importance of work-up (verification) bias correction in assessing the accuracy of SPECT thallium-201 testing for the diagnosis of coronary artery disease. *J Clin Epidemiol* 1996; **49**:735–42.

13. Roger VL, Pellikka PA, Bell MR, Chow CS, Bailey KR, Seward JB. Sex and test verification bias: impact on the diagnostic value of exercise echocardiography. *Circulation* 1997; **95**:405–10.

14. Santana-Boado C, Candell-Riera J, Castell-Conesa J, et al. Diagnostic accuracy of technetium-99m-MIBI myocardial SPECT in women and men. *J Nucl Med* 1998; **39**:751–5.

15. Miller TD, Hodge DO, Christian TF, Milavetz JJ, Bailey KR, Gibbons RJ. Effects of adjustment for referral bias on the sensitivity and specificity of single photon emission computed tomography for the diagnosis of coronary artery disease. *Am J Med* 2002; **112**:290–7.

16. Detrano R, Gianrossi R, Froelicher V. The diagnostic accuracy of the exercise electrocardiogram: a meta-analysis of 22 years of research. *Prog Cardiovasc Dis* 1989; **32**:173–206.

17. Fleischmann KE, Hunink MG, Kuntz KM, Douglas PS. Exercise echocardiography or exercise SPECT imaging: a meta-analysis of diagnostic test performance. *JAMA* 1998; **280**:913–20.

18. Mark DB, Hlatky MA, Harrell FE Jr, Lee KL, Califf RM, Pryor DB. Exercise treadmill score for predicting prognosis in coronary artery disease. *Ann Intern Med* 1987; **106**:793–800.

19. Mark DB, Shaw L, Harrell FE Jr, et al. Prognostic

value of a treadmill exercise score in outpatients with suspected coronary artery disease. *N Engl J Med* 1991; **325**:849–53.

20. Lauer MS, Francis GS, Okin PM, Pashkow FJ, Snader CE, Marwick TH. Impaired chronotropic response to exercise stress testing as a predictor of mortality. *JAMA* 1999; **281**:524–9.

21. Cole CR, Blackstone EH, Pashkow FJ, Snader CE, Lauer MS. Heart-rate recovery immediately after exercise as a predictor of mortality. *N Engl J Med* 1999; **341**:1351–7.

22. Frolkis JP, Pothier CE, Blackstone EH, Lauer MS. Frequent ventricular ectopy after exercise as a predictor of death. *N Engl J Med* 2003; **348**:781–90.

23. Kwok Y, Kim C, Grady D, Segal M, Redberg R. Meta-analysis of exercise testing to detect coronary artery disease in women [comment]. *Am J Cardiol* 1999; **83**:660–6.

24. Barolsky SM, Gilbert CA, Faruqui A, Nutter DO, Schlant RC. Differences in electrocardiographic response to exercise of women and men: a non-Bayesian factor. *Circulation* 1979; **60**:1021–7.

25. Chae SC, Heo J, Iskandrian AS, Wassereben V, Cave V. Identification of extensive thallium-201 myocardial scintigraphy in women by exercise single-photon emission computed tomographic (SPECT) thallium imaging. *J Am Coll Cardiol* 1993; **21**:1305–11.

26. Chikamori T, Hirakawa K, Seo H, et al. Diagnostic significance of exercise-induced ST-segment depression in the lateral limb leads in patients with suspected coronary artery disease. *Am J Cardiol* 1995; **76**:513–16.

27. Ellestad MH, Crump R, Surber M. The significance of lead strength on ST changes during treadmill stress tests. *J Electrocardiol* 1995; **25**(Suppl):31–4.

28. Friedman TD, Greene AC, Iskandrian AS, Hakki A, Kane SA, Segal BL. Exercise thallium-201 myocardial scintigraphy in women: correlation with coronary arteriography. *Am J Cardiol* 1982; **49**:1632–7.

29. Hlatky MA, Pryor DB, Harrell FE, Califf RM, Mark DB, Rosati RA. Factors affecting sensitivity and specificity of exercise electrocardiography. *Am J Med* 1984; **77**:64–71.

30. Hung J, Chaitman BR, Lam J, et al. Noninvasive diagnostic test choices for the evaluation of coronary artery disease in women: a multivariate comparison of cardiac fluoroscopy, exercise electrocardiography and exercise thallium myocardial perfusion scintigraphy. *J Am Coll Cardiol* 1984; **4**:8–16.

31. Marwick TH, Anderson T, Williams MJ, et al. Exercise echocardiography is an accurate and cost-efficient technique for detection of coronary artery disease in women. *J Am Coll Cardiol* 1995; **26**:335–41.

32. Masini M, Picano E, Lattanzi F, Distante A, L'Abbate A. High dose dipyridamole echocardiography test in women: correlation with exercise electrocardiography test and coronary arteriography. *J Am Coll Cardiol* 1988; **12**:682–5.

33. Morise AP, Diamond GA, Detrano R, Bobbio M. Incremental value of exercise electrocardiography and thallium-201 testing in men and women for the presence and extent of coronary artery disease. *Am Heart J* 1995; **130**:267–76.

34. Pratt CM, Francis MJ, Divine GW, Young JB. Exercise testing in women with chest pain. *Chest* 1989; **95**:139–44.

35. Richardson MT, Holly RG, Amsterdam EA, Wang MQ. The value of ten common exercise tolerance test measures in predicting coronary disease in symptomatic females. *Cardiology* 1995; **86**:243–8.

36. Robert AR, Melin JA, Detry J. Logistic discriminant analysis improves diagnostic accuracy of exercise testing for coronary artery disease in women. *Circulation* 1991; **83**:1202–9.

37. Sawada SG, Ryan T, Fineberg NS, Armstrong WF, Judson WE, McHenry PL. Exercise echocardiographic detection of coronary artery disease in women. *J Am Coll Cardiol* 1989; **14**:1440–7.

38. Severi S, Picano E, Michelassi C, et al. Diagnostic and prognostic value of dipyridamole echocardiography in patients with suspected coronary artery disease. *Circulation* 1994; **89**:1160–73.

39. Sketch MH, Mohiuddin SM, Lynch JD, Zencka AE, Runco V. Significant sex differences in the correlation of electrocardiographic exercise testing and coronary arteriograms. *Am J Cardiol* 1975; **36**:169–73.

40. Guiteras P, Chaitman BR, Waters DD, et al. Diagnostic accuracy of exercise ECG lead systems in clinical subsets of women. *Circulation* 1982; **65**:1465–74.

41. Weiner DA, and Principle Investigators. Accuracy of cardiomyography during exercise testing: results of a multicenter study. *J Am Coll Cardiol* 1985; **6**:502–9.

42. Weiner DA, Ryan TJ, McCabe CH, et al. Exercise stress testing. Correlations among history of angina, ST-segment response and prevalence of coronary artery disease in the Coronary Artery Surgery Study (CASS). *N Engl J Med* 1979; **301**:230–5.

43. Pratt CM, Francis MJ, Divine GW, Young JB. Exercise testing in women with chest pain: are there additional exercise characteristics that predict true positive test results? *Chest* 1989; **95**:139–44.

44. Okin PM, Kligfield P. Gender-specific criteria and performance of the exercise electrocardiogram. *Circulation* 1995; **92**:1209–16.

45. Morise AP, Dalal JN, Duval RD. Value of a simple measure of estrogen status for improving the diagnosis of coronary artery disease in women. *Am J Med* 1993; **94**:491–6.

46. Cerqueira MD. Diagnostic testing strategies for coronary artery disease: special issues related to gender. *Am J Cardiol* 1995; **75**:52–60D.

47. Shaw LJ, Hachamovitch R, Redberg RF. Current evidence on diagnostic testing in women with suspected coronary artery disease: choosing the appropriate test. *Cardiol Rev* 2000; **8**:65–74.

48. Snader CE, Marwick TH, Pashkow FJ, Harvey SA, Thomas JD, Lauer MS. Importance of estimated functional capacity as a predictor of all-cause mortality among patients referred for exercise thallium single-photon emission computed tomography: report of 3,400 patients from a single center. *J Am Coll Cardiol* 1997; **30**:641–8.

49. Miller TD, Roger VL, Milavetz JJ, et al. Assessment of the exercise electrocardiogram in women versus men using tomographic myocardial perfusion imaging as the reference standard. *Am J Cardiol* 2001; **87**:868–73.

50. Morise AP, Diamond GA. Comparison of the sensitivity and specificity of exercise electrocardiography in biased and unbiased populations of men and women. *Am Heart J* 1995; **130**:741–7.

51. Jaffe MD. Effect of estrogens on postexercise electrocardiogram. *Br Heart J* 1976; **38**:595–9.

52. Bokhari S, Bergmann SR. The effect of estrogen compared with estrogen plus progesterone on the exercise electrocardiogram. *J Am Coll Cardiol* 2002; **40**:1092–6.

53. Morise AP, Beto R. The specificity of exercise electrocardiography in women grouped by estrogen status. *Int J Cardiol* 1997; **60**:55–65.

54. Buchthal SD, den Hollander JA, Merz CN, et al. Abnormal myocardial phosphorus-31 nuclear magnetic resonance spectroscopy in women with chest pain but normal coronary angiograms [comment]. *N Engl J Med* 2000; **342**:829–35.

55. Panting JR, Gatehouse PD, Yang G-Z, et al. Abnormal subendocardial perfusion in cardiac syndrome X detected by cardiovascular magnetic resonance imaging. *N Engl J Med* 2003; **346**:1948–53.

56. Alexander KP, Shaw LJ, Shaw LK, Delong ER, Mark DB, Peterson ED. Value of exercise treadmill testing in women [published erratum appears in *J Am Coll Cardiol* 1999; **33**:289]. *J Am Coll Cardiol* 1998; **32**:1657–64.

57. Weiner DA, Ryan TJ, Parsons L, et al. Long-term prognostic value of exercise testing in men and women from the Coronary Artery Surgery Study (CASS) registry. *Am J Cardiol* 1995; **75**:865–70.

58. Morise AP, Lauer MS, Froelicher VF. Development and validation of a simple exercise test score for use in women with symptoms of suspected coronary artery disease. *Am Heart J* 2002; **144**:818–25.

59. Roger VL, Jacobsen SJ, Pellikka PA, Miller TD, Bailey KR, Gersh BJ. Prognostic value of treadmill exercise testing: a population based study in Olmsted County, Minnesota. *Circulation* 1998; **98**:2836–41.

60. Blair SN, Kohl HW, Paffenbarger RS, Clark DG, Cooper KH, Gibbons LW. Physical fitness and all-cause mortality, a prospective study of healthy men and women. *JAMA* 1989; **262**:2395–401.

61. Gulati M, Pandey DK, Arnsdorf MF, et al. Exercise capacity and the risk of death in women: the St James Women Take Heart Project. *Circulation* 2003; **108**:1554–9.

62. Mora S, Redberg RF, Cui Y, et al. Ability of exercise testing to predict cardiovascular and all-cause death in asymptomatic women: a 20-year follow-up of the lipid research clinics prevalence study. *JAMA* 2003; **290**:1600–7.

63. Klocke FJ, Baird MG, Bateman TM, et al. ACC/AHA/ASNC guidelines for the clinical use of cardiac radionuclide imaging: a report of the American College of Cardiology/American Heart Association Task Force on Practice Guidelines (ACC/AHA/ASNC Committee to Revise the 1995 guidelines for the Clinical Use of Radionuclide Imaging) 2003 [http://www.acc.org/clinical/guidelines/radio/mi_fulltext.pdf].

64. Hanley PC, Zinsmeister AR, Clements IP, Bove AA, Brown ML, Gibbons RJ. Gender-related differences in cardiac response to supine exercise assessed by radionuclide angiography. *J Am Coll Cardiol* 1989; **13**:624–9.

65. Ababneh AA, Sciacca RR, Kim B, Bergmann SR. Normal limits for left ventricular ejection fraction and volumes estimated with gated myocardial perfusion imaging in patients with normal exercise test results: influence of tracer, gender, and acquisition camera. *J Nucl Cardiol* 2000; **7**:661–8.

66. Rozanski A, Nichols K, Yao SS, Malhotra S, Cohen R, DePuey EG. Development and application of normal limits for left ventricular ejection fraction and volume measurements from 99mTc-sestamibi myocardial perfusion gated SPECT. *J Nucl Med* 2000; **41**:1445–50.

67. Kane GC, Hauser MF, Behrenbeck TR, Miller TD, Gibbons RJ, Christian TF. Impact of gender on rest Tc-99m sestamibi-gated left ventricular ejection fraction. *Am J Cardiol* 2002; **89**:1238–41.

68. Gibbons RJ, Lee KL, Cobb FR, Jones RH. Ejection fraction response to exercise in patients with chest

pain and normal coronary arteriograms. *Circulation* 1981; **64**:952–7.

69. Higginbotham MB, Morris KG, Coleman E, Cobb FR. Sex-related differences in normal cardiac response to upright exercise. *Circulation* 1984; **70**:357–66.

70. Detrano R, Janosi A, Lyons KP, Marcondes G, Abbassi N, Froelicher VF. Factors affecting senstivity and specificity of a diagnostic test: the exercise thallium scintigram. *Am J Med* 1988; **84**:699–710.

71. Friedman TD, Greene AC, Iskandrian AS, Hakki AH, Kane SA, Segal BL. Exercise thallium-201 myocardial scintigraphy in women: correlation with coronary angiography. *Am J Cardiol* 1982; **49**:1632–7.

72. Hung J, Chaitman BR, Lam J, et al. Noninvasive diagnostic test choices for the evaluation of coronary artery disease in women; a multivariate comparison of cardiac fluoroscopy, exercise electrocardiography and exercise thallium myocardial perfusion scintigraphy. *J Am Coll Cardiol* 1984; **4**:8–16.

73. Osbakken MD, Okada RD, Boucher CA, Strauss HW, Pohost GM. Comparison of exercise perfusion and ventricular function imaging: an analysis of factors affecting the diagnostic accuracy of each technique. *J Am Coll Cardiol* 1984; **3**:272–83.

74. Iskandrian AE, Heo J, Nallamothu N. Detection of coronary artery disease in women with use of stress single-photon emission computed tomography myocardial perfusion imaging. *J Nucl Cardiol* 1997; **4**:329–35.

75. Taillefer R, DePuey EG, Udelson JE, Beller GA, Latour Y, Reeves F. Comparative diagnostic accuracy of Tl-201 and Tc-99m sestamibi SPECT imaging (perfusion and ECG gated SPECT) in detecting coronary artery disease in women. *J Am Coll Cardiol* 1997; **29**:69–77.

76. Chae SC, Heo J, Iskandrian AS, Wasserleben V, Cave V. Identification of extensive coronary artery disease in women by exercise single-photon emission computed tomographic (SPECT) thallium imaging. *J Am Coll Cardiol* 1993; **21**:1305–11.

77. Van Train KF, Maddahi J, Berman DS, et al. Quantitative analysis of tomographic stress thallium-201 myocardial scintigrams: a multicenter trial. *J Nucl Med* 1990; **31**:1168–79.

78. Travin MI, Katz MS, Moulton AW, Miele NJ, Sharaf BL, Johnson LL. Accuracy of dipyridamole SPECT imaging in identifying individual coronary stenosis and multivessel disease in women versus men. *J Nucl Cardiol* 2000; **7**:213–20.

79. Ho YL, Wu CC, Huang PJ, et al. Assessment of coronary artery disease in women by dobutamine stress echocardiography: comparison with stress thallium-201 single-photon emission computed tomography and exercise electrocardiography. *Am Heart J* 1998; **135**:655–62.

80. Elhendy A, van Domburg RT, Bax JJ, et al. Noninvasive diagnosis of coronary artery stenosis in women with limited exercise capacity: comparison of dobutamine stress echocardiography and 99mTc sestamibi single-photon emission CT. *Chest* 1998; **114**:1097–104.

81. Amanullah AM, Kiat H, Friedman JD, Berman DS. Adenosine technetium-99m sestamibi myocardial perfusion SPECT in women: diagnostic efficacy in detection of coronary artery disease. *J Am Coll Cardiol* 1996; **27**:803–9.

82. Kong BA, Shaw L, Miller DD, Chaitman BR. Comparison of accuracy for detecting coronary artery disease and side-effect profile of dipyridamole thallium-201 myocardial perfusion imaging in women versus men. *Am J Cardiol* 1992; **70**:168–73.

83. Iskandrian AS, Heo J, Nguyen T, et al. Assessment of coronary artery disease using single-photon emission computed tomography with thallium-201 during adenosine-induced coronary hyperemia. *Am J Cardiol* 1991; **67**:1190–4.

84. Hansen CL, Crabbe D, Rubin S. Lower diagnostic accuracy of thallium-201 SPECT myocardial perfusion imaging in women: an effect of smaller chamber. *J Am Coll Cardiol* 1996; **67**:69–77.

85. Hansen CL, Kramer M, Rastogi A. Lower accuracy of Tl-201 SPECT in women is not improved by size-based normal data bases or wiener filtering. *J Nucl Cardiol* 1999; **6**:177–82.

86. Taillefer R, DePuey EG, Udelson JE, Beller GA, Benjamin C, Gagnon A. Comparison between the end-diastolic images and the summed images of gated 99mTc-sestamibi SPECT perfusion study in detection of coronary artery disease in women. *J Nucl Cardiol* 1999; **6**:169–76.

87. Goodgold HM, Rehder JG, Samuels LD, Chaitman BR. Improved interpretation of exercise Tl-201 myocardial perfusion scintigraphy in women: characterization of breast attenuation artifacts. *Radiology* 1987; **165**:361–6.

88. DePuey EG, Rozanski A. Using gated technetium-99m-sestamibi SPECT to characterize fixed myocardial defects as infarct or artifact. *J Nucl Med* 1995; **36**:952–5.

89. Smanio PE, Watson DD, Segalla DL, Vinson EL, Smith WH, Beller GA. Value of gating of technetium-99m sestamibi single-photon emission computed tomographic imaging. *J Am Coll Cardiol* 1997; **30**:1687–92.

90. Hendel RC, Corbett JR, Cullom SJ, DePuey EG,

Garcia EV, Bateman TM. The value and practice of attenuation correction for myocardial perfusion SPECT imaging: a joint position statement from the American Society of Nuclear Cardiology and the Society of Nuclear Medicine. *J Nucl Cardiol* 2002; **9**:135–43.

91. Mieres JH, Shaw LJ, Hendel RC, et al. A report of the American Society of Nuclear Cardiology task force on women and heart disease (writing group on perfusion imaging in women). *J Nucl Cardiol* 2003; **10**:95–101.

92. Machecourt J, Longere P, Pagret D, et al. Prognostic value of thallium 201–single photon emission computed tomographic myocardial perfusion imaging according to extent of myocardial defect. Study in 1,926 patients with follow-up at 33 months. *J Am Coll Cardiol* 1994; **23**:1096–106.

93. Kamal AM, Fattah AA, Pancholy S, et al. Prognostic value of adenosine single-photon emission computed tomographic thallium imaging in medically treated patients with angiographic evidence of coronary artery disease. *J Nucl Cardiol* 1994; **1**:1254–61.

94. Stratman HG, Tamesis BR, Younis LT, Wittry MD, Miller DD. Prognostic value of dipyridamole technetium-99m sestamibi myocardial tomography in patients with stable chest pain who are unable to exercise. *Am J Cardiol* 1994; **73**:647–52.

95. Stratman HG, Williams GA, Wittry MD, Chaitman BR, Miller DD. Exercise technetium 99m sestamibi tomography for cardiac risk stratification of patients with stable chest pain. *Circulation* 1994; **89**:615–22.

96. Heller GV, Herman SD, Travin MI, Baron JI, Santos-Ocampo C, McClellan JR. Independent prognostic value of intravenous dipyridamole with technetium-99m sestamibi tomographic imaging in predicting cardiac events and cardiac-related hospital admissions. *J Am Coll Cardiol* 1995; **26**:1202–8.

97. Pancholy S, Fattah A, Kamal A, Ghods M, Heo J, Iskandrian AS. Independent and incremental prognostic value of exercise thallium single-photon emission tomographic imaging in women. *J Nucl Cardiol* 1995; **2**:110–16.

98. Hachamovitch R, Berman D, Kiat H, et al. Effective risk stratification using exercise myocardial perfusion single-photon emission computed tomography SPECT in women: gender-related differences in prognostic nuclear testing. *J Am Coll Cardiol* 1996; **28**:34–44.

99. Geleijnse M, Elhendy A, Domburg RT, Cornel JH, Reijs AE, Fioretti PM. Prognostic significance of normal dobutamine–atropine stress sestamibi scintigraphy in women with chest pain. *Am J Cardiol* 1996; **77**:1057–61.

100. Travin M, Duca M, Kline G, Herman SD, Demus DD, Heller GV. Relation of gender to physician use of test results and prognostic value of technetium 99m myocardial single-photon emission computed tomography scintigraphy. *Am Heart J* 1997; **134**:78–82.

101. Geleijnse ML, Elhendy A, van Domburg RT, et al. Cardiac imaging for risk stratification with dobutamine–atropine stress testing in patients with chest pain. Echocardiography, perfusion scintigraphy, or both? *Circulation* 1997; **96**:137–47.

102. Boyne TS, Koplan BA, Parsons WJ, Smith WH, Watson DD, Beller GA. Predicting adverse outcome with exercise SPECT technetium-99m-sestamibi imaging in patients with suspected or known coronary artery disease. *Am J Cardiol* 1997; **79**:270–4.

103. Olmos LI, Dakik H, Gordon R, et al. Long-term prognostic value of exercise echocardiography compared with exercise 201 Tl, ECG, and clinical variables in patients evaluated for coronary artery disease. *Circulation* 1998; **98**:2679–86.

104. Alkeylani A, Miller DD, Shaw LJ, et al. Influence of race on the prediction of cardiac events with stress technetium-99m sestamibi tomographic imaging in patients with stable angina pectoris. *Am J Cardiol* 1998; **81**:293–7.

105. Miller TD, Christian TF, Clements IP, Hodge DO, Gray DT, Gibbons RJ. Prognostic value of exercise thallium-201 imaging in a community population. *Am Heart J* 1998; **135**:663–70.

106. Amanullah AM, Berman DS, Erel J, et al. Incremental prognostic value of adenosine myocardial perfusion single-photon emission computed tomography in women with suspected coronary artery disease. *Am J Cardiol* 1998; **82**:725–30.

107. Marwick TM, Shaw LJ, Lauer MS, et al., on behalf of END Study Group. The noninvasive prediction of cardiac mortality in men and women with known or suspected coronary artery disease. *Am J Med* 1999; **106**:172–8.

108. Gibbons RJ, Hodge DO, Berman DS, et al. Long-term outcome of patients with intermediate-risk exercise electrocardiograms who do not have myocardial perfusion defects on radionuclide imaging. *Circulation* 1999; **100**:2140–5.

109. Vanzetto G, Ormezzano O, Farget D, Comet M, Denis B, Machecourt J. Long-term additive prognostic value of thallium-201 myocardial perfusion imaging over clinical and exercise stress test in low to intermediate risk patients: study in 1137 patients with 6 year follow-up. *Circulation* 1999; **100**:1521–7.

110. Soman P, Parsons A, Lahiri N, Lahiri A. The prognostic value of a normal Tc-99m sestamibi SPECT study

in suspected coronary artery disease. *J Nucl Cardiol* 1999; **6**:252–6.

111. Groutars RG, Verzijbergen JF, Muller AJ, et al. Prognostic value and quality of life in patients with normal rest thallium-201/stress technetium 99m–tetrofosmin dual isotope myocardial SPECT. *J Nucl Cardiol* 2000; **7**:333–41.

112. Galassi AR, Azzarelli S, Tomaselli A, et al. Incremental prognostic value of technetium-99m–tetrofosmin exercise myocardial perfusion imaging for predicting outcomes in patients with suspected of known coronary artery disease. *Am J Cardiol* 2001; **88**:101–6.

113. Ho K-T, Miller TD, Christian TF, Hodge DO, Gibbons RJ. Prediction of severe coronary artery disease and long-term outcome in patients undergoing vasodilator SPECT. *J Nucl Cardiol* 2001; **8**:438–44.

114. Berman DS, Kang X, Hayes SW, et al. Adenosine myocardial perfusion single-photon emission computed tomography in women compared with men. Impact of diabetes mellitus on incremental prognostic value and effect on patient management. *J Am Coll Cardiol* 2003; **41**:1125–33.

115. Miller TD, Roger VL, Hodge DO, Hopfenspirger MR, Bailey KR, Gibbons RJ. Gender differences and temporal trends in clinical characteristics, stress test results, and use of invasive procedures in patients undergoing evaluation for coronary artery disease. *J Am Coll Cardiol* 2001; **38**:690–7.

116. Amanullah AM, Berman DS, Hachamovitch R, Kiat H, Kang X, Friedman JD. Identification of severe or extensive coronary artery disease in women by adenosine technetium-99m sestamibi SPECT. *Am J Cardiol* 1997; **80**:132–7.

117. Douglas PS, Ginsburg GS. The evaluation of chest pain in women. *N Engl J Med* 1996; **334**:1311–15.

118. Marwick TH, Anderson T, Williams MJ, et al. Exercise echocardiography in an accurate and cost-efficient technique for detection of coronary artery disease in women. *J Am Coll Cardiol* 1995; **26**:335–41.

119. Kim C, Kwok YS, Saha S, Redberg RF. Diagnosis of suspected coronary artery disease in women: a cost-effective analysis. *Am Heart J* 1999; **137**:1019–27.

120. Poornima IG, Miller TD, Christian TF, Hodge DO, Bailey KR, Gibbons RJ. Utility of myocardial perfusion imaging in patients with low-risk treadmill scores. *J Am Coll Cardiol* 2004; **43**:194–9.

11

Diagnostic procedures: stress echocardiography

P. Rachael James and John Chambers

Introduction

Coronary heart disease (CHD) remains the most common cause of death in the Western world. The initial assessment of a patient with chronic chest pain usually centers around the characteristics of the pain, the coronary risk profile, and the results of noninvasive testing. An exercise electrocardiogram (exercise test) is still routine[1] because it is quick, inexpensive and widely available. However, a substantial number of patients are unable to exercise because of orthopedic, neurologic, respiratory, or peripheral vascular disease. Furthermore, the resting electrocardiogram may preclude interpretation of the ST segment, for example, if there is left bundle branch block, pre-excitation or left ventricular hypertrophy. By contrast, stress echocardiography maintains its efficacy in these situations.[2–4]

Even in patients who are able to exercise, exercise electrocardiography has a sensitivity of only 40–60% for predicting coronary disease at subsequent angiography. Sensitivity is particularly low for single-vessel disease,[4] in the presence of Q waves,[5] and in women.[6,7] Stress echocardiography is more accurate in all these situations.[8] It is indicated as a class I primary investigation in women where there is a high clinical suspicion of CHD.[9]

Stress echocardiography is now used for the prediction of CHD and also for the evaluation of known coronary artery stenoses, the detection of viable myocardium in patients with impaired left ventricular function (contractile reserve), pre-opera-

> **Box 11.1 Uses of stress echocardiography**
>
> Nondiagnostic exercise treadmill test
> Inability to exercise
> Physiological significance of known coronary artery stenoses
> Risk stratification post myocardial infarction
> Evaluation of aortic stenosis with impaired left ventricular function (low-flow low-gradient aortic stenosis)
> Risk stratification pre-noncardiac surgery (e.g. vascular)
> Evaluation of contractile reserve
> Assessment of mitral valve disease

tive cardiac risk stratification for noncardiac surgery, and in the assessment of valvular disease (Box 11.1).

Stress echocardiography in coronary heart disease (see also Chapters 14 and 18)

Ischemia

Myocardial ischemia leads to abnormal wall motion before there are changes in the surface electrocardiogram.[10] Chest discomfort may not occur, but if it does, it is at the end of this 'ischemic cascade' (Fig. 11.1).[11] This explains why echocardiography is more

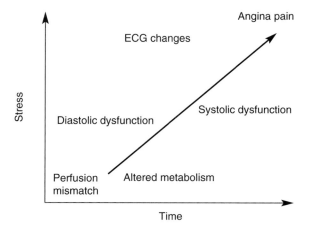

Figure 11.1
Schematic representation of the ischemic cascade, depicting the hierarchy of change which results from reduced perfusion: diastolic dysfunction precedes systolic dysfunction (and the development of a new regional wall motion abnormality), with electrocardiogram (ECG) change and angina as late events.

accurate than electrocardiography for the diagnosis of CHD. This principle was first understood by Tennant and Wiggers in 1935,[12] although stress echocardiography was not described until the 1970s.[13–15] The sensitivity and specificity of stress echocardiography are around 90% (Table 11.1).[4,16–24]

Table 11.1 Sensitivity and specificity of stress echocardiography for the detection of CHD

Reference	No. of patients	Sensitivity (%)	Specificity (%)
Exercise bicycle			
Ryan[4]	309	91	78
Hecht[19]	136	94	88
Exercise treadmill			
Marwick[20]	150	84	82
Crouse[21]	228	97	64
Dobutamine			
Marcovitz[22]	141	96	66
Cohen[23]	52	86	87
Segar[24]	85	95	82

Hibernation

Another application of dobutamine stress echocardiography is in the assessment of myocardial viability in patients with significant left ventricular impairment secondary to chronic ischemia.[25] Prolonged or frequently recurring ischemia and hypoperfusion lead to irreversible tissue damage, fibrosis, and systolic impairment which will not improve with revascularization. However, not all poorly contracting myocardium is permanently damaged and systolic function may improve in response to a restoration in blood supply. Such tissue is termed 'hibernating'[26,27] and it can exhibit temporary improvement in function when stimulated by low-dose dobutamine (typically 5–20 µg/kg/min), reverting to its impaired state with higher doses. The evidence of myocardial viability with stress echocardiography predicts which patients will recover systolic function following revascularization,[28] irrespective of the pattern of resting perfusion.[29] The biphasic response is strongest in predicting functional improvement, while continuous improvement in systolic function with dobutamine does not predict recovery.[30] Furthermore, the detection of viable hibernating myocardium has been shown to have long-term positive prognostic value provided that this is treated. Untreated viability carries a worse prognosis than scarred myocardium.[31,32]

Stress echocardiography and gender

Traditionally women have been largely excluded from studies of noninvasive testing in CHD, despite the condition causing a significant number of premature deaths in women in the Western world. The use of conventional treadmill testing has recognized difficulties in women, but few studies have specifically addressed gender-based differences in the risk stratification of CHD. Despite the fact that there was no gender difference in the false-positive rate of treadmill testing in the large series obtained from the Coronary Artery Surgery Study (CASS), several other studies reported a lower sensitivity and specificity of treadmill exercise testing in women.[7,33–36] There are many problems with exercise testing in women.

Sensitivity is influenced by the lower exercise tolerance of women and increased likelihood of a submaximal heart rate response, together with Bayesian factors which include a lower probability of CHD in women.[37] In addition, false-positive treadmill tests in the female population are not uncommon and may be related to the lower pre-test likelihood of CHD and the higher prevalence of conditions such as hypertension which also result in ST segment changes.[38] Myocardial perfusion imaging is also not without difficulties in women: the sensitivity has been shown to be reduced[39] and anterior wall artifact can arise due to breast attenuation.[40]

Stress echocardiography, using exercise, is more accurate in the diagnosis of CHD in women than conventional treadmill testing.[2,41] Furthermore, the use of exercise or pharmacologic stress echocardiography in women, at low or intermediate pre-test likelihood for CHD, is a new class IIa indication for echocardiography in the recently revised guidelines for echocardiography.[9] The sensitivity of stress echocardiography in women is in the order of 75–93% with a specificity of 82–92%,[17,18,42] which is similar to populations unselected by gender. A positive stress echocardiogram, in women with known or suspected CHD, has significant prognostic value[43] and has been found to yield superior prognostic information when compared with treadmill testing.[44] Furthermore, a negative stress echocardiogram can re-stratify women who had intermediate probability of CHD, into a low-risk population.[45]

How to perform a stress echocardiogram

Choosing the stressor

The initial choice is between exercise and pharmacologic stress. Treadmill exercise is relatively simple to perform, but image acquisition may be difficult due to respiratory artifact. In addition, rapidly resolving wall motion abnormalities may be missed during the time it takes to reposition the patient. Supine bicycle exercise is limited by posture and movement. Many laboratories, therefore, use pharmacologic stress,

usually employing the synthetic catecholamine dobutamine. Dobutamine has predominantly β_1-adrenergic activity and a short plasma half-life of approximately 2 minutes. At low doses, dobutamine increases myocardial contractility but the ensuing increase in oxygen demand is met or exceeded by a concomitant increase in coronary blood flow, due to active vasodilatation. At higher doses, contractility increases further and the heart rate then rises until ischemia develops in the presence of significant coronary stenoses.[46] The concentration of dobutamine necessary to produce such an abnormality is related to the degree of coronary artery stenosis.[46,47] Additional α- and β_2-adrenoreceptor activity tends to have a moderate effect on the systemic vascular resistance.

Other laboratories use vasodilators such as adenosine or dipyridamole, although these agents are contraindicated in patients with a history of bronchospasm. Diagnostic accuracy is similar among all stress modalities[48] (Table 11.1). The choice of stressor depends on the indication for the study, patient characteristics, and individual preference and expertise. A study to detect myocardial viability is usually performed with dobutamine. Younger, fitter patients are often best suited to exercise. Patients with implanted permanent pacemakers can undergo stress echocardiography by incrementally increasing the pacing rate using a standard programmer.

Performing a dobutamine stress echocardiogram

The procedure requires a minimum of two people, usually a doctor and a sonographer. For a diagnostic test, β-adrenergic blockers are withdrawn for at least 48 hours pre-procedure, although for assessment of contractile reserve this is not mandatory.[49] An intravenous cannula is inserted and standard monitoring attached (noninvasive automated blood pressure and electrocardiogram) and a baseline scan is undertaken with the patient in the left lateral decubitus position. Second harmonic imaging is usually used routinely,[50–52] with or without an intravenous contrast agent[53] to enhance endocardial definition, particularly for the free wall of the left ventricle.

Parasternal long-axis, parasternal short-axis, apical four-chamber and apical two-chamber views are generally used and are recorded digitally using a stress package, allowing subsequent split-screen analysis. A five-stage dobutamine protocol is used in many institutions. Dobutamine is usually infused initially at 5 μg/kg/min and increased, at 3-minute intervals, to 10, 20, 30, 40 μg/kg/min. If, despite 40 μg/kg/min dobutamine, the target heart rate is not attained, atropine is administered at peak stress. The addition of atropine serves to increase the sensitivity of dobutamine stress echocardiography, particularly in patients with less severe CHD.[54] For a study assessing contractile reserve to detect hibernation, 5-minute stages up to a dose 10 μg/kg/min are usually used and thereafter 3-minute stages. Side effects are not uncommon with dobutamine, but are usually mild (Box 11.2). Occasionally, a profound vasovagal reaction can occur necessitating the administration of atropine with or without intravenous fluids. A sudden drop in blood pressure during dobutamine stress echocardiography does not have the same adverse significance as in conventional treadmill testing[55,56] and hypotension may be related to the development of dynamic left ventricular outflow tract obstruction.[57] The safety of stress echocardiography is comparable to other stress testing modalities and the incidence of serious arrhythmia or myocardial infarction (MI) is rare.[58–60] However, resuscitation equipment and emergency drugs such as intravenous beta-blockers and fluids must be available.

Reporting the stress echocardiogram

Split-screen analysis permits direct comparison of each view at differing stages of the test, for example, parasternal long-axis images are displayed at rest,

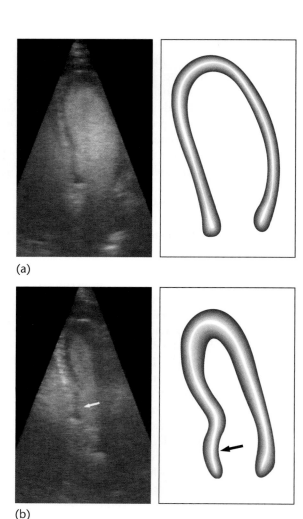

(a)

(b)

Figure 11.2
An apical two-chamber view, with myocardial contrast, during peak dose dobutamine in diastole (a) and systole (b). There is hypokinesia during systole of the mid and basal segments of the inferior wall (white arrow).

alongside images at low- and high-dose dobutamine. This aids the detection of new regional wall motion abnormalities (Fig. 11.2). For analysis a segmental model of the left ventricle, for instance that recommended by the American Society of Echocardiography (Fig. 11.3), is used.[24,61] The normal response to stress is increased wall motion, which encompasses both inward motion of the endocardium and wall thickening. Of these, wall

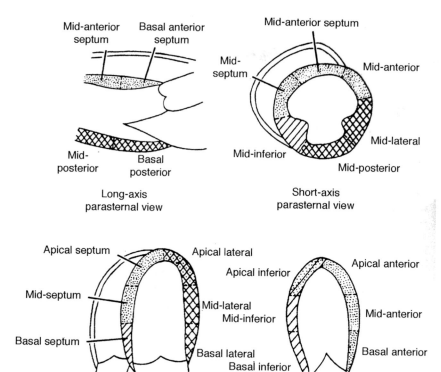

Figure 11.3
The segmentation of the left ventricle by arterial territory. Dobutamine stress echocardiography: correlation with coronary lesion severity as determined by quantitative angiography. Reproduced from reference 24 with permission of the American College of Cardiology.

Left anterior descending distribution
Right coronary artery distribution
Circumflex distribution
Left anterior descending/circumflex overlap
Left anterior descending/right coronary artery overlap

thickening is the more reliable since endocardial motion may be affected by adjacent segments or by gross cardiac motion within the chest cavity. A segment should only be reported if at least 50% of the endocardium can be seen clearly. Each of these segments is graded both at rest and at peak stress, or at the time of any perceived change, either qualitatively or using a scoring system as shown below:

• 1 = normal/hyperkinetic

• 2 = hypokinetic (<50% of the usual inward motion)
• 3 = akinetic (absence of inward motion or thickening)
• 4 = dyskinetic (motion out of phase)
• 5 = paradoxical (motion 180° out of phase; this is often omitted in more modern scoring schedules).

The individual scores are added together and divided by the total number of segments reported, to give a wall motion score index. The normal response to stress is increased wall thickening and consequent hyperkinesis. Myocardial ischemia is defined by the development of hypokinesis, dyskinesis, or akinesis. If wall motion remains unchanged and neither hypokinesis nor hyperkinesis develops, there is a diagnostic dilemma. Many authors interpret this as an ischemic response[21,62] but it may in fact be normal[63,64] and if over-reported it naturally reduces the specificity of the test.[22,65] Over-interpretation of minor wall motion deterioration involving solely the mid or basal inferoposterior segments should be avoided since these are known to be less specific for coronary artery disease.[66,67] Some groups also use evidence of abnormal diastolic filling to enhance sensitivity during dobutamine stress echocardiography. The E-wave velocity of early filling on the transmitral Doppler inflow assessment falls with the onset of ischemia and can be readily assessed during stress imaging.[68]

Stress echocardiography in valve disease (see also Chapter 33)

Low-flow low-gradient aortic stenosis

The hemodynamic assessment of patients with significant aortic stenosis and a normal or mildly hypodynamic left ventricle is usually straightforward. However, difficulties can arise when the ventricular function is severely impaired resulting in low pressure gradients as usually defined by:

- left ventricular ejection fraction <40%
- mean transaortic pressure difference <30 mmHg
- effective orifice area by the continuity equation <1.0 cm^2.

In this group surgical mortality is high (21%) with only 50% of patients surviving for 4 years.[69] Dobutamine stress echocardiography can be particularly helpful to risk stratify patients in this situation and discern low-flow low-gradient aortic stenosis from more minor stenosis with impaired left ventricular systolic function from another cause, e.g. CHD or cardiomyopathy. Usually a maximum dose of

10 μg/kg/min or at most 20 μg/kg/min dobutamine is used. In general, severe aortic stenosis is associated with a relatively large rise in mean pressure difference and a relatively small rise in orifice area. By contrast, moderate stenosis is associated with a small rise in mean pressure difference and a larger rise in effective orifice area. Severe stenosis is present if the mean gradient rises to 30 mmHg or more at any time during dobutamine infusion, as long as the effective orifice area is no greater than 1.2 cm^2.

However, surgical results in patients with low-flow aortic stenosis depend less on the grade of stenosis than on the ability of the left ventricle to recover.[70–72] Therefore, the most important observation during dobutamine infusion is whether the ventricle improves. If the systolic velocity integral reliably increases by >20%, the surgical mortality is relatively lower and the mid-term outlook relatively better than if there is no such increase. Surgical mortality is 5–7% in patients with flow reserve and 32–33% in those without flow reserve.[70,71] Survival at 5 years is 88% after surgery in the presence of flow reserve, but between 10 and 25% if there is no reserve.[72]

Mitral stenosis and regurgitation

Exercise echocardiography, using Doppler, is an accepted and clinically established tool for the evaluation of mitral valve disease. In mitral stenosis, dynamic exercise may precipitate an abrupt increase in the trans-mitral gradient and pulmonary artery pressures.[73–75] It can be particularly helpful in evaluating those patients with moderate mitral stenosis, calculated at rest, with apparently disproportionate symptoms on exercise.[76] Recently, dobutamine stress echocardiography has been used to identify patients with rheumatic mitral stenosis at increased risk of adverse cardiac events and to yield important prognostic information.[77]

Exercise echocardiography has also been used to assess mitral regurgitation. Pulmonary artery pressure and the grade of mitral regurgitation may both be greater on exercise than at rest.[78,79] In addition, there is increasing interest in the role of exercise echocardiography in the evaluation of subclinical left ventricular dysfunction in chronic mitral regurgitation.[79]

Future developments in stress echocardiography

Long-axis function

Long-axis excursion is a measure of the function of longitudinally or spirally arranged fibers in the subendocardial and subepicardial layers of the myocardium, which are responsible for the ventricle becoming more spherical during isovolumetric contraction. The larger intermediate layer of transversely arranged fibers causes ejection of blood during systole. The subendocardial fibers are at greater risk from ischemia than the intermediate layers, so that longitudinal dysfunction precedes transverse dysfunction in patients with CHD, hypertension, mitral valve disease, and dilated cardiomyopathy.[80–83]

Measures of long-axis function using M-mode are more sensitive than wall motion analysis and may allow localization of the coronary stenosis.[83,84] More recently, tissue Doppler has been used to assess delay and velocity of contraction of the mitral annulus. Myocardial velocity, measured using real-time pulsed-wave Doppler, starts to fall progressively after 5 seconds of ischemia[85] and velocities are also low where there is myocardial scarring. A recent study reported sensitivities of 80–93%, depending on the artery stenosed, with specificities of 80–82%.[86] Tissue Doppler has also been used for the evaluation of myocardial viability.[87,88] However, there are drawbacks associated with this methodology,[89] which relate to the influence of factors, other than ischemia, on myocardial velocities such as the movement of adjoining segments with rotation of the heart. Future developments with myocardial strain and strain-rate may overcome these limitations,[90] but they currently remain very much a research tool.

Three-dimensional echocardiography

Commercially available systems now allow rapid acquisition of real-time, transthoracic three-dimensional (3D) datasets. Despite lower frame rate and line density than in two dimensions, estimates of left ventricular mass and volumes are more accurate.[91,92] Since wall motion abnormalities are three-dimensional, it is likely that the technique will also prove superior during stress echocardiography although, to date, limited information exists.[93]

Myocardial contrast echocardiography

Despite the use of second harmonic imaging, which has improved endocardial definition, suboptimal endocardial visualization still occurs and hampers image interpretation. However, trans-pulmonary intravenous contrast agents for blood pool opacification can dramatically improve image quality, endocardial border delineation, and confidence for the interpretation of regional wall motion.[94,95] The use of contrast agents is now widespread, with administration either by bolus or infusion.

Conclusion

Stress echocardiography, either pharmacological or exercise, is of similar sensitivity and specificity to nuclear scintigraphy and has become a well established, noninvasive tool in the investigation of CHD. It is portable, does not require ionizing radiation and is particularly applicable to women, being devoid of some of the constraints of conventional exercise electrocardiography. In women stress echocardiography is more accurate and yields superior prognostic information when compared with exercise electrocardiography. Unlike nuclear scintigraphy, dobutamine stress echocardiography can also risk stratify patients with low-flow low-pressure aortic stenosis, providing important information on surgical mortality and late survival. Exercise stress echocardiography can be used to assess mitral regurgitation and mitral stenosis.

Stress echocardiography has not been as widely disseminated as it deserves because of the need for a training set of at least 100 studies, the need for modern machines (particularly if contrast is being used), and the problem of subjective scoring. These are gradually being resolved with second harmonic imaging and other advances including 3D imaging, new contrast agents and objective techniques such as tissue Doppler. Stress echocardiography still requires highly specialized teams to both perform and interpret a study. However, the benefits are great when compared with exercise electrocardiographic testing and the technique should be routine in all large hospitals with a sizable cardiac workload.

References

1. McNeer JF, Margolis JR, Lee KL, et al. The role of the exercise test in the evaluation of patients for ischemic heart disease. *Circulation* 1978; **57**:64–70.

2. Marwick TH, Anderson T, Williams MJ, et al. Exercise echocardiography is an accurate and cost-efficient technique for the detection of coronary artery disease in women. *J Am Coll Cardiol* 1995; **26**:335–41.

3. Mairesse GH, Marwick TH, Arnese M, et al. Improved identification of coronary artery disease in patients with left bundle branch block by use of dobutamine stress echocardiography and comparison with myocardial perfusion tomography. *Am J Cardiol* 1995; **76**:321–5.

4. Ryan T, Segar DS, Sawada SG, et al. Detection of coronary artery disease with upright bicycle exercise echocardiography. *J Am Soc Echocardiogr* 1993; **6**:186–97.

5. Castellanet MJ, Greenberg PS, Ellestad MH. Comparison of S-T segment changes on exercise testing with angiographic findings in patients with prior myocardial infarction. *Am J Cardiol* 1978; **42**:29–35.

6. Weiner DA, Ryan TJ, Parsons L, et al. Long-term prognostic value of exercise testing in men and women from the Coronary Artery Surgery Study (CASS) registry. *Am J Cardiol* 1995; **75**:865–70.

7. Sketch MH, Mohiuddin SM, Lynch JD, et al. Significant sex differences in the correlation of electrocardiographic exercise testing and coronary arteriograms. *Am J Cardiol* 1975; **36**:169–73.

8. Barasch E, Wilansky S. Dobutamine stress echocardiography in clinical practice. *Tex Heart Inst J* 1994; **21**:202–10.

9. ACC/AHA/ASE 2003 guideline update for the clinical application of echocardiography: summary article. A report of the American College of Cardiology/ American Heart Association task force on practice guidelines (ACC/AHA/ASE committee to update the 1997 guidelines for the clinical application of echocardiography). *Circulation* 2003; **108**:1146–62.

10. Sugishita Y, Koseki S, Matsuda M, et al. Dissociation between regional myocardial dysfunction and ECG changes during myocardial ischemia induced by exercise in patients with angina pectoris. *Am Heart J* 1983; **106**:1–8.

11. Nesto RW, Kowalchuk GJ. The ischemic cascade: temporal sequence of hemodynamic, electrocardiographic and symptomatic expressions of ischemia. *Am J Cardiol* 1987; **57**:23–30C.

12. Tennant R, Wiggers CJ. The effect of coronary occlusion on myocardial contraction. *Am J Physiol* 1935; **112**:351–61.

13. Kraunz RF, Kennedy JW. Ultrasonic determination of left ventricular wall motion in normal man. Studies at rest and after exercise. *Am Heart J* 1970; **79**:36–43.

14. Wann LS, Faris JV, Childress RH, et al. Exercise cross sectional echocardiography in ischemic heart disease. *Circulation* 1979; **60**:1300–8.

15. Mason SJ, Weiss JL, Weisfeldt ML, et al. Exercise echocardiography: detection of regional wall motion abnormalities during ischaemia. *Circulation* 1979; **59**:50–9.

16. Ling LH, Pellikka PA, Mahoney DW, et al. Atropine augmentation in dobutamine stress echocardiography: role and incremental value in a clinical practice setting. *J Am Coll Cardiol* 1996; **28**:551–7.

17. Dionisopoulos PN, Collins JD, Smart SC, et al. The value of dobutamine stress echocardiography for the detection of coronary artery disease in women. *J Am Soc Echocardiogr* 1997; **10**:811–17.

18. Ho YL, Wu CC, Huang PJ, et al. Assessment of coronary artery disease in women by dobutamine stress echocardiography: comparison with stress thallium-201 single-photon-emission computed tomography and exercise electrocardiography. *Am Heart J* 1998; **135**:655–62.

19. Hecht HS, DeBord L, Sotomayor N, et al. Supine bicycle stress echocardiography; peak exercise imaging is superior to postexercise imaging. *J Am Soc Echocardiogr* 1993; **6**:265–71.

20. Marwick TH, Nemec JJ, Pashkow FJ, et al. Accuracy and limitations of exercise echocardiography in a routine clinical setting. *J Am Coll Cardiol* 1992; **19**:74–81.

21. Crouse LJ, Harbrecht JJ, Vacek JL, et al. Exercise echocardiography as a screening test for coronary

artery disease and correlation with coronary arteriography. *Am J Cardiol* 1991; **67**:1213–18.

22. Marcovitz PA, Armstrong WF. Accuracy of dobutamine stress echocardiography in detecting coronary artery disease. *Am J Cardiol* 1992; **69**:1269–73.

23. Cohen JL, Ottenweller JF, George AK, et al. Comparison of dobutamine and exercise echocardiography for detecting coronary artery disease. *Am J Cardiol* 1993; **72**:1226–31.

24. Segar DS, Brown SE, Sawada SG, et al. Dobutamine stress echocardiography; correlation with coronary lesion severity as determined by quantitative angiography. *J Am Coll Cardiol* 1992; **19**:1197–202.

25. Vanoverschelde JL, Pasquet A, Gerber B, et al. Pathophysiology of myocardial hibernation. Implications for the use of dobutamine echocardiography to identify myocardial viability. *Heart* 1999; **82** (Suppl 3):III1–7.

26. Braunwald E, Rutherford J. Reversible ischemic left ventricular dysfunction: evidence for 'hibernating myocardium'. *J Am Coll Cardiol* 1986; **8**:1467–70.

27. Rahimtoola S. The hibernating myocardium. *Am Heart J* 1989; **117**:211–21.

28. Cigarroa CG, de Filippi CR, Bricker ME. Dobutamine stress echocardiography identifies hibernating myocardium and predicts recovery of left ventricular function after coronary revascularisation. *Circulation* 1993; **88**:430–6.

29. Senior R, Lahiri A. Dobutamine echocardiography predicts functional outcome after revascularisation in patients with dysfunctional myocardium irrespective of the perfusion pattern on resting thallium-201 imaging. *Heart* 1999; **82**:668–73.

30. Afridi I, Kleiman NS, Raizner AE, et al. Dobutamine echocardiography in myocardial hibernation: optimal dose and accuracy in predicting recovery of ventricular function after coronary angioplasty. *Circulation* 1995; **91**:663–70.

31. Alfridi I, Grayburn PA, Panza JA, et al. Myocardial viability during dobutamine echocardiography predicts survival in patients with coronary artery disease and severe left ventricular dysfunction. *J Am Coll Cardiol* 1998; **32**:921–6.

32. Merluzin J, Cerny J, Frelich M, et al. Prognostic value of the amount of dysfunctional but viable myocardium in revascularised patients with coronary artery disease and left ventricular dysfunction. *J Am Coll Cardiol* 1998; **32**:912–20.

33. Hung J, Chaitman BR, Lam J, et al. Noninvasive diagnostic test choices for the evaluation of coronary artery disease in women: a multivariate comparison of cardiac fluoroscopy, exercise electrocardiography and exercise thallium myocardial perfusion scintigraphy. *J Am Coll Cardiol* 1984; **4**:8–16.

34. Guiteras P, Chaitman BR, Waters DD, et al. Diagnostic accuracy of exercise ECG lead systems in clinical subsets of women. *Circulation* 1982; **65**:1465–74.

35. Linhart JW, Laws JG, Satinsky JD. Maximum treadmill exercise electrocardiography in female patients. *Circulation* 1974; **50**:1173–8.

36. Shaw LJ, Miller DD, Romers JC, et al. Gender differences in the noninvasive evaluation and management of patients with suspected coronary artery disease. *Ann Intern Med* 1994; **120**:559–66.

37. Diamond GA, Forrester JS. Analysis of probability as an aid in the clinical diagnosis of coronary artery disease. *N Engl J Med* 1979; **300**:1350–8.

38. Schlant RC, Friesinger GC, Leonard JJ. Clinical competence in exercise testing. *J Am Coll Cardiol* 1990; **16**:1061–5.

39. Chae SC, Heo J, Iskandrian AS, et al. Identification of extensive coronary artery disease in women by exercise single-photon emission computed tomographic (SPECT) thallium imaging. *J Am Coll Cardiol* 1993; **21**:1305–11.

40. Stolzenberg J, Kaminsky J. Overlying breast tissue as cause of false-positive thallium scans. *Clin Nucl Med* 1978; **3**:229.

41. Williams MJ, Marwick TH, O'Gorman D, et al. Comparison of exercise echocardiography with an exercise score to diagnose coronary artery disease in women. *Am J Cardiol* 1994; **74**:435–8.

42. Takeuchi M, Sonoda S, Miura Y, et al. Comparative diagnostic value of dobutamine stress echocardiography and stress thallium-201 single-photon-emission computed tomography for detecting coronary artery disease in women. *Coron Artery Dis* 1996; **7**:831–5.

43. Cortigiani L, Dodi C, Paolini EA, et al. Prognostic value of pharmacological stress echocardiography in women with chest pain and unknown coronary artery disease. *J Am Coll Cardiol* 1998; **32**:627–32.

44. Heupler S, Mehta R, Lobo M, et al. Prognostic implications of exercise echocardiography in women with known or suspected coronary artery disease. *J Am Coll Cardiol* 1997; **30**:414–20.

45. Davar JI, Brull DJ, Bulugahipitiya S, et al. Prognostic value of negative dobutamine stress echo in women with intermediate probability of coronary artery disease. *Am J Cardiol* 1999; **83**:100–2.

46. Leong-Poi H, Rim S-J, Le E, et al. Perfusion versus function: the ischemic cascade in demand ischemia. Implications of single versus multivessel stenosis. *Circulation* 2002; **105**:987–92.

47. Santiago P, Vacek JL, Rosamond TL. Dobutamine stress echocardiography: clinical utility, and predictive value at various infusion rates. *Am Heart J* 1994; **128**:804–8.

48. Picano E, Bedetti G, Varga A, et al. The comparable diagnostic accuracies of dobutamine-stress and dipyridamole-stress echocardiographies: a meta-analysis. *Coron Artery Dis* 2000; **11**:151–9.

49. Zaglavara T, Haaverstad R, Cumberledge B, et al. Dobutamine stress echocardiography for the detection of myocardial viability in patients with left ventricular dysfunction taking β blockers: accuracy and optimal dose. *Heart* 2002; **87**:329–35.

50. Senior R, Soman P, Khattar RS, et al. Improved endocardial visualization with second harmonic imaging compared with fundamental two-dimensional echocardiographic imaging. *Am Heart J* 1999; **138**:163–8.

51. Yu EH, Sloggett CE, Iwanochko RM, et al. Feasibility and accuracy of left ventricular volumes and ejection fraction determination by fundamental, tissue harmonic, and intravenous contrast imaging in difficult-to-image patients. *J Am Soc Echocardiogr* 2000; **13**:216–24.

52. Hoffmann R, Marwick TH, Poldermans D, et al. Refinements in stress echocardiographic techniques improve inter-institutional agreement in interpretation of dobutamine stress echocardiograms. *Eur Heart J* 2002; **23**:821–9.

53. Hundley WG, Kizilbash AM, Afridi I, et al. Administration of an intravenous perfluorocarbon contrast agent improves echocardiographic determination of left ventricular volumes and ejection fraction: comparison with cine magnetic resonance imaging. *J Am Coll Cardiol* 1998; **32**:1426–32.

54. Geleijnse ML, Fioretti PM, Roelandt JR. Methodology, feasibility, safety and diagnostic accuracy of dobutamine stress echocardiography. *J Am Coll Cardiol* 1997; **30**:595–606.

55. Marcovitz PA, Bach DS, Mathias W, et al. Paradoxic hypotension during dobutamine stress echocardiography; clinical and diagnostic implications. *J Am Coll Cardiol* 1993; **21**:1080–6.

56. Dubach P, Froelicher VF, Klein J, et al. Exercise-induced hypotension in a male population: criteria, causes and prognosis. *Circulation* 1988; **78**:1380–7.

57. Pellikka PA, Oh JK, Bailey KR, et al. Dynamic intraventricular obstruction during dobutamine stress echocardiography: a new observation. *Circulation* 1992; **86**:1429–32.

58. Mertes H, Sawad SG, Ryan T. Symptoms, adverse effects, and complications associated with dobuta-mine stress echocardiography: experience in 1118 patients. *Circulation* 1993; **88**:15–19.

59. Secknus M, Marwick TH. Evolution of dobutamine echocardiography protocols and indications: safety and side effects in 3011 studies over 5 years. *J Am Coll Cardiol* 1997; **29**:1234–40.

60. Pellikka PA, Roger VL, Oh JK, et al. Stress echocardiography. Part II. Dobutamine stress echocardiography: techniques, implementation, clinical applications, and correlations. *Mayo Clin Proc* 1995; **70**:16–27.

61. American Society of Echocardiography committee on standards (subcommittee on quantitation of two-dimensional echocardiograms). Recommendations of quantification of the left ventricle by two-dimensional echocardiography. *J Am Soc Echocardiogr* 1989; **2**:358–67.

62. Sawada SG, Segar DS, Ryan T, et al. Echocardiographic detection of coronary artery disease during dobutamine infusion. *Circulation* 1991; **103**:2724–30.

63. Martin TW, Seaworth JF, Johns JP, et al. Comparison of adenosine, dipyridamole, and dobutamine in stress echocardiography. *Ann Intern Med* 1992; **116**:190–6.

64. Marangelli V, Iliceto S, Piccinni G, et al. Detection of coronary artery disease by digital stress echocardiography: comparison of exercise, transesophageal atrial pacing and dipyridamole echocardiography. *J Am Coll Cardiol* 1994; **24**:117–24.

65. Roger VL, Pelllika PA, Oh JK, et al. Identification of multivessel coronary artery disease by exercise echocardiography. *J Am Coll Cardiol* 1994; **24**:109–14.

66. Bach DS, Muller DWM, Gros BJ, et al. False positive dobutamine stress echocardiograms: characterization of clinical, echocardiographic and angiographic findings. *J Am Coll Cardiol* 1994; **24**:928–33.

67. Carstensen S, Ali SM, Stensgaard-Hansen FV, et al. Dobutamine–atropine stress echocardiography in asymptomatic healthy individuals: the relativity of stress-induced hyperkinesias. *Circulation* 1995; **92**:3453–63.

68. El-Said EM, Roelandt JRTC, Fioretti PM, et al. Abnormal left ventricular early diastolic filling during dobutamine stress Doppler echocardiography is a sensitive indicator of significant coronary artery disease. *J Am Coll Cardiol* 1994; **24**:1618–24.

69. Connolly HM, Oh JK, Schaff HV, et al. Severe aortic stenosis with low transvalvular gradient and severe left ventricular dysfunction. *Circulation* 2000; **101**:1940–6.

70. Nishimura RA, Grantham JA, Connolly HM, et al. Low-output, low-gradient aortic stenosis in patients with depressed left ventricular systolic function: the

clinical utility of the dobutamine challenge in the catheterization laboratory. *Circulation* 2002; **106**:809–13.

71. Monin J-L, Quere JP, Monchi M, et al. Low-gradient aortic stenosis: operative risk stratification and predictors for long-term outcome: a multicenter study using dobutamine stress haemodynamics. *Circulation* 2003; **108**:319–24.

72. Monin J, Monchi M, Gest V, et al. Aortic stenosis with severe left ventricular dysfunction and low trans-valvular pressure gradients. Risk stratification by low-dose dobutamine echocardiography. *J Am Coll Cardiol* 2001; **37**:2101–7.

73. Sagar KB, Wann LS, Paulson WJ, et al. Role of exercise Doppler in isolated mitral stenosis. *Chest* 1987; **92**:27–30.

74. Leavitt JI, Coats MH, Falk RH. Effects of exercise on transmitral gradient and pulmonary pressure in patients with mitral stenosis or a prosthetic mitral valve: a Doppler echocardiographic study. *J Am Coll Cardiol* 1991; **17**:1520–6.

75. Tunick PA, Friedberg RS, Gargiulo A, et al. Exercise Doppler echocardiography as an aid in clinical decision making in mitral valve disease. *J Am Soc Echocardiogr* 1992; **5**:225–30.

76. Belgi A, Yalcinkaya S, Umuttan D, et al. Echo-cardiographic predictors of hemodynamic response and significance of dyspnea development in patients with mitral stenosis during dobutamine stress echocardiography. *J Heart Valve Dis* 2003; **12**:482–7.

77. Reis G, Motta MS, Barbosa MM, et al. Dobutamine stress echocardiography for noninvasive assessment and risk stratification of patients with rheumatic mitral stenosis. *J Am Coll Cardiol* 2004; **43**:393–401.

78. Tischler MD, Battle RW, Saha M, et al. Observations suggesting a high incidence of exercise-induced severe mitral regurgitation in patients with mild rheumatic mitral valve disease at rest. *J Am Coll Cardiol* 1995; **24**:128–33.

79. Armstrong GP, Griffin BP. Exercise echocardio-graphic assessment in severe mitral regurgitation. *Coron Artery Dis* 2000; **11**:23–30.

80. Henein MY, Priestley K, Davarashvili T, et al. Early changes in left ventricular subendocardial function after successful coronary angioplasty. *Br Heart J* 1993; **69**:501–6.

81. Henein MY, Gibson DG. Suppression of left ventricu-lar early diastolic filling by long axis asynchrony. *Br Heart J* 1995; **73**:151–7.

82. Henein MY, Gibson DG. Abnormal subendocardial function in restrictive left ventricular disease. *Br Heart J* 1994; **72**:237–42.

83. Alam M, Hoglund C, Thorstrand C, et al. Atrioventricular plane displacement in severe conges-tive heart failure following dilated cardiomyopathy or myocardial infarction. *J Intern Med* 1990; **228**: 569–75.

84. Mishra MB, Lythall DA, Chambers JB. A comparison of wall motion analysis and systolic left ventricular long axis function during dobutamine stress echocar-diography. *Eur Heart J* 2002; **23**:579–85.

85. Derumeaux G, Ovize M, Loufoua J, et al. Doppler tissue imaging quantitates regional wall motion during myocardial ischaemia and reperfusion. *Circulation* 1998; **97**:1970–7.

86. Madler CF, Payne N, Wilkenshoff U, et al. Non-invasive diagnosis of coronary artery disease by quantitative stress echocardiography: optimal diagnostic models using off-line tissue Doppler in the MYDISE study. *Eur Heart J* 2003; **24**:1584–94.

87. Rambaldi R, Poldermans D, Bax JJ, et al. Doppler tissue velocity sampling improves diagnostic accuracy during dobutamine stress echocardiography for the assessment of viable myocardium in patients with severe left ventricular dysfunction. *Eur Heart J* 2000; **21**:1091–8.

88. Cain P, Khoury V, Short L, et al. The usefulness of quantitative echocardiographic techniques to predict recovery of regional and global left ventricular function after acute myocardial infarction. *Am J Cardiol* 2003; **91**:391–6.

89. Marwick TH. Quantitative techniques for stress echocardiography: dream or reality? *Eur J Echocardiography* 2002; **3**:171–6.

90. Voigt JU, Exner B, Schmiedehausen K, et al. Strain-rate imaging during dobutamine stress echocardio-graphy provides objective evidence of inducible ischemia. *Circulation* 2003; **107**:2120–6.

91. Qin JX, Shiota T, McCarthy PM, et al. Real-time three-dimensional echocardiographic study of left ventricular function after infarct exclusion surgery for ischaemic cardiomyopathy. *Circulation* 2000; **102**: III101–6.

92. Qin JX, Shiota T, Thomas JD. Determination of left ventricular volume, ejection fraction, and myocardial mass by real-time three-dimensional echocardiogra-phy. *Echocardiography* 2000; **17**:781–6.

93. Sugeng L, Kirkpatrick J, Lang RM, et al. Biplane stress echocardiography using a prototype matrix-array transducer. *J Am Soc Echocardiogr* 2003; **16**:724–31.

94. Rainbird AJ, Mulvagh SL, Oh JK, et al. Contrast dobutamine stress echocardiography: clinical practice assessment in 300 consecutive patients. *J Am Soc Echocardiogr* 2001; **14**:378–85.

95. Hundley WG, Kizilbash AM, Alfridi I, et al. Administration of an intravenous perfluorocarbon contrast agent improves echocardiographic determination of left ventricular volumes and ejection fraction: comparison with cine magnetic resonance imaging. *J Am Coll Cardiol* 1998; **32**:1426–32.

12

The role of CMR and PET in women

Anna John, Almut Mahnke and Sanjay Prasad

Introduction

The diagnosis of cardiac diseases in women can often be difficult. As a group, cardiac problems are frequently underdiagnosed and undertreated. In recent years, there have been tremendous advances in our imaging ability to detect disease of both ischemic and nonischemic etiology. Many of these newer techniques are very safe, noninvasive, and offer much better resolution than more established imaging modalities, with detailed anatomic and functional data. Two of the most important recent techniques are cardiovascular magnetic resonance (CMR) and positron emission tomography (PET). We will discuss their applications in assessment of coronary heart disease (CHD), cardiomyopathy, and structural disease such as congenital heart disease (Table 12.1). Integral to their use is an understanding of how both techniques work. This guides the decision as to when to request these investigations and also determines their strengths and limitations.

Background

Fundamental principles of CMR

Magnetic resonance imaging (MRI) has been widely used to image the brain and other stationary organs within the body. More recently there has been much

Table 12.1 The diagnostic value of PET, CMR, and echocardiography according to indication

Indication	CMR	PET	Echo-cardiography
Coronaries	++	−	+
Perfusion	++	+++	+
Viability	+++	++	++
Congenital/morphology	+++	−	++
Left ventricle function/mass	+++	−	++
Metabolism	+/−	+++	−
Tissue characterization	+++	+	+
Valves	++	−	+++

+++, high diagnostic value; ++, good diagnostic value; +, some diagnostic value; +/−, little diagnostic value; −, no diagnostic value.

excitement as regards its clinical cardiovascular applications, largely as a result of software and hardware advances that enable high temporal and spatial resolution imaging and that permit tracking of the cardiac cycle – known as gating. The term cardiovascular magnetic resonance (CMR) is used to refer to MRI of the heart and great vessels.

MRI is based on the phenomenon of the resonance of atomic nuclei. Hydrogen, as present in fat and water, is the simplest and most abundant element in the human body and comprises a proton nucleus and a single electron – it can therefore also be referred to simply as a proton. Protons can be likened to the planet earth, spinning on its axis, with

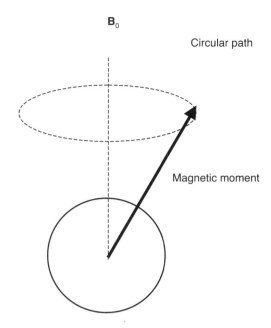

B₀

Circular path

Magnetic moment

Figure 12.1
Protons have a positive electric charge. As protons spin around an axis an electric current is created which in turn induces a magnetic field.

a north–south pole (Fig. 12.1). As such they behave like a small bar magnet. Under normal circumstances, these hydrogen proton 'bar magnets' spin in the body with their axes randomly aligned. When the body is placed in a strong magnetic field, such as an MRI scanner, the protons' axes all line up. This uniform alignment creates a magnetic vector oriented along the axis of the MRI scanner. When additional energy (in the form of a radio wave) is applied to the magnetic field, the magnetic vector is deflected. The radio wave frequency that causes the hydrogen nuclei to resonate is dependent on the strength of the magnetic field. The strength can be altered electronically from head to toe using a series of gradient electric coils. By altering the local magnetic field by these small increments, different slices of the body will resonate as different frequencies are applied. When the radiofrequency source is switched off, the magnetic vector returns to its resting state, and this causes a signal (also a radio wave) to be emitted. It is this emitted signal that is used to create the MR images. Receiver coils are used around the body part under investigation to act as aerials to improve their detection. The intensity of the received signal is then plotted on a gray scale and cross-sectional images are built up. Multiple transmitted radiofrequency pulses can be used in sequence to emphasize particular tissues or abnormalities. Different tissues (such as fat and water) have different relaxation times when the transmitted radiofrequency pulse is switched off and can be identified separately. An MR examination is thus made up of a series of pulse sequences. Contrast among tissues depends on proton density, magnetic relaxation times of the protons and magnetic susceptibility effects. MRI scanners come in different field strengths, usually between 0.5 and 3.0 Tesla (T). Most clinical CMR is currently performed at 1.5 T. The two main types of sequence used in CMR are gradient echo (GE) and spin echo (SE) imaging techniques. GE techniques lead to blood and fat both appearing white. They enable the acquisition of high-quality cine images which can be used to identify myocardial function as well as abnormal flow patterns. Most SE techniques lead to blood appearing black, while fat appears white. They are useful for high-resolution anatomic as opposed to functional imaging. CMR consists of applying these sequences and their variants to determine cardiac physiology, anatomy, metabolism, tissue characterization, and vascular angiography. Image acquisition is multiplanar and no geometric assumptions are made, unlike for example 2D echocardiography, so that measurements are very accurate and reproducible.

Most diseases manifest themselves by an increase in water content, so MRI is a sensitive test for the detection of disease. There are no known biologic hazards of MRI because, unlike X-ray and computed tomography, MRI uses radiation in the radiofrequency range which is found all around us and does not damage tissue as it passes through.

Modern CMR scanners incorporate ultrafast technology which allows real-time imaging (up to 50 frames per second). Most scans are gated to the electrocardiogram (ECG), and in some cases also to the respiratory cycle using diaphragmatic monitoring techniques. Magnetic resonance (MR) contrast agents are used in conjunction with some select MRI sequences such as MR angiography and viability assessment, as will be discussed later.

Positron emission tomography

PET is a unique noninvasive imaging technique, which can produce 3D images of the heart, brain, or other organs. It can help in the diagnosis and management of cancers, certain brain disorders, and heart disease. Molecules, which interact with the body's own metabolic pathways, are labelled with small amounts of radioactivity so that after intravenous (IV) introduction, they can be traced and localized within a certain tissue of the patient. The radionuclides used in PET emit positrons, which react with electrons in the surrounding tissues. During this process, both positron and electron are annihilated, and two photons with an energy of 511 keV are emitted in opposite directions, where they impinge on detectors opposing each other in the detector ring of the scanner. Events are recorded only when signals from both detectors are produced simultaneously. This is called coincidence detection. PET scanners used for human imaging have an intrinsic resolution of approximately 5 mm.

PET has two major advantages over the more common nuclear tests. First, the images are less likely to be distorted by body habitus (e.g. large breasts, obesity), so abnormal results are more reliable. Second, it is an excellent tool for determining whether portions of the heart muscle are still viable (living and functioning). The scan can also measure how well those viable portions are functioning after a myocardial infarction (MI) or other event in which there is a lack of oxygen-rich blood to the heart muscle. PET scanning is not as readily available as more conventional nuclear imaging because of its greater cost and the need for a cyclotron device, which produces necessary isotopes on site. PET uses attenuation correction to correct for artifacts caused by soft tissue such as breast tissue.

Clinical applications

Coronary heart disease

Cardiovascular magnetic resonance

CHD in women continues to be a major public health problem that represents a leading cause of death and disability.[1] CHD is the main cause of heart failure and one of the leading causes of death in developed countries.[2,3] Due to improved treatment and extended survival of these patients, the prevalence of CHD and heart failure as a sequel is rising. However, women with angina have a lower probability of being referred to a specialist[4] and are less likely to be offered revascularization[5] than men. Further inequalities exist in secondary care where women do not receive the same standard of investigations, and interventional and drug treatments.[6,7] The WISE (Women's Ischemia Syndrome Evaluation) investigators found that a classification of 'typical' angina missed 65% of the women who actually had CHD. There is thus an important need to develop and test ways to improve the use of existing diagnostic methods and new ways to diagnose CHD in women. There is also a great requirement for early detection by noninvasive screening techniques.

CMR offers different techniques to assess the presence and the severity of CHD (Table 12.2). These include measurement of ventricular function, viability assessment, perfusion and visualization of coronary arteries directly. Diagnosis of ventricular dysfunction is an important starting point. CMR is considered the gold standard for the measurement of ventricular function and mass and allows the assessment of regional wall motion. Planimetry of a short-axis stack of the left ventricle from the base to apex in systole and diastole allows determination of the left ventricular end-diastolic and systolic volumes,

---

Box 12.1 Practical aspects of CMR and PET scans

CMR
Time of scan ~45–60 minutes
Intravenous peripheral line required if contrast to be given
Electrocardiogram monitoring
Hemodynamic monitoring if any stress agent given
Outpatient study

PET
Time of scan ~2 hours
Intravenous peripheral line
Hemodynamic monitoring often used
Outpatient study

Table 12.2 Current indications for cardiac magnetic resonance

Indications	Class
Rest RV/LV function/ejection fraction	I
Assessment of myocardial viability	IIa
Detection of myocardial ischemia	
Dobutamine stress	IIa
Myocardial perfusion	IIb
Phosphorus-31 myocardial spectroscopy	Research
Diagnosis of hypertrophic cardiomyopathy	
ARVD	IIa
HCM	I
DCM	I
Evaluation of valvular heart disease	IIa
Congenital heart disease	
Shunts	IIa
Pericardial disease	
Differentiate constrictive and restrictive pericarditis	I
Coronary arteries	IIb
Aortic dissection	I

RV, right ventricle; LV, left ventricle; ARVD, arrythmogenic right ventricular dysplasia; HCM, hypertrophic cardiomyopathy; DCM, dilated cardiomyopathy.
Adapted from reference 8 with permission from Lippincott, Williams and Wilkins.

ejection fraction, and stroke volume. In addition, by knowing the density of myocardium plus the volume of tissue, left ventricular mass can be accurately determined. Wall motion abnormalities are identified in two-chamber, four-chamber, and short-axis cine sequences of the entire left ventricle. According to Baer et al. an end-diastolic wall thickness of <5.5 mm suggests non-viable myocardium.[9]

There is much interest in the role of MR coronary angiography (MRCA) to directly visualize coronary arteries (Fig. 12.2). Potentially, this could offer a noninvasive means of assessing vessels for stenoses without the attendant risks seen with X-ray angiography and importantly without the need for exposure to ionizing radiation. Kim et al. were able to reliably exclude triple-vessel and left main stem disease in a multicenter trial, with a high negative predictive value, a sensitivity of 100%, specificity of 85%, and an accuracy of 87%. However, imaging resolution of disease in more distal epicardial coronary arteries was limited, so that overall accuracy was only 72%.[10] While this is encouraging, it is not yet sufficient or robust enough for standard clinical

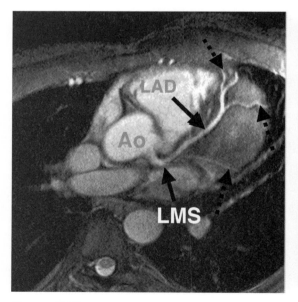 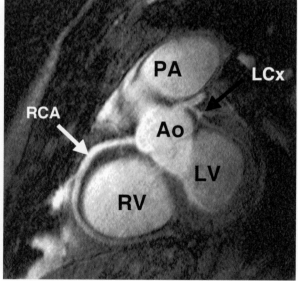

Figure 12.2
Magnetic resonance coronary angiography showing left coronary artery system (left panel; LAD arrow, left anterior descending; Ao, aorta; LMS arrow, left main stem; dotted arrows, LAD branches) and right coronary artery (right panel; Ao, aorta; RV, right ventricle; LV, left ventricle; PA, pulmonary artery; RCA, right coronary artery; LCx, left circumflex).

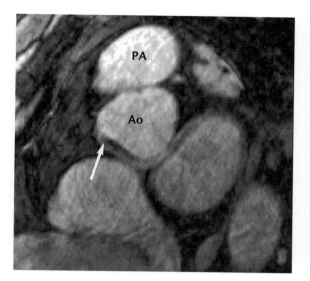 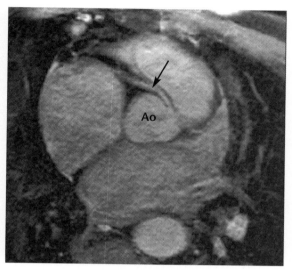

Figure 12.3
Magnetic resonance coronary angiography showing anomalous left coronary artery system and also right coronary artery traversing between aorta (Ao) and pulmonary artery (PA).

application in CHD. MRCA has a current resolution of around 600–900 μm. By contrast, X-ray angiography has a resolution of around 250 μm. MRCA is thus useful to visualize the proximal portion of vessels but not as effective for the mid and distal portions. Metal artifacts generated by coronary stents hinder assessment of in-stent restenosis, although MRCA can be helpful to detect the position of a stent.

On a practical front, the one area where MRCA has an established clinical application is in the assessment of anomalous coronary vessels, where coronary arteries do not arise from their usual sites (Fig. 12.3). MRCA is helpful to identify the actual origin and course of these vessels, particularly their relation to the aorta and pulmonary artery.[11]

In patients with suspected CHD, it is helpful to know how much blood is supplied to each portion of the myocardium – particularly in relation to coronary artery territories. This could also be used to assess the significance of coronary lesions. CMR perfusion provides such a technique. A compact bolus of gadolinium (a paramagnetic contrast agent) is given intravenously and continuous images of the heart are taken during the administration. For each coronary territory, the peak intensity and time to peak of the gadolinium are measured as it first passes through the

myocardium to determine the resting perfusion. By then repeating the study with the administration of a stress agent (usually adenosine) to maximally vasodilate coronary vessels, myocardial perfusion reserve can be determined as the ratio of resting and hyperemic perfusion. This technique will also detect fixed and reversible perfusion defects and thus distinguish between infarction and ischemia. The absence of a myocardial perfusion defect on adenosine stress first-pass perfusion can reliably rule out the presence of significant coronary artery disease.[12]

In patients with established CHD and impaired ventricular function, an important issue is to distinguish hibernating myocardium from nonviable myocardium. Function in regions of viable and hibernating myocardium can be improved through revascularization such as angioplasty or bypass surgery. Ventricular function is assessed in each of the 17 segments of the left ventricle at rest. Inotropic stimulation (using low- and high-dose dobutamine) is then given to determine if there is improvement in function in each of these segments. Normal viable myocardium will have good function at rest which is improved with dobutamine; these regions have an adequate blood supply. By contrast, scar tissue due to previous infarction is nonviable and will show impaired function at rest and also with inotropes. These segments will not improve with revascularization. A third important category is so-called hibernating myocardium. This is viable, metabolically active myocardium where function is impaired at rest due to inadequate coronary blood supply to that region. At low-dose dobutamine, there is some improvement in blood supply so that function improves. At higher doses of dobutamine, the coronary supply is unable to meet the myocardial metabolic requirements and myocardial function in that territory deteriorates. Function can be restored in these recruitable segments of myocardium if vascular supply to that territory is improved.[13]

An additional technique used in CMR is to identify scar tissue directly (Fig. 12.4). Gadolinium contrast agent gives a bright enhanced signal intensity on spin-echo CMR images in regions of scarring or fibrosis where it accumulates. Due to its molecular size, it cannot penetrate the cell membrane of normal viable muscle cells. However, it accumulates in the extracellular matrix which is seen in areas of fibrosis and scarring as occurs in chronic MI. In acute infarction, rupture of the cardiomyocyte cell membranes allows the gadolinium to accumulate within the acutely necrotic cells, leading to late enhancement 10–15 minutes after administration (Fig. 12.5).

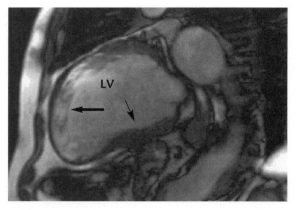

Figure 12.4
CMR in two-chamber view of left ventricle (LV) in a patient with a large anterior infarct. There is significant wall thinning (thick arrow) in a region of infarction compared with normal wall thickness at the basal inferior territory (thin arrow).

Following infarction, the pattern of enhancement always commences in the subendocardium and extends according to the size of infarct towards the epicardium. Thus gadolinium produces a bright signal identifying nonviable tissue. It is given as a simple single, peripheral IV bolus. Late enhancement

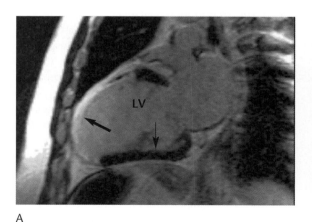

A

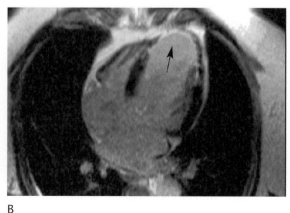

B

Figure 12.5
The CMR scan in two-chamber (panel A) and four-chamber (panel B) views of left ventricle (LV) in a patient with a large anterior myocardial infarction. Images were acquired 15 minutes after intravenous gadolinium and show late enhancement of the anterior wall (A) and the apex (B). These findings are consistent with a transmural infarction, which is unlikely to show any recoverability following revascularization.

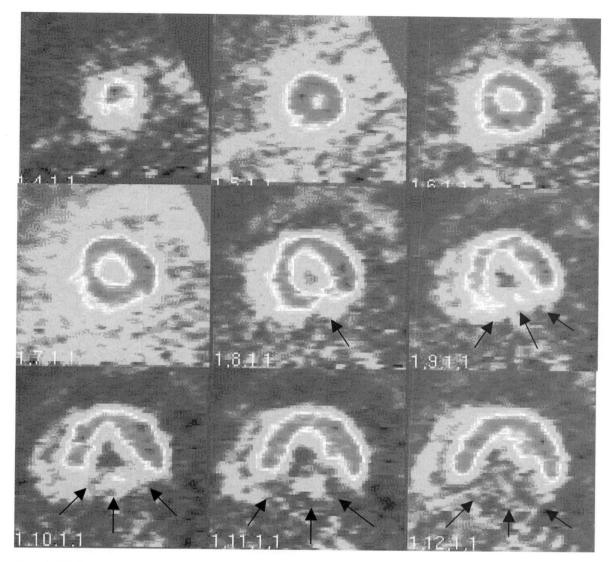

Figure 12.6
FDG-PET images showing left ventricular short axis images in a patient with an inferior myocardial infarction. There is a defect of tracer uptake in the infarcted area (arrow).

viability assessment is the only technique able to show dead alongside viable myocardium. The accuracy of the dobutamine stress test is improved by combination with a gadolinium study. Areas with wall motion abnormalities that improve with low-dose dobutamine, and which either show no gadolinium late enhancement or less than 50% of the transmural wall, can therefore be accurately identi-

fied as dysfunctional but viable hibernating myocardium.[14]

Positron emission tomography

The most commonly used tracer in cardiac PET is fluorine-18-labelled fluorodeoxyglucose (FDG) (Fig. 12.6). It is a glucose analog, which is used to characterize myocardial glucose metabolism throughout the heart. Uptake will be proportional to the amount of viable metabolically active myocardium present. Oxygen-15-labelled water or nitrogen-13-labelled ammonia can be used to separately assess perfusion. In normal regions that have adequate blood supply, there will be a high signal for metabolism and normal perfusion. In scar tissue, both metabolism and perfusion will be absent in proportion to the amount of infarcted myocardium. In viable and hibernating myocardium, perfusion may be normal or slightly reduced; metabolism, however, will be normal. On the basis of current experience and multicenter studies, FDG PET is considered the gold standard for myocardial viability assessment.[15] This may change to CMR as more trial data become available.

PET can also be used to detect impairment of myocardial perfusion in high-risk but asymptomatic women in whom coronary angiogram is not justified, such as those with multiple cardiovascular risk factors,[16,17] relatives of patients with CHD[18] and in diabetic patients without symptoms of coronary disease.[19]

FDG studies can also provide information on function, if the images are acquired in a gated fashion. Its uptake into the cardiomyocyte depends strongly on the presence of insulin and the fasting state of the patient. Therefore, many centers perform FDG studies during hyperinsulinemic euglycemic clamp to standardize measurements.[20]

Nonischemic cardiomyopathy

CMR

In dilated cardiomyopathy (DCM), there is dilatation and functional impairment of the left or both ventricles in the absence of an ischemic etiology (Figs 12.7 and 12.8). The usual presentation is with progressive heart failure, and the cause is mostly idiopathic but can also be viral, toxic, or autoimmune. Recognized complications include arrhythmias and sudden death as well as thromboembolism from intra-cardiac thrombi. CMR provides accurate measurement of left ventricle size and function. It facilitates close monitoring of bi-ventricular function so that even small changes in ventricular dimensions or function can be detected.

CMR is superior to 2D techniques such as echocardiography because it allows more accurate description of ventricular geometry, which is particularly important in remodeled ventricles as occurs in DCM. Radionuclide ventriculography is another 3D technique to assess ventricular function; however, its lower spatial resolution as well as the use of ionizing radiation make it less appropriate for frequent follow-up.

In a study of 90 patients with left ventricular dysfunction of both ischemic and nonischemic etiology, CMR incorporating a gadolinium study accurately identified the presence of scar tissue denoting previous infarction in the 30 patients with known CHD. In the 60 patients with normal coronary angiograms, three interesting groups were identified. The majority (66%) showed no gadolinium uptake, suggesting no fibrosis or scarring. In 14%, there was an identical pattern of gadolinium uptake to that seen in CHD. This would imply that the underlying etiology in these patients was actually an ischemic basis rather than idiopathic DCM. The

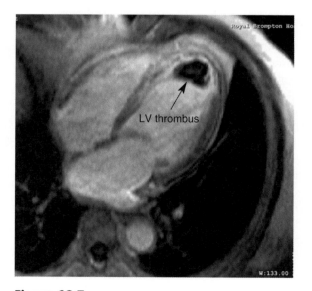

Figure 12.7
CMR scan in four-chamber view of a patient with a large thrombus (arrow). Following gadolinium, nonvascular masses, such as thrombi, do not take up gadolinium and therefore on CMR show a dark (low signal intensity) mass.

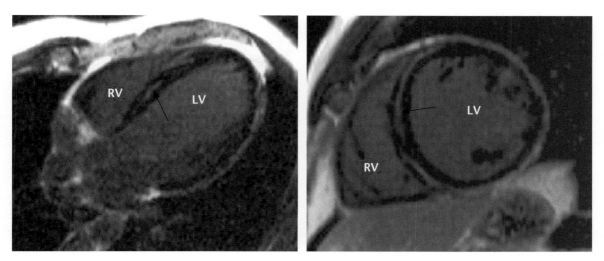

Figure 12.8
CMR of a patient with dilated cardiomyopathy (DCM). In a small proportion of patients with DCM, mid wall fibrosis is seen following gadolinium, which correlates with post-mortem findings. LV, left ventricle; RV, right ventricle.

presence of a normal angiogram in this group suggests that recanalization or an embolic episode is the likely diagnosis. In 20%, there was a pattern of mid-wall hyperenhancement that correlates with the mid-wall fibrosis seen in post-mortem hearts with idiopathic DCM. The distribution is very different from scarring due to infarction. These findings potentially allow noninvasive differentiation between ischemic and idiopathic DCM and may thus make it possible to avoid the use of invasive coronary angiography.[21]

Hypertrophic cardiomyopathy is characterized by left with or without right ventricular hypertrophy and usually involves the interventricular septum (Fig. 12.9). CMR may be used to monitor ventricular function, myocardial mass, and the degree of outflow tract obstruction as well as to detect the degree of myocardial fibrosis. Fibrous degeneration and myocardial disarray have been linked to arrhythmias and sudden cardiac death, and progression into heart failure is a complication.[22–24] Detection of the amount of fibrous tissue correlates with risk factors for sudden cardiac death in patients below 35 years and with progressive disease in older patients. CMR is particularly useful in establishing the diagnosis in apical hypertrophic cardiomyopathy as 2D echocar-

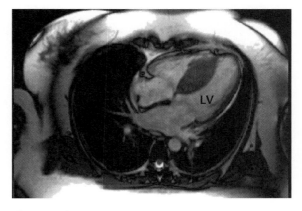

Figure 12.9
CMR of a patient with hypertrophic cardiomyopathy. There is marked thickening of the septum with gross asymmetric hypertrophy. LV, left ventricle.

diography is less effective in visualizing the apex (Fig. 12.10).

Arrhythmogenic right ventricular cardiomyopathy (ARVC) is a rare form of cardiomyopathy associated with ventricular arrhythmias of right ventricular

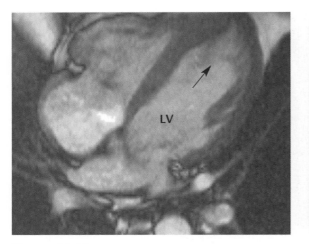 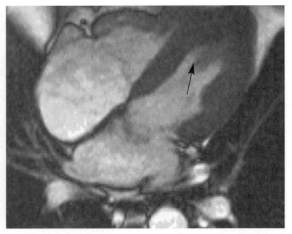

Figure 12.10
CMR scan of a patient with apical hypertrophic cardiomyopathy (left panel in diastole, right panel in systole). There is gross asymmetric apical wall thickening (arrows). LV, left ventricle.

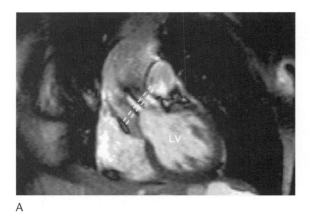

A

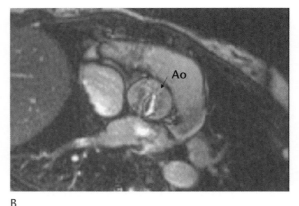

B

Figure 12.11
CMR in left ventricular outflow tract view (A) in a patient with significant aortic stenosis due to a bicuspid aortic valve. Panel B, transverse cut through aortic valve showing bicuspid aortic valve with severely reduced leaflet excursion.

outflow tract origin. It is associated with sudden death[25] and is characterized by fibrofatty replacement of the myocardium, particularly in the right ventricular free wall. Both sexes are equally affected, and inheritance is usually autosomal dominant with incomplete penetrance, but recessive forms have been described.[26] Morphological findings include enlarged ventricular dimensions, aneurysmal dilata-

tion and fibrous or fatty replacement of the myocardium. CMR is ideally suited to address these issues. Unlike in 2D echocardiography, where the right ventricle is difficult to visualize due to its pyramidal shape, unlimited views can be obtained with CMR, and its ability to characterize the composition of tissue by spin-echo can be used to detect fibrosis and fatty deposits in the right ventricle .[27]

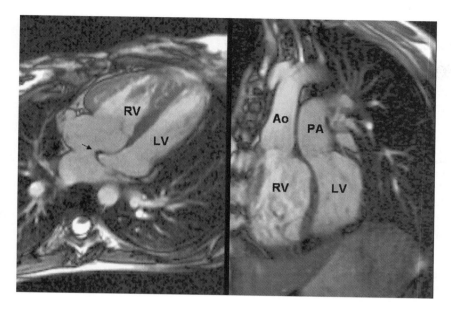

Figure 12.12
CMR in an adult following Mustard operation for transposition of the great arteries. The arrow points to the intra-atrial baffle. Courtesy Dr Philip Kilner.

Positron emission tomography

The use of PET in nonischemic cardiomyopathy is limited mostly to research studies. Abnormal sympathetic function has been described in hypertrophic[28] and arrhythmogenic cardiomyopathy,[29] while perfusion and metabolic abnormalities were found in dilated cardiomyopathy (Fig. 12.13).[30] These findings provide useful information for the under-standing of underlying pathophysiologies; however, in clinical practice, the use of PET is limited to myocardial perfusion.

Secondary left ventricular hypertrophy

Cardiac hypertrophy is a morphological adaptive increase in myocardial mass in response to chronic

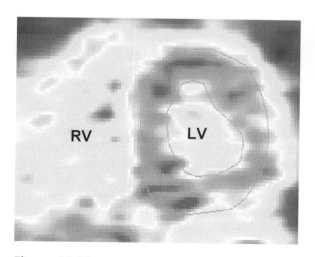
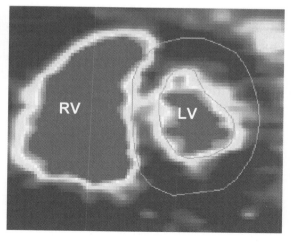

Figure 12.13
Left panel shows an FDG image assessing myocardial metabolism; right panel is a PET perfusion scan with oxygen-15-labelled water. Both short axis orientation.

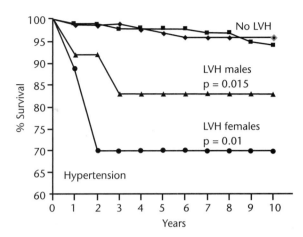

Figure 12.14
Clinical relevance of the left ventricular mass. Females with left ventricular hypertrophy (LVH) due to hypertension have a poorer outcome than their male counterparts. Adapted from reference 36 with permission from American College of Cardiology Foundation.

work overload as in hypertension and aortic stenosis and is a common clinical finding affecting 33% of women over the age of 59 years.[31] Left ventricular hypertrophy (LVH) significantly increases the risk of MI, congestive heart failure, cardiac arrhythmias, and sudden cardiac death (Fig. 12.14).[32–36] Pressure or volume overload results in an increase in myocardial wall stress and hypertrophy may be seen as an attempt to normalize wall stress and oxygen demand. Although initially protective, the increased myocardial mass requires an increase in coronary blood flow to maintain function; thus, ventricular hypertrophy may be associated with myocardial ischemia even with angiographically normal coronary arteries.[37–39]

It is important to treat the underlying cause of LVH aggressively to achieve left ventricular mass regression and to monitor changes in mass and function. CMR can accurately measure left ventricular mass and exclude underlying causes of LVH, e.g. aortic stenosis. PET can be used to assess the myocardial perfusion and perfusion reserve.[40–42]

Atypical chest pain

Atypical chest pain is a common problem in women. Once flow-limiting stenoses have been excluded by X-ray coronary angiography, women with chest pain are frequently managed conservatively with no further treatment or follow-up for their symptoms. However, there is increased awareness that up to 20% of these women have coronary *microvascular* dysfunction and inducible myocardial ischemia.[43] The constellation of angina-like chest pain and a positive exercise test but normal epicardial coronary arteries is termed syndrome X. The pathophysiology remains incompletely understood, but an abnormal myocardial microcirculation has been postulated, hence the synonym microvascular angina. The traditional way of diagnosing microvascular dysfunction is to demonstrate an abnormal flow reserve in a single coronary artery during X-ray angiography, which is not always accurate, as microvascular dysfunction is heterogeneously distributed in the myocardium.[44]

In a study of 20 women with syndrome X, Panting et al. demonstrated a subendocardial hypoperfusion during adenosine infusion associated with chest pain using first-pass myocardial perfusion CMR. These data support the thesis that the chest pain in syndrome X may have an ischemic cause.[45,46]

PET perfusion scanning is also able to assess microvascular dysfunction and provides an alternative diagnostic test in these patients. Comparative trials of CMR and PET in this condition are currently underway.

Valve disease

Echocardiography remains the primary imaging method to assess cardiac valve disease. However, in selected cases such as aortic or pulmonary stenosis, mixed valve disease or suboptimal windows, transthoracic echocardiography may not adequately reflect the degree of valve disease. In these cases (Fig. 12.11), CMR can play a role in the noninvasive assessment, particularly using velocity mapping which has similarities to 2D Doppler but can also be extended into multi-dimensional flow imaging for complex flow dynamics problems.

Mohiaddin et al. investigated the use of CMR phase-shift velocity mapping to assess mitral and pulmonary venous flows, which are important indices in the evaluation of left ventricular diastolic function and in the assessment of mitral valve disease.[47] A similar technique was used by Kilner et al. to evaluate aortic and mitral stenoses. In comparison with Doppler and catheterization measurements, CMR showed good agreement between techniques.[48] Planimetric techniques have also been used successfully by CMR, offering a fast, safe, and noninvasive method to quantify aortic stenosis.[49,50] Imaging of prosthetic valves is safe for all types of valves. PET is not useful in the clinical assessment of cardiac valve disease.

Congenital heart disease

In the assessment of complex congenital heart disease, the advantage of CMR over echocardiography is that it is unlimited in the views that can be acquired. Pulmonary disease or large breasts do not affect the image quality and it is not confined by poor or limited echocardiography windows. Reproducible images with a wide field of view can be acquired of structures such as the right ventricle or the pulmonary arteries, which may be difficult to assess by echocardiography. Its 3D properties allow accurate characterization of the anatomy (Fig. 12.12) – sometimes with the use of contrast-enhanced CMR angiography, which can be used to delineate collaterals or other vascular pathologies such as pulmonary atresia or interruption of the aortic arch. Flow mapping can help identify hemodynamically significant problems including vascular lesions (e.g. pulmonary artery stenosis or coarctation of the aorta) or valvular stenosis (e.g. mitral stenosis with hypertension in the pulmonary vasculature). CMR plays an important role in guiding pregnancy. Assessment of anatomy, right- and left-sided hemodynamics including shunts and shunt volumes as well as operation results can help evaluate whether or not a pregnancy is safe. CMR with its excellent reproducibility also facilitates reliable follow-up to judge disease progression or postoperative results.

Pre-eclampsia

There is little work to date on understanding and characterizing the cardiac changes seen in pre-eclampsia. Potential roles for CMR will be in assessing left ventricular function and size as well as research applications examining endothelial abnormalities characterized by changes in brachial artery reactivity.

Other pathologies

Cardiomyopathy associated with thalassemia

A unique application of CMR has evolved in the management of thalassemia major. In this transfusion-dependent condition, iron overload from transfusions results in cardiac iron accumulation. Chronically, this leads to heart failure, which worldwide is the commonest cause of death in these patients. Iron has paramagnetic properties. Over the last 3 years, by using spin-echo measurements as a surrogate marker for iron estimation in the heart to guide chelation therapy, there has been a sustained 70% fall in mortality. This may translate into a significantly improved survival for these patients, where the average life expectancy is currently only 35.[51,52]

Insulin resistance

Iozzo et al. demonstrated a relationship between type 2 diabetes and myocardial insulin resistance measured with FDG PET, which is independent of the presence of coronary artery disease.[53] Similarly, Paternostro et al. showed insulin resistance in myocardial hypertrophy, which was associated with alterations in the insulin-dependent transmembrane glucose transporters.[54] At present, this application is being assessed in women.

Practical aspects

Adverse effects, limitations, and use in pregnancy

CMR is currently contraindicated in patients with an implanted pacemaker, implantable cardioverter defibrillator device, cerebral clips used for aneurysms, metal deposit in the eye, and spinal operations with metal implants, as well as in patients with severe claustrophobia.

Importantly however, there is a large cohort of patients in whom there is widespread misconception about the safety of CMR. In particular, patients with coronary stents, sternal wires, and all types of prosthetic valves can be safely scanned. Patients with a wide variety of other metal implants such as hip prostheses can also be safely scanned. CMR in pregnancy is considered to be safe in the third trimester. It is probably safe in the second trimester, and limited data exist to support this proposition.[55,56]

Information on MR safety can be found on the following website: http://www.mrisafety.com/. Specialist opinion should always be sought if there is uncertainty about safety in any patient with a metal implant.

Due to its use of ionizing radiation, PET in pregnancy is generally avoided. Although some tracers have a half-life of only minutes, there is no indication to justify a cardiac PET scan during pregnancy. PET scans should also be limited, although not contraindicated, in premenopausal and lactating women.

Comparison with other techniques

Of all cardiovascular imaging techniques, CMR is the most versatile. Its strength is the ability to obtain high-resolution multiplanar images with good tissue characterization. It is superior to nuclear techniques in terms of spatial resolution and the fact that it is free from ionizing radiation.

Compared with echocardiography, CMR has better spatial resolution and is more reproducible and observer-independent, particularly in the assessment of ventricular volumes and geometry, as well as myocardial mass.[57] This is important where an accurate diagnosis is required or for serial assessment pre- and post-treatment. However, echocardiography is cheaper and more accessible. There are no problems in undertaking echocardiography in patients with pacemakers. It is also portable and so can be performed by the bedside. It has the highest temporal resolution of all cardiovascular imaging modalities, and with an experienced examiner provides reasonable assessment of left ventricular function and valve disease. Problems arise in about 20% of patients where suboptimal images are acquired due to factors that interfere with ultrasound penetration, such as obesity or chronic obstructive airways disease, or in patients with large breasts. In addition, considerable inter-observer variability occurs, therefore making follow-up less reliable. Echocardiography is less suited than CMR to accurately assess right ventricular pathology or diseases of the great vessels and other congenital abnormalities. The WISE study has documented low sensitivity of dobutamine echocardiography testing for significant multivessel disease in women with suspected myocardial ischemia and this is an area where CMR may have key strengths.[58]

Imaging of the coronary artery remains difficult due to limitations in temporal and spatial resolution and at present X-ray angiography remains the gold standard.

Compared with single-photon emission computerized tomography (SPECT), PET has a better spatial resolution and thus greater sensitivity. Therefore, usually lower doses of radionuclides are needed to acquire diagnostic images. In addition, attenuation correction, which is necessary to correct for breast artifacts for example, has only very recently become available for SPECT. By contrast, PET is more expensive and requires greater infrastructure and expertise, thus limiting its availability. SPECT cameras are more widely available with lower operational costs and images require less post-acquisition analysis.

Electrocardiography remains a valuable screening tool. Pre-existent pathologies such as previous MI can make interpretation of the ECG difficult, when the baseline ECG is not normal. This is also true for exercise tests that rely on ECG tracings. Particularly in women, the rate of false positive tests is high (some studies suggest as high as 67%). In addition, in many female patients fatigue occurs before sufficient exercise is achieved.[59,60]

When to refer?

A woman should be referred for CMR for:

(1) Accurate diagnosis of left and right ventricular function and size.

(2) Where echocardiography images are suboptimal.

(3) Assessment of cardiomyopathies.

(4) Viability assessment of left ventricular dysfunction and previous Ml.

(5) Perfusion imaging, especially in patients with a false positive exercise test where syndrome X may be a possibility or if there is gross LVH.

(6) Patients with complex valvular lesions.

(7) Presence of congenital abnormalities for diagnosis, monitoring or to assess the hemodynamic status as a baseline, before a pregnancy or if any deterioration in symptoms.

(8) Assessment of pericardial diseases.

(9) Aortic dissection.

Indications for a clinical PET scan are:

(1) Viability assessment and perfusion imaging.

(2) To assess the functional significance of a potentially flow-limiting coronary artery stenosis – particularly in the context of multivessel disease.[61]

(3) In conditions where myocardial perfusion is diffusely impaired due to widespread dysfunction of the coronary microcirculation, such as in hypertrophic cardiomyopathy, syndrome X, or hypertensive heart disease.[62]

Future developments

The application of CMR is likely to expand dramatically. There are a number of key growth areas. Shorter scan times are likely with improved spatial and temporal resolution, especially with the advent of 3-T scanners and parallel imaging techniques. Cardiac MR at 3 T will improve signal to noise, which will benefit viability and perfusion imaging. More real-time imaging with better spatial and temporal resolution due to parallel imaging techniques is being worked on. Improved characterization of coronary angiography and plaque disease (with resolutions closer to 300 μm) will be exciting. Another area of much interest is the use of targeted contrast agents, for instance to visualize vulnerable plaques. Interventional procedures that use the 3D evaluation provided by CMR will be helpful in complex congenital heart disease. Self-gating sequences which obviate the need for ECG leads are promising. Magnetic resonance spectroscopy has potential to detect myocardial ischemia by demonstrating transient reduction in myocardial high-energy phosphates and increases in inorganic phosphate during stress testing.[63]

Recent advances in PET scanner technology should allow the quantification of the transmural distribution of myocardial blood flow. Cardiac adrenoceptors regulation and new potential radioligands for imaging are currently being evaluated.

Conclusion

CMR is a very versatile, noninvasive tool in the diagnosis and follow-up of cardiac disease, which does not involve the use of ionizing radiation. This makes it particularly suitable for imaging of women of childbearing age. It has several key strengths. It has the ability to characterize tissues according to their chemical composition, which is important in diseases of the myocardium such as cardiomyopathies or CHD. It has higher accuracy and reproducibility to measure cardiac function and mass than echocardiography regardless of ventricular geometry, and through the unlimited number of views that can be generated of the heart and the great vessels. In the assessment of coronary lesions, much progress has been made but at this time X-ray angiography still has better spatial resolution. Future developments may overcome this.

The standard clinical application for cardiac PET remains FDG to assess myocardial viability. PET imaging with other tracers which play a major role in the assessment of cardiac metabolism remains an interesting field of ongoing research and may provide further insight into pathophysiological mechanisms of diseases, which are unexplained to date.

Acknowledgments

Thanks to Drs David Dutka, Andrew Elkington, and Mark Westwood for their contributions.

References

1. Misra D. *The Women's Health Data Book: A Profile of Women's Health in the United States*, 3rd edn. Washington, DC: Jacobs Institute of Women's Health and The Henry J. Kaiser Family Foundations, 2001: 69–73.

2. Department of Health. *National Service Framework for Coronary Artery Disease: Modern Standards and Service Models.* London: Stationery Office, 2000.

3. American Heart Association. *Heart Disease and Stroke Statistics—2003 Update.* Dallas, TX: American Heart Association, 2002.

4. Vogels E, Lagro-Janssen A, van Weel C. Sex differences in cardiovascular disease: are women with low socio-economic status at high risk? *Br J Gen Pract* 1999; **49**:963–6.

5. Kee F, Gaffney B, Currie S, et al. Access to coronary catheterisation: fair shares for all? *BMJ* 1993; **307**:1305–7.

6. Spencer I, Unwin N, Pledger G. Hospital investigation of men and women treated for angina. *BMJ* 1995; **310**:1576.

7. McLaughlin T, Soumerai S, Willison D, et al. Adherence to national guidelines for drug treatment of suspected acute myocardial infarction. Evidence of under treatment in women and the elderly. *Arch Intern Med* 1996; **156**:799–805.

8. Pohost GM, Hung L, Doyle M. Clinical use of cardiovascular magnetic resonance. *Circulation* 2003; **108**:647–53.

9. Baer FM, Voth E, Schneider CA, et al. Comparison of low-dose dobutamine–gradient-echo magnetic resonance imaging and positron emission tomography with [18F]fluorodeoxyglucose in patients with chronic coronary artery disease. A functional and morphological approach to the detection of residual myocardial viability. *Circulation* 1995; **91**:1006–15.

10. Kim WY, Danias PG, Stuber M, et al. Coronary magnetic resonance angiography for the detection of coronary stenoses. *N Engl J Med* 2001; **345**:1863–9.

11. Post JC, van Rossum AC, Bronzwaer JG, et al. Magnetic resonance angiography of anomalous coronary arteries. A new gold standard for delineating the proximal course? *Circulation* 1995; **92**:3163–71.

12. Muhling O, Jerosch-Herold M, Nabauer M, et al. Assessment of ischemic heart disease using magnetic resonance first-pass perfusion imaging. *Herz* 2003; **28**:82–9.

13. Nagel E, Lorenz C, Baer F, et al. Stress cardiovascular magnetic resonance: consensus panel report. *J Cardiovasc Magn Reson* 2001; **3**:267–81.

14. Mahrholdt H, Wagner A, Judd RM, et al. Assessment of myocardial viability by cardiovascular magnetic resonance imaging. *Eur Heart J* 2002; **23**:602–19.

15. Dutka DP, Camici PG. Hibernation and congestive heart failure. *Heart Fail Rev* 2003; **8**:167–73.

16. Kaufmann PA, Gnecchi-Ruscone T, di Terlizzi M, et al. Coronary heart disease in smokers: vitamin C restores coronary microcirculatory function. *Circulation* 2000; **102**:1233–8.

17. Kaufmann PA, Gnecchi-Ruscone T, Schafers KP, et al. Low density lipoprotein cholesterol and coronary microvascular dysfunction in hypercholesterolemia. *J Am Coll Cardiol* 2000; **36**:103–9.

18. Sdringola S, Patel D, Gould KL. High prevalence of myocardial perfusion abnormalities on positron emission tomography in asymptomatic persons with a parent or sibling with coronary artery disease. *Circulation* 2001; **103**:496–501.

19. Momose M, Abletshauser C, Neverve J, et al. Dysregulation of coronary microvascular reactivity in asymptomatic patients with type 2 diabetes mellitus. *Eur J Nucl Med Mol Imaging* 2002; **29**:1675–9.

20. Gerber BL, Ordoubadi FF, Wijns W, et al. Positron emission tomography using(18)F-fluoro-deoxyglucose and euglycaemic hyperinsulinaemic glucose clamp: optimal criteria for the prediction of recovery of post-ischaemic left ventricular dysfunction. Results from the European Community Concerted Action Multicenter study on use of (18)F-fluoro-deoxyglucose Positron Emission Tomography for the Detection of Myocardial Viability. *Eur Heart J* 2001; **22**:1691–701.

21. McCrohon JA, Moon JC, Prasad SK, et al. Differentiation of heart failure related to dilated cardiomyopathy and coronary artery disease using gadolinium-enhanced cardiovascular magnetic resonance. *Circulation* 2003; **108**:54–9.

22. Maron BJ, Bonow RO, Cannon RO, et al. Hypertrophic cardiomyopathy: interrrelations of clinical manifestations, pathophysiology, and therapy: parts 1 and 2. *N Engl J Med* 1987; **316**:780–9, 844–52.

23. Moon JC, McKenna WJ, McCrohon JA, et al. Toward clinical risk assessment in hypertrophic cardiomyopathy with gadolinium cardiovascular magnetic resonance. *J Am Coll Cardiol* 2003; **41**:1561–7.

24. Weidman CE, McKenna WJ, Watkins HC, et al. Molecular genetic approaches to diagnosis and management of hypertrophic cardiomyopathy. In: Braunwald E (ed.) *Heart Disease. A Textbook of*

Cardiovascular Medicine. New York: WB Saunders, 1992: 77–83.

25. McKenna WJ, Thiene G, Nava A, et al. Criteria for diagnosis of ARVC. *Br Heart J* 1994; **71**:215–18.

26. Tabib A, Loire R, Chalabreysse L, et al. Circumstances of death and gross and microscopic observations in a series of 200 cases of sudden death associated with arrhythmogenic right ventricular cardiomyopathy and/or dysplasia. *Circulation* 2003; **108**:3000–5.

27. Bluemke DA, Krupinski EA, Ovitt T, et al. MR imaging of arrhythmogenic right ventricular cardiomyopathy: morphologic findings and interobserver reliability. *Cardiology* 2003; **99**:153–62.

28. Hartmann F, Ziegler S, Nekolla S, et al. Regional patterns of myocardial sympathetic denervation in dilated cardiomyopathy: an analysis using carbon-11 hydroxyephedrine and positron emission tomography. *Heart* 1999; **81**:262–70.

29. Wichter T, Schafers M, Rhodes CG, et al. Abnormalities of cardiac sympathetic innervation in arrhythmogenic right ventricular cardiomyopathy: quantitative assessment of presynaptic norepinephrine reuptake and postsynaptic beta-adrenergic receptor density with positron emission tomography. *Circulation* 2000; **101**:1552–8.

30. van den Heuvel AF, van Veldhuisen DJ, van der Wall EE, et al. Regional myocardial blood flow reserve impairment and metabolic changes suggesting myocardial ischemia in patients with idiopathic dilated cardiomyopathy. *J Am Coll Cardiol* 2000; **35**:19–28.

31. Savage DD, Garrison RJ, Kannel WB, et al. The spectrum of left ventricular hypertrophy in a general population sample: The Framingham Study. *Circulation* 1987; **75** (Suppl 1):I26–33.

32. Cooper RS, Simmons BE, Castaner A, et al. Left ventricular hypertrophy is associated with worse survival independent of ventricular function and number of coronary arteries severely narrowed. *Am J Cardiol* 1990; **65**:441–5.

33. Kannel WB. Prevalence and natural history of electro-cardiographic left ventricular hypertrophy. *Am J Med* 1983; **75** (Suppl 3A):4–11.

34. Kannel WB. Left ventricular hypertrophy as a risk factor for arterial hypertension. *Eur Heart J* 1992; **13** (Suppl D):82–8.

35. Levy D, Garrison RJ, Savage DD, et al. Prognostic implications of echocardiographically determined left ventricular mass in the Framingham heart study. *N Engl J Med* 1990; **322**:1561–6.

36. Sullivan J, Vander Zwag RV, el-Zeky F, et al. Left ventricular hypertrophy: effect on survival. *J Am Coll Cardiol* 1993; **22**:508–13.

37. Pichard AD, Gorlin R, Smith H, et al. Coronary flow studies in patients with left ventricular hypertrophy of the hypertensive type. Evidence for an impaired coronary vascular reserve. *Am J Cardiol* 1981; **47**:547–53.

38. Opherk D, Mall G, Zebe H, et al. Reduction of coronary reserve: a mechanism for angina pectoris in patients with arterial hypertension and normal coronary arteries. *Circulation* 1984; **69**:1–7.

39. Marcus ML, Doty DB, Hiratzka LF, et al. A mechanism for angina pectoris in patients with aortic stenosis and normal coronary arteries. *N Engl J Med* 1982; **307**:1362–7.

40. Malik AB, Abe T, O'Kane H, et al. Cardiac function, coronary flow and oxygen consumption in stable left ventricular hypertrophy. *Am J Physiol* 1973; **225**:186–91.

41. O'Keefe DD, Hoffman JIE, Cheitlin R, et al. Coronary blood flow in experimental canine left ventricular hypertrophy. *Circ Res* 1978; **43**:43–51.

42. McAinsh AM, Turner MA, O'Hare D, et al. Cardiac hypertrophy impairs recovery from ischaemia because there is a reduced reactive hyperaemic response. *Cardiovasc Res* 1995; **30**:113–21.

43. Reis SE, Holubkov R, Conrad Smith AJ, et al. Coronary microvascular dysfunction is highly prevalent in women with chest pain in the absence of coronary artery disease: results from the NHLBI WISE study. *Am Heart J* 2001; **141**:735–41.

44. Marroquin OC, Holubkov R, Edmundowicz D, et al. Heterogeneity of microvascular dysfunction in women with chest pain not attributable to coronary artery disease: implications for clinical practice. *Am Heart J* 2003; **145**:628–35.

45. Panting JR, Gatehouse PD, Yang G-Z, et al. Abnormal subendocardial perfusion in cardiac syndrome X detected by cardiovascular magnetic resonance imaging. *N Engl J Med* 2002; **346**:1948–53.

46. Bottcher M, Botker HE, Sonne H, et al. Endothelium-dependent and -independent perfusion reserve and the effect of L-arginine on myocardial perfusion in patients with syndrome X. *Circulation* 1999; **99**:1795–801.

47. Mohiaddin RH, Amanuma M, Kilner PJ, et al. MR phase-shift velocity mapping of mitral and pulmonary venous flow. *J Comput Assist Tomogr* 1991; **15**:237–43.

48. Kilner PJ, Manzara CC, Mohiaddin RH, et al. Magnetic resonance jet velocity mapping in mitral and aortic valve stenosis. *Circulation* 1993; **87**:1239–48.

49. John AS, Dill T, Brandt RR, et al. Magnetic resonance to assess the aortic valve area in aortic stenosis: how

does it compare to current diagnostic standards? *J Am Coll Cardiol* 2003; **42**:519–26.

50. Friedrich MG, Schulz-Menger J, Poetsch T, et al. Quantification of valvular aortic stenosis by magnetic resonance imaging. *Am Heart J* 2002; **144**:329–34.

51. Anderson LJ, Wonke B, Prescott E, Holden S, Walker JM, Pennell DJ. Comparison of effects of oral deferiprone and subcutaneous desferrioxamine on myocardial iron concentrations and ventricular function in beta-thalassaemia. *Lancet* 2002; **360**:516–20.

52. Westwood MA, Sheppard MN, Awogbade M, Ellis G, Stephens AD, Pennell DJ. Myocardial biopsy and T2* magnetic resonance in heart failure due to thalassaemia. *Br J Haematol* 2005; **128**:2.

53. Iozzo P, Chareonthaitawee P, Dutka D, et al. Independent association of type 2 diabetes and coronary artery disease with myocardial insulin resistance. *Diabetes* 2002; **51**:3020–4.

54. Paternostro G, Pagano D, Gnecchi-Ruscone T, et al. Insulin resistance in patients with cardiac hypertrophy. *Cardiovasc Res* 1999; **42**:246–53.

55. Michel SC, Rake A, Keller TM, et al. Fetal cardiographic monitoring during 1.5-T MR imaging. *Am J Roentgenol* 2003; **180**:1159–64.

56. Baker PN, Johnson IR, Harvey PR, et al. A three-year follow-up of children imaged in utero with echoplanar magnetic resonance. *Am J Obstet Gynecol* 1994; **170**:32–3.

57. Bellenger NG, Burgess Ml, Ray SG, et al. Comparison of left ventricular ejection fraction and volumes in heart failure by echocardiography, radionuclide ventriculography and cardiovascular magnetic resonance; are they interchangeable? *Eur Heart J* 2000; **21**:1387–96.

58. Lewis JF, McGorray SP, Pepine CJ. Assessment of women with suspected myocardial ischemia: review of findings of the Women's Ischemia Syndrome Evaluation (WISE) Study. *Curr Womens Health Rep* 2002; **2**:110–14.

59. Sketch MH, Mohiuddin SM, Lynch JD, et al. Significant sex differences in the correlation of electrocardiographic exercise testing and coronary arteriograms. *Am J Cardiol* 1975; **36**:169–73.

60. Sullivan AK, Holdright DR, Wright CA, et al. Chest pain in women: clinical, investigative, and prognostic features. *BMJ* 1994; **308**:883–6.

61. Uren NG, Melin JA, De Bruyne B, et al. Relation between myocardial blood flow and the severity of coronary-artery stenosis. *N Engl J Med* 1994; **330**:1782–8.

62. Choudhury L, Rosen SD, Patel D, et al. Coronary vasodilator reserve in primary and secondary left ventricular hypertrophy. A study with positron emission tomography. *Eur Heart J* 1997; **18**:108–16.

63. Buchthal SD, den Hollander JA, Merz CN, et al. Abnormal myocardial phosphorus-31 nuclear magnetic resonance spectroscopy in women with chest pain but normal coronary angiograms. *N Engl J Med* 2000; **342**:829–35.

13

Diagnostic procedures: electron beam tomography and multislice computed tomography

Leslee J. Shaw and Paolo Raggi

Introduction

Although prevention strategies have resulted in marked declines in cardiovascular disease (CVD) mortality, women have not matched the 35–50% reductions noted for men.[1–4] The third report from the National Cholesterol Education Program (NCEP) emphasizes using global risk scores or multifactorial risk assessment to identify intermediate- to high-risk individuals who will benefit from aggressive risk reduction programs.[3] This method of targeting risk integrates multiple risk factors, such as age, gender, hypertension, smoking, and hyperlipidemia, into a 10-year estimate of coronary heart disease (CHD) death or nonfatal myocardial infarction (MI).[5] The NCEP risk calculator is based upon data from the Framingham study cohort and defines low, intermediate, and high risk as 10-year event rates of <6%, 6–20%, and >20%.[3] Data presented at the 34th Bethesda Conference on atherosclerotic imaging demonstrate that fewer women than men are categorized as intermediate to high risk, which is considered the optimal risk category for screening for subclinical disease.[6,7]

Recent reports further suggest that an alarmingly large number of women who are characterized as low risk have evidence of subclinical disease.[8–11] Thus, standard risk factors account for a lower explanatory variation in outcome in women than men. Indeed, published literature suggests that, on average, only 60% of the variation in outcome in women can be explained using traditional cardiac risk factors (e.g. the Framingham risk score).[8–12] Due to the disparity in risk factor prevalence and the associated prognosis, outcome estimation is challenging in women.

As a consequence, recent research has aimed at the development of imaging and other markers of subclinical disease to improve outcome stratification in women.[11] The focus of this chapter is the use of tomographic techniques, with electron beam tomography (EBT) or multislice computed tomography (MSCT) to measure calcification in the major coronary arteries as a measure of the global plaque burden and attendant CVD risk.

Cardiovascular epidemiology and screening asymptomatic individuals

There has been recent interest in techniques applied to screening for atherosclerosis to further accelerate the already marked reductions in mortality realized over the past few decades with aggressive risk factor modification strategies. Despite the marked reduction in cardiovascular event rates during the past 30 years, sudden cardiac death remains the leading cause of death in the industrialized world[7,13–16] and the rate of nonfatal MI has continued to rise.[17] The overall incidence rate of sudden cardiac death is one per 1000 individuals in the US. Although the relative risk is highest for patients with left ventricular dysfunction or prior MI, asymptomatic individuals with several risk factors (i.e. those at intermediate–high Framingham risk) suffer the largest absolute number of events in the population. Hence, the latter should likely become the focus of intensive preventive efforts as well. Although the incidence of fatal MI is higher in men, evidence suggests that a greater frequency of asymptomatic women as compared with men present with acute MI or sudden cardiac death as their initial presentation for CHD.[2,6,7]

The historic perspective in population-based risk reduction efforts has been based on reducing the burden of sudden cardiac death by reducing the prevalence of coronary artery disease in the population at-large. This was most often attempted by offering general lifestyle advice to the population. More recent efforts have extended beyond population-based efforts to the identification of the asymptomatic high-risk or vulnerable patients. This has stimulated an ongoing debate about the value of cardiovascular screening in asymptomatic subjects, as the overall event rates are exceedingly low in this population. Despite the apparent low risk in previously asymptomatic women, acute MI or sudden cardiac arrest occurs as the presenting event more often in women than in men.[18] Thus, further risk reduction in asymptomatic females must consider the option of cardiovascular screening with goals similar to those of lung and breast cancer screening efforts. In essence, early detection may lead to improved survival and can, therefore, be cost-effective when applied to populations of women.[19]

Defining the effectiveness of atherosclerotic imaging as a screening tool

A screening test utilized in the assessment of prognosis should be considered effective under the following criteria: (1) it is highly accurate in determining the likelihood that an asymptomatic person has the condition; (2) the results are reliable and consistent when applied across population subsets; and (3)

early intervention is likely to have a beneficial impact on population disease incidence. In addition to these commonly applied criteria, the recent Bethesda Conference on atherosclerosis imaging further recommended that an imaging modality must also provide incremental value to the assessment of risk above and beyond the office-based risk assessment (e.g. Framingham risk score) that may also include low-cost laboratory tests (e.g. high sensitivity C-reactive protein).[7] In the area of asymptomatic screening, controversy exists regarding the added value of imaging, with some investigators reporting negative results and others reporting positive results. For example, in the Rotterdam study,[20] carotid intima-media thickness did not improve the estimation of stroke or MI over traditional risk factor assessment, while in the study by Shaw et al.[21] coronary artery calcium was reported to improve the receiver operating characteristics curves for the estimation of mortality.[7,20–22]

Defining measures of subclinical disease

Coronary artery calcification is one measure of subclinical disease that may also be defined as a presymptomatic state. Other indicators of subclinical disease include markers such as inflammatory mediators (e.g. high sensitivity C-reactive protein), abnormal brachial artery reactivity, retinal artery narrowing, and increased carotid intima-media thickness. In addition to coronary calcium measurements, among the various imaging modalities to assess the presence of subclinical disease, research has focused on ankle brachial index, brachial reactivity, retinography, and carotid intima-media thickness.[9,10,23,24] There is increasing interest in the application of magnetic resonance-based techniques for the detection and evaluation of atherosclerotic plaque in vivo, although these approaches are still in their preliminary phases of development.[1,25,26] (See also Chapter 12).

EBT and MSCT scanning are being applied with increasing frequency for the screening of asymptomatic individuals with the purpose of refining the assessment of cardiovascular risk and providing imaging-based incremental prognostic information above traditional risk factors. The sole purpose of cardiovascular screening of asymptomatic individuals is the detection of subclinical disease and ensuing intervention prior to symptomatic presentation. The desired benefit, but ultimately the challenge of screening asymptomatic persons is the avoidance of costly, symptomatic care. However, long-term economic data are, as yet, unavailable to clearly define the societal burden of widespread screening.[19] In a recent review of atherosclerosis imaging modalities, the 34th Bethesda Conference as well as other societal guidelines and position statements have supported the utility of screening intermediate-risk individuals.[19] Currently, EBT and MSCT techniques are most commonly applied in the US for this purpose. In addition to risk assessment, the measurement of coronary artery calcium has been used to assess progression/regression of disease burden using primary prevention strategies (e.g. statin therapy).[27–30]

Detecting coronary artery calcification

Coronary artery calcification is common and increases with age. The prevalence of significant coronary calcification (i.e. score >400) in women ranges from 5% in a middle-aged population to approximately 50% in an elderly cohort.[8,31,32] Coronary calcification occurs as part of the development of atherosclerosis. Indeed, it does not occur in a normal vessel wall but is part of the natural evolution of advancing atherosclerotic plaques and appears to be due to an active process of calcification.[31]

Generally, coronary artery calcification occurs earlier in a man's life (at about the second or third decade), while it takes place about 10 years later in women. The extent of coronary calcification is strongly related to the degree of atherosclerotic disease burden but does not correlate with angiographic stenosis severity.[31] Despite its lack of correlation with angiographic disease or its more prominent occurrence in advanced plaques, recent data show that coronary calcification is a strong estimator of adverse events including all-cause and cardiac

mortality as well as nonfatal MI.[21,33] In the recent report from the South Bay Heart Watch study, patients at intermediate risk (but not low risk) benefited most from referral to coronary calcium screening.

Assessing risk versus estimating obstructive disease

Establishing the societal value of screening includes setting higher standards for imaging performance that includes the estimation of major adverse cardiac events. Determining the prognostic value of a test is different from calculating the diagnostic sensitivity and specificity of a procedure. The aim of the latter approach is to identify a culprit obstructive lesion; for screening, there is no such 'gold standard' test. The detection of subclinical disease through screening of asymptomatic individuals must provide value in terms of risk detection and linking to the initiation of life-saving therapies. This strategy of estimating outcome has been similarly applied to other screening procedures for lung and breast cancer.[19]

Methodology of electron beam and multislice computed tomography

EBT scanning to detect and quantify coronary artery calcification was introduced about 15 years ago and for a long time remained the only method available to screen for coronary artery calcification. At the time of its introduction, this new CT methodology provided a solution to the dilemma of imaging an organ in constant movement such as the heart. Indeed, mechanical CT scanners of older design were unable to overcome the motion artifact produced by a beating heart. In the EBT design, there are no moving mechanical parts like in the traditional computerized axial tomography equipment. Instead, a beam of electrons is projected against a tungsten ring and the impact of the electrons against the tungsten causes the release of an X-ray fan. This fan is rapidly accelerated along the 210° arc of the ring and a rotation can be accomplished in 50–100 msec, while the typical rotational speed of a traditional mechanical CT is about 800–1000 msec. Serial transaxial images are then obtained at 100-msec intervals using slices of 3 mm thickness. Breath-holding sequences, triggered by the electrocardiogram at 40–80% of the R-R interval, are required to minimize artifact due to respiratory motion. Using this technique, epicardial coronary arteries can be easily visualized since they lie surrounded by epicardial fat.[21,34] Coronary calcification can be easily identified because of its high CT density (attenuation), measured in Hounsfield units. Specifically, coronary artery calcification is defined by a lesion density exceeding 130 Hounsfield units and covering a minimum of 3–4 pixels in surface. EBT scanning has much shorter imaging times than other CT scanners.

The EBT design, therefore, allows for the acquisition of images of the heart at very high speed (high temporal resolution),[34] but it offers a lower spatial resolution compared with the slower mechanical CT scanners.

More recently, MSCT scanners have been applied to detect coronary artery calcium.[35–38] These scanners use a strictly paired X-ray source and a set of image detectors (variable from two to 64 in the most modern design) revolving in a spiral manner around the patient lying on a radiological cradle. In this design, the pair scanning mechanical parts are moved in a cranial-caudal direction as they spiral around the patient at about 500 msec per rotation while an electrocardiogram is acquired. Of the multiple images obtained at each level, only those showing minimal to no motion are later selected in a retrospective post-processing approach that takes into consideration the phases of the cardiac revolution as indicated by the electrocardiographic recording. The MSCT technology provides better spatial resolution (crisper images) than EBT, but a lower temporal resolution. To minimize motion artifact with MSCT, a resting heart rate below 60–70 beats per minute is desirable.[35–38] For higher heart rate values, patients must receive beta-blocker therapy prior to imaging.[36–39] One of the benefits of MSCT is the volumetric acquisition that allows for minimal gaps between slices. However, a number of reports have noted the higher radiation exposure to the patient.[35–39] Despite the differences between the two modalities, several investigators have reported moderately strong correlative results.[35–38]

Calcium scores are calculated by either the Agatston score[29] or the volume score.[40] The Agatston score is calculated by multiplying the area of calcification by a density coefficient weighted according to the peak attenuation inside the plaque. It is, therefore, a unitless number and is sensitive to both size and density changes in the plaque. More recently, a calcium volume score, calculated on the basis of the interpolation principle and not sensitive to changes in plaque density, has been introduced and applied to track calcification progression and for monitoring of therapeutic intervention with serial CT scans.[27–29] With both scoring systems, total calcium scores are obtained by summing the score of the individual arteries. The prognostic value of these scores has been published in several large observational series and scores have typically been subdivided in several categories such as low (0–10), mild (11–100), intermediate (101–400), moderately high (401–1000), and high (>1000) risk, corresponding to increasing event rates.[21]

Patho-anatomic differences in women

To optimally apply and assimilate the value of EBT or MSCT imaging modalities, it is helpful to consider the sex-based patho-anatomic differences in atherosclerotic diseases. Simplistically, women not only have a smaller body surface area but also have smaller coronary arteries.[8] A number of recent, albeit provocative reports have noted an increasing role of arterial size and the microvasculature in uniquely affecting outcomes in women.[8,23,41–43] Hormonal factors also appear to affect plaque deposition and lead more often to positive remodeling (i.e. greater vascular wall atherosclerotic storage and minimal luminal intrusion).[41] Thus, in women, evidence of vascular wall abnormalities may play a greater role in risk estimation than provocation of myocardial ischemia, especially in the setting of nonobstructive disease. Recent data from the Atherosclerotic Risk in the Community and Beaver Dam Eye studies provided evidence that retinal artery narrowing is predictive of cardiac death and nonfatal MI in women but not men.[23,42,43] From these data it could be estimated that a standard deviation decline in the retinal arteriole-to-venule ratio related to a 37% increase in cardiac event risk.[23] From a large database of over 4000 women screened using EBT, it was concluded that any burden of coronary artery calcium in women carries a greater risk of death than in men with the same extent of disease.[8] In addition to smaller coronary artery size, hypoestrogenemia has been associated with endothelial dysfunction. There is a loss of vascular distensibility in menopausal women. Additionally, evidence of a worse prognosis in women than men has been demonstrated via measurements of arterial vessel wall thickness.[23,40,42] An increase in carotid intima-media thickness is associated with a worse risk of cardiovascular events in women than men.[23,32,33,44–46] Thus, the extent and severity of atherosclerotic imaging abnormalities should be evaluated within the context of smaller arterial size of women.

The results from CT, retinography, and carotid ultrasound studies support the notion that the arterial size and the functional status of the microvasculature disproportionately influence cardiac event risk in women. They further provide support to the growing hypothesis that study of the vasculature structure and function plays an important role in the detection of risk in women.[23,42,43]

Current evidence on the role of screening asymptomatic women

Traditional risk factors, such as age, hypertension, and hyperlipidemia, account for a little more than half of the explanatory variance in outcome. Thus, the concept of added value in defining effectiveness would mean that the addition of any new imaging or laboratory marker must provide incremental prognostic value above the evaluation of traditional risk factors.[6,8–10,23,24] In screening, an expanding body of knowledge has been put forth on the use of inflammatory or conditional markers such as high sensitivity C-reactive protein[9,10] (see also Chapter 9).

For example, in the Women's Health Study, which included nearly 30 000 middle-aged healthy women, C-reactive protein was a more powerful estimator of first cardiovascular event, even when compared with low-density lipoprotein (LDL) cholesterol.[9] Such reports provide insight into the limited utility of traditional risk assessment, especially in female subsets of the population that are more often characterized as low risk.

Evidence on coronary artery calcium providing added value was initially derived from a report in 306 menopausal women where there was no correlation between the extent of coronary calcification and LDL cholesterol.[24] More recently, several reports have noted an incremental value in estimating mortality as well as major adverse cardiac events in large observational cohorts and epidemiologic series that included a sizeable proportion of women.[8–10,23,24]

Incremental value of coronary calcium in risk detection

There are two critical issues in maximizing screening for women: (1) identifying candidates who will achieve a higher incremental value in screening and (2) understanding the importance of vessel size and how it relates to risk assessment. From the South Bay Heart Watch study, the greatest incremental value of imaging was in patients with an intermediate Framingham risk score. This result was predictable and consistent with Bayes theory where post test risk remains low in low-risk individuals. However, of the 1029 individuals screened in the South Bay Watch study, only 82 were women. Despite this low enrollment of women, one may infer that the lack of predictive accuracy in low-risk subsets may have applicability to female cohorts. And, as such, targeted populations for screening should still include intermediate-risk women, at least for now, until further delineation of risk optimized for female cohorts is defined.

From the EBT Research Foundation in Nashville, TN, a total of 10 377 (40% women) asymptomatic individuals were prospectively enrolled in a cohort study to track survival differences at 5 years.[21] In a subset analysis comparing gender differences, Raggi

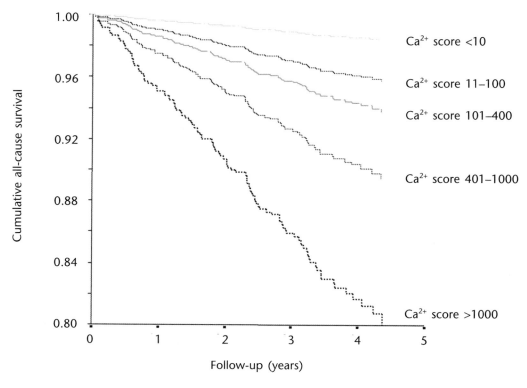

Figure 13.1
Unadjusted all-cause survival from the EBT Research Foundation study in Nashville, TN in 4191 asymptomatic women referred for coronary calcium screening. Event-free survival at 5 years was 99%, 97%, 95%, 90%, and 80%, respectively, for women with calcium scores of 0–10, 11–100, 101–400, 401–1000, and >1000 (p<0.0001). This survival curve was a subset from the report by Shaw et al.[21]

and colleagues noted that for any given calcification extent women had a worse mortality risk as compared with their male counterparts, even after controlling for age and other traditional risk markers as covariates.[8] It appears that, in light of smaller artery size, a given amount of calcification encumbers a greater burden or covers a greater arterial area in women versus men. For women, overall unadjusted 5-year survival ranged from 98% to 80% for those with calcium scores ranging from 0–10 to >1000 (Fig. 13.1, p<0.0001). By comparison, overall survival for men was 99% to 87% for scores ranging from 0–10 to >1000 (p<0.0001). For both women and men, effective risk stratification was possible by the extent of coronary calcification. However, death rates were higher for women, with men achieving

similar event rates at a higher calcium risk. For example, calcium scores of 11–100 were associated with a similar mortality risk in women as that of men with a score of 101–400; the risk associated with a score of 101–400 in women was equivalent to that of a score of 401–1000 in men. Figure 13.2 plots projected 10-year mortality for intermediate and high Framingham risk women and men by their coronary artery calcium measurements. As expected, death rates are worse for high compared with intermediate Framingham risk subsets of women and men. However, women had substantively higher death rates than their male counterparts, especially for scores exceeding 400. In the latter group, diabetic and currently smoking women demonstrated the highest risk of death. Similar to the results noted for

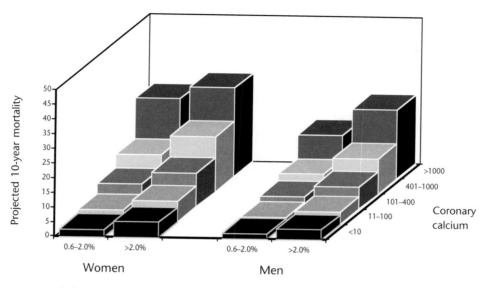

Figure 13.2
Predicted 10-year mortality in women and men by their intermediate or high Framingham risk score and calcium score results. These results were extrapolated from the report by Raggi et al.[8]

retinography and carotid ultrasound, the results appear consistent that traditional risk factors underestimate risk in women and support the utility of additional imaging to delineate vascular atherosclerotic abnormalities.

Although these results may appear controversial, given the differences in body size and arterial diameters, they appear to make reasonable sense. Estimates of variability by gender reveal that a woman's artery is approximately 30% smaller than that of a man.[8] These findings should prompt additional research to create manufacturers' algorithms of gender-tailored scoring systems. But, in lieu of this, physicians should likely be more aggressive in the care of women, especially in the setting of substantial coronary artery calcium accumulation. These results are also consistent with others noting a high risk of events in patients with larger coronary calcium scores.[21,33,47,48] Additionally, these results support the value of atherosclerosis imaging and are in contrast to earlier screening

reports using traditional ischemia testing with treadmill exercise. This latter point may be particularly true for women who have more frequent nonobstructive disease due to hormonally mediated positive remodeling that creates the conditions for potentially larger atherosclerotic disease storage without lumen intrusion. In this case, testing aimed at provoking ischemia would have a poor yield as compared with other modalities that identify vascular abnormalities of wall thickness and calcification or overall vessel narrowing.

Conclusions

There are several compelling points on the use of imaging as screening tools for CVD in women. First, the Framingham or other global risk scores, derived using traditional risk factors, are less reliable in women. The identification of risk in women can be

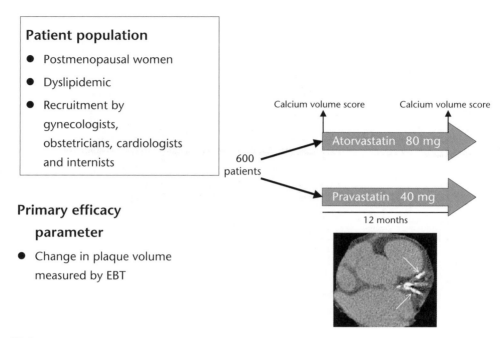

Figure 13.3
Diagram of the inclusion criteria, treatment strategy, and primary outcome for the Beyond Endorsed Lipid Lowering with EBT Scanning (BELLES) trial. EBT, electron beam tomography.

effectively guided by the use of an additional laboratory or imaging test. Although it is uncertain, at this time, whether C-reactive protein will become the screening test of choice, there appears to be a growing body of evidence supporting the utility of coronary artery calcium measurements as a risk assessment tool in asymptomatic women. Recent evidence suggests a synergy of evidence of inflammation and calcification in risk assessment[49] and, as such, additional research is needed to clarify the role of blood versus imaging markers for asymptomatic risk detection. Secondly, further evidence of vascular wall abnormalities appears to uniquely guide risk assessment in women, in large part due to smaller artery size in females. Thirdly, there are compelling reasons why the use of imaging can be a potent motivator for risk modification strategies for patients, and evidence of coronary calcification has been reported to encourage dietary and other lifestyle changes.[50]

Future research is needed to provide gender-specific algorithms tailored to anatomic differences between women and men. An example of such a study is the Beyond Endorsed Lipid Lowering with EBT Scanning (BELLES) trial, currently nearing completion. An ongoing trial is utilizing EBT technology to compare the effectiveness of aggressive versus moderate lipid-lowering therapy on progression of coronary artery calcification. In the presence of disappointing results with menopausal estrogen therapy, statins remain the mainstay of primary as well as secondary prevention of cardiovascular events in women. The end-points of this study include both evidence of atherosclerosis disease progression as well as control of traditional lipid levels and several nontraditional lipoproteins and measurement of other markers of risk (e.g. C-reactive protein). The trial is of particular interest since it involved gynecologists as well as primary care physicians, internists, and cardiologists as recruiting physicians in an attempt to enhance awareness of coronary artery disease-related issues in women in

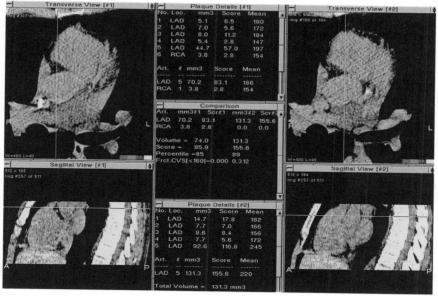

Figure 13.4

Comparative scans at baseline and after 12 months of a single patient treated with statins. The top left and right panels show the initial and follow-up scans in the axial view, while the bottom panels show sagittal views obtained at the same times. The central insert shows an increase in calcium score from a baseline value of 85.9 to 155.6.

as large a group of physicians as possible.[51] Figure 13.3 shows the design of the study and Fig. 13.4 a comparative scan in one of the patients enrolled in the study. Note the almost doubling of the calcium score in the central insert (from 85.9 to 155.6) at the end of 1 year of follow-up.

References

1. Fletcher GF. Preventive cardiology: How can we do better? *J Am Coll Cardiol* 2002; **40**:584–7.

2. Benjamin EJ, Smith SC Jr, Cooper RS, Hill MN, Luepker RV. Task force #1 – magnitude of the prevention problem: opportunities and challenges. 33rd Bethesda Conference. *J Am Coll Cardiol* 2002; **40**:588–603.

3. Executive summary of the third report of the National Cholesterol Education Program (NCEP) expert panel on detection, evaluation, and treatment of high blood cholesterol in adults (Adult Treatment Panel III). *JAMA* 2001; **285**:2486–97.

4. Grundy SM, Pasternak R, Greenland P, Smith S Jr, Fuster V. AHA/ACC scientific statement: Assessment of cardiovascular risk by use of multiple-risk-factor assessment equations: a statement for healthcare professionals from the American Heart Association and the American College of Cardiology. *J Am Coll Cardiol* 1999; **34**:1348–59.

5. http://hin.nhlbi.nih.gov/atpiii/calculator.asp [accessed January 22, 2004].

6. Pasternak RC, Abrams J, Greenland P, Smaha LA, Wilson PW, Houston-Miller N. 34th Bethesda Conference: Task force #1 – Identification of coronary heart disease risk: is there a detection gap? *J Am Coll Cardiol* 2003; **41**:1863–74.

7. Redberg RF, Vogel RA, Criqui MH, Herrington DM,

Lima JA, Roman MJ. 34th Bethesda Conference: Task force #3 – What is the spectrum of current and emerging techniques for the noninvasive measurement of atherosclerosis? *J Am Coll Cardiol* 2003; **41**:1886–98.

8. Raggi P, Shaw LJ, Berman DS, Callister TQ. Gender-based differences in the prognostic value of coronary calcification. *J Womens Health* 2004; **13**:273–83.

9. Ridker PM, Rifai N, Rose L, Buring JE, Cook NR. Comparison of C-reactive protein and low-density lipoprotein cholesterol levels in the prediction of first cardiovascular events. *N Engl J Med* 2002; **347**:1557–65.

10. Ridker PM, Buring JE, Shih J, Matias M, Hennekens CH. Prospective study of C-reactive protein and the risk of future cardiovascular events among apparently healthy women. *Circulation* 1998; **98**:731–3.

11. Wong TY, Klein R, Sharrett AR, et al. Retinal arteriolar narrowing and risk of coronary heart disease in men and women. The Atherosclerosis Risk in Communities Study. *JAMA* 2002; **287**:1153–9.

12. Sharrett AR, Ballantyne CM, Coady SA, et al. Coronary heart disease prediction from lipoprotein cholesterol levels, triglycerides, lipoprotein(a), apolipoproteins A-I and B, and HDL density subfractions: The Atherosclerosis Risk in Communities (ARIC) Study. *Circulation* 2001; **104**:1108–13.

13. Priori SG, Aliot E, Blomstrom-Lundqvist C, et al. Task Force on sudden cardiac death of the European Society of Cardiology. *Eur Heart J* 2001; **22**:1374–450.

14. Naghavi M, Libby P, Falk E, et al. From vulnerable plaque to vulnerable patient: a call for new definitions and risk assessment strategies: Part II. *Circulation* 2003; **108**:1772–8.

15. Naghavi M, Libby P, Falk E, et al. From vulnerable plaque to vulnerable patient: a call for new definitions and risk assessment strategies: Part I. *Circulation* 2003; **108**:1664–72.

16. Schmermund A, Schwartz RS, Adamzik M, et al. Coronary atherosclerosis in unheralded sudden coronary death under age 50: histo-pathologic comparison with 'healthy' subjects dying out of hospital. *Atherosclerosis* 2001; **155**:499–508.

17. Rosamond WD, Chambless LE, Folsom AR, et al. Trends in the incidence of myocardial infarction and in mortality due to coronary heart disease, 1987 to 1994. *N Engl J Med* 1998; **339**:861–7.

18. http://americanheart.org/downloadable/heart/1072969766940HSStats2004Update.pdf [accessed January 15, 2004].

19. Mark DB, Shaw LJ, Lauer MS, O'Malley PG, Heidenreich P. 34th Bethesda Conference: Task force #5 – Is atherosclerosis imaging cost effective? *J Am Coll Cardiol* 2003; **41**:1906–17.

20. del Sol AI, Moons KG, Hollander M, et al. Is carotid intima-media thickness useful in cardiovascular disease risk assessment? The Rotterdam Study. *Stroke* 2001; **32**:1532–8.

21. Shaw LJ, Raggi P, Schisterman E, Berman DS, Callister TQ. Prognostic value of cardiac risk factors and coronary artery calcium screening for all-cause mortality. *Radiology* 2003; **228**:826–33.

22. Detrano RC, Wong ND, Doherty TM, et al. Coronary calcium does not accurately predict near-term future coronary events in high-risk adults. *Circulation* 1999; **99**:2633–8.

23. Wong TY, Klein R, Sharrett AR, et al. Retinal arteriolar narrowing and risk of coronary heart disease in men and women: the Atherosclerosis Risk in Communities Study. *JAMA* 2002; **287**:1153–9.

24. Hecht HS, Superko HR. Electron beam tomography and National Cholesterol Education Program guidelines in asymptomatic women. *J Am Coll Cardiol* 2001; **37**:1506–11.

25. Wilson PWF, Kauppila LI, O'Donnell CJ, et al. Abdominal aortic calcific deposits are an important predictor of vascular morbidity and mortality. *Circulation* 2001; **103**:1529–34.

26. Jaffer FA, O'Donnell CJ, Larson MG, et al. Age and sex distribution of subclinical aortic atherosclerosis – a magnetic resonance imaging examination of the Framingham heart study. *Arterioscler Thromb Vasc Biol* 2002; **22**:849.

27. Callister TQ, Raggi P, Cooil B, Lippolis NJ, Russo DJ. Effect of HMG-CoA reductase inhibitors on coronary artery disease as assessed by electron beam computed tomography. *N Engl J Med* 1998; **339**:1972–7.

28. Budoff MJ, Lane KL, Bakhsheshi H, et al. Rates of progression of coronary calcium by electron beam tomography. *Am J Cardiol* 2000; **86**:8–11.

29. Achenbach S, Ropers D, Pohle K, et al. Influence of lipid-lowering therapy on the progression of coronary artery calcification: a prospective evaluation. *Circulation* 2002; **106**:1077–82.

30. Raggi P, Cooil B, Shaw LJ, et al. Progression of coronary calcification on serial electron beam tomography scanning is greater in patients with future myocardial infarction. *Am J Cardiol* 2003; **92**:827–9.

31. O'Rourke RA, Brundage BH, Froelicher VF, et al. American College of Cardiology/American Heart Association Expert Consensus document on electron-beam computed tomography for the diagnosis and prognosis of coronary artery disease. *Circulation* 2000; **102**:126–40.

32. Newman AB, Naydeck BL, Sutton-Tyrrell K, Feldman A, Edmundowicz D, Kuller LJ. Coronary artery calcification in older adults to age 99: prevalence and risk factors. *Circulation* 2001; **104**:2679–84.

33. Greenland P, LaBree L, Azen SP, Doherty TM, Detrano RC. Coronary artery calcium combined with Framingham score for risk prediction in asymptomatic individuals. *JAMA* 2004; **291**:210–15.

34. Agatston AS, Janowitz AS, Hildner FJ, Zusmer NR, Viamonte M Jr, Detrano R. Quantification of coronary artery calcium using ultrafast computed tomography. *J Am Coll Cardiol* 1990; **15**:827–32.

35. Becker C, Jakobs T, Aydemir S, et al. Helical and single slice conventional versus electron beam CT for quantification of coronary artery calcification. *Am J Roentgenol* 2000; **174**:543–7.

36. Knez A, Becker C, Becker A, et al. New generation computed tomography scanners are equally effective in determining coronary calcium compared to electron beam CT in patients with suspected CAD. *Circulation* 1998; **98**:I-655A.

37. Nasir K, Budoff MJ, Post WS, et al. Electron beam CT versus helical CT scans for assessing coronary calcification: current utility and future directions. *Am Heart J* 2003; **146**:969–77.

38. Horiguchi J, Nakanishi T, Ito K. Quantification of coronary artery calcium using multidetector CT and a retrospective ECG-gating reconstruction algorithm. *Am J Roentgenol* 2001; **177**:1429–35.

39. Knez A, Becker CR, Becker A, et al. Determination of coronary calcium with multi-slice spiral computed tomography: a comparative study with electron-beam CT. *Int J Cardiovasc Imaging* 2002; **18**:295–303.

40. Callister TQ, Cooil B, Raya S, Lippolis NJ, Russo DJ, Raggi P. Coronary artery disease: improved reproducibility of calcium scoring with an electron beam-CT volumetric method. *Radiology* 1998; **208**:807–14 (Comment: *Radiology* 1998; **208**:571–2).

41. Burke AP, Farb A, Malcolm GT, Liang Y, Smialek J, Virmani R. Effects of risk factors on the mechanism of acute thrombosis and sudden coronary death in women. *Circulation* 1998; **97**:2110–16.

42. Bressler NM. Retinal arteriolar narrowing and risk of coronary heart disease. *Arch Ophthalmol* 2003; **121**:113–14.

43. Wong TY, Klein R, Klein BE, Meuer SM, Hubbard LD. Retinal vessel diameters and their associations with age and blood pressure. *Invest Ophthalmol Vis Sci* 2003; **44**:4644–50.

44. Hoff JA, Chomka EV, Krainik AJ, Daviglus M, Rich S, Kondos GT. Age and gender distributions of coronary artery calcium detected by electron beam tomography in 35,246 adults. *Am J Cardiol* 2001; **87**:1335–9.

45. Chambless LE, Folsom AR, Clegg LX, et al. Carotid wall thickness is predictive of incident clinical stroke: the Atherosclerosis Risk in Communities (ARIC) study. *Am J Epidemiol* 2000; **151**:478–87.

46. Barzilay JI, Spiekerman CF, Kuller LH, et al. Prevalence of clinical and isolated subclinical cardiovascular disease in older adults with glucose disorders: the Cardiovascular Health Study. *Diabetes Care* 2001; **24**:1233–9.

47. Raggi P, Callister TQ, Cooil B, et al. Identification of patients at increased risk of first unheralded acute myocardial infarction by electron-beam computed tomography. *Circulation* 2000; **101**:850–5.

48. Wayhs R, Zelinger A, Raggi P. High coronary artery calcium scores pose an extremely elevated risk for hard events. *J Am Coll Cardiol* 2002; **39**:225–30.

49. Park R, Detrano R, Xiang M, et al. Combined use of computed tomography coronary calcium scores and C-reactive protein levels in predicting cardiovascular events in nondiabetic individuals. *Circulation* 2002; **106**:2073–7.

50. Wong NG, Detrano RC, Diamond G, et al. Does coronary artery screening by electron beam computed tomography motivate potentially beneficial lifestyle behaviors? *Am J Cardiol* 1996; **78**:1220–3.

51. Raggi P, Callister TQ, Davidson M, et al. Aggressive versus moderate lipid-lowering therapy in postmenopausal women with hypercholesterolemia – rationale and design of the Beyond Endorsed Lipid Lowering with EBT Scanning (BELLES) trial. *Am Heart J* 2001; **141**:722–6.

14

Stable angina pectoris (recognition and management)

Graham Jackson

Introduction

Chronic stable angina is by definition chronic and stable.[1] Unlike acute coronary syndromes there is time available to optimize management.[2] Optimal therapy is not the same as maximal therapy, as the latter may involve an overly aggressive strategy which is not evidence-based. Recent publications have added perspective to the role of medical therapy, percutaneous coronary intervention and coronary artery bypass graft (CABG) surgery with the need to see them as complementary strategies rather than competing alternatives.[3,4] What emerges is the low event rate (mortality and nonfatal infarction of less than 3% per year) whichever treatment is adopted, which means that a less aggressive interventional approach, in women for example, need not reflect treatment bias but good medical practice. Similarly, as women present at an older age a more conservative and quality of life-driven approach in the elderly may incorrectly seem to be gender bias. Focusing on perceived bias could well be counterproductive whereas concentrating on educating women about coronary heart disease (CHD); its prevention, recognition and treatment; is much more likely to lead to better care overall. While we need to make health-care professionals aware of the problem of CHD in women and its mode of presentation, we also need to communicate with women so that they come forward for evaluation.

Several chapters will discuss risk reduction (see Chapters 2–9) and diagnostic evaluation (see Chapters 10–13), so I will use three real case histories to illustrate the challenges in diagnosis and therapy. Just as evidence-based medicine takes us from belief (hypothesis) to proof (trial results), so we need to translate theory into reality. Though often believed to be a menopausal problem, the first two cases illustrate the need to be alert and wary of atypical and typical symptoms in all women, irrespective of age and menopausal status.

Case one – the atypical

As angina is a symptom of a disease process rather than a disease itself, the correct interpretation of symptoms is paramount in making the diagnosis.[5] It is well recognized that women have more atypical chest pain than men and therefore may need direct questions to tease out an effort-induced relationship which is the classical anginal presentation.[6,7]

A 37-year-old premenopausal insulin-dependent diabetic of 18 years duration visited her family doctor complaining of an ache in the chest for the previous 6 weeks. Thinking it was heartburn she had been using over-the-counter antacids from her local pharmacy. The 'heartburn' was not related to exercise in a clear or consistent way. However, after developing a numbness confined to her left arm which she noticed when climbing stairs and inclines she sought advice because she had read a newspaper article about CHD in women which included a piece

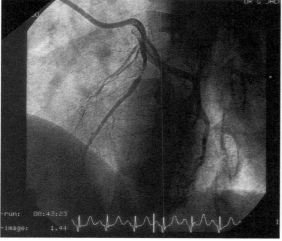

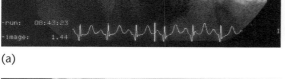

(a)

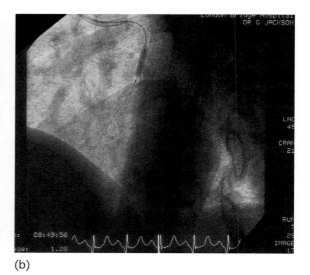

(b)

Figure 14.1
(a) A discrete left anterior descending stenosis; (b) stent being deployed; (c) excellent result.

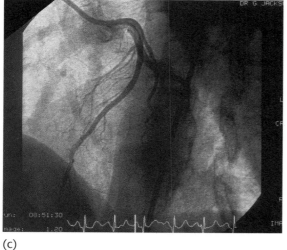

(c)

on numbness in the arms being a possible symptom. Her family doctor felt that the pain was muscular as it was localized to the left arm and he recommended anti-inflammatory agents. He wanted to wait and see how she responded but, because of her diabetes, he decided to refer her for a cardiac opinion which she requested as she was concerned.

When seen in the cardiac clinic she reported a usually active lifestyle without limitation. She was married with two young sons, a lifelong nonsmoker and not overweight (body mass index 24 kg/m²). She had never been hypertensive and there was no family history of vascular disease. Examination was essen-

tially normal with no added heart sounds or murmurs and the blood pressure was 130/80 mmHg. A 12-lead resting electrocardiogram (ECG) was normal and a fasting cholesterol 177 mg/dl.

The story was unconvincing and the only risk factor was diabetes (which was well controlled), yet this is often the management dilemma – is this an anxious young mother who needs reassurance or should we dig deeper? Direct questioning is important and essential when faced with an atypical story given that diabetes is a cardiovascular risk equivalent irrespective of other risk factors. When asked to imagine walking up an incline she said that of late she

Table 14.1 Characteristics of typical and atypical cardiac pain

Typical	Atypical	Women
Tightness	Sharp (not severe)	At rest
Pressure	Knife-like	During sleep
Weight	Stabbing	Stress
Constriction	'Like a stitch'	Jaw, teeth,
Ache	'Like a needle'	arms, neck,
Dull	Pricking feeling	shoulders,
Squeezing feeling	Shooting	back,
Crushing	Can walk around with it	abdomen
'Like a band'	Continuous: 'It's there all day'	
Breathless (tightness)	Located in left chest, abdomen, back or arm in absence of mid-chest pain	
Retrosternal	Unrelated to exercise	
Precipitated by exertion or emotion	Not relieved by rest or nitroglycerin	
Promptly relieved by rest or nitroglycerin	Relieved by antacids; characterized by palpitations without chest pain	

had been a little short of breath. Further probing and the breathlessness sensation became a tightness across the chest relieved by slowing down or stopping. She did not admit to pain at rest but had woken on one occasion 4 weeks previously with pain at the time of a vivid dream. An ischemic story was unfolding and the episode of nocturnal pain, although not recent, was worrying. She was commenced on diltiazem and aspirin, and in view of her young age and my slight anxiety about the night pain, urgent angiography was arranged. Beta-blockers were not used as she occasionally had hypoglycemic episodes and, except for perspiration, they can be masked by beta-blockers.

Angiography revealed a single proximal left anterior descending (LAD) coronary artery stenosis which was successfully stented (Fig. 14.1). She has been symptom-free now for 4 years. With regard to long-term risk reduction, she is taking aspirin, a statin, and an angiotensin-converting enzyme (ACE) inhibitor. Her low-density lipoprotein (LDL) cholesterol is less than 80 mg/dl.

Lesson one – the story

Women more frequently present with atypical chest pain (Table 14.1). This may be due to the increased prevalence of less common causes of ischemia, such

as cardiac syndrome X (see Chapter 15) and non-ischemic syndromes such as mitral valve prolapse, which is frequently associated with atypical pain after rather than during exercise.

The Coronary Artery Surgery Study (CASS) classified symptoms according to three criteria: (1) substernal chest discomfort, (2) precipitated by effort and (3) relieved by rest or glyceryl trinitrate within 10 minutes.[8] Angina was considered typical if all three criteria were present, atypical if any two and nonanginal if only one criterion was present. Of interest, the probability of coronary disease prevalence could be predicted from age, sex, symptom characteristics and Framingham risk factors as accurately as from noninvasive testing. Women have a lower CHD incidence than men but symptoms still predict prevalence (Table 14.2).[9] As women become older their CHD symptoms become more like those

Table 14.2 Chest pain characteristics and the prevalence of significant coronary heart disease in women and men

Angina	Women (%)	Men (%)
Definite	68	95
Possible/probable	30	71
Atypical	6	18

From reference 9.

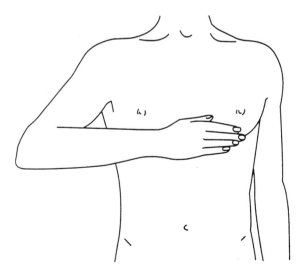

Figure 14.2
Patient may draw flat of hand across chest to indicate central, retrosternal pain that spreads.

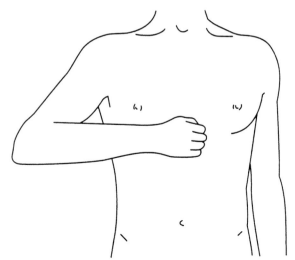

Figure 14.3
Clenched fist in the center vividly illustrating constriction or tightness felt.

of men, so it is important in younger women to have a high index of suspicion and to be aware of the differences and difficulties in the interpretation of the history. To some extent the presentation may be influenced by a woman's perception of a reduced chance of CHD ('it's a man's disease') and priorities within the family, rather than for herself.

Women with chronic stable angina when compared with men are more likely to experience symptoms at rest, during sleep and under emotional stress. Symptoms may be felt more outside the classical central chest location and include the jaw, teeth, arms, neck and shoulders, back and abdomen.[6] The inside of the arm is more likely to be cardiac, the outside muscular.[5] The symptom itself may be different in women who more often complain of breathlessness (blamed on weight), which is their perception of tightness, recent fatigue, perspiration, and palpitations.

In premenopausal women, diabetes is the great leveler with regard to risk, being present in 10% of women sustaining a myocardial infarction and only 2% of normal controls.[10] It is therefore especially important to assess the history in diabetics and to be alert to the potential problem of CHD in otherwise

unlikely candidates. I firmly believe that leading the patient can help establish the diagnosis:

- 'What do you mean by breathlessness – do you feel tight or are you just winded?'
- 'Imagine you are walking up an incline – what happens?'
- 'Has your husband/partner commented that you have slowed down recently?'

It is always important to watch the hand movements as shown in Figs 14.2–14.4, and to take seriously the visit which ends with 'and by the way doctor ...'. Taking a good history and assessing cardiovascular risk is the most important initial step in evaluating any patient and it relies on old-fashioned clinical acumen and taking the time to listen.

Case two – the unlikely

Health-care workers over time and based on epidemiological studies recognize the unlikely or frequent presence of CHD in various racial groups.

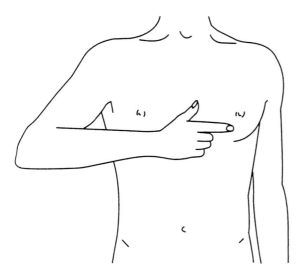

Figure 14.4
Patient almost never points to the pain as if localized.

Asians are particularly vulnerable, especially if diabetic, whereas Afro-Caribbean women rarely develop CHD, particularly if premenopausal; their chest pains often relate to hypertensive left ventricular hypertrophy.[11,12]

A 43-year-old Afro-Caribbean lady was referred by her family doctor because of chest pain. She had just registered with his practice and he noted that she was hypertensive (160/110 mmHg) on lisinopril 15 mg daily. He added atenolol and gave her a trial of glyceryl trinitrate, which she found effective. He referred her for a cardiac assessment. The symptoms were surprisingly typical for ischemia with tightness in the chest on effort for over 12 months. She had noticed the symptoms particularly on steep hills and when she was over-excited or stressed. The pain radiated to the inside of both arms, and to the left more than the right. She was a nonsmoker and her cholesterol was 225 mg/dl with triglycerides 90 mg/dl, high-density lipoprotein (HDL) cholesterol 105 mg/dl, and LDL 100 mg/dl – not a high-risk profile. Her resting ECG was normal and her echocardiogram showed mild left ventricular hypertrophy but good left ventricular function. Her blood pressure was 150/80 mmHg. She was not overweight.

Her only risk factor was hypertension but her symptoms were very suspicious even though she would be considered a very unlikely candidate for CHD. An exercise ECG was performed and was terminated at 4 minutes 11 seconds by chest tightness and anterior ST segment elevation (Fig. 14.5). Her treatment was changed to atenolol 100 mg and amlodipine 5 mg daily and aspirin commenced. Urgent angiography identified a critical origin LAD stenosis (Fig. 14.6) and she underwent coronary artery bypass grafting (CABG) with the left internal mammary artery anastomosed to the LAD and saphenous vein to the diagonal branch. There was no evidence of atheroma beyond the stenosis.

She made a full recovery but needed considerable psychological support and rehabilitation. She has returned to her responsible position in the financial world. A postoperative treadmill exercise ECG (Bruce protocol) was normal at 6 minutes 18 seconds. Her blood pressure is 128/74 mmHg and she is taking atenolol 100 mg, perindopril 4 mg, indapamide 1.5 mg, atorvastatin 20 mg, and aspirin 75 mg daily. Her baseline lipid profile has been improved with a target LDL cholesterol less than 78 mg/dl.

Lesson two – the tests

It is important to restate that angina is a clinical diagnosis which is supported by further investigations. If a woman has a typical pain and an abnormal ECG at rest, the diagnosis is straightforward. However, the resting ECG is usually normal or equivocal. A classic history and a normal resting ECG suggest good left ventricular function.

A woman with chest pain which is atypical will be unlikely to have CHD in the absence of risk factors. In contrast, a woman with typical chest pain and one or two major risk factors will be more likely to have CHD. Where there are doubts regarding the diagnosis or when overall risk of a subsequent event has to be evaluated, noninvasive testing should be performed. However, as the prevalence of CHD in women is lower than in men, the value of noninvasive testing will be lower but a normal test at a good workload for the same reason will almost certainly rule out CHD.[9,13]

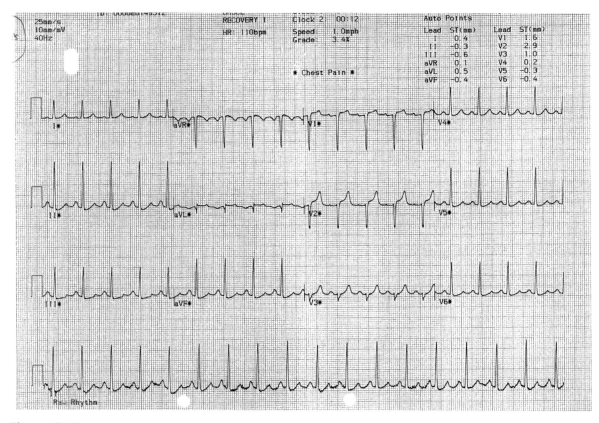

Figure 14.5
Exercise-induced ST elevation at a low workload of 4 minutes 11 seconds.

The exercise ECG is more accurate in detecting CHD when the prevalence is high, leading to a low false-positive rate for CHD but a higher false-negative rate. This means that, when compared with men, women will have a higher false-positive and lower false-negative rate because of their lower overall prevalence of CHD. However, the exercise ECG is widely available, inexpensive, and easy to perform. Interpretation should include exercise duration, hemodynamic response, symptoms at a given workload, and ST-T changes. A normal test at less than 6 minutes of the Bruce treadmill protocol would be inconclusive, whereas a normal test at a good workload (over 9 minutes) rules out significant CHD. The sensitivity (positive for disease) averages 61% and specificity (excluding CHD) 70%.[14]

If a test is inconclusive or when a woman cannot exercise adequately, stress echocardiography or

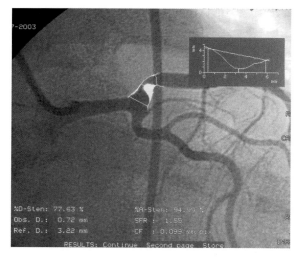

Figure 14.6
Critical left anterior descending stenosis in case 2.

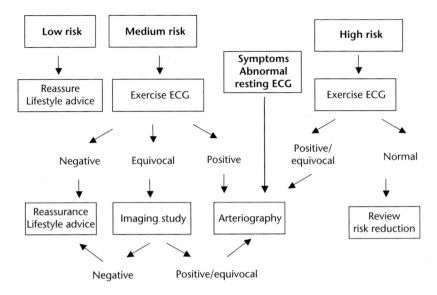

Figure 14.7

An approach to the management of coronary heart disease in women. *Low risk* The estimated risk of CHD is less than 20%. Women are likely to be younger, with atypical pain and no risk factors of significance. *Moderate risk* Risk is 20–80%. A mixture of typical and atypical pain. One major risk factor. *High risk* More than 80% likelihood of CHD. Typical pain. Two major risk factors.

nuclear (single-photon emission computed tomography – SPECT) imaging will provide diagnostic information and improve diagnostic accuracy. Stress echocardiography has a sensitivity of 86% and specificity of 79% and SPECT 78% and 64%, respectively.[14] The test selection decision will depend on the expertise in individual cardiac centers.

Cost, accuracy, and availability are major issues. These issues have to be set in the context of the low event rate in stable angina patients (there is time to evaluate thoroughly) and the major advances in medical therapy, buying both time and symptomatic improvement.[2,3] In Fig. 14.7 an approach to testing is summarized based on baseline risk. All women being evaluated should also have a fasting lipid profile and blood glucose as well as lifestyle assessments (smoking, blood pressure, exercise).

Case three – the classical

'This lady came to see me complaining of tightness in her upper chest and neck walking uphill. She is normally very fit and well but I was concerned lest these symptoms were due to coronary heart disease' – wrote the family doctor about his 73-year-old patient.

The story went back over 2 months with a discomfort in the chest, shoulders, and neck brought on by effort (especially hills) and relieved by rest. She said the symptoms had worsened in terms of decreased ability rather than pain severity. She was on no medication and had stopped smoking 14 years ago. Examination revealed a blood pressure of 180/90 mmHg but was otherwise normal. She wanted to go on holiday so a treadmill exercise ECG was arranged to try to assess severity and risk. She was able to exercise for 7 minutes 52 seconds of the standard Bruce protocol, stopping because of typical symptoms and inferolateral ST depression of 1 mm (Fig. 14.8). Although positive, because of the reasonable workload and ST depression of less than 2 mm, immediate angiography was deferred and she was allowed to go on holiday taking atenolol 50 mg, aspirin 75 mg, and atorvastatin 20 mg as well as a glyceryl trinitrate spray.

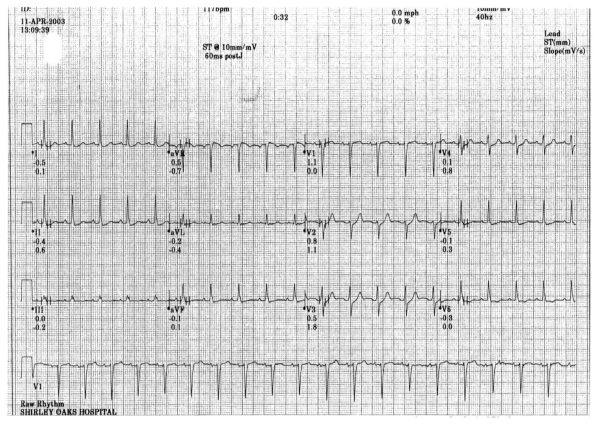

Figure 14.8
Inferolateral ST changes in case 3. Typical borderline changes in a woman.

On return she had benefited from the beta-blockade but was still unacceptably limited by angina. After discussing the options she decided to undergo coronary angiography, which identified good left ventricular function, a 70% proximal and long 90% mid LAD stenosis and a 70% lesion in a large first diagonal vessel. The right coronary artery had two lesions of 80 and 99%. Her baseline cholesterol of 243 mg/dl (triglycerides 90 mg/dl, HDL cholesterol 73 mg/dl, and LDL cholesterol 154 mg/dl) was reduced to 150 mg/dl (triglycerides 95 mg/dl, HDL 53 mg/dl, LDL 78 mg/dl). Her symptoms and prognostically important CHD meant that CABG surgery was the best therapeutic option and this was successfully performed using the left internal mammary artery and two vein grafts.

Postoperatively she completed a rehabilitation program and is now symptom-free, cycling 10 miles a day. She continues on aspirin and a statin as well as atenolol 25 mg daily, but was unable to tolerate an ACE inhibitor, developing facial swelling.

The lesson: management overview

An equal opportunity killer needs equal opportunity management.[11] The only difference between women and men should be their hormones. Although angina may present differently, the disease process and risk factors are the same. Stable angina by definition is stable. Much has been made of gender bias, which assumes that a difference in access to any form of therapy (absolute access or speed of access) means that a particular therapy and management approach is the best available. This blanket philosophy excludes good clinical judgment. If we assume that men with mild-to-moderate stable angina are more likely than women to be referred for coronary angiography and coronary intervention, we would have to be sure this was a superior form of therapy to medical management. There is no evidence to support this view.[2,3] Optimizing medical care and more carefully following the invasive route would then be to a woman's advantage.

At face value many might believe that a less aggressive approach results in gender bias in terms of investigation and treatment of CHD. However, when we consider age at presentation and extent of disease (women are generally older and have more extensive disease) plus other complicating factors (more women are diabetic) it may be that the management of women is being more carefully tailored to their clinical status at that time. Age is an important factor in management because women live longer than men and decision-making for the elderly may be more focused on quality of life and the wish not to be a burden on others, rather than purely avoiding death as an end-point and following any invasive option offered.[15] Thus, so-called gender bias needs to be controlled for age bias by the woman herself as well as her physician. Resources in health care may also dictate the options available, with less for the elderly, meaning less for women. However, different health-care systems may differentially limit health care for the elderly, leading to a solely age-biased restriction which is an unacceptable and unethical policy. The only gender bias that is a real concern is the reluctance of women to recognize that it is not a question of 'will' they get CHD but 'when' will they get CHD. Our focus should be on educating women – they are different but not that different – rather than chastising ourselves about their management.

Women benefit as much as men from lipid-lowering therapy, aspirin and/or clopidogrel, ACE inhibitors or angiotensin II antagonists, percutaneous coronary intervention and CABG surgery.[1,15] Increased interventional or surgical risks are related to small vessel size and disease extent (i.e. they are stable.

lesion, not gender, specific) and co-morbidities, such as diabetes. On the medical side women are more vulnerable to the ACE inhibitor cough (especially Chinese women) and cold extremities from beta-blockers.

Women are less likely to attend cardiac rehabilitation programs, which offer valuable secondary prevention, post-CABG or post-percutaneous transluminal coronary angioplasty. Women who do attend have high drop-out rates.[16] Women return to work less frequently and take longer to recover in general than men. This may reflect the lack of appropriate advice for women and begs the question as to whether rehabilitation tailored to women's needs may be more successful. As women live longer than men they more often live alone and may be afraid to venture out in large cities, particularly if rehabilitation classes or meetings take place outside daylight hours. The importance of social community support is self-evident and, if put in place, may help improve attendance rates.

Mortality rates and risk factors for CHD in African American women exceed those for white women. African American women are twice as likely as white women to have diabetes and three times as likely to die as a result. Fifty per cent are obese and one in three is hypertensive. The increasing risk factors contribute to the heart disease excess, reinforcing the importance of education about a healthy lifestyle. There is also an increased risk in the Asian population, perhaps because of an increased prevalence of insulin resistance.[10]

Conclusion

In this chapter I have used three of my patients to illustrate the way women with stable angina may present and how they should be evaluated. If treatment bias exists it is inexcusable. The management of stable angina is about risk reduction, risk stratification, and risk management. There is time to do all three because of the low yearly event rate. We are driven by statistics and relative risk but statistics are composed of individuals who have an absolute risk. Every aspect of our care has to be individualized and the objective clearly defined – the over-eighties may get symptom relief from surgery but what is the stroke risk and are they really on optimal medical therapy for symptom relief?

I have concerns about women living alone and in fear of going out, which is why rehabilitation and advice must include community nursing visits. There will always be the intellectually arrogant in our profession but it remains our duty to educate them in the hope that they will recognize the real rather than theoretical needs of women with CHD and stable angina. This book will be read by health-care professionals and will be an important reference source, but to experience the benefits of modern therapy women must present earlier in the disease process. It is unclear why they do not – perhaps their priorities are their families rather than themselves so their own health is not given the attention it should receive. It is our challenge to raise awareness and from this fairness in treatment – to do this we need the help of politicians, opinion leaders, and importantly the media and most of all, women themselves.

References

1. Gibbons RJ, Abrams J, Chatterjee K, et al. ACC/AHA 2002 Guidelines update for the management of patients with chronic stable angina – summary article. *J Am Coll Cardiol* 2003; **41**:159–68.

2. Jackson G. Stable angina – medical therapy gives us time to optimise management. *Int J Clin Pract* 2004; **58**:107–8.

3. Rihal CS, Raco DL, Gersh BJ, Yusuf S. Indications for coronary artery bypass surgery and percutaneous coronary intervention in chronic stable angina. *Circulation* 2003; **108**:2439–45.

4. Henderson RA, Pocock SJ, Clayton TC, et al. Seven year outcome in the RITA-2 trial: coronary angioplasty versus medical therapy. *J Am Coll Cardiol* 2003; **42**:1161–70.

5. Jackson G. Diagnosing chest pain. *Pract Cardiovasc Risk Manag* 2004; **2**:2–4.

6. Douglas PS, Ginsberg GS. The evaluation of chest pain in women. *N Engl J Med* 1996; **334**:1311–15.

7. Sullivan AK, Holdright DR, Wright CA, et al. Chest pain in women: clinical, investigative and prognostic features. *BMJ* 1994; **308**:883–6.

8. Weiner DA, Ryan TJ, McCabe CH, et al. Exercise stress testing. Correlations among history of angina, ST-segments response and prevalence of coronary artery disease in the Coronary Artery Surgery Study (CASS). *N Engl J Med* 1979; **301**:230–5.

9. Redberg RF, Shaw LJ. Diagnosis of coronary artery disease in women. *Prog Cardiovasc Dis* 2003; **46**:239–58.

10. Lerner D, Kannel W. Patterns of coronary heart disease morbidity and mortality in the sexes: a 26 year follow up of the Framingham population. *Am Heart J* 1986; **111**:383–90.

11. Jackson G. Coronary artery disease and women. *BMJ* 1994; **309**:555–7.

12. Bhatmagor D, Anand IS, Durrington PN, et al. Coronary risk factors in people from the Indian subcontinent in West London and their siblings in India. *Lancet* 1995; **345**:405–9.

13. Pepine CJ, Balaban RS, Bonow RO, et al. Women's Ischaemic Syndrome Evaluation: diagnosis of stable ischaemia and ischaemic heart disease. *Circulation* 2004; **109**:e44–6.

14. Kwok Y, Kim C, Grady D, et al. Meta-analysis of exercise testing to detect coronary artery disease in women. *Am J Cardiol* 1999; **83**:660–6.

15. Task Force of the European Society of Cardiology. Management of stable angina pectoris. *Eur Heart J* 1997; **18**:394–413.

16. Gallagher R, McKinley S, Dracup K. Predictors of women's attendance at cardiac rehabilitation programmes. *Prog Cardiovasc Nurs* 2003; **18**:121–6.

15
Cardiac syndrome X

Juan Carlos Kaski

Introduction

Cardiac syndrome X, a condition characterized by angina-like chest pain, a positive electrocardiographic response to stress testing, and completely normal coronary arteriograms, is relatively common and affects over 20% of angina patients undergoing diagnostic coronary arteriography.[1] Interestingly, there is a high prevalence of perimenopausal and menopausal women with cardiac syndrome X and, although the reasons for this are not firmly established, estrogen deficiency may be responsible. Low estrogen has been suggested to play a role in the pathogenesis of the condition mainly, but not exclusively, via endothelial dysfunction. The term cardiac syndrome X encompasses heterogeneous subjects and a diversity of pathogenic mechanisms. Although myocardial ischemia is certainly a potential mechanism, it is objectively found in only a relatively small proportion of syndrome X patients. In recent years, however, with the advent of more sensitive techniques it has been possible to identify subgroups of patients with documented myocardial ischemia. Other mechanisms, both cardiac and noncardiac, have also been identified. This chapter summarizes the clinical characteristics of patients with cardiac syndrome X and focuses mainly on pathogenic and diagnostic aspects of the syndrome as well as relevant aspects of its management.

Clinical characteristics

Exercise-induced chest pain, ST segment depression typically suggestive of transient myocardial ischemia, and normal coronary angiograms are the diagnostic hallmarks of cardiac syndrome X.[1,2] The characteristics of the chest pain in these patients are similar to those of patients with obstructive coronary artery disease.[3] On closer scrutiny, however, exertional chest pain in cardiac syndrome X tends to occur with lesser degrees of activity and to be longer in duration and less responsive to the administration of sublingual nitrates.[3] In a proportion of patients the chest pain and ST segment depression occur at rest and can, in some cases, mimic unstable angina or nonST elevation myocardial infarction (MI).[1,3] Chest pain in syndrome X patients is commonly severe and frightening, but unlike angina in a large proportion of coronary heart disease (CHD) patients, it is not necessarily associated with echocardiographic left ventricular dysfunction.[4-6] Myocardial perfusion scan results are, however, suggestive of abnormal coronary blood supply in many cases.[7] Risk factors for CHD, including hyperlipidemia, smoking, obesity, and family history, are similarly present in syndrome X and the general population. Patients with systemic hypertension and those with diabetes mellitus are generally excluded from syndrome X series[8] but the reasons for doing so may need

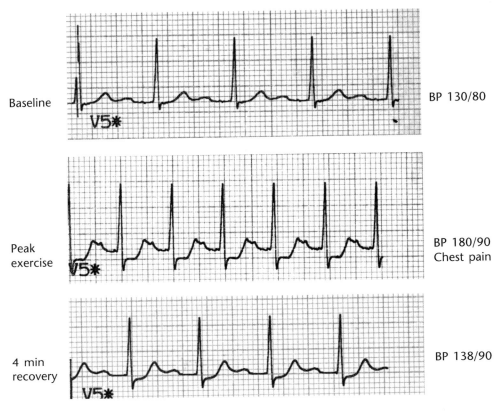

Figure 15.1
Illustrative example of ST segment depression during treadmill exercise stress testing in a patient with cardiac syndrome X.

revision. Differential diagnoses include mainly noncardiac causes such as esophageal dysmotility, fibromyalgia, and costochondritis. Coronary artery spasm as typically seen in patients with variant angina can be ruled out with the use of provocative tests and 24-hour ambulatory ECG monitoring. The latter will often show transient ST segment elevation in patients with epicardial coronary artery spasm, a finding that is rare in cardiac syndrome X and practically limited to individuals with microvascular spasm.[9]

As with chest pain, electrocardiogram (ECG) changes seen during stress testing are also similar in patients with syndrome X and patients with CHD[10] (Fig. 15.1). However, there are differences such as that ischemia-like ST segment depression develops at a higher heart rate–blood pressure product and post-

exercise ST segment depression recovery time is faster in syndrome X patients than in CHD patients.[10] Patients with syndrome X also have ST segment changes during continuous ambulatory ECG monitoring, which are, as with stress testing responses, indistinguishable from those seen in CHD patients[11] (Fig. 15.2). The circadian distribution of ST segment depression episodes is also similar in CHD and syndrome X patients, with most of the episodes of ST depression coinciding with times of increased physical activity.[11] Although the majority of episodes of ST segment depression are associated with tachycardia, a significant proportion occurs in the absence of an increased heart rate.[11] As mentioned earlier, ST segment elevation is rarely observed during pain in syndrome X patients, although some patients with microvascular spasm

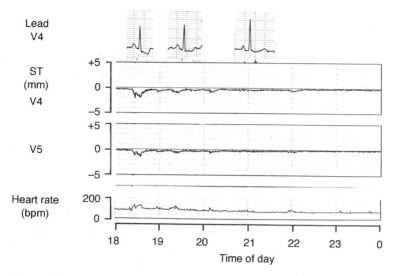

Figure 15.2
In patients with cardiac syndrome X, ST segment changes during continuous ambulatory electrocardiogram monitoring are often associated with increases of heart rate.

have been shown to have episodes of ST segment elevation similar to those seen in variant angina pectoris.[9]

Microvascular dysfunction

A large proportion of patients with cardiac syndrome X have abnormal vasodilatory coronary blood flow responses and an increased reactivity of the coronary microcirculation to vasoconstrictor stimuli.[12] Thus the term 'microvascular angina' has been used to indicate that the ischemia-like symptoms and ST segment shifts seen in cardiac syndrome X may be caused by coronary microcirculatory abnormalities.[12] The precise cause of this abnormality is not known but endothelial dysfunction has been shown to play a role.[13] The endothelium produces a variety of complex vasoactive molecules that contribute to the stability of vascular tone through complex interactions. An imbalance in the production and/or release of these substances can lead to abnormal vasomotor responses, i.e. abnormal vasodilator responses and/or increased vasoreactivity. Plasma levels of endothelin-1 (ET-1), a potent vasoconstrictor peptide produced by the endothelial cell, are raised in patients with chest pain and normal coronary arteries compared with normal controls.[14] Moreover, a significant relationship exists between baseline plasma ET-1 levels and abnormal coronary vascular responses in patients with cardiac syndrome X.[15,16] Cox et al.[15] observed that subjects with higher ET-1 levels had impaired vasodilator responses during atrial pacing compared with patients with normal ET-1 concentrations. These findings suggest that endothelial dysfunction, with an imbalance of vasoconstrictor and vasodilator forces, is a possible cause of microvascular angina in patients with cardiac syndrome X. Coronary endothelial dysfunction both at the microcirculatory and systemic levels has been demonstrated by Egashira et al.[13] and Lekakis et al.,[17] respectively. Moreover, Zeiher et al.[18] and Hasdai et al.[19] have shown that coronary endothelial dysfunction correlates with abnormal myocardial perfusion in patients with chest pain and normal or mildly diseased coronary arteries. Of interest, abnormal thallium myocardial perfusion scans are found in at least one-third of cardiac syndrome X patients. Heterogeneous myocardial perfusion and/or true myocardial ischemia may be responsible for the abnormality. Heterogeneous perfusion of the myocardium is common in patients with chest pain and normal coronary angiograms and suggestive of microcirculatory abnormalities.[20]

Nonischemic mechanisms

Although intuitively, myocardial ischemia is a plausible mechanism of cardiac syndrome X, camps are divided as to the true role of ischemia in syndrome X. The fact that long-term prognosis is good in cardiac syndrome X,[21,22] the observation of normal echocardiographic responses during stress testing,[5,6] and the lack of 'objective' documentation of ischemia in the majority of patients[3,23] contribute to the controversy. In the majority of patients with chest pain and normal coronary angiograms symptoms appear to be noncardiac in origin and investigators believe that the presence of chest pain in these patients may be explained by noncardiac mechanisms such as esophageal dysmotility,[24] musculoskeletal chest pain syndromes,[1] increased pain perception and the release of algogenic substances,[25,26] and psychological abnormalities.[27]

Abnormal pain perception

It has been suggested that cardiac syndrome X may be attributed to a general abnormality of nociception.[28,29] In the past, reports[11] have shown that during ambulatory Holter monitoring >50% of episodes of ischemic ST segment depression were associated with chest pain in syndrome X patients compared with a much lower proportion in patients with chronic stable angina, which was in the range of 30%. Moreover, a large proportion of chest pain episodes in these studies[11] occurred in the absence of ECG changes and these angina attacks were often severe and long-lasting. Studies of pain threshold in cardiac syndrome X patients showed a significantly lower threshold and tolerance values for forearm ischemia and electrical skin stimulation compared with CHD patients and control subjects.[30] Also, several studies have shown that catheter manipulation within the

right heart as well as pacing and intracoronary contrast medium injection in the left ventricle provoked chest pain in syndrome X patients similar to their usual angina-like chest pain.[30–32] Moreover, injection of adenosine, an arteriolar vasodilator with algogenic properties, caused angina in a significantly larger proportion of patients with chest pain and normal coronary arteries, than in controls and CHD patients.[33–35] Similar results were obtained with the administration of epinephrine.[36]

Although these studies provide evidence of an increased cardiac and systemic sensitivity to painful stimuli in syndrome X, the mechanisms underlying this abnormal response remain unknown. Several hypotheses have been proposed to explain this phenomenon, including increased sympathetic activity (for which there is ample evidence in syndrome X), excessive release of algogenic substances, abnormal activation of pain receptors within the heart, and abnormal processing of visceral afferent neural impulses in the peripheral and/or central nervous system.[25,26,37–42]

Psychological abnormalities

It has been suggested that cardiac syndrome X, as we see it now, is similar or equivalent to that commonly observed among soldiers at war and related to environmental stress.[43] In the first half of the twentieth century American researchers coined the term 'neurocirculatory asthenia' to describe an equivalent condition observed outside war scenarios.[44] Despite some similarities it is most unlikely that cardiac syndrome X, as defined in this chapter, and neurocirculatory asthenia are similar entities.

Numerous reports indicate that patients with chest pain and normal coronary angiograms have psychological abnormalities, including anxiety disorders, depression, and hypochondria.[27,45–48] Panic disorders, anxiety and depression are among the most commonly identified diagnoses. Among patients presenting with acute chest pain – 75% of whom were discharged with a diagnosis of noncardiac chest pain – panic disorder went unrecognized in 98% of cases.[46,47] In a study, panic disorders and depression were diagnosed in about one-third of patients presenting with chest pain, but the prevalence in those with and without myocardial ischemia was similar (20% vs 17%). Of interest, in both groups the psychiatric diagnoses predicted higher rates of recurrence of acute chest pain in the subsequent year. Panic disorder and unexplained physical symptoms, including chest pain, are associated with increased use of medical services.[49] Whether conclusions regarding a high prevalence of psychological morbidity in cardiac syndrome X can be safely applied to the various categories of patients that appear to be encompassed by the syndrome is, in my view, quite unlikely. Selection bias, the possibility that psychological abnormalities in these patients are secondary to the uncertainty caused by an ill-defined condition that could in their view cause MI and death, and inadequate reassurance by the managing physician, can account for the findings in many of the published series. A proportion of patients, however, particularly those that have been reported in studies carried out by researchers in the field of psychiatry or psychological medicine, are likely to have primary psychological abnormalities, perhaps reflecting some degree of referral bias. Psychiatric disorders identified in these selected study populations require specialist management.

Myocardial ischemia

Myocardial ischemia, albeit elusive, has been documented in subsets of cardiac syndrome X patients. Crake et al.[50] showed reduced coronary sinus blood oxygen saturation in patients with typical exertional chest pain and normal coronary arteries. Exercise-induced myocardial lactate production, an objective metabolic marker of myocardial ischemia, has been shown to occur in patients with cardiac syndrome X.[51] In a study by Rosano et al.,[23] approximately 30% of syndrome X patients showed ischemic pH changes in the coronary sinus during stress-induced chest pain, similar to those of patients with documented CHD. Whereas thallium-201 myocardial perfusion studies are abnormal in over 30% of cardiac syndrome X patients,[7,52] stress echocardiograms are normal in these patients.[5,6] The negative findings during stress echocardiography have been explained by the presence of mild and patchy myocardial ischemia that is unable to cause wall motion abnormalities. Objective evidence of myocardial ischemia has also been found by Buffon et al.,[53] who reported high levels of markers of ischemia-reperfusion injury during pacing stress in cardiac syndrome X patients.

Two recent independent reports using magnetic resonance spectroscopy[54] and imaging[55] showed a decrease in the phosphocreatine:ATP ratio during handgrip exercise suggestive of myocardial ischemia, and subendocardial hypoperfusion during the intravenous administration of adenosine, respectively. These findings strongly support the role of myocardial ischemia in the genesis of cardiac syndrome X.

The role of estrogen deficiency in cardiac syndrome X (see also Chapter 25)

The high prevalence of women with cardiac syndrome X is intriguing.[1,56] Syndrome X women are often perimenopausal or menopausal[57] and have symptoms of ovarian insufficiency such as hot flushes and migraine. The clinical and gynecological features of female patients with syndrome X have been reported elsewhere.[57,58] There is a high incidence of hysterectomy and signs of ovarian insufficiency in syndrome X women, suggesting that estrogen deficiency could be at least one of the pathogenic mechanisms in a large proportion of syndrome X patients.[58] Estrogen deficiency is a recognized cause of endothelial dysfunction and studies in healthy women have shown an impairment of endothelial function coinciding with the onset of the menopause.[59] 17β-Estradiol deficiency is known to be associated with vasomotor instability and decreased arterial blood flow velocity in humans.[60,61] The acute administration of 17β-estradiol has been shown to improve coronary endothelial function in menopausal women with syndrome X.[62]

Of interest, abnormal ET-1 levels correlate with microvascular angina in menopausal women with syndrome X and Webb et al.[63] have shown that short-term estradiol administration decreases coronary ET-1 levels in menopausal women with CHD. The administration of exogenous estradiol increases peripheral blood flow in otherwise normal menopausal women.[64] In menopausal women, forearm vasodilatation induced by acetylcholine was potentiated by acute local administration of intravenous estradiol,[65] further suggesting that steroid hormones in these women may modulate endothelium-dependent responses in the peripheral circulation. Coronary vasodilatation by 17β-estradiol has been shown to improve endothelial dysfunction[66] and exercise tolerance[67] in menopausal women and to prevent myocardial ischemia in women with CHD.[68,69]

As discussed earlier, excessive release of adenosine or increased sensitivity to it may be responsible for chest pain in syndrome X. Estrogen may alter both adenosine production and the sensitivity of cardiac receptors to adenosine. Recent animal data have shown female/male differences in pain sensitivity.[70] These differences were abolished by ovariectomy and re-established after estrogen replacement therapy.[70] This may explain why clinical studies with 17β-estradiol[71] have reported improved angina symptoms in women with cardiac syndrome X, despite a lack of improvement in exercise-induced ST segment changes. 17β-Estradiol has also been reported to improve ST segment depression in cardiac syndrome X patients.[72] Thus there are a number of mechanisms that could explain the alleviation of chest pain by estrogen, without necessarily having to invoke antiischemic actions.

Management of cardiac syndrome X

Overall, prognosis regarding survival is good in patients with chest pain and normal coronary arteries, but quality of life is poor in many patients. As expected, however, in the small number of patients who have microvascular angina as a secondary phenomenon due to amyloidosis or other systemic conditions that cause microvascular obstruction, prognosis may be poor and directly related to the outcome of the primary disease.[73] Prognosis is also impaired in patients presenting with left bundle branch block, who frequently develop dilated cardiomyopathy during long-term follow-up.[74]

Kaski and Valenzuela[75] have recently reviewed treatment options available for patients with syndrome X and American Heart Association/American College of Cardiology treatment guidelines for acute chest pain associated with normal coronary arteries have recently been issued. A practical approach to patient management has also been discussed by Kaski.[76] It is important to stress that treatment should be tailored to the individual patient needs and, if possible, at tackling the prevailing pathogenic mechanism.

In patients with documented myocardial ischemia and those in whom an association between ST segment shifts and chest pain can be established, calcium channel blockers and β-adrenergic blockers are usually effective.[75] Although it has been suggested that nitrates may be less effective in syndrome X than in CHD patients, approximately 50% of patients show an excellent response to sublingual nitrate administration.[3] Little evidence is available in relation to the efficacy of other antianginal medications, or metabolic modulators, in syndrome X.

Providing appropriate analgesic treatment for chest pain is of paramount importance in this setting, particularly in patients with increased pain sensitivity, whether or not ischemia has been documented. Improving chest pain will most certainly result in improved quality of life in practically every instance. Aminophylline,[77–79] an antagonist of adenosine receptors, and imipramine,[80,81] an antidepressant with analgesic properties, have been shown to improve symptoms in patients with chest pain and normal coronary angiograms. Techniques such as transcutaneous electrical nerve stimulation and spinal cord stimulation can offer good pain control in specific subsets of patients,[82–84] but as with other interventions in syndrome X, studies in larger numbers of patients are lacking. Involving pain management specialists is of vital importance in patients with refractory forms of chest pain.

Psychiatric specialist management is required and it has been shown to be beneficial in a substantial number of patients with well-defined psychological abnormalities.[45] Studies in this field support the role of a structured cognitive behavioral approach for the management of syndrome X, particularly in patients with nonischemic chest pain[85] in whom antianginal and other measures are ineffective.

A major effort should be devoted to aggressively tackle risk factors for CHD, initially in the form of lifestyle modifications, as an effective intervention to improve endothelial dysfunction. The use of statins has recently been shown to improve both exercise capacity and endothelial function in syndrome X patients.[86] Syndrome X patients have an impaired exercise capacity despite normal skeletal muscle function and it has been suggested that this abnormality may be caused by both physical deconditioning and low exertional pain threshold.[87] Eriksson et al.[87] found that physical training improves pain threshold and endothelial function and also delays the onset of exertional pain. Physical training may be a valuable therapeutic intervention in patients with typical exertional chest pain and normal coronary angiograms.

Estrogen therapy (see also Chapter 26)

As discussed in the preceding section, estrogen administration has been shown to have beneficial effects in preventing angina attacks in patients with cardiac syndrome X. Hormone therapy has been used for treatment of women with syndrome X with relatively good results, particularly regarding pain control.[70] Estrogens antagonize the effects of adenosine, improve endothelial function, and dilate the coronary vasculature. However, there are problems at present with the long-term use of at least some forms of estrogen therapy, as controlled clinical trials have suggested that the risk of developing cardiovascular disease, as well as that of breast cancer, may be increased in women taking hormone therapy. Thus although estrogen has the potential to confer cardiovascular protection, it can also cause harm.[88,89] In view of this the US Preventive Services Task Force has suggested that routine menopausal hormone therapy should not currently be advised for the prevention of chronic conditions[88] and similar recommendations could be made for syndrome X patients. However, in very specific cases where a direct relationship can be established between estrogen deficiency and symptoms, short-term courses of hormone therapy may be useful to control chest pain. Women obviously should be informed regarding their individual risk/benefit ratios in relation to this therapy.

Conclusions

The prevalence of cardiac syndrome X is higher in women than in men. In a large proportion of these patients the symptoms are likely to be noncardiac in origin. However, myocardial ischemia is the pathogenic mechanism in a proportion of syndrome X patients. Microvascular endothelial dysfunction may play an important role in the genesis of myocardial ischemia. Estrogen deficiency is likely to contribute to the syndrome through endothelial dysfunction and effects on pain threshold. Exogenous estrogen administration may have a beneficial effect in syndrome X patients but its use is currently limited by recent findings of an adverse effect in large trials of hormone therapy.

References

1. Kaski JC. Cardiac syndrome X and microvascular angina. In: Kaski JC (ed.) *Chest Pain with Normal Coronary Angiograms: Pathogenesis, Diagnosis and Management.* London: Kluwer Academic Publishers, 1999: 1–12.
2. Kemp HG Jr. Left ventricular function in patients with the anginal syndrome and normal coronary arteriograms. *Am J Cardiol* 1973; **32**:375–6.
3. Kaski JC, Rosano GM, Collins P, et al. Cardiac syndrome X: clinical characteristics and left ventricular function. Long-term follow-up study. *J Am Coll Cardiol* 1995; **25**:807–14.
4. Arbogast R, Bourassa MG. Myocardial function during atrial pacing in patients with angina pectoris and normal coronary arteriograms. Comparison with patients having significant coronary artery disease. *Am J Cardiol* 1973; **32**:257–63.
5. Nihoyannopoulos P, Kaski JC, Crake T, et al. Absence

of myocardial dysfunction during stress in patients with syndrome X. *J Am Coll Cardiol* 1991; **18**:1463–70.

6. Panza JA, Laurienzo JM, Curiel RV, et al. Investigation of the mechanism of chest pain in patients with angiographically normal coronary arteries using transesophageal dobutamine stress echocardiography. *J Am Coll Cardiol* 1997; **29**:293–301.

7. Tweddel AC, Martin W, Hutton I. Thallium scans in syndrome X. *Br Heart J* 1992; **68**:48–50.

8. Kaski JC. Syndrome X: a heterogeneous syndrome. In: Kaski JC (ed.) *Angina Pectoris with Normal Coronary Arteries: Syndrome X.* Massachusetts: Kluwer Academic, 1999: 1–12.

9. Mohri M, Koyanagi M, Egashira K, et al. Angina pectoris caused by coronary microvascular spasm. *Lancet* 1998; **351**:1165–9.

10. Gavrielides S, Kaski JC, Galassi AR, et al. Recovery-phase patterns of ST segment depression in the heart rate domain cannot distinguish between anginal patients with coronary artery disease and patients with syndrome X. *Am Heart J* 1991; **122**:1593–8.

11. Kaski JC, Crea F, Nihoyannopoulos P, et al. Transient myocardial ischaemia during daily life in patients with syndrome X. *Am J Cardiol* 1986; **58**:1242–7.

12. Cannon RO III, Epstein SE. 'Microvascular angina' as a cause of chest pain with angiographically normal coronary arteries. *Am J Cardiol* 1988; **61**:1338–43.

13. Egashira K, Inou T, Hirooka Y, et al. Evidence of impaired endothelium-dependent coronary vasodilatation in patients with angina pectoris and normal coronary angiograms. *N Engl J Med* 1993; **328**:1659–64.

14. Kaski JC, Cox ID, Crook JR, et al. Differential plasma endothelin levels in subgroups of patients with angina and angiographically normal coronary arteries. *Am Heart J* 1998; **136**:412–17.

15. Cox ID, Botker HE, Bagger JP, et al. Elevated endothelin concentrations are associated with reduced coronary vasomotor responses in patients with chest pain and normal coronary arteriograms. *J Am Coll Cardiol* 1999; **34**:455–60.

16. Kolasinska-Kloch W, Lesniak W, Kiec-Wilk B, et al. Biochemical parameters of endothelial dysfunction in cardiological syndrome X. *Scand J Clin Lab Invest* 2002; **62**:7–13.

17. Lekakis JP, Papamichael CM, Vemmos CN, et al. Peripheral vascular endothelial dysfunction in patients with angina pectoris and normal coronary arteriograms. *J Am Coll Cardiol* 1998; **31**:541–6.

18. Zeiher AM, Krause T, Schachinger V, et al. Impaired endothelium-dependent vasodilation of coronary resistance vessels is associated with exercise-induced myocardial ischaemia. *Circulation* 1995; **91**:2345–52.

19. Hasdai D, Gibbons RJ, Holmes DR Jr, et al. Coronary endothelial dysfunction in humans is associated with myocardial perfusion defects. *Circulation* 1997; **96**:3390–5.

20. Galassi AR, Crea F, Araujo LI, et al. Comparison of regional myocardial blood flow in syndrome X and one-vessel coronary artery disease. *Am J Cardiol* 1993; **72**:134–9.

21. Pasternak RC, Thibault GE, Savoia M, et al. Chest pain with angiographically insignificant coronary arterial obstruction. Clinical presentation and long-term follow-up. *Am J Med* 1980; **68**:813–17.

22. Kemp HG, Kronmal RA, Vlietstra RE, et al. Seven year survival of patients with normal or near normal coronary arteriograms: a CASS registry study. *J Am Coll Cardiol* 1986; **7**:479–83.

23. Rosano GM, Kaski JC, Arie S, et al. Failure to demonstrate myocardial ischaemia in patients with angina and normal coronary arteries. Evaluation by continuous coronary sinus pH monitoring and lactate metabolism. *Eur Heart J* 1996; **17**:1175–80.

24. De Caestecker JS. Esophageal chest pain. In: Kaski JC (ed.) *Chest Pain with Normal Coronary Angiograms*, 1st edn. Massachusetts: Kluwer Publishers, 1999: 33–47.

25. Maseri A, Crea F, Kaski JC, Crake T. Mechanisms of angina pectoris in syndrome X. *J Am Coll Cardiol* 1991; **17**:499–506.

26. Rosano GMC, Lindsay DC, Poole-Wilson PA. Syndrome X: a hypothesis for cardiac pain without ischaemia. *Cardiologia* 1991; **36**:885–95.

27. Bass C, Wade C. Chest pain with normal coronary arteries: a comparative study of psychiatric and social morbidity. *Psychol Med* 1984; **14**:51–61.

28. Rosen SD, Uren NG, Kaski JC, et al. Coronary vasodilator reserve, pain perception, and sex in patients with syndrome X. *Circulation* 1994; **90**:50–60.

29. Chauhan A, Mullins PA, Thuraisingham SI, et al. Abnormal cardiac pain perception in syndrome X. *J Am Coll Cardiol* 1994; **24**:329–35.

30. Turiel M, Galassi AR, Glazier JJ, Kaski JC, Maseri A. Pain threshold and tolerance in women with syndrome X and women with stable angina pectoris. *Am J Cardiol* 1987; **60**:503–7.

31. Cannon RO III, Quyyumi AA, Schenke WH, et al. Abnormal cardiac sensitivity in patients with chest pain and normal coronary arteries. *J Am Coll Cardiol* 1990; **16**:1359–66.

32. Shapiro LM, Crake T, Poole-Wilson PA. Is altered cardiac sensation responsible for chest pain in

patients with normal coronary arteries? Clinical observation during cardiac catheterisation. *BMJ* 1988; **296**:170–1.

33. Lagerqvist B, Sylven C, Hedenstrom H, et al. Intravenous adenosine but not its first metabolite inosine provokes chest pain in healthy volunteers. *J Cardiovasc Pharmacol* 1990; **16**:173–6.

34. Lagerqvist B, Sylven C, Waldenstrom A. Lower threshold for adenosine-induced chest pain in patients with angina and normal coronary angiograms. *Br Heart J* 1992; **68**:282–5.

35. Lagerqvist B, Sylven C, Beermann B, et al. Intracoronary adenosine causes angina pectoris like pain – an inquiry into the nature of visceral pain. *Cardiovasc Res* 1990; **24**:609–13.

36. Eriksson B, Svedenhag J, Martinsson A, et al. Effect of epinephrine infusion on chest pain in syndrome X in the absence of signs of myocardial ischemia. *Am J Cardiol* 1995; **75**:241–5.

37. Cannon RO, Benjamin SB. Chest pain as a consequence of abnormal visceral nociception. *Dig Dis Sci* 1993; **38**:193–6.

38. Rosen SD, Paulesu E, Wise RJ, et al. Central neural contribution to the perception of chest pain in cardiac syndrome X. *Heart* 2002; **87**:513–19.

39. Rosano GM, Ponikowski P, Adamopoulos S, et al. Abnormal autonomic control of the cardiovascular system in syndrome X. *Am J Cardiol* 1994; **73**:1174–9.

40. Galassi AR, Kaski JC, Crea F, et al. Heart rate response during exercise testing and ambulatory ECG monitoring in patients with syndrome X. *Am Heart J* 1991; **122**:458–63.

41. Gulli G, Cemin R, Pancera P, et al. Evidence of parasympathetic impairment in some patients with cardiac syndrome X. *Cardiovasc Res* 2001; **52**:208–16.

42. Lanza GA, Giordano A, Pristipino C, et al. Abnormal cardiac adrenergic nerve function in patients with syndrome X detected by [123I] metaiodobenzyl-guanidine myocardial scintigraphy. *Circulation* 1997; **96**:821–6.

43. Wood P. Da Costa's syndrome (or effort syndrome). *BMJ* 1941; **I**:813–18.

44. Craig HR, White PD. Etiology and symptoms of neurocirculatory asthenia. Analysis of 100 cases, with comments on prognosis and treatment. *Arch Intern Med* 1934; **53**:633–48.

45. Klimes I, Mayou RA, Pearce MJ, Coles L, Fagg JR. Psychological treatment for atypical non-cardiac chest pain: a controlled evaluation. *Psychol Med* 1990; **20**:605–11.

46. Fleet RP, Beitman BD. Unexplained chest pain: when is it panic disorder? *Clin Cardiol* 1997; **20**:187–94.

47. Fleet RP, Dupuis G, Marchand A, Burelle D, Beitman BD. Detecting panic disorder in emergency department chest pain patients: a validated model to improve recognition. *Ann Behav Med* 1997; **19**:124–31.

48. Potts SG, Bass CM. Psychological morbidity in patients with chest pain and normal or near-normal coronary arteries: a long-term follow-up study. *Psychol Med* 1995; **25**:339–47.

49. Katon W. Panic disorder: relationship to high medical utilization, unexplained physical symptoms, and medical costs. *J Clin Psychiatry* 1996; **57** (Suppl 10): 11–18; discussion 19–22.

50. Crake T, Canepa-Anson R, Shapiro L, et al. Continuous recording of coronary sinus oxygen saturation during atrial pacing in patients with coronary artery disease or with syndrome X. *Br Heart J* 1988; **59**:31–8.

51. Hutchison SJ, Poole-Wilson PA, Henderson AH. Angina with normal coronary arteries: a review. *Q J Med* 1989; **72**:677–88.

52. Legrand V, Hodgson JM, Bates ER, et al. Abnormal coronary flow reserve and abnormal radionuclide exercise test results in patients with normal coronary angiograms. *J Am Coll Cardiol* 1985; **6**:1245–53.

53. Buffon A, Rigattieri S, Santini SA, et al. Myocardial ischemia-reperfusion damage after pacing-induced tachycardia in patients with cardiac syndrome X. *Am J Physiol Heart Circ Physiol* 2000; **279**:H2627–33.

54. Buchthal SD, den Hollander JA, Merz CN, et al. Abnormal myocardial phosphorus-31 nuclear magnetic resonance spectroscopy in women with chest pain but normal coronary angiograms. *N Engl J Med* 2000; **342**:829–35.

55. Panting JR, Gatehouse PD, Yang GZ, et al. Abnormal subendocardial perfusion in cardiac syndrome X detected by cardiovascular magnetic resonance imaging. *N Engl J Med* 2002; **346**:1948–53.

56. Likoff W, Segal BL, Kasparian H. Paradox of normal selective coronary arteriograms in patients considered to have unmistakable coronary heart disease. *N Engl J Med* 1967; **276**:1063–6.

57. Rosano GM, Collins P, Kaski JC, et al. Syndrome X in women is associated with oestrogen deficiency. *Eur Heart J* 1995; **16**:610–14.

58. Kaski JC. Overview of gender aspects of cardiac syndrome X. *Cardiovasc Res* 2002; **53**:620–6.

59. Hayward CS, Kelly RP, Collins P. The roles of gender, the menopause and hormone replacement on cardiovascular function. *Cardiovasc Res* 2000; **46**:28–49.

60. Kronenberg F, Cote LJ, Linkie DM, Dyrenfurth I, Downey JA. Menopausal hot flushes: thermoregulatory, cardiovascular and circulating catecholamine and LH changes. *Maturitas* 1984; **6**:31–43.

61. Ginsburg J, Hardiman P. The peripheral circulation in the menopause. In: Ginsburg J (ed.) *The Circulation in the Female*. Carnforth, UK: Parthenon Publishing, 1989: 99–115.

62. Lieberman EH, Gerhard MD, Uehata A, et al. Oestrogen improves endothelium-dependent, flow-mediated vasodilation in postmenopausal women. *Ann Intern Med* 1994; **12**:936–41.

63. Webb CM, Ghatei MA, McNeill JG, Collins P. 17β-Estradiol decreases endothelin-1 levels in the coronary circulation of postmenopausal women with coronary artery disease. *Circulation* 2000; **102**:1617–22.

64. Volterrani M, Rosano GMC, Coats A, Beale C, Collins P. Estrogen acutely increases peripheral blood flow in postmenopausal women. *Am J Med* 1995; **99**:119–22.

65. Gilligan DM, Badar DM, Panza JA, Quyyumi AA, Cannon RO 3rd. Acute vascular effects of estrogen in postmenopausal women. *Circulation* 1994; **90**:786–91.

66. Roque M, Heras M, Roig E, et al. Short-term effects of transdermal estrogen replacement therapy on coronary vascular reactivity in postmenopausal women with angina pectoris and normal results on coronary angiograms. *J Am Coll Cardiol* 1998; **31**:139–43.

67. Webb CM, Rosano GMC, Collins P. Oestrogen improves exercise-induced myocardial ischaemia in women. *Lancet* 1998; **351**:1556–7.

68. Rosano GMC, Sarrel PM, Poole-Wilson PA, Collins P. Beneficial effect of oestrogen on exercise-induced myocardial ischaemia in women with coronary artery disease. *Lancet* 1993; **342**:133–6.

69. Alpasian M, Shimokawa H, Kuroiwa-Matsumoto M, Harasawa Y, Takeshita A. Short-term estrogen administration ameliorates dobutamine-induced myocardial ischemia in postmenopausal women with coronary artery disease. *J Am Coll Cardiol* 1997; **30**:1466–71.

70. Mogil JS, Sternberg WF, Kest B, Marek P, Liebeskind JC. Sex differences in the antagonism of stress-induced analgesia: effects of gonadectomy and oestrogen replacement. *Pain* 1993; **53**:17–25.

71. Rosano GMC, Peters NS, Lefroy DC, et al. 17β-Estradiol therapy lessens angina in postmenopausal women with syndrome X. *J Am Coll Cardiol* 1996; **28**:1500–5.

72. Albertsson PA, Emanuelsson H, Milsom I. Beneficial effect of treatment with transdermal estradiol-17-β on exercise-induced angina and ST segment depression in syndrome X. *Int J Cardiol* 1996; **54**:13–20.

73. Al Suwaidi J, Velianou JL, Gertz MA, et al. Systemic amyloidosis presenting with angina pectoris. *Ann Intern Med* 1999; **131**:838–41.

74. Opherk D, Schuler G, Wetterauer K, et al. Four-year follow-up study in patients with angina pectoris and normal coronary arteriograms ('syndrome X'). *Circulation* 1989; **80**:1610–16.

75. Kaski JC, Valenzuela Garcia LF. Therapeutic options for the management of patients with cardiac syndrome X. *Eur Heart J* 2001; **22**:283–93.

76. Kaski JC. Pathophysiology and management of patients with chest pain and normal coronary arteriograms (cardiac syndrome X). Clinician update. *Circulation* 2004; **109**:568–72.

77. Elliott PM, Krzyzowska-Dickinson K, Calvino R, et al. Effect of oral aminophylline in patients with angina and normal coronary arteriograms (cardiac syndrome X). *Heart* 1997; **77**:523–6.

78. Emdin M, Picano E, Lattanzi F, et al. Improved exercise capacity with acute aminophylline administration in patients with syndrome X. *J Am Coll Cardiol* 1989; **14**:1450–3.

79. Yoshio H, Shimizu M, Kita Y, et al. Effects of short-term aminophylline administration on cardiac functional reserve in patients with syndrome X. *J Am Coll Cardiol* 1995; **25**:1547–51.

80. Cannon RO III, Quyyumi AA, Mincemoyer R, et al. Imipramine in patients with chest pain despite normal coronary angiograms. *N Engl J Med* 1994; **330**:1411–17.

81. Cox ID, Schwartzman RA, Atienza F, et al. Angiographic progression in patients with angina pectoris and normal or near normal coronary angiograms who are restudied due to unstable symptoms. *Eur Heart J* 1998; **19**:1027–33.

82. Mannheimer C, Carlsson CA, Emanuelsson H, et al. The effects of transcutaneous electrical nerve stimulation in patients with severe angina pectoris. *Circulation* 1985; **71**:308–16.

83. Chauhan A, Mullins PA, Thuraisingham SI, et al. Effect of transcutaneous electrical nerve stimulation on coronary blood flow. *Circulation* 1994; **89**:694–702.

84. Eliasson T, Albertsson P, Hardhammar P, et al. Spinal cord stimulation in angina pectoris with normal coronary arteriograms. *Coron Artery Dis* 1993; **4**:819–27.

85. Mayou RA, Bryant BM, Sanders D, et al. A controlled trial of cognitive behavioural therapy for non-cardiac chest pain. *Psychol Med* 1997; **27**:1021–31.

86. Kayikcioglu M, Payzin S, Yavuzgil O, et al. Benefits of statin treatment in cardiac syndrome-X1. *Eur Heart J* 2003; **24**:1999–2005.

87. Eriksson BE, Tyni-Lenne R, Svedenhag J. Physical training in syndrome X: physical training counteracts deconditioning and pain in syndrome X. *J Am Coll Cardiol* 2000; **36**:1619–25.

88. Paoletti R, Wenger N K. Review of the international position on women's health and menopause, a comprehensive approach. *Circulation* 2003; **107**:1336–9.

89. Mosca L, Appel LJ, Benjamin EJ, et al. Evidence-based guidelines for cardiovascular disease prevention in women. *Circulation* 2004; **109**:672–92.

16
Silent ischemia in women

C. Noel Bairey Merz

Introduction

Silent ischemia is defined as evidence of myocardial ischemia in patients with coronary artery disease in the absence of angina or anginal-equivalent symptomatology. Prior study has documented the clinical[1–3] and prognostic[4–6] implications of silent ischemia experienced during daily life, evidenced by transient asymptomatic ST segment depression on ambulatory electrocardiographic (ECG) monitoring in populations of women and men.

Evidence suggests that women with coronary heart disease (CHD) have a worse prognosis than men.[7,8] Notably, recent data indicated that sudden cardiac death is increasing disproportionately in women compared with men,[9] a marked change in trends from previous decades. Although older age and more adverse risk factor profiles among women with CHD may account for some of this adverse prognosis, recent study has demonstrated that the most evident and largest sex difference in prognosis lies among relatively young, premenopausal women compared with relatively young men.[10] These differences do not appear attributable to baseline risk factors or treatment,[10] and long-term follow-up has demonstrated that the adverse prognostic difference for younger women with CHD is persistent.[11] Because silent ischemia likely plays a role in sudden cardiac death, as well as CHD prognosis, examination of silent ischemia in women is relevant.

Prevalence and prognosis of silent ischemia

The majority of investigations with regard to silent ischemia in both general and CHD populations have been performed in men. The largest study in general subjects, performed exclusively in men, demonstrated a 25% prevalence of ambulatory ECG ischemia, with the majority (92%) of episodes being silent.[12] Among this general population, not overtly diseased men, the presence of silent ischemia was associated with a fourfold increase in cardiac events (p = 0.005).[12] While women were included in two smaller general population studies,[13,14] the study results were not reported by gender.

Among CHD subjects, approximately half demonstrate ambulatory ischemia, with the majority of episodes (73–94%) again being silent.[1–3] While most of these studies included women, they typically represented less than 20% of the total study population, and the results have not been reported stratified by gender. Essentially all studies demonstrated that the presence of ambulatory ischemia predicts adverse cardiac events with risk ratios ranging from 2.7 to 8.1.[4–6]

Other investigations have shown that mental stress-induced ischemia, which is often silent, is independently associated with significantly higher rates of fatal and nonfatal cardiac events and predicts cardiac events above that of exercise-induced ischemia.[15–18]

Mechanisms of silent ischemia

The mechanisms that participate in the triggering of silent ischemia episodes and the determinants of silent ischemia are relatively well investigated. Ambulatory myocardial ischemia during daily life typically occurs at relatively lower heart rate thresholds than exercise stress testing thresholds, suggesting that abnormalities in coronary vasomotor tone (vasoconstriction or a lack of appropriate vasodilation) play a role. Additionally, earlier studies have documented that increases both in heart rate[19] and blood pressure[20] are commonly observed before the onset of ambulatory silent ischemia episodes in patients with CHD, indicating that issues both of coronary blood supply and demand contribute mechanistically to trigger silent ischemia. Other work has demonstrated that strenuous exercise, anger, and smoking[21] are common daily activity determinants of these increases in heart rate and blood pressure that trigger silent ischemia episodes. Essentially none of these studies has examined results stratified by gender.

Mental stress testing offers an opportunity to further explore the pathophysiology of low heart rate myocardial ischemia, similar to that observed during activities of daily living. Work by our group[22] and others[23,24] has demonstrated that mental stress-induced, low heart rate myocardial ischemia is prevalent in approximately half of CHD patients with exercise-induced ischemia. Mental stress-induced ischemia is more likely to be clinically silent, and most often observed in patients with hyperreactive hemodynamic responses to both exercise and mental stress tests. Yeung et al.[25] also confirmed that abnormalities of vasomotor tone, specifically endothelial dysfunction, are mechanistically involved, again confirming that both abnormalities of coronary blood supply and demand are involved in silent ischemia pathophysiology.

Psychophysiological work has further explored mechanistic pathways. Burg and co-workers[23] demonstrated that patients with CHD and mental stress-induced myocardial ischemia were distinguished by a psychological profile consistent with emotional reactivity to social interaction and mental provocation, with anger as the predominant affective state. Rutledge and co-workers[26] further documented that psychosocial risk factors, such as high baseline levels of stress and hostility, predicted smaller treatment benefit in terms of silent ischemia frequency in response to anti-ischemia therapy. Again, the results of these studies have not been reported stratified by gender.

Sex differences in silent ischemia pathophysiology

The hemodynamic mechanisms and triggers of silent ischemia appear to differ between women and men. Cardiovascular reactivity, defined as the difference in variables such as heart rate and blood pressure between periods of rest and during stimulus, has been demonstrated to be a risk factor for atherosclerosis,[27] a marker for accelerated atherosclerosis (measured by carotid intimal-media thickness),[28] and a predictor of future cardiac events.[29] We have demonstrated that elevated blood pressure surges measured during mental stress[30] and during daily life[31] can trigger ischemia in CHD patients. Elevated cardiovascular reactivity reflects an abnormal arterial vasomotor response, and may indirectly therefore be a marker for endothelial dysfunction.

Further work has suggested that women may be disproportionately affected by endothelial dysfunction via sex-specific hormonal mechanisms. In 100 subjects studied with mental stress, we demonstrated that women had overall greater cardiovascular reactivity than men, particularly menopausal women[32] (Fig. 16.1). Stoney and colleagues[33] had previously demonstrated that these sex differences are not accompanied by differences in serum catecholamines, but negatively correlate with serum estradiol levels, suggesting that lower estrogen levels play a role in elevating cardiovascular reactivity among menopausal women. Importantly, cardiovascular stress responses appeared to be greatly enhanced among women of menopausal age (none were taking hormone therapy) compared with premenopausal women or men, especially with regard to blood pressure, in our study (Fig. 16.1). Although our observed enhanced cardiovascular reactivity among the menopausal women was not associated with a greater frequency of induced

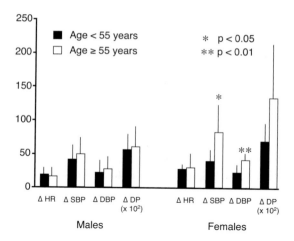

Figure 16.1
Mean values ± standard deviation for Δ heart rate (ΔHR, expressed as bpm), Δ systolic blood pressure (ΔSBP, expressed as mmHg), Δ diastolic blood pressure (ΔDBP, expressed as mmHg), and Δ double product (ΔDP, calculated as Δ [heart rate × systolic blood pressure]) for males <55 years (n = 38) and ≥55 years (n = 46), and for females <55 years (n = 6) and ≥55 years (n = 10). Reproduced from reference 32 with permission from Elsevier.

myocardial ischemia in our relatively small data set,[32] we could not discount the possibility that this enhanced hemodynamic stress response may have an adverse effect in terms of triggering cardiac events.

Further study from our laboratory in this area has documented that defensive hostility is significantly linked with ambulatory silent ischemia in women, but not in men.[34] Because prior study has linked hostility with elevated cardiovascular reactivity,[35] these data suggest that the elevated cardiovascular stress responses observed in menopausal women may be a determinant of silent ischemia in women.

Mechanisms of anginal symptoms

Multiple mechanisms likely contribute to the genesis of anginal symptoms (or lack thereof) associated with myocardial ischemia, including physiological and psychological variables. Ambulatory and mental

stress-induced ischemia are frequently associated with relatively low heart rate physical activities combined with relatively high mental activities.[20] Sheps and co-workers[36] have demonstrated that mental stress testing produces increased cardiovascular reactivity and increases in plasma β-endorphin levels that are significantly correlated with higher pain thresholds. These elevated endorphins may explain why myocardial ischemia is most often silent during mental stress testing, as well as possibly during daily activities. Further sex-stratified analyses of these data indicated that women had significantly lower pain thresholds (e.g. they felt more pain) than men, and that they had significantly lower blood beta-endorphin levels than the men, potentially explaining their lower pain thresholds.[37] Additional factors likely contribute to the expression of angina symptoms in women. Overall in the general population, women experience more anginal chest pain than men,[38] yet paradoxically have less age-adjusted coronary artery disease.[39,40] Indeed, the relatively high prevalence of angina combined with the relatively lower prevalence of angiographic CHD results in anginal symptoms having a lower predictive value for CHD in women.[38] Notably, however, women with angina have a higher cardiovascular risk factor profile,[38] and are at greater risk for CHD events,[41] than women without angina, such that symptoms cannot be dismissed in women.

A number of hypotheses have been suggested to explain the relative excess of anginal chest pain in women compared with men that is in excess of the prevalence of CHD. Previous work has explored whether reporting bias might explain the phenomenon, whereby women more frequently report a variety of nonspecific symptoms.[42] However, Nicholson and co-workers[38] were unable to find evidence to support this. A second hypothesis suggested is that the increased angina observed in women is due to psychological stress and somatization.[43] Again, previous work has been unable to support this concept, suggesting rather that any psychological distress is secondary to the experience of the angina symptoms.[44] A possible contributing mechanism is that of somatic awareness, whereby women with a greater body awareness may perceive and report angina, as well as other bodily symptoms. Indeed, multiple lines of evidence indicate that female animals[45] and women[46] have higher body awareness and lower pain thresholds, potentially related to estrogen levels.[47]

A final explanation for the excess of anginal chest pain experienced by women in the absence of coronary artery disease suggests an abnormality of the coronary microvasculature related to cardiac syndrome X.[48–51] As described in Chapter 15, syndrome X is characterized by angina and evidence of myocardial ischemia in the absence of obstructive coronary artery disease. While earlier work has implicated a variety of putative mechanisms, most recent data from the National Heart, Lung, and Blood Institute-sponsored Women's Ischemia Syndrome Evaluation (WISE) study[52] have documented the presence of metabolic myocardial ischemia in a significant proportion of these women,[53] supporting the concept of microvascular dysfunction with inadequate vasomotor reserve leading to myocardial ischemia in the absence of obstructive coronary artery disease. Thus, angina symptoms are relatively more nonspecific in women than in men.

Furthermore, we have demonstrated a clear uncoupling of ambulatory ischemia and symptoms, such that both the majority of episodes of ambulatory ischemia are silent (asymptomatic), and the majority of ambulatory anginal symptoms reported by subjects are not accompanied by evidence of ischemia.[54] It is clear that anginal symptoms are a relatively insensitive and nonspecific marker of myocardial ischemia in both women and men. Notably, however, while both women and men can have silent ischemia in the ambulatory setting, women are more likely, compared with men, to have angina with and without myocardial ischemia in the absence of obstructive coronary artery disease.

Efficacy of treatment for silent ischemia in women

We[30] and others[55–64] have demonstrated the effect of anti-ischemic therapy on silent ischemia in populations of women and men with CHD. Overall, beta-blockers are effective in reducing the relatively high heart rate-associated ischemia, whereas long-acting calcium channel agents and nitrates are effective in reducing the relatively low heart rate-associated ischemia. Although most of these studies included women, women represented a minority population (<20%) in essentially all of the studies, and none of the studies stratified their results by gender.

The relationship between anti-ischemic therapy for silent ischemia and improvement in cardiac events has been studied in several trials.[62,63,65,66] Pepine and co-workers found that atenolol significantly reduced daily life ischemia and was associated with reduced risk for adverse outcomes (p <0.001) in 306 asymptomatic and mildly symptomatic patients compared with placebo in the Atenolol Silent Ischemia Study Trial (ASIST).[63] Stone and co-workers in the Asymptomatic Cardiac Ischemia Pilot (ACIP) trial found significantly reduced cardiac events at 1-year follow-up in 558 patients with ischemia using angina-guided therapy (32% reduction), ischemia-guided therapy (31% reduction), and revascularization (18% reduction) (p <0.003).[65] A randomized trial of atenolol versus nifedipine versus the combination in 682 subjects was negative for significant differences in cardiac event reduction,[66] and a randomized trial of bisoprolol versus nifedipine in 520 subjects demonstrated a significantly greater event reduction (33%) in the nifedipine group compared with the bisoprolol group (22%) (p <0.03).[62] None of these trials reported their outcomes stratified by gender.

Notably, lipid-lowering has been demonstrated to reduce ambulatory ischemia. The Regression Growth Evaluation Study (REGRESS) tested pravastatin versus placebo in 768 men with CHD and stable angina, and both the occurrence and duration of ischemic episodes were significantly reduced in the pravastatin group.[67] Andrews and colleagues also demonstrated similar effects with lovastatin compared with placebo in 40 women and men;[68] however, the results were not stratified by gender. The ongoing Study Assessing Goals in the Elderly (SAGE) is testing the hypothesis that 80 mg of atorvastatin is superior to 40 mg of pravastatin in reducing ambulatory ischemia in over 800 older women and men.[69] While a variety of mechanisms may contribute to this beneficial effect, lipid-lowering clearly improves endothelial function, a key determinant of ambulatory ischemia.[70] Our earlier work demonstrating more adverse cardiovascular reactivity in older, menopausal women[32] suggests that lipid-lowering-related endothelial function improvement may be particularly efficacious for women. While these studies have been underpowered to examine the impact on cardiovascular events, the large Heart Protection Study (HPS) demonstrated significant reductions in cardiovascular mortality and morbidity in women using 40 mg of daily simvastatin.[71]

Conclusions

Sudden cardiac death is on the rise in women, and women with established CHD face a more adverse prognosis, particularly relatively young (under 55 years) women, compared with age-matched men. Previous studies have documented the clinical and prognostic implications of silent ischemia experienced during daily life, evidenced by transient asymptomatic ST segment depression on ambulatory ECG monitoring in populations of women and men. While essentially none of these studies has stratified the results by gender, evaluation of the pathophysiologic triggers of silent ischemia suggests that women with lower estrogen levels may disproportionately suffer with silent ischemia due to enhanced cardiovascular reactivity and possibly endothelial dysfunction. Notably, anginal symptoms are both insensitive and nonspecific for the presence of myocardial ischemia in daily life in women and men. Women also have a higher prevalence of angina, greater somatic awareness, and lower pain thresholds than men, as well as more myocardial ischemia in the absence of obstructive coronary artery disease (microvascular disease). Outcome studies have documented reductions in cardiac events by treatment of silent ischemia using beta-blockers and calcium channel agents. Statin lipid-lowering therapy has been established as efficacious for reducing ambulatory ischemia in men; an ongoing study of atorvastatin in elderly women and men is testing aggressive versus moderate lipid-lowering for reducing ambulatory ischemia. These data suggest that further evaluation of silent ischemia in women may provide important understanding into sex-specific gaps in CHD outcomes, as well as point toward effective treatments for women for the reduction of CHD morbidity and mortality.

References

1. Stern S, Tzivoni D. Early detection of silent ischemic heart disease by 24-hour ECG monitoring of active subjects. *Br Heart J* 1974; **36**:481–6.
2. Schang SJ, Pepine CJ. Transient asymptomatic ST segment depression during daily activity. *Am J Cardiol* 1977; **39**:396–402.
3. Mulcahy D, Keegan J, Crean P, et al. Silent myocardial ischemia in chronic stable angina: a study of frequency and characteristics in 150 patients. *Br Heart J* 1988; **60**:417–23.
4. Mark DB, Hlatky MA, Califf RM, et al. Painless exercise ST deviation on the treadmill: long term prognosis. *J Am Coll Cardiol* 1989; **14**:885–8.
5. Miranda CP, Lehmann KG, Lachterman B, et al. Comparison of silent and symptomatic ischemia during exercise testing in men. *Ann Intern Med* 1991; **114**:645–56.
6. Laukkanen JA, Kurl S, Lakka TA, et al. Exercise-induced silent myocardial ischemia and coronary morbidity and mortality in middle-aged men. *J Am Coll Cardiol* 2001; **38**:72–9.
7. Tofler GH, Stone PH, Muller JE, et al. Effects of gender and race on prognosis after myocardial infarction: adverse prognosis for women, particularly black women. *J Am Coll Cardiol* 1987; **9**:473–82.
8. Greenland P, Reicher-Reiss H, Goldbourt U, Behar S. In-hospital and 1-year mortality in 1524 women after myocardial infarction: comparison with 4315 men. *Circulation* 1991; **83**:484–91.
9. http://cdc.gov/mmwr/preview/mmwrhtml/mm5106a3.htm [accessed June 15, 2002].
10. Vaccarino V, Parsons L, Every NR, Barron HV, Krumholz HM, for the National Registry of Myocardial Infarction 2 Participants. Sex-based differences in early mortality after myocardial infarction. *N Engl J Med* 1999; **341**:217–25.
11. Vaccarino V, Krumholz HM, Yarzebski J, Gore JM, Goldberg RJ. Sex differences in 2-year mortality after

hospital discharge for myocardial infarction. *Ann Intern Med* 2001; **134**:173–81.

12. Hedblad B, Juul-Moller S, Svensson K, et al. Increased mortality in men with ST segment depression during 24 h ambulatory long-term ECG recording: results from prospective population study 'Men born in 1914,' from Malmo, Sweden. *Eur Heart J* 1989; **10**:149–58.

13. Quyyumi AA, Wright CH, Fox K. Ambulatory electrocardiographic ST segment changes in healthy volunteers. *Br Heart J* 1983; **50**:60–4.

14. Deanfield JE, Ribiero P, Oakley K, et al. Critical analysis of ST-segment changes in normal subjects: implications from ambulatory monitoring in angina pectoris. *Am J Cardiol* 1984; **54**:1321–5.

15. Jain D, Burg M, Soufer R, et al. Prognostic implications of mental stress-induced silent left ventricular dysfunction in patients with stable angina pectoris. *Am J Cardiol* 1995; **76**:31–5.

16. Jiang W, Babyak M, Krantz DS, et al. Mental stress-induced myocardial ischemia and cardiac events. *JAMA* 1996; **275**:1651–6.

17. Krantz DS, Santiago HT, Kop WJ, et al. Prognostic value of mental stress testing in coronary artery disease. *Am J Cardiol* 1999; **84**:1292–7.

18. Sheps DS, McMahon RP, Becker L, et al. Mental stress-induced ischemia and all-cause mortality in patients with coronary artery disease. Results from the Psychophysiological Investigations of Myocardial Ischemia Study. *Circulation* 2002; **105**:1780–4.

19. Panza D, Diodati JG, Callahan TS, et al. Role of increases of heart rate in determining the occurrence and frequency of myocardial ischemia during daily life in patients with stable coronary artery disease. *J Am Coll Cardiol* 1992; **20**:1092–8.

20. Deedwania PC, Nelson JR. Pathophysiology of silent myocardial ischemia during daily life: hemodynamic evaluation by simultaneous electrocardiographic and blood pressure monitoring. *Circulation* 1990; **82**:1296–304.

21. Gabbay FH, Krantz DS, Kop WJ, et al. Triggers of myocardial ischemia during daily life in patients with coronary artery disease: physical and mental activities, anger and smoking. *J Am Coll Cardiol* 1996; **27**:585–92.

22. Rozanski A, Bairey CN, Krantz DS, et al. Mental stress and silent myocardial ischemia in coronary artery disease patients. *N Engl J Med* 1988; **318**:1005–12.

23. Burg MM, Jain D, Soufer R, et al. Role of behavioral and psychological factors in mental stress-induced silent left ventricular dysfunction in coronary artery disease. *J Am Coll Cardiol* 1993; **22**:440–8.

24. Specchia F, Falcone C, Traversi E, et al. Mental stress as a provocative test in patients with various clinical syndromes of coronary heart disease. *Circulation* 1991; **83** (Suppl II):II-108–14.

25. Yeung AC, Vekshtein VI, Krantz DS, et al. The effect of atherosclerosis on the vasomotor response of coronary arteries to mental stress. *N Engl J Med* 1991; **325**:1551–6.

26. Rutledge T, Linden W, Davies RF, et al. Psychological risk factors may moderate pharmacological treatment effects among ischemia heart disease patients. *Psychosom Med* 1999; **61**:834–40.

27. Manuck SB, Kaplan JR, Clarkson TB. Behaviorally induced heart rate reactivity in atherosclerosis in cynomolgus monkeys. *Psychosom Med* 1983; **45**:95–108.

28. Kamarck TW, Everson SA, Kaplan GA, et al. Exaggerated blood pressure responses during mental stress are associated with enhanced carotid atherosclerosis in middle-aged Finnish men. Findings from the Kuopio Ischemic Heart Disease Study. *Circulation* 1997; **96**:3842–8.

29. Sparrow D, Tifft CP, Rosner B, Weiss S. Postural changes in diastolic blood pressure and the risk of myocardial infarction: The Normative Aging Study. *Circulation* 1984; **70**:533–7.

30. Bairey Merz CN, Krantz DS, DeQuattro V, Berman DS, Rozanski A. Effect of beta-blockade on low heart rate-related ischemia during mental stress. *J Am Coll Cardiol* 1991; **17**:1388–95.

31. Deedwania PC, Nelson JR. Pathophysiology of silent myocardial ischemia during daily life. Hemodynamic evaluation by simultaneous electrocardiographic and blood pressure monitoring. *Circulation* 1990; **82**:1296–304.

32. Bairey Merz CN, Kop W, Krantz DS. Helmers KF, Berman DS, Rozanksi A. Cardiovascular stress response and coronary artery disease in women: evidence of an adverse postmenopausal effect. *Am Heart J* 1998; **135**:881–7.

33. Stoney CM, Matthews KA, McDonald RH, Johnson CA. Sex differences in lipid, lipoprotein, cardiovascular, and neuroendocrine responses to acute stress. *Psychophysiology* 1988; **25**:645–56.

34. Helmers KF, Krantz DS, Bairey Merz CN, et al. Defensive hostility: relationship to multiple markers of cardiac ischemia in patients with coronary disease. *Health Psychol* 1995; **14**:202–9.

35. Williams RB Jr. Coronary-prone behaviors, hostility, and cardiovascular health: implications for behavioral and pharmacological interventions. In: Orth-Gomer K, Schneiderman N (eds). *Behavioral Medicine*

Approaches to Cardiovascular Disease Prevention. Mahwah, NJ: Lawrence Erlbaum Associates, 1996: 161–8.

36. Sheps DS, Ballenger MN, DeGent GE, et al. Psychological responses to a speech stressor: correlation of plasma beta-endorphin levels at rest and after psychological stress with thermally measured pain threshold in patients with coronary artery disease. *J Am Coll Cardiol* 1995; **25**:1499–503.

37. Sheps DS, Kaufmann PG, Sheffield D, et al. Sex differences in chest pain in patients with documented coronary artery disease and exercise-induced ischemia: results from the PIMI study. *Am Heart J* 2001; **142**:864–71.

38. Nicholson A, White IR, Macfarlane P, et al. Rose questionnaire angina in younger men and women: gender differences in the relationship to cardiovascular risk factors and other reported symptoms. *J Clin Epidemiol* 1999; **52**:337–46.

39. Wenger NK, Speroff L, Packard B. Cardiovascular health and disease in women. *N Engl J Med* 1993; **329**:247–56.

40. US Department of Commerce, Economics and Statistics Administration, Bureau of the Census. *Statistical Abstract of the United States: 1992*, 112th edn. Washington, DC: US Government Printing Office, 1992.

41. Murabito JM, Anderson KM, Kannel WB, et al. Risk of coronary heart disease in subjects with chest discomfort: The Framingham Heart Study. *Am J Med* 1990; **89**:297–302.

42. Freedland KE, Carney RM, Krone RJ, et al. Psychological factors in silent myocardial ischaemia. *Psychosom Med* 1991; **53**:13–24.

43. Mayou R. Medically unexplained physical symptoms. *BMJ* 1991; **303**:534–5.

44. Stansfeld SA, Davey Smith G, Marmot MG. Association between physical and psychological morbidity in the Whitehall II Study. *J Psychosom Res* 1993; **37**:227–38.

45. Kepler KL, Standifer KM, Paul D, et al. Gender effects and central opioid analgesia. *Pain* 1991; **45**:87–94.

46. Gear RW, Gordon NC, Heller PH, et al. Gender differences in analgesic response to the kappa-opioid pentazocine. *Neurosci Lett* 1996; **205**:207–9.

47. Fillingim RB, Maixner W, Girdler SS, et al. Ischemic but not thermal pain sensitivity varies across the menstrual cycle. *J Psychosom Med* 1997; **59**:512–20.

48. Cannon RO 3rd, Epstein SE. 'Microvascular angina' as a cause of chest pain with angiographically normal coronary arteries. *Am J Cardiol* 1988; **61**:227–38.

49. Egashira K, Inou T, Hirooka Y, et al. Evidence of impaired endothelium-dependent coronary vasodilation in patients with angina pectoris and normal angiograms. *N Engl J Med* 1993; **328**:1659–64.

50. Rosen SD, Uren NG, Kashi JC, et al. Coronary vasodilator reserve, pain perception, and sex in patients with syndrome X. *Circulation* 1994; **90**:50–60.

51. Holdright DR, Lindsay DC, Clarke D, et al. Coronary flow reserve in patients with chest pain and normal coronary arteries. *Br Heart J* 1993; **70**:513–19.

52. Bairey Merz CN, Kelsey SF, Pepine CJ, et al. The Women's Ischemia Syndrome (WISE) Study: protocol design, methodology and feasibility report. *J Am Coll Cardiol* 1999; **33**:1453–61.

53. Buchthal SD, den Hollander JA, Bairey Merz CN, et al. Metabolic evidence of myocardial ischemia by 31-P spectroscopy in women with chest pain but no significant coronary stenoses: pilot phase results from the NHLBI-sponsored WISE study. *N Engl J Med* 2000; **342**:829–35.

54. Krantz DS, Hedges SM, Gabbay FH, et al. The uncoupling of angina and ischemia in ambulatory coronary artery disease patients: daily life triggers differ for chest pain and ST-segment depression. *Am Heart J* 1994; **128**:703–12.

55. Deanfield JE, Detry JRG, Lichtlen PR, Magnani B, Sellier P, Thaulow E. Amlodipine reduces transient myocardial ischemia in patients with coronary artery disease: double-blind Circadian Anti-ischemia Program in Europe (CAPE trial). *J Am Coll Cardiol* 1994; **24**:1460–7.

56. Davies RF, Habibi H, Klinke WP, et al. Effect of amlodipine, atenolol and their combination on myocardial ischemia during treadmill exercise and ambulatory monitoring. *J Am Coll Cardiol* 1995; **25**:619–25.

57. Kawanishi T, Reid C, Morrison B, Rahimtoola S. Response of angina and ischemia to long-term treatment in patients with chronic stable angina: a double-blind randomized individualized dosing trial of nifedipine, propranolol and their combination. *J Am Coll Cardiol* 1992; **19**:409–17.

58. Siu SC, Jacoby RM, Phillips RT, Nesto RN. Comparative efficacy of nifedipine, gastrointestinal therapeutic system versus diltiazem when added to beta-blockers in stable angina pectoris. *Am J Cardiol* 1993; **71**:887–92.

59. Theroux P, Baird M, Juneau M, et al. Effect of diltiazem on symptomatic and asymptomatic episodes of ST-segment depression occurring during daily life and during exercise. *Circulation* 1991; **84**:15–22.

60. Stone PH, Gibson RS, Glasser SP, et al. Comparison

of propanolol, diltiazem and nifedipine in the treatment of ambulatory ischemia in patients with stable angina: differential effects on ambulatory ischemia, exercise performance and anginal symptoms (the ASIS study). *Circulation* 1990; **82**:1962–72.

61. Hill JA, Gonzalez JI, Kolb R, Pepine CJ. Effects of atenolol alone, nifedipine alone and their combination on ambulant myocardial ischemia. *Am J Cardiol* 1991; **67**:671–5.

62. Von Arnim T. Medical treatment to reduce total ischemic burden: Total Ischemic Burden Bisoprolol Study (TIBBS), a multicenter trial comparing bisoprolol and nifedipine – the TIBBS Investigators. *J Am Coll Cardiol* 1995; **25**:231–8.

63. Pepine CJ, Cohn PF, Deedwania PC, et al. Effects of treatment on outcome in mildly symptomatic patients with ischemia during daily life: the Atenolol Silent Ischemia Study (ASIST). *Circulation* 1994; **90**:762–8.

64. Lim R, Dyke L, Dymond DS. Effect on prognosis of abolition of exercise-induced painless myocardial ischemia by medical therapy. *Am J Cardiol* 1992; **69**:733–9.

65. Stone PH, Chaitman BR, McMahon RP, et al, for the ACIP Investigators. Asymptomatic Cardiac Ischemia Pilot (ACIP) study: relationship between exercise-induced and ambulatory ischemia in patients with stable coronary disease. *Circulation* 1996; **94**:1537–44.

66. Dargie HJ, Ford I, Fox KM. Total Ischaemic Burden European Trial (TIBET). Effects of ischaemia and treatment with atenolol, nifedipine SR and their combination on outcome in patients with chronic stable angina. The TIBET Study Group. *Eur Heart J* 1996; **17**:104–12.

67. van Boven AJ, Jukema JW, Zwinderman AH, et al. Reduction of transient myocardial ischemia with pravastatin in addition to the conventional treatment in patients with angina pectoris. *Circulation* 1996; **94**:1503–5.

68. Andrews TC, Raby K, Barry J, et al. Effect of cholesterol reduction on myocardial ischemia in patients with coronary disease. *Circulation* 1997; **95**:324–8.

69. Deedwania PC; Study Assessing Goals in the Elderly Steering Committee and Investigators. Effect of aggressive versus moderate lipid-lowering therapy on myocardial ischemia: the rationale, design, and baseline characteristics of the Study Assessing Goals in the Elderly (SAGE). *Am Heart J* 2004; **148**:1053–9.

70. Forrester JS, Bairey Merz CN, Kaul S. The aggressive LDL lowering controversy. *J Am Coll Cardiol* 2000; **36**:1419–25.

71. Heart Protection Study Collaborative Group. MRC/BHF Heart Protection Study of cholesterol-lowering with simvastatin in 5963 people with diabetes: a randomized placebo-controlled trial. *Lancet* 2003; **361**:2005–16.

17

Acute coronary syndromes – thrombolysis, angioplasty

Annika Rosengren and David Hasdai

Introduction

During the second half of the twentieth century coronary heart disease (CHD) emerged as the single most common cause of death in both women and men in large parts of the industrialized world and is now the leading cause of death worldwide.[1] Acute myocardial infarction (AMI), the irreversible loss of myocardial cells due to acute obstruction of an epicardial coronary vessel, is one of the most important manifestations of coronary disease. Although the incidence of AMI increases sharply with age, women are less prone to develop AMI than men at any given age, with an approximate 9–10-year difference between the sexes[2–6] (Fig. 17.1). The sex difference in mortality and morbidity diminishes with age,

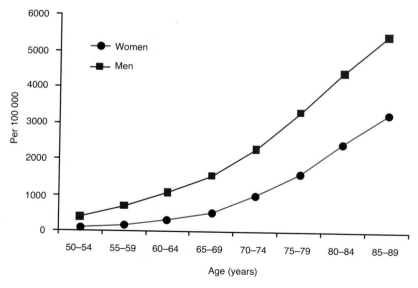

Figure 17.1
Incidence of fatal and nonfatal acute myocardial infarction (AMI) by age and sex. Data from reference 4.

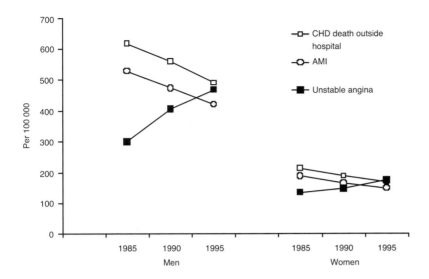

Figure 17.2
Trends in acute coronary heart disease (CHD) mortality and morbidity 1985–1995 in the Minnesota Heart Survey.[12] AMI, acute myocardial infarction.

but even at ages between 75 and 85, the incidence is almost twofold in men compared with women.[4]

One of the more intriguing aspects of coronary disease is the rapid changes in mortality, incidence, and clinical presentation. In many of the established Western market economies there is now a marked reduction in total coronary mortality,[7–9] in out-of-hospital mortality,[10] and also a reduction in the incidence of AMI.[11,12] The reduction in nonfatal events, however, has not been as evident as that for mortality.[11–13] Case severity in AMI seems to be decreasing,[14–16] with infarcts becoming smaller;[17] and there is an increase in the rate of unstable angina pectoris (UAP),[12,18] a milder form of acute coronary disease (Fig. 17.2). Partly, these changes may be attributed to better coronary care[19] but changes in coronary risk factor patterns may play a role.[20]

Trends in CHD vary not only by gender, but also by time period and by type of clinical manifestation under study. With respect to CHD mortality, trends in women have partly been different to those in men, with age-adjusted death rates in the US during the late 1970s and in the 1980s decreasing faster for white men than for white women.[21,22] Later investigations in the US and Finland, however, have shown declines at a similar rate in women and men.[23–25] With respect to nonfatal events, one US study found that the incidence of hospitalized AMI decreased in men but

increased in women and elderly persons.[26] An overall increase in nonfatal hospitalizations in both women and men was reported from two communities in New England.[27] In Sweden, the overall incidence decreased more in men than in women at ages below 65 years, whereas trends in men and women were similar above age 65 years. As a result, the ratio men/women with respect to AMI decreased significantly at ages below 65, with proportionately more younger women with AMI.[18]

CHD and AMI are not the inevitable results of aging; the rapid shifts in incidence and mortality and the large geographical variation appear in response to alterations in lifestyle and risk factors. In Finland, where there has been a dramatic decrease in cardiac mortality over the last three decades, nearly half of the decrease in coronary mortality hazard was associated with changes in risk factors.[28,29] Smoking is probably a stronger risk factor for AMI in middle-aged women than for men, but relative risks associated with serum total cholesterol and blood pressure are similar.[30] However, serum triglycerides, which are strongly related to obesity, have been demonstrated to be a better predictor of future coronary events in women, compared with men.[31] Although speculative, some of the divergence in trends for women and men could reflect changes in lifestyle factors, with less discrepancy in smoking between the sexes, and perhaps also the fact that obesity, which is now increasing worldwide, may be more detrimental to women.

Pathology

AMI is related to acute coronary thrombosis,[32] secondary to coronary atherosclerosis. The relation between atherosclerosis and acute coronary syndromes is complicated. Early post-mortem studies described the absence of a direct relationship between the severity of chronic atherosclerosis and acute coronary syndromes[33] and a review of the molecular bases of the acute coronary syndrome highlighted the concept of the vulnerable atherosclerotic plaque.[34] Rupture of an atherosclerotic plaque is the most common type of plaque complication, accounting for approximately 70% of fatal AMIs and CHD deaths.[35] In some cases, the thrombus instead appears to be superimposed on a de-endothelialized, but otherwise intact, plaque. This type of superficial plaque injury is called 'plaque erosion'. In a case series of 298 consecutive AMI patients dying in hospital, acute coronary thrombi were found in 291 hearts (98%); in 37% of women and 18% of men the plaque substrate for thrombosis was erosion.[36] Erosion of proteoglycan-rich and smooth muscle cell-rich plaques lacking a superficial lipid core or plaque rupture may cause sudden death due to coronary thrombosis. These lesions are more often seen in younger individuals and women.[37] Sex differences in plaque morphology have also been found in post-mortem studies.[38] In an autopsy study of women who had died suddenly from CHD or who had died from noncoronary causes, women older than 50 years of age were much more likely to have a ruptured plaque than were younger premenopausal women, suggesting that that estrogen may have an anti-inflammatory effect on atherosclerotic plaques, resulting in plaque stabilization. Plaque erosion, possibly the major substrate for thrombosis in premenopausal women, may not be inhibited by estrogen.[39]

The development of intravascular ultrasound (IVUS) has offered new possibilities to study plaque morphology in vivo. In a series of women and men with UAP both qualitative and quantitative sex differences in in vivo coronary plaque morphology were detected. Plaques in women appeared less videodense and less often calcified than those in men.[40] Coronary arteries in eight women with documented AMI and angiographically normal or not significantly stenosed vessels were investigated with IVUS. Atherosclerosis was found in all infarct-related arteries.[41] This is important, because women with acute coronary syndrome more often than men have no or nonsignificant angiographic coronary artery stenoses.[42,43] Thus, atherosclerosis is probably the main etiologic factor for AMI even in cases without an angiographically obvious coronary stenosis in the infarct-related vessel.[41]

Differences in clinical characteristics and clinical manifestations (see also Chapters 18 and 19)

Results of studies comparing presenting symptoms in AMI show that women and men, by and large, display the same symptoms. However, some gender differences have been demonstrated in the proportion of symptoms,[44] with women demonstrating more back, jaw, and neck pain, nausea and/or vomiting, dyspnea, palpitations, indigestion, dizziness, fatigue, loss of appetite, and syncope. Men reported more chest pain and diaphoresis. Women and older persons are also over-represented among AMI patients presenting without chest pain.[45] Among patients diagnosed with acute cardiac ischemia, women below 55 years were significantly more likely to be mistakenly discharged from the emergency department.[46] However, in patients seen in the emergency department, typical symptoms also were the strongest predictors of acute coronary syndromes in women.[47] Hence, even though most women with AMI have typical symptoms, slightly more present with less typical symptoms, particularly among the elderly. Coupled with the low incidence in younger women, this may lead to an overall higher propensity to miss AMI cases, both among younger and older women.

Low awareness of CHD among women may lead to not recognizing symptoms and not seeking medical care. Women with AMI tend to present late more

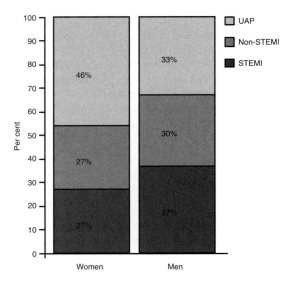

Figure 17.3
Clinical presentation in men and women with acute coronary syndromes in the Global Use of Strategies to Open Occluded Coronary Arteries in Acute Coronary Syndromes study.[43] UAP, unstable angina pectoris; Non-STEMI, acute myocardial infarction without ST elevation; STEMI, acute myocardial infarction with ST elevation.

often than men.[48,49] The proportion of silent AMIs as a proportion of all AMIs has also been demonstrated to be higher in women than in men.[50] An Icelandic study of women found that one-third of all AMIs in women were unrecognized and that the proportion of unrecognized nonfatal AMIs decreased with age.[51] However, in more recent studies the percentage of unrecognized AMIs was slightly lower than previous estimates and similar in women and men.[52]

Clinical manifestations in CHD also differ between women and men. AMI is less often the first manifestation of CHD in women than in men.[2,50,53] In the acute coronary syndrome, there are also differences with respect to type. In a study utilizing data from a clinical trial, a smaller percentage of women than men had AMI with ST elevation (27% vs 37%), and of the patients who presented without ST elevation, fewer women than men had AMI[43] (Fig. 17.3). In the Euro Heart ACS Survey on comparatively unselected patients with acute coronary syndromes

from 103 hospitals in 25 countries, younger but not older women were less likely than men to present with ST elevation, but more likely to be discharged with a diagnosis of UAP.[54] In older patients there were few or no sex differences in clinical presentation or discharge diagnosis. Accordingly, it seems that across the spectrum of acute coronary syndromes, younger, but not older, women may tend to display more UAP and less ST elevation AMI compared with men.

Angiographic findings

Most studies show that women with acute coronary syndromes more commonly have no or only noncritical coronary stenoses compared with men.[42,43,54–57] However, in one study of young AMI survivors three-vessel or left main coronary artery disease was more common in women.[58] In a series of consecutive patients with AMI, 63% of women and 64% of men underwent angiography, with significant coronary artery disease equally prevalent in women and men.[59] In contrast, in the recent Euro Heart ACS survey of over 10 000 patients, women were less likely to undergo angiography, but both older and younger women had less extensive atherosclerosis than men of the same age.[54] The reasons for these inconsistencies are not clear but may result from the selection of candidates for angiography or from low numbers in some studies, resulting in impaired precision in estimates. However, most of the available data seem to indicate less obstructive coronary disease in women with AMI or acute coronary syndromes.

Complications and outcome

The prognosis of women with AMI has been much debated over the last few years. Although prognosis in patients with AMI has improved markedly over recent decades,[60–64] several studies have indicated that women hospitalized with AMI have a higher short-term mortality than men.[65–71] The more advanced age of women at the time of presentation is a major factor contributing to their worse prognosis relative to men[72] and controlling for age and co-morbidity eliminates the association between female gender and increased mortality in several studies.[73–83] However, age is also important in that the effect of sex on short-term mortality may not be the same in younger and older patients. In a large hospital-based US study on 384 878 patients, hospital mortality in women below 50 years was more than twice that for the men.[84] The difference in the mortality rates decreased with increasing age and was no longer significant after the age of 74. This age–sex interaction with respect to short-term mortality in hospitalized AMI cases also has been demonstrated in other studies.[4,85,86] Thus, it seems that among hospitalized cases, younger, but not older, women fare worse after hospitalization for AMI.

Most deaths from CHD, however, occur out of hospital.[4,87,88] Men are more likely to die before hospitalization and studies that have included not only hospital mortality, but also out-of-hospital deaths, have generally found that the higher in-hospital mortality in women was counterbalanced by higher out-of-hospital mortality among men,[4,85,87,89] outweighing the higher mortality in hospitalized cases.

Despite the fact that mortality in women after an AMI may not be very different from that in men, having had an AMI has a disproportionate impact on survival in women because women live longer than men. In women and men aged 65 and over, AMI had a greater impact on mortality in women and significantly narrowed women's typical survival advantage over men.[90]

Reperfusion therapy in women and men with AMI

Current guidelines suggest that reperfusion therapy is indicated in all patients with a history of chest pain or discomfort of less than 12 hours with diagnostic electrocardiographic changes (ST segment elevation or presumably new left bundle branch block), who present within 12 hours, and who have no contraindications.[91] This applies to both women and men. Relevant issues with respect to reperfusion

therapy in women include: (1) whether there is a sex bias in management in AMI, (2) whether benefits of proven therapies are similar in women and men, and (3) whether side effects, particularly with respect to bleeding complications, are similar in women and men. Because fewer women present with ST segment elevation,[43,54] reperfusion therapy will be indicated in a smaller proportion of women, compared with men, with an acute coronary syndrome.

Reports about the use of cardiac procedures and treatments in women and men have produced conflicting results as to whether there is a sex bias in the use of thrombolytic therapy, cardiac catheterization, or revascularization therapies. Studies have demonstrated a marked increase over time in the use of thrombolytic therapy in both women and men, with a greater relative increase observed in women.[92,93] In clinical practice there has been a gender gap in acute treatment of AMI,[93–95] but several studies have shown that this is now no longer apparent.[70,93,96,97] Less use of thrombolytics in women with AMI eligible to receive thrombolytics is, however, still reported.[98,99]

In a recent study, data for patients with ST elevation AMI who did or did not receive thrombolytic therapy were compared.[100] Women were older, but within each age bracket, men were treated more often. Treatment rates decreased with increased prevalence of exclusionary factors, and since both women and the elderly tended to have more such factors, elderly women were treated at a markedly lower rate. However, for patients without contraindications, treatment rates in women and men were similar. In the community-based MITRA (Maximal Individual TheRapy of Acute myocardial infarction) study, women with ST elevation AMI received reperfusion therapy less often than men, and the percentage of patients who were eligible for thrombolysis and received no reperfusion was higher in women.[5] In a study of US Medicare patients with AMI with strict eligibility criteria for reperfusion therapy, independent differences according to sex in the use of reperfusion therapy were, however, minimal.[97] Other than differences in age and co-morbidity, the reason for these discrepancies is not clear, but differences in physicians' perceptions of possible benefits of thrombolytic therapy in women and men are probably important.

An early overview of randomized controlled trials concluded that thrombolysis in AMI reduces mortality in both women and men, although women may have a reduced mortality benefit compared with men.[101] In patients below 76 years with ST elevation AMI, all of whom presented within 6 hours and were treated with thrombolytic therapy, there were no sex differences in in-hospital mortality after adjustment for age and other factors.[102] Women have been demonstrated not to differ significantly from men with regard to early infarct-related artery patency rates, reocclusion after thrombolytic therapy, or ventricular functional response to injury/reperfusion.[68]

In younger women, there has been concern that thrombolysis could cause complications during menstruation. Although no statistically significant increase in bleeding risk during menstruation was demonstrated in one clinical trial, where only 12 of over 10 000 women were menstruating, it was suggested that there may still be a clinically significant increase in the risk of moderate bleeding.[103] Nevertheless, there is now general consensus that the life-saving benefit of thrombolytic therapy for AMI should generally not be withheld because of active menstruation. Pregnancy, a very rare condition among women with AMI, is considered to be a relative contraindication to thrombolysis.[91]

A second concern that has been raised with respect to women and thrombolysis is the increase in risk of cerebral bleeding reported from clinical trials.[104,105] The reason for this is not clear, but might be due to smaller body size. However, in the study by White et al., the increase in risk persisted after controlling for body weight.[104] Possibly, with the introduction of weight-adjusted heparin regimes as adjunctive treatments for thrombolysis, the incidence of this complication among women will be reduced.

Angioplasty in AMI

The role of primary percutaneous intervention (PCI) during the early hours of ST elevation AMI is defined as angioplasty and/or stenting without prior or concomitant fibrinolytic therapy. PCI is an alternative to thrombolysis in patients with contraindica-

tions to thrombolytic therapy, or who are in cardiogenic shock, and is the preferred mode of reperfusion therapy when the appropriate skills and resources are immediately available.[91]

Few studies have compared whether the effect of direct angioplasty in AMI is similar in women and men, but an early meta-analysis of reperfusion and revascularization strategies in patients with CHD concluded that angioplasty resulted in greater procedural morbidity, but similar, if not better long-term outcomes in women.[101] Of studies conducted in patients treated with primary angioplasty for AMI, success and outcomes were similar in women and men in two US studies,[106,107] apart from a lower incidence of documented restenosis in women.[106] In a more recent US study that investigated outcome in a consecutive series of patients with AMI treated with a reperfusion strategy largely based on PCIs, women had a similar outcome to men, despite their older age and higher prevalence of diabetes.[6] In an Italian study, the results of outcome analysis in nonselected patients suggested that sex is not an independent predictor of mortality after primary angioplasty for AMI, and that the benefit of primary stenting is similar in women and men.[108] A recent study which evaluated sex differences in the relative benefit of direct angioplasty versus thrombolytic therapy found that the relative benefit of angioplasty to thrombolysis for the treatment of AMI appeared to be similar in women and men.[109] In contrast, another study that sought to determine whether the higher in-hospital mortality in women after AMI reported in some studies was due to less aggressive treatment also found significantly higher in-hospital mortality in women in a series where all were treated with primary angioplasty, and where procedural success and complication rates were similar.[110]

In acute coronary syndromes without ST elevation, it is currently recommended that in high-risk patients, which includes those who fulfill current criteria for AMI, coronary angiography should be performed.[111] The FRISC-II invasive trial compared the long-term effects of an early invasive versus noninvasive strategy, in terms of death and AMI and the need for repeat hospital admissions and late revascularization procedures in patients with unstable CHD.[112] The beneficial effect of an early invasive strategy was limited to the men; risk of future events was not reduced among the women, partly because women did worse after coronary artery bypass graft (CABG) surgery.[113] The authors speculated that the poor outcome in women who underwent surgery could be due to selection of high-risk patients. Also men subjected to CABG surgery had unexpectedly low mortality.

In patients undergoing coronary stenting for stable or unstable angina, women were found to present a lower risk of angiographic restenosis, as well as need for reintervention.[114] From the available data concerning angioplasty and coronary stenting, there is currently no indication that women should be treated any differently from men. Additionally, women may have a small advantage over men concerning the risk of restenosis.

Conclusions

In women, as well as in men, AMI arises as a complication of coronary atherosclerosis. The incidence and mortality increase sharply with age in both sexes, and risk factors are to a large extent similar, although women may be more susceptible to the effects of smoking and obesity. In large parts of the world, CHD is the most important single cause of death in both women and men. The main sex difference with respect to AMI is that onset in women is later in life, with greater co-morbidity. After AMI, the prognosis is by and large similar; however, women stand to lose more because of their longer life expectancy. Younger women have higher in-hospital mortality compared with younger men, but this is partly due to the fact that more men die outside hospital. Younger women also less often have ST elevation AMI, and women consistently seem to have less obstructive angiographic lesions, consistent with slightly different pathophysiology, with less obstructive thrombus in women. At older ages, there is little sex difference in hospital mortality or the proportion of ST elevation AMI. Given the differences in clinical presentation, reperfusion therapy is not quite as frequently indicated in women as in men. However, where reperfusion is indicated, thrombolysis or angioplasty seem to be equally effective in women and men.

References

1. Murray CJ, Lopez AD. Mortality by cause for eight regions of the world: Global Burden of Disease Study. *Lancet* 1997; **349**:1269–76.
2. Lerner DJ, Kannel WB. Patterns of coronary heart disease morbidity and mortality in the sexes: a 26-year follow-up of the Framingham population. *Am Heart J* 1986; **111**:383–90.
3. Maynard C, Litwin PE, Martin JS, Weaver WD. Gender differences in the treatment and outcome of acute myocardial infarction. Results from the Myocardial Infarction Triage and Intervention Registry. *Arch Intern Med* 1992; **152**:972–6.
4. Rosengren A, Spetz CL, Koster M, Hammar N, Alfredsson L, Rosen M. Sex differences in survival after myocardial infarction in Sweden; data from the Swedish National Acute Myocardial Infarction Register. *Eur Heart J* 2001; **22**:314–22.
5. Heer T, Schiele R, Schneider S, et al. Gender differences in acute myocardial infarction in the era of reperfusion (the MITRA registry). *Am J Cardiol* 2002; **89**:511–17.
6. Mehilli J, Kastrati A, Dirschinger J, et al. Sex-based analysis of outcome in patients with acute myocardial infarction treated predominantly with percutaneous coronary intervention. *JAMA* 2002; **287**:210–15.
7. Sans S, Kesteloot H, Kromhout D. The burden of cardiovascular diseases mortality in Europe. Task Force of the European Society of Cardiology on Cardiovascular Mortality and Morbidity Statistics in Europe. *Eur Heart J* 1997; **18**:1231–48.
8. Wilhelmsen L, Rosengren A, Johansson S, Lappas G. Coronary heart disease attack rate, incidence and mortality 1975–1994 in Goteborg, Sweden. *Eur Heart J* 1997; **18**:572–81.
9. Peltonen M, Asplund K. Age–period–cohort effects on ischaemic heart disease mortality in Sweden from 1969 to 1993, and forecasts up to 2003. *Eur Heart J* 1997; **18**:1307–12.

10. Capewell S, MacIntyre K, Stewart S, et al. Age, sex, and social trends in out-of-hospital cardiac deaths in Scotland 1986–95: a retrospective cohort study. *Lancet* 2001; **358**:1213–17.

11. Rosen M, Alfredsson L, Hammar N, Kahan T, Spetz CL, Ysberg AS. Attack rate, mortality and case fatality for acute myocardial infarction in Sweden during 1987–95. Results from the national AMI register in Sweden. *J Intern Med* 2000; **248**:159–64.

12. McGovern PG, Jacobs DR Jr, Shahar E, et al. Trends in acute coronary heart disease mortality, morbidity, and medical care from 1985 through 1997: the Minnesota heart survey. *Circulation* 2001; **104**:19–24.

13. Volmink JA, Newton JN, Hicks NR, Sleight P, Fowler GH, Neil HA. Coronary event and case fatality rates in an English population: results of the Oxford myocardial infarction incidence study. The Oxford Myocardial Infarction Incidence Study Group. *Heart* 1998; **80**:40–4.

14. Dauerman HL, Lessard D, Yarzebski J, Furman MI, Gore JM, Goldberg RJ. Ten-year trends in the incidence, treatment, and outcome of Q-wave myocardial infarction. *Am J Cardiol* 2000; **86**:730–5.

15. Goff DC Jr, Howard G, Wang CH, et al. Trends in severity of hospitalized myocardial infarction: the atherosclerosis risk in communities (ARIC) study, 1987–1994. *Am Heart J* 2000; **139**:874–80.

16. Hellermann JP, Reeder GS, Jacobsen SJ, Weston SA, Killian JM, Roger VL. Longitudinal trends in the severity of acute myocardial infarction: a population study in Olmsted County, Minnesota. *Am J Epidemiol* 2002; **156**:246–53.

17. Salomaa V, Miettinen H, Palomaki P, et al. Diagnostic features of acute myocardial infarction – changes over time from 1983 to 1990: results from the FINMON-ICA AMI Register Study. *J Intern Med* 1995; **237**:151–9.

18. Rosengren A, Thelle DS, Koster M, Rosen M. Changing sex ratio in acute coronary heart disease: data from Swedish national registers 1984–99. *J Intern Med* 2003; **253**:301–10.

19. Tunstall-Pedoe H, Vanuzzo D, Hobbs M, et al. Estimation of contribution of changes in coronary care to improving survival, event rates, and coronary heart disease mortality across the WHO MONICA Project populations. *Lancet* 2000; **355**:688–700.

20. Kuulasmaa K, Tunstall-Pedoe H, Dobson A, et al. Estimation of contribution of changes in classic risk factors to trends in coronary-event rates across the WHO MONICA Project populations. *Lancet* 2000; **355**:675–87.

21. Sempos C, Cooper R, Kovar MG, McMillen M. Divergence of the recent trends in coronary mortality for the four major race–sex groups in the United States. *Am J Public Health* 1988; **78**:1422–7.

22. Gillum RF. Trends in acute myocardial infarction and coronary heart disease death in the United States. *J Am Coll Cardiol* 1994; **23**:1273–7.

23. Salomaa V, Ketonen M, Koukkunen H, et al. Trends in coronary events in Finland during 1983–1997. The FINAMI study. *Eur Heart J* 2003; **24**:311–19.

24. Rosamond WD, Chambless LE, Folsom AR, et al. Trends in the incidence of myocardial infarction and in mortality due to coronary heart disease, 1987 to 1994. *N Engl J Med* 1998; **339**:861–7.

25. Rosamond WD, Folsom AR, Chambless LE, Wang CH. Coronary heart disease trends in four United States communities. The Atherosclerosis Risk in Communities (ARIC) study 1987–1996. *Int J Epidemiol* 2001; **30** (Suppl 1):S17–22.

26. Roger VL, Jacobsen SJ, Weston SA, et al. Trends in the incidence and survival of patients with hospitalized myocardial infarction, Olmsted County, Minnesota, 1979 to 1994. *Ann Intern Med* 2002; **136**:341–8.

27. Derby CA, Lapane KL, Feldman HA, Carleton RA. Sex-specific trends in validated coronary heart disease rates in southeastern New England, 1980–1991. *Am J Epidemiol* 2000; **151**:417–29.

28. Jousilahti P, Vartiainen E, Tuomilehto J, Pekkanen J, Puska P. Effect of risk factors and changes in risk factors on coronary mortality in three cohorts of middle-aged people in eastern Finland. *Am J Epidemiol* 1995; **141**:50–60.

29. Vartiainen E, Puska P, Pekkanen J, Tuomilehto J, Jousilahti P. Changes in risk factors explain changes in mortality from ischaemic heart disease in Finland. *BMJ* 1994; **309**:23–7.

30. Njolstad I, Arnesen E, Lund-Larsen PG. Smoking, serum lipids, blood pressure, and sex differences in myocardial infarction. A 12–year follow-up of the Finnmark Study. *Circulation* 1996; **93**:450–6.

31. Sharrett AR, Ballantyne CM, Coady SA, et al. Coronary heart disease prediction from lipoprotein cholesterol levels, triglycerides, lipoprotein(a), apolipoproteins A-I and B, and HDL density subfractions: The Atherosclerosis Risk in Communities (ARIC) Study. *Circulation* 2001; **104**:1108–13.

32. DeWood MA, Spores J, Notske R, et al. Prevalence of total coronary occlusion during the early hours of transmural myocardial infarction. *N Engl J Med* 1980; **303**:897–902.

33. Buja LM, Willerson JT. Clinicopathologic correlates of acute ischemic heart disease syndromes. *Am J Cardiol* 1981; **47**:343–56.

34. Libby P. Molecular bases of the acute coronary syndromes. *Circulation* 1995; **91**:2844–50.

35. Naghavi M, Libby P, Falk E, et al. From vulnerable plaque to vulnerable patient: a call for new definitions and risk assessment strategies: Part I. *Circulation* 2003; **108**:1664–72.

36. Arbustini E, Dal Bello B, Morbini P, et al. Plaque erosion is a major substrate for coronary thrombosis in acute myocardial infarction. *Heart* 1999; **82**:269–72.

37. Farb A, Burke AP, Tang AL, et al. Coronary plaque erosion without rupture into a lipid core. A frequent cause of coronary thrombosis in sudden coronary death. *Circulation* 1996; **93**:1354–63.

38. Mautner SL, Lin F, Mautner GC, Roberts WC. Comparison in women versus men of composition of atherosclerotic plaques in native coronary arteries and in saphenous veins used as aortocoronary conduits. *J Am Coll Cardiol* 1993; **21**:1312–18.

39. Burke AP, Farb A, Malcom G, Virmani R. Effect of menopause on plaque morphologic characteristics in coronary atherosclerosis. *Am Heart J* 2001; **141** (2 Suppl):S58–62.

40. Sheifer SE, Arora UK, Gersh BJ, Weissman NJ. Sex differences in morphology of coronary artery plaque assessed by intravascular ultrasound. *Coron Artery Dis* 2001; **12**:17–20.

41. al-Khalili F, Svane B, Di Mario C, et al. Intracoronary ultrasound measurements in women with myocardial infarction without significant coronary lesions. *Coron Artery Dis* 2000; **11**:579–84.

42. Hochman JS, McCabe CH, Stone PH, et al. Outcome and profile of women and men presenting with acute coronary syndromes: a report from TIMI IIIB. TIMI Investigators. Thrombolysis in Myocardial Infarction. *J Am Coll Cardiol* 1997; **30**:141–8.

43. Hochman JS, Tamis JE, Thompson TD, et al. Sex, clinical presentation, and outcome in patients with acute coronary syndromes. Global Use of Strategies to Open Occluded Coronary Arteries in Acute Coronary Syndromes IIb Investigators. *N Engl J Med* 1999; **341**:226–32.

44. Devon HA, Zerwic JJ. Symptoms of acute coronary syndromes: are there gender differences? A review of the literature. *Heart Lung* 2002; **31**:235–45.

45. Canto JG, Shlipak MG, Rogers WJ, et al. Prevalence, clinical characteristics, and mortality among patients with myocardial infarction presenting without chest pain. *JAMA* 2000; **283**:3223–9.

46. Pope JH, Aufderheide TP, Ruthazer R, et al. Missed diagnoses of acute cardiac ischemia in the emergency department. *N Engl J Med* 2000; **342**:1163–70.

47. Milner KA, Funk M, Arnold A, Vaccarino V. Typical symptoms are predictive of acute coronary syndromes in women. *Am Heart J* 2002; **143**:283–8.

48. Gurwitz JH, McLaughlin TJ, Willison DJ, et al. Delayed hospital presentation in patients who have had acute myocardial infarction. *Ann Intern Med* 1997; **126**:593–9.

49. Sheifer SE, Rathore SS, Gersh BJ, et al. Time to presentation with acute myocardial infarction in the elderly: associations with race, sex, and socioeconomic characteristics. *Circulation* 2000; **102**:1651–6.

50. Murabito JM, Evans JC, Larson MG, Levy D. Prognosis after the onset of coronary heart disease. An investigation of differences in outcome between the sexes according to initial coronary disease presentation. *Circulation* 1993; **88**:2548–55.

51. Jonsdottir LS, Sigfusson N, Sigvaldason H, Thorgeirsson G. Incidence and prevalence of recognised and unrecognised myocardial infarction in women. The Reykjavik Study. *Eur Heart J* 1998; **19**:1011–18.

52. Boland LL, Folsom AR, Sorlie PD, et al. Occurrence of unrecognized myocardial infarction in subjects aged 45 to 65 years (the ARIC study). *Am J Cardiol* 2002; **90**:927–31.

53. Orencia A, Bailey K, Yawn BP, Kottke TE. Effect of gender on long-term outcome of angina pectoris and myocardial infarction/sudden unexpected death. *JAMA* 1993; **269**:2392–7.

54. Rosengren A, Wallentin L, Gitt KA, Behar S, Battler A, Hasdai D. Sex, age and clinical presentation of acute coronary syndromes. *Eur Heart J* 2004; **25**:663–7.

55. Mueller C, Neumann FJ, Roskamm H, et al. Women do have an improved long-term outcome after non-ST-elevation acute coronary syndromes treated very early and predominantly with percutaneous coronary intervention: a prospective study in 1,450 consecutive patients. *J Am Coll Cardiol* 2002; **40**:245–50.

56. Johansson S, Bergstrand R, Schlossman D, Selin K, Vedin A, Wilhelmsson C. Sex differences in cardioangiographic findings after myocardial infarction. *Eur Heart J* 1984; **5**:374–81.

57. Glaser R, Herrmann HC, Murphy SA, et al. Benefit of an early invasive management strategy in women with acute coronary syndromes. *JAMA* 2002; **288**:3124–9.

58. Negus BH, Willard JE, Glamann DB, et al. Gender-related differences in coronary angiograms of young survivors of myocardial infarction. *Am J Cardiol* 1994; **74**:814–15.

59. Kilaru PK, Kelly RF, Calvin JE, Parrillo JE. Utilization of coronary angiography and revascularization after acute myocardial infarction in men and women risk stratified by the American College of Cardiology/

American Heart Association guidelines. *J Am Coll Cardiol* 2000; **35**:974–9.

60. Naylor CD, Chen E. Population-wide mortality trends among patients hospitalized for acute myocardial infarction: the Ontario experience, 1981 to 1991. *J Am Coll Cardiol* 1994; **24**:1431–8.

61. Abildstrom SZ, Rasmussen S, Rosen M, Madsen M. Trends in incidence and case fatality rates of acute myocardial infarction in Denmark and Sweden. *Heart* 2003; **89**:507–11.

62. Abrahamsson P, Dellborg M, Rosengren A, Wilhelmsen L. Improved long-term prognosis after myocardial infarction 1984–1991. *Eur Heart J* 1998; **19**:1512–17.

63. Abrahamsson P, Rosengren A, Dellborg M. Improved long-term prognosis for patients with unstable coronary syndromes 1988–1995. *Eur Heart J* 2000; **21**:533–9.

64. Gottlieb S, Goldbourt U, Boyko V, et al. Mortality trends in men and women with acute myocardial infarction in coronary care units in Israel. A comparison between 1981–1983 and 1992–1994. For the SPRINT and the Israeli Thrombolytic Survey Groups. *Eur Heart J* 2000; **21**:284–95.

65. Greenland P, Reicher-Reiss H, Goldbourt U, Behar S. In-hospital and 1-year mortality in 1,524 women after myocardial infarction. Comparison with 4,315 men. *Circulation* 1991; **83**:484–91.

66. Becker RC, Terrin M, Ross R, et al. Comparison of clinical outcomes for women and men after acute myocardial infarction. The Thrombolysis in Myocardial Infarction Investigators. *Ann Intern Med* 1994; **120**:638–45.

67. Kudenchuk PJ, Maynard C, Martin JS, Wirkus M, Weaver WD. Comparison of presentation, treatment, and outcome of acute myocardial infarction in men versus women (the Myocardial Infarction Triage and Intervention Registry). *Am J Cardiol* 1996; **78**:9–14.

68. Woodfield SL, Lundergan CF, Reiner JS, et al. Gender and acute myocardial infarction: is there a different response to thrombolysis? *J Am Coll Cardiol* 1997; **29**:35–42.

69. Gottlieb S, Harpaz D, Shotan A, et al. Sex differences in management and outcome after acute myocardial infarction in the 1990s: a prospective observational community-based study. Israeli Thrombolytic Survey Group. *Circulation* 2000; **102**:2484–90.

70. Hanratty B, Lawlor DA, Robinson MB, Sapsford RJ, Greenwood D, Hall A. Sex differences in risk factors, treatment and mortality after acute myocardial infarction: an observational study. *J Epidemiol Community Health* 2000; **54**:912–16.

71. Marrugat J, Sala J, Masia R, et al. Mortality differences between men and women following first myocardial infarction. RESCATE Investigators. Recursos Empleados en el Sindrome Coronario Agudo y Tiempo de Espera. *JAMA* 1998; **280**:1405–9.

72. Nohria A, Vaccarino V, Krumholz HM. Gender differences in mortality after myocardial infarction. Why women fare worse than men. *Cardiol Clin* 1998; **16**:45–57.

73. Bueno H, Vidan MT, Almazan A, Lopez-Sendon JL, Delcan JL. Influence of sex on the short-term outcome of elderly patients with a first acute myocardial infarction. *Circulation* 1995; **92**:1133–40.

74. Dittrich H, Gilpin E, Nicod P, Cali G, Henning H, Ross J Jr. Acute myocardial infarction in women: influence of gender on mortality and prognostic variables. *Am J Cardiol* 1988; **62**:1–7.

75. Robinson K, Conroy RM, Mulcahy R, Hickey N. Risk factors and in-hospital course of first episode of myocardial infarction or acute coronary insufficiency in women. *J Am Coll Cardiol* 1988; **11**:932–6.

76. Jenkins JS, Flaker GC, Nolte B, et al. Causes of higher in-hospital mortality in women than in men after acute myocardial infarction. *Am J Cardiol* 1994; **73**:319–22.

77. Karlson BW, Herlitz J, Hartford M. Prognosis in myocardial infarction in relation to gender. *Am Heart J* 1994; **128**:477–83.

78. Mahon NG, McKenna CJ, Codd MB, O'Rorke C, McCann HA, Sugrue DD. Gender differences in the management and outcome of acute myocardial infarction in unselected patients in the thrombolytic era. *Am J Cardiol* 2000; **85**:921–6.

79. Coronado BE, Griffith JL, Beshansky JR, Selker HP. Hospital mortality in women and men with acute cardiac ischemia: a prospective multicenter study. *J Am Coll Cardiol* 1997; **29**:1490–6.

80. Malacrida R, Genoni M, Maggioni AP, et al. A comparison of the early outcome of acute myocardial infarction in women and men. The Third International Study of Infarct Survival Collaborative Group. *N Engl J Med* 1998; **338**:8–14.

81. Herman B, Greiser E, Pohlabeln H. A sex difference in short-term survival after initial acute myocardial infarction. The MONICA-Bremen Acute Myocardial Infarction Register, 1985–1990. *Eur Heart J* 1997; **18**:963–70.

82. Hasdai D, Porter A, Rosengren A, Behar S, Boyko V, Battler A. Effect of gender on outcomes of acute coronary syndromes. *Am J Cardiol* 2003; **91**:1466–9, A6.

83. Fiebach NH, Viscoli CM, Horwitz RI. Differences between women and men in survival after myocardial

infarction. Biology or methodology? *JAMA* 1990; **263**:1092–6.

84. Vaccarino V, Parsons L, Every NR, Barron HV, Krumholz HM. Sex-based differences in early mortality after myocardial infarction. National Registry of Myocardial Infarction 2 Participants. *N Engl J Med* 1999; **341**:217–25.

85. MacIntyre K, Stewart S, Capewell S, et al. Gender and survival: a population-based study of 201,114 men and women following a first acute myocardial infarction. *J Am Coll Cardiol* 2001; **38**:729–35.

86. Demirovic J, Blackburn H, McGovern PG, Luepker R, Sprafka JM, Gilbertson D. Sex differences in early mortality after acute myocardial infarction (the Minnesota Heart Survey). *Am J Cardiol* 1995; **75**:1096–101.

87. Tunstall-Pedoe H, Morrison C, Woodward M, Fitzpatrick B, Watt G. Sex differences in myocardial infarction and coronary deaths in the Scottish MONICA population of Glasgow 1985 to 1991. Presentation, diagnosis, treatment, and 28-day case fatality of 3991 events in men and 1551 events in women. *Circulation* 1996; **93**:1981–92.

88. White AD, Rosamond WD, Chambless LE, et al. Sex and race differences in short-term prognosis after acute coronary heart disease events: the Atherosclerosis Risk In Communities (ARIC) study. *Am Heart J* 1999; **138**:540–8.

89. Sonke GS, Beaglehole R, Stewart AW, Jackson R, Stewart FM. Sex differences in case fatality before and after admission to hospital after acute cardiac events: analysis of community based coronary heart disease register. *BMJ* 1996; **313**:853–5.

90. Vaccarino V, Berkman LF, Krumholz HM. Long-term outcome of myocardial infarction in women and men: a population perspective. *Am J Epidemiol* 2000; **152**:965–73.

91. Van de Werf F, Ardissino D, Betriu A, et al. Management of acute myocardial infarction in patients presenting with ST-segment elevation. The Task Force on the Management of Acute Myocardial Infarction of the European Society of Cardiology. *Eur Heart J* 2003; **24**:28–66.

92. Yarzebski J, Col N, Pagley P, Savageau J, Gore J, Goldberg R. Gender differences and factors associated with the receipt of thrombolytic therapy in patients with acute myocardial infarction: a community-wide perspective. *Am Heart J* 1996; **131**:43–50.

93. Johanson P, Abrahamsson P, Rosengren A, Dellborg M. Time-trends in thrombolytics: women are catching up. *Scand Cardiovasc J* 1999; **33**:39–43.

94. Maynard C, Althouse R, Cerqueira M, Olsufka M, Kennedy JW. Underutilization of thrombolytic therapy in eligible women with acute myocardial infarction. *Am J Cardiol* 1991; **68**:529–30.

95. Clarke KW, Gray D, Keating NA, Hampton JR. Do women with acute myocardial infarction receive the same treatment as men? *BMJ* 1994; **309**:563–6.

96. Maynard C, Beshansky JR, Griffith JL, Selker HP. Influence of sex on the use of cardiac procedures in patients presenting to the emergency department. A prospective multicenter study. *Circulation* 1996; **94** (9 Suppl):II93–8.

97. Canto JG, Allison JJ, Kiefe CI, et al. Relation of race and sex to the use of reperfusion therapy in Medicare beneficiaries with acute myocardial infarction. *N Engl J Med* 2000; **342**:1094–100.

98. Barron HV, Bowlby LJ, Breen T, et al. Use of reperfusion therapy for acute myocardial infarction in the United States: data from the National Registry of Myocardial Infarction 2. *Circulation* 1998; **97**:1150–6.

99. Grace SL, Abbey SE, Bisaillon S, Shnek ZM, Irvine J, Stewart DE. Presentation, delay, and contraindication to thrombolytic treatment in females and males with myocardial infarction. *Womens Health Issues* 2003; **13**:214–21.

100. Kaplan KL, Fitzpatrick P, Cox C, Shammas NW, Marder VJ. Use of thrombolytic therapy for acute myocardial infarction: effects of gender and age on treatment rates. *J Thromb Thrombolysis* 2002; **13**:21–6.

101. Eysmann SB, Douglas PS. Reperfusion and revascularization strategies for coronary artery disease in women. *JAMA* 1992; **268**:1903–7.

102. Lincoff AM, Califf RM, Ellis SG, et al. Thrombolytic therapy for women with myocardial infarction: is there a gender gap? Thrombolysis and Angioplasty in Myocardial Infarction Study Group. *J Am Coll Cardiol* 1993; **22**:1780–7.

103. Karnash SL, Granger CB, White HD, Woodlief LH, Topol EJ, Califf RM. Treating menstruating women with thrombolytic therapy: insights from the global utilization of streptokinase and tissue plasminogen activator for occluded coronary arteries (GUSTO-I) trial. *J Am Coll Cardiol* 1995; **26**:1651–6.

104. White HD, Barbash GI, Modan M, et al. After correcting for worse baseline characteristics, women treated with thrombolytic therapy for acute myocardial infarction have the same mortality and morbidity as men except for a higher incidence of hemorrhagic stroke. The Investigators of the International Tissue Plasminogen Activator/Streptokinase Mortality Study. *Circulation* 1993; **88**:2097–103.

105. Gurwitz JH, Gore JM, Goldberg RJ, et al. Risk for intracranial hemorrhage after tissue plasminogen activator treatment for acute myocardial infarction. Participants in the National Registry of Myocardial Infarction 2. *Ann Intern Med* 1998; **129**:597–604.

106. Vacek JL, Rosamond TL, Kramer PH, et al. Sex-related differences in patients undergoing direct angioplasty for acute myocardial infarction. *Am Heart J* 1993; **126**:521–5.

107. Stone GW, Grines CL, Browne KF, et al. Comparison of in-hospital outcome in men versus women treated by either thrombolytic therapy or primary coronary angioplasty for acute myocardial infarction. *Am J Cardiol* 1995; **75**:987–92.

108. Antoniucci D, Valenti R, Moschi G, et al. Sex-based differences in clinical and angiographic outcomes after primary angioplasty or stenting for acute myocardial infarction. *Am J Cardiol* 2001; **87**:289–93.

109. Tamis-Holland JE, Palazzo A, Stebbins AL, et al. Benefits of direct angioplasty for women and men with acute myocardial infarction: results of the Global Use of Strategies to Open Occluded Arteries in Acute Coronary Syndromes Angioplasty (GUSTO II-B) Angioplasty Substudy. *Am Heart J* 2004; **147**:133–9.

110. Vakili BA, Kaplan RC, Brown DL. Sex-based differences in early mortality of patients undergoing primary angioplasty for first acute myocardial infarction. *Circulation* 2001; **104**:3034–8.

111. Bertrand ME, Simoons ML, Fox KA, et al. Management of acute coronary syndromes in patients presenting without persistent ST-segment elevation. *Eur Heart J* 2002; **23**:1809–40.

112. Wallentin L, Lagerqvist B, Husted S, Kontny F, Stahle E, Swahn E. Outcome at 1 year after an invasive compared with a non-invasive strategy in unstable coronary-artery disease: the FRISC II invasive randomised trial. FRISC II Investigators. Fast Revascularisation during Instability in Coronary artery disease. *Lancet* 2000; **356**:9–16.

113. Lagerqvist B, Safstrom K, Stahle E, Wallentin L, Swahn E. Is early invasive treatment of unstable coronary artery disease equally effective for both women and men? FRISC II Study Group Investigators. *J Am Coll Cardiol* 2001; **38**:41–8.

114. Mehilli J, Kastrati A, Bollwein H, et al. Gender and restenosis after coronary artery stenting. *Eur Heart J* 2003; **24**:1523–30.

18

Acute coronary syndromes

Douglas C. Morris

Introduction

Acute coronary syndromes (ACS) include unstable angina, non-Q-wave myocardial infarction (MI), Q-wave MI, and sudden cardiac death. While these conditions are somewhat arbitrarily differentiated into distinct clinical entities (i.e. the presence or absence of specific cardiac markers distinguish unstable angina from a non-Q-wave MI), in a pathophysiologic sense they are very much the same process. The signal event in the vast majority of ACS (70–80%) is the fissuring or rupture of a coronary plaque. The disruption-prone plaque in the coronary artery is typically a modestly stenotic, lipid-laden plaque with a thin fibrous cap. The plaque disruption sets off a cascade of reactions that culminates in thrombus formation. The thrombus, in turn, compromises to various degrees the lumen of the coronary artery. The culmination of this event depends upon the size and stability of the thrombus, the speed and strength of the body's inherent thrombolytic action, and the adequacy of collateral flow to the region of myocardium served by the vessel in question. In a minority of patients with an ACS, there is no plaque disruption but only a superficial erosion of a markedly stenotic and fibrotic plaque. Thrombus formation in such cases may be triggered by systemic factors, such as smoking, cocaine, or diabetes, especially in patients whose diabetes is poorly controlled.[1]

Prevalence of ACS

Unstable angina is the most likely consequence of plaque rupture. Approximately 1.4 million patients are hospitalized annually in the US with a non-ST-segment elevation ACS. The majority of these patients present with unstable angina.[2] The estimated number of yearly admissions for acute ST-segment elevation MIs is 350 000. Fifty percent of patients with an acute MI are assumed to die suddenly before their arrival at the hospital.

Initial classification of ACS

The initial classification and treatment of ACS is predicated upon the presence or absence of ST-segment elevation on the 12-lead electrocardiogram (ECG). ST-segment elevation ACS typically reflect complete and persistent occlusion of a coronary artery. Total occlusion of a coronary artery immediately provokes myocardial necrosis which progresses inexorably across the myocardium in a 'wavefront' or, perhaps a better analogy, in a forest-fire type of pattern from the subendocardial to the subepicardial region.[3] Non-ST-segment elevation ACS are generally characterized by subtotal coronary occlusion or transient complete occlusion with spontaneous lysis of the occluding thrombus or embolization of a

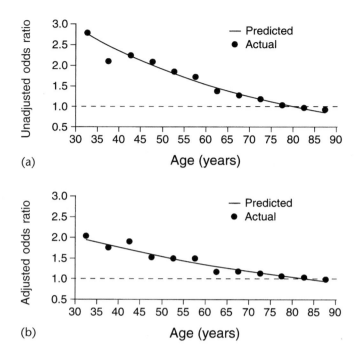

(a)

(b)

Figure 18.1
Odds ratio for death during hospitalization for myocardial infarction in women as compared with men according to age. The unadjusted odds ratios (a) were derived from the model that included sex, age, the interaction between sex and age, and the year of discharge. The adjusted odds ratios (b) were derived from the model that also included race, insurance status, medical history, and severity of clinical abnormalities at admission, type of management in the first 24 hours after admission, and time to presentation. Reproduced from reference 5 with permission from Massachusetts Medical Society.

portion of the atherosclerotic plaque. The embolus generally comprises microparticulate atheromatous material and may contain platelet thrombi. Microvascular obstruction may be a sequela of this embolization.

Gender differences in ACS

Women with an ACS are older and have significantly higher rates of diabetes, hypertension, and prior congestive heart failure.[4] Data from one registry suggested that diabetes is more common only in the younger woman with coronary atherosclerotic heart disease (less than 65 years).[5] Women also have significantly lower rates of prior MI and are less likely to have smoked. Besides these differences in risk factors and co-morbid conditions, there are notable gender differences in the presentation of ACS. The ECG remains the cornerstone for the early diagnosis of acute myocardial ischemia in both sexes. ST-segment changes appear within seconds of the ischemic insult in approximately 60%

of patients. Women are significantly less likely to present with an ST-segment elevation MI than men but are more likely to present with unstable angina. Furthermore, among patients with a definite MI, women are less likely than men to have a Q-wave infarction. ST-segment depression is prognostically important for both women and men. T-wave inversion without elevation of biochemical markers is more common in women. This ECG finding is known to be less specific for coronary atherosclerotic heart disease. The ECG is inconclusive in approximately 40% of all patients and even more commonly nondiagnostic in women.[6] Women with unstable angina have higher rates of angiographically insignificant stenoses (30.5% vs 13.9%).[4] The follow-up event rate in women with non-ST-segment elevation MI and unstable angina is no worse than for men. The risk for early death following an ST-segment elevation MI is higher in women, but this difference decreases with increasing age. Among women less than 50 years of age the early mortality rate (in-hospital) is more than twice that for men but by age 75 the gender difference is insignificant (Fig. 18.1).[5]

Therapy of ACS (see also Chapter 17)

The primary goal of therapy in the ST-segment elevation MI is the rapid restoration of blood flow through the occluded coronary artery in order to halt the progression of necrosis and thereby salvage left ventricular myocardium, limit the infarct size, and improve survival. Conversely, the primary goal of therapy in the patient with the nonocclusive thrombus is to maintain coronary blood flow by preventing or limiting further thrombus formation. Therapy in this heterogeneous group is also directed towards reduction in myocardial ischemia by reducing myocardial oxygen demand and improving coronary blood flow either via collateral vessels or by improved patency of the culprit vessel.

ST-segment elevation ACS

Reperfusion therapy directed at the occluded infarct-related artery is the cornerstone of therapy for the ST-segment elevation MI. While not universally applicable, this therapy should be entertained in every patient with an ST-segment elevation MI. If such an approach seems ill-advised or contraindicated, the reasons should be documented in the medical record. Unfortunately, the available evidence suggests that approximately one-third of patients who are eligible for reperfusion are not offered this therapy.[7] Women are less likely to receive reperfusion therapy than men (odds ratio = 0.88; 95% confidence interval (CI) = 0.83–0.92).[7] This difference does not necessarily represent a gender bias, as patients who have diabetes, those who present later, and those older than 75 years of age also were less likely to receive reperfusion therapy. All of these characteristics are more often seen in the female patient.

The megatrials of thrombolytic therapy have consistently demonstrated a marked improvement in survival with this therapy – 28.4% mortality reduction in ASSET,[8] 49.4% in AIMS,[9] 22.6% in GISSI,[10] and 29.8% in ISIS-2.[11] The Fibrinolytic Therapy Trialists collaborative group performed a comprehensive overview of nine trials of thrombolytic therapy and found an 18% reduction in short-term mortality. The subset of 45 000 patients

with ST-segment elevation or bundle branch block had an even more impressive 25% reduction.[12]

The success of the reperfusion therapy is tied to the adequacy of the restored blood flow, the temporal delay encountered in restoring flow, and the permanence of the patency. The importance of the adequacy of coronary blood flow is established in the Global Use of Strategies to Open Occluded Coronary Arteries (GUSTO)-I angiographic substudy. Following thrombolytic therapy, the 30-day mortality rate was 4.4% in patients with normal flow in the infarct-related artery, 7.4% in the patients who had slow flow, and 8.9% in patients with no flow.[13] Those patients with higher Thrombolysis in MI (TIMI) flow grades 90 minutes after receiving a thrombolytic agent had better ventricular function and regional wall motion in the regions supplied by the infarct-related artery. The critical significance of the temporal delay in treatment is demonstrated in the analysis of the 58 600 patients in the Fibrinolytic Therapy Trial. The maximal effectiveness of fibrinolytic therapy was achieved when therapy was initiated in the first hour following symptom onset (65 lives saved/1000 treated patients). The survival benefit of therapy administered in the subsequent hour was reduced by 50% (37 lives saved/1000 treated patients). Furthermore, only 10 lives per 1000 patients were saved in those treated between 6 and 12 hours.[14] Additional evidence for the benefit of early reperfusion is provided by the Seattle prehospital fibrinolysis trial (MITI) which demonstrated a sevenfold reduction in mortality rate in patients treated before 70 minutes after symptom onset as compared with patients treated later.[15] Recognition of the critical importance that the first hour plays in the beneficial impact of fibrinolytic treatment is underscored by the 'golden hour' metaphor.

Bleeding, particularly intracranial hemorrhage, is the most feared complication of this therapy and the threat responsible for most of the failure to treat. The pooled data from the ECSG, GISSI, TAMI, TIMI, and ISAM investigators suggest an overall incidence of intracranial hemorrhage of 0.75%. The following four clinical variables are, however, associated with an increased risk of intracranial hemorrhage: age older than 65 years, weight less than 70 kg, hypertension on admission, and the use of tissue plasminogen activator (t-PA) rather than streptokinase. Women are more likely to fulfill the first two criteria and, therefore, more prone to develop intracranial hemorrhage with thrombolytic therapy. The risk of intracranial hemorrhage can be predicted based upon the number of risk factors present (no risk factors yields an incidence of 0.26%, one risk factor yields 0.96%, two risk factors yields 1.32%, and three risk factors yields 2.17%).[16]

The limitations posed by thrombolytic therapy are the inability to restore normal coronary flow in 40–50% of patients (TIMI-3 flow restored in 54% with accelerated tPA in GUSTO-I), the occurrence of reocclusion leading to recurrent MI in 5–15% of patients, a 1–2% risk of intracranial hemorrhage with a 40% mortality and a contraindication to thrombolysis in 15–20% of the patients.[17] While not universally available, primary angioplasty has been demonstrated to confer benefits in terms of restoring normal coronary flow (more than 90% vs 54%), saving more lives (20–30 fewer deaths out of 1000 patients treated or a 34% reduction in mortality), less reocclusion (a 47% reduction in nonfatal reinfarction), and causing fewer strokes (10 per 1000 patients treated).[18–21] While PCI is clearly superior to thrombolytics at all time points following an acute ST-segment MI, thrombolytics are, nevertheless, extremely effective in the first hour after the onset of the infarction (the 'golden hour'). The relative benefits of PCI as compared with thrombolysis persist in all clinically important subgroups, including women. The absolute benefits of PCI are greater in proportion to baseline risk, such as in the elderly, diabetics, patients with prior infarction, acute anterior infarction, or patients who receive treatment later after the onset of symptoms.[22] Attempts to enhance the efficacy of thrombolytics by employing more potent or higher-dose agents or augmenting the thrombolytic with an antithrombotic agent have been hampered by an increased risk of intracranial bleeding.

Non-ST-segment ACS

The use of anticoagulant and antiplatelet agents is the mainstay of therapy in these patients, most of whom have developed a nonocclusive thrombus in the infarct-related artery. The primary aims of therapy are to prevent progression of a subtotal coronary thrombus to a total coronary occlusion, alleviate myocardial ischemia, and promote stabilization of the atherosclerotic plaque. Due to their paradoxical prothrombotic potential, thrombolytic agents are not appropriate therapy in non-ST-segment elevation ACS.

Aspirin is the standard antiplatelet therapy used in patients with an ACS. Aspirin inhibits platelet cyclooxygenase by irreversible acetylation, thereby preventing the formation of thromboxane A2, one of the agonists of platelet activation. The use of aspirin is predicated upon the repeated demonstration of a reduction of death or MI in the patient with unstable angina given aspirin for various time intervals (Table 18.1).[23–28] The Antithrombotic Trialists' Collaboration overview noted a 46% reduction in vascular events (8.0% vs 13.3%, p <0.0001) in the unstable angina patients treated with aspirin.[27] Women seem to derive as much benefit as men in trials involving patients at high risk of vascular events.[29] The unresolved issue in these studies is the length of time that the antiplatelet therapy should be continued. There is a rationale for long-term antiplatelet therapy following an episode of acute myocardial ischemia based upon an event rate of approximately 6–8% per year over a 2-year follow-up.[30] In addition, angioscopic studies have shown that coronary thrombi may still be present for up to 30 days following an acute coronary event despite the use of antithrombotic agents.[31] A longer duration of therapy may, therefore, be required to allow for passivation or stabilization of the culprit lesion. Despite the use of aspirin, the risk of subsequent vascular events persists (5–10% in the first week and approximately 20% at 40 days).[32]

Ticlopidine and clopidogrel effectively inhibit platelet aggregation by antagonizing the platelet ADP receptor. While they are both clinically effective, the use of ticlopidine is limited by its potential to cause severe neutropenia and thrombocytopenia. The effectiveness of clopidogrel in reducing ischemic events in patients with atherosclerotic disease was first demonstrated in the Clopidogrel versus Aspirin in Patients at Risk of Ischemic Events (CAPRIE) trial.[33] While this trial found that clopidogrel was more effective than aspirin (8.7% relative reduction in comparison with aspirin), a greater benefit is offered by the joint administration of the two drugs. The enhanced

Table 18.1 Randomized trials of acetylsalicylic acid in unstable angina[28]

Trial (ref.)	Treatment	Follow-up	Aspirin	Control	Relative risk reduction	p Value
Veterans Affairs Study, 1983[23]	ASA 325 mg daily vs placebo	3 months	311/625 (5.0%)	65/641 (10.1%)	41%	0.004
Canadian Study, 1985[24]*	ASA 325 mg 4 times daily or control	18 months (mean)	29/276 (10.5%)	41/279 (14.6%)	30%*	0.072
Montreal Heart Study, 1988[25]	ASA 650 mg first dose then 325 mg twice daily for 6 days or placebo	6 days	6/243 (2.5%)	15/236 (6.4%)	63%	0.04
RISC, 1990[26]	ASA 75 mg for 3 months or placebo	13 months	26/399 (6.5%)	68/397 (17%)	64%	0.0001
Antithrombotic Trialists' Collaboration Meta-analysis[27]†	Various regimens vs placebo/untreated control	Various	8.0%	13.3%	46%	<0.0001

ASA, acetylsalicylic acid; RISC, Research on InStability in Coronary artery disease.
*Intention to treat analysis is presented. Mortality alone was reduced by 43%, p = 0.035.
†Endpoint reported is vascular death, myocardial infarction, or stroke.
Reproduced from reference 28 with permission from Elsevier.

benefit of combination therapy was established in the Clopidogrel in Unstable angina Recurrent Events (CURE) trial. This study demonstrated a 20% relative risk reduction in the composite endpoint of myocardial, stroke, or cardiovascular death (9.3% vs 11.4%; p = 0.00009).[34] In both the CURE and CREDO trials, the CI for the female subgroup results crosses unity. Neither of these studies, however, is adequately powered for gender subgroup analysis. Furthermore, the reductions were consistently noted in all components of the composite endpoint. The benefit of clopidogrel became apparent as early as 2 hours after administration of a 300-mg loading dose. The drug also afforded a significant incremental reduction of 18% in the composite endpoint between 1 month and 1 year. When the CURE results were stratified according to the TIMI risk score, the greatest absolute benefit was observed in the high-risk patients.[34] These data would argue for the immediate administration of clopidogrel in the patient with an ACS and continuation of this therapy for at least 1 year. The argument against its immediate administration is that the use of glycoprotein IIb/IIIa (GPIIb/IIIa) inhibitors is probably equally effective early after an ischemic event

coupled with a trend toward an increase in major bleeding in patients receiving clopidogrel immediately prior to coronary artery bypass graft (CABG) surgery.[28] The immediate use of clopidogrel prior to cardiac catheterization would render urgent surgery more risky.

Unfractionated heparin is the standard anticoagulant in the treatment of the ACS but the data supporting its use are not convincing without the concomitant use of aspirin. Even the combination of agents is not completely effective. Those patients in the recent ACS trials treated with unfractionated heparin and aspirin alone had a 30-day MI and death rate of 7.7–15.7%.[35]

The options available for further reduction in event rates are the replacement of unfractionated heparin with low-molecular-weight heparin or the addition of a GPIIb/IIIa inhibitor to the heparin and aspirin combination. Low-molecular-weight heparin provides several clinical advantages over unfractionated heparin, namely, a more predictable anticoagulant effect, a longer plasma half-life, subcutaneous administration in fixed doses without monitoring of the partial thromboplastin time (PTT), and a lower incidence of side effects including heparin-induced thrombocytopenia. The clinical superiority of enoxaparin in the management of non-ST-segment elevation ACS has been suggested by two major double-blinded, randomized, placebo-controlled trials – The Efficacy and Safety of Subcutaneous Enoxaparin in Non-Q-wave Coronary Events (ESSENCE) and the phase IIb Thrombolysis in Myocardial Infarction (TIMI-IIB). A prospectively planned meta-analysis of these two studies found a significant reduction in the composite endpoint of death or MI with enoxaparin compared with unfractionated heparin at 43 days (7.1% vs 8.6%; p = 0.02). If angina leading to urgent revascularization was included as part of the composite endpoint (admittedly a soft endpoint), event rates were 15.6% versus 18.8%, respectively (p = 0.0005). The variability in PTT levels associated with unfractionated heparin suggests that the better outcomes seen with enoxaparin may lie with more predictable anticoagulation.[36] While enoxaparin was significantly more effective than unfractionated heparin in several subgroups (for example, age >65, long-term aspirin use) there was no subgroup analysis based on gender reported. A cautionary note before completely accepting the premise that low-molecular-weight heparins are preferable in non-ST-segment elevation ACS is the failure of two large trials (FRIC and FRAXIS) to show a benefit of other low-molecular-weight heparins (admittedly different agents than enoxaparin) over unfractionated heparin (Fig. 18.2).[36] Enoxaparin does provide effective anticoagulation comparable to unfractionated heparin during PCI, as demonstrated in the NICE-1 and NICE-4 study groups.[39]

The addition of a GPIIb/IIIa inhibitor to heparin and aspirin has been demonstrated in a pooled analysis of the PRISM-PLUS, PURSUIT, and CAPTURE trials to provide a 34% relative reduction in death or MI rate during 24–48 hours of medical management.[40] A gender difference in platelet response and reactivity has been suggested, including a greater sensitivity of the platelets of women to aggregating stimuli. Women might derive a greater benefit from a platelet inhibitor because of this enhanced platelet reactivity. The clinical trials have been somewhat inconsistent in this regard. The pooled analysis of the EPIC, EPILOG, and

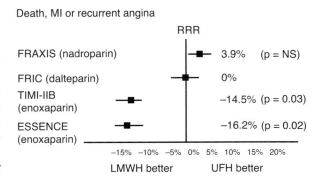

Death, MI or recurrent angina

Figure 18.2
Meta-analysis of low-molecular-weight heparin (LMWH) trials in unstable angina/non-ST-segment elevation myocardial infarction (MI). ESSENCE, Efficacy and Safety of Subcutaneous Enoxaparin in Non-Q-wave Coronary Events; FRAXIS, FRAXiparine in Ischemic Syndromes; FRIC, Fragmin In unstable Coronary artery disease; RRR, relative risk ratio; TIMI, Thrombolysis In Myocardial Infarction; UFH, unfractionated heparin. Adapted from reference 38 with permission from Thieme Publishers, 2004.

EPISTENT trials demonstrated equivalent treatment benefit from abciximab in women and men.[41] Likewise, the ESPRIT study established that eptifibatide offered similar protection among women and men. Data from the PURSUIT trial suggested that eptifibatide treatment provided less protection and greater bleeding risk in women.[42] In contrast to the pooled analysis of the PRISM-PLUS, PURSUIT and CAPTURE trials, the GUSTO-IV ACS trial found that abciximab afforded no benefit to those patients with ACS who were treated conservatively. This discrepancy is perhaps related to suboptimal platelet inhibition with abciximab either due to inadequate initial dosing or an inadequate infusion rate resulting in declining serum concentrations. A more substantial benefit seems to be provided by coupling glycoprotein IIb/IIIa inhibition therapy with early PCI. The relative risk reduction in the 30-day death or MI rate in patients undergoing early PCI in the PURSUIT, PARAGON B, and PRISM-PLUS trials was 31%, 35%, and 42%, respectively, as compared with 6%, 7%, and 12% reductions in patients not undergoing PCI.[43] The small-molecule GPIIb/IIIa inhibitors are the only ones recommended by the American College of Cardiology (ACC)/American Heart Association (AHA) guidelines for 'upstream use' in non-ST-segment elevation ACS.[40]

Data from the CRUSADE (Can Rapid Risk Stratification of Unstable Angina Patients Suppress Adverse Outcomes with Early Implementation of the American College of Cardiology/American Heart Association Guidelines) National Quality Improvement Initiative were examined for sex differences in the treatment and outcomes of patients with non-ST-segment ACS. Despite presenting with higher risk characteristics and having higher unadjusted in-hospital risks for death, reinfarction, heart failure, stroke and transfusion, women were treated less aggressively than men. They were less likely to receive acute heparin, ACE inhibitors, and glycoprotein IIb/IIIa inhibitors and were less likely to receive aspirin, ACE inhibitors and statins at discharge.[44]

Targeting adjunctive therapy in ACS

The most efficacious application of these GPIIb/IIIa agents is not only as 'upstream therapy' prior to PCI but to also target their use for select subsets of patients. The group which has been repeatedly shown to benefit the most from either GPIIb/IIIa inhibitors or low-molecular-weight heparin are those patients who present with an elevated troponin (>0.1 ng/ml). Patients with non-ST-segment elevation ACS who are troponin-positive at admission are at the highest risk of in-hospital death and MI. Furthermore, angiographic studies show that these patients are more likely to have an active plaque with thrombus in the culprit vessel.[45] In the CAPTURE study, which randomized patients with refractory angina prior to angioplasty to abciximab or placebo, those patients with a positive troponin-T demonstrated a beneficial effect of GPIIb/IIIa inhibition, while those who were troponin-T-negative had no treatment effect. Likewise, a retrospective analysis of the patients enrolled in the PRISM study revealed that those patients given tirofiban and aspirin who were troponin-positive had fewer ischemic events than those who were given heparin and aspirin.

Those patients who were troponin-negative had no treatment effect. In the PARAGON-B study the treatment benefit of adding a GPIIb/IIIa inhibitor to aspirin and intravenous heparin was limited almost exclusively to the troponin-positive patients.[45] Other markers of high risk include age over 65 years, diabetes, ST-segment deviation on the presenting ECG, and chronic aspirin therapy.[46] In the TIMI-II registry, ST-segment deviation of at least 0.5 mm was an independent predictor of death or MI at 1 year. A retrospective analysis of the patients enrolled in GUSTO II confirmed that a poorer prognosis was associated with ST-segment depression.[47] New or presumably new T-wave inversion on admission ECGs did not confer increased risk compared with no ECG changes in the TIMI-III registry. Holmvang and associates in the TRIM substudy found an independent risk for subsequent MI or death in patients with unstable angina and T-wave inversions in five or more leads.[48]

Recent studies have explored the possibility that plasma markers of inflammation may serve as predictors of increased cardiovascular risk. Most of the attention has focused on C-reactive protein (CRP). Liuzzo and associates found that patients with unstable angina with CRP levels >3 mg/l had a higher rate of death, MI, and need for revascularization than those with lower CRP levels.[49] CRP has also been shown to be predictive of future adverse events even in patients with a negative troponin-T. The CRP levels do not change after angioplasty in patients with normal pre-procedural levels, but they increase after angioplasty in unstable patients with elevated baseline CRP.[50]

Other novel inflammatory markers which have been suggested to have cardiovascular risk prediction include myeloperoxidase, pregnancy-associated plasma protein A, and interleukin-6. The clinical applicability of any of these markers depends upon its ability to independently predict risk beyond conventional tools, its susceptibility to be reduced by specific therapies, and the cardiovascular consequences of the marker being reduced. Of all the inflammatory markers, CRP comes the closest to meeting these requirements.[50] The appropriate level for defining a high CRP remains undefined.

The investigators in the CAPTURE trial used a threshold of 10 mg/l while most studies have settled

Table 18.2 The TIMI risk score for UA/NSTEMI[51]

Characteristics	Points
Historical	
Age ≥65 years	1
≥3 risk factors for CAD	1
Known CAD (stenosis ≥50%)	1
Aspirin use in past 7 days	1
Presentation	
Recent (≤24 h) severe angina	1
ST-segment deviation ≥0.5 mm	1
↑Cardiac markers	1
Risk score = total points	(0–7)

CAD, coronary artery disease; NSTEMI, non-ST-segment elevation myocardial infarction; TIMI, Thrombolysis In Myocardial Infarction; UA, unstable angina.
Reproduced from reference 51 with permission from Elsevier.

upon a cut-off of 3 mg/l. A simple risk score (TIMI risk score) has also been derived to use as a prognostication scheme to determine a patient's risk of death and ischemic events (Table 18.2).[51] In the test cohort, the ischemic event rates rose precipitously as the risk score increased as follows: 4.7% for a score of 0/1, 8.3% for a score of 2, 13.2% for a score of 3, 19.9% for a score of 5, and 40.9% for a score of 6/7 (Fig. 18.3).[52] Rather than trying to remember a particular risk score, a logical approach to the use of more aggressive therapy (low-molecular-weight heparin or GPIIb/IIIa inhibitors) would be to reserve it for two particular groups of patients. The first is patients at higher risk of recurrent ischemia, namely, troponin-positive, angina-associated ST-segment deviation or diffuse T-wave inversion, or those with prior aspirin use. The second is patients in whom a recurrent ischemic event might more likely prove to be fatal, namely, the elderly, the diabetic, those with a previous Q-wave infarction, or those whose angina was associated with either heart failure or hypotension.

Abciximab and the small-molecule GPIIb/IIIa inhibitors have been found to be equally efficacious in women and men. In these studies the women were older and had more co-morbidities, but no gender

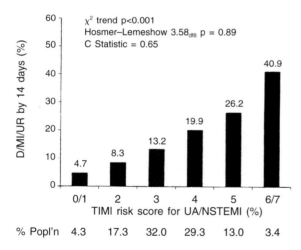

Figure 18.3
Rates of all-cause mortality (D), myocardial infarctions (MI), and severe recurrent ischemia leading to urgent revascularization (UR) through 14 days among patients randomized to unfractionated heparin in the Thrombolysis In Myocardial Infarction (TIMI) IIB trial, with patients stratified by the TIMI risk score. NSTEMI, non-ST-segment elevation myocardial infarction; % Popl'n, percent of overall trial population with that TIMI risk score; UA, unstable angina. Adapted from reference 52.

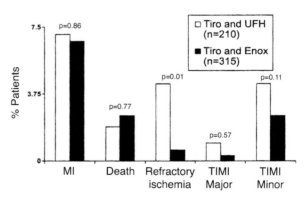

Figure 18.4
Clinical event rates in the ACUTE II trial. ACUTE, Antithrombotic Combination Using Tirofiban and Enoxaparin; enox, enoxaparin; MI, myocardial infarction; TIMI, Thrombolysis In Myocardial Infarction; tiro, tirofiban. Reproduced from reference 53 with permission from Lippincott, Williams and Wilkins.

differences were noted in the clinical outcome for PCI. The women did, however, experience more bleeding problems.[41,42]

The assumption might be that a combination of enoxaparin and GPIIb/IIIa inhibitors would be the most effective therapy for non-ST-segment elevation ACS. Such an approach has been investigated, but only to a limited degree. The Antithrombotic Combination Using Tirofiban and Enoxaparin (ACUTE II) trial found no difference in clinical events and bleeding between the group receiving enoxaparin and the one receiving unfractionated heparin (Fig. 18.4).[53]

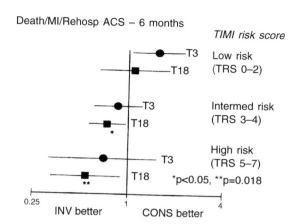

Death/MI/Rehosp ACS – 6 months

Figure 18.5
Comparison of event rates in the Thrombolysis In Myocardial Infarction (TIMI) IIIB versus Treat Angina with Aggrastat and determine Cost of Therapy with an Invasive or Conservative Strategy (TACTICS) TIMI-18 trials stratified by TIMI risk score (TRS). ACS, acute coronary syndromes; CONS, conservative; Intermed, intermediate; INV, invasive; MI, myocardial infarction; Rehosp, rehospitalization. Reproduced from reference 57 with permission from Lippincott, Williams and Wilkins.

Interventional versus conservative treatment for patients with non-ST-elevation ACS (see also Chapter 17)

Once the patient has been risk stratified and administered the appropriate anticoagulant and antiplatelet agents, the therapy to follow has been somewhat contentious. The AHA/ACC guidelines endorse an invasive strategy for patients at high risk, but allow that either an invasive strategy or a conservative strategy is appropriate for patients at moderate or low risk. The initial trials (VANQWISH and TIMI IIIB) found no clinical advantage of an interventional strategy (angiography-driven) over a conservative strategy (ischemia-driven or symptom-driven).[54,55] This lack of benefit in TIMI IIIB applied to women as well as the total group. The subsequent FRISC II study, however, demonstrated a 21% relative reduction in the 6-month MI and death rate with the interventional approach.[56] This benefit of the invasive approach was not, however, evident in the women. The most recent trials in this regard, the TACTICS TIMI-18 and RITA 3, confirmed and extended the results of FRISC II. TACTICS TIMI-18 demonstrated a superior outcome using the invasive strategy in the intermediate-risk and high-risk patients. The latter group demonstrated an impressive 10% absolute reduction in ischemic events (Fig. 18.5).[57] In this study, the benefit of the invasive approach was similar in women and men but the benefit in women was primarily confined to women with markers of increased risk. Among the risk markers, troponin-T had a greater predictive value

for benefit than ST-segment changes or TIMI risk score.[58] At 4 months in RITA 3, 9.6% of the patients in the intervention group and 14.5% in the conservative group (p = 0.001) had died, sustained an MI, or experienced refractory angina. This difference was primarily due to a halving of refractory angina in the intervention group.[59] It should be noted that this benefit of intervention was not evident in women. The authors of the study urge caution in such subgroup analysis.

Much of the advantage offered by the invasive approach in these later studies is due to the advent of coronary stenting and development of adjunctive therapy (GPIIb/IIIa inhibition, thienopyridines). In addition there were design flaws in the earlier studies. In TIMI IIIB and VANQWISH the treatment strategies were not well separated. In TIMI IIIB at 1 year 64% of the invasive group had undergone revascularization versus 58% in the conservative group. Similarly, in VANQWISH the percentages were 44%

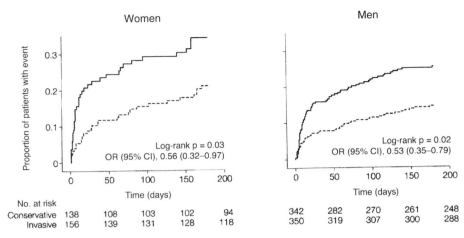

Figure 18.6
Death, myocardial infarction, and rehospitalization for acute coronary syndrome in women and men with elevated troponin T-levels from the TACTICS TIMI-18 study groups separated by treatment strategy. Median follow-up time 180 days for both men and women. OR, odds ratio; CI, confidence interval. Reproduced from reference 58 with permission.

versus 33% at 23 months. Furthermore, in this study many of the deaths occurred in patients who were assigned to intervention but never received the intervention.[59]

Since women with ACS are more likely than men to have either angiographically normal coronary arteries (25% in TIMI IIIB) or single-vessel disease, they are less likely as a group to benefit from an invasive approach. Furthermore, the lack of benefit is at least partly attributable to a higher CABG-related mortality in women. There appears to be no difference in the outcome for PCI as a treatment for ACS in women and men. This increased risk of CABG in women is usually attributable to women being older and having more co-morbid conditions.[60] Conversely, Vaccarino and associates found that younger women undergoing CABG were at higher risk of death than comparably aged men, but that this difference decreased with age. While these young women had more co-morbid conditions than their male counterparts, especially diabetes; these conditions explained less than 30% of the mortality difference.[61] Since medical management fails as often in women as in men and the success rate of PCI is high and the complication rate is low, an early invasive approach seems to be a reasonable strategy in women

as well as men (Fig. 18.6).[62] In both groups the therapy should be tailored to the risk level. The high-risk patients (rest angina and ST-segment depression or elevated cardiac markers) and intermediate-risk patients (class III or IV exertional angina, diabetes or diffuse deep T-wave inversions) warrant an early invasive approach. The low-risk patients (absence of above findings) can be treated with a 'selective invasive strategy'. This strategy includes aggressive pharmacologic therapy including aspirin, clopidogrel, beta-blockers, statins, and angiotensin-converting enzyme inhibitors and provocative testing. Coronary angiography is used in those patients with either recurrent spontaneous angina or objective evidence of stress-induced myocardial ischemia. There are, however, proponents of a routine early invasive strategy in all patients with ACS. The proponents of this approach would make a distinction between coronary angiography per se and angiography leading to PCI. This early invasive approach avoids lengthy delays by immediate discharge of patients with normal coronary angiograms or minimal disease and early surgery for left main or triple-vessel disease. The ambiguities sometimes associated with noninvasive testing can also be avoided. These physicians would argue that coronary anatomy is the most definitive means of tailoring therapy. In this regard, it should be noted that the invasive approach in the troponin-negative group in TACTICS TIMI-18 caused no added harm to the patients[63,64] No randomized clinical trial, however, has evaluated such an approach.

The optimal timing of PCI in the early invasive strategy (whether routine or selective) is not established. The TACTICS TIMI-18 data support PCI between 2 and 3 days post-event. Clinically, PCI is frequently performed with 24 hours of symptom onset.

References

1. Takano M, Mizuno K, Okamatsu K, et al. Mechanical and structural characteristics of vulnerable plaques: analysis by coronary angioscopy and intravascular ultrasound. *J Am Coll Cardiol* 2001; **38**:99–104.
2. Braunwald E, Antman EM, Beasley JW, et al. ACC/AHA guidelines for the management of patients with unstable angina and non-ST-segment elevation myocardial infarction. A report of the American College of Cardiology/American Heart Association Task Force on Practice Guidelines (Committee on the Management of Patients with Unstable Angina). *J Am Coll Cardiol* 2000; **36**:970–1062.
3. Reimer KA, Lowe JE, Rasmussen MM, et al. The wave-front phenomenon of ischemic cell death. I. Myocardial infarct size vs duration of coronary occlusion in dogs. *Circulation* 1977; **56**:786–94.
4. Hochman JS, Tamis JE, Thompson TD, et al. Sex, clinical presentation, and outcome in patients with acute coronary syndromes. *N Engl J Med* 1999; **341**:226–32.
5. Vaccarino V, Parsons L, Every NR, Hal V, Krumholz HM. Sex-based differences in early mortality after myocardial infarction. *N Engl J Med* 1999; **341**:217–25.
6. Rouan GW, Lee TH, Cook EF, et al. Clinical characteristics and outcome of acute myocardial infarction in patients with initially normal or nonspecific electrocardiograms: a report from the Multicenter Chest Pain Study. *Am J Cardiol* 1989; **64**:1087–92.
7. Barron HV, Bowlby LJ, Breen T, et al. Use of reperfusion therapy for acute myocardial infarction in the United States: data from the National Registry of Myocardial Infarction 2. *Circulation* 1998; **97**:1150–6.
8. Wilcox RG, Von der Lippe G, Olsson CG, et al. Trial of tissue plasminogen activator for mortality reduction in acute myocardial infraction (ASSET). *Lancet* 1988; **2**:525–30.
9. AIMS Trial Study Group. Effect of intravenous APSAC on mortality after acute myocardial infarction: preliminary report of a placebo-controlled clinical trial. *Lancet* 1988; **1**:545–9.
10. Gruppo Italiano per lo Studio della Streptochinasi nell'Infarto Miocardico (GISSI). Effectiveness of intravenous thrombolytic treatment in acute myocardial infarction. *Lancet* 1986; **1**:397–401.
11. ISIS-2 (Second international study of infarct survival) Collaborative group. Randomized trial of intravenous streptokinase, oral aspirin. Both or neither among 17,187 cases of suspected acute myocardial infarction: ISIS-2. *Lancet* 1988; **2**:349–60.
12. Fibrinolytic Therapy Trialists (FTT) Collaborative Group. Indications for fibrinolytic therapy in suspected acute myocardial infarction: collaborative overview of early mortality and major morbidity results from all randomized trials of more than 1000 patients. *Lancet* 1994; **343**:311–22.
13. The GUSTO Angiographic Investigators. The effects of tissue plasminogen activator, streptokinase, or both on coronary-artery patency, ventricular function, and survival after acute myocardial infarction. *N Engl J Med* 1993; **329**:1615–22.
14. Boersma E, Maas AC, Deckers JW, et al. Early thrombolytic treatment in acute myocardial infarction: reappraisal of the golden hour. *Lancet* 1996; **348**:771–5.
15. Weaver WD, Cerqueira M, Hallstrom AP, et al. Prehospital initiated vs hospital initiated thrombolytic therapy: the Myocardial Infarction Triage and Intervention Trial. *JAMA* 1993; **270**:1211–16.
16. Simoons ML, Maggioni AP, Knatterud G, et al. Individual risk assessment for intracranial haemorrhage during thrombolytic therapy. *Lancet* 1993; **342**:1523–8.
17. Grech ED, Ramsdale DR. Acute coronary syndrome: ST segment elevation myocardial infarction. *BMJ* 2003; **326**:1379–81.
18. Ghali WA, Donaldson CR, Knudtson ML, et al. Rising to the challenge: transforming the treatment of ST-

segment elevation myocardial infarction. *Can Med Assoc J* 2003; **169**:35–7.

19. Grines CL, Serruys P, O'Neill WW. Fibrinolytic therapy: is it a treatment of the past? *Circulation* 2003; **107**:2538–42.

20. Keeley EC, Boura JA, Grines CL. Primary angioplasty versus intravenous thrombolytic therapy for acute myocardial infarction: a quantitative review of 23 randomised trials. *Lancet* 2003; **361**:13–20.

21. Weaver WD, Simes RJ, Betriu A, et al. Comparison of primary coronary angioplasty and intravenous thrombolytic therapy for acute myocardial infarction. *JAMA* 1997; **278**:2093–8.

22. PCAT collaborators. Primary coronary angioplasty compared with intravenous thrombolytic therapy for acute myocardial infarction: six-month followup and analysis of individual patient data from randomized trials. *Am Heart J* 2003; **145**:47–57.

23. Lewis HD, Davis J, Archibald D, et al. Protective effects of aspirin against acute myocardial infarction and death in men with unstable angina. *N Engl J Med* 1983; **309**:396–403.

24. Cairns J, Gent M, Singer J, et al. Aspirin, sulfinpyrazone, or both in unstable angina. *N Engl J Med* 1985; **313**:1369–75.

25. Theroux P, Ouimet H, McCans J, et al. Aspirin, heparin or both to treat unstable angina. *N Engl J Med* 1988; **319**:1105–11.

26. The RISC Group. Risk of myocardial infarction and death during treatment with low dose aspirin and intravenous heparin in men with unstable coronary artery disease. *Lancet* 1990; **336**:827–30.

27. Antithrombotic Trialists' Collaboration. Collaborative meta-analysis of randomized trials of antiplatelet therapy for prevention of death, myocardial infarction, and stroke in high risk patients. *BMJ* 2002; **324**:71–86.

28. Mehta SR, Yusuf S. Short and long-term oral antiplatelet therapy in acute coronary syndromes and percutaneous coronary intervention. *J Am Coll Cardiol* 2003; **41**:79S–88S.

29. Antithrombotic Trialists' Collaboration. Collaborative overview of randomized trials of antiplatelet therapy I: prevention of death, myocardial infarction, and stroke by prolonged antiplatelet therapy in various categories of patients. *BMJ* 1994; **308**:81–106.

30. Cronin L, Yusuf S, Flather M, et al. OASIS registry 2-year follow-up: outcomes in patients with unstable angina or myocardial infarction without ST segment elevation admitted to hospitals with or without catheterization facilities. *Eur Heart J* 2000; **21**:247.

31. Van Belle E, Lablanche JM, Bauters C, et al. Coronary angioscopic findings in the infarct-related vessel within 1 month of acute myocardial infarction: natural history and the effect of thrombolysis. *Circulation* 1998; **90**:26–30.

32. Flather MD, Weitz JI, Yusuf S, et al. Reactivation of coagulation after stopping infusions of recombinant hirudin and unfractionated heparin in unstable angina and myocardial infarction without ST elevation: results of a randomized trial. OASIS Pilot Study Investigators. *Eur Heart J* 2000; **21**:1473–81.

33. The CAPRIE Steering Committee. A randomized, blinded trial of clopidogrel versus aspirin in patients at risk of ischaemic events. *Lancet* 1996; **348**:1329–39.

34. The CURE Investigators. Effects of clopidogrel in addition to aspirin in patients with acute coronary syndromes without ST segment elevation. *N Engl J Med* 2001; **345**:494–502.

35. Kong DF, Califf RM, Miller DP, et al. Clinical outcomes of therapeutic agents that block the platelet glycoprotein IIb/IIIa integrin in ischemic heart disease. *Circulation* 1998; **98**:2829–35.

36. Cohen M. The role of low-molecular-weight heparin in the management of acute coronary syndromes. *J Am Coll Cardiol* 2003; **41**:55S–61S.

37. Eikelboom JW, Anand SS, Malmberg K, et al. Unfractionated heparin and low-molecular-weight heparin in acute coronary syndrome without ST elevation: a meta-analysis. *Lancet* 2000; **355**:1936–42.

38. Cohen M. Low molecular weight heparins in the management of unstable angina/non-Q-wave myocardial infarction. *Semin Thromb Hemost* 1999; **25** (Suppl 3):113–21.

39. Kereiakes DJ, Grines C, Fry E. Enoxaparin and abciximab adjunctive pharmacotherapy during percutaneous coronary intervention. *J Invasive Cardiol* 2001; **13**:272–8.

40. Cannon C. Small molecule glycoprotein IIb/IIIa receptor inhibitors as upstream therapy in acute coronary syndromes: insights from the TACTICS TIMI-18 trial. *J Am Coll Cardiol* 2003; **41**:43S–8S.

41. Cho L, Topol EJ, Balog C, et al. Clinical benefit of glycoprotein IIb/IIIa blockade with abciximab is independent of gender: pooled analysis from EPIC, EPILOG and EPISTENT trials. *J Am Coll Cardiol* 2000; **36**:381–6.

42. Fernandes LS, Tcheng JE, O'Shea JC, et al. Is glycoprotein IIb/IIIa antagonism as effective in women as in men following percutaneous coronary intervention? Lessons from the ESPRIT study. *J Am Coll Cardiol* 2002; **40**:1085–91.

43. Chew DP, Moliterno DJ. A critical appraisal of

platelet glycoprotein IIb/IIIa inhibition. *J Am Coll Cardiol* 2000; **36**:2028–35.

44. Blomkalns AL, Chen AY, Hochman JS, et al., for the CRUSADE Investigators. Gender disparities in the diagnosis and treatment of non-ST-segment elevation acute coronary syndromes: large-scale observations from the CRUSADE (Can Rapid Risk Stratification of Unstable Angina Patients Suppress Adverse Outcomes with Early Implementation of the American College of Cardiology/American Heart Association Guidelines) National Quality Improvement Initiative. *J Am Coll Cardiol* 2005; **45**:832–7.

45. Newby LK, Ohman EM, Christenson RH, et al. Benefit of glycoprotein IIb/IIIa inhibition in patients with acute coronary syndromes and troponin T-positive status: the PARAGON-B troponin T substudy. *Circulation* 2001; **103**:2891–902.

46. Alexander JH, Harrington RA, Tuttle RH, et al. Prior aspirin use predicts worse outcomes in patients with non-ST-elevation acute coronary syndromes. *J Am Cardiol* 1999; **83**:1147–51.

47. Savonitto S, Ardissino D, Granger CB, et al. Prognostic value of the admission electrocardiogram in acute coronary syndromes. *JAMA* 1999; **281**:707–13.

48. Holmvang L, Clemmenson P, Wagner G, et al. Admission standard electrocardiogram for early risk stratification in patients with unstable coronary artery disease not eligible for acute revascularization therapy. A TRIM substudy. ThRombin Inhibition in Myocardial Infarction. *Am Heart J* 1999; **137**:24–33.

49. Liuzzo G, Biasucci LM, Gallimore JR, et al. The prognostic value of C-reactive protein and serum amyloid a protein in severe unstable angina. *N Engl J Med* 1994; **331**:417–24.

50. Blake GJ, Ridker PM. C-reactive protein and other inflammatory risk markers in acute coronary syndromes. *J Am Coll Cardiol* 2003; **41**:37S–42S.

51. Sabatine MS, Antman EM. The thrombolysis in myocardial infarction risk score in unstable angina/non-ST-segment elevation myocardial infarction. *J Am Coll Cardiol* 2003; **41** (Suppl):89S–95S.

52. Antman EM, Cohen M, Bernink PJ, et al. The TIMI risk score for unstable angina/non-ST elevation MI: a method for prognostication and therapeutic decision making. *JAMA* 2000; **284**:835–42.

53. Cohen M. Anti-thrombotic combination using tirofiban and enoxaparin: the ACUTE II study. *Circulation* 2000; **102**:II-826.

54. Boden WE, O'Rourke MH, Crawford MH, et al. The Veterans Affairs non-Q-wave infarction strategy: outcomes in patients with acute non-Q-wave myocardial randomly assigned to an invasive as compared with a conservative management strategy. *N Engl J Med* 1998; **338**:1785–92.

55. TIMI IIIB Investigators. Effects of tissue plasminogen activator and a comparison of early invasive and conservative strategies in unstable angina and non-Q-wave myocardial infarction: results of the TIMI IIIB Trial. *Circulation* 1994; **89**:1545–56.

56. FRISC II Investigators, Wallentin L, Lagerqvist B, Husted S, et al. Outcome at 1 year after an invasive compared with a non-invasive strategy in unstable coronary-artery disease: the FRISC II invasive randomized trial. *Lancet* 2000; **356**:9–16.

57. Sabatine MS, Cannon CP, Murphy SA, DiBattiste PM, Demopoulos LA, Braunwald E. Implications of upstream GP IIb/IIIa inhibition and stenting in the invasive management of UA/NSTEMI: a comparison of TIMI IIIB and TACTICS TIMI-18. *Circulation* 2001; **104** (Suppl II):II549.

58. Glaser R, Herrmann HC, Murphy SA, et al. Benefit of an early invasive management strategy in women with acute coronary syndromes. *JAMA* 2002; **288**:3124–9.

59. RITA investigators, Fox KA, Poole-Wilson PA, Henderson RA, et al. Interventional versus conservative treatment for patients with unstable angina or non-ST-elevation myocardial infarction: the British Heart Foundation RITA 3 randomised trial. *Lancet* 2002; **360**:743–51.

60. Lagerqvist B, Safstrom K, Stgahle E, et al. Is early invasive treatment of unstable coronary disease equally effective for both women and men? *J Am Coll Cardiol* 2001; **38**:41–8.

61. Vaccarino V, Abramson JL, Veledar E, et al. Sex differences in hospital mortality after coronary artery bypass surgery: evidence for a higher mortality in younger women. *Circulation* 2002; **105**:1176–81.

62. Hochman JS, McCabe CH, Stone PH, et al. Outcome and profile of women and men presenting with acute coronary syndromes: a report from TIMI IIIB. *J Am Coll Cardiol* 1997; **30**:141–8.

63. Boden WE. 'Routine invasive' versus 'selective invasive' approaches to non-ST-segment elevation acute coronary syndromes management in the post-stent/platelet inhibition era. *J Am Coll Cardiol* 2003; **41**:113S-22S.

64. McKay RG. 'Ischemia-guided' versus 'early invasive' strategies in the management of acute coronary syndrome/non-ST-segment elevation myocardial infarction. *J Am Coll Cardiol* 2003; **41**:96S–102S.

19

Percutaneous coronary interventions in women

Alexandra J. Lansky, Ricardo Costa, Ecatarina Critea and Patricia Ward

Introduction

More than 1 million percutaneous coronary interventions (PCIs) are performed annually in the United States with an estimated 36% performed in women, and approximately 45–50% using intracoronary stents and more recently drug-eluting stents.[1] This chapter will review our current understanding of gender-based referral patterns for PCI, as well as the risks and outcomes associated with coronary interventions in women according to specific interventional devices and the presenting clinical syndromes. This is in accordance with the recently published American Heart Association Consensus Statement on percutaneous coronary intervention and adjunctive pharmacotherapy in women.[2]

Referral patterns for diagnostic angiography and coronary intervention

Despite the greater number of women with cardiovascular disease (CVD) in the US, women appear to be referred for diagnostic catheterization less frequently than men. This was demonstrated in an analysis of 82 782 women and men hospitalized with a diagnosis of coronary heart disease (CHD) in 1987, which found that women underwent coronary angiography less often than men.[3] Another study of 840 patients (47% female) with an initial positive noninvasive test for CHD demonstrated that cardiac catheterization was performed in 33.8% of women compared with 45% men (p = 0.007).[4] In contrast, another large study of 3669 patients (36% female) found no gender difference in referral for angiography after an abnormal thallium scan,[5] while other trials have found that the gender difference in referral disappears after adjustment for differences in clinical characteristics.[6,7] Suggested reasons for referral differences have included the older age of women, the greater risk profile, and the lower predictive accuracy of noninvasive testing. The fact remains that in interventional clinical trials, in investigator-driven consecutive registries, in industry-generated market utilization reports, and in post market surveillance registries, women are consistently under-represented compared with men (30% women vs 70% men) despite women's higher prevalence of CHD. Perhaps the most convincing evidence for a gender difference in referral for cardiac catheterization was a controlled study of 720 primary health-care providers, who reviewed scripted videotapes of actors describing the same chest pain symptoms by actors of varying gender and race.[8] This study suggests that the patient's race and sex influenced the physician's decision to refer for cardiac catheterization. Black women were significantly less likely to be referred for cardiac catheterization than white men (odds ratio (OR) = 0.4, 95% confidence interval (CI) 0.2–0.7, p = 0.004). In contrast, most contemporary studies find that once women are referred and undergo cardiac catheterization, revascularization rates and practices are similar to those for men.[9–11] Compared with men, however, women tend to be referred more for PCI than coronary artery bypass grafting (CABG) but this is explained by their reduced incidence of multivessel disease.

Pathophysiologic considerations in the gender disparities in mortality after PCI (see also Chapter 17)

Numerous studies now indicate that despite continued improvements in device technology and the overall improvement in outcomes of women over time following PCI, women consistently tend to have a higher mortality and worse outcomes than men (Tables 19.1–19.3).[12–33] The heightened mortality appears to represent a complex interplay of clinical factors such as delayed onset of disease, older age, comorbidities at the time of presentation, delays in presentation, and other lesion-specific factors.[34–45] Adjustments for such factors in clinical trials and registries are not always consistent nor do they necessarily eradicate differences in outcome.[18,24,46,47] Other factors including humoral factors and angiographic findings specific to women such as smaller vessel caliber, susceptibility to more frequent intimal dissections,[25,48] and perforations following PCI[49] are also thought to account for some of the observed differences in outcome.

Table 19.1 Registries of elective PCI with increased in-hospital mortality for women versus men

Study/registry*	Device/setting	In-hospital mortality	Adjusted OR (95% CI)
ACC-NCDR[12] 1998–2000 n = 100 292 34% female	PCI 54% elective 41% urgent/emergency	Men 1.2% Women 2.0% p <0.0001	
Lansky[13] 1991–1996 n = 7372 28% female	Elective NDA	Men 0.66% Women 1.39% p <0.01	2.28 (1.15–4.55)
Watanabe[14] 1997 n = 82 783 35% female	Elective stents	Men 0.5% Women 1.1% p <0.0001	1.65 (1.33–2.04)
Malenka[15] 1989–1995 n = 12 232 29% female	NDA UA mostly	Men 0.7% Women 1.64% p <0.001	1.64 (1.09–2.47)
Alfonso[17] 1990–1997 n = 981 16% female	Elective stent	Men 2.0% Women 6.0% p = 0.01	RR 2.9 (1.2–7.4)
Bell[18] 1993 n = 3557 27% female	PTCA	Men 2.7% Women 4.2% p = 0.005	1.51 (1.0–2.29) p = 0.05 No difference if corrected for BSA
NHLBI[20] 1985–1986 n = 2136 26% female	PTCA	Men 0.3% Women 2.6% p <0.001	4.53 (1.39–14.7)
Mehilli[21] 1992–1998 n = 4264 24% female	PCI	Death, MI at 30 days Men 3.1% Women 1.9% p <0.001	2.02 (1.27–3.19)

PCI, percutaneous coronary intervention; OR, odds ratio; CI, confidence interval; NDA, new device angioplasty; UA, unstable angina; PTCA, percutaneous transluminal coronary angioplasty; AMI, acute myocardial infarction; RR, relative risk; BSA, body surface area.
*See reference for explanation of study/registry acronym.

Table 19.2 Registries of elective PCI with similar in-hospital mortality for women versus men

Study/registry*	Device	In-hospital mortality	Adjusted OR (95% CI)
Welty[19] 1989–1995 n = 5989 35% female	PTCA 55–63% UA 8% AMI	Men 0.52% Women 1.2% p = 0.017	0.72 (0.39–1.32)
Malenka[15] 1994–1999 n = 33 666 33% female	PCI	Men 1.1% Women 1.2% p = 0.1	1.24 (0.96–1.6)
NHLBI[22] 1997–1998 n = 2524 35% female	PCI	Men 1.3% Women 2.2% p NA	1.60 (0.76–3.35)
Trabattoni[23] 1992–1998 n = 1100 15% female	Stent	Men 0.7%? Women 1.0% p = NS	NA
Weintraub[24] 1980–1991 n = 10 785 2845 female	PTCA	Men 0.1% Women 0.7% p <0.001	1.74 (0.39–7.69)
McEniery[25] 1987 n = 3696 26% female	PTCA	Men 0.09% Women 0.3% p = NS	NA
Arnold[26] 1994 n = 5000 1274 female	PTCA	Men 0.3% Women 1.1% p = 0.001	1.08 (0.81–1.45) Corrected for BSA
Bell[27] 1995 n = 3027 29% female	PTCA	Men 1.1% Women 1.4% p = NS	0.94 (0.76–1.15)
NACI[28] 1996 n = 2855 34% female	NDA Stents, laser, rotablator	Men 1.1% Women 1.4% p = NS	1.02 (0.87–1.2)
NCN[29] 1994–1997 n = 109 708 33% female	PCI 40% stent 8% atherectomy	Men 1.0% Women 1.8% p <0.001	1.07 (0.92–1.24)
Bell[30] 1988–1992 n = 291 21% female	DCA	Men 1.7% Women 1.6% p = NS	

PCI, percutaneous coronary intervention; OR, odds ratio; CI, confidence interval; PTCA, percutaneous transluminal coronary angioplasty; NDA, new device angioplasty; DCA, directional coronary atherectomy; NS, not significant; MI, myocardial infarction; BSA, body surface area.
*See reference for explanation of study/registry acronym.

Gender and the age paradox

After PCI, the higher complication rates facing women have been attributed largely to older age and other unfavorable clinical characteristics.[28,50] For instance, after PCI, the hazard of death has been reported to increase by 65% with every 10-year increase in age.[50] The heightened mortality risk associated with increasing age applies equally to women and men. At the lower end of the age spectrum, however, while the prevalence of CVD is low among young premenopausal women (only 7–9% of patients undergoing coronary revascularization are aged 40 years or less),[51,52] the consequences of

Table 19.3 Late mortality for women and men after elective PCI

Study/registry*	Device/setting	Late mortality	Adjusted OR (95% CI)
NHLBI[22] 1997–1998 n = 2524 35% female	PCI Case mix	Men 4.3% Women 6.5% p = 0.02 Follow-up: 1 year	RR 1.26 (0.85–1.87)
NHLBI[20] 1985–1986 n = 2136 26% female	PTCA Case mix	Men 6.6% Women 10.8% p = 0.001 Follow-up: 5 years	1.20 (0.84–1.73)
Bell[18] 1993 n = 3027 27% female	PTCA Consecutive	Men 27.0% Women 22.0% p = 0.06 Follow-up: 10 years	0.94 (0.76–1.15)
Lansky[13] 1991–1996 n = 7372 28% female	NDA	Men 3.3% Women 4.4% p <0.02 Follow-up: 1 year	NS
Mehilli[21] 1992–1998 n = 4264 24% female	PCI for CAD	Men 4.5% Women 5.2% Death/MI Men 5.9% Women 6.1% Follow-up: 1 year	2.02 (1.27–3.19)
Weintraub[24] 1980–1991 n = 10 785 26% female	PTCA	Men 8.0% Women 5.0% p = 0.0002 Follow-up: 5 years	1.08 (0.84–1.39)
NACI[28] 1990–1994 n = 2855 34% female	NDA Stents, laser, rotablator Elective	Men 5.7% Women 5.9% p = NS Follow-up: 1 year	Women had lower rate than men of repeat TVR
CAVEAT[31] 1995 n = 512 25% female	DCA	Men 0.95% Women 1.4% p = NS Follow-up: 1 year	
BOAT[32] 1998 n = 989 24% female	DCA (+ PTCA)	Men 1.2% Women 0.8% p = NS Follow-up: 1 year	
STARS[33] 1998 n = 1965 29% female	Stent	Men 0% Women 0% p = NS Follow-up: 9 months	

PCI, percutaneous coronary intervention; OR, odds ratio; CI, confidence interval; PTCA, percutaneous transluminal coronary angioplasty; NDA, new device angioplasty; CAD, coronary artery disease; DCA, directional coronary atherectomy; MI, myocardial infarction; NS, not significant; RR, relative risk; TVR, target vessel revascularization.
*See reference for explanation of study/registry acronym.

premature CHD have been shown to be significantly worse for young women than for age-matched men. This has been shown after myocardial infarction (MI),[53] after CABG surgery,[54] and after PCI.[55] In one study, young women (<40 years) with premature CHD requiring PCI had an exaggerated incidence of diabetes compared with men (38% vs 10%, p <0.001), explaining in part the worse outcomes observed in women in this series; the 1-year death and Q-wave MI rate following elective PCI in women was 7.9% versus 0.8% in men (p < 0.01).[55]

Gender and diabetes

Diabetes has been shown to be a particularly strong risk factor for CHD in women,[56–59] and is associated with a heightened cardiovascular mortality in young adults.[58,59] In one report, diabetic women younger than 55 years with no other risk factors for CHD had a 16-fold higher risk of dying from CHD than did women without diabetes.[59] Insights from intravascular ultrasound studies have shown that insulin-treated diabetic patients develop 'impaired arterial remodeling' compared with nondiabetics, and thus have a higher propensity for developing luminal obstruction for any given amount of plaque deposition.[60,61] The combination of impaired remodeling and small vessel caliber in the diabetic female population may prove to be a combination leading to early lumen compromise and more symptomatic coronary disease, and may in part explain why such a preponderance of women with diabetes become symptomatic and require PCI.[61,62] The more diffuse nature of the atherosclerosis process in the diabetic patients, as well as the impaired vasodilator relaxation associated with diabetes in the otherwise healthy premenopausal woman,[63] could also explain the higher ischemic burden and complication rates in the younger female population.

Gender and vessel size

Previous angiographic and necropsy studies have demonstrated that women generally have smaller caliber vessels than men, a difference attributed to women's smaller body size in some[62] but not all studies.[61,64,65] In a study using intravascular ultrasound in women and men with chronic anginal syndromes and de novo, noncomplex native coronary artery lesions, the target lesion and reference segment external elastic membrane dimensions, lumen, and plaque + media cross-sectional areas were smaller in women than men; however, these quantitative differences were entirely attributable to differences in body surface area.[61] Thus, differences in outcome following revascularization may be related in part to vessel caliber. In a series of 5000 angioplasty patients from the Cleveland Clinic, the increased in-hospital mortality for women (1.1% vs 0.3%, p = 0.001) was no longer significant after correcting for differences in body surface area.[61] The 1986 National Heart, Lung, and Blood Institute (NHLBI) percutaneous transluminal coronary angioplasty (PTCA) Registry, which adjusted for clinical differences among women and men (including body surface area), found that gender was not an independent predictor of outcome.[18,24,46,47] Similarly, in a recent pooled analysis of five interventional trials of 3982 patients, the 1-year mortality for women was higher (1.7% vs 0.8%, p <0.05). By multivariate analysis age was the only predictor of 6-month mortality, and not gender, vessel size, or body surface area.[66] Finally, acute complications in women associated with coronary interventions may reflect the complications associated with intervention in small vessels. Specifically, women are susceptible to more frequent intimal dissections[25,26,48] and perforations[49] following PCI. The higher mortality associated with a smaller body surface area is presumably due to higher associated procedural complications such as dissections and perforations; however, specific cause and effect have yet to be elucidated. In a large registry of patients undergoing new device angioplasty,[13] women had smaller vessel size than men (2.66 ± 0.60 mm vs 2.81 ± 0.64 mm, p = 0.0008); however, in contrast to other angiographic studies where differences in mortality were abolished after correcting for differences in body surface area or vessel caliber,[64,65] this study still identified women as having an inherent increased risk of mortality after coronary intervention.

Gender and lesion morphology

Findings of the International Atherosclerosis Project and others have indicated that cardiovascular morbidity and mortality vary with the extent of coronary artery disease,[67,68] and with the overall plaque burden.[69,70] There have been no systematic angiographic or pathologic studies performed to identify potential differences in gender-related lesion morphology. A published series based on diagnostic intravascular ultrasound imaging of lesions requiring PCI found that lesion characteristics including calcium and eccentricity were similar in women and men.[61] Calcium was present with similar frequency (71% vs 72%) and with similar magnitude (total arc of calcium, arc of superficial calcium, arc of reference segment calcium, length of lesion calcium) in women and in men, and a similar percentage of lesions were eccentric (44% in women vs 48% in men, p = 0.4771). Plaque burden, especially reference segment plaque burden, was also similar in women and men. When normalized for the proximal reference, the lesion external elastic membrane cross-sectional area was similar in women and in men. Coupled with the lack of gender-related differences in lesion and reference segment plaque burden, this finding suggests that adaptive remodeling response (the increase in arterial cross-sectional area in response to plaque accumulation) is similar in women and men.[61]

Beyond morphology

Although no obvious gender-based differences in lesion morphology have been identified, differences in plaque response to hormonal or thrombogenic stimuli may be present. Epidemiologic studies support the protective effect of endogenous estrogen in premenopausal women. This may be mediated in part by its effect on the coagulation system. Women taking estrogen have lower fibrinogen levels and higher factor VII levels,[71] both known to be associated with atherosclerosis.[72] Women of any age with a family history of early CHD demonstrate hyperreactive platelet aggregation. Upon activation, platelets obtained from women bind to a greater number of fibrinogen molecules.[73] Thus, some of the gender-related differences in coronary atherosclerosis may be attributed to differences in atherogenic stimuli after estrogen withdrawal rather than to differences in plaque morphology.

Results after conventional elective coronary angioplasty

In the 1985 NHLBI PTCA Registry, female gender was identified as an independent predictor of early complications and mortality following angioplasty.[74] In contemporary series, women undergoing balloon angioplasty continue to have higher in-hospital mortality than men, despite marked improvements in procedural success rates[12–20,24,47] (Table 19.1). Gender differences of in-hospital outcomes influence hospitalization costs,[75] and may be contributing in part to the frequent referral bias and the less aggressive diagnostic evaluation of women with coronary syndromes.[76–79] As angioplasty techniques have evolved, the outcome of women undergoing coronary intervention has been redefined in an effort to change referral patterns of women with CHD. The greatest impact of new devices, including newer-generation balloons, atherectomy, thrombectomy, and laser devices, has been an overall improvement in procedural and angiographic success rates. With the original balloon angioplasty devices available before 1985, procedural success ranged from 60 to 70%, increasing to 80–90% after 1985[46,47,74,80,81] and above 90% with the availability of new device angioplasty techniques in both women and men. While women continued to have a higher mortality than men with new device interventions,[15,21–30] the in-hospital mortality rates in women undergoing new device angioplasty (<1.5%) were reduced compared with previously reported rates (up to 4.1%) associated with balloon angioplasty alone[46,47,74,81] (Tables 19.1 and 19.2).[12–20] A recent evaluation of 33 666 consecutive patients undergoing PCI in New England from 1994 to 1999 showed that concurrent with the changing practice of coronary intervention, the outcomes have improved for both women and men, without significant differences in mortality between genders.[15]

During long-term follow-up after balloon and new device angioplasty (Table 19.3), mortality differences tend to persist for women, but are generally attributable to co-morbid factors. In a registry of new device angioplasty which included 7372 patients,[13] the mortality at 1 year remained higher for women than men (4.39% vs 3.26%, p = 0.018); independent predictors of mortality included diabetes mellitus, unstable angina at the time of intervention, prior MI, but not gender. The overall rates of revascularization and major adverse clinical events at 1 year were lower in women, and male gender was actually an independent risk for increased follow-up events. Late clinical outcomes of women with new device angioplasty are favorable compared with historical balloon angioplasty series (Table 19.3).[13,18,20–22,24,28,31–33,46,47] Despite the slight increase of in-hospital cardiac mortality in women compared with men, the use of 'new device' angioplasty, although rarely used in current interventional practice, is a safe and effective treatment strategy for women with symptomatic CHD.

Restenosis in women

In general, gender differences in angiographic restenosis rates have not been well defined, partly due to the under-representation and small samples of women in prospective trials with systematic angiographic follow-up and partly due to the paucity of published gender-based data from such trials. Paradoxically, registry data have generally reported women to have similar or lower target vessel revascularization rates to men after balloon angioplasty[13,21,25–27,47,81] and stenting,[82–84] despite their consistently smaller vessel size and higher prevalence of diabetes mellitus; factors that are typically associated with higher restenosis and revascularization rates after coronary interventions.[30,84–88] In the absence of systematic angiographic and clinical follow-up, this paradoxical finding is of uncertain clinical significance, either reflecting a true reduction in the need for repeat revascularization in women or a potential referral bias, in which women are less likely, due to differences in symptoms or noninvasive test results or other reasons, to be referred or readmitted for subsequent revascularization.

Results after elective stenting in women

Compared with balloon angioplasty and new devices, intracoronary stents have improved the acute procedural success and in-hospital outcomes of patients undergoing PCI by lowering the rates of vessel closure, in conjunction with reducing the long-term restenosis rates.[89,90] Consequently, in recent years, stent implantation for elective PCI has become the treatment modality of choice and is used in 80–90% of interventional cases in the US. Lesions that are not appropriate for stenting are seldom encountered, and small vessel caliber no longer precludes stent use, as stents are now available for the lower range of coronary vessel sizes including 2.0 mm, 2.5 mm, and 2.75 mm diameters. While no specific gender-based comparisons were performed (or at least published) in the earlier randomized clinical trials comparing stent implantation to balloon angioplasty, the superiority of stenting was demonstrated at all ranges of vessel sizes including vessels smaller than 3.0 mm in diameter, especially relevant to the female population undergoing PCI, and the benefits have therefore been presumed to be generalizable to women.[91] A pooled analysis of seven prospective investigation device exemption (IDE) stent trials was performed that included 7171 patients (2179 women and 4992 men) undergoing elective stenting with a tubular slotted stent design.[16] Outcomes from this pooled analysis were compared based on gender. The inclusion and exclusion criteria were similar in all trials included in the pooled analysis (elective stenting of focal native coronary lesions requiring no more than two stents of 3.0–4.0 mm diameter range). In this series women were older (66 vs 61 years, p = 0.001), had more hypertension (67% vs 53%, p = 0.001), and diabetes (27% vs 18%, p = 0.001) than men and had significantly smaller vessel size (2.90 ± 0.49 mm vs 3.03 ± 0.54 mm, p = 0.001). Despite the higher frequency of risk factors, women had a similar unadjusted in-hospital mortality to men (0.28% women vs 0.14% men, p = not significant (NS)). There was no difference in other complications such as peri-procedural MI or need for CABG surgery. At 1 year however the mortality risk was higher in women than in men (2.25% vs 1.44%, p = 0.015), a difference that was no longer significant after adjusting for differences in co-morbid conditions (OR = 1.2, p = 0.383). In addition, there was no difference in target vessel revascularization between the genders 1 year after stenting (12% women vs 11% men). Thus in the setting of elective stenting with 3.0–4.0 mm devices, the short- and long-term outcomes are comparable across gender and appear generalizable to women.

Subsequent post-approval registries comparing gender-based outcomes after coronary stenting in a broader range of lesion and patient subsets have demonstrated mixed results in women: some with superior outcomes[14] and others with worse outcomes than men.[83] In a study from the Nationwide Inpatient Sample, 118 548 angioplasties performed in 1997 were examined based on gender and use of stents. Among the 59% of patients undergoing stenting, the in-hospital mortality after elective stenting was higher in women (1.1% vs 0.5%, p <0.0001), as was the need for CABG surgery (1.5% vs 1.0%, p <0.0001); these differences were maintained even after multivariate adjustment of differences in risk factors. While the overall outcomes have improved in patients who receive stents, some studies show that female gender remains an independent predictor of mortality compared with men.[83] In another registry of elective coronary stenting in 1001 women and 3263 men, the 30-day combined endpoint of death and MI was 3.1% in women and 1.8% in men (p = 0.02) (OR 2.02, 95% CI 1.27–3.19). At 1 year the death and MI rate was similar for women and men (5.8% vs 6.0% women, p = 0.77). In this study the strongest risk factor in predicting a worse outcome at 30 days was the presence of diabetes in women and older age in men.[84]

In general, while acute and long-term mortality may still be somewhat higher in women than in men undergoing stenting, outcomes have significantly improved in women and the established benefits of elective stenting appear to be generalizable to women.

Results of drug-eluting stents in women

With the recent approval of the Sirolimus-eluting Cyper Stent (Cordis, Johnson and Johnson) based on the SIRIUS trial[92] and the Paclitaxel-eluting TAXUS stent (Boston Scientific) based on the TAXUS IV trial,[93] crude estimates of market penetration approach 60%. Both the Sirius trial and the TAXUS IV trials have demonstrated that the overall benefi-

cial effects of these devices in reducing restenosis are generalizable to the female patient.

The TAXUS IV trial randomized 1314 patients to the TAXUS stent (477 men and 185 women) versus the EXPRESS bare metal stent (477 men and 180 women). Women in the TAXUS group were older, had more hypertension, diabetes, baseline renal insufficiency, unstable angina, and prior congestive heart failure, and fewer women were smokers compared with men. At 9 months women treated with TAXUS had a higher rate of target lesion revascularization (TLR) (6% vs 1.9%, p = 0.007) and target vessel revascularization (TVR) (3.2% vs 8.7%, p = 0.003) compared with TAXUS-treated men. Female gender was not an independent predictor of either TLR (OR 1.72, 95% CI 0.68, 4.37) or TVR (OR 0.89; 95% CI 0.41–1.97). Important independent predictors of TVR included reference vessel diameter (OR 0.36, 95% CI 0.14–0.91, p = 0.03), diabetes (OR 2.54, 95% CI 1.28–5.07, p = 0.008), and body surface area (OR 0.13, 95% CI 0.02–0.84, p = 0.321). In the angiographic subset, restenosis rates were similar for women and men.

There were no sex differences in short- or long-term mortality. For women, treatment with the TAXUS stent reduced restenosis by 71% (8.2% TAXUS vs 29.6% control, p = 0.001) compared with the bare metal stent, and the only independent predictor of restenosis at follow-up for women was randomization to the TAXUS stent (OR 0.42 95% CI 0.11–0.74, p = 0.010). The TAXUS trial demonstrates that the overall beneficial effects of the TAXUS stent in reducing restenosis are generalizable to female patients.

In contrast to the previously mentioned published registry results that generally show lower revascularization rates in women than men, the higher TVR rates in women relative to men in TAXUS IV were independently adjudicated ischemia-driven TVR rates in the setting of a controlled trial with systematic clinical and angiographic follow-up, thus eliminating the potential for referral bias. Based on regression analysis, the independent predictors of TVR were not sex-specific but the consequence of confounders in women including a 42% higher frequency of diabetes, the smaller body surface area and small vessel size; parameters known to increase the risk of revascularization.

Table 19.4 Invasive versus conservative strategy for UA/NSTEMI

Study*	Setting	Endpoint	Overall result	Results in men	Results in women	Comment
TACTICS TIMI 18[94] 2001 n = 2220 34% female	UA/NSTEMI PCI 4–48 h inv	Death, MI, rehospitalization at 30 days	Inv: 7.4% Cons: 10.5% (p = 0.009) 6 months Inv: 15.9% Cons: 19.4% OR = 0.78 (0.62–0.97) p = 0.025	6 months Inv: 15.3% Cons: 19.4% OR = 0.64 (0.47–0.88)	Inv: 17.0% Cons: 19.6% 6 months Inv: 17.0% Cons: 19.6% OR = 0.72 (0.47–1.11)	
RITA 3[95] 2002 n = 1810 38% female	NSTE-ACS	Death, MI, refractory angina at 4 months	Inv: 9.6% Cons: 14.5% p = 0.001	Inv: 8.8% Cons: 17.3%	Inv: 9.6% Cons: 10.9% p = NS	Benefit greater in women with high troponin-T levels OR = 0.47 (0.26–0.83)
		Death, MI at 1 year	Inv: 7.6% Cons: 8.3% p = 0.6	Inv: 7.0% Cons: 10.1	Inv: 8.6%% Cons: 5.1%	
FRISC II[96] 1999 n = 2457 30% female	PCI after 6 days med treatment. No routine GPs	Death, MI at 6 months	Inv: 9.4% Cons: 12.1% p = 0.03		Inv: 10.5% Cons: 8.3% OR = 1.26 (0.80–1.97)	Gender interaction p = 0.011
		Death, MI at 1 year	Inv: 10.4% Cons: 14.1% p = 0.005	Inv: 9.6% Cons: 15.8% p <0.001	Inv: 12.4% Cons: 10.5%	
TIMI IIIB[97] 1995 n = 1423 34% female	UA/NQMI Randomized to tPA or placebo	Death, MI at 1 year	Inv: 12.2% Cons: 10.8% p = 0.4	Death at 6 weeks Inv: 2.6% Cons: 1.4%	Death at 6 weeks Inv: 2% Cons: 4.4% (p = NS)	Benefit not sustained at 1 year
				MI at 6 weeks Inv: 5.5% Cons: 6.0%	MI at 6 weeks Inv: 4.4% Cons: 5.2%	

UA, unstable angina; NSTEMI, non-ST-segment elevation myocardial infarction; PCI, percutaneous coronary intervention; inv, invasive; NSTE, non-ST-segment elevation; ACS, acute coronary syndrome; NQMI, non-Q-wave myocardial infarction; tPA, tissue plasminogen activator; MI, myocardial infarction; cons, conservative; OR, odds ratio; NS, not significant.
*See reference for explanation of study/registry acronym.

Treatment of acute coronary syndromes in women (see also Chapters 17 and 18)

In the context of acute coronary syndromes (ACS) defined as unstable angina or nonST elevation MI, the optimal strategy for the treatment of women remains controversial (Table 19.4).[94–97] The TACTICS TIMI-18 (Treat Angina with Aggrastat and determine Cost of Therapy with an Invasive or Conservative Strategy – Thrombolysis in Myocardial Infarction 18) study showed that women benefited from an aggressive early invasive strategy with glycoprotein IIb/IIIa inhibitor use, early catheterization, and coronary intervention with stenting when necessary.[94] The TACTICS TIMI-18 trial randomly assigned 2220 patients (757 women and 1463 men) to an early invasive treatment with cardiac catheterization within 48 hours of presentation versus a conservative medical strategy with catheterization and revascularization when necessary. In this study, women assigned to the early invasive strategy had a lower rate of death, MI or rehospitalization for ACS (OR 0.72, 95% CI 0.47–1.11) than men. The benefit of the invasive treatment was even greater among women with elevated troponin-T levels (OR 0.47, 95% CI 0.26–0.83). The benefits of early invasive interventional treatment (within 24 hours) of women presenting with ACS was corroborated in a registry of 1450 patients, where the death and MI rates at a mean of 20 months were superior in women compared with men (7% vs 10.5%, OR 0.65, 95% CI 0.42–0.99).[98] In contrast, the Fragmin and Fast Revascularization during Instability in Coronary heart disease (FRISC II) trial, which compared an early invasive strategy with catheterization within 7 days to a conservative strategy, did not demonstrate benefit of the early invasive strategy in women, whereas it did in the male patients.[96] FRISC II enrolled 2457 patients (749 women and 1708 men). There was no difference in the 12-month death and MI rate for women in the invasive versus noninvasive groups (12.4% vs 10.5%, p = NS), in contrast to the favorable effect in the invasively treated group of men (9.6% vs 15.8%, p <0.001). The difference between women and men was significant (women did worse with invasive treatment compared with men (p = 0.008). Perhaps the delayed timing of intervention (7 days) in the invasive

arm of the FRISC II study compared with TACTICS TIMI-18 (<48 hours) may explain some of the disparity in outcomes for women. Nonetheless evidence would suggest that women presenting with nonST segment elevation MI benefit from an early aggressive interventional strategy.[95,97]

Primary angioplasty for acute MI in women

The primary angioplasty in acute myocardial infarction (PAMI) trial,[99] which randomized 395 patients (73% men and 27% women) to angioplasty or thrombolysis with tissue plasminogen activator, was the first randomized trial to directly compare the outcomes of primary PTCA to thrombolyis and to demonstrate the benefit of primary angioplasty in women. As in all other studies, women in PAMI were older (66 vs 58 years old, p <0.001), had more hypertension (54% vs 39%, p = 0.005), and diabetes (19% vs 10%, p = 0.03), and on average presented to the emergency room 1 hour later than male patients (3.8 vs 2.9 hours, p = 0.0004). Overall, the in-hospital mortality was significantly greater for women than men (9.3% vs 2.8%, p = 0.005), as was the rate of hemorrhagic stroke (2.8% vs 0.3%, p = 0.03). The high death rate among women was mainly attributable to the use of thrombolytic therapy (14% lytic vs 4.0% PTCA, p = 0.07), and there were no strokes among women treated with PTCA. These findings and other nonrandomized studies of primary angioplasty strongly support this modality as the preferred treatment for women with acute MI (AMI).

In 'real world' clinical practice, important differences between women and men undergoing primary coronary intervention for AMI have been identified (Table 19.5).[14,15,86,100–103] A total of 1044 patients (317 women and 727 men) underwent primary angioplasty for AMI in the state of New York in 1995.[101] Women had more hypertension (59% vs 44%, p <0.05), more diabetes (19% vs 14%, p <0.05), and more peripheral vascular disease (9.5% vs 5.5%, p <0.05). Men were more likely to be treated sooner (within 6 hours of symptom onset) than women (74% vs 63%, p <0.05); women had more cardiogenic shock and hemodynamic instability than men (25% vs 17%, p <0.05) and a significantly higher in-

Table 19.5 Mortality rates for women and men after primary PCI for acute myocardial infarction

Study/registry*	Device/setting	In-hospital mortality	Adjusted OR (95% CI)
ACC-NCDR[100] 1998–2001 n = 59 792 32% female	PCI	Men 3.1% Women 5.4% p <0.01	1.32 (1.19–1.46)
Watanabe[14] 1997 n = 36 765 36% female	Stents	Men 2.0% Women 4.0% p <0.0001	1.47 (1.23–1.75)
CARS[101] 1995 n = 1044 30% female	PCI	Men 2.3% Women 7.9% p <0.05	2.33 (1.2–4.6) p = 0.02
Late mortality Mehilli[21] 1995–2000 n = 1937 26% female	PCI + lytics	Men 12.9% Women 13.8% Follow-up: 1 year	HR after age adjustment 0.65 (0.49–0.8) p = 0.004
CADILLAC[86] 1997–1999 n = 2082 27% female	Balloon vs stent	Men 3.0% Women 7.8% p <0.0001 Follow-up: 1 year	1.04 (0.49–2.19) p = 0.9
Stent-PAMI[102] 1999 (pub date) n = 900 30% female	Balloon vs stent	Men 2.0% Women 7.9% p <0.0002 Follow-up: 6 months	
Antoniucci[103] 1995–1999 n = 1019 23% female	PTCA + stent	Men 7.0% Women 12.0% p = 0.03 Follow-up: 6 months	1.05 (0.65–1.72) p = 0.7

PCI, percutaneous coronary intervention; OR, odds ratio; CI, confidence interval; AMI, acute myocardial infarction; PTCA, percutaneous transluminal coronary angioplasty; HR, hazard ratio; BSA, body surface area.
*See reference for explanation of study/registry acronym.

hospital mortality (7.9% vs 2.3%, p <0.05). The differences in mortality persisted even after adjustment for all these differences (OR 2.3, 95% CI 1.2–4.6). Thus, while primary angioplasty is preferred over thrombolysis, women still experience greater delays and have a worse outcome than men.

Outcomes after primary stenting in women

Primary balloon angioplasty has been shown to improve outcomes in women;[99] however, mortality and restenosis rates remain high.[101,104] Whether further improvement of outcomes in women can be achieved with contemporary interventional techniques including stent implantation and glycoprotein IIb/IIIa inhibitors has been the focus of recent study.

The Stent PAMI Trial was the first randomized clinical trial to evaluate the use of primary stenting for AMI compared with conventional primary angioplasty.[106] Nine hundred patients (70% men, 30% men) were randomized to the heparin-coated stent (n = 452) versus PTCA (n = 448). While the primary endpoint of the study favored the heparin-coated stent with a reduction in major adverse events (17% vs 24%, p <0.01), mortality at 1 year tended to be higher in patients treated with primary stenting (5.8% vs 3.0%, p = 0.54). For women, mortality after 6 months was significantly worse than for men (7.6% vs 1.9%, p <0.0001), and the highest mortality was among women treated with stent implantation.[105] Thus based on the results of stent PAMI, the optimal treatment for women with AMI remained primary angioplasty rather than the heparin-coated stent.

The subsequent CADILLAC trial,[102,106] a trial of 2665 patients with AMI randomized to the MultiLink stent (Guidant, Santa Clara, CA) or PTCA, and abciximab or placebo, demonstrated that primary stenting with or without the glycoprotein IIb/IIIa inhibitor abciximab is the optimal reperfusion strategy for patients presenting with AMI. A gender-based analysis of the CADILLAC trial demonstrated that women had a higher mortality than men at 30 days and 1 year, independent of interventional modality and despite higher baseline and final TIMI grade 3 flow rates.[107] A multivariate analysis confirmed that the prevalence of higher risk factors (e.g. diabetes, hypertension, and hyperlipidemia) in the female population only partially explained the poor outcomes of women: female gender was an independent predictor of 1-year major adverse cardiac events (MACE) and death. Despite the worse outcome for women, the study also demonstrated that primary stent implantation resulted in better clinical and angiographic outcomes for women, independent of abciximab use. The MultiLink stent reduced the incidence of ischemic target revascularization by 9.6% and major adverse cardiac events by 9% in women compared with PTCA without any impact on death, MI, or stroke. The conclusions of the CADILLAC trial are therefore generalizable to the female patient population as well: stent implantation should be considered the optimal reperfusion strategy for women presenting with AMI. Despite the improvement in outcomes with stent compared with traditional PTCA, women with AMI still have a relatively poor prognosis with a higher risk of mortality and MACE both short- and long-term, independent of elevated baseline risk factors, compared with men (Table 19.5). Considering the prevalence of MI in the female population, a continued search for new adjunctive approaches is required to address the gender gap in AMI outcomes.

Vascular complications

Based on studies from the 1990s, vascular complications were three to four times more frequent in women than men, likely due to the aggressive anticoagulation regimen and the infrequent use of weight-adjusted heparin dosing at the time (Table 19.6).[12,15,18,19,21,22,27,28,30–32,103] In addition, sheath size has rarely been adjusted during intervention in female patients despite the smaller body size. This practice has now evolved with use of smaller sheath sizes due to the smaller profile of newer third- and fourth-generation devices. With the advent of adjunctive pharmacology with glycoprotein IIb/IIIa inhibitors, weight-adjusted heparin is now an accepted practice. Whether these changes in practice have made an impact on vascular complication rates requires further study. This complication adds significantly to the hospitalization duration and costs and studies evaluating adjustments of sheath size to body size and weight-adjusted anticoagulation regimens are needed to determine the best strategy to minimize this complication.

Conclusions

Coronary disease is the leading cause of mortality for women in the US and has been since the turn of the century. Most studies comparing the outcomes after coronary intervention of women and men have demonstrated worse outcomes in women, with approximately 30% of this difference attributable to delayed presentation and the associated risk factors in women. Much of the focus of published studies in women has been comparisons to outcomes in men, and the generally worse outcomes may have led, to a certain extent, to the treatment disparities facing women. Clinical trials focusing on treatment alternatives in women have demonstrated improvements in outcomes with advances in technologies and contemporary therapies such as stenting and drug-

Table 19.6 Vascular complications in women and men after PCI

Study/registry*	Device/setting	Vascular complications
NHLBI[22] 1997–1998 n = 2524 35% female	PCI Case mix	Men 2.6% Women 5.0% p ≤0.001
NHLBI[20] 1985–1986 n = 2136 26% female	PTCA Case mix	Men 2.3% Women: 4.4% p <0.05
Lansky[13] 1991–1996 n = 7372 28% female	NDA	Men 2.4% Women 3.8% p <0.001
Alfonso[17] 1990–1997 n = 981 16% female	Stent	Men 2.0% Women 7.0% p <0.01
Welty[19] 1989–1995 n = 5989 35% female	PTCA 55–63% UA 8% AMI	Men 0.6% Women 1.6% p <0.001
Antoniucci[103] 1995–1999 n = 1019 23% female	PTCA + stent for AMI	Men 3.0% Women 6.0% p = 0.01
Trabattoni[23] 1992–1998 n = 1100 15% female	Elective stent	Men 3.5% Women 9.3% p <0.004
NACI[28] 1996 n = 2855 34% female	NDA Stents, laser, rotablator Elective	Men 1.5% Women 4.0% p <0.05
NCN[29] 1994–1997 n = 109 708 33% female	PCI 40% stent 8% atherectomy	Men 2.7% Women 5.4% p <0.001
CAVEAT[31] 1995 n = 512 25% female	DCA	Men 5.8% Women 10.8% p = 0.003
BOAT[32] 1998 n = 989 24% female	DCA vs PTCA	Men 0.8% Women 2.5% p = 0.05
STARS[33] 1998 n = 1965 29% female	Stent	Men 2.8% Women 7.8% p <0.001

PCI, percutaneous coronary intervention; PTCA, percutaneous transluminal coronary angioplasty; NDA, new device angioplasty; UA, unstable angina; AMI, acute myocardial infarction; DCA, directional coronary atherectomy.
*See reference for explanation of study/registry acronym.

eluting stents, achieving excellent results in this population. All efforts should be focused on the proper screening, prevention, diagnosis, and referral for treatment of women with CHD in order to impact the increasing mortality trends facing this high-risk population.

References

1. American Heart Association. *Heart Disease and Stroke Statistics*: *2004 Update*. Dallas, TX: American Heart Association, 2003.

2. Lansky AJ, Hochman JS, Ward PA, et al. Percutaneous coronary intervention and adjunctive pharmacotherapy in women. A statement for health care professionals from the American Heart Association. *Circulation* 2005; **111**:940–53.

3. Ayanian JZ, Epstein AM. Differences in the use of procedures between women and men hospitalized for coronary disease. *N Engl J Med* 1991; **325**:221–5.

4. Shaw LJ, Miller DD, Romeis JC, Kargl D, Younis LT, Chaitman BR. Gender differences in the noninvasive evaluation and management of patients with suspected coronary heart disease. *Ann Intern Med* 1994; **120**:559–66.

5. Lauer MS, Pashkow FJ, Snader CE, Harvey SA, Thomas JD, Marwick TH. Gender and referral for coronary angiography after treadmill thallium testing. *Am J Cardiol* 1996; **78**:278–83.

6. Mark DB, Shaw LK, DeLong ER, Califf RM, Pryor DB. Absence of sex bias in the referral of patients for cardiac catheterization. *N Engl J Med* 1994; **330**:1101–6.

7. Wong Y, Rodwell A, Dawkins S, Livesey SA, Simpson IA. Sex differences in investigation results and treatment in subjects referred for investigation of chest pain. *Heart* 2001; **85**:149–52.

8. Schulman KA, Berlin JA, Harless W, et al. The effect of race and sex on physicians' recommendations for cardiac catheterization. *N Engl J Med* 1999; **340**:618–26.

9. Roeters van Lennep JE, Zwinderman AH, Roeters van Lennep HW, et al. Gender differences in diagnosis and treatment of coronary heart disease from 1981 to 1997. No evidence for the Yentl syndrome. *Eur Heart J* 2000; **21**:911–18.

10. Bell MR, Berger PB, Holmes DR Jr, Mullany CJ, Bailey KR, Gersh BJ. Referral for coronary artery revascularization procedures after diagnostic coronary angiography: evidence for gender bias? *J Am Coll Cardiol* 1995; **25**:1650–5.

11. Ghali WA, Faris PD, Galbraith PD, et al. Sex differences in access to coronary revascularization after cardiac catheterization: importance of detailed clinical data. *Ann Intern Med* 2002; **136**:723–32.

12. Anderson HV, Shaw RE, Brindis RG, et al. A contemporary overview of percutaneous coronary interventions. The American College of Cardiology-National Cardiovascular Data Registry (ACC-NCDR). *J Am Coll Cardiol* 2002; **39**:1096–103.

13. Lansky AJ, Mehran R, Dangas G, et al. New-device angioplasty in women: clinical outcome and predictors in a 7,372-patient registry. *Epidemiology* 2002; **13** (3 Suppl):S46–51.

14. Watanabe CT, Maynard C, Ritchie JL. Comparison of short-term outcomes following coronary artery stenting in men versus women. *Am J Cardiol* 2001; **88**:848–52.

15. Malenka K, Wennberg DE, Quinton HA, et al. Gender related changes in the practice and outcomes of percutaneous coronary intervention in Northern New England from 1994 to 1999. *J Am Coll Cardiol* 2002; **40**:2092–101.

16. Lansky AJ, Popma JJ, Mehran R, et al. Tubular slotted stents: a 'breakthrough therapy' for women undergoing coronary interventions. Pooled results from the STARS, ACSENT, SMART, and NIRVANA randomized clinical trials. *J Am Coll Cardiol* 1999; **33**:58A.

17. Alfonso F, Hernandez R, Banuelos C, et al. Initial results and long-term clinical and angiographic outcome of coronary stenting in women. *Am J Cardiol* 2000; **86**:1380–3.

18. Bell MR, Holmes DR, Berger PB, Garratt KN, Bailey KR, Gersh BJ. The changing in-hospital mortality of women undergoing percutaneous transluminal coronary angioplasty. *JAMA* 1993; **269**:2091–5.

19. Welty FK, Lewis SM, Kowalker W, Shubrooks SJ Jr. Reasons for higher in-hospital mortality >24 hours after percutaneous transluminal coronary angioplasty in women compared with men. *Am J Cardiol* 2001; **88**:473–7.

20. Kelsey SF, Miller DP, Holubkov R, et al. Results of percutaneous transluminal coronary angioplasty in patients greater than or equal to 65 years of age (from the 1985 to 1986 National Heart, Lung, and Blood Institute's Coronary Angioplasty Registry). *Am J Cardiol* 1990; **66**:1033–8.

21. Mehilli J, Kastrati A, Dirschinger J, Bollwein H, Neumann FJ, Schomig A. Differences in prognostic factors and outcomes between women and men undergoing coronary artery stenting. *JAMA* 2000; **284**:1799–805.

22. Jacobs AK, Johnston JM, Haviland A, et al. Improved outcomes for women undergoing contemporary percutaneous coronary intervention. *J Am Coll Cardiol* 2002; **39**:1608–14.

23. Trabattoni D, Bartorelli AL, Montorsi P, et al. Comparison of outcomes in women and men treated with coronary stent implantation. *Catheter Cardiovasc Interv* 2003; **58**:20–8.

24. Weintraub WS, Wenger NK, Kosinski AS, et al. Percutaneous transluminal coronary angioplasty in women compared with men. *J Am Coll Cardiol* 1994; **24**:81–90.

25. McEniery PT, Hollman J, Knezinek V, et al. Comparative safety and efficacy of percutaneous transluminal coronary angioplasty in men and in women. *Cathet Cardiovasc Diagn* 1987; **13**:364–71.

26. Arnold AM, Mick MJ, Piedmonte MR, Simpfendorfer C. Gender differences for coronary angioplasty. *Am J Cardiol* 1994; **74**:18–21.

27. Bell MR, Grill DE, Garratt KN, Berger PB, Gersh BJ, Holmes DR. Long-term outcome of women compared with men after successful coronary angioplasty. *Circulation* 1995; **91**:2876–81.

28. Robertson T, Kennard E, Mehta S, et al. Influence of gender on in-hospital clinical and angiographic outcomes and on one-year follow-up in the new approaches to coronary intervention (NACI) registry. *Am J Cardiol* 1997; **80**:26K–39K.

29. Foley DP, Melkert R, Serruys PW. Influence of coronary vessel size on renarrowing process and late angiographic outcome after successful balloon angioplasty. *Circulation* 1994; **90**:1239–51.

30. Bell MR, Garratt KN, Bresnahan JF, Holmes DR Jr. Immediate and long-term outcome after directional coronary atherectomy: analysis of gender differences. *Mayo Clin Proc* 1994; **69**:723–9.

31. Omoigui NA, Califf RM, Pieper K, et al. Peripheral vascular complications in the Coronary Angioplasty Versus Excisional Atherectomy Trial (CAVEAT-I). *J Am Coll Cardiol* 1995; **26**:922–30.

32. Baim DS, Cutlip DE, Sharma SK, et al. Final results of the Balloon vs Optimal Atherectomy Trial (BOAT). *Circulation* 1998; **97**:322–31.

33. Leon MB, Baim DS, Popma JJ, et al. A clinical trial comparing three antithrombotic-drug regimens after coronary-artery stenting. Stent Anticoagulation Restenosis Study Investigators. *N Engl J Med* 1998; **339**:1665–71.

34. Wingard DL, Cohn BA, Kaplan GA, Cirillo PM, Cohen RD. Sex differentials in morbidity and mortality risks examined by age and cause in the same cohort. *Am J Epidemiol* 1989; **130**:601–10.

35. Lerner DJ, Kannel WB. Patterns of coronary heart disease morbidity and mortality in sexes: a 26-year follow-up of the Framingham population. *Am Heart J* 1986; **111**:383–90.

36. Wenger NK. Gender, coronary heart disease, and coronary bypass surgery. *Ann Intern Med* 1990; **112**:557–8.

37. Greenland P, Reicher-Reiss H, Goldburt U, Behar S, Investigators and the Israeli SPRINT. In hopital and 1 year mortality in 1,524 women after myocardial infarction. Comparison with 4,315 men. *Circulation* 1991; **83**:484–91.

38. Vaccarino V, Krumholz HM, Berkman LF, Horwitz RI. Sex differences in mortality after myocardial infarction. Is there evidence for an increased risk for women? *Circulation* 1995; **91**:1861–71.

39. Becker RC, Terrin M, Ross R, et al. Comparisons of clinical outcomes for women and men after acute myocardial infarction. *Ann Intern Med* 1994; **120**:638–45.

40. Goldberg RJ, Gorak EJ, Yarzebski J, et al. A community wide perspective of sex differences and temporal trends in the incidence and survival rates after acute myocardial infarction and out-of-hospital deaths caused by coronary heart disease. *Circulation* 1993; **87**:1947–53.

41. Wong ND, Cupples LA, Ostfeld AM, Levy D, Kannel WB. Risk factors for long term coronary prognosis after initial myocardial infarction: the Framingham study. *Am J Epidemiol* 1989; **130**:469–80.

42. Pohjola S, Siltman P, Romo M. Five year survival of 728 patients after acute myocardial infarction: a community study. *Br Heart J* 1980; **43**:176–83.

43. Tofler GH, Stone PH, Muller JE, et al. Effect of gender and race on prognosis after myocardial infarction: adverse prognosis for women, particularly black women. *J Am Coll Cardiol* 1987; **9**:473–82.

44. Dittrich H, Gilpin E, Nicod P, Cali G, Henning H, Ross J Jr. Acute myocardial infarction in women: influence of gender on mortality and prognostic variables. *Am J Cardiol* 1988; **62**:1–7.

45. Kornowski R, Goldburt U, Boyko V, Behar S. Clinical predictors of reinfarction among women and men after a first myocardial infarction. *Cardiology* 1995; **86**:163–8.

46. Welty FK, Mittleman MA, Healy RW, Muller JE, Shubrooks SJ Jr. Similar results of percutaneous transluminal coronary angioplasty for women and men with postmyocardial infarction ischemia. *J Am Coll Cardiol* 1994; **23**:35–9.

47. Kelsey SF, James M, Holubkov R, Cowley MJ, Detre KM. Results of percutaneous transluminal coronary angioplasty in women. 1985–1986 National Heart, Lung, and Blood Institute's Coronary Angioplasty Registry. *Circulation* 1993; **87**:720–7.

48. Ilia R, Bigham H, Brennan J, Cabin H, Cleman M,

Remetz M. Predictors of coronary dissection following percutaneous transluminal coronary balloon angioplasty. *Cardiology* 1994; **85**:229–34.

49. Ellis SG, Ajluni S, Arnold AZ, et al. Increased coronary perforation in the new device era. Incidence, classification, management, and outcome. *Circulation* 1994; **90**:2725–30.

50. Taddei CF, Weintraub WS, Douglas JS Jr, et al. Influence of age on outcome after percutaneous transluminal coronary angioplasty. *Am J Cardiol* 1999; **84**:245–51.

51. Kofflard MJ, de Jaegere PP, van Domburg R, et al. Immediate and long-term clinical outcome of coronary angioplasty in patients aged 35 years or less. *Br Heart J* 1995; **73**:82–6.

52. Stone GW, Ligon RW, Rutherford BD, McConahay DR, Hartzler GO. Short-term outcome and long-term follow-up following coronary angioplasty in the young patient: an 8-year experience. *Am Heart J* 1989; **118**:873–7.

53. Vaccarino V, Parsons L, Every NR, Barron HV, Krumholz HM. Sex-based differences in early mortality after myocardial infarction. National Registry of Myocardial Infarction 2 Participants. *N Engl J Med* 1999; **341**:217–25.

54. Lytle BW, Kramer JR, Golding LR, et al. Young adults with coronary atherosclerosis: 10 year results of surgical myocardial revascularization. *J Am Coll Cardiol* 1984; **4**:445–53.

55. Lansky AJ, Mehran R, Dangas G, et al. Comparison of differences in outcome after percutaneous coronary intervention in men-vs-women less than 40 years of age. *Am J Cardiol* 2004; **93**:916–19.

56. Barrett-Connor E, Cohn B, Wingard D, Edelstein S. Why is diabetes mellitus a stronger risk factor for fatal ischemic heart disease in women than in men? *JAMA* 1991; **265**:627–31.

57. Brezinka V, Padmos I. Coronary heart disease risk factors in women. *Eur Heart J* 1994; **15**:1571–84.

58. Vaccarino V, Parsons L, Every NR, Barron HV, Krumholz HM. Impact of history of diabetes mellitus on hospital mortality in women and men with first acute myocardial infarction. The National Registry of Myocardial Infraction 2 Participants. *Am J Cardiol* 2000; **85**:1486–9.

59. DeStefano F, Newman J. Comparison of coronary heart disease mortality risk between black and white people with diabetes. *Ann Intern Med* 2001; **134**:173–81.

60. Kornowski R, Mintz GS, Kent KM, et al. Increased restenosis in diabetes mellitus after coronary interventions is due to exaggerated intimal hyperplasia. A serial intravascular ultrasound study. *Circulation* 1997; **95**:1366–9.

61. Kornowski R, Lansky A, Mintz G, et al. Comparison of women and men in cross-sectional area luminal narrowing, quantity of plaque, and lumen location in coronary arteries by intravascular ultrasound in patients with stable angina pectoris. *Am J Cardiol* 1997; **79**:1601–5.

62. Dodge, JT, G Brown, EL Bolson, Dodge HT. Lumen diameter of normal human coronary arteries. Influence of age, sex, anatomic variation, and left ventricular hypertrophy or dilation. *Circulation* 1992; **86**:232–46.

63. Di Carli MF, Afonso L, Campisi R, et al. Coronary vascular dysfunction in premenopausal women with diabetes mellitus. *Am Heart J* 2002; **144**:711–18.

64. MacAlpin RN, Abbasi AS, Grollman JH, Eber L. Human coronary artery size during life: a cine arteriographic study. *Radiology* 1973; **108**:567–76.

65. Roberts CS, Roberts WC. Cross-sectional area of the proximal portions of the three major epicardial coronary arteries in 98 necropsy patients with different coronary events: relationship to heart weight, age, and sex. *Circulation* 1980; **62**:953–9.

66. Cantor WJ, Miller JM, Hellkamp AS, et al. Vessel size, body surface area, and outcomes following percutaneous coronary intervention in women. *Am Heart J* 2002; **144**:297–302.

67. Deupree RH, Fields RI, McMahan CA, Strong JP. Atherosclerotic lesions and coronary heart disease: key relationships in necropsied cases. *Lab Invest* 1973; **28**:252–62.

68. Daoud AS, Florentin RA, Goodale F. Diffuse coronary atherosclerosis versus isolated plaques in the etiology of myocardial infarction. *Am J Cardiol* 1964; **13**:69–74.

69. Goffman JW. The quantitative nature of the relationship of coronary atherosclerosis and coronary heart disease. *Cardiol Digest* 1969; **4**:28–38.

70. Kagan AR, Vemura K. Atherosclerosis of the aorta and coronary arteries in five towns. Material and methods. *Bull World Health Organ* 1976; **53**:485–645.

71. Nabulsi AA, Folsom AR, White A. Association of hormone-replacement therapy with various cardiovascular risk factors in post-menopausal women. *N Engl J Med* 1993 **328**:1069–75.

72. Meade TW, Mellows S, Brozovic M. Haemostatic function and ischaemic heart disease: principal results of the Northwick Park heart study. *Lancet* 1986; **2**:533–7.

73. Roberts JW, Goldshmidt-Clermont PJ, Bray P, et al. Effect of gender on thrombogenic factors in asympto-

matic people at high risk for coronary heart disease. *Circulation* 1994; **90** (Suppl I):I-283

74. Cowley MJ, Mullin SM, Kelsey SF, et al. Sex differences in early and long-term results of coronary angioplasty in the NHLBI PTCA Registry. *Circulation* 1985; **71**:90–7.

75. Paul SD, Eagle KA, Guidry U, et al. Do gender-based differences in presentation and management influence predictors of hospitalization costs and length of stay after an acute myocardial infarction? *Am J Cardiol* 1995; **76**:1122–5.

76. Behar S, Gottlieb S, Hod H, et al. Influence of gender in the therapeutic management of patients with acute myocardial infarction in Israel. The Israeli Thrombolytic Survey Group. *Am J Cardiol* 1994; **73**:438–43.

77. Chiriboga DE, Yarzebski J, Goldberg RJ, et al. A community-wide perspective of gender differences and temporal trends in the use of diagnostic and revascularization procedures for acute myocardial infarction. *Am J Cardiol* 1993; **71**:268–73.

78. Giacomini MK. Gender and ethnic differences in hospital-based procedure utilization in California. *Arch Intern Med* 1996; **156**:1217–24.

79. Kudenchuk PJ, Maynard C, Martin JS, Wirkus M, Weaver WD. Comparison of presentation, treatment, and outcome of acute myocardial infarction in men versus women (the Myocardial Infarction Triage and Intervention Registry). *Am J Cardiol* 1996; **78**:9–14.

80. Ruygrok PN, de Jagere PP, van Domburg RT, van den Brand MJ, Serruys PW, de Feyter PJ. Women fare no worse than men 10 years after attempted coronary angioplasty. *Cathet Cardiovasc Diagn* 1996; **39**:9–15.

81. Keelan ET, Nunez BD, Grill DE, Berger PB, Holmes DR, Bell MR. Comparison of immediate and long-term outcome of coronary angioplasty performed for unstable angina and rest pain in women and men. *Mayo Clin Proc* 1997; **72**:5–12.

82. Lansky AJ. Outcomes of percutaneous and surgical revascularization in women. *Prog Cardiovasc Dis* 2004; **46**:305–19.

83. Mehilli J, Kastrati A, Bollwein H, et al. Gender and restenosis after coronary artery stenting. *Eur Heart J* 2003; **24**:1523–30.

84. Moriel M, Feld S, Almagor Y, et al. Results of coronary artery stenting in women versus men: single center experience. *Isr Med Assoc J* 2003; **5**:398–402.

85. Fishman RF, Kuntz RE, Carrozza JP, et al. Long-term results of directional coronary atherectomy: predictors of restenosis. *J Am Coll Cardiol* 1992; **20**:1101–10.

86. Carrozza JP Jr, Kuntz RE, Levine MJ, et al. Angiographic and clinical outcome of intracoronary stenting: immediate and long-term results from a large single-center experience. *J Am Coll Cardiol* 1992; **20**:328–37.

87. Kuntz RE, Safian RD, Carroza JP, Fishman RF, Mansour M, Baim DS. The importance of the acute luminal diameter in determining restenosis after coronary atherectomy or stenting. *Circulation* 1992; **86**:1827–35.

88. Dussaillant GR, Mintz GS, Pichard AD, et al. Small sent size and intimal hyperplasia contribute to restenosis: a volumetric intravascular ultrasound analysis. *J Am Coll Cardiol* 1995; **26**:720–4.

89. Fishman D, Leon MB, Baim D, et al. A randomized comparison of coronary stent placement and balloon angioplasty in the treatment of coronary disease. *N Engl J Med* 1994; **331**:496–501.

90. Serruys P, de Jaeger P, Kiemeneji F, et al. A comparison of balloon expandable-stent implantation with balloon angioplasty in the treatment of coronary heart disease. *N Engl J Med* 1994; **331**:489–95.

91. Savage M, Fishman D, Rake R, et al. Efficacy of coronary stenting versus balloon angioplasty in small coronary arteries. *J Am Coll Cardiol* 1997; **31**:307–11.

92. Moses JW, Leon MB, Popma JJ, et al. Sirolimus-eluting stents versus standard stents in patients with stenosis in a native coronary artery. *N Engl J Med* 2003; **349**:1315–23.

93. Stone GW, Ellis SG, Cox DA, et al. A polymer-based, paclitaxel-eluting stent in patients with coronary heart disease. *N Engl J Med* 2004; **350**:221–31.

94. Glaser R, Herrmann HC, Murphy SA, et al. Benefit of an early invasive management strategy in women with acute coronary syndromes. *JAMA* 2002; **288**:3161–4.

95. Fox KA, Poole-Wilson PA, Henderson RA, et al. Interventional versus conservative treatment for patients with unstable angina or non-ST-elevation myocardial infarction: the British Heart Foundation RITA 3 randomised trial. Randomized Intervention Trial of unstable Angina. *Lancet* 2002; **360**:743–51.

96. Lagerqvist B, Safstrom K, Stahle E, et al. Is early invasive treatment of unstable coronary heart disease equally effective for both women and men? FRISC II study group investigators. *J Am Coll Cardiol* 2001; **38**:41–8.

97. Hochman JS, McCabe CH, Stone PH, et al. Outcome and profile of women and men presenting with acute coronary syndromes: a report from TIMI IIIB. TIMI Investigators. Thrombolysis in Myocardial Infarction. *J Am Coll Cardiol* 1997; **30**:141–8.

98. Mueller C, Neumann FJ, Roskamm H, et al. Women do have improved long-term outcome after non-ST elevation acute coronary syndromes treated very early and predominantly with percutaneous coronary

intervention: a prospective study in 1450 consecutive patients. *J Am Coll Cardiol* 2002; **40**:245–50.

99. Stone GW, Grines CL, Browne KF, et al. Implication of recurrent ischemia after reperfusion therapy in acute myocardial infarction: a comparison of thrombolytic therapy and primary angioplasty. *J Am Coll Cardiol* 1995; **26**:66–72.

100. Beinart SC, Vaccarino V, Abramson JL, Hewitt K, Weintraub WS. Effect of gender according to age on in-hospital mortality in patients with acute myocardial infarction in the ACC-National Cardiovascular Data Registry. *J Am Coll Cardiol* 2003; **41** (Suppl A):540 [abstr].

101. Vakili BA, Kaplan RC, Brown DL. Sex-based differences in early mortality of patients undergoing primary angioplasty for first acute myocardial infarction. *Circulation* 2001; **104**:3034–8.

102. Stone GW, Garcia E, Giambartolomei A, et al. The powerful interaction between age and gender in determining short-term mortality after mechanical reperfusion therapy in acute myocardial infarction – insights from the PAMI stent randomized trial. *Circulation* 1998; **98**:785 [abstr].

103. Antoniucci D, Valenti R, Moschi G, et al. Sex-based differences in clinical and angiographic outcomes after primary angioplasty or stenting for acute myocardial infarction. *Am J Cardiol* 2001; **87**: 289–93.

104. Zijlstra F, Hoorntje JC, de Boer MJ, et al. Long-term benefit of primary angioplasty as compared with thrombolytic therapy for acute myocardial infarction. *N Engl J Med* 1999; **341**:1413–19.

105. Grines CL, Cox DA, Stone GW, et al., for the Stent Primary Angioplasty in Myocardial Infarction Study Group. Coronary angioplasty with or without stent implantation for acute myocardial infarction. *N Engl J Med* 1999; **34**:1949–56.

106. Stone GW, Grines CL, Cox DA, et al. Comparison of angioplasty with stenting, with or without abciximab, in acute myocardial infarction. *N Engl J Med* 2002; **346**:957–66.

107. Lansky AJ, Grines C, Desai K, et al. Primary stenting optimizes the outcome of women with acute myocardial infarction: results from the CADILLAC trial. *J Am Coll Cardiol* 2002; **39**:39 [abstr].

20

Coronary artery bypass graft surgery

Fred H. Edwards

Introduction

During the time when coronary artery bypass graft (CABG) surgery was first gaining widespread acceptance, several prominent heart centers found an increased operative mortality in women undergoing the procedure.[1-5] Over the following years, this finding has been substantiated in numerous studies.[6-13] Initially this gender difference in CABG mortality was attributed to the smaller coronary vessels of women and the attendant technical difficulty in creating anastomoses to these small vessels.[5,11,14-16] In more recent years, this logic has been challenged and other explanations have been offered. In particular, it has been shown that women present for CABG with more compelling co-morbid conditions as compared with men,[7-11,17,18] women are less likely to receive internal mammary artery (IMA) conduits,[8,11,17-22] and women receive fewer bypass grafts overall.[8,17,21,22] Several groups have reported a referral bias causing women to present for revascularization at a later stage in the disease process as compared with men.[6,17,18,23-25]

While some have investigated reasons for the excess mortality in women, others have challenged the true existence of this excess mortality. Of the groups reporting higher unadjusted CABG mortality rates in women, several have shown that statistical risk adjustment reveals an insignificant difference in mortality between risk-matched men and women.[11-13,26] Still other groups have shown no significant gender difference in mortality even when using raw, unadjusted data.[17,21,22,27]

These facts illustrate the extraordinarily controversial nature of gender issues in coronary artery surgery. Fortunately, the welcome rise in scientific and public interest in women's health over the last decade has done much to address these important controversies. While some aspects remain unresolved, there are some facts that have emerged to become well-accepted in all quarters.

Consistent observations

1. CABG is performed less frequently in women

Virtually all CABG series report a predominantly male population. Typically women make up between 20% and 30% of the CABG population. In the largest reported series, the Society of Thoracic Surgeons National Cardiac Surgery Database (STS Database) found that women made up 28% of the 344 913 patients undergoing CABG from 1994 through 1996.[8]

In the United States over the last two decades more women than men have died each year from cardiovascular disease.[28] That more men than women undergo CABG and percutaneous coronary revascularization,[21] then, seems counter-intuitive and invites speculation that revascularization may be underutilized in women. In spite of the increased awareness of the benefits of CABG in women, there has been little change in the proportion of women undergoing the procedure. O'Rourke et al.[29] examined the large experience of the Northern New England Cardiovascular Disease Study Group and found that the percentage of women undergoing CABG ranged from 26.6% in 1987–1989 to 27.7% in 1993–1997. On the other hand, Abramov et al.[22] found a modest increase in the proportion of women undergoing CABG, with a rise from 14% in 1989 to just over 20% in 1998.

2. In CABG patients, there are consistent gender differences in cardiac risk factors

There is universal agreement that gender differences exist in cardiac risk factors, and there is a striking consistency in the nature of those differences.

Coronary artery disease

Most authorities have found that women present with fewer diseased coronary vessels as compared with their male counterparts.[8,9,13,22,30] This logically accounts for at least part of the reason why women receive fewer bypass grafts than men.[8,21,22] Offsetting this observation, however, is the suggestion that women are actually less likely to have significant distal coronary disease.[31]

Left ventricular function

In spite of the fact that women generally have an increased incidence of co-morbidity, most studies show that the ejection fraction (EF) in women is higher than that of men undergoing CABG.[8,9,13,22,31] Logically, this might be at least partially attributable to the lesser degree of coronary insufficiency in women, but that has not been firmly established. Paradoxically, even though women generally have

higher EFs, women undergoing CABG consistently manifest more accentuated symptoms of congestive heart failure than men.[8,9,11,22,26,27,30–32] There have been no formal investigations of this paradox, but it may be important to note that at least one study[29] showed that women had higher left ventricular end-diastolic pressures in the face of better EF as compared with men.

3. In CABG patients, there are consistent gender differences in extra-cardiac risk factors

In the last decade, virtually every major study confirmed that women undergoing CABG have a higher incidence of diabetes mellitus. As compared with the male population, the female CABG population consistently has more than a 40% increase in the incidence of diabetes.[8,9,12,13,22,26] The association of diabetes with adverse postoperative outcomes is well known in many surgical specialties, but the sequelae in CABG operations are particularly devastating. There is a clear association with operative mortality[8,11,33] as well as mediastinitis and soft tissue wound infections.

The need for nonelective surgery is also considerably more common in women than in men. Once again, this seems paradoxical, since women generally have less coronary artery disease on preoperative angiography. There is some thought that there may be a gender difference in plaque physiology or endothelial dysfunction to account for plaque instability,[28] but this has not been fully investigated.

A less consistent, but common finding in most series is that tobacco abuse is more prevalent in the male population. Likewise, most studies report that the female population presenting for CABG is older than the male population.[32]

4. There is an inverse relationship between body surface area and CABG operative mortality

The issue of body surface area (BSA) has been central to discussions of gender differences in CABG surgery. Smaller coronary arteries unquestionably make for a more difficult anastomosis, thereby raising the probability of technical error and graft closure. This resultant compromised revascularization could then lead to ischemic events which would adversely impact operative mortality. An analysis from the STS Database[8] has shown convincingly that BSA was inversely related to operative mortality for a large multi-institutional population. The mortality of the smallest patients was approximately twice that of the largest patients. In that study, women had a higher operative mortality for each BSA group except for BSA <1.8 m[2], where there was a minimal difference in mortality between men and women.

Others have confirmed the inverse relationship between mortality and BSA.[11,15,16,29] There is little question that this relationship exists, but it may be simplistic to extrapolate this fact to conclude that women, being smaller, must have small coronary arteries and so are predisposed to graft failure. A recent study[31] found that women are no more likely than men to have native coronary vessels less than 1.5 mm in diameter. Furthermore, it appears that there may be only a minimal gender difference in CABG mortality when the procedure is performed without cardiopulmonary bypass (CPB).[18,34–36] Off-pump CABG (OPCAB) anastomoses are more technically demanding than those associated with conventional CABG. If, in fact, women generally have more challenging anastomoses then the more difficult OPCAB procedures would magnify the difference in outcomes. This has not been observed, thereby arguing against coronary size as a major factor.

5. Women have suboptimal use of bypass conduits

In virtually all major series,[8,11,13,17,18,21,22] women are less likely to receive an IMA conduit as compared with men. This is a particularly important observation, since the use of at least one IMA is unequivocally associated with both in-hospital and long-term improvement in CABG mortality.[37,38] The fact that this conduit is used less frequently in women clearly predisposes the female population to increased risk. There appears to be no satisfactory explanation for the underutilization of IMA grafts in women, except

possibly for the fact that women are more likely to undergo urgent and emergency operations.

Women also receive a fewer number of bypass grafts as compared with men.[8,11,13,17,18,21,22] This has often been attributed to differences in coronary vessel size and quality, but from the discussion above, one might challenge this explanation as being overly simplistic.

Outcomes of coronary artery bypass graft surgery

Operative mortality

Operative mortality has long been the central focus of gender issues in CABG surgery. For over two decades, numerous groups have sought to determine whether women undergoing CABG have a greater chance of dying than men. In the last decade, most physicians have come to recognize the essential need for some form of risk stratification to allow valid comparisons of risk-matched CABG patients. Accordingly, the question in the current era has become: among statistically risk-matched patients undergoing CABG, do women have a greater chance of dying than men? In a strictly biostatistical sense, the issue is whether gender is an independent risk factor for CABG operative mortality.

To examine this question, it is appropriate to focus on the more current studies of CABG surgery. Changes in the patient population as well as changes in operative technique indicate that it is probably not valid to extrapolate findings from reports earlier than the mid-1980s to the present clinical milieu. These early reports, however, did serve a valuable purpose in alerting the cardiovascular community to the possibility of an increased risk for women undergoing CABG. In response, several studies were initiated to specifically investigate this issue.

The 1992 study of the New York state experience[39] showed that gender was a significant independent predictor of CABG mortality for both crude and adjusted results. The following year O'Connor et al., using the Northern New England Cardiovascular Disease Study Group data,[11] reported that unadjusted mortality was higher for women (7.1% in women vs 3.3% for men), but when BSA was used in risk adjustment, sex was no longer significantly associated with mortality. In 1995 Carey et al.[12] found that the unadjusted mortality for women was higher than for men, but after adjusting for the presence of diabetes, there was no gender difference in mortality. The same year, Mickleborough et al.[17] published the first major series showing no gender difference in adjusted or nonadjusted CABG mortality. In contrast to most other reports, the female population in that study did not demonstrate an increase in the need for urgent surgery. Also contrasting with most other reports, the operations were performed by one surgeon.

In 1997 Hammar et al.[13] reported a large experience from Sweden. Findings were consistent with the O'Connor[11] study, in that the unadjusted mortality in women was approximately twice that of men, but after risk adjustment there was no significant difference in operative mortality. The Society of Thoracic Surgeons presented their experience from the STS Database in a 1998 report.[8] This was by far the largest reported population, consisting of 344 914 patients, of whom 97 153 were women. This study found that women carried a significantly higher risk of CABG mortality regardless of whether results were crude or adjusted for significant risk factors. This is the only report that subdivided the risk spectrum to examine specific risk categories. In so doing, it was found that at the very high risk categories, the gender difference in mortality was not significant. For all other categories, gender was an independent predictor of CABG operative mortality.

In 1998 Jacobs et al.[27] reported the experience from the Bypass Angioplasty Revascularization Investigation (BARI) study. The unadjusted operative mortality was almost identical for both women and men. It should be mentioned that the BARI population is a very select group that is not representative of all patients undergoing CABG. On the other hand, the demographic profile of women in the BARI trial is quite similar to that of most other studies. In a 1999 publication[21] from a single center, Aldea et al. also found no gender difference in adjusted or unadjusted CABG mortality. Importantly, the women in this report received IMA conduits in more than 90% of operations. This is in contrast to the typical IMA usage of around 60–75% for women. Another study in which there was no gender difference in unadjusted

mortality was published by Abramov et al.[22] the following year. It should be noted, however, that the mortality rate was 50% higher in women: 2.7% in women versus 1.8% in men (p = 0.09).

These reports by Jacobs, Aldea, and Abramov et al. suggested a trend toward diminishing gender differences in CABG mortality. Subsequent reports,[10,26] however, have once again shown significant differences in crude mortality. A particularly important 2002 study by Vaccarino et al.[9] examined the relationship between age and CABG mortality. In this report, the overall mortality in women was 5.3% as compared with the 2.9% male mortality. In patients more than 60 years old the sex difference in mortality was considerably less pronounced (p <0.001). Younger women carried a particularly high risk, with those less than 50 years of age having more than three times the mortality of men in the same age group. It is noteworthy that Carey et al.[12] also found that younger women carried a higher risk compared with more elderly women undergoing CABG. Since age is a universally accepted risk factor for CABG mortality, older women will tend to lie at the high-risk part of the risk spectrum. This age relationship, then, may contribute to the STS observation[8] that women at high risk have minimal gender differences in operative mortality.

In summary, three reports[11,13,26] found that adjusted mortality rates show no gender difference. All three of these reports noted a higher operative mortality in women when unadjusted data were analyzed. There are four reports[17,21,22,27] which found that crude, unadjusted mortality rates showed no gender difference. The study based on the BARI trial[27] focuses on a very select population, while another of these studies[21] differs from the typical experience in that a very high use of IMA conduits was employed in women. The other two studies[17,22] are overlapping reports from a single prestigious Canadian university.

A total of eight reports[8–13,26,39] found either crude or adjusted mortality to be higher in women. After a variety of risk adjustment techniques were brought into play, three of these studies[11,13,26] found no gender difference in mortality, while two others[8,39] demonstrated statistically significant gender differences.

With the typical CABG population seen in North America, it appears that the female population will generally have a greater operative risk than the male population. When risk-matched groups of men and women are compared, however, the published evidence regarding CABG outcome is evenly divided and therefore inconclusive.

Operative morbidity

The scientific evidence is also divided as to whether women have a higher complication rate following CABG. Woods et al. found that women had a significantly higher probability of postoperative morbidity,[26] but Aldea et al. found that there was no gender difference in complication rates.[21] Several reports indicate that compared with men, women experience a longer postoperative hospitalization,[22,26,40] require more prolonged ventilatory support,[40,41] and have higher rates of neurologic complications.[22,41] Others report no gender difference in neurologic complications[17,21] and there is at least one report of higher neurologic complications in men.[26]

The role of gender in the specific type of complication acquired is controversial, but it does seem clear that women and men respond differently once a complication has developed. When women get a major postoperative complication, they are more likely to die from it than men with same complication.[10,11] This seems to be particularly true for postoperative pump failure.

In the current era of CABG surgery approximately 15% of patients will be readmitted within 6 weeks after discharge. There is some evidence that women are more likely to be readmitted within 6–8 weeks.[28,42–45] This should be regarded as a delayed complication[42] of significant importance, but the wide variation in discharge and readmission criteria make this complication difficult to assess. In the study of the New York heart surgery centers by Hannan et al.,[42] female gender was an independent predictor of readmission, but Stuer et al.[43] found that after risk adjustment women were no more likely than men to require readmission.

Long-term results

In the 1980s several studies reported better long-term results for men. The graft patency rate was higher for men and men also had greater relief of angina.[2,46] On the other hand, there was no demonstrable gender difference in survival. In separate reports from the mid-1990s Hammar et al.[13] and Davis et al.[47] have confirmed that observation. Carey et al. found that women had lower survival rates at 10 years after surgery, but when diabetes was taken into account the gender differences disappeared.[12] More recent studies have found that women actually have a survival advantage over men at 5 years when risk adjustment is carried out.[22,27] There appears to be general agreement that women receive good long-term clinical benefits from CABG and that their results are at least as good as their male counterparts.[18]

Approaches to risk reduction

Certainly there are some lingering controversies in this field, but the attention devoted to gender issues in the last decade has shed light on valuable ways to improve surgical care for women undergoing CABG.

1. Improve referral practices

Some evidence suggests the existence of a referral bias in which women present for CABG at a later stage and therefore with more disease than men.[6,17,18,23–25] Presumably this bias arises from the misconception that women receive less benefit and have worse outcomes than men.[6,17,21,26] Tobin et al.[24] reported that, even after a positive stress test, women were ten times less likely than men to undergo coronary catheterization. Women are also less likely to undergo catheterization after myocardial infarction, despite having more angina than men.[48] Some, however, believe that there is only an apparent bias and that referral differences can be explained by statistical analysis of clinical variables.[49] Regardless of whether the differences are real or apparent, it does seem important to carefully examine local referral patterns. Increased awareness both in the health-care community and the lay public[18] can have a beneficial impact on referrals so that women in need of CABG can have earlier and safer surgical treatment.

2. Ensure optimal glucose control in diabetic patients (see also Chapter 3)

Diabetes is a well-recognized risk factor for CABG operative mortality and long-term complications. The great majority of studies show that diabetes is 40–50% more common in women than men undergoing CABG.[8,9,12,22,26] Importantly, the adverse clinical impact of diabetes is more pronounced in diabetic women than in diabetic men.[50] Traditionally, surgeons treating diabetic patients intentionally allowed blood glucose levels to fall in the 200–300 mg/dl range, with the specific intent of avoiding the devastating sequelae of profound hypoglycemia. Recent studies, however, have shown that hyperglycemia in the first two postoperative days is the single most important predictor of mediastinitis after cardiac surgery.[51,52] There is good evidence that this complication can be minimized by more strict control of blood glucose. Perioperative continuous intravenous insulin infusions to maintain blood glucose levels below 200 mg/dl in postoperative diabetic patients have been shown to significantly reduce the incidence of mediastinitis.[51,52]

3. Tailor anesthetic and sedation medications (see also Chapter 39)

Drugs used for anesthesia and immediate postoperative sedation are often dosed without regard for body weight,[53] thereby inducing a relatively larger pharmacologic load in the smaller female population. This practice is particularly concerning when one notes that women require more prolonged postoperative ventilation than men.[40,53] Duration of time on the ventilator is directly related to a number of serious complications including pneumonia, sternal dehiscence, mediastinitis, and the need for long-term ventilatory support. Avoidance of oversedation should minimize the problem of prolonged ventilation and its associated complications.

4. Optimize thyroxine treatment for women with hypothyroidism

Zindrou and colleagues[54] found a CABG mortality rate of 16.7% in women requiring thyroid replacement therapy. The operative mortality for hypothyroid men did not differ from euthyroid men. In women an inverse relationship between CABG operative mortality and both levothyroxine dose and free thyroxine concentration was found, but that relationship was not present in men. More aggressive perioperative therapy to treat the hypothyroid state in women may well minimize the very high CABG mortality seen in this subset of patients.

5. Consider preoperative hormone replacement therapy?

Given the potential serious complications associated with hormone replacement therapy (HRT), it does not seem advisable to administer this preparation to patients undergoing CABG. Nevertheless, it should be mentioned that a 2002 study from the Texas Heart Institute found that female sex without HRT was an independent risk factor for CABG operative mortality.[55] Women not receiving HRT experienced a 6.7% mortality, while women receiving HRT had a 2.3% mortality (p <0.01). The mortality was 2.7% for men. Another study[56] found that CABG mortality for women treated with HRT was significantly better than that of women not treated (2.7% vs 7.4%), but HRT was not a significant predictor of mortality in multivariate analysis.

6. Maximize use of the internal mammary artery

The IMA clearly confers both a short- and long-term protective effect that significantly enhances survival.[37,38] In spite of this well-known fact, women are less likely to receive an IMA graft.[8,11,13,17,18,21,22] There is no rational explanation for this practice. IMA size is approximately equal in women and men, so the technical challenge in creating an anastomosis should not be a consideration. Even when urgent and emergency operations are being performed, it is quite safe to use the IMA. Perhaps the only time[17] to avoid use of the IMA is when confronted with a soft, friable sternum that predisposes to sternal dehiscence. This should be distinctly uncommon.

Aldea and his colleagues[21] used an IMA conduit in 91% of women undergoing CABG. This is one of the very few studies that found no gender difference in either crude or adjusted operative mortality.

7. Minimize intraoperative anemia

Women have lower hematocrit levels than men presenting for CABG.[21,57–59] This is significant since even mild anemia is associated with some increased risk of postoperative death.[58] Furthermore, the smaller body size of women results in greater intraoperative hemodilution from the pump prime solution. The combination of these two factors often results in low hematocrit values during CPB. Recent studies confirm that women are significantly more likely than men to have very low hematocrit values during CPB.[58,59] There is compelling evidence that these low hematocrit levels during bypass are strongly associated with operative mortality and other postoperative complications.[58,59] Both DeFoe et al.[58] and Habib et al.[59] suggest that a major portion of the excess mortality observed in women may be due to the more profound intraoperative anemia seen in women.

Since low intraoperative hematocrit values are associated with an increase in postoperative complications, efforts should be made to raise the red blood cell concentration. This may be accomplished by standard hemoconcentration methods, perhaps augmented by modified ultrafiltration. Habib et al.[59] suggest minimizing the pump prime volume by direct alterations of the pump circuitry. More liberal use of blood transfusions during CPB should be considered as well.

8. Consider the use of off-pump surgical revascularization

There is some evidence to suggest that women may have better outcomes with OPCAB procedures than with conventional CABG surgery.[8,34–36] Brown et al.[35] found that women undergoing conventional CABG had an operative mortality that was 42% higher than a risk-matched group of women undergoing OPCAB (p <0.05). In a retrospective review of 413 patients,[34] Athanasiou found that female gender was not a predictor of OPCAB operative mortality. Capdeville

et al.[36] also found no statistically significant gender difference in OPCAB mortality, even though the mortality was more than three times higher in women (3.3% in women vs 0.8% in men).

While OPCAB surgery seems to offer some promise, it should be mentioned that patient selection has not been rigorously controlled in any study to date. As pointed out by Brown et al., there are clear indications in their study[35] that the female on-pump group had a higher severity of illness index than the female OPCAB group. It should also be mentioned that there is no major gender difference in outcomes associated with valve surgery,[60] which argues against a major role for the pump itself.

Observed trends

Certainly the past decade has seen an unprecedented interest in gender-specific issues associated with CABG. Although many issues remain controversial, we can now see that many other issues have become well accepted. In particular, we know that CABG is an effective means of revascularization for women. We also know that unadjusted CABG mortality is often higher for women, that women receive a fewer number of bypass grafts, and that the IMA is used less often in women. Now that there is greater awareness of these facts, one might logically ask whether

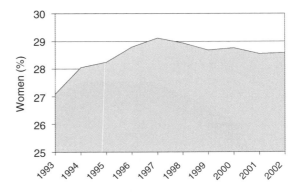

Figure 20.1
Percent of women undergoing coronary artery bypass graft surgery in the Society of Thoracic Surgeons National Cardiac Surgery Database.

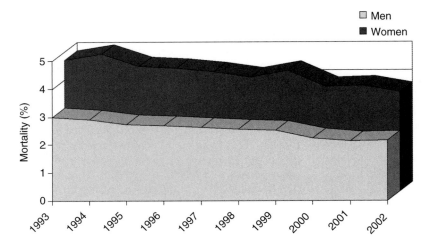

Figure 20.2
Trends in operative mortality from coronary artery bypass graft surgery and gender differences in the Society of Thoracic Surgeons National Cardiac Surgery Database.

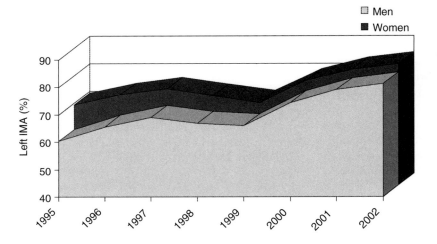

Figure 20.3
Left internal mammary artery (IMA) usage trends and gender differences in the Society of Thoracic Surgeons National Cardiac Surgery Database.

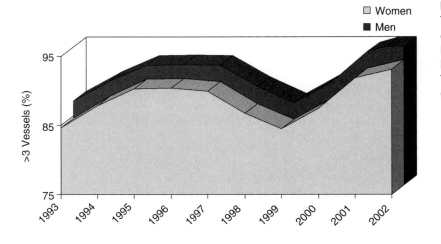

Figure 20.4
Trends and gender differences for patients having three or more vessels bypassed in the Society of Thoracic Surgeons National Cardiac Surgery Database.

there has been a change in outcomes or practice patterns.

A review of data from the STS National Cardiac Surgery Database offers some insight regarding trends over the last decade. Over 1.5 million patients were included in this trend analysis. As shown in Fig. 20.1, the proportion of women undergoing CABG gradually increased from 1993 through 1998, but has been unchanged since then. Figure 20.2 shows that the unadjusted CABG operative mortality for women has fallen from 4.70% to 3.54% over the last decade. In spite of these improved results in women, however, the operative mortality remains approximately 50% higher than in men undergoing CABG.

Figure 20.3 shows that women receive a left IMA graft much more often than in the past. The left IMA was used in 60.54% of women in 1995, while 81.16% of women received left IMA bypasses in 2002. Since IMA usage has been clearly associated with improved CABG mortality, one may logically conclude that the increased use of mammary grafting in women has made some contribution to improved outcomes in women.

In virtually all reports, women have received a fewer number of bypass grafts than men. Figure 20.4 shows that this finding is true for a national population as well. There does, however, appear to be a trend toward progressively more bypass grafts in women. In 1993, 84.6% of women received three or more bypasses. This has progressively risen to 93% in 2002, but women still receive slightly fewer grafts on average compared with men.

These moderately encouraging trends from the STS Database imply some change in practice patterns over the last 10 years. It is not possible to conclude that these changes are the direct result of increased awareness of gender-specific issues, but it does seem likely that the enormous number of published articles have had – and will continue to have – a salutary impact on the practice of surgical revascularization in women.

References

1. Tyras DH, Barner HB, Kaiser GC, Codd JE, Laks H, Willman VL. Myocardial revascularization in women. *Ann Thorac Surg* 1978; **25**:449–35.
2. Loop FD, Golding LR, MacMillan JP, Cosgrove DM, Lytle BW, Sheldon WC. Coronary artery surgery in women compared with men: analysis of risk and long term results. *J Am Coll Cardiol* 1983; **1**:383–90.
3. Gardner TJ, Horneffer PJ, Gott VL, et al. Coronary artery bypass grafting in women. *Ann Surg* 1985; **201**:780–4.
4. Richardson JV, Cyrus RC. Reduced efficacy of coronary artery bypass grafting in women. *Ann Thorac Surg* 1986; **42**:S16–21.
5. Fisher LD, Kennedy JW, Davis KB, et al. Association of sex, physical size, and operative mortality after coronary artery bypass in the Coronary Artery Surgery Study (CASS). *J Thorac Cardiovasc Surg* 1982; **84**:334–41.
6. Khan SS, Nessim S, Gray R, et al. Increased mortality of women in coronary artery bypass surgery: evidence for referral bias. *Ann Intern Med* 1990; **112**:561–7.
7. Edwards FH, Clark RE, Schwartz M. Coronary artery bypass grafting: The Society of Thoracic Surgeons National Database experience. *Ann Thorac Surg* 1994; **57**:12–19.
8. Edwards FH, Carey JS, Grover FL, Bero JW, Hartz RS. Impact of gender on coronary bypass operative mortality. *Ann Thorac Surg* 1998; **66**:125–31.
9. Vaccarino V, Abramson JL, Veledar E, Weintraub WS. Sex differences in hospital mortality after coronary artery bypass surgery. *Circulation* 2002; **105**:1176–81.
10. Zitser-Gurevich Y, Simchen E, Galai N, Mandel M. Effect of perioperative complications on excess mortality among women after coronary bypass: the Israeli Coronary Bypass Graft study (ISCAB). *J Thorac Cardiovasc Surg* 2002; **123**:517–24.
11. O'Connor GT, Morton JR, Diehl MJ, et al. Differences between men and women in hospital mortality associated with coronary artery bypass graft surgery. *Circulation* 1993; **88**:2104–10.
12. Carey JS, Cukingnan RA, Singer LKM. Health status after myocardial revascularization: inferior status in women. *Ann Thorac Surg* 1995; **59**:112–17.
13. Hammar N, Sandberg E, Larsen FF, Ivert T. Comparison of early and late mortality in men and women after isolated coronary artery bypass graft surgery in Stockholm, Sweden 1980 to 1989. *J Am Coll Cardiol* 1997; **29**:659–64.

14. Golino A, Panza A, Jannelli G, et al. Myocardial revascularization in women. *Tex Heart Inst J* 1991; **18**:194–8.

15. Schwann TA, Habib RH, Zacharias A, et al. Effects of body size on operative, intermediate, and long-term oucomes after coronary artery bypass operation. *Ann Thorac Surg* 2001; **71**:521–31.

16. O'Connor NJ, Morton JR, Birkmeyer JD, Olmstead EM, O'Connor GT. Effect of coronary artery diameter in patients undergoing coronary bypass surgery. *Circulation* 1996; **93**:652–5.

17. Mickleborough LL, Takagi Y, Maruyama H, Sun Z, Mohamed S. Is sex a factor in determining operative risk for aortocoronary bypass graft surgery? *Circulation* 1995; **92** (Suppl II):II80–II84.

18. Lawton JS, Brister SJ, Petro KR, Dullum M. Surgical revascularization in women: unique intraoperative factors and considerations. *J Thorac Cardiovasc Surg* 2003; **126**:936–8.

19. Dignan RJ, Yeh T, Dyke CM, Lutz HA, Wechsler AS. The influence of age and sex on human internal mammary artery size and reactivity. *Ann Thorac Surg* 1992; **53**:792–7.

20. Kurlansky PA, Traad EA, Galbut DL, Singer S, Zucher M, Ebra G. Coronary bypass surgery in women: a long-term comparative study of quality of life after bilateral internal mammary artery grafting in men and women. *Ann Thorac Surg* 2002; **74**:1517–25.

21. Aldea GS, Gaudiani JM, Shapira OM, et al. Effect of gender on postoperative outcomes and hospital stays after coronary artery bypass grafting. *Ann Thorac Surg* 1999; **67**:1097–103.

22. Abramov D, Tamariz MG, Sever JY, et al. The influence of gender on the outcome of coronary artery bypass surgery. *Ann Thorac Surg* 2000; **70**:800–6.

23. Steingart RM, Packer M, Hamm P, et al. Sex differences in the management of coronary artery disease. *N Engl J Med* 1991; **325**:226–30.

24. Tobin JN, Wassertheil S, Wexler JP, et al. Sex bias in considering coronary bypass surgery. *Ann Intern Med* 1987; **107**:19–25.

25. Bergelson BA, Tommaso CL. Gender differences in clinical evaluation and triage in coronary artery disease. *Chest* 1995; **108**:1510–13.

26. Woods SE, Noble G, Smith JM, Hasselfeld K. The influence of gender in patients undergoing coronary artery bypass graft surgery: an eight year prospective hospitalized cohort study. *J Am Coll Surg* 2003; **196**:428–34.

27. Jacobs AK, Kelsey SF, Brooks MM, et al. Better outcome for women compared with men undergoing coronary revascularization: a report from the Bypass Angioplasty Revascularization Investigation (BARI). *Circulation* 1998; **98**:1279–85.

28. Wenger NK. Is what's good for the gander good for the goose? *J Thorac Cardiovasc Surg* 2003; **126**:929–31.

29. O'Rourke DJ, Malenka DJ, Olmstead EM, et al. Improved in-hospital mortality in women undergoing coronary artery bypass grafting. *Ann Thorac Surg* 2002; **71**:507–11.

30. Haan CK, Chiong JR, Coombs LP, Edwards FH, Geraci SA. Comparison of risk profiles and outcomes in women versus men > 75 years of age undergoing coronary artery bypass grafting. *Am J Cardiol* 2003; **91**:1255–8.

31. Mickleborough LL, Carson S, Ivanov J. Gender differences in quality of distal vessels: effect on results of coronary artery bypass grafting. *J Thorac Cardiovasc Surg* 2003; **126**:950–8.

32. Jacobs AK. Coronary revascularization in women in 2003: sex revisited. *Circulation* 2003; **107**:375–7.

33. Szabo Z, Hakanson E, Svedjeholm R. Early postoperative outcome and medium-term survival in 540 diabetic and 2239 nondiabetic patients undergoing coronary artery bypass grafting. *Ann Thorac Surg* 2002; **74**:712–19.

34. Athanasiou T, Al-Ruzzeh A, Del Stanbridge R, et al. Is the female gender an independent predictor of adverse outcome after off-pump coronary artery bypass grafting? *Ann Thorac Surg* 2003; **75**:1153–60.

35. Brown PP, Mack MJ, Simon AW, et al. Outcomes experience with off-pump coronary artery bypass surgery in women. *Ann Thorac Surg* 2002; **74**:2113–20.

36. Capdeville M, Chamogeogarkis T, Lee JH. Effect of gender on outcomes of beating heart operations. *Ann Thorac Surg* 2001; **72**:S1022–5.

37. Edwards FH, Clark RE, Schwartz M. The impact of internal mammary artery conduits on operative mortality in coronary revascularization. *Ann Thorac Surg* 1994; **57**:27–32.

38. Leavitt BJ, O'Connor GT, Olmstead EM, et al. Use of the internal mammary artery graft and in-hospital mortality and other adverse outcomes associated with coronary artery bypass grafting. *Circulation* 2001; **103**:507–12.

39. Hannan EL, Bernard HR, O'Donnell JF. Gender differences in mortality rates for coronary artery bypass surgery. *Am Heart J* 1992; **123**:866–72.

40. Butterworth J, James R, Prielipp R, Cerese J, Livingston J, Burnett D. Female gender associates with increased duration of intubation and length of stay after coronary artery surgery. *Anesthesiology* 2000; **92**:414–24.

41. Shroyer ALW, Coombs LP, Peterson ED, et al. The Society of Thoracic Surgeons: 30-day operative mortality and morbidity risk models. *Ann Thorac Surg* 2003; **75**:1856–65.

42. Hannan EL, Racz MJ, Walford G, et al. Predictors of readmission for complications of coronary artery bypass graft surgery. *JAMA* 2003; **290**:773–80.

43. Steuer J, Blomqvist P, Granath F, et al. Hospital readmission after coronary artery bypass grafting: are women doing worse? *Ann Thorac Surg* 2002; **73**: 1380–6.

44. Stewart RD, Campos CT, Jennings B, et al. Predictors of 30-day hospital readmission after coronary artery bypass. *Ann Thorac Surg* 2000; **70**:169–74.

45. Vaccarino V, Lin ZQ, Kasl SV, et al. Gender differences in recovery after coronary artery bypass surgery. *J Am Coll Cardiol* 2003; **41**:307–14.

46. Johnson WD, Kayser KL, Pedraza PM. Angina pectoris and coronary artery bypass surgery: patterns of prevention and recurrence in 3105 consecutive patients followed up to 11 years. *Am Heart J* 1984; **108**:1190–7.

47. Davis KB, Chaitman B, Ryan T, Bittner V, Kennedy JW. Comparison of 15-year survival for men and women after initial medical or surgical treatment for coronary artery disease: a CASS registry study. *J Am Coll Cardiol* 1995; **25**:1000–9.

48. Steingart RM, Packer M, Hamm P, et al. Sex differences in the management of coronary artery disease. *N Engl J Med* 1991; **325**:226–30.

49. Ghali WA, Faris PD, Galbraith D, et al. Sex differences in access to coronary revascularization after cardiac catheterization: importance of detailed clinical data. *Ann Intern Med* 2002; **136**:723–32.

50. Thomas JL, Braus PA. Coronary artery disease in women – a historical perspective. *Arch Intern Med* 1998; **158**:333–7.

51. Zerr KJ, Furnary AP, Grunkemeier GL, et al. Glucose control lowers the risk of wound infection in diabetics after open heart operations. *Ann Thorac Surg* 1997; **63**:356–61.

52. Furnary AP, Zerr KJ, Grunkemeier GL, Starr AS. Continuous intravenous insulin infusion reduces the incidence of deep sternal wound infection in diabetic patients after cardiac surgical procedures. *Ann Thorac Surg* 1999; **67**:352–62.

53. Koch CG, Mangano CM, Schwann N, Vaccarino V. Is it gender, methodology, or something else? *J Thorac Cardiovasc Surg* 2003; **126**:932–5.

54. Zindrou D, Taylor KM, Bagger JP. Excess coronary artery bypass mortality among women with hypothyroidism. *Ann Thorac Surg* 2002; **74**:2121–5.

55. Nussmeier NA, Marino MR, Vaughn WK. Hormone replacement therapy is associated with improved survival in women undergoing coronary artery bypass grafting. *J Thorac Cardiovasc Surg* 2002; **124**:1225–9.

56. Shackelford DP, Daniels S, Hoffman MK, Chitwood R. Estrogen therapy in women undergoing coronary artery bypass grafting. Effect on surgical complications. *Obstet Gynecol* 2000; **95**:732–5.

57. Utley JR, Wilde EF, Leyland SA. Intraoperative blood transfusion is a major risk factor for coronary artery bypass grafting in women. *Ann Thorac Surg* 1995; **60**:570–4.

58. DeFoe GR, Ross CS, Olmstead EM, et al. Lowest hematocrit on bypass and adverse outcomes associated with coronary artery bypass grafting. *Ann Thorac Surg* 2001; **71**:769–76.

59. Habib RH, Zacharias A, Schwann TA, Riordan CJ, Durham SJ, Shah A. Adverse effects of low hematocrit during cardiopulmonary bypass in the adult: should current practice be changed? *J Thorac Cardiovasc Surg* 2003; **125**:1438–50.

60. Edwards FH, Peterson ED, Coombs LP, et al. Prediction of operative mortality after valve replacement surgery. *J Am Coll Cardiol* 2001; **37**;885–92.

21
Cardiac rehabilitation for women

Barry A. Franklin, Amy Fowler, Laxmi Mehta and Kavitha Chinnaiyan

Introduction

In 1995, Falk and associates,[1] using the combined data from four previous studies, demonstrated that nearly 90% of acute myocardial infarctions (MIs) involve coronary artery sites with <70% obstruction in the months to years before infarction. Thus, coronary occlusion and acute MI most frequently evolve from mild-to-moderate stenoses, especially less obstructive plaques that are more lipid-rich and vulnerable to rupture. Contemporary studies suggest that the nature of plaque determines the risk of acute cardiovascular events, and that inflammation, plaque rupture, and thrombosis represent the final common pathway for acute coronary syndromes (ACS).[2] These findings suggest a new paradigm in the treatment of patients with coronary heart disease (CHD) and explain why it has been difficult to demonstrate a reduction in cardiovascular events in most studies examining coronary artery bypass graft (CABG) surgery or percutaneous transluminal coronary angioplasty (PTCA). Although revascularization procedures are highly effective at relieving signs and/or symptoms of myocardial ischemia, such interventions are unlikely to prevent plaque rupture at sites that appear non-obstructive on coronary angiography.

Individuals who experience an acute coronary event are at increased risk of subsequent coronary events, regardless of treatment. Although the degree of left ventricular dysfunction and residual myocardial ischemia largely determines the risk of future cardiac events,[3] risk status can be influenced by numerous interventions and lifestyle changes (Fig. 21.1). Multicenter clinical trials have confirmed that mortality from acute MI can be decreased by approx-

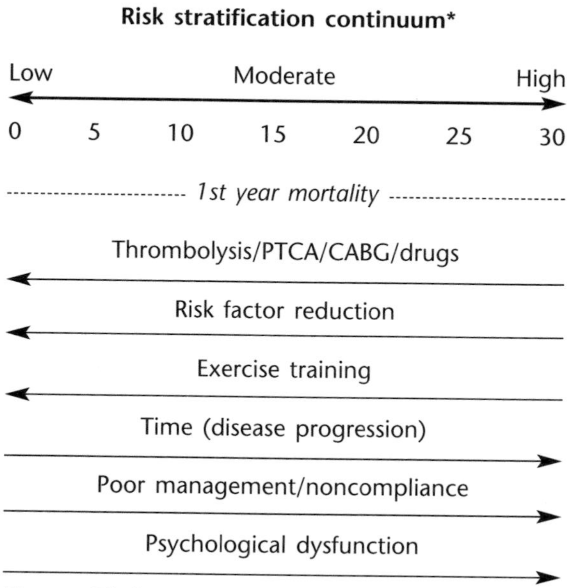

Risk stratification continuum*

Figure 21.1
Variables that may potentially influence the patient's risk status (i.e. low, moderate, high). PTCA, percutaneous transluminal coronary angioplasty; CABG surgery, coronary artery bypass graft surgery. *Based on extent of myocardial ischemia and left ventricular dysfunction.

imately 25% with early thrombolytic reperfusion,[4] emergent PTCA,[5] or both. Selected patients at moderate-to-high risk may experience a reduction in ischemic signs/symptoms and recurrent cardiac events from elective PTCA or CABG surgery; however, the escalating number of 'repeat' coronary revascularization procedures highlights the palliative nature of these interventions. For patients with symptomatic CHD who are not candidates for percutaneous or surgical revascularization, enhanced external counterpulsation therapy, involving a treatment series of modified blood pressure cuffs wrapped around the lower extremities, has been effective in reducing angina and improving functional capacity.[6,7]

Aggressive risk factor interventions aimed at smoking cessation, lipid modification, and exercise training, and efficacious drugs – including beta-blockers, aspirin or other platelet active agents, angiotensin-converting enzyme inhibitors, lipid-lowering agents (i.e. statins) and, more recently, a recombinant ApoA-1 Milano/phospholipid complex (ETC-216) – have produced regression or limitation of progression of coronary atherosclerosis, as verified by coronary angiography or intravascular ultrasound, and significant reductions in initial and recurrent nonfatal and fatal cardiovascular events.[8–9] Recent studies suggest that an intensive lipid-lowering statin regimen provides greater protection against death or major cardiovascular events than does a standard regimen, and that patients with ACS benefit from early and continued lowering of low-density lipoprotein (LDL) cholesterol to levels substantially below current target recommendations.[10–11] In contrast, time (disease progression), poor patient management or compliance, and psychological dysfunction,[12] manifested as anger/hostility, depression, chronic stress, or social isolation, can lead to increased risk and a poor prognosis.

Meta-analyses of randomized, controlled clinical trials conducted in the early 1980s on post-MI patients showed that exercise-based cardiac rehabilitation decreased cardiovascular-related and all-cause mortality by 20–24% (Fig. 21.2),[13–15] especially as a component of multifactorial rehabilitation (i.e. 26% reduction in mortality vs 15% in exercise-only trials),[16] with no difference in the rate of nonfatal recurrent cardiac events. Although it has been suggested that contemporary pharmacotherapies,

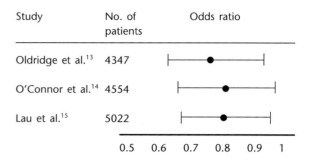

Figure 21.2
Meta-analyses of the effects of exercise-based cardiac rehabilitation on all-cause mortality after myocardial infarction.

thrombolytics, and revascularization procedures, which markedly decrease early post-infarction mortality, may diminish the impact of adjunctive cardiac rehabilitation programs on survival, three recent reports provide the best evidence to date that mortality benefits of exercise-based cardiac rehabilitation persist in modern cardiology.[17–19]

In the United States alone, more than 500 000 women die of cardiovascular disease (CVD) each year, exceeding the number of deaths in men and the next seven causes of death in women combined.[20] Moreover, mortality after acute MI is higher among women than men.[21] Many of these deaths occur in African American and Hispanic women who, unfortunately, also have the lowest awareness of their risk factors and excess mortality. Recently, an expert panel/writing group from the American Heart Association (AHA) provided evidence-based recommendations for the prevention of CVD in women (Fig. 21.3).[20] Lifestyle interventions such as smoking cessation, regular physical activity, cardiac rehabilitation, a heart-healthy diet, and weight maintenance (or reduction) were given Class I status (i.e. strongly recommended) for all women because of their potential to reduce major risk factors and the development or progression of CVD. Because a mere 11–20% of patients with CHD participate in group or home-based cardiac rehabilitation programs,[16] and the ratio of men to women referred is approximately 4:1, it appears that less than 5% of all women with CHD have the opportunity to realize the benefits that cardiac rehabilitation programs have to

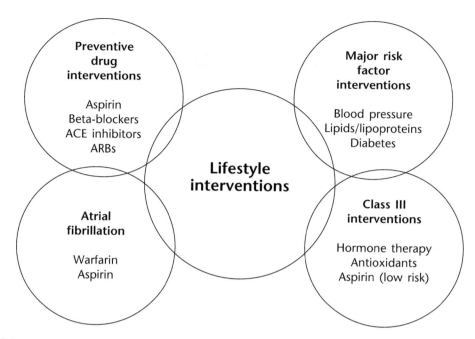

Figure 21.3
Clinical recommendations for the prevention of cardiovascular disease in women are grouped into the following categories: lifestyle interventions, major risk factor interventions, atrial fibrillation/stroke prevention, preventive drug interventions, and a Class III category where routine intervention for cardiovascular disease prevention is not recommended. ACE, angiotensin-converting enzyme; ARB, angiotensin-receptor blocker.

offer.[22] These findings, and other reports, highlight the vast underutilization of these services, especially in older adults and women.[23,24]

This chapter addresses the available data on gender differences (and similarities) in exercise-based cardiac rehabilitation, with specific reference to the initial clinical profile and referral patterns, exercise testing, barriers to program participation, strategies to enhance enrollment and adherence, considerations regarding fitness and mortality, outcomes in intensive, long-term multidisciplinary interventions, and special considerations for women.

Initial patient profile: women versus men

After an acute MI, women report receiving less counseling from their health-care providers than their male counterparts.[25,26] These deficiencies encompass return to work issues, resumption of household activities, and sexual activity.[26] After coronary revascularization, physician referrals to cardiac rehabilitation are also less likely to be received by women. Women report receiving little to no support from health-care professionals and, less frequently, spousal encouragement to participate in cardiac rehabilitation programs as compared with men.[25]

Women entering outpatient cardiac rehabilitation programs are generally older,[23,26–29] have a higher prevalence of coexisting illness,[27] more traditional CHD risk factors,[27] and a lower exercise capacity.[27] Psychologically, women also have lower quality of life and self-efficacy scores,[27,30] more anxiety[30,31] and depression,[32] and greater social isolation.[31] Women are also more likely to have a prior history of diabetes mellitus and hypertension.[27,29,33] Some studies have shown a higher prevalence[33] of cigarette smoking in women while others have shown a lower

Table 21.1 Comparison of peak exercise test responses of men and women entering cardiac rehabilitation programs (mean ± standard deviation)

Variable	Men* (n = 170)	Women* (n = 50)	Men† (n = 37)	Women† (n = 17)
METs	5.5 ± 2.0	4.1 ± 1.7	5.7 ± 1.4‡	4.6 ± 1.4‡
HR (beats/min)	123‡	105‡	128 ± 22	130 ± 20
% HR max	74 ± 12	64 ± 12	84‡	87‡
SBP (mmHg)	174‡	164‡	161 ± 24	166 ± 22
HR × SBP	$21.4 ± 5.3 × 10^3$	$17.2 ± 4.3 × 10^3$	$19.5 ± 6.6 × 10^3$	$21.3 ± 6.3 × 10^3$
RER	–	–	1.05 ± 0.13	1.06 ± 0.14
Ventilation (l/min)	–	–	62 ± 18	44 ± 15
No. with angina	15 (9%)	5 (10%)	–	–
No. with ST ↓ (≥ 1mm)	15 (9%)	0 (0%)	–	–

METs, metabolic equivalents (1 MET = 3.5 ml/kg/min); HR, heart rate; SBP, systolic blood pressure; HR × SBP, rate–pressure product; RER, respiratory exchange ratio (VCO_2/VO_2); ST ↓, ST segment depression.
*Data from reference 33.
†Data from reference 23.
‡Value calculated based on available data.

prevalence.[29] Women are also significantly more obese,[27] with a higher total cholesterol,[27,29,33,34] LDL cholesterol[27,34] and high-density lipoprotein (HDL) cholesterol[27,33,34] as compared with men. Fewer women are employed or married at the time of enrollment into cardiac rehabilitation programs.[28,29,33] Thus, the clinical profiles of women and men entering cardiac rehabilitation programs differ markedly. The differences may be partially attributed to gender, as well as more advanced age, selective referral bias of women with coexisting debilitating diseases, and varied social support systems.

Exercise testing

Two widely cited reports provide a comparison of exercise test responses in similarly aged women and men entering cardiac rehabilitation programs (Table 21.1). At baseline, women were less aerobically fit than men (p <0.05), 4.6 ± 1.4 metabolic equivalents (METs) versus 5.7 ± 1.4 METs and 4.1 ± 1.7 METs versus 5.5 ± 2.0 METs, corresponding to 84% and 75% of the values of their gender-matched counterparts, respectively.[23,33] Older women were comparable to older men in attaining physiologic evidence of a true maximal effort, as reflected by peak respiratory exchange ratios.[23] More recently, Lavie et al.[27] reported that the resting heart rate, resting systolic

blood pressure, and peak rate–pressure product were similar in women and men entering an exercise-based cardiac rehabilitation program. Women had a lower peak heart rate (126 ± 25 bpm vs 135 ± 25 bpm, p = 0.05) and were less aerobically fit (4.9 ± 1.4 METs vs 6.6 ± 1.9 METs, p <0.001).[27] Two investigations found no difference in the frequency of angina between women and men during baseline exercise testing.[33,35] However, a higher incidence of ischemic ST segment depression during exercise testing has been reported by some in men,[33,36] whereas other studies found no difference.[34] Total exercise treadmill time was also lower in women (5.7 ± 2.2 min vs 7.0 ± 3.3 min, p = 0.0007).[36] Kligfield and associates[37] reported a lower heart rate recovery in women compared with men (9.6 ± 5.4 bpm vs 13.6 ± 6.0 bpm, p <0.01) during submaximal exercise testing.

Suboptimal adherence: barriers to program participation

Only 11–38% of all eligible coronary patients are referred for outpatient cardiac rehabilitation,[16] and on average less than 25% of these patients actually participate in formal programs.[24,38] Regardless of gender, adherence rates to multidisciplinary cardiac rehabilitation programs decline over time.

Approximately 25–50% of participants drop out within the first 6 months and up to 90% drop out by the end of the first year.[38–40] Although data on compliance and attendance rates of women in these programs are conflicting, women's referral rates to outpatient cardiac rehabilitation programs are indeed lower than their male counterparts.[25,29,41] Ades et al.[23] found that the strength of the referring physician's recommendation for participation was the most influential factor in cardiac rehabilitation entry; moreover, physicians were less likely to emphasize cardiac rehabilitation to their women patients.

Numerous factors may explain lack of enrollment and high drop-out rates for both women and men, including: cost (e.g. limited or no insurance reimbursement); inconvenient program hours or facility location (e.g. excessive travel time); schedule conflicts; concomitant family demands; co-morbid illnesses; exercise-related symptomatology; or combinations thereof.[42,43] Other variables that may influence adherence to exercise-based rehabilitation include leisure-time physical activity, blue-collar employment, smoking status, and occupational activity.[33,44]

Women are faced with several unique barriers to participation that may account for their lower enrollment and potential differences in attendance and drop-out rates. The role of caregiver is traditionally and typically the woman's – maintaining the home, caring for children, an older spouse and/or family member. Women are also more likely to live alone and are less likely to own and drive a vehicle.[23,33] Some women may feel uncomfortable participating in a male-dominated program, whereas others may be reluctant to participate due to lack of prior physical activity experience.[42] Many programs offer classes geared to the majority of their clientele, that is, middle-aged to older men, and few programs provide specific exercise or educational offerings for women.[45] Postcoronary women also tend to increase their activity levels sooner and to a greater extent than men, primarily by undertaking housework at an earlier stage in their recovery.[46,47] Thus, they may not feel that they need a structured rehabilitation program to enhance their exercise tolerance for activities of daily living. Men, in contrast, tend to increase their activity levels later, generally by walking in home-based or medically supervised cardiac rehabilitation programs.[46,48,49]

Strategies to enhance exercise adherence

According to Prochaska and DiClemente, interventions designed to empower patients to initiate and maintain lifestyle modifications should be based on their particular stage of readiness for change (Fig. 21.4).[50] Their transtheoretical model includes six stages of intentional behavior change that occur over time: precontemplation – does not intend to take action in the next 6 months; contemplation – intends to take action in the next 6 months; preparation – has taken some behavioral steps and intends to take action in the next 30 days; action – has changed behavior for less than 6 months; and maintenance – has changed behavior for more than 6 months.[51,52]

To effectively assist and maximally empower patients to initiate and maintain lifestyle modifications,

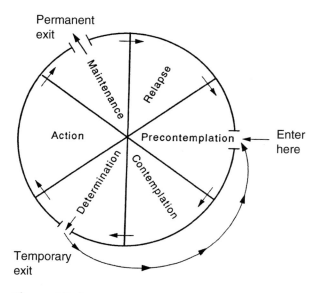

Figure 21.4
Progressive stages of readiness for behavior change, with specific reference to temporary and permanent exits and relapse. Adapted from reference 50.

strategies employed by cardiac rehabilitation professionals and physicians should be appropriate for the individual's stage of readiness for change. For example, while the precontemplator may need consciousness raising, the contemplator may require a critical analysis of the 'pros and cons' of becoming more physically active. Similarly, exploring alternative action plans, providing specific instructions (how tos), offering positive personal feedback, and halting relapse may be employed for the contemplation, preparation, action, and maintenance phases, respectively.

Research and empiric experience suggest that selected exercise program modifications and motivational strategies may enhance a participant's interest and enthusiasm as well as long-term adherence (Box 21.1).[53] Additionally, adherence in women may be improved by emphasizing the importance of their participation to the well-being of their spouse and/or family, providing a formal smoking cessation program as part of treatment, and enlisting help for childcare and some responsibilities at home, when feasible.[33] Cigarette smoking[54,55] and lack of spousal support[56] (Fig. 21.5) have been reported to have a negative impact on adherence to exercise therapy in

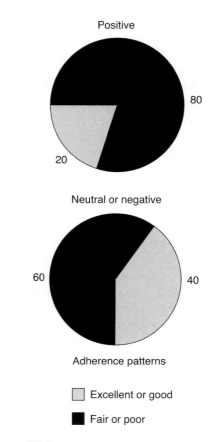

Figure 21.5
Relation of wife's attitudes to husband's adherence to an exercise training program. Adapted from reference 56.

men after MI. Interestingly, men are often accompanied to the exercise rehabilitation sessions by their wives, whereas the converse is rarely true.[57]

Physical conditioning: considerations regarding fitness and mortality (see also Chapter 7)

Although regular physical activity and improved cardiorespiratory fitness are widely believed to be

---

Box 21.1 Strategies to enhance long-term exercise adherence

- Minimize musculoskeletal injuries with a moderate exercise prescription
- Encourage group participation
- Emphasize variety and enjoyment in the exercise program
- Incorporate a 'personalized' positive approach to participants and realistic goal setting
- Employ periodic fitness testing, including lipid/lipoprotein profiling and body composition assessment, to evaluate patient progress
- Recruit spouse support in promoting the exercise program
- Encourage participant documentation of daily exercise achievements through progress charts or logs
- Provide music during exercise sessions
- Recognize individual accomplishments through extrinsic rewards (e.g. T-shirts, trophies, certificates)
- Provide well-trained, highly motivated, and enthusiastic exercise leaders

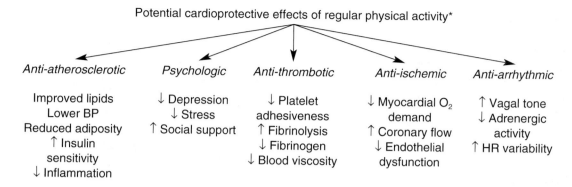

Figure 21.6
Lifestyle and/or structured interventions to increase physical activity and cardiorespiratory fitness may provide multiple mechanisms to reduce nonfatal and fatal cardiovascular events. *Moderate-to-vigorous exercise intensities (i.e. ≥55% HR max, ≥12–13 rating of perceived exertion (6–20 scale)). BP, blood pressure; HR, heart rate.

cardioprotective, a recent meta-analysis concluded that these variables had significantly different relationships to heart disease.[58] The risk decreased linearly with increasing levels of physical activity; in contrast, there was a precipitous drop in risk as one moved from the lowest to the second lowest fitness category. Beyond this fitness demarcation, the reductions in relative risk paralleled those observed with increasing physical activity, but were nearly twice as great for cardiorespiratory fitness. Thus, extremely low aerobic fitness warrants consideration as a separate risk factor.

Previous studies in persons without known CHD have identified a low level of aerobic fitness as an independent risk factor for all-cause and cardiovascular mortality.[59] Recently, Kavanagh and associates extended these data to men[60] and women[61] with established CHD who were referred for exercise-based cardiac rehabilitation. A single-center design obtained data on 2380 women (59.7 ± 9.5 years), including 1052 after MI, 620 after CABG surgery procedures, and 708 with proven CHD, who underwent cardiopulmonary exercise testing. The follow-up ranged from 0.4 to 25 years (median, 4.5 years). Directly measured peak oxygen uptake ($\dot{V}O_2$ peak) on a cycle ergometer at program entry proved to be a powerful predictor of cardiovascular and all-cause mortality. Values ≥13 ml/kg/min (3.7 METs) conferred a 50% reduction in cardiac mortality. Moreover, the magnitude of the advantage of well

conserved aerobic fitness was relatively independent of gender: the $\dot{V}O_2$ peak cut-off point above which there was a marked benefit in prognosis (13 ml/kg/min in women vs 15 ml/kg/min in men), as well as the 1 ml/kg/min advantage in $\dot{V}O_2$ peak when treated as a continuous variable (10% lowering of cardiac mortality in women vs 9% in men). The investigators concluded that even a small, training-induced increase in aerobic power may make a major difference, not only in functional capacity, but in survival outcome as well.

Contemporary guidelines suggest that individuals should engage in ≥30 minutes of moderate-intensity physical activity such as brisk walking on most, and preferably all, days of the week.[62] Randomized trials have now shown that a lifestyle approach to physical activity among previously sedentary persons is feasible and has similar effects on aerobic fitness, body composition, and coronary risk factors as compared with a traditional structured exercise program.[63,64] In a recent randomized trial of men with stable CVD and an angiographically documented stenosis amenable to PTCA, a 12–month exercise training program compared with PTCA resulted in superior event-free survival and exercise capacity at lower costs.[65] There are multiple mechanisms by which moderate-to-vigorous physical activity, improved aerobic fitness, or both, may decrease morbidity and mortality rates associated with CVD (Fig. 21.6), including anti-atherosclerotic, anti-ischemic, anti-arrhythmic, anti-thrombotic, and psychosocial effects.[66]

Intensive, long-term, multidisciplinary interventions

Recent studies have shown that aggressive modification of coronary risk factors, particularly abnormal lipids/lipoproteins, may slow, halt, and even reverse coronary atherosclerosis in patients with documented CHD.[67] Recognition of multiple risk factors can identify women at increased risk for the progression of atherosclerosis and acute cardiac events.[68] Therapeutic lifestyle changes may include a low-fat and low-cholesterol diet, exercise training, weight control or weight loss, smoking cessation, stress reduction, and medications to favorably alter lipoprotein profiles.[69–71] Although most studies enrolled only men, selected trials that included women are summarized below, with specific reference to gender differences or similarities, when reported (see also Chapter 4).

The Heart Protection Study

The Heart Protection Study (HPS) compared simvastatin versus placebo in patients at high risk for CHD. Only patients 40–80 years of age for whom the clinical evidence did not indicate a clear course of action were included in the study.[72] Approximately 20 000 patients were randomized to receive either a fixed dose of simvastatin (40 mg/day) or a matching placebo. Antioxidant vitamin therapy (600 mg α-tocopherol, 250 mg ascorbic acid, 20 mg β-carotene) was also included with a matching placebo. Compliance and cross-over rates from the control population were monitored during the study.[73]

Previous studies using antioxidant therapy have reported conflicting results.[74–76] Despite the hypothetical attractiveness of antioxidant therapy in reducing the risks of CHD, the vitamin therapy arm in the HPS demonstrated no effect on morbidity or mortality. On the other hand, simvastatin significantly decreased all-cause mortality by 13% (p = 0.0003), with a significant 17% reduction (p <0.0001) in deaths attributed to any vascular cause. Women and men benefited comparably. Statin therapy as an intervention to reduce overall coronary risk in women had been inadequately studied in previous prevention trials. The LIPID and the AFCAPS/TexCAPS trials found that women and men benefitted equally with statin therapy.[77,78] The HPS, with a total of 5082 women, provided a sizable database to analyze the impact of statin therapy on vascular event rates in a population stratified by gender. A 24% reduction in major vascular events was achieved in both women and men, suggesting a beneficial role of statin therapy, regardless of sex.

UCSF Arteriosclerosis Specialized Center of Research Intervention Trial

The University of California School of Medicine, San Francisco (UCSF) Arteriosclerosis Specialized Center of Research Intervention Trial examined the effects on coronary atherosclerosis of reducing cholesterol levels with diet and a combined drug program in patients with heterozygous familial hypercholesterolemia (average total cholesterol = 373 mg/dl) and LDL cholesterol levels above 200 mg/dl.[79] Quantitative angiography was performed at baseline and about 2 years later in the 72 patients who completed the trial (41 women and 31 men). Improvements in angiographic findings and LDL levels in women were at least as great as those observed in men.

To date, approximately 18 serial angiographic trials have reported the effects of lowering LDL cholesterol on the progression of coronary atherosclerosis.[80] Nearly 12% of the 4100 individuals randomized to these trials were women. Subjects who achieved LDL cholesterol lowering in these trials were approximately twice as likely to demonstrate regression, 1.5 times more likely to demonstrate stabilization, and half as likely to demonstrate progression of coronary artery atherosclerosis relative to the placebo-treated subjects.[81] For the most part, major clinical outcome benefits were achieved with only very modest angiographic changes.

The Monitored Atherosclerosis Regression Study

The Monitored Atherosclerosis Regression Study (MARS) was a double-blind, placebo-controlled, randomized trial that tested whether lowering LDL cholesterol level with diet plus lovastatin (40 mg twice daily) would slow the rate of progression and/or cause regression of coronary lesions on quantitative angiography in patients with CHD.[82] Participants included 247 men and 23 women, with total cholesterol levels ranging from 190 to 295 mg/dl and angiographically documented CHD. In the group receiving lovastatin, the total cholesterol level decreased by 32%, and the LDL cholesterol decreased by 38%. Follow-up angiography after 2 years revealed that the average luminal narrowing increased by 0.9% in the placebo recipients and decreased by 4.1% in lovastatin recipients (p = 0.005). There was no reported difference in per-patient outcomes between women and men.

The Scandinavian Simvastatin Survival Study

In the Scandinavian Simvastatin Survival Study (4S) trial, 4444 patients (3617 men, 827 women) with angina pectoris or previous MI and mild-to-moderate hypercholesterolemia (range, 213–309 mg/dl) were randomly assigned to simvastatin or placebo.[83] After a median follow-up of 5.4 years, the probability that a woman would escape a major coronary event was 77.7% in the placebo group and 85.1% in the simvastatin group, corresponding to a relative risk of 0.65 (Table 21.2). Thus, simvastatin reduced the risk of major coronary events in women by about the same extent as it did in men. This was the first trial to show that cholesterol-lowering per se reduced major coronary events in women.

Special considerations
Muscle mass and strength

The Framingham Study found that essentially half of women over age 65 cannot lift 10 pounds. Fortunately, more recent studies have demonstrated that older adults who perform progressive resistance exercise or weight training can improve their strength at any age.

Resistance training has been shown to be safe and effective in increasing muscle strength and endurance in clinically stable coronary patients.[84] Cardiac demands during activities of daily living, such as carrying groceries, are attenuated as a result of the decreased rate–pressure product at any given load.[85,86] Ades et al.,[87] in a study of 42 post coronary women over the age of 65, found that resistance training over a 6-month period resulted in improvements in balance, endurance, coordination, flexibility, and strength-related activities such as carrying groceries and lifting luggage.

Fiatarone and associates[88] conducted a randomized, placebo-controlled trial comparing four groups: lower-body resistance exercise, a multivitamin nutritional supplement, both interventions combined, and neither (control group) in 100 frail nursing home residents (63 women, 37 men; age = 87.1 ± 0.6 years, mean ± standard error of the mean) over a 10-week period. Exercisers demonstrated improved muscle strength (113 ± 8%), which was unrelated to age and sex, increased gait velocity (11.8 ± 3.8%), augmented stair-climbing power (28.4 ± 6.6%) and increased cross-sectional thigh muscle area (2.7 ± 1.8%) compared with nonexercisers who showed little or no change in these variables. These were unrelated to age and sex. Multivitamin supplementation without concomitant exercise had no effect on these outcome measures. The improvements in the exercisers translated to an increased ability to perform activities of daily living.

Table 21.2 Major coronary events in women and men on simvastatin versus placebo

Major coronary event	Number (%) of patients		
	Placebo	Simvastatin	Relative risk* (95% CI)
Women	91 (21.7)	59 (14.5)	0.65 (0.47–0.91)
Men	531 (29.4)	371 (20.5)	0.66 (0.58–0.76)

*Calculated by Cox regression analysis; CI, confidence interval.
Adapted from the Scandinavian Simvastatin Survival Study.[83]

Bone density

Osteoporosis, characterized by low bone mass and a gradual deterioration of bone tissue which result in amplified bone fragility, is inevitable as people age and predisposes them to an increased risk of fracture. Primary osteoporosis often occurs following menopause in women and in older men. Secondary osteoporosis is a result of medications or other diseases. Osteoporosis is linked to approximately 1.5 million fractures annually in the United States, including approximately 700 000 vertebral fractures, 300 000 hip fractures, 250 000 distal forearm fractures, and 250 000 fractures at other sites.[89,90] The lifetime risk of major fractures is 40% for white women and 13% for white men aged 50 years and older. Following a hip fracture, there is a 10–20% mortality over the subsequent 6 months; moreover, 50% of victims will be unable to walk without assistance, and 25% will require long-term care. Thus, unless preventive interventions are taken now, a catastrophic global epidemic of osteoporosis seems inevitable.

One-third to one-half of all menopausal women and nearly half of all persons over the age of 75 years will be affected by osteoporosis. Risk factors associated with osteoporosis include female gender, increased age, Caucasian or Asian race, low body weight and body mass index, maternal or personal history of fractures, estrogen deficiency, cigarette smoking, excessive consumption of alcohol or caffeine, and diets low in calcium and/or high in fiber. Late menarche, early menopause, amenorrhea, and anorexia are other variables associated with low bone mineral density. Predictors of future fracture risk not only include a low bone mineral density, but also a history of falls, low physical function, and/or impaired cognition or vision.[91–94]

Prevention and treatment of osteoporosis is multifactorial, including adequate nutritional supplementation, regular exercise, and various medications which either stimulate bone formation (fluoride, anabolic steroids) or inhibit bone resorption (menopausal hormone therapy, calcitonin, and bisphosphonates). Calcium is the primary nutrient for attaining peak bone mass and for preventing and treating osteoporosis. Calcium intake for adults should be maintained at 1000–1500 mg per day.

Because vitamin D enhances calcium absorption, it should be taken in conjunction with calcium. The recommended intake of vitamin D is 400–600 IU daily.

Estrogen, a constituent of hormone therapy (HT), increases bone mineral density in older menopausal women and younger perimenopausal women.[95] A meta-analysis of HT research has demonstrated that estrogen given for 2 years to menopausal women resulted in an increase in bone mineral density of 6.8% in the spine and 4.1% at the femoral neck.[96] The Women's Health Initiative trial, the largest and most comprehensive study to date, demonstrated that estrogen–progesterone therapy and estrogen therapy increased bone mineral density in healthy menopausal women, which resulted in fewer fractures of the hip, vertebrae, and wrist. Despite the positive effects on bone mineral density, HT has significant negative effects on CVD and breast cancer.[97] Since the publication of this study, there has been an increased interest in alternative options to treating osteoporosis. In particular, researchers are examining selective estrogen receptor modulators, such as raloxifene. The Multiple Outcomes of Raloxifene Evaluation (MORE) trial demonstrated a reduction in vertebral fractures with raloxifene despite a relatively modest increase in bone mineral density.[98]

Studies have shown that regular physical activity, especially resistance and weight-bearing exercise, is associated with a higher peak bone mass. Weight-bearing exercise such as walking, jogging, or aerobic dance stimulates the formation of new bone (or at least helps to maintain bone density) by placing added, regular stress on the spine and skeletal system. Exercise also helps prevent further bone loss in women who are already affected.[94] Clinical trials have demonstrated a reduction in falls with regular exercise, due to improvements in dynamic balance and strength.[99]

Although calcium intake is strongly recommended in preventing osteoporosis, it should be combined with other therapeutic interventions. In a recent study of 40–65-year-old menopausal women, in which all subjects received 800 mg of calcium supplements daily, patients were randomized to exercise or no exercise for 1 year. Women who exercised and used HT increased measurements of bone density in the femoral neck, trochanteric and lumbar spine by 1–2%.[100] Recent studies have also shown that aerobic exercise is associated with maintaining lumbar spine bone mineral density in menopausal women[101] and that resistance training helps preserve lumbar, femoral, and radial bone mineral density.[102]

In summary, women should not assume that nutritional supplements, various drugs (e.g. HT), or exercise alone will prevent bone loss. Osteoporosis is multifactorial and requires coordination of pharmacologic and nonpharmacologic interventions to be successful.

Menopause

The cessation of menstrual function – menopause – generally occurs between the ages of 45 and 55 years. The accompanying metabolic, physical, and emotional changes are associated with an increased risk of several health problems and chronic diseases, including osteoporosis and CHD.[103] The most common physical symptoms are sudden heat sensations (hot flashes), cold shivers, and dry skin. Others report an increase in body weight and fat stores and reduced exercise tolerance. Emotional problems may include anxiety, depression, and irritability. Although some of the physical and emotional problems may be attributed to the hormonal changes of menopause, others may be due to aging or medical problems that existed before menopause.

Approximately 10–15 years after the drop in estrogen level associated with menopause, the incidence of CHD in women rises dramatically. This may be attributed, at least in part, to the associated changes in lipids and lipoproteins. After menopause, a woman's cholesterol and triglyceride levels increase; HDL cholesterol generally decreases by approximately 10 mg/dl, and LDL cholesterol increases to exceed that of her age-matched male counterparts.[104] Indeed, the Framingham Study has documented a 10-fold increase in the incidence of coronary events after the age of 55 years for women.[105]

Women in cardiac rehabilitation programs may derive considerable benefit from regular exercise, which has been shown to favorably modify many of the adverse physiologic and psychologic changes that are associated with the decrease in estrogen production at menopause. For example, regular aerobic exercise may improve confidence and self-image, reduce depression and anxiety, decrease the frequency and severity of hot flashes, and positively contribute to the management of stress, quality of sleep, and bone mineralization.[94] Menopausal women with heart disease who participate in a cardiac rehabilitation program may derive even greater lipid/lipoprotein benefits over long periods of time as compared with men.[106]

Hormone therapy (see also Chapters 25 and 26)

Until recently, numerous observational studies and meta-analyses had strongly suggested that menopausal HT, with or without progestin, reduced the risk of symptomatic atherosclerotic CHD. This had been reported in both primary and secondary prevention settings.[107–109] Thus, it was unexpected when the Heart and Estrogen/progestin Replacement Study (HERS) showed no overall effect of 4.1 years of estrogen plus progestin therapy for secondary prevention of CHD in menopausal women.[110] Since then, five additional trials confirmed the overall null effects observed in HERS.[111]

The Women's Health Initiative randomized controlled trial

The Women's Health Initiative (WHI) was designed to focus on defining the risks and benefits of strategies that could potentially reduce the incidence of heart disease, breast and colorectal cancer, and fractures in healthy menopausal women. The hormone trial was divided into two arms – the estrogen/progestin versus placebo intervention[112] and the estrogen-only versus placebo component.[113]

In the first arm, menopausal women (n = 16 608) with an intact uterus were enrolled, and participants received conjugated equine estrogen, 0.625 mg/day, plus medroxyprogesterone acetate, 2.5 mg/day, in one tablet (n = 8506) or placebo (n = 8102).[112] The primary outcome was CHD, with a planned duration of 8.5 years. The trial was stopped prematurely at an average follow-up of 5.2 years, when the health risks

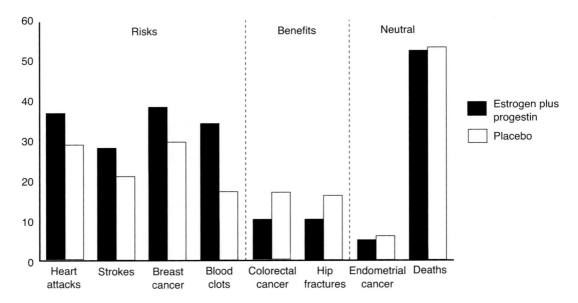

Figure 21.7
Results from the Women's Health Initiative, comparing hormone replacement therapy (estrogen plus progestin) versus placebo in 16 608 menopausal women, with specific reference to risks versus benefits in a variety of chronic diseases and medical conditions.[112] The figure shows the number of cases per year in 10 000 women. 'Neutral' indicates no clear benefit or risk.

exceeded the health benefits. Blood lipid levels showed greater reductions in LDL cholesterol (−12.7%) and increases in HDL cholesterol (7.3%) and triglycerides (6.9%) with estrogen plus progestin relative to placebo. Resting systolic blood pressure was, on average, 1.0 mmHg higher in women taking estrogen plus progestin at 1 year, rising to 1.5 mmHg at 2 years and beyond.

The rate of coronary events was increased by 29% for women taking estrogen plus progestin relative to placebo (37 vs 30 cases per 10 000 women). Most of the excess was in nonfatal MI. Total CVD, including events requiring hospitalization, was increased by 22% in the estrogen plus progestin group. Kaplan–Meier estimates of cumulative hazards for CHD indicated that differences between the treatment groups became apparent soon after randomization. The rate of strokes, breast cancer, and blood clots was also higher in women taking estrogen plus progestin (Fig. 21.7). No significant differences were observed in the incidence of endometrial cancer and all-cause mortality. Estrogen plus progestin

increased bone mineral density and reduced the risk of fracture in healthy menopausal women (hazard ratio, 0.76; 95% confidence interval, 0.69–0.83). The effect did not differ in women stratified by age, body mass index, smoking status, history of falls, personal or family history of fracture, total calcium intake, past use of HT, or bone mineral density.

The estrogen-alone component of the WHI randomized menopausal women (n = 10 739), aged 50–79 years, with prior hysterectomy, including 23% of minority race/ethnicity, to receive either 0.625 mg/day of conjugated equine estrogen or placebo.[113] The intervention phase of the trial was terminated early as estrogen increased the risk of stroke, reduced the risk of hip and other fractures, and did not significantly affect the incidence of CHD (the primary outcome) or overall mortality. It was concluded that conjugated equine estrogen should not be recommended for chronic disease prevention in menopausal women.

Based on these results, the AHA recently updated its earlier recommendations[114,115] regarding the role of HT in the primary and secondary prevention of CVD in menopausal women. Interventions categorized as Class III, which are considered either not useful and/or potentially harmful, include that: combined estrogen plus progestin HT should not be initiated or continued to prevent CVD in menopausal women; and, other forms of menopausal HT (e.g. unopposed estrogen) should not be initiated or continued to prevent CVD in menopausal women.[20]

Musculoskeletal complications

Certain modes of exercise (e.g. jogging, step aerobics) may be inappropriate for some menopausal women, especially those with decreased bone density, balance problems, or both. Low estrogen and calcium levels may markedly increase the incidence of partial or complete stress fractures that result from recurrent microtrauma. Consequently, the exercise prescription may require modification to reduce the potential for injury.

Excessive intensity (>90% $\dot{V}O_2$ max), frequency (≥5 days/week) or duration (≥45 minutes/session) of training in men offers little additional gain in aerobic capacity, yet the incidence of orthopedic injury increases substantially (Fig. 21.8).[116] Previously, we described the effects of a 12-week, moderate-intensity walk-jog physical conditioning program on the incidence of injury in lean-to-normal weight (n = 13) and obese (n = 23) middle-aged women.[117] Jogging speed was individually adjusted to correspond to the heart rate at 75% $\dot{V}O_2$ max; however, it was reduced if musculoskeletal trauma so dictated. Eleven women, four from the normal weight and seven from the obese group, sustained leg and foot injuries severe enough to cause either a reduction of training intensity or a temporary discontinuation of conditioning. Nine of the 11 injuries (82%) occurred during the first 6 weeks of the training regimen. Although a greater number of obese women were injured during the conditioning program, the injury percentage in each group was identical (30%). The anticipated lack of mobility in the obese women, which was expected to result in numerous orthopedic complications, was apparently negated by the exercise prescription, which was based on a percent-

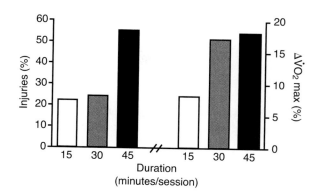

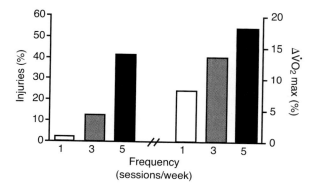

Figure 21.8
Relationship between frequency and duration of exercise training, percentage improvement in aerobic capacity (Δ$\dot{V}O_2$ max), and the incidence of orthopedic injury. Above an exercise duration of 30 minutes/session, or a frequency of three sessions/week, additional improvement in $\dot{V}O_2$ max is small, yet the injury rate increases disproportionately. Adapted from reference 116.

age of aerobic capacity. Collectively, these data suggest that normal-weight and moderately obese women experience no greater incidence of exercise-related musculoskeletal injury than their male counterparts, if they are trained at a comparable exercise intensity.

Attention to warm-up, proper walking shoes, and training on appropriate terrain (avoiding hard and uneven surfaces) should aid in decreasing attrition due to injury. Novice female exercisers may also need education about the value of a good sports brassiere, with wide shoulder straps, breathable fabrics, seamless cups, ample armholes, covered hooks or fasteners, and limited vertical stretch.[94] A recommended program for beginners is to *accumulate* 30 minutes or more of mild-to-moderate physical activity on most, and preferably all, days of the week.[118] Recent studies have shown that intermittent exercise, accumulated in 8–10-minute bouts throughout the day, results in similar health-fitness benefits as a comparable period of continuous exercise.[119–121]

Stress urinary incontinence

Up to 30% of girls and women aged 15–64 years experience stress urinary incontinence (SUI), or the involuntary loss of urine during physical exertion.[122] Unfortunately, this potentially embarrassing but relatively common condition may decrease a woman's desire and motivation to exercise, decreasing adherence. In a small percentage of cases, varying the type or intensity of activity can attenuate the incontinence. More often, however, treatment options such as absorbent pads, pelvic floor muscle training (PFMT), medication, devices, or surgical interventions may be considered.

Most commonly, urology and urogynecology specialists recommend PFMT as a first-line treatment of SUI. PFMT, also known as Kegel exercises, often results in variable short-term cure or improvement rates, depending on the patient's compliance to the prescribed regimen and the quality of instruction. Other conservative options for SUI are intravaginal and intraurethral devices that are appropriate for women who are not surgical candidates or whose incontinence is related only to physical exertion.[123] Intravaginal devices, similar to a sanitary tampon, act by increasing the outflow resistance whereas intraurethral devices directly prevent urine leakage. Both devices may be inserted and removed at the patient's discretion.

Surgical options for SUI are numerous and varied. Techniques include: injectable periurethral bulking agents which increase tissue bulk around the urethra; laparoscopic colposuspension that lifts the bladder neck and urethra that have dropped abnormally low into the pelvic area; and tension-free vaginal tape involving placing a mesh-like tube under the urethra to return it to its normal position.

Pharmacologic options for the treatment of SUI are limited in terms of safety and efficacy. Recently pilot studies utilizing duloxetine, a combined serotonin and norepinephrine reuptake inhibitor, have demonstrated significant improvement in urinary incontinence with a low incidence of adverse side effects.[124,125] These preliminary results suggest that duloxetine may become a first-line treatment for mild-to-moderate stress urinary incontinence.[125]

Conclusions

Women are less likely to participate in formal cardiac rehabilitation programs and, when they do, their baseline physiologic and psychologic profiles may differ markedly from their male counterparts. Those who enter rehabilitation programs are generally older, have more anxiety and depression, lower self-efficacy, greater stress at home, a higher prevalence of traditional coronary risk factors, more coexisting illness, lower exercise tolerance, increased symptoms and more advanced CVD than men. Moreover, women are faced with numerous gender-specific barriers to participation that may account for their lower enrollment, poorer attendance, and higher drop-out rates. On the other hand, women who participate in exercise-only or intensive, multidisciplinary interventions, despite poorer compliance than men, demonstrate comparable or even greater improvements in functional capacity, coronary risk, and psychosocial well-being. This may be attributed, at least in part, to their greater coronary risk profile and lower cardiorespiratory fitness at program entry (i.e. improvement in women and men generally shows an inverse relation with these variables). The challenge for physicians and allied health professionals is to enroll increasing numbers of women, at an earlier stage of their disease, in home-based or group cardiac rehabilitation programs that are designed to circumvent or attenuate barriers to participation and adherence, so that many more women may realize the benefits that secondary prevention can provide.

References

1. Falk E, Shah PK, Fuster V. Coronary plaque disruption. *Circulation* 1995; **92**:657–71.

2. Libby P. Atherosclerosis: the new view. *Sci Am* 2002; **286**:46–55.

3. DeBusk RF, Blomqvist CG, Kouchoukos NT, et al. Identification and treatment of low-risk patients after acute myocardial infarction and coronary-artery bypass graft surgery. *N Engl J Med* 1986; **314**:161–6.

4. Simoons ML, Serruys PW, van den Brand M, et al. Early thrombolysis in acute myocardial infarction: limitation of infarct size and improved survival. *J Am Coll Cardiol* 1986; **7**:717–28.

5. Grines CL, Browne KF, Marco J, et al. A comparison of immediate angioplasty with thrombolytic therapy for acute myocardial infarction. *N Engl J Med* 1993; **328**:673–9.

6. Arora RR, Chow TM, Jain D, et al. The multicenter study of enhanced counterpulsation (MUST-EECP): effect of EECP on exercise-induced myocardial ischemia and anginal episodes. *J Am Coll Cardiol* 1999; **33**:1833–40.

7. Ochoa AB, Franklin BA. Enhanced external counterpulsation therapy: a noninvasive approach to treating heart disease. *Am J Med Sports* 2003; **5**:194–8.

8. Franklin BA, Kahn JK. Delayed progression or regression of coronary atherosclerosis with intensive risk factor modification: effects of diet, drugs, and exercise. *Sports Med* 1996; **22**:306–20.

9. Nissen SE, Tsunoda T, Tuzcu EM, et al. Effect of recombinant ApoA-1 Milano on coronary atherosclerosis in patients with acute coronary syndromes: a randomized controlled trial. *JAMA* 2003; **290**:2292–300.

10. Cannon CP, Braunwald E, McCabe CH, et al. Intensive versus moderate lipid lowering with statins after acute coronary syndromes. *N Engl J Med* 2004; **350**:1495–504.

11. Nissen SE, Tuzcu EM, Schoenhagen P, et al. REVERSAL Investigators. Effect of intensive compared with moderate lipid-lowering therapy on progression of coronary atherosclerosis: a randomized controlled trial. *JAMA* 2004; **291**:1071–80.

12. Williams RB, Barefoot JC, Schneiderman N. Psychosocial risk factors for cardiovascular disease: more than one culprit at work. *JAMA* 2003; **290**:2190–2.

13. Oldridge NB, Guyatt GH, Fisher ME, Rimm AA. Cardiac rehabilitation after myocardial infarction: combined experience of randomized clinical trials. *JAMA* 1988; **260**:945–50.

14. O'Connor GT, Buring JE, Yusuf S, et al. An overview of randomized trials of rehabilitation with exercise after myocardial infarction. *Circulation* 1989; **80**:234–44.

15. Lau J, Antman EM, Jimenez-Silva J, Kupelnick B, Mosteller F, Chalmers TC. Cumulative meta-analysis of therapeutic trials for myocardial infarction. *N Engl J Med* 1992; **327**:248–54.

16. Wenger NK, Foelicher ES, Smith LK, et al. *Cardiac Rehabilitation*. Clinical Practice Guideline No. 17. AHCPR Pub. No. 96-0672. Rockville, MD: US Department of Health and Human Services, Public Health Service, Agency for Health Care Policy and Research and National Heart, Lung, and Blood Institute, October 1995.

17. Taylor RS, Brown A, Ebrahim S, et al. Exercise-based rehabilitation for patients with coronary heart disease: systematic review and meta-analysis of randomized controlled trials. *Am J Med* 2004; **116**:682–92.

18. Smart N, Marwick TH. Exercise training for heart failure patients: a systematic review of factors that improve patient mortality and morbidity. *Am J Med* 2004; **116**:693–706.

19. Piepoli MF, Davos C, Francis DP, Coats AJ, ExTraMATCH Collaborative. Exercise training meta-analysis of trials in patients with chronic heart failure (ExTraMATCH). *BMJ* 2004; **328**:189–91.

20. Mosca L, Appel LJ, Benjamin EJ, et al. Evidence-based guidelines for cardiovascular disease prevention in women. *Circulation* 2004; **109**:672–93.

21. American Heart Association. *Heart Disease and Stroke Statistics – 2004 Update*. Dallas, TX: American Heart Association, 2003.

22. Froelicher VF, Herbert W, Myers J, Ribisl P. How cardiac rehabilitation is being influenced by changes in health care delivery. *J Cardiopulm Rehabil* 1996; **16**:151–9.

23. Ades PA, Waldmann ML, Polk DM, Coflesky JT. Referral patterns and exercise response in the rehabilitation of female coronary patients aged $\geq$ 62 years. *Am J Cardiol* 1992; **69**:1422–5.

24. Ades PA, Waldmann ML, McCann WJ, Weaver SO. Predictors of cardiac rehabilitation participation in older coronary patients. *Arch Intern Med* 1992; **152**:1033–5.

25. Caulin-Glaser T, Blum M, Schmeizl R, Prigerson HG, Zaret B, Mazure CM. Gender differences in referral to cardiac rehabilitation programs after revascularization. *J Cardiopulm Rehabil* 2001; **21**:24–30.

26. Hamilton GA, Seidman RN. A comparison of the recovery period of women and men after an acute myocardial infarction. *Heart Lung* 1993; **22**:308–15.

27. Lavie CJ, Milani RV. Effects of cardiac rehabilitation and exercise training on exercise capacity, coronary risk factors, behavioral characteristics and quality of life. *Am J Cardiol* 1995; **75**:340–3.

28. Richardson LA, Buckenmeyer PJ, Bauman BD, Rosneck JS, Newman I, Josephson RA. Contemporary cardiac rehabilitation: patient characteristics and temporal trends over the past decade. *J Cardiopulm Rehabil* 2000; **20**:57–64.

29. Thomas RJ, Houston N, Lamendola C, et al. National survey on gender differences in cardiac rehabilitation programs. *J Cardiopulm Rehabil* 1996; **16**:402–12.

30. Schuster PM, Waldron J. Gender differences in cardiac rehabilitation patients. *Rehabil Nurs* 1991; **16**:248–53.

31. Brezinka V, Dusseldorp E, Maes S. Gender differences in psychosocial profile at entry into cardiac rehabilitation. *J Cardiopulm Rehabil* 1998; **18**:445–9.

32. Rankin SH. Differences in recovery from cardiac surgery: a profile of male and female patients. *Heart Lung* 1990; **19**:481–5.

33. Cannistra LB, Balady GJ, O'Malley CJ, Weiner DA, Ryan TJ. Comparison of the clinical profile and outcome of women and men in cardiac rehabilitation. *Am J Cardiol* 1992; **69**:1274–9.

34. O'Farrell P, Murray J, Huston P, et al. Sex differences in cardiac rehabilitation. *Can J Cardiol* 2000; **16**:319–25.

35. Balady GJ, Jette D, Scheer J, Downing J. Changes in exercise capacity following cardiac rehabilitation in patients stratified according to age and gender. *J Cardiopulm Rehabil* 1996; **16**:38–46.

36. Frishman WH, Gomberg-Maitland M, Hirsch H, et al. Differences between male and female patients with regard to baseline demographics and clinical outcomes in the Asymptomatic Cardiac Ischemia Pilot (ACIP) Trial. *Clin Cardiol* 1998; **21**:184–90.

37. Kligfield P, McCormick A, Chai A, Jacobson A, Feuerstadt P, Hao SC. Effect of age and gender on heart rate recovery after submaximal exercise during cardiac rehabilitation in patients with angina pectoris, recent acute myocardial infarction, or coronary bypass surgery. *Am J Cardiol* 2003; **92**:602–3.

38. Oldridge NB. Cardiac rehabilitation exercise programme; compliance and compliance-enhancing strategies. *Sports Med* 1988; **6**:42–55.

39. Balady GJ, Fletcher BJ, Froelicher ES, et al. American Heart Association Medical/Scientific Statement: Position statement: Cardiac rehabilitation programs: A statement for health care professionals from the American Heart Association. *Circulation* 1994; **90**:1602–10.

40. Radtke KL. Exercise compliance in cardiac rehabilitation. *Rehabil News* 1989; **14**:182–6.

41. Plach SK. Women and cardiac rehabilitation after heart surgery: patterns of referral and attendance. *Rehabil Nurs* 2002; **27**:104–9.

42. Conn VS, Taylor SG, Abele PB. Myocardial infarction survivors: age and gender differences in physical health, psychosocial states and regimen adherence. *J Adv Nurs* 1991; **16**:1026–34.

43. Oldridge NB, Ragowski B, Gottlieb M. Use of outpatient cardiac rehabilitation services: factors associated with attendance. *J Cardiopulm Rehabil* 1992; **12**:25–31.

44. Hamm LF, Leon AS. Exercise training for the coronary patient. In: Wenger NK, Hellerstein HK (eds). *Rehabilitation of the Coronary Patient*, 3rd edn. New York: Churchill Livingstone, 1993: 367–402.

45. Durstine JL, Thomas RJ, Miller NH, et al. Women and cardiac rehabilitation programming. Read before the Vth World Congress of Cardiac Rehabilitation, Bordeaux, France, July 5–8, 1992.

46. Boogard, MAK, Briody ME. Comparison of the rehabilitation of men and women postmyocardial infarction. *J Cardiopulm Rehabil* 1985; **5**:649–51.

47. Hamilton GA, Seidman RN. A comparison of the recovery period for women and men after an acute myocardial infarction. *Heart Lung* 1993; **22**:308–15.

48. Boogard MAK. Rehabilitation of the female patient after myocardial infarction. *Nurs Clin North Am* 1984; **19**:433–40.

49. Parchert MA, Creason N. The role of nursing in the rehabilitation of women with cardiac disease. *J Cardiovasc Nurs* 1989; **3**:57–64.

50. Prochaska J, DiClemente C. Transtheoretical therapy, toward a more integrative model of change. *Psychother Theory Res Pract* 1982; **19**:276–88.

51. Velicer WF, Prochaska J, Fava JL, Norman GJ, Redding CA. Smoking cessation and stress management: applications of the transtheoretical model of behavior change. *Homeostasis* 1998; **38**:216–33.

52. Burbank PM, Reibe D, Padula CA, Nigg C. Exercise and older adults: changing behavior with the transtheoretical model. *Orthop Nurs* 2002; **21**:51–63.

53. Franklin BA. Program factors that influence exercise adherence: practical adherence skills for the clinical staff. In: Dishman RK (ed). *Exercise Adherence*. Champaign, IL: Human Kinetics, 1988: 237–58.

54. Oldridge NB, Wicks JR, Hanley C, Sutton JR, Jones NL. Noncompliance in an exercise rehabilitation program for men who have suffered a myocardial infarction. *Can Med Assoc J* 1978; **111**:361–4.

55. Waites TF, Watt EW, Fletcher GF. Comparative functional and physiologic status of active and drop-out coronary bypass patients of a rehabilitation program. *Am J Cardiol* 1983; **51**:1087–90.

56. Heinzelman F, Bagley R. Response to physical activity programs and their effects on health behavior. *Public Health Rep* 1970; **85**:905–11.

57. O'Callaghan WG, Teo KK, O'Riordan J, Webb H, Dolphin T, Horgan JH. Comparative response of male and female patients with coronary artery disease to exercise rehabilitation. *Eur Heart J* 1984; **5**:649–51.

58. Williams PT. Physical fitness and activity as separate heart disease risk fators: a meta-analysis. *Med Sci Sports Exerc* 2001; **33**:754–61.

59. Franklin BA. Survival of the fittest: evidence for high-risk and cardioprotective fitness levels. *Curr Sports Med Rep* 2002; **1**:257–9.

60. Kavanagh T, Mertens DJ, Hamm LF, et al. Prediction of long-term prognosis in 12,169 men referred for cardiac rehabilitation. *Circulation* 2002; **106**:666–71.

61. Kavanagh T, Mertens DJ, Hamm LF, et al. Peak oxygen intake and cardiac mortality in women referred for cardiac rehabilitation. *J Am Coll Cardiol* 2003; **42**:2139–43.

62. Thompson PD, Buchner D, Piña IL, et al. Exercise and physical activity in the prevention and treatment of atherosclerotic cardiovascular disease. *Circulation* 2003; **107**:3109–16.

63. Dunn AL, Marcus BH, Kampert JB, Garcia ME, Kohl HW 3rd, Blair SN. Comparison of lifestyle and structured interventions to increase physical activity and cardiorespiratory fitness: a randomized trial. *JAMA* 1999; **281**:327–34.

64. Andersen RE, Wadden TA, Bartlett SJ, Zemel B, Verde TJ, Franckowiak SC. Effects of lifestyle activity vs structured aerobic exercise in obese women: a randomized trial. *JAMA* 1999; **281**:335–40.

65. Hambrecht R, Walther C, Möbius-Winkler S, et al. Percutaneous coronary angioplasty compared with exercise training in patients with stable coronary artery disease. A randomized trial. *Circulation* 2004; **109**:1371–8.

66. Franklin BA, de Jong A, Kahn JK, McCullough PA. Fitness and mortality in the primary and secondary prevention of coronary artery disease: does the effort justify the outcome? *Am J Med Sports* 2004; **6**:23–7.

67. Gould KL, Ornish D, Scherwitz L, et al. Changes in myocardial perfusion abnormalities by positron emission tomography after long-term, intense risk factor modification. *JAMA* 1995; **274**:894–901.

68. Rackley CE. Strategies for the prevention of atherosclerotic progression in women. *Cardiol Rev* 2002; **10**:119–25.

69. Haskell WL, Alderman EL, Fair JM, et al. Effects of intensive multiple risk factor reduction on coronary atherosclerosis and clinical cardiac events in men and women with coronary artery disease: The Stanford Coronary Risk Intervention Project (SCRIP). *Circulation* 1994; **89**:975–90.

70. Ornish D, Brown SE, Scherwitz LW, et al. Can lifestyle changes reverse coronary heart disease? The Lifestyle Heart Trial. *Lancet* 1990; **336**:129–33.

71. Farmer JA, Gotto AM. The Heart Protection Study: expanding the boundaries for high-risk coronary disease prevention. *Am J Cardiol* 2003; **92** (Suppl):3i–9i.

72. MRC/BHF Heart Protection Study Collaborative Group. MRC/BHF Heart Protection Study of cholesterol-lowering therapy and of antioxidant vitamin supplementation in a wide range of patients at increased risk of coronary heart disease death: early safety and efficacy experience. *Eur Heart J* 1999; **20**:725–41.

73. Heart Protection Study Collaborative Group (HPSCG). MRC/BHF Heart Protection Study of cholesterol lowering with simvastatin in 20,536 high-risk individuals: a randomized placebo-controlled trial. *Lancet* 2002; **360**:7–22.

74. Yusuf S, Sleight P, Pogue J, Bosch J, Davies R, Dagenais G. Effects of an angiotensin-converting enzyme inhibitor, ramipril, on cardiovascular events in high risk subjects. The Heart Outcomes Prevention Evaluation Study Investigators. *N Engl J Med* 2000; **342**:145–53.

75. Brown BG, Zhao XQ, Chait A, et al. Simvastatin and niacin, antioxidant vitamins, or the combination for the prevention of coronary disease. *N Engl J Med* 2001; **345**:1583–92.

76. Stephens NG, Parsons A, Schofield PM, Kelly F, Cheeseman K, Mitchinson MJ. Randomised controlled trial of vitamin E in patients with coronary disease: Cambridge Heart Antioxidant Study (CHAOS). *Lancet* 1996; **347**:781–6.

77. The Long-term Intervention with Pravastatin in Ischaemic Disease (LIPID) Study Group. Prevention of cardiovascular events and death with pravastatin in patients with coronary artery disease and a broad range of initial cholesterol levels. *N Engl J Med* 1998; **339**:1349–57.

78. Downs JR, Clearfield M, Weis S, et al. Primary prevention of acute coronary events with lovastatin in men and women with average cholesterol levels: results of the AFCAPS/TexCAPS. Air Force/Texas Coronary Atherosclerosis Prevention Study. *JAMA* 1998; **279**:1615–22.

79. Kane JP, Malloy MJ, Ports TA, Phillips NR, Diehl JC, Havel RJ. Regression of coronary atherosclerosis during treatment of familial hypercholesterolemia with combined drug regimens. *JAMA* 1990; **264**:3007–12.

80. Hodis HN, Mack, WJ, Lobo R. Antiatherosclerosis interventions in women. *Am J Cardiol* 2002; **90** (Suppl):17F–21F.

81. Blankenhorn DH, Hodis HN. Duff Memorial Lecture: Arterial imaging and atherosclerosis reversal. *Arterioscler Thromb* 1994; **14**:177–92.

82. Blankenhorn DH, Azen SP, Kramsch DM, et al. Coronary angiographic changes with lovastatin therapy. The Monitored Atherosclerosis Regression Study (MARS). The MARS Research Group. *Ann Intern Med* 1993; **119**:969–76.

83. Scandinavian Simvastatin Survival Study Group. Randomised trial of cholesterol lowering in 4444 patients with coronary heart disease: the Scandinavian Simvastatin Survival Study (4S). *Lancet* 1994; **344**:1383–9.

84. Pollock ML, Franklin BA, Balady GJ, et al. AHA Science Advisory. Resistance exercise in individuals with and without cardiovascular disease: benefits, rationale, safety and prescription. *Circulation* 2000; **101**:828–33.

85. McCartney N, McKelvie RS, Martin J, Sale DG, MacDougall JD. Weight-training-induced attenuation of the circulatory response of older males to weight training. *J Appl Physiol* 1993; **74**:1056–60.

86. Franklin BA, Swain DP, Shephard RJ. New insights in the prescription of exercise for coronary patients. *J Cardiovasc Nurs* 2003; **18**:116–23.

87. Ades PA, Savage PD, Cress ME, Brochu M, Lee NM, Poehlman ET. Resistance training on physical performance in disabled older female cardiac patients. *Med Sci Sports Exerc* 2003; **35**:1265–70.

88. Fiatarone MA, O'Neill EF, Ryan ND, et al. Exercise training and nutritional supplementation for physical frailty in very elderly people. *N Engl J Med* 1994; **330**: 1769–75.

89. US Congress Office of Technology Assessment. *Hip Fracture Outcomes in People Age 50 and Over – Background Paper*. OTA-BP-H-120. Washington, DC: US Government Printing Office, 1994.

90. Riggs BL, Melton LJ. The worldwide problem of osteoporosis: insights afforded by epidemiology. *Bone* 1995; **17** (5 Suppl):505S–11S.

91. Agency for Healthcare Research and Quality. *Osteoporosis in Postmenopausal Women: Diagnosis and Monitoring*. Evidence Report/Technology Assessment No. 28. AHRQ Publication No. 01-E031.

Rockville, MD: Agency for Healthcare Research and Quality, 2001.

92. Albrand G, Munoz F, Sornay-Rendu E, DuBoeuf F, Delmas PD. Independent predictors of all osteoporosis-related fractures in healthy postmenopausal women: the OFELY study. *Bone* 2003; **32**:78–85.

93. Franklin BA, Munnings F. Rejuvenation through exercise, 1996 Encyclopedia Britannica. *Medical and Health Annual* 1995; 253–8.

94. Stuhr RM, Agostini R. Exercise and women's issue. In: Peterson JA, Bryant CX (eds). *The Fitness Handbook*, 2nd edn. St Louis: Wellness Bookshelf, 1995: 245–58.

95. Writing Group for the PEPI. Effects of hormone therapy on bone mineral density: results from the Postmenopausal Estrogen/Progestin Interventions (PEPI) Trial. *JAMA* 1996; **276**:1389–96.

96. Wells G, Tugwell P, Shea B, et al. Meta-analyses of therapies for postmenopausal osteoporosis. V. Meta-analysis of the efficacy of hormone replacement therapy in treating and preventing osteoporosis in postmenopausal women. *Endocr Rev* 2002; **23**:529–39.

97. Cauley JA, Robbins J, Chen Z, et al. Effects of estrogen plus progestin on risk of fracture and bone mineral density: the Women's Health Initiative Randomized Trial. *JAMA* 2003; **290**:1729–38.

98 Delmas PD, Ensrud K, Adachi J, et al. Efficacy of raloxifene on vertebral fracture risk reduction in postmenopausal women with osteoporosis: four-year results from a randomized clinical trial. *J Clin Endocrinol Metab* 2002; **87**:3609–17.

99. Carter ND, Khan KM, McKay HA, et al. Community-based exercise program reduces risk factors for falls in 65- to 75-year old women with osteoporosis: randomized controlled trial. *Can Med Assoc J* 2002; **167**:997–1004.

100. Going S, Lohman T, Houtkooper L, et al. Effects of exercise on bone mineral density in calcium-replete postmenopausal women with and without hormone replacement therapy. *Osteoporos Int* 2003; **14**:637–43.

101. Kelly GA. Aerobic exercise and lumbar spine bone mineral density in postmenopausal women: a meta-analysis. *J Am Geriatr Soc* 1998; **46**:143–52.

102. Kelly GA, Kelley KS, Tran ZV. Resistance training and bone mineral density in women. *Am J Phys Med Rehabil* 2001; **80**:65–77.

103. Kannel WB. Metabolic risk factors for coronary heart disease in women: perspective from the Framingham Study. *Am Heart J* 1987; **114**:413–19.

104. Judelson D. Gender differences in evaluation and management of coronary disease. *Cardiovasc Dis Chest Pain* 1994; **10**:1–8.

105. Lerner DJ, Kannel WB. Patterns of coronary heart disease morbidity and mortality in the sexes: a 26-year follow-up of the Framingham population. *Am Heart J* 1986; **111**:383–90.

106. Warner JG Jr, Brubaker PH, Zhu Y, Morgan TM, Ribisl PM, Miller HS. Long-term (5-year) changes in HDL cholesterol in cardiac rehabilitation patients. Do sex differences exist? *Circulation* 1995; **92**:773–7.

107. Stampfer MJ, Colditz GA, Willett WC, et al. Postmenopausal estrogen therapy and cardiovascular disease. Ten-year follow-up from the Nurses Health Study. *N Engl J Med* 1991; **325**:756–62.

108. Sullivan JM, El-Zeky F, Vander Zwaag R, Ramanathan KB. Effect on survival of estrogen replacement therapy after coronary artery bypass grafting. *Am J Cardiol* 1997; **79**:847–50.

109. Newton KM, LaCroix AZ, McKnight B, et al. Estrogen replacement therapy and prognosis after first myocardial infarction. *Am J Epidemiol* 1997; **145**:269–77.

110. Hulley S, Grady D, Bush T, et al. Randomized trial of estrogen plus progestin for secondary prevention of coronary heart disease in postmenopausal women. Heart and Estrogen/progestin Replacement Study (HERS) Research Group. *JAMA* 1998; **280**:605–13.

111. Herrington DM, Klein KP. Randomized clinical trials of hormone replacement therapy for treatment or prevention of cardiovascular disease: a review of the findings. *Atherosclerosis* 2003; **166**:203–12.

112. Writing Group for the Women's Health Initiative Investigators. Risks and benefits of estrogen plus progestin in healthy postmenopausal women. Principal results from the Women's Health Initiative randomized controlled trial. *JAMA* 2002; **288**:321–33.

113. Writing Group for the Women's Health Initiative Investigators. Effects of conjugated equine estrogen in postmenopausal women with hysterectomy. The Women's Health Initiative randomized controlled trial. *JAMA* 2004; **291**:1701–12.

114. Smith SC, Blair SN, Bonow RO, et al. AHA/ACC guidelines for preventing heart attack and death in patients with atherosclerotic cardiovascular disease: 2001 update. A statement for healthcare professionals from the American Heart Association and the American College of Cardiology. *Circulation* 2001; **104**:1577–9.

115. Pearson TA, Blair SN, Daniels SR, et al. AHA guidelines for primary prevention of cardiovascular disease and stroke: 2002 update: consensus panel guide to comprehensive risk reduction for adult patients without coronary or other atherosclerotic vascular diseases. *Circulation* 2002; **106**:388–91.

116. Pollock ML, Gettman LR, Milesis CA, Bah MD, Durstine L, Johnson RB. Effects of frequency and duration of training on attrition and incidence of injury. *Med Sci Sports* 1977; **9**:31–6.

117. Franklin BA, Lussier L, Buskirk ER. Injury rates in women joggers. *Phys Sports Med* 1979; **7**:105–13.

118. Pate RR, Pratt M, Blair SN, et al. Physical activity and public health. A recommendation from the Centers for Disease Control and Prevention and the American College of Sports Medicine. *JAMA* 1995; **273**:402–7.

119. Debusk RF, Stenestrand J, Sheehan M, Haskell WL. Training effects of long versus short bouts of exercise in healthy subjects. *Am J Cardiol* 1990; **65**:1110–13.

120. Jakicic JM, Wing RR, Butler BA, Robertson RJ. Prescribing exercise in multiple short bouts versus one continuous bout: effects on adherence, cardiorespiratory fitness, and weight loss in overweight women. *Int J Obes Relat Metab Disord* 1995; **19**:893–901.

121. Murphy MH, Hardman AE. Training effects of short and long bouts of brisk walking in sedentary women. *Med Sci Sports Exerc* 1998; **30**:152–7.

122. Balmforth J, Cardozo LD. Trends toward less invasive treatment of female stress urinary incontinence. *Urology* 2003; **62**:52–60.

123. Vierhout ME, Lose G. Preventive vaginal and intra-urethral devices in the treatment of female urinary stress incontinence. *Curr Opin Obstet Gynecol* 1997; **9**:325–8.

124. Newman DK. Stress urinary incontinence in women. *Am J Nurs* 2003; **103**:46–55.

125. Schuessler B, Baessler K. Pharmacologic treatment of stress urinary incontinence: expectations for outcomes. *Urology* 2003; **62**:31–8.

Part 2
Pregnancy/Hormonal Therapies

22

Cardiac disease and cardiac surgery in pregnancy

Marla A. Mendelson

Cardiac physiology during pregnancy, labor and delivery

The expected hemodynamic changes of pregnancy may complicate the course of pregnancy, labor, delivery, or postpartum recovery in women with heart disease. This chapter focuses on women with valvular, congenital, aortic, myocardial or arrhythmic disease who require medical or surgical treatment during pregnancy. Disease-specific potential risks have to be identified and treated to help facilitate a successful pregnancy. The literature regarding cardiovascular complications of pregnancy is replete with numerous case reports and expanded case reports which will be cited when significant potential issues are highlighted.

Hemodynamic alterations expected during pregnancy result from a physiologic 40% increase in blood volume with a 40–50% increase in cardiac output.[1] These changes begin in early pregnancy, peaking at about 20 weeks' gestation (Table 22.1). Plasma volume increases more than the erythrocyte volume, resulting in relative anemia of pregnancy. Augmented cardiac preload may not be tolerated by women with obstructive cardiac lesions such as mitral or aortic stenosis or with impaired ventricular function. Women with normal pulmonary compliance can accommodate the additional blood volume and preload burden. If pulmonary vascular hypertension is present, right-sided heart failure or right-

Table 22.1 Cardiovascular changes of pregnancy by trimester

Trimester	Expected cardiovascular changes
1	• Cardiac output begins to rise as stroke volume increases • Peripheral vasodilation begins
2	• Cardiac output maximal at 30–50% baseline • Minute ventilation increases causing tachypnea • Physiologic anemia of pregnancy • Blood pressure decreases
3	• Heart rate accelerates to maintain increased cardiac output • Uterine compression of inferior vena cava in supine position
Labor and delivery	• Uterine contractions cause bolus of 'fluid' into general maternal circulation • Pain causes tachycardia
Postpartum	• Fluid shifts occur over 24–48 hours • Hemodynamic changes may not resolve for 6–12 weeks

to-left shunting within the heart causes hypoxia and increases the risk of maternal mortality.

Beginning in early pregnancy systemic blood pressure decreases as systemic vascular resistance declines due to peripheral vasodilation decreasing cardiac afterload. This decrease in the mean aortic pressure and widening of the pulse pressure is maximal in the second trimester. Mitral and aortic regurgitation may improve with afterload reduction. In the supine position, the gravid uterus compresses the inferior vena cava, acutely decreasing preload and causing supine hypotension or syncope.[2] Increases in heart rate and stroke volume are attenuated in the left lateral decubitus position during both pregnancy and labor, when hemodynamic fluctuations may be deleterious for women with specific cardiac lesions.

Hemodynamic changes of labor and delivery may pose potential problems for the woman with heart disease. For example, with each uterine contraction of labor, there is a transient bolus of fluid into the intravascular space augmenting cardiac output by 15–20%, with a 10% increase in mean systemic arterial blood pressure. A reflex bradycardia may occur. These changes are attenuated in the left lateral decubitus position.[2] Pain and anxiety stimulate the sympathetic nervous system, causing a rise in blood pressure and heart rate. The prolonged Valsalva maneuver required during pushing may increase blood pressure and afterload, potentially complicating aortic disease. Epidural anesthesia should be instituted slowly with adequate, carefully controlled rehydration to prevent marked fluctuations in blood pressure. Vasodilation from anesthesia may result in a marked hypotension; after vigorous fluid resuscitation, the woman with obstructive valvular disease or a cardiomyopathy may develop pulmonary edema. Electrocardiographic monitoring for arrhythmia facilitates rapid intervention for tachyarrhythmias. Hemodynamic monitoring with a pulmonary artery catheter can help avoid excessive fluid administration while maintaining adequate perfusion pressure during labor and delivery in the setting of severe valvular stenosis or left ventricular dysfunction; this should continue into the early postpartum period because rapid volume shifts may have adverse hemodynamic effects. Endocarditis prophylaxis at the time of labor and delivery is considered optional for an uncomplicated vaginal or cesarean delivery.[3]

The safety of breastfeeding while taking medications required during the postpartum period should be carefully evaluated with the pediatrician. For example, heparin is not secreted in breast milk, and warfarin apparently is inactive. No major hemody-namic differences have been observed in women who breastfeed. Hemodynamic changes usually resolve by 6 weeks postpartum but may take up to 12 weeks.[4]

Valvular heart disease (see also Chapters 32 and 33)

In the past, rheumatic heart disease was the major cause of valvular heart disease in women of childbearing age. Currently it is less common in developed countries, but remains a problem in the Third World. It remains an important issue for women who emigrate to North America or Europe and present during pregnancy. In recent years congenital valvular heart disease is increasingly recognized at birth, during childhood, or in adulthood.[5] Valvular heart disease in women is associated with increased risk of cardiovascular complications, preterm delivery, intrauterine growth retardation, and lower birth weight.[6]

Mitral valve disease

Historically, mitral stenosis was the most common rheumatic valvular lesion diagnosed during pregnancy.[5] In mitral stenosis, pulmonary venous hypertension develops, the right ventricle dilates and right ventricular dysfunction with tricuspid regurgitation occurs. Expanded stroke volume and increased heart rate may cause symptoms for the first time during pregnancy. Left atrial enlargement increases the risk of atrial fibrillation and left atrial thrombus formation in the hypercoagulable pregnant patient. If atrial fibrillation occurs, therapeutic anticoagulation is required to prevent systemic embolization, although the specific drug used during pregnancy remains controversial.[7,8] Poor cardiac output or atrial fibrillation with an increased ventricular rate may compromise blood flow to the uterus; infants born to mothers with mitral stenosis had lower birth weights.[6] During pregnancy, it is important to continue rheumatic fever prophylaxis with daily penicillin.[7]

Mitral stenosis can be confirmed and monitored during pregnancy by two-dimensional and Doppler echocardiography to determine left atrial size,

Table 22.2 Cardiac diagnostic testing during pregnancy

Indication	Testing	Safety issues
Arrhythmia detection	Electrocardiogram	Safe
	Holter	Safe
	Event monitor	Safe
Arrhythmia provocation	Stress testing	Heart-rate-limited
Diagnosis of valvular heart disease	Doppler echocardiography	Safe
Assess cardiac anatomy and function	Doppler echocardiography	Safe
	Magnetic resonance imaging	After 18 weeks' gestation
Detection of intra-atrial thrombus	Transesophageal echocardiography	Sedation required
Diagnosis of aortic dissection	Transesophageal echocardiography	See above
	Computed tomography	Radiation risk
Detection of ischemia	Stress testing	Heart-rate-limited
	Radionuclide imaging	Contraindicated
	Cardiac catheterization and angiography	Radiation risk, requires abdominal shielding

ventricular function, and severity of stenosis (Table 22.2). Pulmonary artery pressure can be estimated by the velocity of the tricuspid regurgitation jet and the transmitral gradient as assessed with Doppler echocardiography. The transmitral gradient by echocardiography may appear higher due to the increased cardiac output and velocity of blood flow in the latter half of pregnancy and may translate into a smaller calculated valve area.[9] Thrombi of the left atrial appendage are best visualized with transesophageal echocardiography.

The major risks during pregnancy are atrial fibrillation, embolic events, and pulmonary edema. Women with mild symptoms may respond to limitations of physical activity and restricted dietary sodium. Cardioselective β-adrenergic blockade may help maintain sinus rhythm or slow the heart rate in atrial fibrillation.[10] β-Adrenergic blockade in pregnancy carries the risk of fetal bradycardia, congestive heart failure, bronchospasm, central nervous system effects, nausea, diarrhea, abdominal discomfort, and hypoglycemia (Table 22.3). These drugs pass through the placenta and are secreted in breast milk.[10] Adverse fetal affects, described when the mother has been treated for hypertension, include intrauterine growth restriction, maternal or fetal bradycardia, delayed neonatal breathing, neonatal hypoglycemia, and neonatal hyperbilirubinemia. Atrial fibrillation with hemodynamic

compromise necessitates electrical cardioversion after adequate systemic anticoagulation.[11] Adenosine, a naturally occurring substance with a brief half-life, may be administered acutely to treat paroxysmal supraventricular tachycardia.[12] Calcium channel blockers, such as verapamil and diltiazem, can be used orally. Pulmonary edema is treated with diuretics and digoxin for left ventricular dysfunction or rate control (Table 22.3).[7]

Percutaneous, trans-septal mitral balloon valvuloplasty has been performed in pregnant women with symptoms of heart failure refractory to medical therapy to forestall the need for surgical valve replacement.[13–17] In one series there were no deleterious radiation effects to the child after 5 years.[17] Balloon mitral valvuloplasty is contraindicated if significant mitral regurgitation or a left atrial thrombus is present. Cardiac surgery (see below) is indicated in women with symptoms despite medical therapy and if balloon valvuloplasty is not an option.

Mitral regurgitation occurs due to mitral valve prolapse, prior endocarditis, ruptured chordae tendineae, rheumatic disease, or as part of congenital cardiac disease. Mitral regurgitation with mitral prolapse maybe part of the Marfan syndrome (see below). Pregnancy is well tolerated with mitral regurgitation with normal left ventricular function. With decreased systemic vascular resistance, the severity of mitral regurgitation may decrease during

Table 22.3 Common cardiovascular medications in pregnancy

Drug and indication	Reported risks in pregnancy	FDA class
Anticoagulant and antiplatelet agents for prevention of thrombus and prosthetic valve dysfunction; thrombolytics		
Warfarin	Teratogenic, embryopathy, contraindicated	X
Heparin*	Bleeding, osteoporosis, thrombocytopenia, prosthetic valve thrombosis	B/C
Aspirin	Bleeding, early ductus closure	C/D
Streptokinase; tissue plasminogen activator	Bleeding, allergy	C
β-Adrenergic blockers for arrhythmias, mitral stenosis, coronary heart disease or valvular dysfunction		
Metoprolol	Unknown	C
Atenolol	Intrauterine growth restriction	D
Propranolol	Intrauterine growth restriction, bradycardia, hypoglycemia, respiratory depression	C
Esmolol	Fetal bradycardia	C
Inotropic agents for ventricular dysfunction		
Digoxin	Probably safe; dosing may vary	C
Dopamine	Unknown	C
Dobutamine	Unknown	B
Amrinone	Unknown	C
Diuretics for congestive heart failure or pulmonary edema		
Thiazide	Volume depletion, neonatal jaundice, thrombocytopenia	C/D
Furosemide	Volume depletion	C
Vasodilators for valvular disease or ventricular dysfunction		
Nitrates	Hypotension	C
Sodium nitroprusside	Cyanide toxicity	C
Angiotensin-converting enzyme inhibitors†	Contraindicated, oligohydramnios, neonatal anuria	D
Hydralazine	Fetal distress with decrease in blood pressure rate, thrombocytopenia	C
Calcium channel blockers for arrhythmias, hypertension or coronary spasm		
Diltiazem, verapamil, nifedipine, amlodipine	Unknown, possible uterine effects	C
Antiarrhythmic agents for supraventricular or ventricular arrhythmias		
Adenosine	Bradycardia, transient asystole	C
Verapamil	Uterine effects	C
Quinidine	Oxytotic at toxic doses, fetal thrombocytopenia, VIII cranial nerve toxicity	C
Procainamide	Unknown	C
Lidocaine	Fetal central nervous system and cardiac toxicity	B/C
Amiodarone	Maternal or fetal thyroid disorder	D
Sotolol	QT prolongation, torsade de pointes, few data available, see β-adrenergic blockers	D
Flecainide, propafenone	Limited information	C

FDA, US Food and Drug Administration.
*Unfractionated and low-molecular-weight forms.
†Risk applies to angiotensin-receptor blockers.

pregnancy; the characteristic 'click' of mitral valve prolapse may not be auscultated as pregnancy progresses. Severe mitral regurgitation with limited exercise capacity may require mitral valve repair prior to conception.

Aortic valve disease

Aortic stenosis may be due to rheumatic disease, a congenitally bicuspid aortic valve, or prior endocarditis.[18] A bicuspid aortic valve may be clinically silent but when stenotic, symptoms may first develop during pregnancy. As in mitral stenosis, the increase in cardiac output, stroke volume, and heart rate of pregnancy may cause congestive heart failure.[19] Mild to moderate aortic stenosis may be well tolerated. In severe aortic stenosis, clinical symptoms of chest pain, syncope, or dyspnea often appear after 20 weeks' gestation when cardiac output is maximal. Echocardiography defines the anatomy of the valve and left ventricular size and function. Doppler echocardiography measures the valve gradient and quantifies regurgitation. The gradient across the aortic valve increases during pregnancy because the velocity of blood flow rises: there may be an increased gradient during pregnancy without progression of stenosis. Congenital aortic stenosis is associated with an increased risk of congenital heart disease in the offspring.[20]

Women with severe aortic stenosis, a valve area less than 1.0 cm^2, should be discouraged from becoming pregnant, especially if symptomatic with reduced functional capacity. If moderate aortic stenosis is identified prior to pregnancy, it may be best to proceed with pregnancy before the stenosis progresses and surgery is required. A woman of childbearing age may have had a Ross procedure for aortic valve disease in which the pulmonic valve is placed in the aortic position and a homograft replaces the pulmonic valve, obviating the need for long-term anticoagulation; she should tolerate pregnancy well.[21] Postoperative complications of the Ross procedure include pulmonic graft stenosis and neo-aortic insufficiency. Palliative percutaneous balloon aortic valvuloplasty has been described during pregnancy when symptoms develop in the second or third trimester.[22,23] Radiation exposure should be minimal with abdominal lead shielding. Surgical intervention

(discussed below) may be required if medical management fails or the patient is not a candidate for percutaneous valvuloplasty.[24,25] The choice of valve replacement in a woman of childbearing age remains controversial; porcine valve replacement to avoid long-term anticoagulation will necessitate reoperation because the porcine valve has an estimated life-span of 7–10 years.[8,26] A mechanical valve requires full, therapeutic anticoagulation which complicates future pregnancies, posing risks to both mother and fetus.[27]

During labor and delivery, a hemodynamic monitoring catheter may help in the management of severe aortic stenosis by maintaining adequate cardiac filling pressures while avoiding excessive preload and pulmonary edema.

Anesthetic agents that cause significant vasodilation should be used with care to avoid increasing the gradient across the aortic valve. Prophylactic antibiotics for endocarditis are optional in this patient population for a normal uncomplicated vaginal delivery.

Aortic regurgitation may be due to rheumatic fever, endocarditis, vasculitis, aortic dilation, Marfan syndrome, or a congenitally bicuspid aortic valve. Mild or moderate aortic regurgitation with normal ventricular size and function is well tolerated during pregnancy. With the decrease in systemic vascular resistance, the murmur of aortic regurgitation may diminish as pregnancy progresses. Severe aortic regurgitation with left ventricular dilation and decreased left ventricular function may worsen with the additional volume load of pregnancy. Ideally medications are not used in the first trimester, but if afterload reduction is necessary, after 13 weeks' gestation, hydralazine should be used for vasodilation instead of angiotensin-converting enzyme (ACE) inhibitors, which are contraindicated in the second and third trimester of pregnancy (see Table 22.3). Antibiotic prophylaxis at the time of labor and delivery is optional. Aortic regurgitation due to active endocarditis during pregnancy may require surgery if the infection cannot be controlled or if hemodynamic deterioration occurs despite medical therapy.[7]

Tricuspid valve disease

Rheumatic tricuspid stenosis is usually associated with mitral and/or aortic valve involvement. This is often well tolerated, even when intervention has been required for mitral or aortic disease.[28] Congenital tricuspid atresia is most often diagnosed and repaired during childhood.

Tricuspid valve regurgitation is often associated with complex congenital cardiac disease, often after surgical repair. In general, tricuspid regurgitation is well tolerated during pregnancy unless it is secondary to a cardiomyopathy or as a sequela of congenital heart disease such as tetralogy of Fallot. Severe tricuspid valve regurgitation due to prior endocarditis is rare but has been associated with illicit intravenous drug use.

Pulmonic valve disease

Pulmonic valvar stenosis is most often congenital in origin and in adults is usually of mild or moderate severity. There is no increased risk in pregnancy if the woman is asymptomatic and has normal exercise tolerance.[29] Severe pulmonic stenosis may necessitate percutaneous balloon valvuloplasty, optimally performed prior to pregnancy. The woman with severe pulmonic stenosis may become symptomatic with the increased preload of pregnancy and develop secondary tricuspid regurgitation. Pulmonic stenosis is often associated with other congenital heart lesions such as tetralogy of Fallot and may be present years after surgery. Branch pulmonary artery stenosis may cause an increased gradient across the pulmonic valve at echocardiography and if severe, may require percutaneous stent placement. Pulmonic regurgitation is well tolerated during pregnancy if right ventricular function is normal and tricuspid regurgitation minimal.[29,30]

Prosthetic valves

The use of porcine homograft or bioprosthetic valves may eliminate the need for anticoagulation in the aortic position but not in the mitral position.[31,32] Valve deterioration has been described during the teen years and young adulthood, but these changes appear to be independent of pregnancy.[33–35] A woman with a bioprothesis should be evaluated prior to a planned pregnancy.[36]

Thromboembolic events, bleeding, and endocarditis are the major risks for a woman with a mechanical prosthetic valve during pregnancy.[27,37–41] Other risks include heart failure, atrial fibrillation, and prosthetic valve thrombosis and dysfunction.[39,40] The estimated risk of valve thrombosis varies between 4 and 14% despite anticoagulation. Emergent thrombolysis with streptokinase or tissue plasminogen activator during pregnancy has been described.[40] Concerns have been raised as to whether multiple cutaneous heparin injections can provide adequate anticoagulation for a mechanical prosthetic heart valve.[26,27,38,39,41–46] Heparin, a large molecule, does not cross the placenta. Maternal risks with heparin include osteoporosis, thrombocytopenia, and bleeding. Subcutaneous administration should be changed to intravenous administration near the time of delivery to allow more precise control, especially when cesarean section is required.[46,47] Low-molecular-weight heparin may be easier to administer throughout pregnancy, but has been studied only in women at risk for thromboembolic events.[47–49] The use of low-molecular-weight heparin for prosthetic valve anticoagulation during pregnancy has been questioned after reports of maternal death despite adequate anticoagulation.[46,48–50]

Warfarin sodium offers reliable, therapeutic anticoagulation but crosses the placenta and has an associated embryopathy including nasal hypoplasia, saddle nose, and stippled epiphysis.[8,32,51] A Canadian study assessed the risk of embryopathy as 6.4%.[38] The risk was increased when the warfarin dose was greater than 5 mg.[52] Warfarin has been associated with a high rate of spontaneous abortion and still-birth.[32,53,54] Administered in the second and third trimesters, warfarin has been associated with serious central nervous system defects, including optic atrophy, Dandy–Walker malformation, and agenesis of the corpus collosum. Hemorrhagic complications may occur in the neonatal period.

Congenital heart disease (see also Chapter 32)

Common congenital heart diseases in the adult include atrial and ventricular septal defects, patent ductus arteriosus, and coarctation of the aorta.

Unrepaired complex cyanotic congenital heart disease rarely presents in the adult; usually palliation or surgical repair has occurred. After surgery, residual heart disease and/or surgical sequelae may include tachyarrhythmias, heart block, valvular stenosis or regurgitation, ventricular dysfunction or vascular abnormalities. These should be assessed and treated prior to conception.[29,55,56] Pregnancy is contraindicated when there is significant pulmonary hypertension, as there is a 50% risk of maternal mortality.[30,56] Maternal hemodynamics and medications directly affect fetal outcome. Maternal cyanosis is associated with higher incidence of abortion, stillbirth, and small-for-gestational-age babies.[57]

The risk of congenital heart disease in the offspring of women with congenital heart disease is between 3.7 and 16.1% compared with the general population.[20,55,58,59] Paternal congenital heart disease confers a risk estimated from 2.1 to 14%.[20,55] Fetal echocardiography at 22 weeks' gestation can identify most major cardiac malformations to help anticipate and treat problems in the neonatal period.[60]

Common congenital heart lesions in adults

Atrial septal defect, ventricular septal defect, patent ductus arteriosus

Atrial septal defect, secundum type, is one of the most common congenital heart lesions in adults and is more common than primum or sinus venosus atrial septal defects.[55,61] The ostium primum defect usually is detected and closed during childhood; however, an intracardiac shunt or regurgitation through the mitral valve may be present in adults. An uncorrected atrial septal defect may be complicated by pulmonary hypertension. During pregnancy, as systemic blood pressure falls below that of the elevated right-sided pressure, the interatrial shunt reverses and cyanosis results.[30] Therefore severe pulmonary hypertension is a contraindication to pregnancy. A woman with unrepaired atrial septal defect is at risk for paradoxical emboli if undergoing prolonged bed rest and requires anticoagulation for the prevention of deep venous thrombosis. Secundum atrial septal defects are currently closed by catheter-based devices.

Pregnancy should be delayed 6 months after the procedure to allow for endothelialization of the device. A repaired atrial septal defect without associated pulmonary hypertension does not confer increased risk in pregnancy and antibiotic prophylaxis at delivery is not indicated.[3] The risk of atrial arrhythmias may persist despite prior surgery or device closure. Patients with right-to-left shunting should have filters placed on all vascular accesses.

Ventricular septal defect is the most common congenital heart anomaly identified at birth; it is less common in adults as it may close spontaneously within the first 5 years of life. Aortic regurgitation may be present as the aortic leaflet prolapses into a membranous ventricular septal defect.[55] Rarely, pulmonary hypertension occurs. This is a high-risk lesion for endocarditis, but antibiotic prophylaxis is optional for an uncomplicated vaginal delivery.[3] After closure of the ventricular septal defect, there may be residual shunting from multiple muscular defects. Residual shunting or pulmonary hypertension can be confirmed by Doppler echocardiography during pregnancy. After surgical closure, pregnancy is not of increased risk if pulmonary pressures are normal, but there is significant maternal risk if pulmonary hypertension is present (see Eisenmenger's syndrome below).[30]

When diagnosed during childhood, a patent ductus arteriosus is usually ligated; it is rarely detected during adulthood. Elevation of pulmonary artery pressure and potential reversal of shunt with profound systemic hypotension pose the same theoretic risks as the septal defects.[55] Previous repair, normal pulmonary pressures, and preserved left ventricular function bode well for pregnancy.

Eisenmenger's complex is the hemodynamic consequence of a shunt lesion that has caused severe pulmonary vascular disease. Right ventricular pressure is increased, resulting in right-to-left shunting of deoxygenated blood. Cyanosis develops with digital clubbing and polycythemia. Pregnancy is contraindicated in women with Eisenmenger's syndrome, as there is a maternal mortality rate up to 50%.[30,55] A recent series of experiences from three referral centers reported a maternal mortality of 27%.[62] During pregnancy right ventricular enlargement may result in heart failure or arrhythmia. Right-to-left shunting may increase, worsening hypoxemia.[63] For women presenting in the first trimester of pregnancy, termination should be considered for the sake of maternal health. Later in pregnancy, termination can pose substantial risk and should be monitored carefully.[57]

Pregnant women with Eisenmenger's syndrome should limit their physical activities, avoid the supine position in later pregnancy, and possibly receive prophylactic anticoagulation.[64] At the time of labor and delivery, there should be a hemodynamic monitoring catheter to follow the fluid status and intracardiac pressures.[65,66] Oxygen saturation should be followed, and oxygen administered through labor, delivery, and in the postpartum period.[64] The risk to the mother appears to be increased with cesarean section.[67] The fetal mortality can exceed 40% even if the mother survives. Prematurity and low birth weight have been correlated with the severity of maternal cyanosis.[57,68]

Complex cyanotic congenital heart disease

Tetralogy of Fallot, the most common cyanotic congenital heart disease, includes a large ventricular septal defect, infundibular pulmonic stenosis, right ventricular hypertrophy, and an overriding aorta.[55] In unrepaired tetralogy of Fallot there is bi-directional shunting through the ventricular septal defect. As systemic vascular resistance decreases throughout pregnancy, there is increased right-to-left shunting and hypoxia occurs. The severity of cyanosis could worsen with a dramatic fall in systemic blood pressure after hemorrhage or profound vasodilation.[30,55] Prolonged Valsalva maneuvers, as pushing of the second stage of labor, may further decrease systemic blood flow, favoring right-to-left shunting and worsening cyanosis.

Pregnancy should be well tolerated after correction of tetralogy of Fallot with mild, residual tricuspid regurgitation, pulmonic stenosis or regurgitation.[30,69] Preconception Doppler echocardiography can determine baseline pulmonary pressures and valvular abnormalities. Significant pulmonary regurgitation and/or right ventricular outflow tract obstruction causing right ventricular dilatation and dysfunction may necessitate surgery prior to conception.[70] Holter monitoring can document supraventricular or ventricular arrhythmias if symptoms of palpitations,

near-syncope, or syncope arise. Antiarrhythmic medication is continued through pregnancy if clinically indicated; there are limited case reports of treatment during pregnancy using most agents (see Table 22.3), but some are contraindicated, e.g. US Food and Drug Administration (FDA) Class D.

Ebstein's anomaly is characterized by distal displacement of the septal leaflet of the tricuspid valve into the right ventricle with atrialization of the right ventricle. If severe, it is typically treated in childhood. Women of childbearing age may be relatively asymptomatic, with a less severe form. Tricuspid regurgitation often is present, and there may be an atrial septal defect or a patent foramen ovale. Cyanosis can occur in the adult and worsen with exercise, fatigue, or exposure to cold. An observational report of women with Ebstein's anomaly found that pregnancy outcome correlated with preconception maternal cardiac status.[71] Tricuspid regurgitation may increase during pregnancy; the right ventricle could enlarge and possibly fail. Cyanosis may appear for the first time as systemic blood pressure falls, promoting right-to-left shunting through an atrial septal defect or a patent foramen ovale. These patients may have an accessory bypass tract, the Wolff–Parkinson–White syndrome, facilitating a supraventricular tachycardia.[71] Limited data are available regarding pregnancy after tricuspid valve reconstruction, but the risk of complications during pregnancy depends on the degree of residual tricuspid regurgitation, right ventricular function, and presence of arrhythmia. Tricuspid regurgitation may increase with the prolonged Valsalva maneuver of pushing in the second stage of labor.

There have been case reports of women of childbearing age with severe complex cyanotic congenital heart disease who have undergone successful pregnancies.[72-83] An uncomplicated pregnancy is associated with normal or near-normal pulmonary artery pressures, normal systemic ventricular function, and absence of cyanosis.[79] Electrophysiologic sequelae such as bradyarrhythmias, heart block, supraventricular arrhythmias, or ventricular arrhythmias necessitate the continuation of antiarrhythmic therapy during pregnancy. Women with tricuspid atresia, single ventricle, or double outlet right ventricle may have undergone a Fontan procedure, a conduit to direct venous blood to the pulmonary artery. Although they may have a subnormal response to exercise and limited cardiac reserve, there are reports of successful pregnancies.[81] Potential complications include atrial fibrillation/flutter, peripheral edema, hepatomegaly, and ascites.[82]

D-Transposition of the great arteries occurs when the aorta arises from the right ventricle and the pulmonary artery from the morphologic left ventricle. Previously, this was repaired by an atrial switch (Mustard or Senning procedure) to redirect incoming venous flow to the appropriate ventricle. After the Mustard repair, the morphologic right (systemic) ventricle must withstand the additional blood volume load of pregnancy and if dilated, may not return to original size and function after pregnancy. Atrial arrhythmias or heart block may occur years after the atrial switch operation and complicate pregnancy. Normal functional capacity, sinus rhythm, and an intact repair contribute to a favorable outcome of pregnancy.[77,78,80] Women currently approaching childbearing age will have undergone the arterial switch (Jatene) procedure to reattach the great vessel to the appropriate ventricle and re-implant the coronary arteries. Pregnancy has not yet been reported in survivors of the arterial switch procedure surgery.

L-Transposition of the great vessels, characterized by the aorta arising from the morphologic right ventricle receiving blood from the left atrium and the pulmonary artery arising from a morphologic left ventricle, may be present in relatively asymptomatic adults.[55] Cardiac complications of L-transposition of the great arteries include heart block, systemic A-V valve regurgitation and systemic ventricular failure. A report of 22 patients with 60 pregnancies noted congestive heart failure during pregnancy related to severe systemic A-V valve regurgitation.[83] Other reported complications included toxemia, endocarditis, cyanosis, cerebrovascular accident, and myocardial infarction (MI) in a patient with anomalous coronary artery anatomy.[83,84] Heart block may limit cardiac adaptation to the hemodynamic changes of pregnancy.[84]

Aortic disease

Aortic disease may be congenital, as a coarctation of the aorta, or part of the Marfan syndrome.[85]

Hormonal changes mediate smooth muscle relaxation within the aortic wall and pregnant women may be more susceptible to aortic dilation, dissection, and rupture in the last trimester of pregnancy.[86] However, a recent study did not find increased incidence of aortic disease in women during pregnancy.[87]

Coarctation of the aorta, a focal narrowing of the distal aortic arch or descending aorta, typically after the left subclavian artery, usually is diagnosed during childhood. In adults, it may be complicated by hypertension, aortic disease, or arteritis and it is associated with a bicuspid aortic valve, ventricular septal defect, or patent ductus arteriosus.[55] Coarctation of the aorta is associated with aneurysms of the circle of Willis which may manifest as intracranial hemorrhage. After childhood repair, preconception evaluation should determine significant restenosis (gradient >20 mmHg) or hypertension requiring medication. In the setting of unrepaired coarctation of the aorta, there is theoretical concern as to whether uteroplacental perfusion is adequate. Hypertension may worsen during pregnancy and pre-eclampsia may occur.[88,89] There have been reports of aortic dissection during pregnancy.[86,88]

Marfan syndrome, a rare connective tissue disorder, has autonomic dominant genetic transmission with a high degree of penetrance. Clinical manifestations include skeletal, ocular, pulmonary, and cardiovascular abnormalities. Aortic dilatation may first manifest in young adulthood with aortic dissection, aortic rupture, or aortic valve regurgitation.[90–93] Myxomatous changes of the aortic or mitral valve result in leaflet prolapse and valvular regurgitation. Women with Marfan syndrome considering pregnancy must be aware that there is the 50% risk of offspring inheriting the syndrome and that there is increased risk of aortic rupture and dissection in the third trimester.[90–93] Hormonally mediated changes in the aortic wall with high estrogen levels may interfere with collagen deposition in the media and predispose to aneurysm formation or dissection.[7] Pyeritz reported that 20 of 32 women with Marfan syndrome with aortic dilatation died of aortic dissection during or shortly after pregnancy. Pregnancy should be discouraged if the aortic diameter exceeds 4.0 cm by echocardiography.[92,93] Noninvasive imaging with transesophageal echocardiography, computed tomography, or magnetic resonance imaging can evaluate aortic size before or during pregnancy, or if aortic dissection is suspected.

Medical therapy of the aortic dissection includes intravenous β-adrenergic blockade and sodium nitroprusside infusion to control blood pressure. Sodium nitroprusside, a potent vasodilator, is also used in pregnancy for hypertensive crisis unresponsive to conventional therapy. It is metabolized to cyanide and thiocyanate and crosses the placenta, raising concern as to its potential fetal toxicity. In animal studies, fetal deaths occurred during administration of very high (25 mg/kg/min) doses, but no such effects were observed with standard therapeutic doses (less than 10 mg/kg/min). Therefore, maternal cyanide levels have to be monitored during extended therapy. Adverse maternal effects include flushing, hypotension, and cyanide toxicity. Surgical intervention is indicated for ascending aortic dissection, as in the nonpregnant patient.[94] Continuation of prophylactic β-adrenergic blockade in the woman with Marfan syndrome or aortic dilation is recommended to prevent aortic dilation during pregnancy.[90]

Coronary heart disease (see also Chapters 14 and 18)

Despite their age, young women may have coronary heart disease (CHD) related to long-standing diabetes mellitus, hypercholesterolemia, hypertension, prior thoracic radiation, or cigarette smoking. CHD suspected during pregnancy or in the preconception evaluation of a woman at risk can be diagnosed by stress echocardiography. Exercise may be heart-rate-limited during pregnancy, but combining cardiac ultrasound with submaximal exercise improves the diagnostic yield. Radionuclide agents should not be used during pregnancy unless absolutely necessary. If cardiac catheterization is deemed necessary during pregnancy for a clinical indication, it should be performed with abdominal shielding (see Table 22.2). Angina and MI rarely occur during pregnancy, but in women at risk, chest pain evaluation must consider CHD.[95] CHD may become symptomatic during pregnancy. Coronary artery spasm may cause angina in the presence of normal coronary arteries, throm-

boembolic events may occur in the hypercoaguable pregnant patient, or coronary dissection may occur.[96–99] The medical management of symptomatic CHD during pregnancy should be similar to the nonpregnant state (see Table 22.3). Selective β-adrenergic blockers, indicated for ischemic disease, hypertension, or arrhythmia, should be continued throughout pregnancy. Atenolol (FDA Class D) should be changed to metoprolol (FDA Class C) during pregnancy. Nitrates should be reserved for symptomatic control of angina because of potential headache, dizziness, weakness, or postural hypotension. Calcium channel blockers may be used for vasospasm. These agents may cause significant hypotension, peripheral edema, and constipation. Low-dose aspirin may be tolerated, although there are risks of bleeding during pregnancy and premature closure of the ductus arteriosus. Intravenous heparin can be used in the patient with unstable angina. There have been rare anecdotal reports of percutaneous transluminal coronary angioplasty (PTCA) and coronary artery bypass graft (CABG) surgery performed during pregnancy[24,25,100] (see below).

MI has been reported during pregnancy or in the postpartum period.[95,101] The women tend to be older, and may have pre-eclampsia. Other case reports suggest that coronary artery thromboembolism may cause the infarct. Coronary artery dissection has also been described as an etiology.[96–98] Medical therapy should be as in the nonpregnant state, although thrombolytic therapy should be avoided and direct angioplasty is preferred.[100] Aspirin should be administered.

During labor, women with symptomatic CHD should continue medications, unless contraindicated, and receive supplemental oxygen. Nitrates and the esmolol may be administered intravenously. Vaginal delivery is preferred; cesarean section is reserved for obstetric indications. There have been case reports of women who have had successful pregnancies after MI and even anecdotal experience with pregnancy after CABG surgery.[102] After CABG surgery, aspirin is continued to maintain graft patency. Lipid-lowering medications, such as niacin, gemfibrozil, lovastatin, pravastatin, simvastatin, or atorvastatin, should not be continued during pregnancy.[103] Normal functional capacity, the absence of angina, and normal ventricular reserve are the best predictors of favorable pregnancy outcome in women with CHD.

Myocardial disease (see also Chapters 29, 30 and 32)

Although rare, women of childbearing age may have acquired systolic or diastolic myocardial dysfunction from a viral myocarditis, prior peripartum cardiomyopathy, prior chemotherapy and/or chest radiation, severe hypertensive disease, or advanced valvular heart disease. It is crucial to evaluate women before conception to assess functional reserve. Women with a history of myocarditis but with normal cardiac function at rest and a normal response to exercise off medications may have a successful pregnancy. Pregnancy is contraindicated in women with symptoms of congestive heart failure occurring with minimal activity or at rest.[104] A dilated left ventricle may further enlarge with pregnancy, as it is unknown whether the heart will revert to normal size and function after the pregnancy; as normally occurs. Preconception evaluation includes assessment of prescribed medications: for example, ACE inhibitors are contraindicated during pregnancy and should be discontinued either before conception or as soon as possible in the first trimester. Abrupt discontinuation of medication may worsen the patient's clinical status. Hydralazine is used during pregnancy for hypertension or vasodilatation. Risks may include reflex tachycardia and hypotension.

Augmented preload during pregnancy in the patient with cardiomyopathy poses the risk of pulmonary edema, usually after the 20th week of gestation. Limitation of dietary salt intake, restriction of physical activity, digoxin, and hydralazine should be instituted when clinically indicated (see Table 22.3). Digoxin can be used during pregnancy to improve systolic function, although the volume of distribution is increased, and higher levels may be required. Diuretic therapy should be reserved for congestive heart failure or pulmonary edema. β-Adrenergic blockers at low doses are instituted once pulmonary edema has resolved. Pregnancy is a hypercoagulable state, and prophylactic anticoagulation may be considered in women who are not ambulatory. When severe pulmonary edema occurs, intravenous inotropic agents, such as dopamine, dobutamine, or amrinone, may be required but may cause tachycardia and ventricular ectopy. They are used in a critical care setting often in conjuction with hemodynamic monitoring (Swan–Ganz catheter). Amrinone, a vasodilator and inotropic agent, administered intravenously has risks of thrombocytopenia, arrhythmia, and hypotension. These women are at risk of developing atrial fibrillation or ventricular ectopy. Amiodarone, a potent anti-arrhythmic with a prolonged half-life, is often needed. It has been associated with maternal and fetal thyroid dysfunction as well as with maternal pulmonary and dermatologic complications (Table 22.3).

Invasive hemodynamic monitoring helps to maintain intracardiac filling pressures during labor and delivery. The impaired ventricle is dependent on adequate preload; however, excessive preload results in pulmonary edema. Fluid shifts may occur after delivery, so the catheter should remain in place for 24–48 hours.

Hypertrophic cardiomyopathy, characterized by myocardial thickening, decreased ventricular compliance and diastolic dysfunction, may be present in women of childbearing age, either idiopathic or secondary to hypertension.[105–109] There is asymmetric hypertrophy of the septum or global, left ventricular hypertrophy. In idiopathic hypertrophic subaortic stenosis, there is asymmetric septal hypertrophy and abnormal mitral valve motion with mitral regurgitation. Women require adequate volume; therefore, the increased preload of pregnancy is not a problem. However, theoretically the decrease in afterload with systemic vasodilation may be problematic. Atrial fibrillation may occur; with the loss of the atrial component of ventricular filling, pulmonary edema may result. Although women present with heart failure and excessive volume overload, inotropic agents such as digoxin should be avoided.[107] Sympathomimetic agents for tocolysis may increase heart rate, further decreasing outflow from the heart and must be used with caution. During the second stage of labor, the Valsalva maneuver should be avoided. Women who require β-adrenergic blockade therapy to prevent the risk of sudden death should continue this medication throughout pregnancy.[107]

Women with cardiomyopathy may have undergone cardiac transplantation for congenital heart disease, hypertrophic cardiomyopathy, postpartum cardiomyopathy, or the presence of a cardiac tumor.[110–114] There have been case reports of successful deliveries after cardiac transplantation and after combined heart–lung transplantation.[110,112–114] The transplanted heart is denervated, although contracting normally. Preconception evaluation should assess cardiac function with echocardiographic stress testing and the absence of rejection should be established by biopsy. Blood pressure should be well controlled throughout pregnancy as hypertension may worsen.[110,112] Immunosuppressive agents must be continued, although fetal complications have been reported with prednisone and cyclosporine.[114–116] Cyclosporine levels must be monitored to avoid toxicity.[115,116] Periodic assessment for rejection with myocardial biopsy may be required. Breastfeeding is discouraged in women taking immunosuppressive agents.[115]

Cardiac arrhythmias (see also Chapter 37)

Palpitations commonly occur during pregnancy representing an awareness of the normal, expected increase in heart rate, isolated premature beats, or a life-threatening arrhythmia. Symptoms occurring at rest or throughout the day should be evaluated to detect significant supraventricular or ventricular arrhythmias by Holter monitoring or event monitoring (Table 22.2). If an arrhythmia is detected during pregnancy, cardiac function should be evaluated by echocardiography. Stress testing is rarely indicated to provoke arrhythmias but may prove useful in the preconception evaluation of the woman with a history of cardiac arrhythmias to determine the need to continue medication during the pregnancy. Other contributing etiologies such as anemia, hyperthyroidism, or drug effect should be considered. Often decongestants, thought safe during pregnancy, may precipitate arrhythmias.

Supraventricular arrhythmias during pregnancy are common; however, symptoms are usually not diagnostic.[12] Atrial fibrillation is rare and is usually associated with underlying hypertensive heart disease, valvular heart disease, hyperthyroidism, pulmonary embolism, pericardial disease, or following cardiac surgery.[117] Intravenous adenosine is used acutely to control rate and convert supraventricular rhythms.[12,118,119] Long-term rhythm control may require cardioselective beta-blockade.[118,119] Verapamil and diltiazem have been used in pregnancy but little information is available.[118,119] For intractable, hemodynamically significant supraventricular arrhythmias, radiofrequency ablation has been used when indicated, with abdominal lead shielding.[117]

Ventricular arrhythmias may be due to caffeine, cocaine, decongestants, or underlying structural heart disease. Women with the long QT syndrome may be at risk for ventricular tachycardia and beta-blockade should be continued during pregnancy.[118,120] Once ventricular arrhythmias are identified, structural heart disease must be considered. Specifically, in late pregnancy, ventricular arrhythmias may be a manifestation of peripartum cardiomyopathy. Life-threatening ventricular tachycardia necessitates electrical cardioversion. Amiodarone may be required for atrial fibrillation or ventricular tachycardia if there is insufficient control with beta-blockade (Table 22.3).[121] Anecdotally, women with implantable defibrillators have tolerated pregnancy.

Heart block occurring for the first time during pregnancy is rare. However, women diagnosed with congenital or acquired heart block prior to conception may have a pacemaker. Pacemaker-dependent patients usually tolerate pregnancy well and heart rate adjustments are not usually required.

Cardiac surgery during pregnancy

Cardiac surgery with extracorporeal circulation may be required during pregnancy to preserve maternal health when medical therapy fails or is not the treatment of choice in an unstable patient. Surgery occurs rarely during pregnancy. The only clinical information available is in the form of case reports, expanded case reports and reviews.[24,122–124] Mitral and aortic valve stenosis and/or regurgitation with severe congestive heart failure (New York Heart

Association functional class III or IV) may necessitate surgery. Surgery for prosthetic valve dysfunction due to thrombosis has been described.[123] Indications for operation for endocarditis may be present and surgery may be required despite the pregnancy.[94] Cardiac surgery during pregnancy may be necessary in heart failure associated with atrial or ventricular septal defects, acute aortic dissection, or CABG surgery in the setting of unstable angina.[24,85,124,125] Medical or catheter-based therapies are preferred when appropriate but if the patient remains clinically unstable surgery should be considered, addressing potential risks to both the mother and fetus.

Potential maternal risks of cardiac surgery during pregnancy include air embolism, hypotension, decreased placental perfusion, uterine contraction, neurologic deficit, and death.[24,124,125] Maternal operative death in one series of 13 patients was 13.3% with concomitant fetal loss.[123] In another review, it ranged between 1.5% and 5%.[122]

Specific fetal risks of cardiac surgery during pregnancy include bradycardia, preterm delivery, neurologic deficit, and stillbirth.[124,125] Fetal mortality has been estimated at 20% but in reviews it has ranged from 16% to 33%.[24,94,122,124,125]

Based on the existing case reports, the following recommendations have been proposed. Cardiac surgery is optimally performed in the early third trimester between 24 and 28 weeks because organogenesis is complete. If performed later, it may precipitate preterm labor and delivery.[125] Normothermic cardioplegia has been recommended because hypothermia may initiate uterine contractions and has been associated with higher fetal death rates.[124] High flow rates may preserve adequate uteroplacental perfusion.[24,122,124,125]

References

1. Robson SC, Hunter S, Moore M, et al. Hemodynamic changes during the puerperium: a Doppler and M-mode echocardiography study. *Br J Obstet Gynaecol* 1987; **94**:1028–39.

2. Kinsella SM, Lohmann G. Supine hypotensive syndrome. *Obstet Gynecol* 1994; **83**:774–88.

3. Dajani AS, Taubert KA, Wilson W, et al. Prevention of bacterial endocarditis. *JAMA* 1997; **277**:1794–801.

4. Capeless EL, Clapp JF. When do cardiovascular parameters return to their preconceptive values? *Am J Obstet Gynecol* 1991; **165**:883–6.

5. McFaul PB, Dornan JC, Lamki H, et al. Pregnancy complicated by maternal heart disease: a review of 519 women. *Br J Obstet Gynaecol* 1988; **95**:861–7.

6. Hameed B, Karaalp IS, Tummala PP, et al. The effect of valvular heart disease on maternal and fetal outcome of pregnancy. *J Am Coll Cardiol* 2001; **37**:893–9.

7. Bonow RO, Carabello B, de Leon AC, et al. Guidelines for the management of patients with valvular heart disease: executive summary. A report of the American College of Cardiology/American Heart Association Task Force on Practice Guidelines (Committee on Management of Patients with Valvular Disease). *Circulation* 1998; **98**:1949–84.

8. Hung L, Rahimtoola S. Prosthetic heart valves and pregnancy. *Circulation* 2003; **107**:1240–6.

9. Rokey R, Hsu HW, Moise KJ, et al. Inaccurate noninvasive mitral valve area calculation during pregnancy. *Obstet Gynecol* 1994; **84**:950–5.

10. Narasimhan C, Joseph G, Singh TC. Propranolol for pulmonary edema in mitral stenosis. *Int J Cardiol* 1994; **44**:178–9.

11. Rosemond RL. Cardioversion during pregnancy. *JAMA* 1993; **269**:3167.

12. Elkayam U, Goodwin TM. Adenosine therapy for supraventricular tachycardia during pregnancy. *Am J Cardiol* 1995; **72**:521–3.

13. Mazur W, Parilak LD, Kaluza G, et al. Balloon valvuloplasty for mitral stenosis. *Curr Opin Cardiol* 1999; **14**:95–103.

14. Kalra GS, Arora R, Kahn JA, et al. Percutaneous mitral commissurotomy for severe mitral stenosis during pregnancy. *Cathet Cardiovasc Diagn* 1994; **33**:28–30.

15. Sananes S, Iung B, Vahanian A, et al. Fetal and obstetrical impact of percutaneous balloon mitral commissurotomy during pregnancy. *Fetal Diagn Ther* 1994; **9**:218–25.

16. Nercolini DC, da Rocha Loures Bueno R, Eduardo

Guerios E, et al. Percutaneous mitral balloon valvulo-plasty in pregnant women with mitral stenosis. *Catheter Cardiovasc Interv* 2002; **57**:318–22.

17. Mangione JA, Lourenco RM, dos Santos ES, et al. Long-term follow up of pregnant women after percutaneous mitral valvuloplasty. *Catheter Cardiovasc Interv* 2000; **50**:413–17.

18. Lao TT, Sermer M, MaGee L, et al. Congenital aortic stenosis and pregnancy: a reappraisal. *Am J Obstet Gynecol* 1993; **169**:540–5.

19. Easterling TR, Chadwick HS, Otto CM, et al. Aortic stenosis in pregnancy. *Obstet Gynceol* 1988; **72**:113–18.

20. Whittemore R, Wells JA, Castellsague X. A second-generation study of 427 probands with congenital heart defects and their 837 children. *J Am Coll Cardiol* 1994; **3**:1459–67.

21. Ross DN. The pulmonary autograft: the Ross principle (or Ross procedural confusion). *J Heart Valve Dis* 2000; **9**:174–5.

22. Lao TT, Adelman AG, Sermer M, et al. Balloon valvuloplasty for congenital aortic stenosis in pregnancy. *Br J Obstet Gynaecol* 1993; **100**:1141–2.

23. Banning A, Pearson J, Hall R. Role of balloon dilatation of the aortic valve in pregnancy patients with severe aortic stenosis. *Br Heart J* 1993; **70**:544–5.

24. Becker RM. Intracardiac surgery in pregnant women. *Ann Thorac Surg* 1993; **36**:453–8.

25. Weiss B, von Sugresser L, Alon E, et al. Outcome of cardiovascular surgery and pregnancy. A systematic review of the period 1984–1996. *Am J Obstet Gynecol* 1998; **179**:1643–53.

26. Ayhan A, Yapar EG, Yuce K, et al. Pregnancy and its complications after cardiac valve replacement. *Int J Obstet Gynecol* 1991; **35**:117–22.

27. Marcus-Braun N, Segal D, Merkin M, et al. Anticoagulation in pregnant women with prosthetic heart valve – a new approach for therapy. *Harefuah* 2003; **142**:508–11, 567.

28. Roguin A, Rinkevich D, Milo S, et al. Long-term follow-up of patients with severe rheumatic tricuspid stenosis. *Am Heart J* 1998; **136**:103–8.

29. Perloff JK, Warnes C. Challenges posed by adults with repaired congenital heart disease. *Circulation* 2001; **103**:2637–43.

30. Perloff JK. Congenital heart disease and pregnancy. *Clin Cardiol* 1994; **17**:579–87.

31. Badduke BR, Jamieson WRE, Miyagishima RT, et al. Pregnancy and childbearing in a population with biologic valvular protheses. *J Thorac Cardiovasc Surg* 1991; **102**:179–86.

32. Salazar E, Espinola N, Roman L, Cassonova JM. Effect of pregnancy on the duration of bovine pericardial bioprostheses. *Am Heart J* 1999; **137**:714–20.

33. Jamieson WRE, Miller CD, Akins CW, et al. Pregnancy and bioprostheses: influence on structural valve deterioration, *Ann Thorac Surg* 1995; **60**:S282–7.

34. Avila WS, Rossi EG, Grinberg M, et al. Influence of pregnancy after bioprosthetic valve replacement in young women: a prospective five-year study. *J Heart Valve Dis* 2002; **11**:864–9.

35. North RA, Sadler L, Stewart AW, et al. Long-term survival and valve-related complications in young women with cardiac valve replacements. *Circulation* 1999; **99**:2669–76.

36. Reimold S, Rutherford J. Valvular heart disease in pregnancy. *N Engl J Med* 2003; **349**:52–9.

37. Hanania G, Thomas D, Michel PL. Pregnancy and prosthetic heart valves: a French cooperative retrospective study of 155 cases. *Eur Heart J* 1994; **15**:1651–8.

38. Chan WS, Anand S, Ginsberg JS. Anticoagulation of pregnant women with mechanical heart valves: a systematic review of the literature. *Arch Intern Med* 2000; **160**:191–6.

39. Suri V, Sawhney H, Vasishta K, et al. Pregnancy following cardiac valve replacement surgery. *Int J Gynecol Obstet* 1999; **64**:239–26.

40. Behrendt P, Schwartzkopff B, Perings S, Gerhardt A, Zotz RB, Strauer BE. Successful thrombolysis of St. Jude medical aortic prothesis with tissue-type plasminogen activator in a pregnant woman: a case report. *Cardiol Rev* 2002; **10**:349–53.

41. Roberts N, Ross D, Flint S, Arya R, Blott M. Thromboembolism in pregnant women with mechanical prosthetic heart valves anticoagulated with low molecular weight heparin. *Br J Obstet Gynaecol* 2001; **108**:327–9.

42. Salazar E, Izaguirre R, Verdejo J, Mutchinick O. Failure of adjusted doses of subcutaneous heparin to prevent thromboembolic phenomena in pregnant patients with mechanical cardiac valve protheses. *J Am Coll Cardiol* 1996; **27**:1698–703.

43. Ginsberg JS, Chan WS, Bates SM, et al. Anticoagulation of pregnant women with mechanical heart valves. *Arch Intern Med* 2003; **163**:694–8.

44. Ginsberg J, Greer I, Hirsh J, Use of antithrombotic agents during pregnancy. *Chest* 2001; **119**:122S-31S.

45. Barbour LA, Smith JM, Marlar RA. Heparin levels to guide thromboembolism prophylaxis during pregnancy. *Am J Obstet Gynecol* 1995; **173**:1869–73.

46. Al-Lawati AA, Venkitraman M, Al-Delaime T, et al. Pregnancy and mechanical heart valves replacement;

dilemma of anticoagulation. *Eur J Cardiothor Surg* 2002; **22**:223–7.

47. Laurent P, Dussarat G, Bonal J, et al. Low molecular weight heparins: a guide to their optimum use in pregnancy. *Drugs* 2002; **62**:463–77.

48. Rowan JA, McCowan L, Raudkivi PJ, et al. Enoxaparin treatment in women with mechanical heart valves during pregnancy. *Am J Obstet Gynecol* 2001; **185**:633–7.

49. Lev-Ran O, Kramer A, Gurevitch J, Shapira I, Mohr R. Low-molecular-weight heparin for prosthetic heart valves: treatment failure. *Ann Thorac Surg* 2000; **69**: 264–6.

50. Berndt N, Khan I, Gallo R. A complication in antico-agulation using low-molecular weight heparin in a patient with a mechanical valve: a case report. *J Heart Valve Dis* 2000; **9**:844–6.

51. Hanania G. Management of anticoagulants during pregnancy. *Heart* 2001; **86**:125–6.

52. Cotrufo M, De Feo M, De Santo LS, et al. Risk of warfarin during pregnancy with mechanical valve prostheses. *Obstet Gynecol* 2002; **99**:35–40.

53. Sadler L, McCowan L, White H, et al. Pregnancy outcomes and cardiac complications in women with mechanical, bioprosthetic and homograft valves. *Int J Obstet Gynecol* 2000; **107**:245–53.

54. Born D, Martinez EE, Almeida P, et al. Pregnancy in patients with prosthetic heart valves: the effects of anticoagulation on mother, fetus and neonate. *Am Heart J* 1992; **124**:413–17.

55. Perloff J, Koos B. Pregnancy and congenital heart disease. In: Perloff J, Child J (eds). *Congenital Heart Disease in Adults*. Philadelphia: WB Saunders, 1998: 144–65.

56. Deanfield J, Thaulow E, Warnes C, et al. Management of grown up congenital heart disease. *Eur Heart J* 2003; **24**:1035–84.

57. Sawhney H, Suri V, Vasishta K, et al. Pregnancy and congenital heart disease – maternal and fetal outcome. *Aust N Z J Obstet Gynaecol* 1998; **38**:266–71.

58. Rose V, Gold RJM, Lindsay G, et al. A possible increase in the incidence of congenital heart defects among the offspring of affected parents. *J Am Coll Cardiol* 1985; **6**:376–82.

59. Burn J, Brennan P, Little J, et al. Recurrence risks in offspring of adults with major heart defects: results from first cohort of British collaborative study. *Lancet* 1998; **351**:311–16.

60. Crawford DC, Chita SK, Allan LD. Prenatal detection of congenital heart disease: factors affecting obstetric management and survival. *Am J Obstet Gynecol* 1988; **59**:352–6.

61. Actis Dato GM, Rinaudo P, Revelli A, et al. Atrial septal defect and pregnancy: a retrospective analysis of obstetrical outcome before and after surgical correction. *Minerva Cardioangiol* 1998; **46**:63–8.

62. Daliento L, Somerville J, Presbitero P, et al. Eisenmenger syndrome. Factors relating to deterioration and death. *Eur Heart J* 1998; **19**:1845–55.

63. Lust KM, Boots RJ, Dooris M, et al. Management of labor in Eisenmenger syndrome with inhaled nitric oxide. *Am J Obstet Gynecol* 1999; **181**:419–23.

64. Avila WS, Grinberg M, Snitcowsky R, et al. Maternal and fetal outcome in pregnant women with Eisenmenger's syndrome. *Eur Heart J* 1996; **16**:460–4.

65. Midwall J, Jaffin H, Herman MV, Kupersmith J. Shunt flow and pulmonary hemodynamics during labor and delivery in the Eisenmenger's syndrome. *Am J Cardiol* 1978; **42**:299–303.

66. Pollack KL, Chestnut DH, Wenstron KD. Anesthetic management of a parturient with Eisenmenger's syndrome. *Anesth Analg* 1990; **70**:212–15.

67. Gleicher N, Midwall J, Hochberer D, et al. Eisenmenger's syndrome and pregnancy. *Obstet Gynecol Surv* 1979; **34**:721–41.

68. Whittemore R. Congenital heart disease: its impact on pregnancy. *Hosp Pract* 1983; **180**:65–74.

69. Nissenkorn A, Friedman S, Schonfeld A, et al. Fetomaternal outcome in pregnancies after total correction of the tetralogy of Fallot. *Int Surg* 1984; **69**:125–8.

70. Therrien J, Marx GR, Gatzoulis MA. Late problems in tetralogy of Fallot – recognition, management, and prevention. *Cardiol Clin* 2002; **20**:395–404.

71. Connolly HM, Warnes CA. Ebstein's anomaly: outcome of pregnancy. *J Am Coll Cardiol* 1994; **23**:1194–8.

72. Chuah SY, Hughes J, Rowlands DB. A successful pregnancy in a patient with congenital tricuspid stenosis and a patent ovale foramen. *Int J Cardiol* 1992; **34**:112–14.

73. Hatjis CG, Gibson M, Capeless EL, et al. Pregnancy in a patient with tricuspid atresia. *Obstet Gynecol* 1983; **145**:114–15.

74. Baumann H, Schneider H, Drack G, et al. Pregnancy and delivery by cesarean section in a patient with transposition of the great arteries and single ventricle: case report. *Br J Obstet Gynaecol* 1987; **94**:704–8.

75. Smoleniec JS, Weaver JB. Two vaginal deliveries in a patient with a single ventricle, transposition of the great arteries, and pulmonary stenosis. *J Obstet Gynecol* 1992; **12**:24–6.

76. Stiller RJ, Vintzieos AM, Nochimson DJ, et al. Single ventricle in pregnancy: case report and review of the literature. *Obstet Gynecol* 1984; **64**:18S–20S.

77. Neukermans K, Sullivan TJ, Pitlick PT. Successful pregnancy after the Mustard operation for transposition of the great arteries. *Am J Cardiol* 1988; **62**:838–9.

78. Clarkson PM, Wilson NJ, Neutze JM, et al. Outcome of pregnancy after Mustard operation for transposition of the great arteries with intact ventricular septum. *J Am Coll Cardiol* 1994; **24**:190–3.

79. Presbitero P, Somerville J, Stone S, et al. Pregnancy in cyanotic congenital heart disease. Outcome of mother and fetus. *Circulation* 1994; **89**:2673–6.

80. Genoni M, Jenni R, Hoerstrup SP, et al. Pregnancy after atrial repair for transposition of the great arteries. *Heart* 1999; **81**:276–7.

81. Canobbio MM, Mair DD, Van Der Velde M, Koos BJ. Pregnancy outcomes after the Fontan repair. *J Am Coll Cardiol* 1996; **28**:763–7.

82. Hoare JV, Radford D. Pregnancy after Fontan repair of complex congenital heart disease. *Aust N Z J Obstet Gynaecol* 2001; **41**:464–8.

83. Connolly HM, Grogan M, Warnes CA. Pregnancy among women with congenitally corrected transposition of great arteries. *J Am Coll Cardiol* 1999; **33**:1692–5.

84. Therrien J, Barnes I, Somerville J. Outcome of pregnancy in patients with congenitally corrected transposition of the great arteries. *Am J Cardiol* 1999; **84**:820–4.

85. Uchida T, Ogino H, Ando M, et al. Aortic dissection in pregnant women with the Marfan syndrome. *Kyobu Geka* 2002; **55**:693–6 [in Japanese].

86. Immer FF, Bansi AG, Immer-Bansi AS, et al. Aortic dissection in pregnancy: analysis of risk factors and outcome. *Ann Thorac Surg* 2003; **76**:309–14.

87. Oskoui R, Lindsay J. Aortic dissection in women: 40 years of age and the unimportance of pregnancy. *Am J Cardiol* 1994; **73**:821–3.

88. Saidi AS, Bezold LI, Altman CA, et al. Outcome of pregnancy following intervention for coarctation of the aorta. *Am J Cardiol* 1998; **82**:786–8.

89. Beauchesne LM, Connolly HM, Ammash NM, et al. Coarctation of the aorta: outcome of pregnancy. *J Am Coll Cardiol* 2001; **38**:1728–33.

90. Elkayam U, Ostrzega E, Shotan A, Mehra A. Cardiovascular problems in pregnant women with the Marfan syndrome. *Ann Intern Med* 1995; **123**:117–22.

91. Lipscomb KJ, Smith JC, Clarke B, Donnai P, Harris R. Outcome of pregnancy in women with Marfan's syndrome. *Br J Obstet Gynaecol* 1997; **104**:201–6.

92. Pyeritz RE. Maternal and fetal complications of pregnancy in the Marfan syndrome. *Am J Med* 1981; **71**:784–90.

93. Lind J, Wallenburg HC. The Marfan syndrome and pregnancy: a retrospective study in a Dutch population. *Eur J Obstet Gynecol* 2001; **98**:28–35.

94. Gopal K, Hudson IM, Ludmir J, et al. Homograft aortic root replacement during pregnancy. *Ann Thorac Surg* 2002; **74**:243–5.

95. Roth A, Elkayan U. Acute myocardial infarction associated with pregnancy. *Ann Intern Med* 1996; **125**:751–62.

96. Celik SK, Sagcan A, Altintig A, et al. Primary spontaneous coronary artery dissections in atherosclerotic patients. Report of nine cases with review of the pertinent literature. *Eur J Cardiothorac Surg* 2001; **20**:573–6.

97. McKechnie RS, Patel D, Eitzman D, Rajagopalan S, Murthy T. Spontaneous coronary artery disease in a pregnant woman. *Obstet Gynecol* 2001; **98**:899–902.

98. Esinler I, Yigit N, Ayham A, Kes S, Aytemir K, Acil T. Coronary artery dissection during pregnancy. *Acta Obstet Gynecol Scand* 2003; **82**:194–6.

99. Hameed AB, Tummala PP, Goodwin T, et al. Unstable angina during pregnancy in two patients with premature coronary atherosclerosis and aortic stenosis in association with familial hypercholesterolemia. *Am J Obstet Gynecol* 2000; **182**:1152–5.

100. Sharma GL, Loubeyre C, Morice MC. Safety and feasibility of the radial approach for primary angioplasty in acute myocardial infarction during pregnancy. *J Invasive Cardiol* 2002; **14**:359–62.

101. Donnelly S, McKenna P, Sugrue D. Myocardial infarction during pregnancy. *Br J Obstet Gynaecol* 1993; **100**:781–2.

102. Frenkel Y, Barkai G, Reisen L, et al. Pregnancy after myocardial infarction: are we playing safe? *Obstet Gynecol* 1991; **77**:822–5.

103. Cashin-Hemphill L, Noone M, Abbott JF, et al. Low-density lipoprotein apheresis therapy during pregnancy. *Am J Cardiol* 2000; **88**:202–3.

104. Elkayam U, Tummala PP, Rao K, et al. Maternal and fetal outcomes of subsequent pregnancies in women with peripartum cardiomyopathy. *N Engl J Med* 2001; **344**:1567–71.

105. Schannwell CM, Schmitz L, Schoebel FC, et al. Left ventricular diastolic function in pregnancy in patients with arterial hypertension. A prospective study with M-mode echocardiography and Doppler echocardiography. *Z Kardiol* 2001; **90**:427–36.

106. Schannwell CM, Zimmerman T, Schneppenheim M, et al. Left ventricular hypertrophy and diastolic dysfunction in healthy pregnant women. *Cardiol* 2002; **97**:73–8.

107. Autore C, Conte MR, Piccininno M, et al. Risk associ-

ated with pregnancy in hypertrophic cardiomyopathy. *J Am Coll Cardiol* 2002; **40**:1864–9.

108. Piacenza JM, Kirkorian G, Audra PH, et al. Hypertrophic cardiomyopathy and pregnancy. *Eur J Obstet Gynecol Reprod Biol* 1998; **80**:17–23.

109. Thaman R, Varnava A, Hamid MS, et al. Pregnancy related complications in women with hypertrophic cardiomyopathy. *Heart* 2003; **89**:752–6.

110. Mendelson MA. Cardiac transplantation and pregnancy. In: Gleicher N, Elkayam U, Gall S, et al. (eds). *Principles and Practice of Medical Therapy in Pregnancy*, 3rd edn. Stamford: Appleton & Lange, 1998: 990–5.

111. Bordignon S, Aramayo AM, Nunes e Silva D, et al. Pregnancy after cardiac transplantation. Report of one case and review. *Arq Bras Cardiol* 2000; **75**:515–22.

112. Morini A, Spina V, Aleandri V, et al. Pregnancy after heart transplant: update and case report. *Hum Reprod* 1998; **3**:749–57.

113. Troche V, Ville Y, Fernandez H. Pregnancy after heart or heart–lung transplantation: a series of 10 pregnancies. *Br J Obstet Gynaecol* 1998; **105**:454–8.

114. Cowan SW, Coscia LC, Philips LZ, et al. Pregnancy outcomes in female heart and heart–lung transplant recipients. *Transplant Proc* 2002; **34**:1855–6.

115. Kossoy LR, Herbert CM III, Colston Wentz A. Management of heart transplant recipients: guidelines for the obstetrician–gynecologist. *Am J Obstet Gynecol* 1988; **159**:490–9.

116. Wagoner LE, Taylor DO, Olsen SL, et al. Immunosuppressive therapy, management, and outcome of heart transplant recipients during pregnancy. *J Heart Lung Transplant* 1994; **13**:993–9.

117. Blomstrom-Lundqvist C, Scheinman M, Aliot E, et al. ACC/AHA/ESC Guidelines for the management of patients with supraventricular arrythmias – Executive Summary: A Report of the American College of Cardiology/American Heart Association Task Force on Practice Guidelines and the European Society of Cardiology Committee for Practice Guidelines (Writing Committee to Develop Guidelines for the Management of Patients With Supraventricular Arrhythmias). *J Am Coll Cardiol* 2003; **42**:1493–531.

118. Gowda R, Khan I, Mehta N, Vasavada B, Sacchi T. Cardiac arrhythmias in pregnancy: clinical and therapeutic considerations. *Int J Cardiol* 2003; **88**:129–33.

119. Joglar J, Page R. Antiarrhythmic drugs in pregnancy. *Curr Opin Cardiol* 2001; **16**:40–5.

120. Rashba EJ, Zareba W, Moss AJ, et al. Influence of pregnancy on the risk for cardiac events in patients with hereditary long QT syndrome. *Circulation* 1998; **97**:451–6.

121. Oakley C, Child A, Jung B, et al. Expert consensus document on management of cardiovascular disease during pregnancy: The Task Force on the Management of Cardiovascular Diseases During Pregnancy of the European Society of Cardiology. *Eur Heart J* 2003; **24**:761–81.

122. Mahli A, Izdes S, Coskun D. Cardiac operations during pregnancy: review of factors influencing fetal outcome. *Ann Thorac Surg* 2000; **69**:1622–6.

123. Salazar E, Espinola N, Molina FJ, Reyes A, Barragan R. Heart surgery with cardiopulmonary bypass in pregnant women. *Arch Cardiol Mex* 2001; **71**:20–7.

124. Pomini F, Mercogliano D, Cavalletti C, Caruso A, Pomini P. Cardiopulmonary bypass in pregnancy. *Ann Thorac Surg* 1996; **61**:259–68.

125. Parry A, Westaby S. Cardiopulmonary bypass during pregnancy. *Ann Thorac Surg* 1996; **61**:1865–9.

23
Hypertension in pregnancy

Gregory Y.H. Lip, William Foster and D. Gareth Beevers

Introduction

Hypertension occurs in about 5% of all pregnancies. However, this covers a wide range of conditions that carry different implications for pregnancy outcome and require different management strategies. Raised blood pressure may be a marker of underlying maternal disease or it may be a consequence of the pregnancy itself. Importantly, however, hypertension in pregnancy affects the fetus as well as the mother, and can result in fetal growth retardation and, if severe, both maternal and fetal morbidity and mortality. If recognized early and managed appropriately, many of these complications can be reduced.

Hypertensive diseases in pregnancy, including pre-eclampsia, remain major causes of maternal and fetal mortality in the UK, where the fetal mortality rate is around 2%.[1] In a recent US study, pregnancy-induced hypertension was found to be the underlying cause in 16% of maternal deaths.[2] Although maternal mortality due to hypertension fell markedly until the mid-1980s, eclampsia remains an important cause of a significant number of deaths,[3,4] and there has been no further decrease in mortality since this time.[2] For example, pre-eclampsia is responsible for one-sixth of all maternal deaths[2,5] and a doubling of perinatal mortality.[6] In addition, in one report fetal survival following mid-trimester severe pregnancy-induced hypertension was as low as 13%.[7]

Despite accurate figures on the effects of raised blood pressure, the precise causes of hypertension in pregnancy are unknown, and eclampsia has been referred to as the 'disease of theories'.

Epidemiology

The exact frequency of hypertension in pregnancy depends on a great many variables, including the stage of pregnancy that has been reached. Equally important is the quality of blood pressure measurement. Most large-scale surveys depend on single (and very casual) readings taken by doctors and midwives who have not received special training in blood pressure measurement. Often the mother is anxious and unrelaxed, and the equipment is inadequately maintained with wrong-sized arm cuffs.

Perhaps the most reliable data come from a survey in Oxford by Redman.[8] In a survey of 6000 women in an unselected obstetric population, 0.1% were found to have a blood pressure of 160/100 mmHg or more before the 20th week of pregnancy, and this figure rose to 3.7% when taking the maximum antenatal reading at any stage of pregnancy.[8] The all-too-often quoted threshold of 140/90 mmHg or more was found in 2.0% of women in early pregnancy and in 21.5% of women at some stage (usually very near to term). From the clinical point of view, the higher threshold more closely reflects the level where positive action might be taken by the clinician.[8] Most of the women with raised blood pressure in early pregnancy probably have pre-existing or chronic hypertension. Most with raised pressure in late pregnancy have either pregnancy-induced hypertension or pre-eclampsia. The combined frequency of pre-eclampsia and eclampsia varies between 1% and 6%, depending on parity, with the higher figure being seen in first pregnancies. In specialist hypertension obstetric clinics the figure is, not surprisingly, much higher at 11.9% and 16% for normotensive and hypertensive women respectively.[9]

In the developed world, perinatal mortality is now approaching 10 per 1000 and of these deaths just under half are due to raised blood pressure. Furthermore, maternal mortality is low, at around 50 deaths per million women; about one-fifth of these deaths can be attributed to all hypertensive diseases combined. Most maternal deaths in England and Wales have been reported to be due to eclampsia or pre-eclampsia, with cerebral hemorrhage being the lethal event.[10] In many cases of death (72% in one series) due to eclampsia or pre-eclampsia, the care (diagnosis and management) was considered to have been substandard, with half of the patients who died of eclampsia having had convulsions despite being admitted to the obstetric wards.[10]

Hypertensive syndromes in pregnancy

There have been several attempts at classifying hypertension in pregnancy. However, none is entirely satisfactory – the current classification is based on the International Society for the Study of Hypertension in Pregnancy (ISSHP) recommendations.[11–13]

Pre-existing essential hypertension (see also Chapter 31)

This is otherwise referred to as chronic hypertension, present before the 20th week of pregnancy, where it is assumed the mother had pre-existing hyperten-

sion, although often no data are available. Thus, chronic hypertension refers to long-term hypertension that is not confined to or caused by pregnancy, but may be revealed for the first time during pregnancy, typically toward the end.

The usual 'cause' of chronic hypertension is essential hypertension. However, secondary causes of hypertension, although infrequent, may occur. About 5% of women of childbearing age have chronic pre-existing hypertension, which is usually mild, as defined by the World Health Organization criterion of a blood pressure of >140/90 mmHg. In women in their late 30s and 40s this figure approaches 10%. Mild essential hypertension in pregnancy does not appear to carry a bad prognosis for the mother or fetus and its early treatment does not convincingly prevent the onset of pre-eclampsia.

Secondary hypertension in pregnancy

This is uncommon, but is accounted for by the more frequent causes of secondary hypertension in younger people, such as pheochromocytoma, renal disease, and primary hyperaldosteronism. For example, pheochromocytoma is well described in association with pregnancy and is associated with a poor maternal and fetal outcome. Hypertension associated with renal disease may exacerbate renal impairment, resulting in poor pregnancy outcome, deterioration of renal function across pregnancy, and subsequent subfertility.

Pregnancy-induced hypertension

Pregnancy-induced hypertension usually develops after the 20th week of pregnancy and usually resolves within 10 days of delivery. For diagnosis of pregnancy-induced hypertension to be made, the blood pressure must be documented to be normal both before and after pregnancy.

There have been many definitions of pregnancy-induced hypertension. The ISSHP defines pregnancy-induced hypertension as a single diastolic blood pressure (phase V) of ≥110 mmHg or two readings of ≥90 mmHg at least 4 hours apart occurring after the 20th week of pregnancy. The National High Blood

Pressure Education Program of the US defines pregnancy-induced hypertension as a rise of >15 mmHg diastolic or 30 mmHg systolic compared with readings taken in early pregnancy.[12] A concise clinical definition by Davey and MacGillivray[11] describes the condition as the occurrence of a blood pressure of 140/90 mmHg or more on at least two separate occasions a minimum of 6 hours apart in a woman known to have been normotensive before this time, and in whom the blood pressure has returned to normal limits by the sixth postpartum week. One major disadvantage of these definitions is that they do not accurately take into account pregnancy outcome and imply that there is an abnormality that requires drug treatment. The threshold at which drug treatment is recommended is emphatically not 140/90 mmHg. Many young pregnant women may, in fact, show the blood pressure increase required for the diagnosis of pre-eclampsia without increasing their pressure to 140/90 mmHg,[12] and a recent study has suggested that a blood pressure of 130/80 represents the 95th centile in an outpatient setting, with the 140/90 value representing greater than 2 standard deviations from the mean.[14] Pregnancy-induced hypertension affects up to 25% of women in their first pregnancy and in 10% of subsequent pregnancies. If pregnancy-induced hypertension is mild and does not progress to pre-eclampsia or eclampsia, the prognosis is usually good. However, women who develop hypertension de novo early in the second half of pregnancy are likely to progress to pre-eclampsia, with the development of proteinuria, thrombocytopenia, edema, and the need for early delivery.

Pre-eclampsia

Pregnancy-induced hypertension (blood pressure >140/90 mmHg) after the 20th week of pregnancy, which is associated with proteinuria (>300 mg/l), is often referred to as pre-eclampsia. This commonly occurs in primigravidas in the second half of pregnancy and marks a severe, acute change in the mother's condition. Although pre-eclampsia is defined as presenting after 20 weeks,[12] occasionally it may occur earlier[15] or become evident only after delivery. The incidence of severe proteinuric pre-eclampsia in the UK is of the order of 1 in 20–30 first pregnancies.

The risk factors for pre-eclampsia include fetal-specific and maternal-specific factors, which are further discussed in detail below. For example, pre-eclampsia is more common in primigravidas, those aged under 20 years or over 35 years, or in women with previous severe pre-eclampsia.[16–18] There is also a familial (probably genetic) predisposition to pre-eclampsia.[17,19,20]

Pre-eclampsia is also more common in underweight women and those of short stature, and in women with chronic hypertension, especially if associated with chronic renal disease.[21] Women with chronic hypertension are three to seven times more likely to develop higher blood pressures and proteinuria (often referred to as 'superimposed pre-eclampsia') than normotensive women.

The mother is usually symptomatic, with frontal headaches and visual symptoms (jagged, angular flashes at the periphery of her visual fields, loss of vision in areas) due to cerebral edema. There is often epigastric pain due to hepatic edema and, occasionally, an itch over the mask region of the face.

On examination, the blood pressure may be high, with a sharp increase in proteinuria. Usually hypertension precedes proteinuria[8,22] but the converse is occasionally encountered. The blood pressure is usually unstable at rest,[23] and the circadian rhythm is altered, firstly, with a loss of physiological nocturnal dipping[24] and, in severe cases, 'reverse dipping', with the highest blood pressures seen at night.[22] Early papilledema may be seen on fundoscopy. There may be increased and brisk reflexes and clonus. Edema is a less reliable indicator, as mild pretibial and facial edema are commonly found in normal pregnancy. Urgent antihypertensive and anticonvulsant treatment are needed. It should be noted that pregnancy-induced hypertension, with or without proteinuria, may be superimposed on chronic hypertension.

Eclampsia

Eclampsia is a hypertensive emergency that is associated with a high incidence of both maternal and fetal death. It is a convulsive condition, usually associated with proteinuric pregnancy-induced hypertension, occurring in around 1 pregnancy in 500. Chesley[25] estimates that one-half of cases develop antepartum, one-quarter during delivery, and another one-quarter after delivery.

The condition resembles other forms of hypertensive encephalopathy, with the similar symptoms of headaches, nausea, vomiting, and convulsions. Blood pressures are invariably high and proteinuria >300 mg/l is almost always present. There may be gross edema, and convulsions, if they occur, usually develop in labor or in the puerperium.

Convulsions may be preceded by auras, epigastric pain, apprehension, and hyper-reflexia, although there is little or no warning in many cases. After intense tonic–clonic seizures, the patient may become stuporous or comatose. Another complication common to eclampsia and hypertensive encephalopathy is cortical blindness,[26,27] which results from petechial hemorrhages and focal edema in the occipital cortex.[28] Other complications include pulmonary edema, renal failure, hepatic failure, papilledema, retinal hemorrhages, exudates, and cotton-wool spots, as well as retinal detachment and cerebrovascular accidents.

Etiology and pathogenesis

Genetic factors

There is abundant evidence in favor of familial factors in the pathogenesis of pre-eclampsia. The inheritance is uncertain, but is thought to be a single recessive gene; thus, for pre-eclampsia, the mother must be homozygous for the gene.[20] However, pre-eclampsia does not always affect identical twin sisters, so other factors must be relevant.[29]

There is an increased prevalence of past pre-eclampsia in the mothers but not mothers-in-law of pre-eclamptic women.[30] There is also an increased frequency of pre-eclampsia and eclampsia in the daughters but not daughters-in-law of women who themselves had a well-documented history of eclampsia.[20,31] The frequency of eclampsia was greatest in the daughters if they themselves had been the product of an eclamptic pregnancy.[31] There is a higher incidence if the fetus is male,[32] in oocyte recipients,[33] and in pregnancies from parents of dissimilar ethnic origin.[34] Furthermore, a molecular variant of angiotensinogen,

which has already been implicated in the pathogenesis of nonpregnant hypertension, has been described as being associated with pre-eclampsia.[35]

Pregnancies affected with trisomy 13 are also frequently associated with eclampsia.[36] However, chromosome exclusion studies have suggested that a gene on chromosome 1, 3, 9 or 18 may be implicated.[37] There is also an increased incidence of HLA-DR4 in pre-eclamptic mothers and their babies.[38] In addition, there are reports of an increase in human leukocyte antigen (HLA) homozygosity in the mother,[39] and an increase in HLA compatibility between pre-eclamptic women and their partners.[40] However, other workers have failed to confirm any difference in sex ratio[41] or increased HLA homozygosity or compatibility.[38]

Parity and multiple pregnancies

Pre-eclampsia is more common in primigravidas, and also in women with five or more pregnancies, with a rate of approximately 6%. The condition remains common in second or third pregnancies if they are by a different father.[42]

The incidence of pregnancy-induced hypertension is increased in twin pregnancies, both monozygotic and dizygotic twins. In a case–control study of 187 twin pregnancies, 21% developed a pregnancy-induced hypertensive disorder, compared with 13% of singleton pregnancies, although there was no difference in the incidence of pre-eclampsia.[43]

Previous pre-eclampsia or oral contraceptive-induced hypertension

Mothers with a previous history of pre-eclampsia or oral contraceptive-induced hypertension have an increased risk of developing the condition in subsequent pregnancies.

Ethnic origin

Pre-eclampsia is commoner in black and Asian communities in the UK.[44,45] Also, the risk of pregnancy-induced hypertension is increased 1.9-fold when the parents are of different ethnic origin with greater genetic dissimilarity.[34] However, whether this is due to a true racial difference rather than environmental, genetic or socio-economic factors remains uncertain. There is also evidence of a difference in outcome depending on ethnic origin, with hypertensive Indo-Asians having much worse prognosis than other racial groups in a retrospective cohort of women attending a hypertension obstetric clinic.[46]

Obesity

In the normal pregnancy, the average rate of weight gain is lowest during the first trimester, peaks during the second trimester and slows slightly in the third trimester.[47] In a 10-year survey of all deliveries in San Francisco, maternal height, hypertension, cesarean delivery, and fetal size correlated positively with the rate of gain in each trimester.[47] Maternal obesity, however, has been associated with pre-eclampsia and an increased incidence of essential hypertension.

Socio-economic factors

The incidence of pre-eclampsia is higher in women from low socio-economic status. However, this is likely to be associated with other confounders such as obesity, poor diet, and overcrowding. By contrast, smoking appears to have a protective effect against pre-eclampsia, although it is associated with smaller premature babies, presumably due to a direct effect not mediated by the level of the blood pressure.

Hemodynamics

The primary defect in pregnancy-induced hypertension is thought to be failure of the second wave of trophoblastic invasion during the second trimester. Usually, the trophoblast invades the entire length of the spiral arteries by 22 weeks' gestation, resulting in the transformation of the maternal spiral arteries to floppy, thin-walled vessels, which are unresponsive to hormonal stimuli. This leads to an appreciable fall in peripheral vascular resistance and, thus, a fall in blood pressure.

An abnormality of mid-trimester placentation in pre-eclampsia was first noted over 20 years ago.[48] If the second wave of trophoblastic invasion fails, the peripheral resistance does not fall and the hemodynamic mechanisms are not reset for the increased vascular space of pregnancy. The muscular coats are also retained by the spiral arteries, which are sensitive to circulating pressor agents, especially angiotensin II. At the spiral arteries, the reduced volume of trophoblast leads to an imbalance in the prostacyclin–thromboxane system, leading to an overproduction of thromboxane, and less prostacyclin, which encourages vasospasm of spiral arteries and local platelet aggregation.

The damaged muscular coat and intima of the spiral arteries undergo accelerated atherosclerosis ('acute atherosis') that further narrows and occludes the arterioles, resulting in a further increase in blood pressure and a decrease in perfusion of the intervillous space. These lead to more acute ischemia, with vascular occlusions and placental infarctions. The sequelae include fetal ischemia and hypoxia, resulting in intrauterine growth retardation and, in severe cases, intrauterine death.

It should be noted, however, that while virtually all women with pre-eclampsia show failure of second wave of trophoblastic invasion, not all women with invasion failure become hypertensive, although they do have babies with intrauterine growth retardation.[49] The other point is that although pre-eclampsia may develop suddenly in late pregnancy, or even following delivery, the pathologic process has its origins before 30 weeks, or even earlier.

The renin–angiotensin system

In pregnancy, the high levels of estrogen stimulate the generation of high levels of renin substrate by the liver. Furthermore, various hemodynamic factors activate the release of renin from the kidney and there are also raised levels of renin of ovarian and placental origin. The consequent raised levels of plasma angiotensin II and aldosterone are intimately related to the control of maternal fluid volume homeostasis, renal function, and uterine blood flow.

Pregnant women appear to be relatively resistant to the pressor effects of angiotensin II, possibly due to down-regulation of the angiotensin receptors and activation of endothelium-derived relaxing factors, including the prostaglandins and nitric oxide.[50] There is also now an increasing awareness of the role of noncirculating (local) renin–angiotensin systems, which exert more immediate control of fetoplacental blood flow.

In pregnancy complicated by third-trimester hypertension, there appears to be an increased responsiveness to angiotensin II, which is detectable even before 15 weeks' gestation.[51] Possibly because of this, circulating levels of renin and angiotensin II fall. Thus, there is a paradox that, in normal pregnancy, renin and angiotensin levels are very high in comparison with nonpregnant women, while in hypertensive pregnancies, plasma renin and angiotensin II levels are less 'abnormal'. This paradox may be explained by the increasing importance of local renin systems, as well as the increased sensitivity to angiotensin II, with increased peripheral vascular resistance and a decline in extracellular fluid volume. There is, therefore, inhibition of the renin–angiotensin system, presumably as a result of secondary compensatory changes of hypertension in pregnancy.[52]

It is now also known that there are specific angiotensin (AT_2) receptors on developing cardiovascular tissues in the fetus, although their role is uncertain. Blockade of the renin system by the angiotensin-converting enzyme (ACE) inhibitors is not, however, associated with any specific developmental abnormalities, but does cause oligohydramnios and fetal anuria.[53]

There remain a great many partially understood interactions between the various local and circulating vasodilating and vasoconstricting hormones as well as the mineralocorticoids, estrogens, and progestogens.[54] In pre-eclampsia the rise in blood pressure is in part explained by increased sensitivity to angiotensin II, which may represent an attempt to maintain fetoplacental blood flow through the abnormal nonmuscular spiral arteries. Whatever happens, blocking the renin system is hazardous in pregnancy.

Endothelial dysfunction and lipid peroxides

Endothelial cell dysfunction may be involved in the pathogenesis of pre-eclampsia. With inadequate perfusion of the early trophoblast, there is tissue damage and hypoxia leading to the release of agents (such as lipid peroxides) which perpetuate further vascular endothelial damage. This suggestion is consistent with the findings of high lipid peroxide levels in pre-eclamptic women and their placental tissue.[55,56]

High levels of endothelin-1 have been shown in pre-eclampsia.[57,58] There is also evidence for decreased endothelial-dependent relaxation and prostacyclin metabolism, suggesting that pre-eclampsia involves generalized maternal endothelial dysfunction.[59]

Recent work showing elevated levels of serum asymmetric dimethylarginine and reduced flow-mediated dilatation in women who went on to develop pre-eclampsia adds further support to the concept of endothelial dysfunction preceding development of pre-eclampsia.[60]

Coagulation and hemostasis

In severe pregnancy-induced hypertension, platelets are both consumed and activated, leading to a coagulopathy. Activation of intravascular coagulation and fibrin deposition are likely to be responsible for some of the specific organ damage seen in severe pregnancy-induced hypertension. Increased plasma levels of β-thromboglobulin (an index of platelet activation), thrombin–antithrombin (an index of coagulation), fibronectin and laminin (indices of endothelial damage) have been found up to 4 weeks before the onset of clinical features of pre-eclampsia.[61] The fibrinolytic system may also be involved, as increased levels of maternal plasminogen activator inhibitor have been found.[62]

Normal pregnancy increases levels of fibrin D-dimer, a fibrin degradation product, which is an index of intravascular fibrin turnover and thrombogenesis,[63] with a further increase in levels in patients developing pre-eclampsia.[64,65] The study by Trofatter et al.[66] showed that, when compared with fibrin D-dimer-negative pre-eclamptic women, fibrin D-dimer-positive women had significantly higher blood pressures, prompting delivery, greater proteinuria, more abnormal liver function tests, and higher serum creatinine and urea levels. In particular, fibrin D-dimer-positive women had a greater risk of cesarean section, premature delivery, low birth weight, and low Apgar scores.[66] Testing for fibrin D-dimer levels may, therefore, be useful in early screening and follow-up for a pre-eclamptic coagulopathy and outcome following pregnancy. However, one recent study of such patients did not show any significant change in fibrin D-dimer levels from normal pregnancy,[67] despite previous evidence that pre-eclampsia and eclampsia are associated with a state of increased coagulopathy, as shown by increased levels of fibrin formation, platelet activation, and a decrease in platelet count.[66,68]

A few women develop a more serious complication, often referred to as the HELLP syndrome, which comprises hemolysis, elevated liver enzymes and low platelets.[69] Maternal thrombocytopenia is significantly associated with maternal and perinatal mortality, with an increased risk of eclampsia.[70]

Pre-eclampsia is more common in those with factor V Leiden and other coagulation abnormalities.[71]

Immunologic factors

An immunologic mechanism is supported by the reduced prevalence of pregnancy-induced hypertension in women who have had prior full-term pregnancy[18] or blood transfusion.[72] There is also an increased risk among users of contraceptives that prevent exposure to sperm, suggesting that pregnancy-induced hypertension may be related to initial exposure of the patient to foreign antigen.[73]

One report suggests that the risk of pregnancy-induced hypertension is inversely proportional to the duration of sexual cohabitation before conception.[74] Thus, pregnancy-induced hypertension may be prevented by increasing the duration of sexual cohabitation before first pregnancy with that partner. This finding is consistent with the immunologic hypothesis of pregnancy-induced hypertension: during a protracted sexual relationship women develop an immune response against spermatozoa, which is not found in virgin women or in women using barrier methods of contraception that prevent exposure to spermatozoa.[74]

The effects of pregnancy-induced hypertension on organs other than the placenta are mediated by the hypertension or by the activation of components of the complement system. This causes immune complex deposition on the renal basement membrane, thus allowing protein to leak into the urine.

Angiogenic factors

Various circulating ligands are increased in pre-eclampsia; whether these are markers of the disease process or pathogenic molecules remains unclear. Recent work has found elevated levels of soluble fms-like tyrosine kinase and reduced levels of placental growth factor in women who later developed pre-eclampsia compared with control women.[75]

Recent work from Oxford has looked at syncitiotrophoblast debris in normal pregnancy and pre-eclampsia. Whereas placental debris is shed in normal pregnancy, the burden appears to be higher in pre-eclamptic pregnancies.[76]

Circulating adhesion molecules and metalloproteinases

Another study of different soluble adhesion molecules has found elevated levels of soluble E-selectin and vascular cell adhesion molecule 1 in the serum of women with pre-eclampsia when compared with women with a normal pregnancy.[77]

The matrix metalloproteinases (MMPs) are a group of enzymes which, coupled with their inhibitors, tissue inhibitors of metalloproteinases (TIMPs), tightly regulate turnover of extracellular matrix. It is now fairly well established that the major defect in pre-eclampsia and eclampsia is failure of trophoblastic invasion; this process by its nature must involve turnover of the extracellular matrix, and it is therefore possible that the balance of MMPs and TIMPs may be central to the pathological process in pre-eclampsia and eclampsia. Recent work in women with pregnancy-induced hypertension has shown that the balance of MMPs and TIMPs in such women is different to that seen in pregnant women without hypertension, and in nonpregnant women.[78]

Other factors

Pre-eclampsia is more common in diabetics, and those with hydatiform mole and Rhesus isoimmunization.

Diagnosis

A blood pressure in pregnancy of 140/90 mmHg is traditionally considered to be the dividing line between normality and abnormality. However, normal blood pressure in pregnancy falls during the first trimester, when cardiac output is increasing. This reaches a nadir in mid-pregnancy and increases during the third trimester to prepregnancy levels.[79] Consequently, even women with long-standing hypertension may appear normotensive when first seen in the antenatal clinic. Hence, a woman presenting with a blood pressure of 120/70 mmHg at 12 weeks should be around 110/60 mmHg at 28 weeks. A reading of 130/80 mmHg at this stage can, therefore, be considered to be abnormal.

Blood pressure measurement in pregnancy

The blood pressure should be measured monthly for the first two trimesters and thereafter weekly. If the pressure is above 140/90 mmHg, it should be remeasured after 5 minutes rest in the seated position in a quiet room. Continued high blood pressures require detailed clinical assessment of the patient, and if blood pressure exceeds 160/110 mmHg, inpatient assessment is required.

Measurement of diastolic blood pressure

It is well established that Korotkoff phase V correlates better with directly measured diastolic blood pressures. In an analysis of the world literature of hypertension in pregnancy, there is an increasing tendency to report diastolic phase V values.[80] In some

pregnant women, however, the Korotkoff sounds can be heard even at zero cuff pressure, due to the marked peripheral vasodilatation.[81] In such women, phase IV has to be used, although the median difference between phase IV and phase V readings was only 2.7 mmHg in pregnant women[82] compared with 0.7 mmHg in nonpregnant control subjects. A survey among obstetricians and midwives reported that half favored phase V and half favored phase IV.[83] The universal use of phase V for recording diastolic blood pressure in pregnancy is advocated, unless the K4–K5 difference exceeds 20 mmHg.

As with nonobstetric medicine, the quality of blood pressure measurement is often poor so that clinical decisions are frequently made on the basis of hurried readings obtained in a noisy and unrelaxed environment.

Posture

In the third trimester, obstruction of the venous return by a gravid uterus in a supine woman may reduce cardiac output by 20% or more.[84] Although arterial pressure is maintained by reflex vasoconstriction, systolic blood pressure readings can fall by one-third in 10% of cases.[85] This 'supine hypotension syndrome' may result in symptoms such as restlessness, over-breathing, pallor, and faintness.[85] Thus, blood pressure in the pregnant woman should be measured either when she is lying on her side or in the sitting position.

Clinical management

The aims of clinical management of hypertension in pregnancy are:

(1) To protect the mother from the effects of high blood pressure;
(2) To prevent progression of the disease and the occurrence of eclamptic convulsions;
(3) To minimize the risks to the fetus; and
(4) To deliver the fetus when the risk to the mother or fetus, if the pregnancy continues, outweighs the risks of delivery and prematurity.

The ideal clinical management of hypertension in pregnancy is to detect it early. Each visit to the antenatal clinic should include a blood pressure recording.

Pre-eclampsia

Urgent transfer to a specialized maternity unit with an adequate special care pediatric unit is indicated, together with antihypertensive and anticonvulsant therapy. Diazepam and magnesium sulfate prevent seizures and reduce blood pressure.

Eclampsia

The first line of management is to control the seizures. If at home, the woman should be laid on her side and an airway established. Intravenous diazepam, usually 20–40 mg, is used. Occasionally phenytoin is used to prevent recurrence of seizures. In the US, and increasingly elsewhere, magnesium sulfate is a popular choice as an anticonvulsant in eclampsia, and its use has now been advocated as the optimal first-line drug.[86,87] Intravenous hydralazine is a useful antihypertensive drug of first choice, given as a 5-mg bolus at 20-minute intervals or as an infusion of 25 mg in 500 ml of Hartman's solution, with the dose titrated against the woman's blood pressure. An alternative is an intravenous infusion of labetolol.

If the woman is in labor, or induction is considered, an epidural anesthetic may be helpful, both to lower the blood pressure and to reduce the tendency to seizures by reducing the pain of uterine contractions. However, the ultimate treatment of eclampsia is urgent delivery of the baby.

Investigation

Relevant laboratory investigations are summarized in Table 23.1.

Renal function and electrolytes

Serum urea and electrolytes should be measured at the first antenatal visit and again if blood pressure rises. In severe pre-eclampsia, serum sodium and potassium may fall to low levels due to secondary hyperaldosteronism induced by renal ischemia and hepatic dysfunction. Routine biochemical measurements also assist in detection of primary hyperaldosteronism, with low serum potassium and normal or high normal levels of serum sodium.

Urate

Plasma urate concentrations have been advocated as the only useful biochemical indicator of deterioration. However, measurement of serum urate as an indicator of fetal well-being is only useful in subjects with evidence of specific renal impairment or exceptionally high risk before 36 weeks of pregnancy.[88]

Hematological indices

In severe pre-eclampsia and eclampsia there is a consumptive coagulopathy. A fall in platelet count, with a prolonged prothrombin time and increased fibrin degradation products, indicates severe disease.

Ultrasound scans and cardiotocograph

Fetal monitoring should be undertaken by means of regular ultrasound scanning to detect intrauterine growth retardation. Cardiotocography may be useful, especially when the pregnancy has advanced beyond 30 weeks and the mother is admitted with pregnancy-induced hypertension. Sudden decelerations of fetal heart rate strongly suggest fetal distress, as to a lesser extent does an unresponsive or unvariable fetal heart rate.

Proteinuria

The detection of proteinuria is a crucial part of antenatal care, and when persistent, a 24-hour urine protein excretion should be measured. Occasionally, traces of proteinuria may be due to cystitis or pyelitis in pregnancy, and should be investigated with urine microscopy and culture.

Table 23.1 Laboratory tests in hypertension in pregnancy*

Test	Rationale
Full blood count	Hemoconcentration is found in pre-eclampsia and is an indicator of severity Decreased platelet count suggests severe pre-eclampsia
Blood smear	Signs of microangiopathic hemolytic anemia favor the diagnosis of pre-eclampsia
Urinalysis	If dipstick proteinuria of 11 or more, a quantitative measurement of 24-hour protein excretion is required Hypertensive pregnant women with proteinuria should be considered to have pre-eclampsia until proven otherwise
Biochemistry, including serum creatinine, urate, liver function tests	Abnormal or rising levels suggest pre-eclampsia and are an indicator of disease severity
Lactate dehydrogenase	Elevated levels are associated with hemolysis and hepatic involvement, suggesting severe pre-eclampsia
Serum albumin	Levels may be decreased even with mild proteinuria, perhaps due to capillary leak or hepatic involvement in pre-eclampsia

*Adapted from recommendations of the National High Blood Pressure Education Program Working Group Report on High Blood Pressure in Pregnancy.[10]

Other developments

The monitoring of 24-hour ambulatory blood pressure has been proposed as an alternative to conventional blood pressure measurements in pregnancy. In a prospective comparative study of 99 women, 24-hour ambulatory blood pressure monitoring and conventional blood pressure measurement gave significantly correlated but different values of blood pressure, resulting in a high rate of false-positive and false-negative diagnoses of hypertension.[89] Thus, 24-hour ambulatory blood pressure monitoring cannot replace conventional blood pressure measurement unless a new definition of hypertension in pregnancy using 24-hour ambulatory blood pressure monitoring is established.

Treatment

There is a paucity of good randomized clinical trials of sufficient size or power to provide firm clinical guidelines for the treatment of hypertension in pregnancy.

Recommendations about what level of blood pressure warrants treatment during pregnancy are controversial, especially since blood pressure normally falls to a nadir in the mid-trimester of pregnancy. A general policy is to treat chronic hypertension if blood pressure is consistently >140/90 mmHg after the first trimester, or if blood pressure rises by >30 mmHg systolic or >15 mmHg diastolic above the values prior to pregnancy or during the first trimester. This view can be challenged now it is known that the treatment of mild hypertension confers no benefit to the mother or the fetus. It is, therefore, our policy to treat only diastolic pressures of 100 mmHg or more on repeated measurements. In the absence of any information on the value of reducing systolic pressures, our policy is to withhold drugs unless the systolic pressure persistently exceeds 160 mmHg.

Rest and sedation

Once raised blood pressure is established in a pregnant woman, bed rest has been advocated as central to primary management. However, bed rest has never been shown to be of any value. Two randomized controlled studies in mild-to-moderate hypertension without proteinuria during the last trimester illustrate the lack of benefit of bed rest. Matthews[90] showed no difference in pregnancy outcome between women who were confined to bed rest in hospital and those who led normal lives at home. In the study by Rubin et al.[91] there was an excess of spontaneous premature labor and respiratory distress syndrome in the placebo group despite bed rest in hospital. By contrast, the drug-treated group were able to be sent home, with fewer complications.

However, simply relaxing as inpatients with a regular diet and no medication was sufficient to normalize blood pressure within 5 days in over 80% of women admitted with mild pregnancy-induced hypertension, although many subsequently became hypertensive again (half before labor and half during labor, although 13% remained normotensive throughout the puerperium).[92] In a study by Sibai et al.[93] there was no difference in perinatal outcome among the 200 primigravidas with mild pre-eclampsia who were randomized to hospital rest alone or hospital rest combined with labetolol, although drug therapy was associated with more fetal growth retardation.

Sedatives and tranquilizers should be avoided as they tend to reduce the mother's level of consciousness and they cross the placenta, causing depression of the fetal central and peripheral nervous systems. These drugs do not lower blood pressure and there is little justification for their use. There is an increasing view that bed rest and tranquilizers have no place in modern obstetrics.

Salt restriction

Salt restriction is now known to be hazardous in pregnancy as it may aggravate any plasma volume depletion and underlying renal impairment.[94,95] In a controlled trial of 2019 patients, salt restriction was found to be associated with a twofold increase in perinatal mortality and a higher incidence of eclampsia.[96]

Calcium

Populations with a high dietary calcium intake have a low incidence of pre-eclampsia. Several randomized trials also suggest that calcium supplements reduce the incidence of pre-eclampsia and are associated with a modest reduction in the incidence of high blood pressure,[97] although there is no clear effect on other outcome measures.[98]

Weight reduction

Obesity in pregnancy is often associated with hypertension, with waist circumference up to 16 weeks' gestation predicting pregnancy-induced hypertension.[99] However, calorie restriction from 30 weeks in high-weight-gain primigravidas did not alter the incidence of pre-eclampsia, but instead caused a reduction in birth weight.[100] Mothers should be encouraged to avoid excessive weight gain in pregnancy, but should not be advised to go on strict diets.

Antihypertensive drugs

Antihypertensive drugs are given to protect the mother's circulation, mostly against the risk of stroke. They have little effect on the progression of pregnancy-induced hypertension or the development of pre-eclampsia[9] but they help maintain the pregnancy longer to allow the fetus to become more mature. The benefits to the fetus of pharmacologic treatment also remain controversial. This is particularly so since many of the limited trials have included women with pregnancy-induced hypertension and those with chronic hypertension. As perinatal mortality in the developed world is now around 1%, a prospective trial to prove the value of treatment would need to be conducted on a multicenter basis, involving thousands of patients, and to date this has not proved feasible.

Diuretics

Diuretics are usually of little use, except for relief of acutely painful edema and left ventricular failure. A review of the use of thiazides in the control of uncomplicated hypertension in pregnancy concluded that there was no evidence of an adverse effect, although the incidence of hypertension and edema was reduced.[101] However, diuretics did not prevent pre-eclampsia or reduce perinatal mortality. In addition, thiazides may cause a rise in urate concentration.

If pre-eclampsia is present, however, maternal blood volume is reduced and further reduction by diuretics may decrease the venous return to the heart, cardiac output and blood flow to vital organs; a reduction in plasma volume may also reduce perfusion of the placental bed. Thiazide diuretic use has also been shown to decrease clearance of maternal plasma dehydroandrosterone sulfate, suggesting that there is decreased placental perfusion.[102] Thus, diuretic use in pre-eclampsia might be harmful.

Centrally acting drugs

Probably the most widely used antihypertensive drug in pregnancy is α-methyldopa. High doses of methyldopa can be used to achieve blood pressure control and no long-term adverse effects on mother or fetus have been demonstrated.[103,104] The drug crosses the placenta and is found in amniotic fluid.

In women with chronic hypertension during pregnancy, antihypertensive therapy with methyldopa significantly improved pregnancy outcome, especially with a reduction in mid-trimester abortions.[103] However, methyldopa did not reduce the incidence of superimposed pre-eclampsia. Unwanted side effects including depression, lethargy, sedation, and postural hypotension, may necessitate drug withdrawal in 15% of patients. While there are no reports of methyldopa causing postnatal depression, the possibility of this complication should be borne in mind.

Beta-blockers

Beta-blockers are generally safe and effective antihypertensive drugs in pregnancy. There is no evidence of a teratogenic effect and the drugs are well tolerated by the mother. Together with methyldopa, beta-blockers were considered first-line antihypertensive drugs in pregnancy.

However, there is growing evidence that certain beta-blockers may have adverse effects if used in early pregnancy. For example, in a small prospective, randomized, double-blind, placebo-controlled study from Glasgow, where 29 women with mild essential hypertension were randomized to placebo or atenolol, babies in the atenolol group had significantly lower birth weights than those in the placebo group.[105] A larger retrospective cohort study of hypertensive women showed similar results, with duration of treatment and use earlier in pregnancy particularly associated with lower birth weight;[106] more recent work has compared women taking atenolol with those taking calcium antagonists, and found that atenolol was associated with lower birth weight, but the difference was only apparent if the drugs were taken in the first trimester.[107] Intrauterine growth retardation has previously been ascribed to other beta-blockers, such as propranolol,[108,109] although subsequent prospective studies with propranolol,[91,110] atenolol,[91,110] oxprenolol,[111] and metoprolol[112] in pregnancy-induced hypertension failed to show any difference in average birth weight in mothers given beta-blockers. However, these studies may reflect the late initiation of antihypertensive therapy (for example, at a mean of 33.8 weeks' gestation in the study by Rubin et al.[91]), compared with the use of atenolol in early pregnancy (before 20 weeks' gestation, as in the study by Butters et al.[105] and Paran et al.[109]). The time of initiation of beta-blocker therapy is, therefore, an important consideration in intrauterine growth retardation. Some beta-blockers have also been associated with neonatal hypotension and hypoglycemia.

Labetolol is an increasingly popular beta-blocker (with some alpha-blocking activity) for use in hypertension in pregnancy. For example, in small studies in severe hypertension, labetolol by intravenous infusion (20–160 mg/hour) or intermittent bolus (50–100 mg at 20–30-minute intervals) reduced blood pressure smoothly, although hypotension, oliguria, and bradycardia have been reported in neonates when fetal distress or hypoxia was also present.[113] It has also been suggested that labetolol has specific advantages because of its actions in reducing platelet aggregation[114] and reducing placental vascular resistance.[115] In addition, babies born to women taking labetolol were reported to be up to 500 g heavier than those born to women taking atenolol.[116]

Frishman and Chesner[117] suggest the following guidelines on the use of beta-blockers in pregnancy:

(1) Avoid the use of beta-blockers during the first trimester of pregnancy;
(2) Use the lowest possible beta-blocker dose;
(3) If possible, beta-blocker use should be discontinued 2–3 days prior to delivery, to limit the effects on uterine contractility and to avoid neonatal complications from beta-blockade; and
(4) Use of beta-blockers with β_1 selectivity, intrinsic sympathomimetic activity, or alpha-blocking activity may be preferable as these agents are less likely to interfere with β_2-mediated uterine relaxation and peripheral vasodilatation.

Hydralazine

This second-line antihypertensive drug is widely used in patients with severe hypertension and pre-eclampsia, but only rarely in the first trimester of pregnancy. Although hydralazine crosses the placenta, the only problem with use in late pregnancy is thrombocytopenia.[118] Other adverse effects, such as headache, nausea, and vomiting, may be difficult to distinguish from imminent eclampsia.

Calcium antagonists

Most calcium antagonists are unlicensed for use in pregnancy. However, in one uncontrolled trial, nifedipine (40–120 mg daily) was effective as a second-line agent where beta-blockade or methyldopa was unsuccessful in controlling moderate hypertension.[119] A single open-label study of oral nifedipine in severe hypertension in pregnancy has also shown it to be effective.[120] Nifedipine has the additional property (which is usually an advantage) of relaxing the uterus,[121] although this might in theory cause prolongation of the second stage of labor and postpartum hemorrhage.

Alpha-blockers

Prazosin is safe in pregnancy, with no records of teratogenesis. In a small study comparing prazosin with oxprenolol, there was satisfactory blood pressure control and fetal growth in patients taking prazosin.[122] However, there are no reliable data on the use of the newer, long-acting alpha-blockers, such as doxazosin or terazosin, in pregnancy.

Angiotensin-converting enzyme inhibitors

ACE inhibitors are useful drugs in nonpregnant hypertensive patients, particularly if they have diabetes mellitus or glomerulonephritis. However, these drugs have been associated with spontaneous abortions and fetal abnormalities, mainly skull ossification defects; such drugs are, therefore, contraindicated in pregnancy.[53,123,124] Use of these agents also causes severe disturbance of fetal and neonatal renal function, such as oligohydramnios, pulmonary hypoplasia, and long-lasting neonatal anuria or renal failure.[125]

In patients previously taking ACE inhibitors, and if the drug is stopped in the first trimester of pregnancy, the baby is likely to be born at or near term, with normal birth weight.[124] However, continued treatment with the drug carries a risk of early delivery, low birth weight, and neonatal problems discussed previously.

Aspirin

Many randomized trials have been conducted using low-dose aspirin to prevent pre-eclampsia. The results, although suggestive of some benefit for aspirin use, have some inconsistencies due to the heterogeneous nature of the studies. For example, the early use of low-dose aspirin (150 mg/day) was effective in preventing fetal growth retardation and maternal proteinuria in women with previous fetal growth retardation and/or fetal death or abruptio placentae in at least one pregnancy.[126] However, in the Italian Study of Aspirin in Pregnancy, low-dose aspirin (50 mg/day) did not affect the clinical course or outcome of pregnancy in women at moderate risk of pregnancy-induced hypertension, intrauterine growth retardation, or both.[127] The large Collaborative Low-dose Aspirin Study in Pregnancy (CLASP) found that the use of aspirin at a dose of 60 mg/day was associated with a nonstatistically significant reduction in the incidence of proteinuric pre-eclampsia, with no significant effect on the incidence of intrauterine growth retardation, still-birth or neonatal death.[128] The findings of the CLASP study do not support routine prophylactic or therapeutic administration of aspirin to all women at increased risk of pre-eclampsia, although aspirin may be justified in women judged to be especially liable to early-onset pre-eclampsia requiring very preterm delivery.[128] More recent work has failed to show benefit with aspirin at a dose of 150 mg daily; women at high risk of pre-eclampsia on the basis of impaired uterine artery flow were randomized to aspirin or placebo. There were no significant differences between the two groups in the outcomes (pre-eclampsia, preterm delivery, low birth weight, placental abruption, and perinatal death).[129] The Australasian Society for the Study of Hypertension in Pregnancy recommends use of prophylactic low-dose aspirin from early pregnancy in the following groups:

(1) Women with prior fetal loss after the first trimester, with placental insufficiency;
(2) Women with severe fetal growth retardation in a preceding pregnancy either due to pre-eclampsia or unexplained causes;
(3) Women with severe early-onset pre-eclampsia in a previous pregnancy requiring delivery at or before 32 weeks' gestation.[130]

Aspirin is not indicated routinely for healthy nulliparous women, women with mild chronic hypertension, and women with established pre-eclampsia.[131]

Magnesium

The value of magnesium in the management of eclampsia is well established. It has anticonvulsant effects and some antihypertensive properties, and both intravenous and intramuscular routes of administration have been used successfully.[131] The drug has a rapid onset of action, a nonsedative effect, a wide safety margin and, in instances of toxicity, an antidote exists in the form of calcium gluconate.

However, magnesium remains underutilized, with only 60% of British obstetricians using it as first-

line therapy in eclampsia and 40% in pre-eclampsia.[132] In North America, it is considered the drug of choice for eclampsia.[133,134] The Eclampsia Trial Collaborative Group has reported that magnesium reduced the risk of further convulsions, with less maternal and neonatal morbidity than conventional anticonvulsants.[135] More recent results from the Magpie trial have confirmed the benfits of magnesium, with little or no risk to mother and baby.[87] Prophylactic magnesium therapy has also been shown to reduce the risk of developing eclampsia.[136]

Delivery

The ultimate treatment of pregnancy-induced hypertension and pre-eclampsia, as well as eclampsia, is delivery, especially when the fetus is mature enough for the neonatal facilities available. The worst effects of prolonged renal and cerebral damage are reduced for the mother and the fetus is delivered before being affected by serious chronic hypoxia in utero. Gestation should therefore be allowed to continue until spontaneous labor occurs or the cervix becomes favorable for induction of labor at or near term.

Delivery before term is required in patients with severe, persisting hypertension, with rapid weight gain, a decrease in creatinine clearance, significant proteinuria, evidence of fetal growth retardation, or the development of severe headache, papilledema, hyper-reflexia, scotoma, or right upper quadrant (hepatic) pain.

Hypertensive crises/eclampsia

The only management stratagem which has been shown to be of benefit in hypertensive crises is effective antihypertensive therapy. The antihypertensive used should be given parenterally, although the degree to which blood pressure should be decreased acutely is disputed. Levels of 90–104 mmHg have been suggested by the National High Blood Pressure Education Program Working Group Report.[12]

Hydralazine (40 mg slow intravenously, followed by a further 20–40 mg) is commonly used in the UK as antihypertensive therapy, but magnesium sulfate is now the best option for treatment of both convulsions and hypertension. Diazoxide is recommended for the occasional patient whose hypertension is refractory to hydralazine. Other alternatives that have been used successfully are labetolol and nifedipine. However, nifedipine may potentiate magnesium sulfate, leading to profound hypotension.[137] Diuretics and hyperosmotic agents should be avoided. In addition, sodium nitroprusside should be avoided in view of the possibility of fetal cyanide poisoning.

Delivery should be delayed until seizures are controlled and consciousness is regained. Seizures should be treated with intravenous diazepam, and phenytoin (10 mg/kg intravenously over 20 minutes) given as prophylaxis. Replacement of clotting factors, platelets, and plasma volume (for example, with salt-poor albumin) may be necessary. Using this approach to the management of eclampsia, only one maternal death was reported among 245 consecutive cases of eclampsia, and of those fetuses who were alive when treatment was started and who weighed ≥1800 g at birth, all but one survived.[133]

Postnatal hypertension

Blood pressures rise progressively during the first 5 days after a normal delivery and this may be exaggerated in hypertensive patients.[138] Thus, the signs and symptoms of pre-eclampsia may occur for the first time in the postnatal period, and close blood pressure monitoring and possible antihypertensive therapy are required. Following the pregnancy, all patients with early and/or severe hypertension should be investigated for an underlying cause.

If hypertension is due to pregnancy-induced hypertension alone, blood pressure usually returns to normal after delivery, and antihypertensive therapy can gradually be withdrawn over 2 or 3 days. If the raised blood pressure was due to pre-existing essential hypertension, with or without pre-eclampsia,

antihypertensive therapy should be continued. Methyldopa, which causes depression and tiredness, is best avoided in the puerperium, but other drugs are quite safe. Drug therapy should be minimized in women who are breastfeeding, although the beta-blockers are safe.

Further pregnancy

Mothers who have had pre-eclampsia during a first pregnancy should be forewarned of a 7.5% recurrence risk for their second.[18] A history of spontaneous or induced first-trimester abortion in a first pregnancy does not confer the same relative immunity to severe pre-eclampsia in the subsequent pregnancy.[18] Other causes of hypertension should be considered when a patient develops hypertension in pregnancy, especially if there are any unusual features or the hypertension is severe. For example, patients with undiagnosed coarctation of the aorta may present with hypertension in pregnancy.[139]

If pregnant again, women with previous pre-eclampsia should be targeted for management in a joint antenatal and blood pressure clinic. Chesley[140] found that in 466 later pregnancies in 189 women who had had eclampsia, only 25% had recurrent hypertension and only four had a second episode of eclampsia.

Such women are usually regarded as being more likely to develop essential hypertension in later life and regular screening for hypertension is recommended. However, in a 22–44-year follow-up of patients with previous eclampsia, the long-term prognosis was excellent, with the blood pressure distribution being similar to that of the general population.[141] If a woman with a history of hypertension in pregnancy wishes oral contraceptives, this should not be a contraindication, although careful monitoring is essential. The developmental status of children born to women with pre-eclampsia is usually good.

References

1. Douglas KA, Redman CWG. Eclampsia in the United Kingdom. *BMJ* 1994; **309**:1395–400.

2. Chang J, Elam-Evans LD, Berg CJ, et al. Pregnancy-related mortality surveillance – United States, 1991–1999. *MMWR Surveill Summ* 2003; **52**:1–8.

3. Redman CWG. Eclampsia still kills. *BMJ* 1988; **296**:1209–10.

4. Sachs BP, Brown DAJ, Driscoll SG, et al. Maternal mortality in Massachusetts. Trends and prevention. *N Engl J Med* 1987; **316**:667–72.

5. Kaunitz AM, Hughes JM, Grimes DA, Smith JC, Rochat RW, Kafrissen ME. Causes of maternal mortality in the United States. *Obstet Gynecol* 1985; **65**:605–12.

6. Taylor DJ. The epidemiology of hypertension during pregnancy. In: Rubin PC (ed). *Handbook of Hypertension,* Vol. 10. *Hypertension in Pregnancy.* Amsterdam: Elsevier Science, 1988: 223–40.

7. Sibai BM, Spinnato JA, Watson DL, Lewis JA, Anderson GD. Eclampsia. IV. Neurologic findings and future outcome. *Am J Obstet Gynecol* 1985; **152**:184–92.

8. Redman GWG. Hypertension in pregnancy. In: Swales JD (ed). *Textbook of Hypertension.* Oxford: Blackwell, 1994: 767–84.

9. Lydakis C, Beevers M, Beevers DG, Lip GY. The prevalence of pre-eclampsia and obstetric outcome in pregnancies of normotensive and hypertensive women attending a hospital specialist clinic. *Int J Clin Pract* 2001; **55**:361–7.

10. Department of Health and Social Security. *Report on Confidential Enquiries into Maternal Deaths in England and Wales 1982–84.* London: HMSO, 1986: 10–19.

11. Davey DA, MacGillvray I. The classification and definition of the hypertensive disorders of pregnancy. *Am J Obstet Gynecol* 1988; **158**:892–8.

12. National High Blood Pressure Education Program. National High Blood Pressure Education Program Working Group Report on High Bood Pressure in Pregnancy. *Am J Obstet Gynecol* 1990; **163**:1689–712.

13. Classification of the hypertensive disorders of pregnancy. *Lancet* 1989; **1**:935–6.

14. Oschsenbein-Kolble N, Roos M, Gasser T, Huch R, Huch A, Zimmermann R. Cross sectional study of automated blood pressure measurements throughout pregnancy. *Br J Obstet Gynaecol* 2004; **111**:319–25.

15. Lindheimer MD, Spargo BH, Katz AI. Eclampsia during the 16th week. *JAMA* 1974; **230**:1006–8.

16. Davies AM. Geographical epidemiology of the toxemias of pregnancy. *Isr J Med Sci* 1971; **7**:753–821.

17. Eskenazi B, Fenster L, Sidney S. A multivariate analysis of risk factors for pre-eclampsia. *JAMA* 1991; **266**:237–41.

18. Campbell DM, MacGillivray I, Carr-Hill R. Pre-eclampsia in second pregnancy. *Br J Obstet Gynaecol* 1985; **92**:131–40.

19. Chesley LC, Annito JE, Cosgrove RA. The familial factor in toxemia of pregnancy. *Obstet Gynecol* 1968; **32**:303–11.

20. Chesley LC, Cooper DW. Genetics of hypertension in pregnancy: possible single gene control of pre-eclampsia and eclampsia in the descendants of eclamptic women. *Br J Obstet Gynaecol* 1986; **93**:898–908.

21. Felding CF. Obstetric aspects in women with histories of renal disease. *Acta Obstet Gynecol Scand* 1969; **48** (Suppl 2):1–43.

22. Seligman SA. Diurnal blood pressure variation in pregnancy. *Br J Obstet Gynaecol* 1971; **78**:417–22.

23. Redman CWG, Beilin LJ, Bonnar J. Variability of blood pressure in normal and abnormal pregnancy. *Perspect Nephrol Hypertens* 1976; **5**:53–60.

24. Chesley LC. Vascular reactivity in normal and toxemic patients. *Clin Obstet Gynecol* 1966; **9**:871–81.

25. Chesley LC. *Hypertensive Disorders in Pregnancy.* New York: Appleton-Century Crofts, 1978.

26. Sibai BM, McCubbin JH, Anderson GD, Lipshitz J, Dilts PVJ. Eclampsia. I. Observations from 67 recent cases. *Obstet Gynecol* 1981; **58**:609–13.

27. Liebowitz HA, Hall PE. Cortical blindness as a complication of eclampsia. *Ann Emerg Med* 1984; **13**:365–7.

28. Cunningham FG, Fernandez CO, Hernandez C. Blindness associated with pre-eclampsia and eclampsia. *Am J Obstet Gynecol* 1995; **172**:1291–8.

29. Thornton JG, Sampson J. Genetics of pre-eclampsia. *Lancet* 1990; **336**:1319–20.

30. Sutherland A, Cooper DW, Howie PW, Liston WA, MacGillivray I. The incidence of severe pre-eclampsia amongst mothers and mothers-in-law of pre-eclampsia and controls. *Br J Obstet Gynaecol* 1981; **88**:785–91.

31. Cooper DW, Hill JA, Chesley LC, Bryans CI. Genetic control of susceptibility to eclampsia and pre-eclampsia. *Br J Obstet Gynaecol* 1988; **95**:644–53.

32. Toivanen P, Hirvonen T. Sex ratio of newborns:

preponderance of males in toxemia of pregnancy. *Science* 1970; **170**:187–8.

33. Serhal PF, Craft I. Immune basis for pre-eclampsia: evidence from oocyte recipients. *Lancet* 1987; **2**:744.

34. Alderman BW, Sperling RS, Daling JR. An epidemiological study of the immunogenetic aetiology of pre-eclampsia. *BMJ* 1986; **292**:372–4.

35. Ward K, Hata A, Jeunemaitre X, et al. A molecular variant of angiotensinogen associated with pre-eclampsia. *Nat Genet* 1993; **4**:59–61.

36. Boyd PA, Lindenbaum RH, Redman C. Pre-eclampsia and trisomy 13: a possible association. *Lancet* 1987; **2**:425–7.

37. Hayward C, Livingstone J, Holloway S, et al. An exclusion map for pre-eclampsia: assuming autosomal recessive inheritance. *Am J Hum Genet* 1992; **50**:749–57.

38. Kilpatrick DC, Liston WA, Jazwinska EC, Smart GE. Histocompatibility studies in pre-eclampsia. *Tissue Antigens* 1987; **29**:232–6.

39. Redman CWG, Bodmer JG, Bodmer WF, Beilin LJ, Bonnar J. HLA antigens in severe pre-eclampsia. *Lancet* 1978; **2**:397–9.

40. Jenkins DM, Need JA, Scott JS, Morris H, Pepper M. Human leucocyte antigens and mixed lymphocyte reaction in severe pre-eclampsia. *BMJ* 1978; **1**:542–4.

41. Campbell DM, Carr-Hill R. Fetal sex and pre-eclampsia in primigravidae. *Br J Obstet Gynaecol* 1983; **90**:26–7.

42. Need JA. Pre-eclampsia in pregnancies by different fathers: immunological studies. *BMJ* 1975; **1**:548–9.

43. Santema JG, Koppelaar I, Wallenburg HC. Hypertensive disorders in twin pregnancy. *Eur J Obstet Gynecol Reprod Biol* 1995; **58**:9–13.

44. McVicar J. The effect of race on perinatal mortality. In: Studd J (ed). *Progress in Obstetrics and Gynaecology,* Vol. 1. London: Churchill Livingstone, 1981: 92–104.

45. Terry PB, Condie RG, Settatree RS. Analysis of ethnic differences in perinatal statistics. *BMJ* 1980; **2**:1307–8.

46. Lydakis C, Beevers DG, Beevers M, Lip GY. Obstetric and neonatal outcome following chronic hypertension in pregnancy among different ethnic groups. *Q J Med* 1998; **91**:837–44.

47. Abrams B, Carmichael S, Selvin S. Factors associated with the pattern of maternal weight gain during pregnancy. *Obstet Gynecol* 1995; **86**:170–6.

48. Pijenenborg R, Anthony J, Davey DA, et al. Placental bed spiral arteries in the hypertensive disorders of pregnancy. *Br J Obstet Gynaecol* 1991; **98**:648–55.

49. Sheppard BL, Bonnar J. Ultrasound abnormalities of placental villi in placentas from pregnancies compli-

cated by intrauterine fetal growth retardation: their relation to decidual spiral arterial lesions. *Placenta* 1980; **1**:145–56.

50. Baker PW, Broughton-Pipkin F, Symonds EM. Longitudinal study of platelet angiotensin II binding in normal pregnancy. *Clin Sci* 1992; **83**:89–95.

51. Gant NF, Daley GL, Chand S, Whalley PS, MacDonald PC. A study of angiotensin II pressor response throughout primigravid pregnancy. *J Clin Invest* 1973; **52**:2682–9.

52. Weir RJ, Brown JJ, Fraser R, et al. Plasma renin, renin substrate, angiotensin II and aldosterone in hypertensive disease of pregnancy. *Lancet* 1973; **1**:291–5.

53. Shotan A, Widerhorn J, Hurst A, Elkayam U. Risks of angiotensin-converting enzyme inhibition during pregnancy: experimental and clinical evidence, potential mechanisms and recommendations for use. *Am J Med* 1994; **96**:451–6.

54. Brown MA, Zammit VC, Mitar DA, Whitworth JA. Renin–aldosterone relationships in pregnancy-induced hypertension. *Am J Hypertens* 1992; **5**:366–71.

55. Hubel CA, Roberts JM, Taylor RN, et al. Lipid peroxidation in pregnancy: new perspectives on pre-eclampsia. *Am J Obstet Gynecol* 1989; **161**:1025–34.

56. Wang Y, Walsh SW, Kay HH. Placental lipid peroxides and thromboxane are increased and prostacyclin is decreased in women with pre-eclampsia. *Am J Obstet Gynecol* 1992; **167**:946–9.

57. Taylor RN, Varma M, Teng NN, Roberts JM. Women with pre-eclampsia have higher plasma endothelin levels than women with normal pregnancies. *J Clin Endocrinol Metab* 1990; **71**:1675–7.

58. Schiff E, Ben-Baruch G, Peleg E, et al. Immunoreactive circulating endothelin-1 in normal and hypertensive pregnancies. *Am J Obstet Gynecol* 1992; **166**:624–8.

59. Roberts JM, Taylor RN, Musci TJ, Rodgers GM, Hubel CA, McLaughlin MK. Pre-eclampsia: an endothelial cell disorder. *Am J Obstet Gynecol* 1989; **161**:1200–4.

60. Savvidou MD, Hingorani AD, Tsikas D, Frolich JC, Vallance P, Nicolaides KH. Endothelial dysfunction and raised plasma concentrations of asymmetric dimethylarginine in pregnant women who subsequently develop pre-eclampsia. *Lancet* 2003; **361**: 1511–17.

61. Ballegeer V, Spitz B, Kieckens L, Moreau H, Van Assche A, Collen D. Predictive value of increased plasma levels of fibronectin in gestational hypertension. *Am J Obstet Gynecol* 1989; **161**:432–6.

62. de Boer K, Lecander I, ten Cate JW, Borm JJ, Treffers

PE. Placental-type plasminogen activator inhibitor in pre-eclampsia. *Am J Obstet Gynecol* 1988; **158**:518–22.

63. van Wersch JW, Ubachs JM. Blood coagulation and fibrinolysis during normal pregnancy. *Eur J Clin Chem Clin Biochem* 1991; **29**:45–50.

64. Proietti AB, Johnson MJ, Proietti FA, Repke JT, Bell WR. Assessment of fibrin(ogen) degradation products in pre-eclampsia using immunoblot, enzyme-linked immunosorbent assay, and latex-based agglutination. *Obstet Gynecol* 1991; **77**:696–700.

65. Gaffney PJ, Creighton LJ, Callus M, Thorpe R. Monoclonal antibodies to cross-linked fibrin degradation products (XL-FDP): II. Evaluation in a variety of clinical conditions. *Br J Haematol* 1988; **68**:91–6.

66. Trofatter KF Jr, Howell ML, Greenberg CS, Hage ML. Use of the fibrin D-dimer in screening for coagulation abnormalities in preeclampsia. *Obstet Gynecol* 1989; **73**:435–40.

67. Koh SC, Anandakumar C, Montan S, Ratnam SS. Plasminogen activators, plasminogen activator inhibitors and markers of intravascular coagulation in pre-eclampsia. *Gynecol Obstet Invest* 1993; **35**:214–21.

68. Perry KG, Martin JN. Abnormal hemostasis and coagulopathy in preeclampsia and eclampsia. *Clin Obstet Gynecol* 1992; **35**:338–50.

69. Weinstein L. Syndrome of hemolysis, elevated liver enzymes, and low platelet count: a severe consequence of hypertension in pregnancy. *Am J Obstet Gynecol* 1982; **142**:159–67.

70. Redman CWG, Bonnar J, Beilin L. Early platelet consumption in pre-eclampsia. *BMJ* 1978; **1**:467–9.

71. Agorastos T, Karavida A, Lambropoulos A, et al. Factor V Leiden and prothrombin G20210A mutations in pregnancies with adverse outcome. *J Matern Fetal Neonatal Med* 2002; **12**:267–73.

72. Feeney JG, Tovey LAD, Scott JS. Influence of previous blood-transfusion on incidence of pre-eclampsia. *Lancet* 1977; **1**:874–5.

73. Klonoff-Cohen HS, Savitz DA, Cefalo RC, McCann MF. An epidemiologic study of contraception and pre-eclampsia. *JAMA* 1989; **262**:3143–7.

74. Robillard PY, Hulsey TC, Périanin J, Janky E, Miri EH, Papiernik E. Association of pregnancy-induced hypertension with duration of sexual cohabitation before conception. *Lancet* 1994; **344**:973–5.

75. Levine RJ, Maynard SE, Qian C, et al. Circulating angiogenic factors and the risk of preeclampsia. *N Engl J Med* 2004; **350**:672–83.

76. Sargent IL, Germain SJ, Sacks GP, Kumar S, Redman CW. Trophoblast deportation and the maternal inflammatory response in pre-eclampsia. *J Reprod Immunol* 2003; **59**:153–60.

77. Chaiworapongsa T, Romero R, Yoshimatsu J, et al. Soluble adhesion molecule profile in normal pregnancy and pre-eclampsia. *J Matern Fetal Neonatal Med* 2002; **12**:19–27.

78. Tayebjee MH, Karalis I, Nadar SK, Beevers DG, MacFadyen RJ, Lip GYH. Circulating matrix metalloproteinase-9 (MMP-9) and tissue inhibitors of metalloproteinases -1 and -2 (TIMP-1 & 2) levels in gestational hypertension. *Am J Hypertens* 2004; **17**:762A [abstr].

79. MacGillivray I, Rose GA, Rowe B. Blood pressure survey in pregnancy. *Clin Sci* 1969; **37**:395–407.

80. Zarifis J, Lip GYH, Blackman D, Churchill D, Beevers DG. Measurement of diastolic blood pressure in obstetric research. *Hypertens Pregnancy* 1996; **15**:135–7.

81. Petrie JC, O'Brien ET, Littler WA, de Swiet M. Recommendations on blood pressure measurement. *BMJ* 1986; **293**:610–15.

82. Perry IJ, Stewart BA, Brockwell J, et al. Recording diastolic blood pressure in pregnancy. *BMJ* 1990; **301**:1198.

83. Perry IJ, Wilkinson LS, Shinton RA, Beevers DG. Conflicting views on the measurement of blood pressure in pregnancy. *Br J Obstet Gynaecol* 1991; **98**:241–3.

84. Lees MM, Taylor S, Scott DB, Kerr MG. A study of cardiac output at rest throughout pregnancy. *J Obstet Gynaecol Br Commonw* 1967; **74**:319–27.

85. Holmes F. Incidence of supine hypotensive syndrome in late pregnancy. *J Obstet Gynaecol Br Emp* 1960; **67**:254–8.

86. Saunders N, Hammersley B. Magnesium for eclampsia. *Lancet* 1995; **346**:788–9.

87. Magpie Trial Collaboration Group. Do women with pre-eclampsia, and their babies, benefit from magnesium sulphate? The Magpie Trial: a randomised placebo-controlled trial. *Lancet* 2002; **359**:1877–90.

88. Obiekwe BC, Chard T, Sturdee DW, Cockrill B. Serial measurement of serum uric acid as an indicator of fetal well-being in late pregnancy. *J Obstet Gynaecol* 1984; **5**:17–20.

89. Olofsson P, Persson K. A comparison between conventional and 24-hour automatic blood pressure monitoring in hypertensive pregnancy. *Acta Obstet Gynecol Scand* 1995; **74**:429–33.

90. Matthews DD. A randomized controlled trial of bed rest and sedation or normal activity and non-sedation in the management of non-albuminuric hypertension in late pregnancy. *Br J Obstet Gynaecol* 1977; **84**:108–14.

91. Rubin PC, Butters L, Clark DM, et al. Placebo-

controlled trial of atenolol in treatment of pregnancy-associated hypertension. *Lancet* 1983; **2**:431–4.

92. Cunningham FG, Leveno KJ. Management of pregnancy-induced hypertension. In: Rubin PC (ed). *Handbook of Hypertension*, Vol. 10. *Hypertension in Pregnancy*. Amsterdam: Elsevier Science, 1988: 290–319.

93. Sibai BM, Gonzalez AR, Mabie WC, Moretti M. A comparison of labetolol plus hospitalization versus hospitalization alone in the management of pre-eclampsia remote from term. *Obstet Gynecol* 1987; **70**:323–7.

94. Gallery E. Chronic and secondary hypertension. In: Rubin PC (ed). *Handbook of Hypertension,* Vol. 10. *Hypertension in Pregnancy*. Amsterdam: Elsevier Science, 1988: 202–22.

95. Palomaki JF, Lindheimer MD. Sodium depletion simulating deterioration in a toxemic pregnancy. *N Engl J Med* 1970; **282**:88–9.

96. Robinson M. Salt in pregnancy. *Lancet* 1958; **1**:178–81.

97. Atallah AN, Hofmeyr GJ, Duley L. Calcium supplementation during pregnancy for preventing hypertensive disorders and related problems. *Cochrane Database Syst Rev* 2002; (1):CD001059.

98. Belizan JM, Villar J, Gonzalez L, Campodonico L, Bergel E. Calcium supplementation to prevent hypertensive disorders of pregnancy. *N Engl J Med* 1991; **325**:1399–405.

99. Sattar N, Clark P, Holmes A, Lean ME, Walker I, Greer IA. Antenatal waist circumference and hypertension risk. *Obstet Gynecol* 2001; **97**:268–71.

100. Campbell DM, MacGillivray I. The effect of a low calorie diet or thiazide diuretic on the incidence of pre-eclampsia and on birth weight. *Br J Obstet Gynaecol* 1975; **82**:572–7.

101. Collins R, Yusof S, Peto R. Overview of randomised trials of diuretics in pregnancy. *BMJ* 1985; **290**:17–23.

102. Gant NF, Madden JD, Siteri PK, MacDonald PC. The metabolic clearance rate of dehydroisoandrosterone sulfate. III. The effect of thiazide diuretics in normal and future pre-eclamptic pregnancies. *Am J Obstet Gynecol* 1975; **123**:159–63.

103. Redman CWG, Beilin L, Bonnar J, Ounsted MK. Fetal outcome in trial of antihypertensive treatment in pregnancy. *Lancet* 1976; **2**:753–6.

104. Cockburn J, Moar VA, Ounsted M, Redman CWG. Final report of study on hypertension during pregnancy: the effects of specific treatment on the growth and development of children. *Lancet* 1982; **1**:647–9.

105. Butters L, Kennedy S, Rubin PC. Atenolol in essential hypertension during pregnancy. *BMJ* 1990; **301**:587–9.

106. Lydakis C, Lip GY, Beevers M, Beevers DG. Atenolol and fetal growth in pregnancies complicated by hypertension. *Am J Hypertens* 1999; **12**:541–7.

107. Bayliss H, Churchill D, Beevers M, Beevers DG. Antihypertensive drugs in pregnancy and fetal growth: evidence for 'pharmacological programming' in the first trimester? *Hypertens Pregnancy* 2001; **21**:161–74.

108. Rubin PC. Beta-blockers in pregnancy. *N Engl J Med* 1981; **305**:1323–6.

109. Paran E, Holzberg G, Mazor M, Zmora E, Insler V. Beta-adrenergic blocking agents in the treatment of pregnancy-induced hypertension. *Int J Clin Pharmacol Ther* 1995; **33**:119–23.

110. Rubin PC, Butters L, Low RA, Reid JL. Atenolol in the treatment of essential hypertension during pregnancy. *Br J Clin Pharmacol* 1982; **14**:279–81.

111. Fidler J, Smith V, Fayers P, De Swiet M. Randomised controlled comparative study of methyldopa and oxprenolol in treatment of hypertension in pregnancy. *BMJ* 1983; **286**:1927–30.

112. Wichman K, Ryulden G, Karlberg BE. A placebo controlled trial of metoprolol in the treatment of hypertension in pregnancy. *Scand J Clin Lab Invest* 1984; **169**:90–4.

113. Woods DL, Malan AF. Side effects of labetolol in new born infants. *Br J Obstet Gynaecol* 1983; **90**:876.

114. Walker JJ, Erwin L, Lang G, et al. Labetolol and platelet function in pre-eclampsia. *Lancet* 1982; **2**:279.

115. Lunnell NO, Nylund L, Lewander R, Sarby B. Acute effect of an antihypertensive drug, labetolol, on utero placental blood flow. *Br J Obstet Gynaecol* 1982; **89**:640–4.

116. Lardoux H, Gerard J, Blazquez G, Chouty F, Flouvat BB. Hypertension in pregnancy: evaluation of two beta-blockers, atenolol and labetolol. *Eur Heart J* 1983; **4** (Suppl G):35–40.

117. Frishman WH, Chesner M. Beta-adrenergic blockers in pregnancy. *Am Heart J* 1988; **115**:147–52.

118. Widerlov E, Karlman I, Storsater J. Hydralazine-induced neonatal thrombocytopenia. *N Engl J Med* 1980; **303**:1235.

119. Constantine G, Beevers DG, Reynolds AL, Luesley DM. Nifedipine as a second line antihypertensive drug in pregnancy. *Br J Obstet Gynaecol* 1987; **94**:1136–42.

120. Walters BNJ, Redman CWG. Treatment of severe pregnancy associated hypertension with the calcium antagonist nifedipine. *Br J Obstet Gynaecol* 1984; **91**:330–6.

121. Ulmsten N, Andersson KE, Wingerup L. Treatment of

premature labor with the calcium antagonist nifedipine. *Acta Gynecol* 1980; **229**:1–5.

122. Lubbe WF, Hodge JV. Combined alpha- and beta-adrenoceptor antagonism with prazosin and oxprenolol in control of severe hypertension in pregnancy. *N Z Med J* 1981; **691**:169–72.

123. Pryde PG, Sedman AB, Nugent CE, Barr M. Angiotensin converting enzyme inhibitor fetopathy. *J Am Soc Nephrol* 1993; **3**:1575–82.

124. Are ACE inhibitors safe in pregnancy? *Lancet* 1989; **2**:482–3.

125. Hanssens M, Keirse MJNC, Vankelecom F, Van Assche FA. Fetal and neonatal effects of treatment with angiotensin-converting enzyme inhibitors in pregnancy. *Obstet Gynecol* 1991; **78**:128–35.

126. Uzan S, Beaufils M, Breart G, Bazin B, Capitant C, Paris J. Prevention of fetal growth retardation with low dose aspirin: findings of the EPREDA trial. *Lancet* 1991; **337**:1427–31.

127. Italian Study of Aspirin in Pregnancy. Low-dose aspirin in prevention and treatment of intrauterine growth retardation and pregnancy-induced hypertension. *Lancet* 1993; **341**:396–400.

128. CLASP Collaborative Group. CLASP: a randomised trial of low-dose aspirin for the prevention and treatment of pre-eclampsia among 9364 pregnant women. *Lancet* 1994; **343**:619–29.

129. Yu CK, Papageorghiou AT, Parra M, Palma Dias R, Nicolaides KH. Randomised controlled trial using low-dose aspirin in the prevention of pre-eclampsia in women with abnormal uterine artery Doppler at 23 weeks' gestation. *Ultrasound Obstet Gynecol* 2003; **22**:233–9.

130. Brennecke SP, Brown MA, Crowther CA, et al. Aspirin and prevention of pre-eclampsia. Position statement of the use of low-dose aspirin in pregnancy by the Australasian Society for the Study of Hypertension in Pregnancy. *Aust N Z J Obstet Gynaecol* 1995; **35**:38–41.

131. Sibai BM, Graham JM, McCubbin JH. A comparison of intravenous and intramuscular magnesium sulfate regimes in pre-eclampsia. *Am J Obstet Gynecol* 1984; **150**:728–33.

132. Gülmezoglu AM, Duley L. Use of anticonvulsants in eclampsia and pre-eclampsia: survey of obstetricians in the United Kingdom and Republic of Ireland. *BMJ* 1998; **316**:975–6.

133. Pritchard JA, Cunningham FG, Pritchard SA. The Parkland Memorial Hospital protocol for treatment of eclampsia: evaluation of 245 cases. *Am J Obstet Gynecol* 1984; **148**:951–63.

134. Sibai BM. Eclampsia VI: maternal–perinatal outcome in 254 consecutive cases. *Am J Obstet Gynecol* 1990; **163**:1049–55.

135. The Eclampsia Trial Collaborative Group. Which anticonvulsant for women with eclampsia? Evidence from the Collaborative Eclampsia Trial. *Lancet* 1995; **345**:1445–63.

136. Lucas MJ, Leveno KJ, Cunningham FG. A comparison of magnesium sulfate with phenytoin for the prevention of eclampsia. *N Engl J Med* 1995; **33**:201–6.

137. Waisman GD, Mayorga LM, Cámera MI, Vigolo CA, Matinotti A. Magnesium plus nifedipine: potentiation of hypotensive effect in pre-eclampsia? *Am J Obstet Gynecol* 1988; **159**:308–9.

138. Walters BN, Thompson ME, Lee A, De Swiet M. Blood pressure in the puerperium. *Clin Sci* 1986; **71**:589–94.

139. Dizon-Twonson D, Magee KP, Twickler DM, Cox SM. Coarctation of the abdominal aorta in pregnancy: diagnosis by magnetic resonance imaging. *Obstet Gynecol* 1995; **85**:817–19.

140. Chesley LC. Hypertension in pregnancy: definitions, familial factor and remote prognosis. *Kidney Int* 1980; **18**:234–40.

141. Chesley LC, Annito JE, Cosgrove RA. The remote prognosis of eclamptic women. *Am J Obstet Gynecol* 1976; **125**:509–13.

24
Peripartum cardiomyopathy

Celia M. Oakley

Introduction (see also Chapters 22 and 29)

The sudden onset of heart failure in the puerperium is devastating as it can transform a previously healthy woman to life-threatening illness and a young family from joy to tragedy within days. In less severe cases it has a later and more insidious onset, simulating dilated cardiomyopathy (DCM) except for its temporal relationship to the pregnancy. Although long recognized, the cause was not and still is not fully understood. It was first described in 1937 when it was attributed to 'idiopathic myocardial degeneration'[1] and joined the cardiomyopathies after that neologism was adopted in the 1960s. Myocarditis has been found on endomyocardial biopsy in a high proportion of these patients[2,3] and an autoimmune mechanism is likely.[4]

Since the key early papers from city hospitals in the US by Walsh et al. and by Demakis et al.[5,6] there have been numerous small case studies and reviews which have emphasized the different perspectives of the authors, depending on their geographical source and catchment populations. Reports have come from tertiary referral centers, city hospitals, and rural communities from Europe and the Americas to Nigeria and the Caribbean.[7–15]

Definition (see Box 24.1)

Peripartum cardiomyopathy (PPCM) is defined arbitrarily as unexplained left ventricular systolic dysfunction confirmed echocardiographically and developing in the last month of pregnancy or within 5 months of delivery.[16]

The definition, refined at a workshop held in 1997, aims to exclude patients with previously unsuspected DCM and to include only patients with no previous history of possible myocardial disease. It requires that there be no other identifiable cause for the heart failure and that the left ventricular systolic dysfunction be demonstrated echocardiographically.

Patients with structural heart disease which does not account for left ventricular failure are not immune from developing superimposed peripartum cardiomyopathy. Indeed an already reduced cardiovascular reserve may bring PPCM to light when it might otherwise have remained subclinical in a woman with an otherwise normal heart.[17,18]

Incidence

The true incidence is unknown, as past diagnostic criteria have varied and figures have mainly been derived from referral centers. Milder community-based cases probably go undiagnosed, as may even medically well policed hospital-supervised pregnancies. Even severe cases may not enter the statistics, especially in less well developed areas. Estimated incidence rates vary greatly from 1 in 1485 to 1 in 15 000 live births and the disorder may have greater prevalence in some parts of the world than in others for both ethnic (genetic) and environmental reasons.

A consensus opinion was of an incidence of between 1 in 3000 and 1 in 4000,[19] which gives an estimated 250–300 cases each year in the UK. This would make it far more common than is generally realized. The apparent rarity of PPCM in the developed world and the near certainty of serious under-reporting of it have made it difficult to study.

Box 24.1 Diagnostic criteria

- Development of cardiac failure in the last month of pregnancy or within 5 months of delivery
- Absence of another identifiable cause
- Absence of identifiable heart disease before the last month of pregnancy
- Left ventricular systolic dysfunction demonstrated by echocardiography
- Ejection fraction less than 45% or
- M-mode fractional shortening less than 30% or both and
- End-diastolic dimension more than 2.7 cm/m^2

Etiology (see Box 24.2)

It is believed that PPCM is a distinct entity rather than previously undiagnosed DCM unmasked by the hemodynamic stress of pregnancy. As hemodynamic stress is maximal during pregnancy, the usual onset of PPCM in the puerperium when the circulatory burden has remitted does not suggest exacerbation of pre-existing heart disease. Deterioration and heart failure in DCM develop as cardiovascular work increases and it is most likely to present in the second trimester[20] rather than in the puerperium when hemodynamic changes are receding or may be over. Moreover, the high frequency of myocarditis would not be expected in patients presenting with simple decompensation of pre-existing DCM. However, there seems to be an increased incidence of a positive family history of DCM in patients with PPCM[21–23] and if DCM is an autoimmune disorder (as suggested by the finding of autoantibodies) then an exacerbation at the time of restoration of immune competence after delivery would not be unexpected.

Except for cases of multiple pregnancy, hemodynamic stresses do not explain the patients perceived to be at particular risk in the early papers. Risk factors for PPCM were said to be multiparity, older maternal age, pre-eclampsia, gestational hypertension, and African race, but a high prevalence in Northern Nigeria is explained by local traditional practices with high salt intake and overheating rather than by ethnicity.

The high frequency with which myocarditis is found when biopsies are performed within a month of presentation and the recovery of many patients with PPCM, as in myocarditis occurring outside pregnancy, provide good evidence for a causal role. The real prevalence may be greater as many negative biopsies may have been taken outside the time-frame and histological diagnosis using the Dallas criteria has been inconsistent because of variability of inclusion of patients with 'borderline myocarditis', sampling errors,[24] and particularly as immunohistochemical stains were not included in the criteria. It is probable also that only fulminant cases are biopsied within a month of onset as milder cases tend to have an ill-defined onset.

The cause of the myocarditis remains in contention. Viruses have long been suspected to start the process of inflammation, with immune responses against infected myocytes causing myocyte death and initiating an ongoing autoimmune process against exposed cardiac proteins. But no infective agent has yet been found and infection may not play a part.

The mother exists in an immunosuppressed state during pregnancy and it is postulated that fetal cells may enter the maternal circulation and remain there without rejection.[25] If micro-chimeric hematopoietic cells enter cardiac tissue during the immunosuppressed pregnant state, then recovery of immune competence postpartum and recognition of nonself might well trigger a vigorous autoimmune reaction.[26] Prior exposure to paternal histocompatibility antigens expressed by sperm or previous immunization from earlier pregnancies may also play a role.

Support for abnormal immunologic activity as a possible cause for PPCM comes from the finding of high titers of autoantibodies.[27] Such antibodies have previously been shown to be present in the sera of patients with DCM, but several autoantibodies have been found which were unique to PPCM patients and not found in DCM patients.[4] Other contributing factors may lie in the unique hormonal and micronutrient environment of pregnancy,[28] genetic elements,[29] and infectious agents which lead to breakdown of self-tolerance as well as maladaptive responses to the hemodynamic changes of pregnancy.[30–32]

> **Box 24.2 Classical predisposing factors**
>
> - Multiple pregnancy
> - Multiparity
> - Older maternal age
> - Pre-eclampsia and gestational hypertension
> - African (and African American) race
> - Previous peripartum cardiomyopathy

Diagnosis

Diagnosis rests on identification of new left ventricular dysfunction developing around the time of parturition. The difficulties in early recognition are that many healthy women develop shortness of breath, fatigue, and pedal edema in late pregnancy, symptoms that are common to those of congestive heart failure.

Heart failure

Clinical onset soon after the birth may be with fulminant cardiac failure or sometimes with severe chest pain simulating myocardial infarction (MI). In other cases the onset of symptoms may be more gentle in later weeks or even months postpartum. A typical feature of the heart failure in PPCM, especially in the worst cases, is the frequency of marked fluid retention or even anasarca, which may be blamed on or contributed to by excess fluids administered during cesarean section, although not confined to women who have had a surgical delivery.[33]

Embolism

Embolism is frequent and a stroke or embolus to any site may be the first sign that something is wrong.[34–37] Echocardiography performed routinely to exclude a cardiac source for systemic embolism or as part of the diagnostic work-up for possible pulmonary embolism may show thrombus in one or both ventricles with unsuspected poor function despite absence of cardiac symptoms. This kind of case indicates the huge reserve possessed by the normal heart and the failure of clinicians to pick up physical signs. It emphasizes how blunt an instrument we have in having to rely on patients' perception of unwellness before we suspect a cardiac problem in patients with a less dramatic presentation.

The increased tendency to thromboembolism in PPCM compared with idiopathic DCM is attributable to the hypercoagulable state which exists in pregnancy, with increased concentration of coagulation factors VII, VIII and X and of plasma fibrinogen plus increased platelet adhesiveness. This increases the thrombotic risk imposed by blood stasis consequent upon ventricular dysfunction.

Arrhythmias

Arrhythmias are common and may be the presenting feature.[30] This propensity is in keeping with the tendency for arrhythmias to increase in frequency in pregnancy associated with heightened sympathetic drive. Both supraventricular (Fig. 24.1) and ventricular tachycardia[38] may usher in heart failure, which if not reported early because the mother is busy and distracted may have increased the ventricular dysfunction (tachycardia failure). Indeed the two conditions may blur, with uncertainty remaining even after restoration of sinus rhythm and subsequent recovery as to what part if any was played by PPCM rather than just a vulnerability of the parturient heart (maladaptation). Arrhythmias or emboli precipitated by pregnancy in pre-existing but undiagnosed cardiomyopathies may mimic PPCM.[39]

Chest pain

As in myocarditis outside pregnancy, chest pain may be severe and a presenting feature. Both the pain and the electrocardiogram (ECG) changes can mimic MI,[40] another rare complication of pregnancy which also tends to occur in the postpartum period.

Doubt may still remain after echocardiography, as this too may suggest MI if it shows marked focal

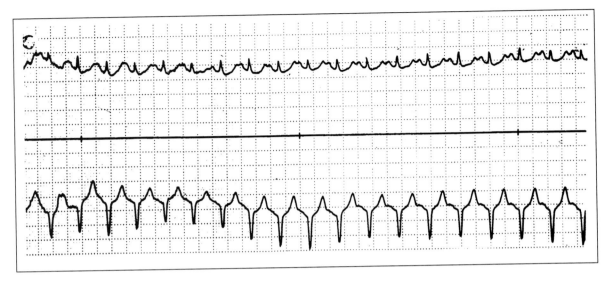

Figure 24.1
Supraventricular tachycardia in the same patient as in Fig. 24.2. She also had bursts of ventricular tachycardia.

akinesia or hypokinesia (as it occasionally does also in acute myocarditis outside pregnancy). It is important to perform coronary angiography for differentiation, as revascularization by percutaneous intervention or even coronary bypass graft surgery may be needed if a dissected or thrombosed coronary artery is shown and a large territory is threatened.

Time of onset of PPCM

We have no idea when the disorder starts. We only know when it causes clinical presentation. Some dyspnea and fatigue is almost universal in late pregnancy, so how would the rare woman with early PPCM be recognized? Abnormal physical signs would be subtle or absent, so early diagnosis would require routine high-tech echocardiographic screening of left ventricular function, a daunting logistic and financial prospect. More feasible would be serial screening of predisposed patients, particularly those with a family history of DCM or PPCM.

Most cases of PPCM do not develop symptoms until the postpartum period and even the most severe cases, those who develop fulminating conges-

tive heart failure during the first days after giving birth, provide no hints that they had been developing the condition during late pregnancy.

Even patients who had been under close observation in hospital because of pre-eclampsia have rarely been suspected of having PPCM before delivery, as cardiac dysfunction is not often recognized or is attributed to their hypertension and systemic illness. Moreover, heart failure in PPCM has a seemingly precipitous onset postnatally, just when delivery has cured most pre-eclamptic and eclamptic patients. Milder cases usually present later in the puerperium with more insidious onset of dyspnea and fatigue, which had at first been attributed to extra work and broken nights.

There is no information about left ventricular function before the recognition of cardiac dysfunction either in the most severe cases with onset of pulmonary edema and anasarca or in the milder ones who had felt quite well after the birth before sliding into failure. Still milder cases must exist and run an unrecognized course.

Family screening should be undertaken if possible, to establish whether any members have subclinical left ventricular dysfunction indicating a genetic tendency to PPCM.

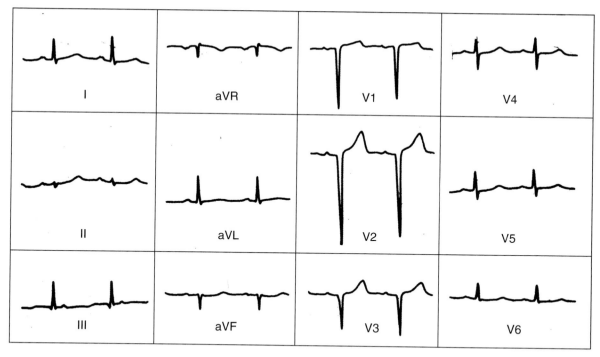

Figure 24.2
Electocardiogram from a patient with peripartum cardiomyopathy who went into severe heart failure 2 days after the birth of twins. It shows sinus rhythm with low voltage in the standard and unipolar leads and QS waves in chest leads V1–V3. Coronary arteriography was normal and the left ventricle showed global hypokinesia. Although at first considered for transplantation, she made a slow but incomplete recovery and became asymptomatic.

Physical examination

Physical examination may reveal an anxious breathless patient with tachycardia, hypotension, raised jugular venous pressure, a third heart sound gallop, sometimes a soft systolic murmur, pulmonary rales, hepatomegaly, and edema. Physical signs in milder cases may be far from obvious and tend to be overlooked in this technological age or attributed to other causes because a heart disorder is not suspected.

Box 24.3 Differential diagnosis

- Pre-existing dilated cardiomyopathy
- Peripartum myocardial infarction (coronary dissection, thrombosis or embolism)
- Ritodrine-induced pulmonary edema (premature delivery)
- Pulmonary embolism – thrombus or amniotic fluid
- Fluid overload (due to overinfusion)

Investigations

Electrocardiogram

The ECG usually shows a sinus tachycardia often with multiple supraventricular or ventricular ectopic beats or bursts of sustained tachycardia. QRS voltage may be low or normal or the QRS may be widened and a frank left bundle branch block pattern is often present. A QS pattern, usually in the chest leads, may suggest MI (Fig. 24.2). T-wave inversion and prolongation of the QTc are frequent. The ECG may be normal in mild cases.

Chest X-ray

The chest X-ray usually shows a large heart and pulmonary venous congestion or frank pulmonary edema. Small pleural effusions are frequent.

Echocardiography

Echocardiography typically shows ventricular dilatation usually affecting both ventricles and marked generalized hypokinesis. Less often the hypokinesis appears to be more focal, bringing the possibility of a coronary artery problem. Mitral and tricuspid valve regurgitation are usual and apical thrombi may be seen in the left or less often in both ventricles. These usually look shaggy, irregular and mobile in early cases. Spontaneous echo contrast is commonly seen due to slow flow. All the indices of contractility are markedly reduced. A pericardial effusion is often present.

Cardiac catheterization and angiocardiography

Cardiac catheterization reveals a raised pulmonary artery wedge pressure but normal or barely raised pulmonary artery pressure, a raised left ventricular end-diastolic pressure and normal coronary arteries on angiography. Left ventricular angiography is better avoided as echochardiography provides all the information. If endomyocardial biopsy is performed it should be from the right ventricle and only if it is free from thrombus.

Laboratory data

Laboratory findings are mostly within normal limits and cardiac enzymes are not usually elevated, but atrial and brain natriuretic peptide are elevated and D-dimer will be raised in patients with intracardiac thrombus.

Treatment

The need for early delivery and its mode should be assessed between obstetricians, anesthetists, and cardiologists in that minority of women with onset antepartum.

The patient should preferably be managed in a cardiac unit so that her condition, cardiac rhythm, blood pressure and ECG, oxygen saturations, electrolytes, and urine output can be appropriately monitored. Conventional treatment for heart failure is needed, with furosemide and spironolactone and angiotensin-converting enzyme (ACE) inhibitors or angiotensin II receptor blockers plus beta-blockers. (ACE or thromboxane A2 inhibitors are contraindicated in patients who have not yet delivered because they cause fetal renal failure; alternative vasodilators should be chosen until after delivery, which should be expedited.) Digoxin should not be given unless atrial fibrillation develops. This is rare and best treated by rapid cardioversion under full heparin cover but only after transesophageal echocardiography has excluded thrombus formation and only then if the arrhythmia has started within the last 24 hours.

Anticoagulant treatment

Anticoagulants should be given to patients with PPCM whether or not intraventricular thrombi have been shown or embolism has occurred. It is uncertain for how long they should be continued but certainly until all thrombus has disappeared, D-dimer is normal, and ventricular function has improved.

Immunosuppressive treatment

Immunosuppressive treatment should be considered in patients with biopsy-documented myocarditis who have failed to respond. The threshold for starting the treatment is arbitrary because of lack of evidence but will be lower in sicker patients in whom the most rapid improvement is sought. The failure of the Myocarditis Treatment Trial to show benefit may have had to do with protocol violation, starting too late in patients with equivocal biopsy results, and the failure to include immunohistological criteria.[41] Women with PPCM were not evaluated. A more recent retrospective study of intravenous immune globulin in women with PPCM suggested greater improvement in ejection fraction in the patients given immune globulin than in those not given it.[42]

The sickest patients will need intravenous inotropic support and should be transferred to a specialist cardiac intensive care unit where a balloon pump or more intensive left ventricular assist can be supplied as a bridge to recovery, with transplantation performed only as a last resort because of the likelihood of eventual improvement. Because of young age and the needs of the newborn and possibly other young children at home, women with PPCM receive top priority for cardiac transplantation.[43] Pulmonary embolism with infarction can be a contraindication to this procedure and full anticoagulation should be maintained right from the time of diagnosis of PPCM.

Prognosis

About a quarter of the published patients died,[6,13] but this obviously excludes milder unrecognized cases and the outlook will be better for patients with access to modern cardiac intensive care and to transplantation if needed. In Brazil half of Avila et al.'s patients improved and a quarter developed DCM.[13] This is one of the largest personal series.

Prognosis depends on whether left ventricular function returns to normal. The sooner this happens the better, but even patients whose improvement (monitored by echocardiography) is delayed longer than the arbitrary 6 months that has been suggested may yet show better function over a more extended period. Even apparently normal function will disguise an inevitable loss of myocytes, because myocytolysis is a basic part of the myocarditis which probably initiates the cardiomyopathy in nearly all patients. Some loss of cardiovascular reserve is therefore inherent in the diagnosis and reduction in contractile reserve has been shown by dopamine challenge even after apparently full recovery.

Rather little information exists concerning recurrence of PPCM if a future pregnancy is undertaken.[44–48] This is because of its rarity and the understandable reluctance of both patients and their cardiologists to take the unknown risk. Single-center experience is necessarily small. The largest comes from Brazil,[44,45] where Avila et al. performed a prospective study in which they compared the outcome of pregnancy in 18 patients with PPCM, 11 of whom had persistent left ventricular dysfunction, with eight who had primary DCM. Deterioration of left ventricular function was not seen in any of those with PPCM whose function had recovered. This good experience was in accordance with that of Albanesi Filho et al. but with not with that of Elkayam whose information on larger numbers had been gathered by questionnaire to all members of the American College of Cardiology. Elkayam et al. described 44 patients who went through subsequent pregnancies.[46,47] It seems that recurrence, while not inevitable, may occur even in patients who appear to have made a full recovery. The recurrence rate was 21% with 0% mortality among 28 patients with complete recovery and 44% with 19% mortality among 16 patients with persistent left ventricular dysfunction. These figures emphasize the risks of subsequent pregnancy, which should be avoided in patients with persistent left ventricular dysfunction and approached with caution even in patients who seem to have made a full recovery. Patients should continue their heart failure therapy for a year after recovery to allow time for optimal remodeling.[48] They should be monitored closely during the next pregnancy and for 6 months after it. Patients whose left ventricular function is borderline should undergo stress echocardiography. Those with a less than favorable response should be advised against embarking on another pregnancy.

No information exists concerning the risk of recurrence in a woman whose partner has changed since the pregnancy complicated by PPCM, or on whether the multiparity which has been associated with increased risk of PPCM would mean increased cardiac damage and greater risk of failure to survive subsequent pregnancy.

Patients whose left ventricular function has not returned to normal should be strongly advised to avoid future pregnancy.

References

1. Gouley BA, McMillan TM, Bellet S. Idiopathic myocardial degeneration associated with pregnancy and especially the puerperium. *Am J Med Sci.* 1937; **19**:185–99.

2. Melvin KR, Richardson PJ, Olsen EG, Daly K, Jackson G. Peripartum cardiomyopathy due to myocarditis. *N Engl J Med* 1982; **307**:731–4.

3. Midvei MG, DeMent SH, Feldman AM, Hutchins GM, Baughman KL. Peripartum myocarditis and cardiomyopathy. *Circulation* 1990; **81**:922–8.

4. Ansari AA, Fett JD, Carraway RE, Mayne AE, Onlamoon N, Sundstrom JB. Autoimmune mechanisms as the basis for human peripartum cardiomyopathy. *Clin Rev Allergy Immunol* 2002; **23**:301–24.

5. Walsh JJ, Burch GE, Black WC, Ferrans VJ, Hibbs RG. Idiopathic myocardiopathy of the puerperium (postpartal heart disease). *Circulation* 1965; **32**: 19–31.

6. Demakis JG, Rahimtoola SH, Sutton GC, et al. Natural course of peripartum cardiomyopathy. *Circulation* 1971; **44**:1053–61.

7. Brockington IF. Postpartum hypertensive heart failure. *Am J Cardiol* 1971; **27**:650–8.

8. Davidson NM, Parry EHO. Peripartum cardiac failure. *Q J Med* 1978; **47**:431–61.

9. Costanzo-Nordin MR, O'Connell JB. Peripartum cardiomyopathy in the 1980s: etiologic and prognostic consideration and review of the literature. *Prog Cardiol* 1989; **2**:225–39.

10. Brown CS, Bertolet BD. Peripartum cardiomyopathy: a comprehensive review. *Am J Obstet Gynecol* 1998; **178**:409–14.

11. Veille JC, Zaccaro D. Peripartum cardiomyopathy: summary of an international survey on peripartum cardiomyopathy. *Am J Obstet Gynecol* 1999; **181**:315–19.

12. Heider AL, Kuller JA, Strauss RA, Wells SR. Peripartum cardiomyopathy: a review of the literature. *Obstet Gynecol Surv* 1999; **54**:526–31.

13. Avila WS, de Carvalho ME, Tschaen CK, et al. Pregnancy and peripartum cardiomyopathy. A comparative and prospective study. *Arq Bras Cardiol* 2002; **79**:484–93.

14. Fett JD, Carraway RD, Dowell DL, King ME, Pierre R. Peripartum cardiomyopathy in the Hospital Albert Schweitzer District of Haiti. *Am J Obstet Gynecol* 2002; **186**:1005–10.

15. Ferrero S, Colombo BM, Fenini F, Abbamonte LH, Arena E. Peripartum cardiomyopathy. A review. *Minerva Ginecol* 2003; **55**:139–51.

16. Pearson GD, Veille J-C, Rahimtoola SH, et al. Peripartum cardiomyopathy: National Heart, Lung and Blood Institute and Office of Rare Diseases (National Institutes of Health) workshop recommendations and review. *JAMA* 2000; **283**:1183–8.

17. Oakley CM, Nihoyannopoulos P. Peripartum cardiomyopathy with recovery in a patient with coincidental Eisenmenger ventricular septal defect. *Br Heart J* 1992; **67**:190–2.

18. Purcell IF, Williams DO. Peripartum cardiomyopathy complicating severe aortic stenosis. *Int J Cardiol* 1995; **52**:163–6.

19. Ventura SJ, Peters KD, Martin JA, Maurer JD. Births and deaths: United States, 1996. *Mon Vital Stat Rep* 1997; **46** (1 Suppl 2):1–40.

20. Chan F, Ngan Kee WD. Idiopathic dilated cardiomyopathy presenting in pregnancy. *Can J Anaesth* 1999; **46**:1146–9.

21. Pierce JA. Familial occurrence of postpartal heart failure. *Arch Intern Med* 1962; **111**:163–6.

22. Massad LS, Reiss CK, Mutch DG, Hasket EJ. Family peripartum cardiomyopathy after molar pregnancy. *Obstet Gynecol* 1993; **81**:886–8.

23. Pearl W. Familial occurrence of peripartum cardiomyopathy. *Am Heart J* 1995; **129**:421–2.

24. Chow LH, Radio LH, Sears TD, McManus BM. Insensitivity of right ventricular endomyocardial biopsy in the diagnosis of myocarditis. *J Am Coll Cardiol* 1989; **14**:915–20.

25. Artlett CM, Jimenez SA, Smith JB. Identification of fetal DNA and cells in skin lesions from women with systemic sclerosis. *N Engl J Med* 1998; **338**:1186–91.

26. Nelson JL. Pregnancy, persistent microchimerism and auto-immune disease. *J Am Med Womens Assoc* 1998; **53**:31–2.

27. Ansari AA, Fett JD, Carraway RE, et al. Autoimmune mechanisms as the basis for human peripartum cardiomyopathy. *Clin Rev Allegy Immunol* 1998; **23**:301–24.

28. Fett JD, Ansari AA, Sundstrom JB, Coombs GF. Peripartum cardiomyopathy; a selenium disconnection and an autoimmune connection. *Int J Cardiol* 2002; **86**:311–16.

29. Fett JD, Sundstrom JB, Etta King M, Ansari AA. Mother–daughter peripartum cardiomyopathy. *Int J Cardiol* 2002; **86**:331–2.

30. Julian DG, Szekely P. Peripartum cardiomyopathy. *Prog Cardiovasc Dis* 1985; **27**:223–46.

31. Mone SM, Sanders SP, Colan SD. Control mechanisms for physiological hypertrophy of pregnancy. *Circulation* 1996; **94**:667–72.

32. Geva T, Mauer MB, Striker L, Kirshon B, Pivarnik JM. Effects of physiological load of pregnancy on left ventricular contractility and remodeling. *Am Heart J* 1997; **133**:53–9.

33. Task Force on the Management of Cardiovascular Diseases During Pregnancy of the European Society of Cardiology. Expert consensus document on management of cardiovascular diseases during pregnancy. *Eur Heart J* 2003; **24**:761–81.

34. Carlson KM, Browning JE, Eggleston MK, Ghjerman RB. Peripartum cardiomyopathy presenting as lower extremity arterial thromboembolism. A case report. *J Reprod Med* 2000; **45**:351–3.

35. Lasinska-Kowara M, Dudziak M, Suchorzewska J. Two cases of peripartum cardiomypathy initially misdiagnosed for pulmonary embolism. *Can J Anaesth* 2001; **48**:773–7.

36. Nishi I, Ishimitsu T, Isiizu T, et al. Peripartum cardiomyopathy and biventricular thrombi. *Circ J* 2002; **66**:863–5.

37. Kaufman I, Bondy R, Benjamin A. Peripartum cardiomyopathy and thromboembolism; anaesthetic management and clinical course of an obese, diabetic patient. *Can J Anaesth* 2003; **50**:161–5.

38. Colombo J, Lawal AH, Bhandari A, Hawkins JL, Atlee JL. Case 1 – 2002 – a patient with severe peripartum cardiomyopathy and persistent ventricular fibrillation supported by a biventricular assist device. *J Cardiothorac Vasc Anesth* 2002; **16**:107–13.

39. Lui CY, Marcus FI, Sobonya RE. Arrhythmogenic right ventricular dysplasia masquerading as peripartum cardiomyopathy with atrial flutter, advanced atrioventricular block and embolic stroke. *Cardiology* 2002; **97**:49–50.

40. Dickfeld T, Gagliardi JP, Marcos J, Russell SD. Peripartum cardiomyopathy presenting as an acute myocardial infarction. *Mayo Clin Proc* 2002; **77**:500–1.

41. Mason JW, O'Connell JB, Herskowitz A, et al. A clinical trial of immunosuppressive therapy for myocarditis. *N Engl J Med* 1995; **333**:269–75.

42. Bozkurt B, Villaneuva FS, Holubkov R, et al. Intravenous immune globulin in the therapy of peripartum cardiomyopathy. *J Am Coll Cardiol* 1999; **34**:177–80.

43. Aziz TM, Burgess MI, Acladious NN, et al. Heart transplantation for peripartum cardiomyopathy: a report of three cases and a literature review. *Cardiovasc Surg* 1999; **7**:565–7.

44. Albanesi Filho FM, da Silva TT. Natural course of subsequent pregnancy after peripartum cardiomyopathy. *Arq Bras Cardiol* 1999; **73**:47–57.

45. de Souza JL JR, de Carvalho Frimm C, Nastari L, Mady C. Left ventricular function after a new pregnancy in patients with peripartum cardiomyopathy. *J Card Fail* 2001; **7**:30–5.

46. Elkayam U, Tummala PP, Rao K, et al. Maternal and fetal outcomes of subsequent pregnancies in women with peripartum cardiomyopathy. *N Engl J Med* 2001; **344**:1567–71.

47. Elkayam U. Pregnant again after peripartum cardiomyopathy: to be or not to be? *Eur Heart J* 2002; **23**:753–6.

48. Baughman KL. Risks of repeat pregnancy after peripartum cardiomyopathy: double jeopardy. *J Card Fail* 2001; **7**:36–7.

25

Sex hormones and normal cardiovascular physiology in women

David M. Herrington and Bonny P. McClain

Introduction (see also Chapters 22 and 26)

Female sex hormones play an important role in virtually every aspect of cardiovascular physiology. During the last two decades the postulated cardioprotective effects of endogenous and exogenous estrogen stimulated interest in a comprehensive review of the effects of the female sex hormones on cardiovascular physiology and disease. The presumption was that careful study of the physiologic effects of estrogen would reveal important mechanisms that could be harvested to provide more efficient and perhaps gender-independent means to maintain vascular health or prevent cardiovascular disease (CVD). More recently, the unexpected findings of neutral or adverse effects of hormone therapy (HT) on cardiovascular risk in randomized clinical trials have called into question previous assumptions about the effects of exogenous estrogen on cardiovascular physiology and their implications for cardiovascular health and disease. Ironically, these dramatic findings continue to provide a mandate to characterize the cardiovascular effects of estrogen in more detail. However, the emphasis has now changed from a focus on potential beneficial mechanisms to possible harmful ones. Unfortunately to date, mechanisms contributing to estrogen-related increases in cardiovascular events in older menopausal women have not been clearly determined. Thus, the current review represents a summary of concepts and information gleaned primarily prior to the major randomized trials of HT, including the Women's Health Initiative (WHI). A few areas of interest have emerged in recent years that add new dimensions to our understanding of the cardiovascular effects of estrogen and offer potential mechanisms to explain the increased risk for myocardial infarction (MI) and stroke observed in WHI. These include new information about the estrogen receptor and how estrogen receptor polymorphisms may modify response to HT. This information is reviewed in the first part of the chapter. This chapter also reviews the effects of the female sex hormones on the central components of cardiovascular physiology including regional and systemic blood flow, blood pressure regulation, cardiac performance, endothelial function, and hemostasis. The emphasis is on the role of these hormones in normal physiology. Their effects on various CVD states such as hypertension or atherosclerosis are discussed in other chapters.

The data presented are limited to the effects of estrogens and progestins. In some circumstances there are important differences between endogenous versus exogenous hormones or naturally occurring versus synthetic sex hormones. However, for the most part estrogens or progestins behave as a class in cardiovascular physiology. Studies of the menstrual cycle, pregnancy, natural or surgical menopause, and estrogen and/or progestin administration provide clues to these class effects. The main exception to this

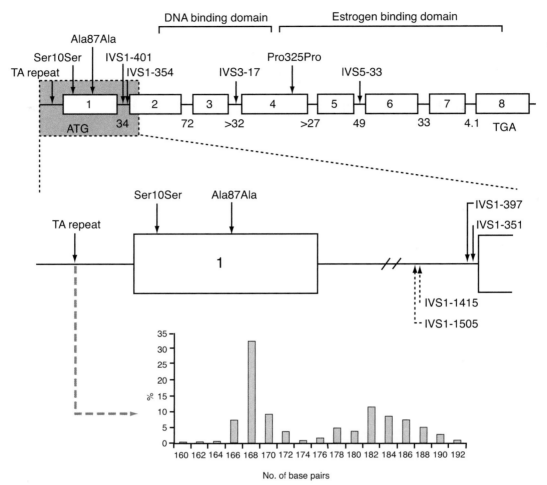

Figure 25.1
Numbered boxes indicate exons, the numbers under each intron indicate the estimated size of the intron, expressed in kilobase pairs. Intronic regions (solid black lines) are not drawn to scale. Vertical arrows indicate single nucleotide polymorphisms and the TA repeat polymorphism (solid indicates previously recognized variants and dashed indicates unpublished variants). The bar chart illustrates the distribution of TA repeats measured in base pairs observed in the women enrolled in the Estrogen Replacement and Atherosclerosis trial. Adapted with permission from reference 2. Copyright © 2002 Massachusetts Medical Society.

rule occurs with high-dose and/or highly potent estrogens and progestins found in oral contraceptives. In this case their effects are more pharmacologic in nature and often different from what is seen in naturally occurring levels or with replacement doses.

What emerges from this review is a unifying concept of estrogen as an agent capable of shifting the balance of vasomotor regulation in favor of vasodilation. In the final section of this chapter, this concept is explored and the implications for normal physiology and maintenance of vascular health are discussed.

ER-α and ER-β gene structure and function

Estrogen receptors are members of the family of steroid hormone receptors that serve as ligand-mediated transcription factors for the activation of a variety of hormone target genes.[1] Two estrogen receptors, ER-α and ER-β, have been identified and characterized. ER-α is a 25-kb gene located on 6q24.1. The classical gene structure is composed of eight exons and seven introns that range in size from 4.1 to 72 kb (Fig. 25.1). ER-β is a smaller protein which nevertheless shares significant homology with ER-α in many of the key functional domains. The 66-kDa protein encoded by ER-α contains both DNA and hormone binding domains as well as several trans-activation factor binding domains that play key roles in modulating ER-α function.[3] The ER-α protein serves as a ligand-mediated transcription factor for a large number of downstream target genes.

Both ER-α and ER-β are expressed in a wide variety of tissues in numerous mammalian species as well as in both women and men, reflecting the breadth of physiologic effects of endogenous and exogenous estrogen. Autoradiographic and biochemical analyses have demonstrated the presence of estrogen and progesterone receptors in several vascular tissues. Cytoplasmic or nuclear estrogen receptors are present in the aortic media and vascular smooth muscle cells of rats,[4–6] rabbit aortic endothelial cells,[7] canine aortic and coronary cytoplasmic preparations,[8,9] vascular smooth muscle cells of muscular and elastic arteries in baboons,[10–12] and in human aortic[13] and coronary[14] smooth muscle cells.[13] There are fewer data on female sex hormone receptors in myocardial tissue. Nonetheless, autoradiographic techniques have demonstrated estrogen receptors in atrial myocardial tissues in rats.[4] Lin et al. identified both cytoplasmic and nuclear estrogen receptors in myocardial tissue from ovariectomized baboons that were receiving estrogen replacement. However, in monkeys not receiving estrogen replacement, no nuclear estrogen receptors were detectable.[12] Similarly, receptors to progesterone have been described in canine vascular tissues,[8] in baboon aorta,[11,12] and in the aorta, coronary and carotid arteries in humans.[14] In the human specimens, progesterone receptors were found throughout the intima, media, and adventitia of the aorta but were localized to the endothelial nuclei of the intima in the coronary and carotid arteries. Progesterone receptors have also been described in baboon[11] and human[15] myocardium. Interestingly, no progesterone receptors were identified in the vessels supplying the uterus, breast, prostate, kidney, or gastrointestinal tract.[15]

Estrogen receptors play important roles in the expression of nitric oxide, endothelial cell adhesion molecules, inflammatory cytokines, and the expression of apolipoprotein AI, the primary protein constituent of high-density lipoprotein (HDL) particles.[16] ER-α, or perhaps a 46-kDa truncation isoform, also plays a role in activation of several kinase-mediated signaling cascades producing a portfolio of rapid nongenomic actions such as activation of endothelial nitric oxide synthase and subsequent increase in bioavailable endothelial nitric oxide.[17] Frequently, binding of the estrogen receptor also results in an increase in synthesis of progesterone receptors which, when bound to progesterone, results in downregulation of estrogen receptor synthesis.[18]

ER-α and ER-β polymorphisms

Several hundred coding region, regulatory region, and intronic single-nucleotide polymorphisms, and short tandem repeat polymorphisms are now known to exist in the human ER-α and ER-β genes. For historical reasons, variants that produce restriction fragment length polymorphisms in ER-α were the first to be recognized and have received the most attention in clinical studies. Of these, the variants associated with the restriction enzymes *PvuII* and *XbaI* have been examined with respect to numerous noncardiovascular but estrogen-sensitive clinical phenotypes, including risk,[19,20] age of onset,[21] and estrogen-receptor[22,23] status in breast cancer, risk of spontaneous abortion,[24,25] bone mineral density,[26–29] and cognitive decline.[30]

ER-α variants affect risk for cardiovascular disease

ER-α variants have been associated with functional, anatomic, and clinical manifestations of coronary disease. Significantly impaired coronary vasodilator responses to intravenous adenosine in men homozygous for the IVS1-397 C allele have been observed.[31] These same subjects also had 60–70% higher levels of autoantibodies to oxidized low-density lipoprotein (ox-LDL) cholesterol, a determinant of impaired coronary endothelial function.[31] Fivefold more coronary atherosclerosis was observed in IVS1-397 C/C homozygotes than those with the IVS1-397 T/T genotype.[32] In addition, an increased incidence of coronary thrombosis was reported among IVS1-397 C/C men compared with IVS1-397 T/T men.[32] Extent of coronary disease has also been associated with the presence of long alleles in the promoter of the TA repeat polymorphism demonstrating more extensive and complicated coronary lesions.[33,34]

A population-based cohort of the Framingham Heart Study reported individuals with the CC genotype of the IVS1-397 T/C variant associated with an increased odds ratio for MI.[35] Additionally, a higher frequency of coronary thrombosis was reported in the CC genotype of the ER-α IVS1-397 T/C variant compared with TT genotype. Additional studies are necessary to determine if the associations reported in the Helsinki Heart Study coronary specimens are applicable to women. In the aggregate these data suggest that ER-α variants may modify risk for atherosclerosis and clinical coronary heart disease (CHD).

ER-α variants alter response to hormone therapy

During the last decade, HT became one of the most frequently prescribed drugs in the United States, touting a highly diversified portfolio of presumed benefits for postmenopausal women. The belief that HT might reduce a woman's risk for CHD contributed considerably to its widespread use. Beginning in 1998, results from a series of randomized clinical trials, including recent data reported by Manson et al.[36] and Hodis et al.,[37] clearly demonstrate that HT does not slow clinical or anatomic progression of established coronary disease, nor does it prevent clinical cardiovascular events in previously healthy women. Indeed, data from the WHI, in conjunction with data from several other clinical endpoint trials, suggest that HT may even increase cardiovascular risk. The clinical implications of the cardiovascular and other data from these trials and revised recommendations concerning HT use have been described previously in detail.[36–38]

Effects of sex hormones on regional and systemic blood flow

The regulation of blood pressure and coronary circulation is influenced by variations in vascular tone. Although this relationship affects the incidence of hypertension and CHD, the direct effects of sex hormones on vasomotor tone have not been well characterized.[39] Not surprisingly, the most readily apparent cardiovascular effects of the female sex hormones involve regulation of vasomotor tone in reproductive organs. Estrogen causes vasodilation in a wide variety of mammalian arteries in reproductive tissues including uterine,[40–45] vaginal,[40] and urethral[40] arterial distributions in animals, and vaginal,[46,47] urethral,[48] uterine,[49] and vulval[50] arterial distributions in women. These effects are consistent with the increased metabolic demands of the reproductive system during pregnancy.

However, the effects of estrogen on regional blood flow are not limited to reproductive organs. Estrogen increases hindleg blood flow in dogs,[51] skin, thyroid, and mammary blood flow in ewes,[52] and hand or forearm blood flow in women.[53,54] Estrogen also increases myocardial perfusion in ewes,[45] and causes coronary vasodilation in isolated perfused hearts[45] and coronary vascular ring preparations from rabbits.[55–57] Estrogen treatment in women with coronary disease delays the onset of ischemia and increases exercise tolerance during treadmill testing.[58] However, it is possible that these effects reflect enhanced endothelial-dependent vasodilator capacity rather than a direct vasodilator effect.

Data from Collins et al. suggest that high-dose estrogen exerts a direct vasodilatory effect through a calcium antagonistic effect.[59] Others have demonstrated that estrogen can hyperpolarize vascular smooth muscle membranes from isolated dog coronaries, an effect that renders them less responsive to vasoconstrictor stimuli.[9] In one study of forearm vascular resistance, physiologic doses of estrogen enhanced the endothelial-independent vasodilator response to nitroprusside[60] but several other studies failed to detect such an effect in monkeys[61,62] or humans.[63,64]

In animals, progestin has been shown to diminish the estrogen-associated increases in genital blood flow.[40-43] Progestin has also been reported to diminish vulval blood flow[47] and induce hand arterial vasospasm in a postmenopausal woman.[54] On the other hand, high levels of progesterone are associated with a direct coronary vasodilating effect in rabbit coronary arteries in vivo.[65]

The effects of estrogen on blood flow in nonreproductive organs suggest a more generalized systemic effect on vascular tone. Indeed, several studies have demonstrated a decrease in systemic vascular resistance associated with either acute[66,67] or chronic estrogen administration[66] in ewes. This effect on systemic vascular resistance resembles the changes that occur in vascular tone during normal human pregnancy.[68-70] The potential mechanisms for this vasodilating effect of estrogen are presented in subsequent sections of this chapter.

Effects of sex hormones on blood pressure

The possible effects of estrogen on blood pressure have been considered for many years.[71] Sexual dimorphism exists for blood pressure in animals[72,73] and in humans,[74] with premenopausal females having lower blood pressure than similar-aged males. In humans, this sexual dimorphism is lost or reversed after menopause.[75,76]

During the menstrual cycle, blood pressure is lowest during the luteal phase at a time when the estrogen level is high.[77-79] Blood pressure also falls significantly during pregnancy coincident with significant increases in total estrogen and progesterone production.[70,80,81] Some cross-sectional studies also suggest that loss of endogenous estrogen at the time of menopause is associated with higher blood pressures,[82,83] and greater increases in blood pressure with age[83] when compared with similar-

aged premenopausal women. However, other studies have failed to detect an influence of menopause on blood pressure.[84,85]

The effects of exogenous estrogen or progestin administration on blood pressure are less clear. Oral contraceptive use is clearly associated with an increase in blood pressure,[71,86-90] and some women become frankly hypertensive.[91] On the other hand, clinical studies and clinical trials of estrogen therapy in menopausal women have shown slight increases,[92,93] slight decreases,[92,94-97] or no difference[98-103] in measures of blood pressure compared with controls. In one report, progesterone alone was reported to lower blood pressure in humans.[104] Because of differences in patient populations, dose and formulation of estrogen, duration of treatment, and presence or absence of simultaneous progestational agents, these studies are difficult to compare. A recent longitudinal observational study of 226 healthy, normotensive menopausal women from the Baltimore Longitudinal Study of Aging reported that increases in systolic blood pressure over time were significantly smaller in menopausal women taking continuous HT than in those not taking HT. These smaller increases in HT users were more evident at older age. Additionally, HT use did not affect diastolic blood pressure, although values did not change significantly over time in either group. None of the variables that might affect blood pressure, such as body mass index, total and HDL cholesterol levels, smoking status, alcohol use, physical activity or a family history of CVD, influenced these effects.[105] However, in the Postmenopausal Estrogen/Progestin Interventions (PEPI) trial, no significant changes in blood pressure were found with unopposed estrogen and various combined hormone regimens.[103]

In summary, physiologic conditions associated with increases in plasma levels of estrogen (and progesterone) such as the premenopause years, the luteal phase of the menstrual cycle and pregnancy are associated with lower blood pressure. In menopausal women, replacement doses of estrogen, with or without progestin, have not consistently demonstrated a similar blood pressure-lowering effect. However, the lack of a clear-cut effect of replacement doses of exogenous estrogen, with or without progestins, on blood pressure in humans does not mean that these hormones have no effect on blood

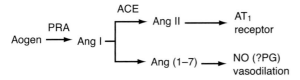

Figure 25.2
Illustration of the basic steps in angiotensin peptide metabolism. Angiotensinogen (Aogen), also referred to as renin substrate, is secreted by the liver. Its conversion to angiotensin I (Ang I) is determined by the plasma renin activity (PRA). Ang I is subsequently converted to angiotensin II (Ang II) by angiotensin-converting enzyme (ACE), or to angiotensin (1–7) (Ang (1–7)). Binding of Ang II to the angiotensin type 1 receptor (AT$_1$) causes vasoconstriction in peripheral arterioles and stimulates aldosterone secretion in the adrenal cortex. Ang (1–7) appears to enhance both nitric oxide (NO)- and prostaglandin (PG)-mediated vasodilator responses in some settings.

pressure regulation. In fact, as will be seen in subsequent sections, there are ample data to suggest that estrogen has counterbalancing effects on vasomotor tone and fluid retention resulting in little or no net change in blood pressure despite significant changes in the balance of vasoconstrictors and vasodilators in favor of vasodilation.

Effects of estrogen on the renin–angiotensin system

The renin–angiotensin system is one of the major determinants of vasomotor tone and sodium and water metabolism in mammalian species. Recent data suggest that the influence of estrogen and progestins on systemic vascular resistance and blood pressure can be partially explained by their gender-specific effects on the renin–angiotensin system.

The first step in angiotensin peptide metabolism is the synthesis of angiotensinogen or renin substrate in the liver (Fig. 25.2). In rats[106–109] and in humans,[91,110] estrogen administration results in significant increases in angiotensinogen. In one study, normal women taking oral contraceptives or ethinyl estradiol

(50 μg) had 2.4-fold higher levels of angiotensinogen than similar women on no HT.[91] The effects of replacement doses of estrogen on angiotensinogen in menopausal women are an active area of interest. An increase in angiotensinogen is also seen during normal pregnancy in women.[111] In rats, renal and hepatic levels of angiotensinogen mRNA are reduced after ovariectomy.[112] Furthermore, the 5' flanking region of both the rat[113] and human[114] angiotensinogen gene contains a sequence with strong homology to other known estrogen responsive elements. Thus, estrogen appears to significantly enhance angiotensinogen expression through a classic steroid hormone control mechanism.

The effects of estrogen on angiotensin peptide metabolism do not stop with angiotensinogen. Estrogen also enhances plasma renin activity in rats,[108] monkeys,[115] and humans,[116] and ovariectomy reduces renal renin and renal and hepatic renin mRNA in rats.[112] The combination of increased substrate and enhanced enzyme activity results in significant increases in angiotensin I synthesis.[108,115,116] Angiotensin I levels are also increased during proestrus and estrus in rats.[117] In contrast, Seely et al. reported a significant increase in angiotensinogen, and decreased active renin and angiotensin-converting enzyme, in menopausal women with conjugated equine estrogen (CEE) regimens of HT.[118]

Despite the estrogen-associated increases in angiotensinogen, plasma renin activity and angiotensin I, these changes do not necessarily translate into a cardiovascular pressor response. In fact, the opposite may occur. In animal models estrogen appears to alter the metabolism of angiotensin I, diverting it away from angiotensin II in favor of angiotensin. This may be accomplished by decreasing angiotensin-converting enzyme, an effect that has been documented in plasma of cynomolgus monkeys,[115] and rats,[119] in the anterior pituitary of rats,[120] and most recently in humans.[118,121–123] Furthermore, estrogens also blunt the actions of any angiotensin II produced by either a downregulation or decrease in sensitivity of angiotensin II receptors. This effect of estrogen is best documented in the central nervous system where angiotensin II receptors in the anterior pituitary are known to vary with the estrus cycle in rats, with the fewest angiotensin II binding sites

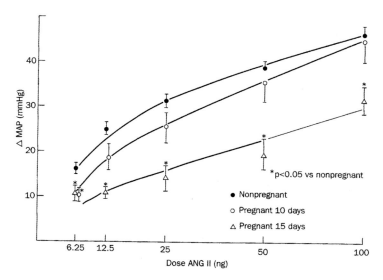

Figure 25.3
Effect of pregnancy in pressor response to angiotensin II (ANG II). Pregnancy results in blunting of the pressor response (MAP, mean arterial pressure) to ANG II at 15 days of pregnancy. Nonpregnant, n = 11; pregnant 10 days, n = 6; pregnant 15 days, n = 6. Data are means ± standard error. Reproduced from reference 130 with permission.

occurring when circulating estrogen levels are high.[120,124] Angiotensin II receptors in the anterior pituitary increase after ovariectomy[120] and decrease with subsequent estrogen replacement.[120,124] Similar effects of estrogen on angiotensin II receptors have been reported in cultured rat aortic smooth muscle cells.[125] These effects may account for the blunted dipsogenic and pressor responses to angiotensin II in estrogen-treated rats,[126] and the resistance to the pressor effect of angiotensin II observed during pregnancy in women.[127,128] Others have reported a decrease in pressor response to angiotensin II in pregnant rats despite no change in receptor number or binding affinity, suggesting other unrecognized mechanisms for attenuating the pressor response to angiotensin II (Fig. 25.3).[129,130]

The diversion of angiotensin I away from angiotensin II towards angiotensin (1–7) which occurs during proestrus[117] or with estrogen administration[119] in rats is also a potentially important cardiovascular effect of estrogen because of the vasodilator properties of angiotensin (1–7).[131,132] Angiotensin (1–7) is a potent stimulator of vasodila-

tor prostaglandin synthesis and release in human and animal vascular smooth muscle.[133,134] Furthermore, angiotensin (1–7) causes a nitric oxide-dependent vasodilator response in canine[135] and porcine[136] coronary arteries, and feline mesenteric and hindquarter vascular beds.[131]

In summary, physiologic levels of estrogen have profound influences on the renin–angiotensin system that, in the aggregate, result in a shift of angiotensin metabolism in favor of vasodilation. This is consistent with the hemodynamic data suggesting an estrogen-associated decrease in systemic vascular resistance. There are few data on the effects of progestins on the renin–angiotensin system at this time.

Sex hormones and regulation of blood volume

The lack of a clear-cut estrogen-associated reduction in blood pressure, despite the vasodilatory properties of estrogen, may be partially due to a concomitant increase in plasma volume. Pregnancy has long been recognized to increase plasma volume.[137] These changes can occur after as little as 6 weeks of pregnancy.[137] Increases in blood volume have also been reported with estrogen replacement in menopausal women[96] and with estrogen administration in sheep[138] and guinea pigs.[139] The estrogen-associated volume expansion is most likely secondary to an effect of estrogen on sodium retention. In rats, sodium excretion varies with the estrus cycle, with sodium retention being greatest when estrogen levels are high.[140] In dogs, estradiol results in sodium retention that is independent of mineralocorticoid activity.[141] In menopausal women, estradiol reduces renal excretion of sodium and water without altering potassium balance, again suggesting that the effects of estrogen are not mediated by an aldosterone-related mechanism.[142] Estrogen- and progesterone-effected changes in plasma volume may also result from adjustments in extracellular fluid distribution in relation to transcapillary fluid dynamics.[143] Thus, the vasodilating properties of estrogen mediated through changes in the renin–angiotensin axis may be offset by a direct effect on volume expansion through enhanced sodium retention. The net result is little or no effect on resting blood pressure. However, the balance between vasodilating and vasoconstricting forces appears to be shifted towards vasodilation.

Sex hormones and cardiac function

Heart rate,[144] end-diastolic volume,[144,145] stroke volume,[68] and cardiac output[68,69,146] all dramatically increase and systemic vascular resistance falls[69] during human pregnancy and during ovulation induction in infertile women,[147] an intervention that replicates endogenous levels of estradiol seen in pregnancy. Similar changes occur during pregnancy in other mammals as well.[139,148,149] These changes begin prior to the development of the hemodynamic demands of the fetus[70,139,144] and correlate with the concomitant increases in serum estradiol.[146]

Increases in cardiac output and stroke volume and reductions in systemic vascular resistance have been reported with estradiol replacement therapy in women,[96,150] nonhuman primates,[151] and other mammalian species.[66,152] However, several recent well designed studies have reported no effect of HT on cardiac function.[153–157] Only one randomized, placebo-controlled study showed a potential favorable effect in mild hypertensive women of combined CEE and medroxyprogesterone acetate (MPA) on hemodynamic load on the heart, measured by echocardiography.[158] Inconsistent findings in previous studies may be the result of variety in the routes of administration, presence or absence of progestogen, varying doses and duration of treatment, and type of progestogen utilized.[159]

The currently available data on the effects of estrogen on human ventricular function are difficult to interpret because of variability in the loading conditions of the heart in the studies conducted to date. Most echocardiographic studies of human pregnancy suggest that ventricular contractility, as measured by ejection fraction, remains essentially unchanged.[68,145,160] However, Eckstein et al. demonstrated that cardiac index and peak aortic flow velocity were significantly reduced in premenopausal women whose estrogen levels were suppressed by a gonadotropin-releasing hormone agonist,[161] suggesting that estrogen has a direct effect on myocardial function. Similarly, late menopausal women were found to have larger end-systolic volumes, and lower peak left ventricular ejection and filling rates than similar early menopausal women.[162] Menopausal estrogen therapy resulted in increases in peak aortic flow velocity and mean aortic acceleration at 10 weeks and 1 year, suggesting an enhanced and maintained cardiac inotropism associated with estrogen replacement.[162] These observations are consistent with animal studies showing decreases in cardiac performance such as stroke work, ejection fraction, and shortening velocity with ovariectomy,[163] and increases in these same parameters with estrogen replacement,[164] or during pregnancy.[165]

The exact mechanism for the estrogen-related increase in inotropism in rat hearts is not known. Some studies report an estrogen-related increase in Ca^{2+}-myosin ATPase resulting in shifts of the expression of myosin isoenzymes.[163,164] Estrogen has also been reported to stimulate rat myocyte guanylate cyclase,[166] and sarcolemmal Na^+–K^+ ATPase.[167] These observa-

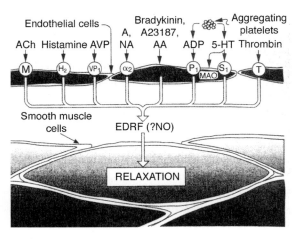

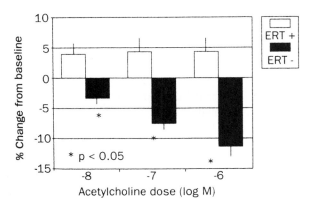

Figure 25.4

Formation of vasoactive factor(s) by vascular endothelium. Various substances may, by activation of specific receptors on endothelial cells, evoke release of relaxing factor(s) (endothelial-derived relaxing factor (EDRF), which is possibly nitric oxide (?NO)) that, in turn, causes relaxation of arterial vessels. ACh, acetylcholine; M, muscarinic receptors; H_2, histaminergic receptors; AVP, arginine vasopressin; VP_1, vasopressinergic receptors; P_1, purinergic receptors; A, adrenaline (epinephrine); NA, noradrenaline (norepinephrine); α_2, α_2-adrenergic receptor; AA, arachidonic acid; ADP, adenosine diphosphate; MAO, monoamine oxidase; 5-HT, 5-hydroxytryptamine (serotonin); S_1, serotonergic receptors; T, thrombin receptors. Reproduced from reference 168 with permission.

Figure 25.5

Plot of mean percent change in coronary diameter in response to serial doses of acetylcholine in menopausal women with mild coronary disease. Vertical lines indicate standard error of the mean. Women who were current users of estrogen replacement therapy (ERT) (n = 4) had significant vasodilator response, whereas women who were not on estrogen (n = 6) had a vasoconstrictor response consistent with endothelial dysfunction. Reproduced from reference 63 with permission.

tions suggest that estrogen is capable of modulating certain aspects of cardiac myocellular function in rats. However, the relevance of these observations for human ventricular function remains unknown.

Effects of sex hormones on endothelial-dependent vasodilator capacity

Normally, arteries dilate when exposed to a variety of chemical and physical stimuli including acetylcholine, histamine, serotonin, adenosine, and increased blood flow.[168,169] These stimuli lead to endothelial cell release of several factors that cause vascular smooth muscle relaxation. Chief among these is endothelial-derived relaxing factor (EDRF) which is thought to be nitric oxide or a closely related compound (Fig. 25.4).[168–170] Atherosclerosis is associated with impaired endothelial-dependent relaxation, presumably due to impaired production or release of EDRF and possibly other endothelial-derived factors.[171] In this case the weak direct vasoconstrictor effect of agents such as acetylcholine or serotonin predominate leading to vasoconstriction.

Estrogen plays an important role in modulating the relationship between various endothelial-dependent vasodilator stimuli and the subsequent vascular smooth muscle cell response in normal as well as atherosclerotic vessels. Estrogen facilitates the normal vasodilator response to acetylcholine in rabbit femoral arteries[172] and porcine coronary arteries[173] in vitro. Williams et al. demonstrated that both chronic[61] and acute (<15 minutes)[62,174] estrogen administration attenuates or reverses the expected coronary vasoconstriction effect of acetylcholine in ovariectomized cynomolgus monkeys with coronary atherosclerosis. Acute and chronic exposure to various forms of estrogen has also been shown to enhance endothelial-dependent vasodilator capacity in the coronary[44,45,63,64,147,175] (Fig. 25.5) and forearm[175–177] arterial distributions of menopausal women with mild atherosclerosis or coronary disease risk factors, as well as in the forearm of healthy menopausal women.[60] These effects have been documented both in the macrovasculature[63,64,175] and in the resistance arterioles.[60,64,175,176] These data suggest that estrogen plays a fundamentally important role in facilitating the synthesis, release, delivery, or response to EDRF or other endothelial-dependent modulations of vasomotor tone. The acute estrogen administration studies suggest that estrogen effects on endothelial function may involve post-translational mechanisms since significant changes can be seen in less than 15 minutes. Progesterone appears to blunt the favorable effect of estrogen on endothelial-dependent vasodilation in canine vascular rings[178] and in coronary arteries of cynomolgus monkeys in vivo.[174]

The exact mechanism(s) through which estrogen exerts its effects on endothelial-dependent vasomotor regulation and responsiveness are unclear. Gisclard and colleagues speculated that estrogen upregulates synthesis of acetylcholine receptors thus facilitating acetylcholine endothelial stimulation of EDRF synthesis and/or release.[172] Estrogen-associated enhancement of muscarinic receptor function has been documented in other mammalian tissues.[179] Treatment with estradiol also results in upregulation of nitric oxide synthase in cultured human aortic endothelial cells.[180] In a transgenic rat model of hypertension, estrogen appears to increase the dependency of basal vasomotor tone on nitric oxide synthesis,[135] a finding also consistent with an estrogen-associated upregulation of nitric oxide synthase. A study of serum nitrate and nitrite levels as a surrogate measure of nitric oxide release demonstrated significant increases during the follicular phase of the menstrual cycle in normal women and during exogenous estradiol-induced follicular development in women undergoing in vitro fertilization.[181]

Other endothelial-derived agents such as prostacyclin (PGI$_2$) and to a lesser extent endothelial-derived hyperpolarizing factor (EDHF) also contribute to endothelial-dependent vasodilation. Prostacyclin is a potent vasodilator[182] with a different mechanism of action for vasodilation than EDRF. Subthreshold levels of PGI$_2$ have been shown to potentiate the vasodilator response to EDRF in porcine coronary arteries.[183] Since estrogen is known to modulate prostanoid metabolism, it may also influence endothelial-dependent vasodilator capacity through an effect on PGI$_2$ synthesis. In high doses, estrogen enhances PGI$_2$ synthesis in human umbilical vessels.[184] Estrogen-induced augmentation of PGI$_2$ synthesis has also been demonstrated in female piglet aortic endothelial cells[185] and rat cultured aortic smooth muscle cells.[186,187] However, indomethacin in a sufficient dose to inhibit PGI$_2$ synthesis did not alter estrogen-enhanced endothelium-dependent vasodilation in rabbit femoral arteries.[172]

Thus, estrogen clearly plays an important role in modulating the nitric oxide pathway responsible for regulating vasomotor responses to various physiologic endothelial stimuli. The effects of progesterone are less clear; however, the small amount of data currently available suggests that it may attenuate the enhancing effect of estrogen. The mechanism(s) through which estrogen exerts its effects are not yet fully understood. In addition to possible effects on muscarinic receptor function and upregulation of nitric oxide synthase, estrogen may also increase the delivery of nitric oxide to the vascular smooth muscle by acting as an antioxidant.

Antioxidant properties of estrogen

Endothelial cells, macrophages, smooth muscle cells, and neutrophils all produce reactive oxygen species capable of peroxidizing endothelial cell membrane phospholipids, causing functional and structural defects in the endothelium. One of the first membrane receptors to fail under oxidative stress is the muscarinic acetylcholine receptor.[188] This observation may explain why endothelial-dependent vasodilator capacity is impaired so early in the atherosclerotic process.[189] The locally produced oxygen radicals may also inhibit endothelial-dependent vasodilator capacity by inactivating EDRF en route from the endothelium to the vascular smooth muscle[190] as well as through a direct vasoconstrictor effect.[191] Thus, shifting the local balance between reactive oxygen species and antioxidant compounds would be expected to have a favorable effect on endothelial-dependent vasodilator function.

Estrogens are known to possess varying degrees of antioxidant activity. Estradiol and estrone have been shown to inhibit peroxidation of methylinoleate by UV radiation[192] and microsomal phospholipid by Fe^{3+}-ADP.[193] Catechol metabolites of estradiol and estrone have also been shown to be potent inhibitors of lipid peroxidation in vivo and in vitro[194,195] and to regenerate α-tocopherol from its oxidized state – tocopheroxyl.[196] Estradiol reduces oxidative modification of LDL in vitro in animals[197–199] and in menopausal women.[200] This capacity of estrogen to act as an antioxidant points to another mechanism through which it could enhance endothelial-dependent vasodilator capacity, and help protect against atherosclerosis.

Effects of sex hormones on hemostasis and thrombosis

The interaction between coagulation factors, platelets, and vascular endothelium generates numerous signals that modulate vascular smooth muscle cell tone, growth, and differentiation, and other aspects of cellular function. Furthermore, thrombosis plays a central role in the development of acute coronary and cerebral syndromes as well as the development of the underlying disease process of atherosclerosis. Therefore, the effects of estrogen and progesterone on the coagulation and fibrinolytic systems and on platelet function are a critical component of cardiovascular physiology. The effects of estrogen on hemostasis and thrombosis are highly dose-dependent. The effects of physiologic levels of estrogen or doses found in replacement therapy are significantly different from those associated with oral contraceptives. Although both pro- and anticoagulant and fibrinolytic effects are seen with all doses, in general the balance is shifted away from thrombosis with low-dose estrogen, and towards thrombosis with high-dose estrogen.

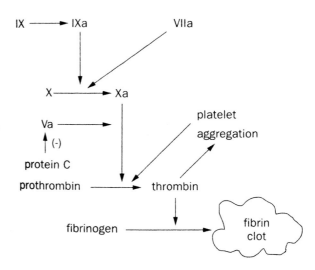

Figure 25.6
Final common pathway for the coagulation cascade. Factor IXa from the intrinsic pathway or factor VIIa from the extrinsic (requiring tissue injury) pathway convert factor X to Xa. Factors Xa, Va, and platelet surface membrane interact to create the prothrombinase complex which cleaves prothrombin to thrombin. Thrombin then activates soluble fibrinogen to form fibrin monomers which then polymerize to form a fibrin clot.

Physiologic changes in endogenous estrogen levels influence various coagulation and fibrinolytic factors. Fibrinogen,[201] α1-antiplasmin,[202] tissue plasminogen activator (tPA),[203] and von Willebrand's factor[204] have all been reported to vary with the menstrual cycle. Pregnancy is accompanied by an increase in fibrinogen and factor VII.[205,206] Plasminogen is also increased during pregnancy, but this is offset by a simultaneous increase in plasminogen activator inhibitors which results in a net gradual decrease in fibrinolytic activity persisting until postpartum.[207,208] Menopause is associated with increases in levels of procoagulant factors VII and fibrinogen, as well as the anticoagulant factor antithrombin III and plasminogen, which promotes fibrinolysis,[209–211] making the net effect of menopause on hemostasis less clear.

The effect of hormone replacement regimens on coagulation (Fig. 25.6) has been studied in some detail. Several large cross-sectional studies and clinical trials have documented that hormone replacement doses of estrogen are associated with small increases in factor VII.[212–215] However, this effect of low-dose estrogen is not observed in women on estrogen replacement combined with low-dose progestins,[212,215–217] or in women on transdermal estrogen, a form of administration that avoids the first-pass stimulatory effects on hepatic protein synthesis.[218] Transient increases in factors IX and X have also been reported in users of menopausal HT.[219] It is possible that some of the estrogen-associated increases in factor VII are due to concomitant increases in triglycerides. Elevated triglycerides are known to increase levels and activation of factor VII.[220,221]

The slight estrogen-associated increase in procoagulant factors is likely offset by anticoagulant effects further down the coagulation cascade. For example, unopposed estrogen replacement is associated with a 5% increase in protein C,[212] the enzyme substrate that degrades factor V and therefore slows the rate of coagulation. In addition, fibrinogen levels have been consistently reported to be lower in users of hormone replacement therapy, either unopposed estrogen or combination therapy.[102,212,214,217] This effect on fibrinogen is particularly intriguing since fibrinogen levels have clearly been shown to be an independent risk factor for cardiovascular events in a number of prospective epidemiologic studies.[222–225] Although some studies have reported a decrease in antithrombin III with opposed[215] and unopposed regimens,[212,215] others have failed to detect such an effect.[226,227]

There are fewer data on the effects of estrogen and progestins on the fibrinolytic system (Fig. 25.7). The most compelling data come from Gebara et al. who demonstrated significantly lower levels of plasminogen activator inhibitor-1 (PAI-1) in menopausal women on hormone replacement compared with nonusers. Similar differences were seen in premenopausal women compared with similar-aged men or menopausal women.[228] These findings are consistent with earlier reports from smaller clinical studies of estrogen[209,227,229] or estrogen plus progestin.[217,229]

Estrogen replacement is also associated with decreased levels of tPA antigen.[228] However, since the vast majority of tPA is complexed with PAI-1, decreased levels of tPA antigen likely still reflect enhanced fibrinolytic capacity because of decreased

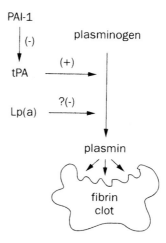

Figure 25.7
The fibrinolytic pathway. Plasminogen is cleaved to plasmin in the presence of a plasminogen activator such as tissue plasminogen activator (tPA). Plasminogen activators can be inhibited by plasminogen activator inhibitors such as plasminogen activator inhibitor-1 (PAI-1). The cleavage of plasminogen to plasmin can also be competitively inhibited by the plasminogen-like moiety found in lipoprotein (a) (Lp(a)). Plasmin is the fibrin-cleaving enzyme responsible for clot dissolution.

PAI-1. Recently, estrogen administration has been related to lower levels of lipoprotein (a) (Lp(a)) in both cross-sectional[212] and prospective studies.[230,231] Lp(a) includes a protein, apolipoprotein (a), which closely resembles plasminogen[232] and can cause competitive inhibition of plasminogen by binding to plasminogen binding sites on the surface of endothelial cells, resulting in decreased fibrinolysis.[233,234] The mechanism for PAI-1 reductions remain unclear.[235,236] Thus, by reducing PAI-1 and Lp(a) and increasing plasminogen, estrogen replacement would be expected to enhance fibrinolysis. Combination CEE and MPA also enhance plasminogen activity,[215,218,226,227] a benefit not seen with estradiol alone.[227]

Estrogen and progesterone also appear to have important effects on platelet function. In vivo estrogen reduces vasopressin-induced calcium uptake in human platelets,[237] platelet adherence to endothelial cell matrix,[238] and epinephrine-induced platelet aggregation.[239] Platelets from women receiving estrogen replacement therapy and platelets from nonusers that were subsequently incubated with estrogen have reduced adrenaline-induced aggregation and ATP release.[239] In rats, ovariectomy increased, and estradiol decreased, platelet aggregation in response to ADP.[240] The addition of progestin to low-dose estrogen does not alter the effects of estrogen on platelet aggregation.[216,239]

There is now clear evidence of increased risk for intravascular clotting including deep venous thrombosis or pulmonary embolus reported in users of HT.[241–244] The precise mechanism that may confer cardiovascular risk in women on HT has not been characterized but research continues to advance our understanding of this critical cornerstone in the cardiovascular health of menopausal women.

In general, the effects of high doses and/or high-potency estrogens, as are found in oral contraceptives, are significantly different from the effects of physiologic or replacement doses of estrogen. Oral contraceptives are known to increase the procoagulant factors V, VII, VIII, IX, X, and fibrinogen[245,246] and decrease the anticoagulant and fibrinolytic components antithrombin III and tPA.[247] Platelet aggregation is also increased by oral contraceptive use.[247] Users of oral contraceptives are at increased risk for vascular events including MI and stroke (especially in smokers and in women over the age of 35 years).[248,249] For deep vein thrombosis, there appears to be a dose-dependent relationship between estrogen and risk.[250] In women on oral contraceptives, the presence of the Leiden factor V mutation increases risk of deep vein thrombosis by 30-fold.[251] This mutation, which occurs in 2% of the general population,[252] leaves factor V resistant to proteolysis by activated protein C and, therefore, increases risk of thrombosis.[221] Thus, by increasing factor V and decreasing its proteolysis, the combination of high-dose estrogen and the Leiden mutation appears to impart significant increased risk for venous thrombosis. Emerging data suggest that genetic variants of key mediators of hemostatic function, i.e. platelets and coagulation factors, contribute to risk for atherothrombosis. Ongoing research is attempting to identify genetic susceptibility factors as potential mediators of this increased risk. The role of these susceptibility factors in CVD risk in HT users may help to identify subgroups of women with genetic predisposition to risk of adverse events and allow the targeting of safer and more effective therapies.

In summary, replacement doses of estrogen appear to inhibit coagulation and platelet aggregation while enhancing fibrinolysis. The small increases in some of the procoagulant factors appear to be offset by increases in their inactivating counterparts and reductions in other elements of the coagulation cascade. In the case of high-dose estrogen, the increases in procoagulant factors appear to dominate, resulting in increased risk of thrombosis. This risk is dramatically enhanced when the normal proteolytic counter-regulatory enzymes are thwarted as in the case of Leiden factor V mutation. These effects on hemostasis have broad implications for cardiovascular physiology. In addition to the obvious impact on propensity for clot formation and the related clinical sequelae, inhibiting platelet-endothelial interactions will also reduce platelet-related signals for vascular smooth muscle contraction and proliferation.

Estrogen as a vasodilator

Clearly, the female sex hormones play an important role in cardiovascular physiology. Their effects, however, are generally mediated through modulation of the other major cardiovascular regulatory systems, rather than through direct effects of the hormones themselves. Nevertheless, by influencing angiotensin peptide, nitric oxide, and prostaglandin metabolism and platelet function and by acting as an antioxidant, estrogen has a profound effect on vasomotor tone and function. In concert, the effects of estrogen in these areas result in a significant shift in the balance of vasodilators and vasoconstrictors in favor of vasodilation. This vasodilator effect of estrogen is not readily clinically apparent because of the concomitant increase in plasma volume resulting from estrogen-associated sodium and water retention. These estrogen-associated vascular changes can be understood teleologically by the need for the female organism to meet the metabolic demands during pregnancy and compensate for the potential blood loss at the time of delivery.

However, this shift in the balance of vasodilator and vasoconstrictor stimuli may also account for some of the protection against chronic vascular disease that is apparent prior to menopause and can possibly be extended through estrogen replacement after menopause. This protection may occur as a result of the general paradigm that acute vasoconstrictors are chronic promoters of vascular smooth muscle cell proliferation; and conversely, acute vasodilators are chronic inhibitors of proliferation.[253] Since vascular smooth muscle cell proliferation is a central component of both hypertension and atherosclerotic vascular disease, estrogen's actions to promote vasodilation could also provide some chronic protection against the development of vascular disease. The array of factors that contribute to increased incidence of cardiovascular disease in men and menopausal women continue to be investigated. Reports from The Heart Estrogen/progestin Replacement Study and WHI do not report a cardioprotective role of HT in hypertensive menopausal women. Emerging data suggest that gender differences in the effects of estrogen on vascular contraction may be a novel research focus. Other chapters will address the effects of estrogen on lipid and carbohydrate metabolism which also account for a large portion of the apparent ability of estrogen to protect against atherosclerosis.

References

1. Herrington DM. Role of estrogen receptor-α in pharmacogenetics of estrogen action. *Curr Opin Lipidol* 2003; **14**:145–50.
2. Herrington DM, Howard TD, Hawkins GA, et al. Estrogen receptor polymorphisms and effects of estrogen replacement on high-density lipoprotein cholesterol in women with coronary disease. *N Engl J Med* 2002; **346**:967–74.
3. Norris JD, Paige LA, Christensen DJ, et al. Peptide antagonists of the human estrogen receptor. *Science* 1999; **285**:744–6.
4. Stumpf WE, Sar M, Aumuller G. The heart: a target organ for estradiol. *Science* 1977; **196**:319–21.
5. Nakao J, Chang WC, Murota SI, Orimo H. Estradiol-binding sites in rat aortic smooth muscle cells in culture. *Atherosclerosis* 1981; **38**:75–80.
6. Lin AL, Shain SA. Estrogen-mediated cytoplasmic and nuclear distribution of rat cardiovascular estrogen receptors. *Arteriosclerosis* 1985; **5**:668–77.
7. Colburn P, Buonassisi V. Estrogen-binding sites in endothelial cell cultures. *Science* 1978; **201**:817–19.
8. Horwitz KB, Horwitz LD. Canine vascular tissues are targets for androgens, estrogens, progestins, and glucocorticoids. *J Clin Invest* 1982; **69**:750–8.
9. Harder DR, Coulson PB. Estrogen receptors and effects of estrogen on membrane electrical properties of coronary vascular smooth muscle. *J Cell Physiol* 1979; **100**:375–82.
10. Lin AL, McGill HC Jr, Shain SA. Hormone receptors of the baboon cardiovascular system. Biochemical characterization of myocardial cytoplasmic androgen receptors. *Circ Res* 1981; **49**:1010–16.
11. Lin AL, McGill HC Jr, Shain SA. Hormone receptors of the baboon cardiovascular system. Biochemical characterization of aortic and myocardial cytoplasmic progesterone receptors. *Circ Res* 1982; **50**:610–16.
12. Lin AL, Gonzalez R Jr, Carey KD, Shain SA. Estradiol-17β affects estrogen receptor distribution and elevates progesterone receptor content in baboon aorta. *Arteriosclerosis* 1986; **6**:495–504.
13. Campisi D, Cutolo M, Carruba G, et al. Evidence for soluble and nuclear site I binding of estrogens in human aorta. *Atherosclerosis* 1993; **103**:267–77.
14. Losordo DW, Kearney M, Kim EA, Jekanowski J, Isner JM. Variable expression of the estrogen receptor in normal and atherosclerotic coronary arteries of premenopausal women. *Circulation* 1994; **89**:1501–10.
15. Ingegno MD, Money SR, Thelmo W, et al. Progesterone receptors in the human heart and great vessels. *Lab Invest* 1988; **59**:353–6.
16. Mendelsohn ME, Karas RH. The protective effects of estrogen on the cardiovascular system. *N Engl J Med* 1999; **340**:1801–11.
17. Russell KS, Haynes MP, Sinha D, Clerisme E, Bender JR. Human vascular endothelial cells contain membrane binding sites for estradiol, which mediate rapid intracellular signaling. *Proc Natl Acad Sci U S A* 2000; **97**:5930–5.
18. Norman A, Litwack G. *Hormones.* Orlando: Academic Press, 1987.

19. Wilson PW, Anderson KM, Harris T, Kannel WB, Castelli WP. Determinants of change in total cholesterol and HDL-C with age: the Framingham Study. *J Gerontol* 1994; **49**:M252–7.

20. Schachter BS, Lehrer S. Risk of miscarriage and a common variant of the estrogen receptor gene. *Am J Epidemiol* 1994; **140**:1144–5.

21. Parl FF, Cavener DR, Dupont WD. Genomic DNA analysis of the estrogen receptor gene in breast cancer. *Breast Cancer Treat Res* 1989; **14**:57–64.

22. Hill SM, Fuqua SA, Chamness GC, Greene GL, McGuire WL. Estrogen receptor expression in human breast cancer associated with an estrogen receptor gene restriction fragment length polymorphism. *Cancer Res* 1989; **49**:145–8.

23. Yaich L, Dupont WD, Cavener DR, Parl FF. Analysis of the PvuII restriction fragment-length polymorphism and exon structure of the estrogen receptor gene in breast cancer and peripheral blood. *Cancer Res* 1992; **52**:77–83.

24. Lehrer S, Sanchez M, Song HK, et al. Oestrogen receptor B-region polymorphism and spontaneous abortion in women with breast cancer. *Lancet* 1990; **335**:622–4.

25. Berkowitz GS, Stone JL, Lehrer SP, Marcus M, Lapinski RH, Schachter BS. An estrogen receptor genetic polymorphism and the risk of primary and secondary recurrent spontaneous abortion. *Am J Obstet Gynecol* 1994; **171**:1579–84.

26. Kobayashi S, Inoue S, Hosoi T, Ouchi Y, Shiraki M, Orimo H. Association of bone mineral density with polymorphism of the estrogen receptor gene. *J Bone Miner Res* 1996; **11**:306–11.

27. Deng HW, Li J, Li JL, et al. Association of estrogen receptor-α genotypes with body mass index in normal healthy postmenopausal Caucasian women. *J Clin Endocrinol Metab* 2000; **85**:2748–51.

28. Sano M, Inoue S, Hosoi T, et al. Association of estrogen receptor dinucleotide repeat polymorphism with osteoporosis. *Biochem Biophys Res Commun* 1995; **217**:378–83.

29. Han K, Choi J, Moon I, et al. Non-association of estrogen receptor genotypes with bone mineral density and bone turnover in Korean pre-, peri-, and postmenopausal women. *Osteoporosis Int* 1999; **9**:290–5.

30. Yaffe K, Lui L-Y, Grady D, Stone K, Morin P. Estrogen receptor 1 polymorphisms and risk of cognitive impairment in older women. *Biol Psychiatry* 2002; **51**:677–82.

31. Lehtimaki T, Laaksonen R, Mattila KM, et al. Oestrogen receptor gene variation is a determinant of coronary reactivity in healthy young men. *Eur J Clin Invest* 2002; **32**:400–4.

32. Lehtimaki T, Kunnas TA, Mattila KM, et al. Coronary artery wall atherosclerosis in relation to the estrogen receptor 1 gene polymorphism: an autopsy study. *J Mol Med* 2002; **80**:176–80.

33. Kunnas TA, Laippala P, Penttila A, Lehtimaki T, Karhunen PJ. Association of polymorphism of human α oestrogen receptor gene with coronary artery disease in men: a necropsy study. *BMJ* 2000; **321**:273–4.

34. Lu H, Higashikata T, Inazu A, et al. Association of estrogen receptor-α gene polymorphisms with coronary artery disease in patients with familial hypercholesterolemia. *Arterioscler Thromb Vasc Biol* 2002; **22**:821–7.

35. Shearman AM, Cupples LA, Demissie S, et al. Association between estrogen receptor α gene variation and cardiovascular disease. *JAMA* 2003; **290**:2263–70.

36. Manson JE, Hsia J, Johnson KC, et al. Estrogen plus progestin and the risk of coronary heart disease. *N Engl J Med* 2003; **349**:523–34.

37. Hodis HN, Mack WJ, Azen SP, et al. Hormone therapy and the progression of coronary-artery atherosclerosis in postmenopausal women. *N Engl J Med* 2003; **349**:535–45.

38. Grady D. Postmenopausal hormones – therapy for symptoms only. *N Engl J Med* 2003; **348**:1835–7.

39. Orshal JM, Khalil RA. Gender, sex hormones, and vascular tone. *Am J Physiol Regul Integr Comp Physiol* 2004; **286**:R233–49.

40. Batra S, Bjellin L, Iosif S, Martensson L, Sjogren C. Effect of oestrogen and progesterone on the blood flow in the lower urinary tract of the rabbit. *Acta Physiol Scand* 1985; **123**:191–4.

41. Resnik R, Brink GW, Plumer MH. The effect of progesterone on estrogen-induced uterine blood flow. *Am J Obstet Gynecol* 1977; **128**:251–4.

42. Anderson SG, Hackshaw BT, Still JG, Greiss FC Jr. Uterine blood flow and its distribution after chronic estrogen and progesterone administration. *Am J Obstet Gynecol* 1977; **127**:138–42.

43. Penney LL, Frederick RJ, Parker GW. 17β-Estimulation of uterine blood flow in oophorectomized rabbits with complete inhibition of uterine ribonucleic acid synthesis. *Endocrinology* 1981; **109**:1672–6.

44. Still JG, Greiss FC. Effects of cis- and trans-clomiphene on the uterine blood flow of oophorectomized ewes. *Gynecol Invest* 1976; **7**:187–200.

45. Magness RR, Rosenfeld CR. Local and systemic

estradiol-17β: effects on uterine and systemic vasodilation. *Am J Physiol* 1989; **256**:E536–42.

46. Semmens JP, Wagner G. Estrogen deprivation and vaginal function in postmenopausal women. *JAMA* 1982; **248**:445–8.

47. Sarrel PM. Ovarian hormones and the circulation. *Maturitas* 1990; **12**:287–98.

48. Versi E, Tapp A, Cardozo L, Montogmery J. Abstracts of the Fifth International Congress on the Menopause 164. 1987.

49. de Ziegler D, Bessis R, Frydman R. Vascular resistance of uterine arteries: physiological effects of estradiol and progesterone. *Fertil Steril* 1991; **55**:775–9.

50. Sarrel PM. Sexuality and menopause. *Obstet Gynecol* 1990; **75** (4 Suppl):26S–30S.

51. Haigh AL, Lloyd S, Pickford M. A relationship between adrenaline and the mode of action of oxytocin and oestrogen on vascular smooth muscle. *J Physiol* 1965; **178**:563–76.

52. Rosenfeld CR, Morriss FH Jr, Battaglia FC, Makowski EL, Meschia G. Effect of estradiol-17β on blood flow to reproductive and nonreproductive tissues in pregnant ewes. *Am J Obstet Gynecol* 1976; **124**:618–29.

53. Volterrani M, Rosano G, Coats A, Beale C, Collins P. Estrogen acutely increases peripheral blood flow in postmenopausal women. *Am J Med* 1995; **99**:119–22.

54. Sarrel PM. Progestogens and blood flow. *Int Proc J* 1989; **1**:266–71.

55. Collins P, Shay J, Jiang C, Moss J. Nitric oxide accounts for dose-dependent estrogen-mediated coronary relaxation after acute estrogen withdrawal. *Circulation* 1994; **90**:1964–8.

56. Jiang C, Sarrel PM, Poole-Wilson PA, Collins P. Acute effect of 17β-estradiol on rabbit coronary artery contractile responses to endothelin-1. *Am J Physiol* 1992; **263**:H271–5.

57. Jiang CW, Sarrel PM, Lindsay DC, Poole-Wilson PA, Collins P. Endothelium-independent relaxation of rabbit coronary artery by 17β-oestradiol in vitro. *Br J Pharmacol* 1991; **104**:1033–7.

58. Rosano GM, Sarrel PM, Poole-Wilson PA, Collins P. Beneficial effect of oestrogen on exercise-induced myocardial ischaemia in women with coronary artery disease. *Lancet* 1993; **342**:133–6.

59. Collins P, Rosano GM, Jiang C, Lindsay D, Sarrel PM, Poole-Wilson PA. Cardiovascular protection by oestrogen – a calcium antagonist effect? *Lancet* 1993; **341**:1264–5.

60. Gilligan DM, Badar DM,·Panza JA, Quyyumi AA, Cannon RO III. Acute vascular effects of estrogen in postmenopausal women. *Circulation* 1994; **90**:786–91.

61. Williams JK, Adams MR, Klopfenstein HS. Estrogen modulates responses of atherosclerotic coronary arteries. *Circulation* 1990; **81**:1680–7.

62. Williams JK, Adams MR, Herrington DM, Clarkson TB. Short-term administration of estrogen and vascular responses of atherosclerotic coronary arteries. *J Am Coll Cardiol* 1992; **20**:452–7.

63. Herrington DM, Braden GA, Williams JK, Morgan TM. Endothelial-dependent coronary vasomotor responsiveness in postmenopausal women with and without estrogen replacement therapy. *Am J Cardiol* 1994; **73**:951–2.

64. Reis SE. Oestrogens attenuate abnormal coronary vasoreactivity in postmenopausal women. *Ann Med* 1994; **26**:387–8.

65. Jiang CW, Sarrel PM, Lindsay DC, Poole-Wilson PA, Collins P. Progesterone induces endothelium-independent relaxation of rabbit coronary artery in vitro. *Eur J Pharmacol* 1992; **211**:163–7.

66. Magness RR, Parker CR Jr, Rosenfeld CR. Systemic and uterine responses to chronic infusion of estradiol-17β. *Am J Physiol* 1993; **265**:E690–8.

67. Naden RP, Rosenfeld CR. Systemic and uterine responsiveness to angiotensin II and norepinephrine in estrogen-treated nonpregnant sheep. *Am J Obstet Gynecol* 1985; **153**:417–25.

68. Vered Z, Poler SM, Gibson P, Wlody D, Perez JE. Noninvasive detection of the morphologic and hemodynamic changes during normal pregnancy. *Clin Cardiol* 1991; **14**:327–34.

69. Mashini IS, Albazzaz SJ, Fadel HE, et al. Serial noninvasive evaluation of cardiovascular hemodynamics during pregnancy. *Am J Obstet Gynecol* 1987; **156**:1208–13.

70. Clapp JF III, Seaward BL, Sleamaker RH, Hiser J. Maternal physiologic adaptations to early human pregnancy. *Am J Obstet Gynecol* 1988; **159**:1456–60.

71. Laragh JH, Sealey JE, Ledingham JG, Newton MA. Oral contraceptives. Renin, aldosterone, and high blood pressure. *JAMA* 1967; **201**:98–102.

72. Ganten U, Schroder G, Witt M, Zimmermann F, Ganten D, Stock G. Sexual dimorphism of blood pressure in spontaneously hypertensive rats: effects of anti-androgen treatment. *J Hypertens* 1989; **7**:721–6.

73. Bachmann J, Feldmer M, Ganten U, Stock G, Ganten D. Sexual dimorphism of blood pressure: possible role of the renin–angiotensin system. *J Steroid Biochem Mol Biol* 1991; **40**:511–15.

74. Data from the Hypertension Detection and Follow-up Program. Race, education and prevalence of hypertension. *Am J Epidemiol* 1977; **106**:351–61.

75. Harlan WR, Hull AL, Schmouder RL, Landis JR,

Thompson FE, Larkin FA. Blood pressure and nutrition in adults. The National Health and Nutrition Examination Survey. *Am J Epidemiol* 1984; **120**:17–28.

76. Landahl S, Bengtsson C, Sigurdsson JA, Svanborg A, Svardsudd K. Age-related changes in blood pressure. *Hypertension* 1986; **8**:1044–9.

77. Dunne FP, Barry DG, Ferriss JB, Grealy G, Murphy D. Changes in blood pressure during the normal menstrual cycle. *Clin Sci (Lond)* 1991; **81**:515–18.

78. Greenberg G, Imeson JD, Thompson SG, Meade TW. Blood pressure and the menstrual cycle. *Br J Obstet Gynaecol* 1985; **92**:1010–14.

79. Kelleher C, Joyce C, Kelly G, Ferriss JB. Blood pressure alters during the normal menstrual cycle. *Br J Obstet Gynaecol* 1986; **93**:523–6.

80. Capeless EL, Clapp JF. Cardiovascular changes in early phase of pregnancy. *Am J Obstet Gynecol* 1989; **161** (6 Pt 1):1449–53.

81. Schwartz J, Freeman R, Frishman W. Clinical pharmacology of estrogens: cardiovascular actions and cardioprotective benefits of replacement therapy in postmenopausal women. *J Clin Pharmacol* 1995; **35**:314–29.

82. Eferakeya AE, Imasuen JE. Relationship of menopause to serum cholesterol and arterial blood pressure in some Nigerian women. *Public Health* 1986; **100**:28–32.

83. Weiss NS. Cigarette smoking and arteriosclerosis obliterans: an epidemiologic approach. *Am J Epidemiol* 1972; **95**:17–25.

84. Hjortland MC, McNamara PM, Kannel WB. Some atherogenic concomitants of menopause: The Framingham Study. *Am J Epidemiol* 1976; **103**:304–11.

85. Matthews KA, Meilahn E, Kuller LH, Kelsey SF, Caggiula AW, Wing RR. Menopause and risk factors for coronary heart disease. *N Engl J Med* 1989; **321**:641–6.

86. Fisch IR, Freedman SH, Myatt AV. Oral contraceptives, pregnancy, and blood pressure. *JAMA* 1972; **222**:1507–10.

87. Kunin CM, McCormack RC, Abernathy JR. Oral contraceptives and blood pressure. *Arch Intern Med* 1969; **123**:362–5.

88. Stern MP, Brown BW, Haskell WL, Farquhar JW, Wehrle CL, Wood PS. Cardiovascular risk and use of estrogens or estrogen-progestagen combinations. *JAMA* 1976; **235**:811–15.

89. Beral V. Cardiovascular-disease mortality trends and oral-contraceptive use in young women. *Lancet* 1976; **2**:1047–52.

90. Briggs E, Mack A, Taylor L, et al. Blood-pressure in women after one year of oral contraception. *Lancet* 1971; **1**:467–70.

91. Shionoiri H, Eggena P, Barrett JD, et al. An increase in high-molecular weight renin substrate associated with estrogenic hypertension. *Biochem Med* 1983; **29**:14–22.

92. Wren BG, Routledge DA. Blood pressure changes: oestrogens in climacteric women. *Med J Aust* 1981; **2**:528–31.

93. Wren BG, Routledge AD. The effect of type and dose of oestrogen on the blood pressure of postmenopausal women. *Maturitas* 1983; **5**:135–42.

94. McKay HD, Lindsay R, Purdie D. Vascular complications of long-term oestrogen therapy. *Front Horm Res* 1977; **5**:174–91.

95. Lind T, Cameron EC, Hunter WM, et al. A prospective, controlled trial of six forms of hormone replacement therapy given to postmenopausal women. *Br J Obstet Gynaecol* 1979; **86** (Suppl 3):1–29.

96. Luotola H. Blood pressure and hemodynamics in postmenopausal women during estradiol-17β substitution. *Ann Clin Res* 1983; **15** (Suppl 38):1–121.

97. von Eiff AW, Lutz HM, Gries J, Kretzschmar R. The protective mechanism of estrogen on high blood pressure. *Basic Res Cardiol* 1985; **80**:191–201.

98. Utian WH. Effect of postmenopausal estrogen therapy on diastolic blood pressure and bodyweight. *Maturitas* 1978; **1**:3–8.

99. Erkkola R, Lammintausta R, Punnonen R, Rauramo L. The effect of estriol succinate therapy on plasma renin activity and urinary aldosterone in postmenopausal women. *Maturitas* 1978; **1**:9–14.

100. Pfeffer RI, Kurosaki TT, Charlton SK. Estrogen use and blood pressure in later life. *Am J Epidemiol* 1979; **110**:469–78.

101. Notelovitz M. Effect of natural oestrogens on blood pressure and weight in postmenopausal women. *S Afr Med J* 1975; **49**:2251–4.

102. Lip GY, Beevers M, Churchill D, Beevers DG. Hormone replacement therapy and blood pressure in hypertensive women. *J Hum Hypertens* 1994; **8**:491–4.

103. The Writing Group for the PEPI Trial. Effects of estrogen or estrogen/progestin regimens on heart disease risk factors in postmenopausal women. The Postmenopausal Estrogen/Progestin Interventions (PEPI) Trial. *JAMA* 1995; **273**:199–208.

104. Rylance PB, Brincat M, Lafferty K, et al. Natural progesterone and antihypertensive action. *BMJ (Clin Res Ed)* 1985; **290**:13–14.

105. Scuteri A, Bos AJ, Brant LJ, Talbot L, Lakatta EG, Fleg JL. Hormone replacement therapy and longitudinal

changes in blood pressure in postmenopausal women. *Ann Intern Med* 2001; **135**:229–38.

106. Chang E, Perlman AJ. Multiple hormones regulate angiotensinogen messenger ribonucleic acid levels in a rat hepatoma cell line. *Endocrinology* 1987; **121**: 513–19.

107. Kunapuli SP, Benedict CR, Kumar A. Tissue specific hormonal regulation of the rat angiotensinogen gene expression. *Arch Biochem Biophys* 1987; **254**:642–6.

108. Nasjletti A, Matsunaga M, Masson GM. Effects of estrogens on plasma angiotensinogen and renin activity in nephrectomized rats. *Endocrinology* 1969; **85**:967–70.

109. Tartagni F, Ambrosioni E, Montebugnoli L, Magnani B. [New method for determination of intralymphocytic sodium]. *G Clin Med* 1979; **60**:500–6.

110. Crane MG, Harris JJ. Estrogens and hypertension: effect of discontinuing estrogens on blood pressure, exchangeable sodium, and the renin–aldosterone system. *Am J Med Sci* 1978; **276**:33–55.

111. Tewksbury DA. Angiotensin-biochemistry and molecular biology. In: Laragh JH, Brenner BM (eds). *Hypertension: Pathophysiology, Diagnosis and Management*. Raven Press, 1990: 1197–216.

112. Chen YF, Naftilan AJ, Oparil S. Androgen-dependent angiotensinogen and renin messenger RNA expression in hypertensive rats. *Hypertension* 1992; **19**:456–63.

113. Feldmer M, Kaling M, Takahashi S, Mullins JJ, Ganten D. Glucocorticoid- and estrogen-responsive elements in the 5'-flanking region of the rat angiotensinogen gene. *J Hypertens* 1991; **9**:1005–12.

114. Clauser E, Gaillard I, Wei L, Corvol P. Regulation of angiotensinogen gene. *Am J Hypertens* 1989; **2** (5 Pt 1):403–10.

115. Brosnihan KB, Weddle D, Anthony MS, Heise CM, Li P, Ferrario CM. Effects of chronic hormone replacement on the renin–angiotensin system in cynomolgus monkeys. *Hypertension* 1997; **15**:715–26.

116. McDonald WJ, Cohen EL, Lucas CP, Conn JW. Renin-renin substrate kinetic constants in the plasma of normal and estrogen-treated humans. *J Clin Endocrinol Metab* 1977; **45**:1297–304.

117. Senanayake P, Martins A, Ganten D, Brosnihan KB. Angiotensin II in the kidney of transgenic hypertensive rat is resistant to the reduced expression of the renin gene. *Hypertension* 1995; **25**:1409.

118. Seely EW, Brosnihan KB, Jeunemaitre X, et al. Effects of conjugated oestrogen and droloxifene on the renin–angiotensin system, blood pressure and renal blood flow in postmenopausal women. *Clin Endocrinol (Oxf)* 2004; **60**:315–21.

119. Brosnihan KB, Li P, Ganten D, Ferrario CM. Estrogen

protects transgenic hypertensive rats by shifting the vasoconstrictor–vasodilator balance of RAS. *Am J Physiol* 1997; **273** (6 Pt 2):R1908–15.

120. Seltzer A, Pinto JE, Viglione PN, et al. Estrogens regulate angiotensin-converting enzyme and angiotensin receptors in female rat anterior pituitary. *Neuroendocrinology* 1992; **55**:460–7.

121. Nogawa N, Sumino H, Ichikawa S, et al. Effect of long-term hormone replacement therapy on angiotensin-converting enzyme activity and bradykinin in postmenopausal women with essential hypertension and normotensive postmenopausal women. *Menopause* 2001; **8**:210–15.

122. Umeda M, Ichikawa S, Kanda T, Sumino H, Kobayashi I. Hormone replacement therapy increases plasma level of angiotensin II in postmenopausal hypertensive women. *Am J Hypertens* 2001; **14**:206–11.

123. Sumino H, Ichikawa S, Ohyama Y, et al. Effects of hormone replacement therapy on serum angiotensin-converting enzyme activity and plasma bradykinin in postmenopausal women according to angiotensin-converting enzyme-genotype. *Hypertens Res* 2003; **26**:53–8.

124. Chen FM, Printz MP. Chronic estrogen treatment reduces angiotensin II receptors in the anterior pituitary. *Endocrinology* 1983; **113**:1503–10.

125. Schiffrin EL, Franks DJ. Effect of steroids on angiotensin II receptors in cultured vascular smooth muscle. *Fed Proc* 1984; **43**:1037.

126. Fregly MJ, Rowland NE, Sumners C, Gordon DB. Reduced dipsogenic responsiveness to intracerebroventricularly administered angiotensin II in estrogen-treated rats. *Brain Res* 1985; **338**:115–21.

127. Abdul-Karim R, Assalin S. Pressor response to angiotonin in pregnant and nonpregnant women. *Am J Obstet Gynecol* 1961; **82**:246–51.

128. Gant NF, Chand S, Whalley PJ, MacDonald PC. The nature of pressor responsiveness to angiotensin II in human pregnancy. *Obstet Gynecol* 1974; **43**:854.

129. Nasjletti A, Matsunaga M, Masson GM. Effects of estrogens on pressor responses to angiotensin and renin. *Proc Soc Exp Biol Med* 1970; **133**:407–9.

130. Paller MS. Mechanism of decreased pressor responsiveness to ANG II, NE, and vasopressin in pregnant rats. *Am J Physiol* 1984; **247**:H100–8.

131. Osei SY, Ahima RS, Minkes RK, Weaver JP, Khosla MC, Kadowitz PJ. Differential responses to angiotensin-(1–7) in the feline mesenteric and hindquarters vascular beds. *Eur J Pharmacol* 1993; **234**:35–42.

132. Benter IF, Diz DI, Ferrario CM. Pressor and reflex sensitivity is altered in spontaneously hypertensive

rats treated with angiotensin-(1–7). *Hypertension* 1995; **26** (6 Pt 2):1138–44.

133. Jaiswal N, Tallant EA, Diz DI, Khosla MC, Ferrario CM. Subtype 2 angiotensin receptors mediate prostaglandin synthesis in human astrocytes. *Hypertension* 1991; **17** (6 Pt 2):1115–20.

134. Tallant EA, Diz DI, Khosla MC, Ferrario CM. Identification and regulation of angiotensin II receptor subtypes on NG108-15 cells. *Hypertension* 1991; **17** (6 Pt 2):1135–43.

135. Brosnihan KB, Li P, Ferrario CM. Angiotensin-(1–7) dilates canine coronary arteries through kinins and nitric oxide. *Hypertension* 1996; **27** (3 Pt 2):523–8.

136. Porsti I, Bara AT, Busse R, Hecker M. Release of nitric oxide by angiotensin-(1–7) from porcine coronary endothelium: implications for a novel angiotensin receptor. *Br J Pharmacol* 1994; **111**:652–4.

137. Lund CJ, Donovan JC. Blood volume during pregnancy. Significance of plasma and red cell volumes. *Am J Obstet Gynecol* 1967; **98**:394–403.

138. Ueda S, Fortune V, Bull BS, Valenzuela GJ, Longo LD. Estrogen effects on plasma volume, arterial blood pressure, interstitial space, plasma proteins, and blood viscosity in sheep. *Am J Obstet Gynecol* 1986; **155**:195–201.

139. Hart MV, Hosenpud JD, Hohimer AR, Morton MJ. Hemodynamics during pregnancy and sex steroid administration in guinea pigs. *Am J Physiol* 1985; **249** (2 Pt 2):R179–85.

140. Christy NP, Shaver JC. Estrogens and the kidney. *Kidney Int* 1974; **6**:366–76.

141. Johnson JA, Davis JO, Baumber JS, Schneider EG. Effects of estrogens and progesterone on electrolyte balances in normal dogs. *Am J Physiol* 1970; **219**:1691–7.

142. Dignam WS, Voskian J, Assali NS. Effects of estrogens on renal hemodynamics and excretion of electrolytes in human subjects. *J Clin Endocrinol Metab* 1956; **16**:1032–42.

143. Stachenfeld NS, Taylor HS. Effects of estrogen and progesterone administration on extracellular fluid. *J Appl Physiol* 2004; **96**:1011–18.

144. Clapp JF III. Maternal heart rate in pregnancy. *Am J Obstet Gynecol* 1985; **152** (6 Pt 1):659–60.

145. Katz R, Karliner JS, Resnik R. Effects of a natural volume overload state (pregnancy) on left ventricular performance in normal human subjects. *Circulation* 1978; **58**:434–41.

146. Ueland K, Metcalfe J. Circulatory changes in pregnancy. *Clin Obstet Gynecol* 1975; **18**:41–50.

147. Veille JC, Morton MJ, Burry K, Nemeth M, Speroff L. Estradiol and hemodynamics during ovulation induction. *J Clin Endocrinol Metab* 1986; **63**:721–4.

148. Metcalfe J, Parer JT. Cardiovascular changes during pregnancy in ewes. *Am J Physiol* 1966; **210**:821–5.

149. Hoversland AS, Parer JT, Metcalfe J. Hemodynamic adjustments in the pygmy goat during pregnancy and early postpartum. *Biol Reprod* 1974; **10**:578–88.

150. Riedel M, Oeltermann A, Mugge A, Creutzig A, Rafflenbeul W, Lichtlen P. Vascular responses to 17β-oestradiol in postmenopausal women. *Eur J Clin Invest* 1995; **25**:44–7.

151. Williams JK, Kim YD, Adams MR, Chen MF, Myers AK, Ramwell PW. Effects of estrogen on cardiovascular responses of premenopausal monkeys. *J Pharmacol Exp Ther* 1994; **271**:671–6.

152. Giraud GD, Morton MJ, Davis LE, Paul MS, Thornburg KL. Estrogen-induced left ventricular chamber enlargement in ewes. *Am J Physiol* 1993; **264** (4 Pt 1):E490–6.

153. Pines A, Fisman EZ, Shapira I, et al. Exercise echocardiography in postmenopausal hormone users with mild systemic hypertension. *Am J Cardiol* 1996; **78**:1385–9.

154. Lee WS, Harder JA, Yoshizumi M, Lee ME, Haber E. Progesterone inhibits arterial smooth muscle cell proliferation. *Nat Med* 1997; **3**:1005–8.

155. Kessel H, Kamp O, Kenemans P, et al. Effects of 15 months of 17β-estradiol and dydrogesterone on systolic cardiac function according to quantitative and Doppler echocardiography in healthy postmenopausal women. *Am J Obstet Gynecol* 2001; **184**:910–16.

156. Vogelvang TE, Mijatovic V, Kamp O, et al. Neither long-term treatment with raloxifene nor hormone replacement therapy modulate cardiac function in healthy postmenopausal women: two randomized, placebo-controlled, 2-year studies. *Am J Obstet Gynecol* 2002; **186**:729–36.

157. Snabes MC, Payne JP, Kopelen HA, Dunn JK, Young RL, Zoghbi WA. Physiologic estradiol replacement therapy and cardiac structure and function in normal postmenopausal women: a randomized, double-blind, placebo-controlled, crossover trial. *Obstet Gynecol* 1997; **89**:332–9.

158. Light KC, Hinderliter AL, West SG, et al. Hormone replacement improves hemodynamic profile and left ventricular geometry in hypertensive and normotensive postmenopausal women. *J Hypertens* 2001; **19**:269–78.

159. Vogelvang TE, van der Mooren MJ, Kamp O, Mijatovic V, Visser CA, Kenemans P. Effects of oral and transdermal low-dose estrogen therapy on echocardiographic parameters of cardiac function. *Fertil Steril* 2003; **80**:546–53.

160. Cole P, Cook F, Plappert T, Saltzman D, St John SM. Longitudinal changes in left ventricular architecture and function in peripartum cardiomyopathy. *Am J Cardiol* 1987; **60**:871–6.

161. Eckstein N, Pines A, Fisman EZ, et al. The effect of the hypoestrogenic state, induced by gonadotropin-releasing hormone agonist, on Doppler-derived parameters of aortic flow. *J Clin Endocrinol Metab* 1993; **77**:910–12.

162. Pines A, Fisman EZ, Ayalon D, Drory Y, Averbuch M, Levo Y. Long-term effects of hormone replacement therapy on Doppler-derived parameters of aortic flow in postmenopausal women. *Chest* 1992; **102**: 1496–8.

163. Schaible TF, Malhotra A, Ciambrone G, Scheuer J. The effects of gonadectomy on left ventricular function and cardiac contractile proteins in male and female rats. *Circ Res* 1984; **54**:38–49.

164. Scheuer J, Malhotra A, Schaible TF, Capasso J. Effects of gonadectomy and hormonal replacement on rat hearts. *Circ Res* 1987; **61**:12–19.

165. Schaible TF, Scheuer J. Comparison of heart function in male and female rats. *Basic Res Cardiol* 1984; **79**:402–12.

166. Shanahan MF, Edwards BM. Stimulation of glucose transport in rat cardiac myocytes by guanosine 3′,5′-monophosphate. *Endocrinology* 1989; **125**:1074–81.

167. Ziegelhoffer A, Dzurba A, Vrbjar N, Styk J, Slezak J. Mechanism of action of estradiol on sodium pump in sarcolemma from the myocardium. *Bratisl Lek Listy* 1990; **91**:902–10.

168. Vanhoutte PM. Endothelium and control of vascular function. State of the Art lecture. *Hypertension* 1989; **13** (6 Pt 2):658–67.

169. Luscher TF, Richard V, Tschudi M, Yang Z. Serotonin and the endothelium. *Clin Physiol Biochem* 1990; **8** (Suppl 3):108–19.

170. Moncada S, Radomski MW, Palmer RM. Endothelium-derived relaxing factor. Identification as nitric oxide and role in the control of vascular tone and platelet function. *Biochem Pharmacol* 1988; **37**:2495–501.

171. Shimokawa H, Flavahan NA, Shepherd JT, Vanhoutte PM. Endothelium-dependent inhibition of ergonovine-induced contraction is impaired in porcine coronary arteries with regenerated endothelium. *Circulation* 1989; **80**:643–50.

172. Gisclard V, Miller VM, Vanhoutte PM. Effect of 17β-estradiol on endothelium-dependent responses in the rabbit. *J Pharmacol Exp Ther* 1988; **244**:19–22.

173. Bell DR, Rensberger HJ, Koritnik DR, Koshy A. Estrogen pretreatment directly potentiates endothe-

lium-dependent vasorelaxation of porcine coronary arteries. *Am J Physiol* 1995; **268** (1 Pt 2):H377–83.

174. Williams JK, Honore EK, Washburn SA, Clarkson TB. Effects of hormone replacement therapy on reactivity of atherosclerotic coronary arteries in cynomolgus monkeys. *J Am Coll Cardiol* 1994; **24**:1757–61.

175. Gilligan DM, Quyyumi AA, Cannon RO III. Effects of physiological levels of estrogen on coronary vasomotor function in postmenopausal women. *Circulation* 1994; **89**:2545–51.

176. Gilligan DM, Badar DM, Panza JA, Quyyumi AA, Cannon RO III. Effects of estrogen replacement therapy on peripheral vasomotor function in postmenopausal women. *Am J Cardiol* 1995; **75**:264–8.

177. Lieberman EH, Gerhard MD, Uehata A, et al. Estrogen improves endothelium-dependent, flow-mediated vasodilation in postmenopausal women. *Ann Intern Med* 1994; **121**:936–41.

178. Miller VM, Vanhoutte PM. Progesterone and modulation of endothelium-dependent responses in canine coronary arteries. *Am J Physiol* 1991; **261** (4 Pt 2):R1022–7.

179. Dohanich GP, Fader AJ, Javorsky DJ. Estrogen and estrogen–progesterone treatments counteract the effect of scopolamine on reinforced T-maze alternation in female rats. *Behav Neurosci* 1994; **108**:988–92.

180. Hishikawa K, Nakaki T, Marumo T, Suzuki H, Kato R, Saruta T. Up-regulation of nitric oxide synthase by estradiol in human aortic endothelial cells. *FEBS Lett* 1995; **360**:291–3.

181. Rosselli M, Imthurn B, Macas E, Keller PJ, Dubey RK. Circulating nitrite/nitrate levels increase with follicular development: indirect evidence for estradiol mediated NO release. *Biochem Biophys Res Commun* 1994; **202**:1543–52.

182. Moncada S, Korbut R, Bunting S, Vane JR. Prostacyclin is a circulating hormone. *Nature* 1978; **273**:767–8.

183. Shimokawa H, Flavahan NA, Lorenz RR, Vanhoutte PM. Prostacyclin releases endothelium-derived relaxing factor and potentiates its action in coronary arteries of the pig. *Br J Pharmacol* 1988; **95**:1197–203.

184. Makila UM, Wahlberg L, Vlinikka L, Ylikorkala O. Regulation of prostacyclin and thromboxane production by human umbilical vessels: the effect of estradiol and progesterone in a superfusion model. *Prostaglandins Leukot Med* 1982; **8**:115–24.

185. Seillan C, Ody C, Russo-Marie F, Duval D. Differential effects of sex steroids on prostaglandin secretion by male and female cultured piglet endothelial cells. *Prostaglandins* 1983; **26**:3–12.

186. Chang WC, Nakao J, Orimo H, Murota S. Stimulation of prostacyclin biosynthetic activity by estradiol in rat aortic smooth muscle cells in culture. *Biochim Biophys Acta* 1980; **619**:107–18.

187. Chang WC, Nakao J, Orimo H, Murota SI. Stimulation of prostaglandin cyclooxygenase and prostacyclin synthetase activities by estradiol in rat aortic smooth muscle cells. *Biochim Biophys Acta* 1980; **620**:472–82.

188. Pearson PJ, Lin PJ, Schaff HV. Global myocardial ischemia and reperfusion impair endothelium-dependent relaxations to aggregating platelets in the canine coronary artery. A possible cause of vasospasm after cardiopulmonary bypass. *J Thorac Cardiovasc Surg* 1992; **103**:1147–54.

189. Vita JA, Treasure CB, Nabel EG, et al. Coronary vasomotor response to acetylcholine relates to risk factors for coronary artery disease. *Circulation* 1990; **81**:491–7.

190. Gryglewski RJ, Palmer RM, Moncada S. Superoxide anion is involved in the breakdown of endothelium-derived vascular relaxing factor. *Nature* 1986; **320**:454–6.

191. Vanhoutte PM, Katusic ZS. Endothelium-derived contracting factor: endothelin and/or superoxide anion? *Trends Pharmacol Sci* 1988; **9**:229–30.

192. Yagi K, Komura S. Inhibitory effect of female hormones on lipid peroxidation. *Biochem Int* 1986; **13**:1051–5.

193. Sugioka K, Shimosegawa Y, Nakano M. Estrogens as natural antioxidants of membrane phospholipid peroxidation. *FEBS Lett* 1987; **210**:37–9.

194. Nakano M, Sugioka K, Naito I, Takekoshi S, Niki E. Novel and potent biological antioxidants on membrane phospholipid peroxidation: 2-hydroxy estrone and 2-hydroxy estradiol. *Biochem Biophys Res Commun* 1987; **142**:919–24.

195. Yoshino K, Komura S, Watanabe I. Effect of estrogens on serum and liver lipid peroxide levels in mice. *J Clin Biochem Nutr* 1987; **3**:233–40.

196. Mukai K, Daifuku K, Yokoyama S, Nakano M. Stopped-flow investigation of antioxidant activity of estrogens in solution. *Biochim Biophys Acta* 1990; **1035**:348–52.

197. Maziere C, Auclair M, Ronveaux MF, Salmon S, Santus R, Maziere JC. Estrogens inhibit copper and cell-mediated modification of low density lipoprotein. *Atherosclerosis* 1991; **89**:175–82.

198. Huber LA, Scheffler E, Poll T, Ziegler R, Dresel HA. 17β-estradiol inhibits LDL oxidation and cholesteryl ester formation in cultured macrophages. *Free Radic Res Commun* 1990; **8**:167–73.

199. Rifici VA, Khachadurian AK. The inhibition of low-density lipoprotein oxidation by 17–beta estradiol. *Metabolism* 1992; **41**:1110–14.

200. Sack MN, Rader DJ, Cannon RO III. Oestrogen and inhibition of oxidation of low-density lipoproteins in postmenopausal women. *Lancet* 1994; **343**:269–70.

201. Turksoy RN, Phillips LL, Southam AL. Influence of ovarian function on the fibrinolytic enzyme system. I. Ovulatory and anovulatory cycles. *Am J Obstet Gynecol* 1961; **82**:1211–15.

202. Wallmo L, Gyzander E, Karlsson K, Lindstedt G, Radberg T, Teger-Nilsson AC. α_2–Antiplasmin and α_2–macroglobulin – the main inhibitors of fibrinolysis – during the menstrual cycle, pregnancy, delivery, and treatment with oral contraceptives. *Acta Obstet Gynecol Scand* 1982; **61**:417–22.

203. Casslen B, Andersson A, Nilsson IM, Astedt B. Hormonal regulation of the release of plasminogen activators and of a specific activator inhibitor from endometrial tissue in culture. *Proc Soc Exp Biol Med* 1986; **182**:419–24.

204. Mandalaki T, Louizou C, Dimitriadou C, Symeonidis P. Variations in factor VIII during the menstrual cycle in normal women. *N Engl J Med* 1980; **302**:1093–4.

205. Foley ME, Isherwood DM, McNicol GP. Viscosity, haematocrit, fibrinogen and plasma proteins in maternal and cord blood. *Br J Obstet Gynaecol* 1978; **85**:500–4.

206. Dalaker K, Prydz H. The coagulation factor VII in pregnancy. *Br J Haematol* 1984; **56**:233–41.

207. Bonnar J, Davidson JF, Pidgeon CF, McNicol GP, Douglas AS. Fibrin degradation products in normal and abnormal pregnancy and parturition. *BMJ* 1969; **3**:137–40.

208. Shaper AG, Macintosh DM, Evans CM, Kyobe J. Fibrinolysis and plasminogen levels in pregnancy and the puerperium. *Lancet* 1965; **2**:706–8.

209. Meilahn EN. Hemostatic factors and risk of cardiovascular disease in women. An overview. *Arch Pathol Lab Med* 1992; **116**:1313–17.

210. Meade TW, Haines AP, Imeson JD, Stirling Y, Thompson SG. Menopausal status and haemostatic variables. *Lancet* 1983; **1**:22–4.

211. Meade TW, Dyer S, Howarth DJ, Imeson JD, Stirling Y. Antithrombin III and procoagulant activity: sex differences and effects of the menopause. *Br J Haematol* 1990; **74**:77–81.

212. Nabulsi AA, Folsom AR, White A, et al. Association of hormone-replacement therapy with various cardiovascular risk factors in postmenopausal women. The Atherosclerosis Risk in Communities Study Investigators. *N Engl J Med* 1993; **328**:1069–75.

213. Meade TW. Clotting factors and ischaemic heart disease: the epidemiologic evidence. In: Meade TW (ed). *Anticoagulants and Myocardial Infarction: A Reappraisal*. New York: John Wiley, 1984: 91–111.

214. Manolio TA, Furberg CD, Shemanski L, et al. Associations of postmenopausal estrogen use with cardiovascular disease and its risk factors in older women. The CHS Collaborative Research Group. *Circulation* 1993; **88**:2163–71.

215. Lobo RA, Pickar JH, Wild RA, Walsh B, Hirvonen E. Metabolic impact of adding medroxyprogesterone acetate to conjugated estrogen therapy in postmenopausal women. The Menopause Study Group. *Obstet Gynecol* 1994; **84**:987–95.

216. Aylward M. Coagulation factors in opposed and unopposed oestrogen treatment at the climacteric. *Postgrad Med J* 1978; **54** (Suppl 2):31–7.

217. Scarabin PY, Plu-Bureau, Bara L, Bonithon-Kopp C, Guize L, Samama MM. Haemostatic variables and menopausal status: influence of hormone replacement therapy. *Thromb Haemost* 1993; **70**:584–7.

218. Alkjaersig N, Fletcher AP, de Ziegler D, Steingold KA, Meldrum DR, Judd HL. Blood coagulation in postmenopausal women given estrogen treatment: comparison of transdermal and oral administration. *J Lab Clin Med* 1988; **111**:224–8.

219. Bonnar J, Haddon M, Hunter DH, Richards DH, Thornton C. Coagulation system changes in postmenopausal women receiving oestrogen preparations. *Postgrad Med J* 1976; **52** (Suppl 6):30–6.

220. Skartlien AH, Lyberg-Beckmann S, Holme I, Hjermann I, Prydz H. Effect of alteration in triglyceride levels on factor VII–phospholipid complexes in plasma. *Arteriosclerosis* 1989; **9**:798–801.

221. Dahlback B, Carlsson M, Svensson PJ. Familial thrombophilia due to a previously unrecognized mechanism characterized by poor anticoagulant response to activated protein C: prediction of a cofactor to activated protein C. *Proc Natl Acad Sci U S A* 1993; **90**:1004–8.

222. Meade TW. Orchidectomy versus oestrogen for prostatic cancer: cardiovascular effects. *BMJ (Clin Res Ed)* 1986; **293**:953–4.

223. Kannel WB, Wolf PA, Castelli WP, D'Agostino RB. Fibrinogen and risk of cardiovascular disease. The Framingham Study. *JAMA* 1987; **258**:1183–6.

224. Yarnell JW, Baker IA, Sweetnam PM, et al. Fibrinogen, viscosity, and white blood cell count are major risk factors for ischemic heart disease. The Caerphilly and Speedwell collaborative heart disease studies. *Circulation* 1991; **83**:836–44.

225. Balleisen L, Schulte H, Assmann G, Epping PH, van de Loo J. Coagulation factors and the progress of coronary heart disease. *Lancet* 1987; **2**:461.

226. Notelovitz M, Kitchens C, Ware M, Hirschberg K, Coone L. Combination estrogen and progestogen replacement therapy does not adversely affect coagulation. *Obstet Gynecol* 1983; **62**:596–600.

227. Notelovitz M, Kitchens CS, Ware MD. Coagulation and fibrinolysis in estrogen-treated surgically menopausal women. *Obstet Gynecol* 1984; **63**:621–5.

228. Gebara OC, Mittleman MA, Sutherland P, et al. Association between increased estrogen status and increased fibrinolytic potential in the Framingham Offspring Study. *Circulation* 1995; **91**:1952–8.

229. Jespersen J, Petersen KR, Skouby SO. Effects of newer oral contraceptives on the inhibition of coagulation and fibrinolysis in relation to dosage and type of steroid. *Am J Obstet Gynecol* 1990; **163** (1 Pt 2): 396–403.

230. Soma M, Fumagalli R, Paoletti R, et al. Plasma Lp(a) concentration after oestrogen and progestagen in postmenopausal women. *Lancet* 1991; **337**:612.

231. van der Mooren MJ, Demacker PN, Thomas CM, Rolland R. Beneficial effects on serum lipoproteins by 17β-oestradiol–dydrogesterone therapy in postmenopausal women; a prospective study. *Eur J Obstet Gynecol Reprod Biol* 1992; **47**:153–60.

232. Mbewu AD, Durrington PN. Lipoprotein (a): structure, properties and possible involvement in thrombogenesis and atherogenesis. *Atherosclerosis* 1990; **85**:1–14.

233. Hajjar KA, Gavish D, Breslow JL, Nachman RL. Lipoprotein(a) modulation of endothelial cell surface fibrinolysis and its potential role in atherosclerosis. *Nature* 1989; **339**:303–5.

234. Miles LA, Fless GM, Levin EG, Scanu AM, Plow EF. A potential basis for the thrombotic risks associated with lipoprotein(a). *Nature* 1989; **339**:301–3.

235. Kooistra T, Bosma PJ, Jespersen J, Kluft C. Studies on the mechanism of action of oral contraceptives with regard to fibrinolytic variables. *Am J Obstet Gynecol* 1990; **163** (1 Pt 2):404–13.

236. Quehenberger P, Kapiotis S, Partan C, et al. Studies on oral contraceptive-induced changes in blood coagulation and fibrinolysis and the estrogen effect on endothelial cells. *Ann Hematol* 1993; **67**:33–6.

237. Raman BB, Standley PR, Rajkumar V, Ram JL, Sowers JR. Effects of estradiol and progesterone on platelet calcium responses. *Am J Hypertens* 1995; **8**:197–200.

238. Miller ME, Dores GM, Thorpe SL, Akerley WL. Paradoxical influence of estrogenic hormones on platelet–endothelial cell interactions. *Thromb Res* 1994; **74**:577–94.

239. Bar J, Tepper R, Fuchs J, Pardo Y, Goldberger S,

Ovadia J. The effect of estrogen replacement therapy on platelet aggregation and adenosine triphosphate release in postmenopausal women. *Obstet Gynecol* 1993; **81**:261–4.

240. Johnson M, Ramey E, Ramwell PW. Androgen-mediated sensitivity in platelet aggregation. *Am J Physiol* 1977; **232**:H381–5.

241. Writing Group for the WHI Investigators. Risks and benefits of estrogen plus progestin in healthy postmenopausal women. Principal results from the Women's Health Initiative randomized controlled trial. *JAMA* 2002; **288**:321–33.

242. Speroff L. The Heart Estrogen/progestin Replacement Study (HERS). *Maturitas* 1998; **31**:9–14.

243. Wenger NK. Cardioprotection for the post-menopausal woman. HERS results and their implications. *Prev Cardiol* 1998; **1**:9–11.

244. Meade TW, Stirling Y, Wilkes H, Mannucci PM. Effects of oral contraceptives and obesity on protein C antigen. *Thromb Haemost* 1985; **53**:198–9.

245. Malm J, Laurell M, Dahlback B. Changes in the plasma levels of vitamin K-dependent proteins C and S and of C4b-binding protein during pregnancy and oral contraception. *Br J Haematol* 1988; **68**:437–43.

246. Bonnar J. Coagulation effects of oral contraception. *Am J Obstet Gynecol* 1987; **157**:1042–8.

247. Rosenberg L, Kaufman DW, Helmrich SP, Miller DR, Stolley PD, Shapiro S. Myocardial infarction and cigarette smoking in women younger than 50 years of age. *JAMA* 1985; **253**:2965–9.

248. Stadel BV. Oral contraceptives and cardiovascular disease. *N Engl J Med* 1981; **305**:672–7.

249. Bottiger LE, Boman G, Eklund G, Westerholm B. Oral contraceptives and thromboembolic disease: effects of lowering oestrogen content. *Lancet* 1980; **1**:1097–101.

250. Vandenbroucke JP, Koster T, Briet E, Reitsma PH, Bertina RM, Rosendaal FR. Increased risk of venous thrombosis in oral contraceptive users who are carriers of the Factor V Leiden mutation. *Lancet* 1994; **344**:1453–7.

251. Griffin JH, Evatt B, Wideman C, Fernandez JA. Anticoagulant protein C pathway defective in majority of thrombophilic patients. *Blood* 1993; **82**:1989–93.

252. Dzau VJ, Gibbons GH. Cell biology of vascular hypertrophy in systemic hypertension. *Am J Cardiol* 1988; **62**:30G–5G.

253. Garg UC, Hassid A. Nitric oxide-generating vasodilators and 8-bromo-cyclic guanosine monophosphate inhibit mitogenesis and proliferation of cultured rat vascular smooth muscle cells. *J Clin Invest* 1989; **83**:1774–7.

26

Menopausal hormone therapy

John C. Stevenson

Introduction

Cardiovascular disease (CVD), of which coronary heart disease (CHD) is the most common, is the major cause of death in women over 60 years of age. Approximately 50% of women develop CHD in their lifetime, 30% die from the disease, and 20% develop a stroke. Yet many women still perceive CVD, particularly CHD, as a male condition, despite the fact that eventually more women than men die from the disease.[1] Women generally perceive breast cancer as the commonest cause of female death, despite the fact that they have more than five times the risk of dying from CHD than from breast cancer.

Gender differences in the presentation of CHD have been identified. Angina pectoris is more common in women than in men,[2] but the onset of the clinical symptoms of CHD in women is generally 7–10 years behind that in men. There are also gender differences in the way that CHD is treated. This is possibly because women tend to be referred at later stages in the disease, so there are fewer opportunities for successful intervention with thrombolytic agents and revascularization procedures.

Gonadal steroids seem to have an important role for the cardiovascular system in women.[3] Premenopausal women rarely develop CHD, but loss of ovarian function leads to a clear increase in the disease.[4] Thus, the menopause is a unique CHD risk factor for women. The menopause is associated with adverse changes in metabolic risk factors for CHD as well as adverse vascular effects.

Since ovarian hormones are thought to protect against CHD, it has long been assumed that hormone replacement therapy (HRT) will do the same. However, this prevailing view needs to be reassessed in the light of the findings from large clinical trials conducted over the past few years.

Risk factors for CHD (see also Chapters 2–9)

CHD is a multifactorial disease, but certain major risk factors can account for the vast majority of myocardial infarctions (MIs). A recent observational study (INTERHEART) of almost 30 000 men and women from different communities and ethnic groups worldwide showed that such risk factors are common to all groups and can predict over 90% of the CHD risk.[5] Lifestyle factors, including smoking, poor diet high in saturated fats and low in fruit and vegetables, physical inactivity, and stress, have an important causal role in the incidence of CHD in all populations, while moderate alcohol consumption appears protective. Genetic and environmental factors are also significant. Metabolic diseases and risk factors, including diabetes mellitus, obesity, dyslipidemia, hypertension, and insulin resistance,

---

Box 26.1 Effect of menopause on risk factors for coronary heart disease

Lipids/lipoproteins
low-density lipoprotein (LDL) cholesterol ↑   high-density lipoprotein (HDL) cholesterol ↓ HDL_2 cholesterol ↓   triglycerides ↑
apolipoprotein AI ↓   apolipoprotein B ↑   apolipoprotein (a) ↑   LDL particle size ↓

Glucose/insulin
pancreatic insulin secretion ↓   insulin elimination ↓

Hemostasis
fibrinogen ↑   factor VII ↑   antithrombin III ↑   plasminogen activator inhibitor-1 ↑

Body composition
android fat ↑   gynoid fat ↓

Vascular function
arterial waveform pulsatility index ↑   endothelial-dependent vasodilatation ↓

---

have a substantial impact on the development of CHD. These risk factors contribute to the development of atherosclerosis and thrombotic complications. Reducing these risk factors can slow the progression of CHD and its clinical complications before, and even after, the occurrence of a cardiovascular event. Loss of ovarian hormones at the menopause has a widespread adverse impact on many of these risk factors.

Effects of menopause on CHD risk factors (Box 26.1)

Loss of ovarian function at the menopause is associated with adverse changes in the lipid profile.[6] There is an increase in total and low-density lipoprotein (LDL) cholesterol and triglycerides, and a decrease in high-density lipoprotein (HDL) and the important HDL_2 subfraction. Disturbances of glucose and insulin metabolism are of major importance in the development of CHD. Insulin resistance, accompanied by compensatory hyperinsulinemia, is a pivotal mechanism in the pathogenesis of CHD. Insulin resistance is associated with low HDL and HDL_2, increased triglycerides and small dense LDL, increased factor VII, decreased tissue plasminogen activator (tPA) and increased plasminogen activator inhibitor-1 (PAI-1), decreased arterial wall compliance and arterial blood flow, increased blood pressure, and increased central adiposity.[7] These adverse CHD risk factors are collec-

tively termed the 'metabolic syndrome', the presence of which is linked to increased CVD risk.[8] Glucose and insulin metabolism are adversely affected by the menopause. Although there is no immediate change in circulating insulin concentrations, this masks a decrease in pancreatic insulin secretion and in insulin elimination.[9] Menopausal women become increasingly insulin-resistant as a result of decreased insulin sensitivity, which results in hyperinsulinemia.[10] Menopause also results in a redistribution of body fat towards an android distribution.[11] Alterations in coagulation factors have also been described at the menopause. Serum fibrinogen, factor VII activity, antithrombin III and PAI-1, which are highly predictive of CHD, are significantly increased after the menopause.[12] Thus, the menopause itself results in the development of a metabolic syndrome in women.[13]

The menopause has adverse effects on arterial function. It is associated with reduced compliance in the carotid artery, as measured by an increase in arterial waveform pulsatility index.[14] Endothelial-dependent vasodilatation is also impaired in menopausal women.[15]

Hormone replacement therapy (see also Chapter 25) (Table 26.1)

HRT comprises estrogen, with or without the addition of a progestogen (Table 26.1). There has

Table 26.1 Different types of hormone replacement therapy (HRT) and routes of administration

Type of HRT	Route of administration
Estrogen	
Conjugated equine estrogens	Oral
17β-Estradiol	Oral/transdermal/ percutaneous/ subcutaneous/ intranasal
Estrone sulfate	Oral
Progestogen	
19-Nortestosterone	
Norgestrel	Oral/transdermal/ intrauterine
Norethisterone acetate (NETA)	Oral/transdermal
Norgestimate	Oral
Desogestrel	Oral
Gestodene	Oral
Dienogest	Oral
C21 progesterone	
Medroxyprogesterone acetate	Oral
Dydrogesterone	Oral
Chlormadinone acetate	Oral
Medrogestone	Oral
Cyproterone acetate	Oral
Drosperinone	Oral
Promegestone	Oral
Trimegestone	Oral
Progesterone	Oral/suppository/ pessary

been recent debate as to whether HRT should be renamed hormonal therapy (HT), but this issue over nomenclature is rather trivial and detracts those without special expertise in hormones from the more important issue of the different types of HRT. In the case of HRT and CHD, there is evidence that a lack of female hormones at least contributes to the development of CHD. Therefore, giving hormones to prevent or treat the disease in adults should be regarded as true replacement therapy, HRT, irrespective of age.

Estrogen

Estrogen is given on a continuous basis, by tablets, skin patches, skin gels, subcutaneous implants or intranasal sprays. Natural estrogens, as opposed to synthetic estrogen derivatives, are preferred for HRT, including 17β-estradiol, estrone sulfate, and conjugated equine estrogens. Estrogens have a wide range of effects on various tissues, and are responsible for all the benefits obtained with HRT. While the effects of different types of estrogens are very similar in some systems, for example in the relief of menopausal symptoms and in the prevention of osteoporosis, their metabolic effects may differ considerably.

Progestogen

Progestogens can be given by tablets and skin patches, and locally by intrauterine systems. Progesterone can be given by tablets, pessaries, and suppositories. The main beneficial action of progestogens is to prevent or reverse estrogen-induced proliferation of endometrial tissue. The addition of a progestogen in HRT is designed to prevent excess endometrial proliferation, hyperplasia, and an increased risk of endometrial cancer, and thus progestogens are not usually given to women who have been hysterectomized. Progestogens may be added cyclically for 12–14 days each month, leading to a regular cyclical withdrawal bleed. This type of HRT is most suitable for women around the time of the menopause, and gives good cycle control with predictable bleeding. They may be given continuously with estrogen in order to induce endometrial atrophy and avoid bleeding completely. This regimen is more likely to be successful in women who are a few years past the menopause and are almost completely devoid of any residual spontaneous ovarian activity. In such women, they may eventually result in amenorrhea in around 80%. There is a wide range of progestogens available worldwide, including 19-nortestosterone derivatives, 19-norpregnane derivatives, and C21 steroids. These vary considerably in their effects, largely due to their differing steroid receptor activities. Thus, as well as binding to the progesterone receptor, they may, or may not, also bind to other receptors, giving additional estrogenic, anti-estrogenic, androgenic, anti-androgenic, glucocorticoid, and anti-mineralocorticoid effects. Again, while the endometrial effects of the different progestogens tend to be similar, their metabolic effects can be quite different.

Thus it can be seen that the metabolic effects of different HRT regimens may vary considerably. These metabolic effects have their impact mainly on the cardiovascular system. Thus, when describing the effects of HRT on CHD risk, it is essential to define which specific HRT regimen is being considered. It must be remembered that the effects of HRT will vary according to the dose of the steroids, the type of steroids, and their route of administration.

Prevention and treatment of CHD in menopausal women

The first step in the prevention of CHD is lifestyle modification. Cessation of smoking, dietary improvement with reduction in saturated fat intake, weight control, and increase in physical activity will contribute to a reduced risk in most people. Antihypertensive therapy is given as appropriate to hypertensive menopausal women. Similarly, aspirin, beta-blockers, lipid-lowering drugs, and angiotensin-converting enzyme (ACE) inhibitors can be administered prophylactically to menopausal women who have established disease or high multifactorial risk of CHD. Finally, revascularization procedures and coronary artery bypass graft surgery are important treatment options for women with CHD.

Effects of HRT on CHD

HRT is another intervention with the potential to prevent CHD in menopausal women. Many epidemiologic studies have shown that estrogen administration to menopausal women results in a reduction in CHD of around 40%, an effect that does not appear to be lost when cyclical progestogen is added for endometrial protection in nonhysterectomized women.[16] However, to date the results of randomized clinical trials have not supported the findings of the observational studies. In order to explain this apparent contradiction, a consideration of the mechanisms by which HRT impacts the cardiovascular system is necessary. HRT has a variety of metabolic effects as well as direct arterial effects, all of which will contribute to its overall impact.

Effects on lipids and lipoproteins

HRT has major effects on lipid and lipoprotein metabolism, which are dependent on the type, dose, and route of administration of therapy (Fig. 26.1).[17]

Total cholesterol levels are reduced by 5–10% within 3 months of use of HRT, irrespective of the type or route of administration of therapy. This effect is maintained during long-term treatment.[18] Oral estrogen lowers LDL cholesterol by upregulating apolipoprotein B_{100} receptors, particularly in the

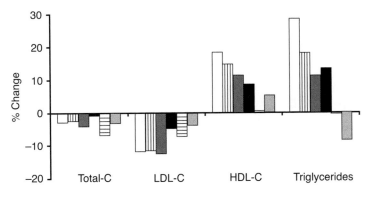

Figure 26.1
Percent change in total cholesterol (total-C), low-density lipoprotein cholesterol (LDL-C), high-density lipoprotein cholesterol (HDL-C), and triglycerides seen with varying doses of conjugated equine estrogens (CEE), oral 17β-estradiol (17β-E_2) and transdermal 17β-estradiol (trans 17β-E_2). Adapted from reference 17.

□ CEE 1.25 mg (n = 268)   ■ 17β-E_2 2 mg (n = 283)   ▤ trans 17β-E_2 0.1 mg (n = 61)

▥ CEE 0.627 mg (n = 1513)   ■ 17β-E_2 1 mg (n = 94)   ▨ trans 17β-E_2 0.05 mg (n = 627)

liver, thereby increasing LDL uptake. HRT appears to cause the greatest magnitude of decrease in LDL in women with the highest baseline levels.[19] HRT may therefore be considered as a lipid-lowering agent in menopausal women with mild to moderate hypercholesterolemia. Transdermal estrogen causes a smaller reduction in LDL levels.[17] The addition of progestogens to estrogen therapy has no obvious adverse effect in terms of lowering of LDL, since they increase LDL production but also increase their clearance.[20] Qualitative changes in LDL that are induced by HRT may also be important for CHD risk. HRT appears to increase the proportion of small dense LDL,[21] but it also increases the clearance of these atherogenic particles from the circulation, so they are less likely to be retained in the arterial wall. Transdermal HRT appears to have no effect on LDL particle size.[22]

Oral estrogen also increases HDL, particularly HDL_2, by decreasing its catabolism through inhibition of hepatic lipase, and increasing hepatic synthesis of apolipoprotein AI. Transdermal estrogen has a less marked effect on HDL levels than oral estrogen,[17] but it does reduce HDL_3, which could theoretically be beneficial for CHD risk.[12] Androgenic progestogens, such as norgestrel and norethisterone acetate (NETA), reverse the HDL-raising effect of estrogen[23,24] because they increase hepatic lipase activity. This effect is regarded as potentially disadvantageous. But since it is not known whether the reduction in HDL reflects any impairment in reverse cholesterol transport, or in remnant clearance, the clinical significance of lowering HDL remains to be determined. In contrast, the less androgenic progestogens have less effect on the estrogen-induced increase in HDL cholesterol. Medroxyprogesterone acetate (MPA) does cause some impedance of the estrogen-induced HDL increase whereas dydrogesterone and micronized progesterone have little effect.[25,26]

Oral estrogen may also reduce lipoprotein (a) (Lp(a)).[17] Lp(a) is of potential importance in atherogenesis. It may enhance the binding and retention of LDL in the subendothelial space, thereby increasing the susceptibility of LDL to oxidation. The reduction of Lp(a) by estrogen could therefore decrease atheroma development and progression. Estrogen also reduces the oxidation, and therefore the atherogenicity, of LDL.[27]

Estrogen also improves the postprandial clearance of atherogenic chylomicron remnants,[28] decreases lipoprotein-induced arterial smooth muscle proliferation, and reduces arterial cholesterol ester influx and hydrolysis.

The effect of estrogen on triglycerides varies considerably according to the type and route of administration of therapy.[17,23] Orally administered conjugated equine estrogens, and to a lesser extent 17β-estradiol, increase triglycerides because of their hepatic first-pass effect on very low-density lipoprotein (VLDL) apolipoprotein B synthesis and secretion. In contrast, transdermally administered estrogen causes a decrease in triglyceride production, which is consistent with the physiologic role of estrogen, and is the preferred route in women with raised triglyceride levels. Depending on their androgenicity, progestogens reduce VLDL secretion and this results in a lowering of triglycerides,[23] an effect which is clearly beneficial. Such an effect is not seen with the nonandrogenic progestogens such as dydrogesterone.[25]

The relative benefits or risks of changing HDL levels compared with changing triglyceride levels with respect to the development of CHD are not yet known. HRT may have the unusual effect of causing both HDL and triglyceride levels to be changed in the same direction (i.e. both increased or both decreased), so the HRT only rarely changes both parameters in a beneficial direction. Whether it is better to have decreased triglycerides at the expense of decreased HDL, or increased HDL with concomitant increased triglycerides is not known.

When all the above HRT-induced changes to lipids and lipoproteins are considered together, it would appear that most HRT combinations are likely to be beneficial overall in terms of CHD risk from lipid changes. In certain individuals, such as patients with dyslipidemia or diabetes, the maximal lipid benefit of HRT can be achieved by tailoring the HRT regimen to provide the desired effect on lipids and lipoproteins.

Effects on glucose and insulin metabolism

In vitro and in vivo studies have shown that pancreatic insulin secretion is increased by estrogen or progestogen, and that insulin resistance is decreased by estrogen, but is increased by progestogen. The effects of estrogens on glucose and insulin metabolism differ according to the preparation. Oral 17β-estradiol appears to improve insulin resistance,[29] whereas alkylated estrogens such as ethinyl estradiol and conjugated equine estrogens may raise insulin levels and impair glucose tolerance.[30] Transdermal 17β-estradiol is fairly neutral in its effects.[31]

The effect of co-administering androgenic progestogens with estrogen on glucose and insulin metabolism is dependent on the route of administration of these steroids. Progestogen addition may modify the effects of estrogen on glucose and insulin metabolism, depending on the type of progestogen used. Testosterone-derived progestogens, such as norgestrel, may increase insulin resistance.[32] NETA given orally may also have a negative effect,[31] but when given transdermally it has little impact.[32] However, with a continuous combined transdermal estradiol/NETA combination, a reduction in fasting insulin with no change in fasting glucose has been observed, which may indicate an improvement in insulin sensitivity.[22] Nonandrogenic progestogens such as dydrogesterone have little adverse effect,[33] although MPA has unwanted effects.

Effects on body fat distribution

The redistribution of body fat from gynoid to android distribution that occurs during the menopause[11] is associated with an increased risk of CHD. HRT does not usually cause a significant increase in weight, and may limit or reverse the increases in android fat distribution in menopausal women.[34]

Effects on hemostasis

Estrogen affects coagulation and fibrinolysis, increasing both pro-coagulant and fibrinolytic activity, but the effects of the menopause are not well documented. The effects of HRT on hemostasis are somewhat complex.[35,36] Estrogen has been shown to reduce PAI-1, antithrombin III, and fibrinogen. Estrogen also inhibits platelet aggregation and increases prostacyclin production by the endothelium and arterial smooth muscle cells. Although certain pro-coagulant factors that are linked with atheroma development are reduced by HRT, oral estrogen also increases thrombogenesis. It is likely that the initiation of estrogen therapy causes a transient imbalance between coagulation and fibrinolysis, thereby causing a short-term increase in risk for both coronary events and venous thromboembolism, which disappears as these processes gradually readjust and come back into a balance. The nonoral administration of estrogen may limit or even avoid this adverse effect.[22,37,38] Progestogens are probably fairly neutral in their effects on hemostasis. No data are available on the effects of HRT in women with coagulopathies, but transdermal estrogen is probably preferable to oral estrogen in these women.

Effects on arterial function

Estrogen receptors are found throughout the arterial tree, and there is strong evidence to suggest that estrogens have direct arterial effects.[39] The overall effects of HRT on arterial function are beneficial. Estrogen reverses the reduction in arterial compliance that occurs in menopausal women, an effect only partially attenuated by the addition of NETA. Reduced resistance to blood flow and increased vessel elasticity may reduce myocardial risk either by reducing the likelihood of acute coronary artery vasospasm or by lessening atheroma formation.[40]

Estrogen causes vasodilatation through a variety of different effects. It decreases vascular tone and reactivity by modulating the release of vasoconstrictors and vasodilators by the vascular endothelium. Estrogen also affects the release of vasoactive substances and neurotransmitters, including histamine, serotonin, and prostaglandins, and adjusts the release of vasoactive neurotransmitters at presynaptic junctions. Postmenopausal estrogen use has been shown to reduce blood pressure,[41] although this effect is small.

The effects of estrogen on arterial function are mediated by various pathways, including endothelium-dependent and calcium-dependent mechanisms, or by other mechanisms, such as reduction in ACE activity. A major vasodilatory effect is mediated by an acute effect on the nitric oxide synthase (NOS) pathway, which leads to increased levels of endothelial nitric oxide synthase (eNOS)[42] and increased production of the potent vasodilator nitric oxide (NO). Estradiol stimulates NO release via endothelial cell surface estrogen receptors, as shown by the addition of physiologic doses of estrogen to human endothelial cells.[43] Estradiol also reduces the release of the potent vasoconstrictor, endothelin-1.[44]

There is also evidence that estrogens act independently of the endothelium, possibly by acting as a calcium antagonist. The arterial vasodilatation produced by the addition of 17β-estradiol to isolated rings of rabbit coronary artery is still evident when the vascular endothelium has been removed.[45] Estrogen modulates calcium channels in the smooth muscle cell membranes of blood vessels and in cardiac myocytes in a dose-dependent manner. It inhibits calcium-induced contraction of the coronary artery, inhibits inward calcium currents and reduces intracellular free calcium in isolated cardiac myocytes.[46] In addition, estrogen activates BK_{Ca} channels to cause coronary artery relaxation.[47]

Arterial function may also be affected by estrogen through changes in the renin–angiotensin system. Patients with enhanced angiotensin-1 conversion, resulting from the deletion allele of the ACE gene polymorphism, have impaired NO release from the vascular endothelium.[48] The ACE gene deletion allele has been associated with CHD, particularly in women.[49] HRT has been shown to reduce circulating ACE activity, an effect of both estrogen and progestogen.[22,50,51]

Inflammatory processes are likely to be involved in atherogenesis and plaque destabilization. HRT lowers the levels of the cell adhesion molecule E-selectin in menopausal women with hypercholesterolemia[52] and in healthy menopausal women.[22,53] Elevated levels of C-reactive protein (CRP), an acute phase protein, are associated with increased CHD risk.[54] Oral HRT increases CRP levels, but the clinical significance of this finding is unclear as it also decreases levels of other inflammatory markers, while transdermal HRT does not have this effect.[55] Abnormal deposition and remodeling of the vascular extracellular matrix are thought to be significant in the development and progression of atheroma. Therapies which regulate and normalize these processes may therefore retard or inhibit atherogen-

esis. Matrix metalloproteinases (MMPs) and tissue inhibitor metalloproteinases (TIMPs) are key in the deposition and remodeling processes. MMPs are zinc-dependent enzymes that degrade components of the extracellular matrix such as collagen and proteoglycans, and have been implicated in the development of CVD.[56] These enzymes may be associated with atheromatous plaque progression and regression and plaque rupture. TIMPs are one of several types of circulating inhibitors of MMPs. The addition of estradiol to cultures of human vascular smooth muscles cells causes a dose-dependent increase in the release of MMPs.[57] Slight increases in MMPs may therefore counteract increased vascular deposition of collagen, whereas high levels of MMPs may promote development of atheroma. The administration of low doses of estrogen may therefore retard or inhibit atheroma development, but too high doses may have a deleterious effect.

Clinical studies of HRT and CHD

Epidemiologic studies

Many epidemiologic studies of different designs, including case–control and cohort studies, have been remarkably consistent in demonstrating a reduction in CHD with HRT use in menopausal women.[58] There have been concerns that the apparent reductions in CHD with HRT reflect a healthy-user bias. Women who choose to use HRT tend to have fewer CHD risk factors, while those with unhealthy lifestyles or pre-existing diseases are often not recommended HRT. However, these biases can be addressed by large studies with cases and controls matched for lifestyle and major risk factors. Such studies have still shown a reduction of CHD risk of about 40%.[16] Observational studies have also demonstrated that estrogen replacement therapy appears beneficial in menopausal women with established CHD. Women sustaining an MI had a better survival if they were current users of HRT,[59] while a 50–80% reduction in the incidence of CHD and an increase in survival over 10 years with HRT have also been reported.[60] The greatest benefit in terms of survival was seen in women with the most severe coronary atheroma.

Randomized clinical trials

Surrogate vascular function endpoint studies

Several studies have assessed the effect of HRT on vascular reactivity in peripheral arteries. Beneficial effects have been demonstrated in several small studies.[61,62] Studies have also been conducted to assess the anti-ischemic effects of acute estrogen therapy on myocardial ischemia induced by a variety of methods.

The acute administration of sublingual 17β-estradiol has been shown to reduce myocardial ischemia in menopausal women with established CHD, as evidenced by a delay in the development of myocardial ischemia on electrocardiogram (ECG) exercise testing and prolongation of overall exercise time compared with placebo.[63] Similarly, short-term intravenous administration of conjugated equine estrogen has been shown to reduce dobutamine-induced myocardial ischemia in menopausal women with CHD.[64] The wall motion index score was improved with estrogen compared with saline. Myocardial ischemia, as reflected by measurement of pH in the coronary sinus during incremental atrial pacing, was also reduced by acute sublingual 17β-estradiol compared with placebo.[65] These studies provide evidence that short-term administration of estrogen could be used as an anti-ischemic agent in menopausal women with CHD.

The effects of chronic estrogen therapy on exercise-induced myocardial ischemia have been assessed in a double-blind, randomized, placebo-controlled cross-over study.[66] Menopausal women with CHD were randomized to receive either placebo patches or transdermal 17β-estradiol. Exercise time to 1-mm ST segment depression on ECG was substantially increased after 4 and 8 weeks of estrogen therapy.

Surrogate atheroma endpoint studies

Randomized trials of HRT effects on atheroma progression have been carried out using both ultra-sound techniques and quantitative coronary angiography. An assessment of atheroma progression can be made by ultrasonic measurement of carotid artery intima-media thickness (IMT). Of the ultrasound randomized clinical trials, one study showed no effect of HRT using oral 17β-estradiol 1 mg plus gestodene 25 μg,[67] but the treatment duration was only 1 year, which may be too short a time to observe an effect. Another study showed trends towards reduction in IMT with HRT after 2 years of treatment, more marked with oral 17β-estradiol 1.5 mg plus cyclical desogestrel 0.15 mg than with conjugated equine estrogens 0.625 mg plus cyclical norgestrel 0.15 mg, but this did not reach statistical significance.[68] In a larger randomized trial of women mainly in the early menopause, a significant reduction in the rate of subclinical atheroma progression was seen in women taking oral 17β-estradiol 1 mg compared with placebo.[69] This effect was not seen when the comparison was made in women who were also receiving lipid-lowering medication, confirming earlier findings from an observational study.[70] In contrast, a sub-study of the Heart and Estrogen/progestin Replacement Study (HERS), which included older menopausal women with established CHD, found no difference in progression of carotid atheroma between conjugated equine estrogens 0.625 mg plus MPA 2.5 mg and placebo.[71]

This latter finding is in agreement with randomized trials using quantitative coronary angiography to document atheroma progression. The effects of estrogen replacement on the progression of coronary artery atherosclerosis (ERA) trial studied menopausal women with coronary artery disease documented by angiography randomized to conjugated equine estrogens 0.625 mg with or without the addition of MPA 2.5 mg or placebo.[72] No significant differences in mean luminal diameter were observed between active treatment and placebo groups after 3.2 years. It is of concern that the ERA study was also unable to demonstrate any beneficial effect of taking statins, or any detrimental effect of being hypertensive or a cigarette smoker. Similar findings were reported in the Women's Angiographic Vitamin and Estrogen (WAVE) trial,[73] which studied menopausal women with established coronary heart disease randomized to the same HRT regimen or placebo. No significant differences in minimum luminal diameter were observed between HRT and placebo groups after 2.8 years. Similarly, no significant differences were found between antioxidant vitamin use and placebo in the same study. Caution must be used in interpreting these angiographic studies, since uncertainties exist regarding the use of lesion area measurement as an endpoint when evaluating the course of coronary artery disease.[74]

Taken overall, studies of atheroma progression suggest that HRT alone may reduce atheroma progression in younger menopausal women who do not have significant atherosclerosis, but it has no measurable effect in older women with established disease. However, it is possible that HRT may still prevent the development of plaques even without effecting changes in IMT.[75]

CHD clinical endpoint studies

The HERS prospective clinical trial of HRT enrolled 2763 postmenopausal women, mean age 67 years, with established CHD who were randomized to receive conjugated equine estrogens 0.625 mg plus MPA 2.5 mg daily or placebo.[76] After a mean of 4 years of follow-up there was no significant difference between the groups in the outcomes of nonfatal MI or cardiac death. However, the interpretation of these results is not straightforward. For example, in the first year after randomization patients in the HRT group had an increased event rate that decreased steadily in the subsequent years, with a statistically significant trend. In the placebo group, the event rate was lower than expected in the first year, with higher rates during further follow-up. It remains unknown if these observations reflect a true pattern of events, or whether such variations may be due to chance. There was in fact an imbalance in the use of statins between the groups, with greater usage in the placebo group. Another major concern about trials of older menopausal women is the starting dose of HRT used,[77] as discussed below.

This pattern of early increase and late decrease in CHD risk seen in HERS has been seen in other secondary prevention studies of HRT. The small Papworth HRT atherosclerosis study (PHASE) randomized trial of transdermal 17β-estradiol with or without transdermal NETA also failed to show

benefit in women with CHD,[78] but again the dose of estradiol used (80 µg per day) was high for the age of the patients. In contrast, a randomized trial using the relatively lower dose of oral estradiol 1 mg daily showed a nonsignificant reduction in coronary deaths during the first 12 months of study, although no breakdown of coronary events was given.[79]

The Women's Health Initiative (WHI) trials of HRT for primary prevention of CHD were conducted in healthy menopausal women aged between 50 and 80 years. In these trials, 16 608 nonhysterectomized women were randomized to either conjugated equine estrogens 0.625 mg plus MPA 2.5 mg daily or placebo, and followed for a mean duration of 5.2 years.[80] Also, 10 739 hysterectomized women were randomized to either conjugated equine estrogens 0.625 mg daily alone or placebo, and followed for a mean duration of 6.8 years.[81] These trials also showed an early increase in clinical coronary events followed by a subsequent decline. Exactly the same estrogen doses were used in these trials in women aged up to 80 years as were used in HERS, ERA, and WAVE.

A common finding of these clinical trials of HRT is an apparent increase in cardiovascular events in the HRT group in the early years of treatment, which appears to diminish in later years (Fig. 26.2). One possible explanation for this observation of 'early harm' is an increase in thrombogenesis, which would be immediate on commencement of the therapy but would also be transient as the hemostatic system of coagulation and fibrinolysis came back into balance. This effect on thrombogenesis would be dose-dependent. Another possibility could be a transient increase in abnormal vascular remodeling with the commencement of HRT, through increases of MMP activity, which again would be dose-dependent. The response of various tissues to different estrogen doses varies with age, both chronological and menopausal, in menopausal women. It is well known that a standard dose of conjugated equine estrogens 0.625 mg causes very little in the way of breast tenderness when commenced in a 50-year-old woman, but can cause profound mastalgia when commenced in a 65-year-old woman. A similar phenomenon is seen in the skeleton, where women aged around 60 years using 17β-estradiol 1 mg daily show the same magnitude of bone density gain as

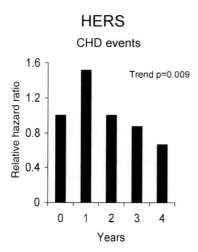

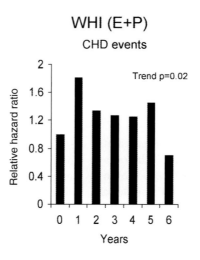

Figure 26.2
Relative hazard ratios of coronary heart disease (CHD) events over time in the Heart and Estrogen/progestin Replacement Study (HERS)[76] and the Women's Health Initiative (WHI) estrogen plus progestogen (E+P) arm.[83] Both studies show significant trends towards reductions over time.

women aged around 50 years using 17β-estradiol 2 mg daily.[82] Older menopausal women appear more sensitive to the effects of estrogens. The use of inappropriately high doses of estrogen in the HERS trial[76] of women of average age 67 years, and in the PHASE trial[78] also of women of average age 67 years, could actually destabilize existing atheromatous plaques, and this effect could have contributed to the early increase in cardiovascular events seen in these studies. Such adverse effects could perhaps have been avoided by the use of lower doses of estrogen. Exactly the same explanation would account for the findings of the WHI trials,[80,81] where the same overall pattern of early harm followed by later reduction was observed. Although the participants in these trials were supposedly free from CHD, the average age of the women was 64 years in the estrogen/progestogen arm, and 65 years in the estrogen-alone arm, and thus varying degrees of atheroma would be present. Yet the starting dose of conjugated equine estrogens was again 0.625 mg.

Paradox between observational and randomized trials of HRT and CHD

Can the discrepancy in the findings of observational studies and randomized trials be explained? With regards to observational studies, they have the disadvantage of being nonrandomized and hence open to selection bias. There is no doubt that users of HRT tend to have fewer cardiovascular risk factors than nonusers. However, large observational studies have sufficient numbers to be able to adjust for such potential confounders. It is therefore not justifiable to dismiss the findings of observational studies purely on the basis of a 'healthy-user' bias. Healthy-user bias would also affect the outcomes of osteoporotic fractures, yet in osteoporosis studies there is no discordance between observational studies and randomized trials. The discrepancy between the results from the observational studies and the randomized clinical trials may be because of differences both in the study populations and in the treatments.

As described above, there are concerns about the dosage of estrogen and the type of progestogen used in the randomized trials. But another critical fact is that the age of the women starting on HRT is around the mid-sixties. Thus the starting dose of HRT used in these trials is inappropriately high for their age. In contrast, women in observational studies, who have themselves chosen to go onto HRT, have mainly done so for the relief of vasomotor symptoms at the menopause. So although in the majority of observational studies, the dose and type of HRT would have been the same as in the randomized trials, namely conjugated equine estrogens 0.625 mg with or without MPA, the starting age would have been around 50 years, some 15 years younger than those in

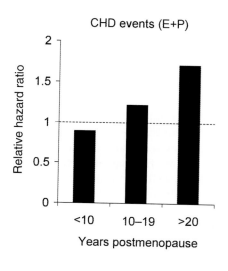

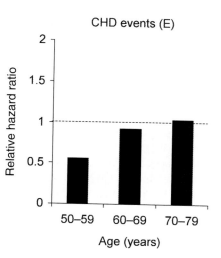

Figure 26.3
Relative hazard ratios of coronary heart disease (CHD) events according to time since menopause in the Women's Health Initiative (WHI) estrogen plus progestogen (E+P) arm,[83] and according to age in the WHI estrogen-alone (E) arm.[81]

the randomized trials. Further support for this concept of different age responses to the same starting dose of estrogen comes from the WHI trials (Fig. 26.3), where in the estrogen-alone arm the risk of CHD was lower in the women aged 50–60 years compared with the later ages.[81] In the estrogen/progestogen arm, this phenomenon was not observed with chronological age but was observed with menopausal age.[83] It has been pointed out that the WHI was not sufficiently powered to demonstrate any reduction in CHD in women aged 50–54 years, the age group most commonly started on HRT for relief of menopausal symptoms.[84]

It has also been speculated that the difference in findings between observational studies and randomized trials is that the age difference means that the younger women in the observational studies have much less likelihood of having diseased arteries when starting on HRT, and that only relatively healthy arteries respond to HRT.[84,85] Studies in primates have shown that early initiation of estrogen therapy is able to inhibit the development of atherosclerosis, but little effect is seen once there is established disease.[85] It could certainly be true that younger menopausal women will respond more favorably to HRT, and these women are not without CHD risk. It has been highlighted that women under age 65 years are more than twice as likely to die from MI than comparably aged men, and that atherosclerosis is already developing in women in their forties and fifties.[86]

However, the notion that there is only a window of opportunity around the menopause transition for commencement of HRT to benefit the cardiovascular system is questionable. There are data from humans, as opposed to the primates, that even diseased arteries will respond favorably to estrogen. Infusion of physiological doses of 17β-estradiol directly into the coronary arteries of women with CHD reversed the vasoconstrictor effect of acetylcholine which occurs in diseased arteries.[87] A second infusion of acetylcholine after the estrogen infusion produced the normal response of vasodilatation and increased blood flow. Furthermore, an estradiol-eluting stent has been shown to reduce restenosis when implanted into diseased coronary arteries.[88] Thus, HRT could still be of benefit to older women with varying degrees of coronary atheroma, provided that the correct starting dose of an appropriate HRT regimen is employed to avoid any early harm and thus reap the later benefit.

Summary

Female CHD is now recognized as one of the major diseases in women, and there is evidence that loss of female sex hormones contributes to its development. There is very sound biological plausibility for beneficial effects of HRT on the cardiovascular system.

Indeed, to suggest that HRT will not benefit the cardiovascular system would require a detailed hypothesis as to how this could occur in the light of the known actions of estrogen, and almost certainly a major revision of our understanding of cardiovascular pathophysiology. Almost all epidemiologic studies have indicated a beneficial effect of HRT on the risk and development of CHD in menopausal women. These findings are largely supported by small clinical studies with a variety of surrogate endpoints. Randomized trials using hard clinical endpoints have failed to show a significant reduction in coronary events from HRT use. This failure may be in part due to the selection of the wrong population in terms of age, but may additionally be due to inappropriate HRT regimens, in terms of dose and possibly type of steroids, being employed. A pattern of early harm followed by later benefit has emerged from these trials. It is plausible that transient adverse effects on thrombogenesis and vascular remodeling are responsible for the early harm, while beneficial effects on metabolic risk factors and arterial function are responsible for the later benefit. It must be appreciated that HRT regimens vary considerably in their metabolic effects, and hence in their cardiovascular effects. Further research is urgently required to define the ideal dose, type, route of administration, and duration of HRT for maximal cardiovascular benefit.

HRT is licensed for use in the relief of menopausal symptoms and the prevention of menopausal osteoporosis, and there is currently nothing more cost-effective for these indications. At present, there is insufficient evidence to justify using HRT solely for the prevention and treatment of CHD in menopausal women.[89] Equally, there is insufficient evidence to justify dismissing HRT as a potential therapy for CHD, or for claiming that it causes overall cardiovascular harm when considering the risks and benefits of HRT use. If HRT use is indicated in women who happen to be at increased CVD risk, it is clearly essential that attention be paid to the starting dose and regimen of steroids used.

Regulatory authorities worldwide have reacted inappropriately to reports of overall harm, rather than benefit, resulting from HRT use. Indeed, the US Food and Drugs Administration (FDA) even issued a 'black box' warning (www.fda.gov). These reactions are largely based on the findings of WHI and the Million Women Study (MWS).[90] It must be remembered that WHI studied women who were not specifically requiring HRT for symptom relief and who were not at increased risk for osteoporosis. These women thus had no indication to take HRT, and in fact the main outcome of the study was that neither benefit nor harm was seen in over 99% of women. This finding is hardly surprising, whereas the overreaction of regulatory authorities is. A small increase in breast cancer diagnosis was seen in the estrogen-progestogen arm, while a small decrease was seen in the estrogen-alone arm. No increase in mortality was seen. MWS was an observational study based on questionnaires completed at study entry and follow-up through the UK National Cancer Registry. The study has been widely criticized because of selection and surveillance biases, and treatment misclassification. Its findings cannot be considered robust, and almost certainly represent a gross overestimation of breast cancer risk. No large prospective randomized trial of HRT risk–benefit has been undertaken in an appropriate population of women who are either requiring menopausal symptom relief or are at increased risk for osteoporosis, and are given an appropriate dose and regimen. In the future, HRT regimens may be devised which prevent CHD, stroke, and dementia, and avoid any increase in breast cancer, stroke, and venous thromboembolism.

References

1. American Heart Association. *Heart Disease and Stroke Statistics – 2003 Update*. Dallas, TX: American Heart Association, 2002.
2. Lerner DJ, Kannel WB. Patterns of coronary heart disease morbidity and mortality in the sexes: a 26-year follow-up of the Framingham population. *Am Heart J* 1986; **111**:383–90.
3. Grady D, Rubin SM, Petitti DB, et al. Hormone

therapy to prevent disease and prolong life in the postmenopausal woman. *Ann Intern Med* 1992; **117**: 1016–37.

4. Gordon T, Kannel WB, Hjortland MC, et al. Menopause and coronary heart disease: the Framingham Study. *Ann Intern Med* 1978; **89**:157–61.

5. Yusuf S, Hawken S, Ounpuu S, et al. Effect of potentially modifiable risk factors associated with myocardial infarction in 52 countries (the INTERHEART study): case–control study. *Lancet* 2004; **364**:937–52.

6. Stevenson JC, Crook D, Godsland IF. Influence of age and menopause on serum lipids and lipoproteins in healthy women. *Atherosclerosis* 1993; **98**:83–90.

7. Godsland IF, Stevenson JC. Insulin resistance: syndrome or tendency? *Lancet* 1995; **346**:100–3.

8. Marroquin OC, Kip KE, Kelley DE, et al. Metabolic syndrome modifies the cardiovascular risk associated with angiographic coronary artery disease in women. *Circulation* 2004; **109**:714–21.

9. Walton C, Godsland IF, Proudler AJ, Wynn V, Stevenson JC. The effects of the menopause on insulin sensitivity, secretion and elimination in non-obese, healthy women. *Eur J Clin Invest* 1993; **23**:466–73.

10. Proudler AJ, Felton CV, Stevenson JC. Ageing and the response of plasma insulin, glucose and C-peptide concentrations to intravenous glucose in postmenopausal women. *Clin Sci* 1992; **83**:489–94.

11. Ley CJ, Lees B, Stevenson JC. Sex- and menopause-associated changes in body-fat distribution. *Am J Clin Nutr* 1992; **55**:950–4.

12. Stevenson JC. Metabolic effects of the menopause and oestrogen replacement. In: Barlow DH (ed.). *Baillière's Clinical Obstetrics and Gynaecology. The Menopause: Key Issues.* London: Ballière Tindall, 1996: 449–67.

13. Spencer CP, Godsland IF, Stevenson JC. Is there a menopausal metabolic syndrome? *Gynecol Endocrinol* 1997; **11**:341–55.

14. Gangar KF, Vyas S, Whitehead M, et al. Pulsatility index in internal carotid artery in relation to transdermal oestradiol and time since menopause. *Lancet* 1991; **338**:839–42.

15. Sanada M, Higashi Y, Nakagawa K, et al. Comparison of forearm endothelial function between premenopausal and postmenopausal women with or without hypercholesterolemia. *Maturitas* 2003; **44**:307–15.

16. Grodstein F, Manson JE, Colditz GA, Willett WC, Speizer FE, Stampfer MJ. A prospective, observational study of postmenopausal hormone therapy and primary prevention of cardiovascular disease. *Ann Intern Med* 2003; **133**:933–41.

17. Godsland IF. Effects of postmenopausal hormone replacement therapy on lipid, lipoprotein, and apolipoprotein (a) concentrations: analysis of studies published from 1974–2000. *Fertil Steril* 2001; **75**:898–915.

18. Whitcroft SI, Crook D, Marsh MS, Ellerington MC, Whitehead MI, Stevenson JC. Long-term effects of oral and transdermal hormone replacement therapies on serum lipid and lipoprotein concentrations. *Obstet Gynecol* 1994; **84**:222–6.

19. Tikkanen MJ, Kuusi T, Vartiainen B, et al. Treatment of postmenopausal hypercholesterolaemia with oestradiol. *Acta Obstet Gynecol* 1979; **88** (Suppl): 83–8.

20. Wolfe BM, Huff MW. Effect of low dosage progestin-only administration upon plasma triglycerides and lipoprotein metabolism in postmenopausal women. *J Clin Invest* 1993; **92**:456–61.

21. van der Mooren MJ, de Graaf J, Demacker PN, et al. Changes in the low-density lipoprotein profile during 17β-oestradiol–dydrogesterone therapy in postmenopausal women. *Metabolism* 1994; **43**:799–802.

22. Stevenson JC, Oladipo A, Manassiev N, Whitehead MI, Guilford S, Proudler AJ. Randomized trial of effect of transdermal continuous combined hormone replacement therapy on cardiovascular risk markers. *Br J Haematol* 2004; **124**:802–8.

23. Crook D, Cust MP, Gangar KF, et al. Comparison of transdermal and oral estrogen/progestin hormone replacement therapy: effects on serum lipids and lipoproteins. *Am J Obstet Gynecol* 1992; **166**:950–5.

24. Spencer C, Crook D, Ross D, Cooper A, Whitehead MI, Stevenson JC. A randomised comparison of the effects of oral versus transdermal 17β-oestradiol, each combined with sequential oral norethisterone acetate, on serum lipoprotein levels. *Br J Obstet Gynaecol* 1999; **106**:948–53.

25. Crook D, Godsland IF, Hull J, Stevenson JC. Hormone replacement therapy with dydrogesterone and oestradiol-17β: effects on serum lipoproteins and glucose tolerance. *Br J Obstet Gynaecol* 1997; **104**: 298–304.

26. The Writing Group for the PEPI Trial. Effects of estrogen or estrogen/progestin regimens on heart disease risk factors in postmenopausal women. The Postmenopausal Estrogen/Progestin Interventions (PEPI) Trial. *JAMA* 1995; **273**:199–208.

27. Sack MN, Rader DJ, Cannon RO. Oestrogen and inhibition of oxidation of low-density lipoproteins in postmenopausal women. *Lancet* 1994; **343**:269–70.

28. Westerveld HT, Kock LAW, van Rijn JM, et al. 17β-Estradiol improves postprandial lipid metabolism in postmenopausal women. *J Clin Endocrinol Metab* 1995; **80**:249–53.

29. Cagnacci A, Soldani R, Carriere PL, et al. Effects of low doses of transdermal 17β-oestradiol on carbohydrate metabolism in postmenopausal women. *J Clin Endocrinol Metab* 1992; **74**:1396–400.

30. Spellacy WN, Buhi WC, Birk SA. The effects of estrogens on carbohydrate metabolism: glucose, insulin and growth hormone studies on one hundred and seventy one women ingesting Premarin, mestranol and ethinyl estradiol for six months. *Am J Obstet Gynecol* 1972; **114**:378–92.

31. Spencer CP, Godsland IF, Cooper AJ, Ross D, Whitehead MI, Stevenson JC. Effects of oral and transdermal 17β-estradiol with cyclical oral norethindrone acetate on insulin sensitivity, secretion, and elimination in postmenopausal women. *Metabolism* 2000; **49**:742–7.

32. Godsland IF, Gangar KF, Walton C, et al. Insulin resistance, secretion, and elimination in postmenopausal women receiving oral or transdermal hormone replacement therapy. *Metabolism* 1993; **42**:846–53.

33. Manassiev NA, Godsland IF, Crook D, Proudler AJ, Whitehead MI, Stevenson JC. Effect of postmenopausal oestradiol and dydrogesterone therapy on lipoproteins and insulin sensitivity, secretion and elimination in hysterectomised women. *Maturitas* 2002; **42**:233–42.

34. Gambacciani M, Ciaponi M, Cappagli B, et al. Body weight, body fat distribution, and hormonal replacement therapy in early postmenopausal women. *J Clin Endocrinol Metab* 1997; **82**:414–17.

35. Winkler UH. Menopause, hormone replacement therapy and cardiovascular disease: a review of haemostaseological findings. *Fibrinolysis* 1992; **6** (Suppl 3):5–10.

36. Stevenson JC. Cardiovascular effects of estrogens. *J Steroid Biochem Mol Biol* 2000; **74**:387–93.

37. Fox J, George AJ, Newton JR, et al. Effect of transdermal oestradiol on the haemostatic balance of menopausal women. *Maturitas* 1993; **18**:55–64.

38. Scarabin P-Y, Oger E, Plu-Bureau G. Differential association of oral and transdermal oestrogen-replacement therapy with venous thromboembolism risk. *Lancet* 2003; **362**:428–32.

39. Stevenson JC. The metabolic and cardiovascular consequences of HRT. *Br J Clin Pract* 1995; **49**:87–90.

40. Marsh MS, Whitehead M, Stevenson J. *Hormone Replacement Therapy and Cardiovascular Disease.* London: Martin Dunitz, 1996.

41. Hassager C, Christiansen C. Blood pressure during oestrogen/progestogen substitution therapy in healthy postmenopausal women. *Maturitas* 1988; **9**: 315–23.

42. Wingrove CS, Garr E, Pickar JH, Dey M, Stevenson JC. Effects of equine oestrogens on markers of vasoactive function in human coronary artery endothelial cells. *Mol Cell Endocrinol* 1999; **150**:33–7.

43. Stefano GB, Prevot V, Beauvillain JC, et al. Cell-surface estrogen receptors mediate calcium-dependent nitric oxide release in human endothelia. *Circulation* 2000; **101**:1594–7.

44. Wingrove CS, Stevenson JC. 17β-Oestradiol inhibits stimulated endothelin-1 release from human vascular endothelial cells. *Eur J Endocrinol* 1997; **137**:205–8.

45. Jiang C, Sarrel P, Lindsay D, et al. Endothelium-independent relaxation of rabbit coronary artery by 17β-oestradiol *in vitro*. *Br J Pharmacol* 1991; **104**:1033–7.

46. Jiang C, Poole-Wilson PA, Sarrel PM, et al. Effect of 17β-oestradiol on contraction, Ca^{2+} current and intracellular free Ca^{2+} in guinea-pig isolated cardiac myocytes. *Br J Pharmacol* 1992; **106**:739–45.

47. White RE, Darkow DJ, Falvo Lang JL. Estrogen relaxes coronary arteries by opening BK_{Ca} channels through a cGMP-dependent mechanism. *Circ Res* 1995; **77**:936–42.

48. Buikema H, Pinto YM, Rooks G, et al. The deletion polymorphism of the angiotensin-converting enzyme gene is related to phenotypic differences in human arteries. *Eur Heart J* 1996; **17**:787–94.

49. Schuster H, Wienker TF, Stremmler U, et al. An angiotensin-converting enzyme gene variant is associated with acute myocardial infarction in women but not in men. *Am J Cardiol* 1995; **76**:601–3.

50. Proudler AJ, Ahmed AIH, Crook D, et al. Hormone replacement therapy and serum angiotensin-converting-enzyme activity in postmenopausal women. *Lancet* 1995; **346**:89–90.

51. Proudler AJ, Cooper A, Whitehead MI, Stevenson JC. Effect of oestrogen-only and oestrogen–progestogen replacement therapy upon circulating angiotensin I-converting enzyme activity in postmenopausal women. *Clin Endocrinol* 2003; **58**:30–5.

52. Koh KK, Cardillo C, Bui MN, et al. Vascular effects of oestrogen and cholesterol lowering therapies in hypercholesterolaemic postmenopausal women. *Circulation* 1999; **99**:354–60.

53. Koh KK, Bui MN, Mincemoyer R, Cannon RO. Effects of hormone therapy on inflammatory cell adhesion molecules in postmenopausal healthy women. *Am J Cardiol* 1997; **80**:1505–7.

54. Pradhan AD, Manson JE, Rossouw JE, et al. Inflammatory biomarkers, hormone replacement therapy, and incident coronary heart disease: prospective analysis from the Women's Health

Initiative observational study. *JAMA* 2002; **288**: 980–7.

55. Post MS, van der Mooren MJ, Stehouwer CD, et al. Effects of transdermal and oral oestrogen replacement therapy on C-reactive protein levels in postmenopausal women: a randomised, placebo-controlled trial. *Thromb Haemostasis* 2002; **88**:605–10.

56. Dollery CM, McEwan JR, Henney AM. Matrix metalloproteinases and cardiovascular disease. *Circ Res* 1995; **77**:863–8.

57. Wingrove CS, Garr E, Godsland IF, et al. 17β-Oestradiol enhances release of matrix metalloproteinase-2 from human vascular smooth muscle cells. *Biochim Biophys Acta* 1998; **1406**:169–74.

58. Stampfer MJ, Grodstein F. Role of hormone replacement in cardiovascular disease. In: Lobo RA (ed). *Treatment of the Postmenopausal Woman: Basic and Clinical Aspects*. New York: Raven Press, 1994: 223–33.

59. Schlipak MG, Angeja BG, Go AS, Frederick PD, Canto JG, Grady D. Hormone therapy and in-hospital survival after myocardial infarction in postmenopausal women. *Circulation* 2001; **104**:2300–9.

60. Sullivan JM, Zwaag RV, Hughes JP, et al. Estrogen replacement therapy and coronary artery disease. *Arch Intern Med* 1990; **150**:2557–62.

61. Gerhard M, Walsh BW, Tawakol A, et al. Estradiol therapy combined with progesterone and endothelium-dependent vasodilation in postmenopausal women. *Circulation* 1998; **98**:1158–63.

62. Higashi Y, Sanada M, Sasaki S, et al. Effect of estrogen replacement therapy on endothelial function in peripheral resistance arteries in normotensive and hypertensive postmenopausal women. *Hypertension* 2001; **37**:651–67.

63. Rosano GM, Sarrel PM, Poole-Wilson PA, et al. Beneficial effect of oestrogen on exercise-induced myocardial ischaemia in women with coronary artery disease. *Lancet* 1993; **342**:133–6.

64. Alpaslan M, Shimokawa H, Kuroiwa-Matsumoto M, et al. Short-term estrogen administration ameliorates dobutamine-induced myocardial ischemia in postmenopausal women with coronary artery disease. *J Am Coll Cardiol* 1997; **30**:1466–71.

65. Rosano GM, Caixeta AM, Chierchia S, et al. Short-term anti-ischemic effect of 17β-estradiol in postmenopausal women with coronary artery disease. *Circulation* 1997; **96**:2837–41.

66. Webb CM, Rosano GM, Collins P. Oestrogen improves exercise-induced myocardial ischaemia in women. *Lancet* 1998; **351**:1556–7.

67. Angerer P, Stork S, Kothny W, Schmitt P, von Schacky C. Effect of oral postmenopausal hormone replacement on progression of atherosclerosis: a randomized, controlled trial. *Arterioscler Thromb Vasc Biol* 2001; **21**:262–8.

68. de Kleijn MJ, Bots ML, Bak AA, et al. Hormone replacement therapy in perimenopausal women and 2-year change of carotid intima-media thickness. *Maturitas* 1999; **32**:195–204.

69. Hodis HN, Mack WJ, Lobo RA, *et al*. Estrogen in the prevention of atherosclerosis. A randomized, double-blind, placebo-controlled trial. *Ann Intern Med* 2001; **135**:939–53.

70. Espeland MA, Applegate W, Furberg CD, Lefkowitz D, Rice L, Hunninghake D. Estrogen replacement therapy and progression of intimal-medial thickness in the carotid arteries of postmenopausal women. ACAPS Investigators. Asymptomatic Carotid Atherosclerosis Progression Study. *Am J Epidemiol* 1995; **142**:1011–19.

71. Byington RP, Furberg CD, Herrington DM, et al. Effect of estrogen plus progestin on progression of carotid atherosclerosis in postmenopausal women with heart disease: HERS B-mode substudy. *Arterioscler Thromb Vasc Biol* 2002; **22**:1692–7.

72. Herrington DM, Reboussin DM, Brosnihan BK, et al. Effects of estrogen replacement on the progression of coronary-artery atherosclerosis. *N Engl J Med* 2000; **343**:522–9.

73. Waters DD, Alderman EL, Hsia J, et al. Effects of hormone replacement therapy and antioxidant vitamin supplements on coronary atherosclerosis in postmenopausal women: a randomized controlled trial. *JAMA* 2002; **288**:2432–40.

74. Brown BG, Zhao XQ, Sacco DE, et al. Lipid lowering and plaque regression: new insights into prevention of plaque disruption and clinical events in coronary disease. *Circulation* 1993; **87**:1781–91.

75. Le Gal G, Gourlet V, Hogrel P, Plu-Bureau G, Touboul PJ, Scarabin PY. Hormone replacement therapy use is associated with a lower occurrence of carotid atherosclerotic plaques but not with intima-media thickness progression among postmenopausal women. The vascular aging (EVA) study. *Atherosclerosis* 2003; **166**:163–70.

76. Hulley S, Grady D, Bush T, et al. Randomized trial of estrogen plus progestin for secondary prevention of coronary heart disease in postmenopausal women. *JAMA* 1998; **280**:605–13.

77. Stevenson JC, Flather M, Collins P. Coronary heart disease in women. *N Engl J Med* 2000; **343**:1891–4.

78. Clarke SC, Kelleher J, Lloyd-Jones H, Slack M, Schofiel PM. A study of hormone replacement

therapy in postmenopausal women with ischaemic heart disease: the Papworth HRT atherosclerosis study. *Br J Obstet Gynaecol* 2002; **109**:1056–62.

79. Cherry N, Gilmour K, Hannaford P, et al. Oestrogen therapy for prevention of reinfarction in postmenopausal women: a randomised placebo controlled trial. *Lancet* 2002; **360**:2001–8.

80. Writing Group for the Women's Health Initiative Investigators. Risks and benefits of estrogen plus progestin in healthy postmenopausal women. *JAMA* 2002; **288**:321–33.

81. Women's Health Initiative Steering Committee. Effects of conjugated equine estrogen in postmenopausal women with hysterectomy. *JAMA* 2004; **291**:1701–12.

82. Lees B, Stevenson JC. The prevention of osteoporosis using sequential low-dose hormone replacement therapy with estradiol-17β and dydrogesterone. *Osteoporosis Int* 2001; **12**:251–8.

83. Manson JE, Hsia J, Johnson KC, et al. Estrogen plus progestin and the risk of coronary heart disease. *N Engl J Med* 2003; **349**:523–34.

84. Naftolin F, Taylor HS, Karas R, et al. The Women's Health Initiative could not have detected cardioprotective effects of starting hormone therapy during the menopause transition. *Fertil Steril* 2004; **81**: 1498–501.

85. Mikkola TS, Clarkson TB. Estrogen replacement therapy, atherosclerosis, and vascular function. *Cardiovasc Res* 2002; **53**:605–19.

86. Wenger NK. You've come a long way, baby. Cardiovascular health and disease in women: problems and prospects. *Circulation* 2004; **109**:558–60.

87. Collins P, Rosano GM, Sarrel PM, et al. 17β-Estradiol attenuates acetylcholine-induced coronary arterial constriction in women but not men with coronary heart disease. *Circulation* 1995; **92**:24–30.

88. Abizaid A, Albertal M, Costa MA, et al. First human experience with the 17β-estradiol-eluting stent. *J Am Assoc Cardiol* 2004; **43**:1118–21.

89. Mosca L, Appel LJ, Benjamin EJ, et al. Evidence-based guidelines for cardiovascular disease prevention in women. *Circulation* 2004; **109**:672–93.

90. Million Women Study Collaborators. Breast cancer and hormone-replacement therapy in the Million Women Study. *Lancet* 2003; **362**:419–27.

27

Polycystic ovary syndrome

Kalpana Lakhani and Paul Hardiman

Introduction

Women with polycystic ovary syndrome (PCOS) typically present to their general practitioner, gynecologist or endocrinologist with menstrual irregularity, infertility, obesity, or androgenic symptoms of hirsutism or acne. Underlying these symptoms however, is a range of endocrine and metabolic abnormalities, which predispose these women to type 2 diabetes and cardiovascular disease (CVD). This view of the syndrome as a multisystem disorder dates back to 1980 when Burghen et al.[1] identified the central role of insulin resistance in women with PCOS. Since that time it has been found to be associated with obesity,[2–5] lipid abnormalities,[6–8] impaired glucose tolerance,[9–11] insulin resistance,[12] hypertension,[7,13] and higher circulating levels of plasminogen activator inhibitor.[14]

Interpretation of studies designed to assess cardiovascular risk markers, morbidity, and mortality in women with PCOS has been hindered by the lack of an agreed definition of the syndrome. Although at least 20% of young women have polycystic ovaries (PCO),[15,16] only between one- and three-quarters of these have symptoms of infertility, menstrual irregularity or hirsutism, consistent with the diagnosis of PCOS.[15–17] The definition used in North America did not include ultrasound features, but used clinical symptoms such as anovulation and/or hyperandrogenism as diagnostic criteria, with endocrine results used to exclude conditions including adult-onset congenital adrenal hyperplasia, hyperprolactinemia, and androgen-secreting neoplasms.[18] By contrast in Europe greater emphasis has been placed on ultrasound diagnosis of PCO which is considered by many to be the essential phenotype.[19] However, a consensus was reached in 2003 in which the syndrome is diagnosed when at least two of the following criteria are met: chronic anovulation, clinical or biochemical hyperandrogenism, ultrasound features of PCO.

The clinical features of the syndrome in relation to coronary heart disease

Signs of hyperandrogenism, hirsutism and acne, have been identified as common features in women with PCOS undergoing cardiac catheterization and are associated with more severe disease.[20] However, since rates of cardiovascular disease are low in premenopausal women and androgen levels in women with PCOS normalize before menopause,[21] so that they are similar to those in healthy women,[22] the association between hyperandrogenemia and coronary heart disease in women with the syndrome is unproven.

The results of the Dutch Breast Cancer Screening Study demonstrated an increased incidence of anovulatory cycles during reproductive years in women who later developed CVD.[23] Data from a large cohort of over 82 000 female nurses in the Nurses Health Study[24] showed that women reporting irregular cycles had an increased risk of fatal and nonfatal coronary heart disease (CHD) compared with women with normal menstrual cycles, even after adjusting for confounding factors including family history and personal exercise history. There was also a nonsignificant increase in overall stroke risk associated with irregular cycles. This study also identified oligomenorrhea and irregular menstrual cycles as risk factors for developing type 2 diabetes mellitus, a major risk factor in itself for CVD, especially in women.[25]

Obesity, one of the features of the original description of the syndrome by Stein and Leventhal,[26] is seen in 35–60% of women with PCOS.[2] Typically this obesity is 'centripetal', related to truncal abdominal fat distribution as demonstrated by an increased waist to hip ratio[3,4] as opposed to the thighs and hips (gluteofemoral fat). Hyperandrogenism is associated with a preponderance of fat localized to truncal abdominal sites.[27] This distribution is seen even with a body mass index (BMI) within normal range[28] and correlates with insulin resistance.[29] Recently, Elting and colleagues[5] reported that obesity, rather than menstrual cycle pattern, is more closely associated with hyperinsulinemia, hyperlipidemia, and hypertension in older women. Epidemiologic studies have shown that this pattern of fat distribution, independent of body weight, is an important predictor of diabetes,[30] hyperinsulinemia,[31] hyperlipidemia,[32] and CVD.[33]

Signs of hyperandrogenism, hirsutism, and acne have been identified as common features in women with PCOS undergoing cardiac catheterization and are associated with more severe disease.[20] However, since rates of CVD are low in premenopausal women and androgen levels in women with PCOS normalize before menopause[21] so that they are similar to those in healthy women,[22] the association between hyperandrogenemia and CHD in women with the syndrome is unproven.

Cardiovascular risk factors in women with PCOS

Glucose intolerance and diabetes mellitus

The link between hyperandrogenemia and abnormal carbohydrate metabolism was first suggested in the early 1920s by Archard and Thiers, who described the phenomenon as 'le diabetes des femmes à barbe'.[34] Fifty years later Kahn and co-workers[35] described the syndrome of insulin resistance in six young women with acanthosis nigricans. Two of these women also had polycystic ovarian morphology, diagnosed by gynecography in one case and on laparoscopy in the other, with hirsutism, primary amenorrhoea, and elevated testosterone levels; one was virilized, although neither of them was obese. This presentation, however, is rare and represents an extreme degree of insulin resistance in PCOS.

An association between hyperandrogenism and hyperinsulinemia was suggested by Burghen et al. in 1980,[1] who reported increased insulin concentrations and a correlation between basal insulin measurements with both testosterone and androstenedione in eight obese PCOS women compared with controls. Chang et al.[36] subsequently reported hyperinsulinemia in nonobese PCOS subjects and insulin resistance has been reported in both lean and obese women with PCOS.[37–39] However, others have failed to demonstrate insulin resistance in nonobese subjects.[37–41] Overall, the prevalence of insulin resistance in women with PCOS in the US is in the range of 30–60%,[12] whereas glucose intolerance is found in 8–40%.[9,10]

Data from several long-term follow-up studies have shown the prevalence of diabetes to be three to seven times higher in PCOS women compared with the general population.[42–45] Similarly in an extension of the only mortality study of women with the syndrome,[43] Wild and colleagues[44] found that diabetes-related morbidity and mortality were higher than expected in the women with PCOS. In a longitudinal study of PCOS women followed for an average of 6.2 years, Norman et al.[46] reported that of those who are initially normoglycemic, 9% develop impaired glucose tolerance (IGT) and 8% noninsulin-dependent diabetes (NIDDM), whereas 54% with of those with IGT at the start develop NIDDM.

Dyslipidemia

As shown in Table 27.1,[6–8,13,47–55] most published studies (including those which included weight-matched controls) have shown a degree of dyslipidemia in women with PCOS. There is, however, less agreement as to which lipid subfractions are

Table 27.1 Summary of lipid profiles in women with polycystic ovary syndrome

Author	Subjects/controls	Total cholesterol	LDL cholesterol	HDL cholesterol	Triglycerides
Wild et al.[6]*		↔	↔	↓	↑
Graf et al.[49]	Lean/lean	↔	↔	↓	↑
Graf et al.[49]	Obese/obese	↔	↔	↓	↔
Mahabeer et al.[48]	Lean/lean	↑	↑	↔	↑
Mahabeer et al.[48]	Obese/obese	↑	↑	↓	↔
Slowinska-Srzednicka et al.[50]	Obese/lean	↔	↔	↓	↑
Conway et al.[7]	Lean/lean	↔	Not measured	↓	↔
Conway et al.[7]	Obese/obese	↔	Not measured	↓	↑
Holte et al.[51]	Lean/lean	↑	↑	↓	↑
Holte et al.[51]	Obese/obese	↔	↔	↔	↔
Talbott et al.[13]*		↑	↑	↓	↑
Norman et al.[52]*		↔	↔	↓	↔
Robinson et al,[53]	Lean/lean	↔	↔	↔	↔
Robinson et al.[53]	Obese/obese	↔	↔	↓	↑
Talbott et al. <40 years[8]		↑	↑	↔	↔
Talbott et al. >40 years[8]		↔	↔	↔	↑
Legro et al.[54]		↔	↔	↔	↔
Mather et al.[55]*		Not measured	↑	↓	↔ After adjusting for lifestyle factors
Legro et al.[47]	Lean/lean	↑	↑	↔	↔
Legro et al.[47]	Obese/obese	↑	↑	↑	↑

LDL, low-density lipoprotein; HDL, high-density lipoprotein; ? ↔, no difference; ↓, decreased; ↑, increased.
*Not stratified by weight.

affected.[7] Nearly half of these studies demonstrate higher levels of triglycerides and low-density lipoprotein (LDL) cholesterol, with slightly more showing reduced high-density lipoprotein (HDL) levels and slightly fewer reporting increased total cholesterol, compared with unaffected controls. On the other hand Legro et al.[47] reported higher levels of HDL in PCOS women compared with controls. As discussed previously, these conflicting results probably reflect differences in the criteria for defining cases and controls and the confounding effects of BMI.

Hypertension

Studies that have examined blood pressure in young women with PCOS have also produced discrepant results. Conway et al.[7] reported higher systolic pressure in young obese women with PCOS compared with women with normal ovaries; however, the latter were not matched for BMI. In the Swedish follow-up study, the prevalence of treated hypertension was three times greater in women with a history of PCOS.[42] Talbott et al.[13] also found higher systolic blood pressure in women with PCOS prior to controlling for the confounding effect of BMI, but not on multivariate analysis after adjusting for BMI. Mahabeer et al.[48] reported higher systolic and diastolic pressures among both lean and obese women with PCOS compared with lean and obese control women. On the other hand, 24-hour blood pressure recording[56] in young PCOS women with matched controls did reveal higher mean and systolic blood pressures. Elting et al.[5] evaluated 346 women (mean age 38.7 years; mean BMI 24.4 kg/m²) with PCOS and reported an increased prevalence of hypertension (2.5-fold) than in a corresponding age group of the Dutch female population.

Other studies with adequately matched controls failed to provide evidence of hypertension in women with PCOS.[57,58] In a recent study in a Czech population, the prevalence of hypertension was not increased among women diagnosed with PCOS on wedge resection performed more than 20 years earlier.[45] Further studies are therefore required to clarify whether PCOS is an independent risk factor for increased blood pressure.

Atherosclerosis

The combination of dyslipidemia and hyperinsulinemia would suggest that PCOS women might have accelerated vascular disease. Wild et al.[20] reported increased rates of hirsutism, central obesity, diabetes, and hypertension in both pre- and postmenopausal women with coronary artery stenosis on cardiac catheterization than in women without such lesions. Guzick and colleagues[59] reported increased intima-media thickness (IMT) in the carotid artery, an indication of subclinical atherosclerosis, in PCOS women compared with control women. Similarly, Talbott et al.[8] in a larger study reported increased IMT in PCOS women aged 45 years or more compared with controls; the difference remained significant after adjusting for age and BMI. However, in younger women aged between 30 and 44 years, no significant difference in IMT was found between those with PCOS and controls, although a higher proportion of those with PCOS had a higher atherosclerotic index (the overall mean of the IMT mean measurements at eight sites) compared with controls. More recently, we have reported a higher prevalence of carotid plaque index (sum of plaque grades across right and left carotid arteries) in PCOS women compared with age-matched controls.[60] Similarly in a study using an automatic arterial wall track system, we reported increased IMT in the common carotid and femoral arteries in young PCOS women compared with controls independent of blood pressure, BMI, and lipid levels.[61] Further evidence of an association with atherosclerosis was provided by Birdsall et al.,[62] who reported that women with ultrasound features of PCO had more coronary artery segments with greater than 50% stenosis and a trend towards greater severity of CHD than women with normal ovaries. Similarly, Christian et al.[63] reported increased coronary artery calcification (odds ratio, 2.52), assessed using electron beam computed tomography in PCOS women aged 30–45 years, who were matched to two control women by age and BMI (odds ratio, 5.5).

Hemodynamic studies

Hemodynamic studies in women with PCOS have largely been confined to the pelvic vasculature. However Prelevic et al. reported decreased flow velocity over the aortic arch[64] and increased forearm blood flow[65] in young women with PCOS compared with age-matched controls. Using pulsed Doppler ultrasound, we found reduced vascular tone in the internal carotid artery[66] in young women with PCOS as well as those with ultrasound features of PCO (but with no clinical or biochemical features of the syndrome) compared with control women with normal ovaries on ultrasound. This decrease was independent of blood pressure, insulin resistance, and other endocrine and metabolic parameters.

There is also evidence of altered vascular responsiveness in PCOS women. We found a paradoxical constrictor response to 5% carbon dioxide, a known vasodilator,[67] in the internal carotid artery in young women with PCOS, as well as in those with ultrasound evidence of PCO with no clinical or biochemical features of the syndrome, compared with control women with normal ovaries on ultrasound. A similar paradoxical constrictor response to glyceryl trinitrite has also been reported in the uterine artery.[68] In obese PCOS women, the impairment of methacholine chloride-induced dilatation correlated directly with insulin resistance and hyperandrogenemia[69] and returned to normal with insulin-sensitizing agents,[70] suggesting endothelial dysfunction in these women.

Impaired viscoelastic properties have been demonstrated in PCOS women. Using an echo-locked arterial wall track system, we found decreased vascular compliance and increased vascular stiffness index in the common and internal carotid arteries[71] in young PCOS women.

Surrogate markers of CVD

Metabolic derangements of PCOS overlap with those of the metabolic syndrome (a combination of glucose intolerance, lipid abnormalities, and hypertension).[72] In a recent study, 22% of women with PCOS were found to have the metabolic syndrome (compared with 8% of the controls) but the prevalence was not significantly increased in women with significant ultrasound features of PCO (disregarding symptoms), compared with those without these features.[73]

The view of PCOS as a condition associated with increased cardiovascular morbidity has been supported by the finding of associations with newer risk markers. Thus levels of plasminogen activator inhibitor-1 and fibrinogen, both of which increase thrombosis and atherogenesis through a number of mechanisms affecting hemostasis, blood rheology, and platelet aggregation, are also increased.[14] Similarly increased levels of endothelin-1, a marker of atherogenesis, have been found in both obese and nonobese women with PCOS.[74] Recently Kelly et al.[75] reported higher levels of C-reactive protein (CRP) in women with PCOS than in controls. The levels were positively correlated with BMI and inversely with insulin sensitivity. This is of interest because CRP may be an independent risk marker for CVD.[76–79] CRP is increased after myocardial infarction and seems to be a predictor of future cardiovascular events.[80] Plasma levels of homocysteine are also significantly increased in PCOS women compared with controls. This increase, which was independent of insulin and lipid profiles,[81] is of interest because hyperhomocysteinemia is associated with early atherosclerosis and is considered another independent risk for cardiovascular mortality.[82] There is, moreover, some evidence of a significant reduction in homocysteine concentrations as a result of exercise in young obese PCOS women.[83]

Cardiovascular mortality

Dahlgren et al.,[42] using a mathematical model, estimated that women with PCOS have a 7.4-fold increased risk of cardiovascular events. Recently, in a cross-sectional study to investigate the relationship between age and metabolic factors on cardiovascular risk, Macut et al.[84] reported that the adolescent (mean age 16.9 years), obese (BMI 35.04 kg/m²), and adult PCOS group (mean age 29.66 years; BMI 34.57 kg/m²) cohorts are at increased risk of CVD in later life.

In the only published study of mortality in PCOS women[43] the diagnosis was based on histological examination of ovarian wedge biopsies; clinical indices such as androgen excess and irregular menstrual cycle were not assessed. In this large study with an average follow-up of 30 years, all-cause mortality was not higher than the national rates for women of the same age. Of the total of 59 deaths, 15 were from circulatory disease (standardized mortality ratio (SMR) 0.83; 95% confidence interval (CI) 0.46–1.36); 13 deaths were from CHD (SMR 1.40; 95% CI 0.75–2.40) and two deaths were from other circulatory disease. Deaths from type 2 diabetes were higher than expected. The authors concluded that women with PCOS do not have increased mortality rates from circulatory disease, although the condition is associated with cardiovascular risk factors. Several reasons have been put forward to explain this surprising finding. Firstly, the diagnosis was based on ovarian morphology, which is not the same as PCOS. Secondly, many records were not retrieved, raising the possibility of selection bias. Thirdly, most of the subjects in this study resided in the south of England, but their mortality rate was compared with national data, thereby failing to take account of regional differences in cardiovascular mortality. It has also been suggested that the cause of death recorded on the death certificate may be misleading in diabetic patients who die from cardiovascular complications. Alternatively, however, the finding of no increase in cardiovascular mortality may be correct, in spite of the associated risk factors, and may be indicative of some protective factor such as increased levels of vascular endothelial growth factor.

Summary

Nearly 70 years since PCOS was first described, and more than 20 years after the link with hyperinsulinemia was reported, the long-term consequences of the syndrome are often overlooked. Insulin resistance is now known to underlie a cluster of cardiovascular risk factors including hypertension, dyslipidemia, and fibrinolytic disturbances. Consequently many doctors recommend cardiovascular risk assessment either for all patients with the syndrome or those they perceive to be at greatest risk, for example women who are also overweight, although the benefits of this strategy have yet to be proven. Aside from measurement of blood pressure, this assessment usually includes a fasting lipid profile and screening for glucose intolerance. For patients in whom these tests reveal hypertension, dyslipidemia or diabetes, treatment should follow standard guidelines, as there is currently no evidence that the relationship of these abnormalities to CVD is any different in women who have PCOS to those who do not. More controversially however, some doctors advocate long-term treatment (with metformin) for all women with PCOS.[85] This practice has been criticized[86] on the basis that an association between increased cardiovascular mortality and PCOS, let alone the benefits of any intervention to prevent this increase, are unproven. On the other hand, it does not seem reasonable to deny women with the syndrome treatment for the next 20 or 30 years that may be required to accumulate this evidence. At the very least doctors, whether gynecologists, endocrinologists, general practitioners or cardiologists, should advise their patients of the current evidence in relation to cardiovascular risk and recommend lifestyle modifications, including a balanced low-calorie, low-carbohydrate diet and regular exercise, as these have been found to attenuate these risk factors in PCOS women. At the same time, researchers in these disciplines must collaborate to quantify the degree of cardiovascular morbidity and mortality associated with PCOS, to assess the feasibility of screening and ultimately the effectiveness of lifestyle modification and pharmacologic treatment for these women.

References

1. Burghen GA, Givens JR, Kitabehi AE. Correlation of hyperandrogenism with hyperinsulinaemia in polycystic ovarian disease. *J Clin Endocrinol Metab* 1980; **50**:113–16.

2. Balen AH, Conway GS, Kaltsas G, et al. Polycystic ovary syndrome: the spectrum of the disorder in 1741 patients. *Hum Reprod* 1995; **10**:2107–11.

3. Evans DJ, Barth JH, Burke CW. Body fat topography in women with androgen excess. *Int J Obes* 1988; **12**:157–62.

4. Pasquali R, Casimirri F, Cantobelli S, et al. Insulin and androgen relationships with abdominal body fat distribution in women with and without hyperandrogenism. *Horm Res* 1993; **39**:179–87.

5. Elting MW, Korsen TJ, Schoemaker J. Obesity, rather than menstrual cycle pattern or follicle cohort size, determines hyperinsulinaemia, dyslipidaemia and hypertension in ageing women with polycystic ovary syndrome. *Clin Endocrinol (Oxf)* 2001; **55**:767–76.

6. Wild RA, Painter PC, Coulson PB, Carruth KB, Ranney GB. Lipoprotein lipid concentrations and cardiovascular risk in women with polycystic ovary syndrome. *J Clin Endocrinol Metab* 1985; **61**:946–51.

7. Conway GS, Agrawal R, Betteridge DJ, Jacobs HS. Risk factors for coronary artery disease in lean and obese women with the polycystic ovary syndrome. *Clin Endocrinol (Oxf)* 1992; **37**:119–25.

8. Talbott E, Clerici A, Berga SL, et al. Adverse lipid and coronary heart disease risk profiles in young women with polycystic ovary syndrome: results of a case–control study. *J Clin Epidemiol* 1998; **51**:415–22.

9. Robinson S, Kiddy D, Gelding SV, et al. The relationship of insulin insensitivity to menstrual pattern in women with hyperandrogenism and polycystic ovaries. *Clin Endocrinol (Oxf)* 1993; **39**:351–5.

10. Dunaif A, Graf M, Mandeli J, Laumas V, Dobrjansky A. Characterization of groups of hyperandrogenic women with acanthosis nigricans, impaired glucose tolerance, and/or hyperinsulinemia. *J Clin Endocrinol Metab* 1987; **65**:499–507.

11. Conway GS, Jacobs HS, Holly JM, Wass JA. Effects of luteinzing hormone, insulin, insulin-like growth factor I and insulin-like growth factor small protein I in polycystic ovary syndrome. *Clin Endocrinol (Oxf)* 1990; **33**:593–603.

12. Dunaif A. Polycystic ovary syndrome. In: Givens JR, Haseltine F, Merriam GR (eds). *Current Issues in Endocrinology and Metabolism.* Cambridge, MA: Blackwell Scientific, 1992: 248–60.

13. Talbott E, Guzick D, Clerici A, et al. Coronary heart disease risk factors in women with polycystic ovary syndrome. *Arterioscler Thromb Vasc Biol* 1995; **15**:821–6.

14. Atiomo WU, Bates SA, Condon JE, Shaw S, West JH,

Prentice AG. The plasminogen activator system in women with polycystic ovary syndrome. *Fertil Steril* 1998; **69**:236–41.

15. Clayton RN, Ogden V, Hodgkinson J, et al. How common are polycystic ovaries in normal women and what is their significance for the fertility of the population? *Clin Endocrinol (Oxf)* 1992; **37**:127–34.

16. Polson DW, Adams J, Wadsworth J, Franks S. Polycystic ovaries – a common finding in normal women. *Lancet* 1988; **1**:870–2.

17. Dunaif A. Insulin resistance and the polycystic ovary syndrome: mechanism and implications for pathogenesis. *Endocr Rev* 1997; **18**:774–800.

18. Zawdaki JK, Dunaif A. Diagnostic criteria for polycsytic ovary syndrome: towards a rational approach. In: Dunaif A, Givens JR, Haseltine F, Merriam GR (eds). *Polycystic Ovary Syndrome*. Boston: Blackwell, 1992: 377–84.

19. Adams J, Franks S, Polson DW, et al. Multifollicular ovaries: clinical and endocrine features and response to pulsatile gonadotropin releasing hormone. *Lancet* 1985; **2**:1375–9.

20. Wild RA, Grubb B, Hartz A, Van Nort JJ, Bachman W, Bartholomew M. Clinical signs of androgen excess as risk factors for coronary artery disease. *Fertil Steril* 1990; **54**:255–9.

21. Winters SJ, Talbott E, Guzick DS, Zborowski JV, McHugh KP. Serum testosterone levels decrease in middle age in women with polycystic ovary syndrome. *Fertil Steril* 2000; **73**:724–9.

22. Davis SR, Burger HG. Clinical review 82: androgens and the postmenopausal women. *J Clin Endocrinol Metab* 1996; **81**:2759–63.

23. Gorgles WJ, van der Graaf Y, Blankenstein MA, Collette HJ, Erkelens DW. Urinary sex hormone excretions in premenopausal women and coronary heart disease: a nested case–referent study in the DOM-cohort. *J Clin Epidemiol* 1997; **50**:275–81.

24. Solomon CG, Hu FB, Dunaif A, et al. Menstrual cycle irregularity and risk for future cardiovascular disease. *J Clin Endocrinol Metab* 2002; **87**:2013–17.

25. Solomon CG, Hu FB, Dunaif A, et al. Long or highly irregular menstrual cycles as a marker for risk of type 2 diabetes mellitus. *JAMA* 2001; **286**:2421–6.

26. Stein IF, Leventhal ML. Amenorrhoea associated with bilateral polycystic ovaries. *Am J Obstet Gynecol* 1935; **29**:181–91.

27. Evans DJ, Hoffman DG, Kalkhoff RK, Kissebah AH. Relationship of androgenic activity in body fat topography, fat cell morphology and metabolic aberrations in premenopausal women. *J Clin Endocrinol Metab* 1983; **57**:304–10.

28. Bringer J, Lefebvre P, Boulet F, et al. Body composition and regional fat distribution in polycystic ovarian syndrome. Relationship to hormonal and metabolic profiles. *Ann N Y Acad Sci* 1993; **687**:115–23.

29. Rebuffe-Scrive M, Cullberg G, Lundberg PA, Lindstedt G, Bjorntorp P. Anthropometric variables and metabolism in polycystic ovarian disease. *Horm Metab Res* 1989; **21**:391–7.

30. Hartz AJ, Rupley DC, Rimm AA. The association of girth measurements with disease in 32,856 women. *Am J Epidemiol* 1984; **119**:71–80.

31. Haffner SM, Fong D, Hazuda HP, Pugh JA, Patterson JK. Hyperinsulinemia, upper body adiposity, and cardiovascular risk factors in non-diabetics. *Metabolism* 1988; **37**:338–45.

32. Freedman DS, Jacobsen SJ, Barboriak JJ, et al. Body fat distribution and male/female differences in lipids and lipoproteins. *Circulation* 1990; **81**:1498–506.

33. Folsom AR, Kaye SA, Sellers TA, et al. Body fat distribution and 5-year risk of death in older women. *JAMA* 1993; **269**:483–7.

34. Archard G, Thiers H. Hirsutes and its link with glycolytic insufficiency (diabetes of the bearded women). *Bull Acad Natl Med* 1921; **86**:51–85.

35. Kahn CR, Flier JS, Bar RS, Archal JA, Gorden P. The syndrome of insulin resistance and acanthosis nigricans. *N Engl J Med* 1976; **294**:739–45.

36. Chang RJ, Nakamura RM, Judd H, Kaplan SA. Insulin resistance in nonobese patients with polycystic ovary syndrome. *J Clin Endocrinol Metab* 1983; **57**:356–9.

37. Plymate SR, Matej LA, Jones RE, Friedl KE. Inhibition of sex hormone-binding globulin production in the human hepatoma (Hep G2) cell line by insulin and prolactin. *J Clin Endocrinol Metab* 1988; **67**:460–4.

38. Dunaif A, Segal KR, Shelley DR, Green G, Dobrjansky A, Licholai T. Evidence for distinctive and intrinsic defects in insulin action in polycystic ovary syndrome. *Diabetes* 1992; **41**:1257–66.

39. Sir-Petermann, T, Angel, B, Maliqueo M, et al. Prevalence of type II diabetes mellitus and insulin resistance in parents of women with polycystic ovary syndrome. *Diabetologia* 2002; **45**:959–64.

40. Holte J, Bergh T, Berne C, Berglund G, Lithell H. Enhanced early insulin response to glucose in relation to insulin resistance in women with polycystic ovary syndrome and normal glucose tolerance. *J Clin Endocrinol Metab* 1994; **78**:1052–8.

41. Rajkhowa M, Bicknell J, Jones M, Clayton RN. Insulin sensitivity in obese and nonobese women with polycystic ovary syndrome – relationship to hyperandrogenaemia. *Fertil Steril* 1994; **61**:605–11.

42. Dahlgren E, Janson PO, Johansson S, Lapidus L, Oden A. Polycystic ovary syndrome and risk for myocardial infarction. Evaluated from a risk factor model based on a prospective population study of women. *Acta Obstet Gynecol Scand* 1992; **71**:599–604.

43. Pierpoint T, McKeigue PM, Isaacs AJ, Wild SH, Jacobs HS. Mortality of women with polycystic ovary syndrome at long-term follow-up. *J Clin Epidemiol* 1998; **51**:581–6.

44. Wild S, Pierpoint T, Jacobs H, McKeigue P. Long-term consequences of polycystic ovary syndrome: results of a 31 year follow-up study. *Hum Fertil (Camb)* 2000; **3**:101–5.

45. Cibula D, Cifkova R, Fanta M, Poledne R, Zivny J, Skibova J. Increased risk of non-insulin dependent diabetes mellitus, arterial hypertension and coronary artery disease in perimenopausal women with a history of the polycystic ovary syndrome. *Hum Reprod* 2000; **15**:785–9.

46. Norman RJ, Masters L, Milner CR, Wang JX, Davies MJ. Relative risk of conversion from normoglycaemia to impaired glucose tolerance or non-insulin dependent diabetes mellitus in polycystic ovary syndrome. *Hum Reprod* 2001; **16**:1995–8.

47. Legro RS, Kunselman AR, Dunaif A. Prevalence and predictors of dyslipidemia in women with polycystic ovary syndrome. *Am J Med* 2001; **111**:607–13.

48. Mahabeer S, Naidoo C, Norman RJ, Jialal I, Reddi K, Joubert SM. Metabolic profiles and lipoprotein lipid concentrations in non-obese and obese patients with polycystic ovarian disease. *Horm Metab Res* 1990; **22**:537–40.

49. Graf M, Richards CJ, Brown V, Meissner L, Dunaif A. The independent effects of hyperandrogenaemia, hyperinsulinaemia, and obesity on lipid and lipoprotein profiles in women. *Clin Endocrinol (Oxf)* 1990; **33**:119–31.

50. Slowinska-Srzednicka J, Zgliczynski S, Wierzbicki M, et al. The role of hyperinsulinemia in the development of lipid disturbances in nonobese and obese women with the polycystic ovary syndrome. *J Endocrinol Invest* 1991; **14**:569–75.

51. Holte J, Bergh T, Berne C, Lithell H. Serum lipoprotein lipid profile in women with the polycystic ovary syndrome: relation to anthropometric, endocrine and metabolic variables. *Clin Endocrinol (Oxf)* 1994; **41**:463–71.

52. Norman RJ, Hague WM, Masters SC, Wang XJ. Subjects with polycystic ovaries without hyperandrogenaemia exhibit similar disturbances in insulin and lipid profiles as those with polycystic ovary syndrome. *Hum Reprod* 1995; **10**:2258–61.

53. Robinson S, Henderson AD, Gelding SV, et al. Dyslipidaemia is associated with insulin resistance in women with polycystic ovaries. *Clin Endocrinol (Oxf)* 1996; **44**:277–84.

54. Legro RS, Blanche P, Krauss RM, Lobo RA. Alterations in low-density lipoprotein and high-density lipoprotein subclasses among Hispanic women with polycystic ovary syndrome: influence of insulin and genetic factors. *Fertil Steril* 1999; **72**:990–5.

55. Mather KJ, Kwan, F, Corenblum B. Hyperinsulinemia in polycystic ovary syndrome correlates with increased cardiovascular risk independent of obesity. *Fertil Steril* 2000; **73**:150–6.

56. Holte JGG, Berne CBTLH. Elevated ambulatory daytime blood pressure in women with polycystic ovary syndrome: a sign of pre-hypertensive state? *Hum Reprod* 1996; **11**:23–8.

57. Zimmermann S, Phillips RA, Dunaif A, et al. Polycystic ovary syndrome: lack of hypertension despite profound insulin resistance. *J Clin Endocrinol Metab* 1992; **75**:508–13.

58. Sampson M, Kong C, Patel A, Unwin R, Jacobs HS. Ambulatory blood pressure profiles and plasminogen activator inhibitor (PAI-1) activity in lean women with and without the polycystic ovary syndrome. *Clin Endocrinol (Oxf)* 1996; **45**:623–9.

59. Guzick DS, Talbott EO, Sutton-Tyrrell K, Herzog HC, Kuller LH, Wolfson SK, Jr. Carotid atherosclerosis in women with polycystic ovary syndrome: initial results from a case–control study. *Am J Obstet Gynecol* 1996; **174**:1224–9.

60. Talbott EO, Guzick DS, Sutton-Tyrrell K, et al. Evidence for association between polycystic ovary syndrome and premature carotid atherosclerosis in middle aged women. *Arterioscler Thromb Vasc Biol* 2000; **20**:2414–21.

61. Lakhani K, Seifalian AM, Hardiman P. Evidence of atherosclerosis in young women with polycystic ovary syndrome. *Hum Reprod* 2003; **18** (Suppl 1):25 [abstr].

62. Birdsall MA, Farquhar CM, White HD. Association between polycystic ovaries and extent of coronary artery disease in women having cardiac catheterization. *Ann Intern Med* 1997; **126**:32–5.

63. Christian RC, Behrenbeck T, Fitzpatrick LA. Clinical hyperandrogenism and body mass index predict coronary calcification in premenopausal women with polycystic ovary syndrome (PCOS). *Endocr Soc Abstracts* 2000: 400.

64. Prelevic GM, Beljic T, Balint-Peric L, Ginsburg J. Cardiac flow velocity in women with the polycystic ovary syndrome. *Clin Endocrinol (Oxf)* 1995; **43**:677–81.

65. Prelevic GM, Wood J, Okolo S, Ginsburg J. Peripheral blood flow in young women with the polycystic ovary syndrome. *J Endocrinol* 1996; **151** (Suppl):13 [abstr].

66. Lakhani K, Constantinovici N, Purcell WM, Fernando R, Hardiman P. Internal carotid artery haemodynamics in women with polycystic ovaries. *Clin Sci (Lond)* 2000; **98**:661–5.

67. Lakhani K, Constantinovici N, Purcell WM, Fernando R, Hardiman P. Internal carotid-artery response to 5% carbon dioxide in women with polycystic ovaries. *Lancet* 2000; **356**:1166–7.

68. Lees C, Jurkovic D, Zaidi J, Campbell S. Unexpected effect of a nitric oxide donor on uterine artery Doppler velocimetry in oligomenorrheic women with polycystic ovaries. *Ultrasound Obstet Gynecol* 1998; **11**:129–32.

69. Steinberg HO, Chaker H, Leaming R, Johnson J, Brechtel G, Baron AD. Obesity/insulin resistance is associated with endothelial dysfunction: implications for the syndrome of insulin resistance. *J Clin Invest* 1996; **97**:2601–10.

70. Paradisi G, Steinberg HO, Hempfling A, et al. Polycystic ovary syndrome is associated with endothelial dysfunction. *Circulation* 2001; **103**:1410–15.

71. Lakhani K, Seifalian AM, Hardiman P. Impaired carotid viscoelastic properties in women with polycystic ovaries. *Circulation* 2002; **106**:81–5.

72. Reaven GM. Pathophysiology of insulin resistance in human disease. *Physiol Rev* 1995; **75**:473–86.

73. Atiomo MU, Mikhlides DP, Morris R, Hardiman P. Ultrasound features of polycystic ovaries (PCO) and metabolic syndrome X. *Bioscientifica – Endocrine Abstracts* 2002; **3**:117.

74. Diamanti-Kandarakis E, Spina G, Kouli C, Migdalis I. Increased endothelin-1 levels in women with polycystic ovary syndrome and the beneficial effect of metformin therapy. *J Clin Endocrinol Metab* 2001; **86**:4666–73.

75. Kelly CC, Lyall H, Petrie JR, Gould GW, Connell JM, Sattar N. Low grade chronic inflammation in women with polycystic ovarian syndrome. *J Clin Endocrinol Metab* 2001; **86**:2453–5.

76. Tracy RP, Lemaitre RN, Psaty BM, et al. Relationship of C-reactive protein to risk of cardiovascular disease in the elderly. Results from the Cardiovascular Health Study and the Rural Health Promotion Project. *Arterioscler Thromb Vasc Biol* 1997; **17**:1121–7.

77. Ridker PM, Hennekens CH, Buring JE, Rifai N. C-reactive protein and other markers of inflammation in the prediction of cardiovascular disease in women. *N Engl J Med* 2000; **342**:836–43.

78. Rifai N, Ridker PM. Proposed cardiovascular risk assessment algorithm using high-sensitivity C-reactive protein and lipid screening. *Clin Chem* 2001; **47**:28–30.

79. Pepys MB, Berger A. The renaissance of C reactive protein. *BMJ* 2001; **322**:4–5.

80. Lagrand WK, Visser CA, Hermens WT, et al. C-reactive protein as a cardiovascular risk factor: more than an epiphenomenon? *Circulation* 1999; **100**:96–102.

81. Loverro G, Lorusso F, Mei L, Depalo R, Cormio G, Selvaggi L. The plasma homocysteine levels are increased in polycystic ovary syndrome. *Gynecol Obstet Invest* 2002; **53**:157–62.

82. Blacher J, Benetos K, Kirzin JM, Malmajec A, Guize L, Safer ME. Relation of plasma total homcysteine to cardiovascular mortality in French population. *Am J Cardiol* 2002; **15**:591–5.

83. Randeva HS, Lewandowski KC, Drzewoski J, et al. Exercise decreases plasma total homocysteine in overweight young women with polycystic ovary syndrome. *J Clin Endocrinol Metab* 2002; **87**:4496–501.

84. Macut D, Micic D, Cvijovic G, et al. Cardiovascular risk in adolescent and young adult obese females with polycystic ovary syndrome (PCOS). *J Pediatr Endocrinol Metab* 2001; **14** (Suppl 5):1353–9.

85. Nestler JE. Should patients with polycystic ovarian syndrome be treated with metformin: an enthusiatic endorsement. *Hum Reprod* 2002; **17**:1950–3.

86. Harborne L, Fleming R, Lyall H, Norman J, Sattar N. Descriptive review of the evidence for the use of metformin in polycystic ovary syndrome. *Lancet* 2003; **361**:1894–901.

Part 3
Heart Failure

28
Diastolic dysfunction

Dalane W. Kitzman and Jalal K. Ghali

Introduction

One of the most profound sex-related differences in cardiovascular disease (CVD) is in heart failure, where systolic function is severely reduced in most men but is preserved in most women. The marked sex difference in diastolic heart failure (DHF) may be due, at least in part, to altered responses to chronic hypertension, aging, and menopause. This chapter discusses the pathophysiology, diagnosis, prognosis, and therapy of this important disorder in older women.

Epidemiology

In contrast to the decline in overall CVD over the past two decades, the rate of congestive heart failure (CHF) in the US is increasing dramatically.[1] In the Cardiovascular Health Study (CHS), a population-based observational study of cardiovascular risk in the elderly, CHF prevalence increased in women from 4.1% at age 70 years to 14.3% at age 85 years (Fig. 28.1).[2] During 6 years of follow-up, the incidence of CHF in CHS was 10.6/1000 person-years at age 65 and was 42.5/1000 person-years at age ≥80 years.[3] Women who develop heart failure, particularly those in the older age range, frequently have preserved left ventricular (LV) systolic function,

a syndrome commonly termed diastolic heart failure. In the population-based Olmsted Community project, records were reviewed from all patients during a 1-year period in whom an assessment of LV ejection fraction (EF) was obtained within 3 weeks of a new diagnosis of CHF.[4] A normal EF was found in 43% of patients and this phenomenon increased with age (Fig. 28.2).[4] Other large population-based

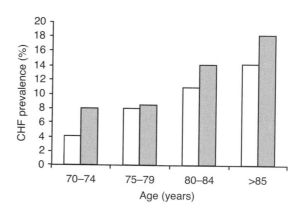

Figure 28.1
Prevalence of congestive heart failure (CHF) versus age in elderly men (dark bars) and women (light bars) in the Cardiovascular Health Study. Even in an older cohort such as this, CHF prevalence increased with age. Adapted from reference 2 with permission from Excerpta Medica, Inc.

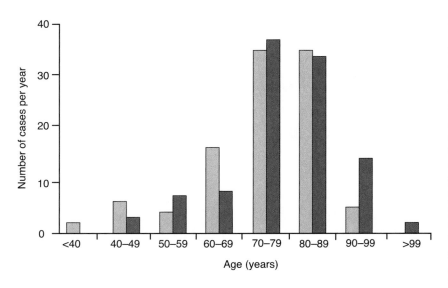

Figure 28.2
Numbers of patients in Olmsted County, Minnesota hospitalized with congestive heart failure (CHF) in 1991 versus age with normal (dark bars) and reduced (light bars) ejection fraction. Note that CHF with a normal ejection fraction is absent in the youngest group (age <40 years) in contrast to the oldest group (age >99), where it comprises essentially all patients. Adapted from reference 4 with permission.

reports have found the prevalence of normal EF among those with heart failure to be even higher, well over 50%.[2,5–10]

There is a remarkable sex-related difference in DHF. In the cross-sectional analysis of CHS, 67% of elderly women with prevalent CHF had a normal EF, whereas this finding was present in only 42% of men (Fig. 28.3).[2] During the longitudinal analysis of 6-year follow-up in CHS, over 90% of women who developed heart failure had normal systolic function.[3] Because women significantly outnumber men in the older population, the population-attributable risk of reduced systolic function was relatively small compared with those with normal systolic function.[3] Other large population-based reports, including the Framingham Heart Study,[5] the Strong Heart Study of American Indians,[7] the Helsinki Ageing Study,[8] and large Medicare studies,[9,10] have found a similarly profound sex differential in this disorder. Thus, the typical person with heart failure living in the community is an older woman with normal LV systolic function and systolic hypertension. This contrasts significantly with the typical patient seen in referral heart failure clinics, who is a middle-aged man with severely reduced systolic function and coronary heart disease (CHD) (Table 28.1).[11] Indeed, as one editorial declared, DHF is predominantly a disorder of older women.[12]

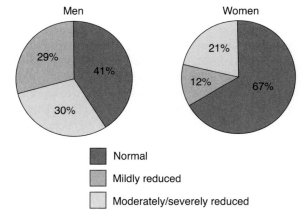

Figure 28.3
Left ventricular ejection fraction by gender among community-dwelling elderly with congestive heart failure in the Cardiovascular Health Study. Reproduced from reference 2 with permission.

Pathophysiology

Relatively few data are available regarding the pathophysiology of DHF, and even fewer regarding women specifically. Sex-related differences in normal LV function may contribute to the female

Table 28.1 Heart failure in older versus middle-aged patients

Characteristic	Elderly	Middle-aged
Prevalence	6–18%	<1%
Gender	Predominantly women	Predominantly men
Etiology	Hypertension	Coronary heart disease
LV systolic function	Normal	Impaired
Co-morbidities	Multiple	Few

LV, left ventricular.
Adapted from reference 11.

preponderance of DHF. Three large population-based studies – Framingham, CHS, and HyperGEN (Hypertension Genetic Epidemiology Network) – have reported that Doppler LV diastolic filling velocities are significantly different in women compared with men, with increased early and atrial filling velocities in women.[13] Women, particularly older women, also tend to have higher LVEFs, independent of their smaller chamber size.[14,15]

The female left ventricle in mammals has a distinctly different response to pressure load, such as is typical of systemic hypertension, compared with males. HyperGEN showed that the deceleration time of early diastolic flow and isovolumic relaxation time were lengthened in hypertensive women compared with men, independent of all other factors, indicative of decreased myocardial relaxation.[13] Furthermore, a report from the Losartan Intervention for Endpoint reduction in hypertension (LIFE) study showed that EF and fractional shortening were on average 2–3 percentage points higher in hypertensive women than in men. It was first observed in hypertensive subjects in the Framingham study that the pattern of hypertrophic remodeling in women was concentric whereas in men it was eccentric. This sex-related difference in hypertensives has since been reported in several other studies, including HyperGEN[16] and LIFE.

Douglas et al.[17] performed a key study that confirmed and explained these sex differences observed in humans. Using aortic banding to create a model of chronic LV pressure overload in male and female rats, they showed that male rats responded with LV dilation and modest wall thickening (eccentric hypertrophy) with resultant increased wall stress and decreased LV contractility. The female rats, on the other hand, increased their LV wall thickness and maintained a normal chamber size (concentric hypertrophy), and thereby enjoyed near-normal wall stress, and normal (even a trend toward supranormal) contractility. As a result, the female rats were able to continue to generate substantially higher systolic pressures, despite the excess afterload. Several other studies have shown similar overall results.[18–20]

Large population-based studies have consistently shown that the strongest, most common risk factor for the development of heart failure is systolic hypertension. Combining this key point with the findings of the Douglas study provides a cohesive explanation for the divergent manifestations of heart failure in women versus men (Table 28.1). The male left ventricle is less able to tolerate a pressure load, and in the presence of chronic systolic hypertension becomes dilated with thin walls and a depressed EF. The female left ventricle is able to tolerate the pressure load better by developing concentric hypertrophy, allowing it to maintain normal LV size and EF. However, the long-term cost of this adaptation is impaired LV diastolic function. This may help to explain the higher prevalence of DHF in women, and why men tend to develop systolic heart failure (SHF), whereas women tend to develop DHF. This unifying concept, while theoretical, is supported by a broad array of evidence. Another potential contributor to this phenomenon is the earlier onset of CHD in men. Although not widely appreciated, these concepts are pivotal to understanding the pathophysiology of heart failure in women and the elderly.

The above interplay between LV remodeling and pressure load has been shown in rodent models to be influenced substantially by estrogen and androgen,

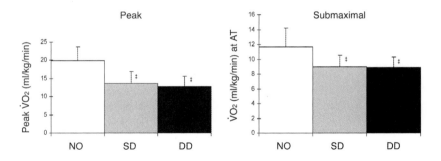

Figure 28.4

Exercise oxygen consumption ($\dot{V}O_2$) during peak exhaustive exercise (left panel) and during submaximal exercise at the ventilatory anaerobic threshold (AT, right panel) in age-matched normal subjects (NO), elderly patients with heart failure due to systolic dysfunction (SD), and elderly patients with heart failure with normal systolic function, presumed diastolic dysfunction (DD) (men and women combined). Exercise capacity is severely reduced in patients with diastolic heart failure compared with normals ($p < 0.001$) and to a similar degree as in those with systolic heart failure. Overall, peak exercise $\dot{V}O_2$ was 33% lower in the women compared with the men (not shown). ‡Indicates a statistically significant difference ($p < 0.01$) between the designated group compared with NO. Adapted from data in reference 25.

and to be related to sex differences in cardiac angiotensin-converting enzyme (ACE) expression.[21]

In addition to these sex-related changes, there are a number of normal age-related changes in cardiovascular structure and function that are likely relevant to the development of DHF. These include increased arterial and myocardial stiffness, decreased diastolic myocardial relaxation, increased LV mass, decreased peak contractility, reduced myocardial and vascular responsiveness to β-adrenergic stimulation, decreased coronary flow reserve, and decreased mitochondrial response to increased demand for adenosine triphosphate (ATP) production.[11] Consequently, insults from acute myocardial ischemia/infarction, poorly controlled hypertension, atrial fibrillation, iatrogenic volume overload, and pneumonia, that would be tolerated in younger patients, can cause acute CHF in older women.[11]

These normal age-related changes result in decreased cardiovascular reserve which confers an approximately 1% per year decline in maximal exercise oxygen consumption.[22] In addition, women have different cardiovascular physiologic responses to exercise than men, particularly in heart rate and stroke volume, independent of age and body size.[22–24]

Exercise intolerance, manifested as exertional dyspnea and fatigue, is the primary symptom in chronic heart failure. While the pathophysiology of exercise intolerance in SHF as it presents in middle-aged men has been intensively examined, few studies have examined the pathophysiology of exercise intolerance in DHF. In a recent study, maximal exercise testing with expired gas measures was performed in three groups of older subjects: SHF, DHF, and age-matched controls.[25] In comparison to the normal controls, peak exercise oxygen consumption, an objective measure of exercise capacity, was severely reduced in the patients with DHF and to a similar degree as those with SHF (Fig. 28.4).[25] In addition, submaximal exercise capacity, as measured by the ventilatory anaerobic threshold, was similarly reduced in DHF and SHF patients, and this was accompanied by a reduced health-related quality of life.[25]

Two studies have examined the central (cardiac) and peripheral (vascular) components of the exercise response in order to determine the mechanism(s) of the severely reduced exercise capacity in DHF. In the first, using invasive cardiopulmonary exercise testing, it was demonstrated that severe exercise intolerance was related to an inability to increase stroke volume via the Frank–Starling mechanism despite severely increased LV filling pressure, indicative of diastolic dysfunction (Fig. 28.5).[26] This

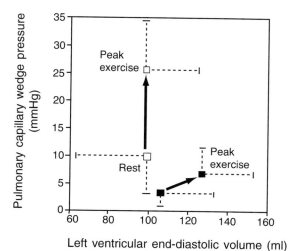

Figure 28.5

Left ventricular (LV) diastolic function (men and women combined) assessed by invasive cardiopulmonary exercise testing in patients with heart failure and normal systolic function (open boxes) and age-matched normals (closed boxes). Pressure–volume relation was shifted upward and leftward at rest. In the patients with exercise, LV diastolic volume did not increase despite marked increase in diastolic (pulmonary wedge) pressure. Due to diastolic dysfunction, failure of the Frank–Starling mechanism resulted in severe exercise intolerance. Reproduced from reference 26 with permission from American College of Cardiology Foundation.

resulted in severely reduced exercise cardiac output and early lactate formation that appeared to be responsible for the severely reduced exercise capacity and associated chronic exertional symptoms.

The second study indicated that decreased aortic distensibility, likely due to the combined effects of aging- and hypertension-induced thickening and remodeling of the thoracic aortic wall, may be an important contributor to exercise intolerance in chronic DHF. Magnetic resonance imaging and maximal exercise testing with expired gas analysis were performed in a group of elderly patients with isolated DHF and in age-matched healthy subjects. The patients with DHF had increased pulse pressure and thoracic aortic wall thickness and markedly decreased aortic distensibility, which correlated closely with their severely decreased exercise capacity (Figs 28.6 and 28.7).[27]

As discussed above, several lines of evidence suggest that systemic hypertension plays an important role in the genesis of DHF. In animal models, diastolic dysfunction develops early in systemic hypertension, and LV diastolic relaxation is very sensitive to increased afterload.[28–33] Increased afterload may impair relaxation, leading to increased LV filling pressures, decreased stroke volume, and symptoms of dyspnea and congestion.[31] Nearly all (88%) DHF patients have a history of chronic systemic hypertension.[2,34,35] In addition, severe systolic hypertension is usually present during acute exacerbations (pulmonary edema).[36–38]

The role of ischemia in DHF is uncertain. It would seem likely that it is a significant contributor in many cases. It had been hypothesized that patients found to have a normal EF following an episode of CHF may merely have had transiently reduced systolic function and/or ischemia at the time of the acute exacerbation. In order to address this question, an echocardiogram was performed at the time of presentation in 38 consecutive patients with acute hypertensive pulmonary edema and was repeated again about 3 days later after resolution of pulmonary edema and control of hypertension.[38] The LVEF and wall motion score index at follow-up were similar to that found during the acute echocardiogram. Furthermore, of those who had LVEF ≥50% at follow-up (n = 18), all but two had LVEF ≥50% acutely, and in those two cases, the LVEF was >40%, above the level which would be expected to cause acute heart failure on the basis of primary systolic dysfunction (Fig. 28.8). These data suggest that marked transient systolic dysfunction and overt ischemia do not play a primary role in most patients who present with acute CHF in the presence of severe systolic hypertension and are subsequently found to have a normal EF.[38] Further, they support the concept that acute pulmonary edema in these patients is most likely due to an exacerbation of diastolic dysfunction caused by severe systolic hypertension. The data also suggest that the EF measurement from an echocardiogram performed in follow-up accurately reflects that during an episode of acute pulmonary edema.[38]

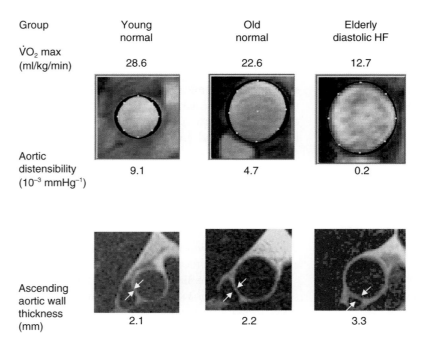

Group	Young normal	Old normal	Elderly diastolic HF
$\dot{V}O_2$ max (ml/kg/min)	28.6	22.6	12.7
Aortic distensibility (10^{-3} mmHg^{-1})	9.1	4.7	0.2
Ascending aortic wall thickness (mm)	2.1	2.2	3.3

Figure 28.6
Data and magnetic resonance images from representative subjects from healthy young, healthy elderly, and elderly patients with diastolic heart failure (men and women combined). Maximal exercise oxygen consumption ($\dot{V}O_2$ max), aortic distensibility at rest, and ascending aortic wall thickness. Patients with diastolic heart failure have severely reduced exercise tolerance ($\dot{V}O_2$ max) and aortic distensibility and increased aortic wall thickness. Reproduced from reference 27 with permission.

In a related study, 3-year follow-up was performed in 46 patients who initially presented with acute hypertensive pulmonary edema.[37] The majority had a normal EF. Of those who were referred clinically for coronary angiography (n = 38), 33 had obstructive epicardial coronary artery disease, and 19 underwent revascularization. However, of these 19, by 6 months follow-up, nine had been hospitalized with recurrent pulmonary edema and one had died. Severe systolic hypertension was nearly uniformly present at the time of recurrent pulmonary edema.[37] These two studies suggest that severe systolic hypertension may play a pivotal role in the pathogenesis of acute exacerbations of DHF.

Neurohormonal activation likely plays an important role in the pathophysiology of DHF as it does in patients with SHF. In a group of patients with primary DHF, Clarkson et al. showed that atrial natriuretic peptide and brain natriuretic peptide (BNP) were substantially increased and there was an exaggerated response during exercise,[39] a pattern similar to that described in patients with SHF. In the study described above,[25] BNP was significantly increased in patients with DHF compared with normal controls, but not as severely as in those with SHF. Norepinephrine, however, was increased to a similar degree as in SHF.

The role of genetic predisposition in the genesis of DHF in the elderly is not known. Diastolic LV relaxation is significantly modulated by β-adrenergic stimulation via phospholamban and, to a lesser extent, cardiac troponin-I, both of which are substantially under genetic control. Furthermore, data from the HyperGEN study have shown significant heritability of hypertension,[40] LV mass,[41] and Doppler diastolic filling,[42] all factors that likely play a role in DHF in the elderly. The genetic basis of familial hypertrophic cardiomyopathy, which has substantial phenotypic similarities to isolated DHF in the elderly, has been described.[43,44] It is noteworthy that in that disorder, the phenotype may not be expressed for 30–50 years.

Diagnosis and clinical features (see also Chapter 29)

While the distinction between heart failure due to systolic dysfunction versus diastolic dysfunction can

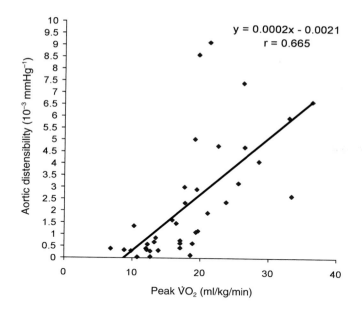

Figure 28.7
A close relationship between peak $\dot{V}O_2$ and proximal aortic distensibility in a group of 30 subjects (men and women combined; 10 healthy young, 10 healthy old, and 10 elderly patients with diastolic heart disease). Each symbol represents the data from one participant.
Reproduced from reference 27 with permission from The American College of Cardiology Foundation.

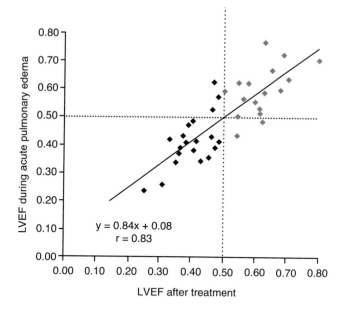

Figure 28.8
Left ventricular ejection fraction (LVEF) measured during acute pulmonary edema and at follow-up, 1–3 days after treatment (men and women combined). Nearly all patients found to have normal EF (>50%; lighter dots) at follow-up also had normal EF during acute pulmonary edema. Reproduced from reference 38 with permission.

be assisted by demographics and clinical signs,[45] evaluation of new-onset heart failure in an elderly patient should include an imaging test, usually an echocardiogram. This will not only assess systolic function, but will also exclude unexpected but important diagnoses, such as aortic stenosis, severe valvular regurgitation, large pericardial effusion, hypertrophic obstructive cardiomyopathy, and cardiac amyloidosis. Unfortunately, a definitive noninvasive measure is not available for diastolic dysfunction. Doppler LV diastolic filling indexes and particularly the newer tissue Doppler techniques[46] can provide helpful supplementary information, but their role in the clinical diagnosis of the DHF syndrome is unclear and their independent discriminatory power in unselected populations is not known.

Diagnostic criteria from the European Study Group on Diastolic Heart Failure[47] include: signs and symptoms of CHF, a normal or at most mildly reduced LVEF, and evidence of abnormal diastolic function. Subsequent work by Vasan and Levy,[48] and Gandhi et al.,[38] suggests that DHF diagnosis can usually be made without the mandate for measurement of EF at the time of the acute event. Invasive measures of diastolic function are impractical, and not feasible in most circumstances. Furthermore two studies by Zile et al. suggest that measures of diastolic function, invasive or otherwise, are not necessary for the diagnosis of DHF, since nearly all patients who meet the other criteria for DHF will have diastolic dysfunction.[49,50] Thus, the original European criteria have undergone substantial modification, primarily by simplification as a result of the above progress in our understanding of the syndrome of DHF.[51–53] In addition to positive inclusion criteria, care should be taken to exclude other causes for the signs and symptoms suggesting heart failure.[54] Finally, patients with heart failure, a normal EF, and no other explanation for their symptoms have the more 'pure' diagnosis of *isolated* DHF. In CHS, this subgroup comprised 42% of the patients with CHF and a normal EF.[2] Typical patients with isolated DHF are women, and often have high normal or supernormal EF (70% or more), normal or small LV chamber size, thick walls with concentric hypertrophy, and no segmental wall motion abnormalities.

Because active myocardial ischemia can present as heart failure, particularly in the elderly, and has independent prognostic and therapeutic implications, a stress test is often indicated, or in the case of concomitant severe or unstable angina, coronary angiography.

Recent studies suggest that rapid BNP assays could aid in the diagnosis of heart failure, particularly in the emergency setting, and may help in judging disease severity.[20] However, as expressed in the American College of Cardiology/American Heart Association guidelines, the role of BNP assays in the routine evaluation and management of heart failure

patients remains to be defined.[20] Furthermore, it is unclear what diagnostic value such assays may have in chronic stable heart failure patients. It is underappreciated that among healthy subjects, women have significantly different ranges of BNP, and that BNP is affected by age as well.[55,56] Further, since BNP appears to be increased in DHF as well as systolic failure,[39] it will likely not be helpful in discriminating between these two disorders.[25]

Prognosis

The severity of exercise intolerance and the frequency of hospitalization appear to be similar in patients with SHF versus DHF.[25,57–60] This high rate of hospitalization is associated with poor quality of life and high health-care costs.[61,62] The annual mortality rate for *diastolic* heart failure in the Framingham Study was 8.9% per year, a rate about twofold higher than in nested case–controls, although it was only half that reported for *systolic* heart failure (19.6%).[5] Similar results were found in CHS.[6] However, in *hospitalized* patients, mortality is similar with DHF and SHF (Fig. 28.9).[4,57,58,63,64] An important observation in the CHS was that, given the higher prevalence among the elderly, the population-attributable

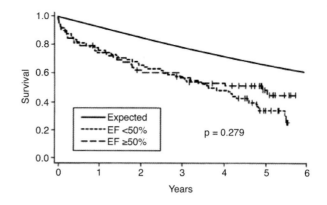

Figure 28.9
Survival of patients admitted with congestive heart failure by ejection fraction (EF) (men and women combined). Reproduced from reference 4 with permission.

mortality in patients with DHF is actually higher than SHF, highlighting the public health implications of DHF in the elderly.[6]

Along with age, gender is an important predictor of mortality in persons with heart failure, and prognosis appears to be better in women than in men.[3,8,65] Not all of the sex-related difference in heart failure outcome is mediated by the difference in the proportion of each gender that has SHF versus DHF.[66]

Management

Our literature base regarding therapy of DHF is embarrassingly scant.[53,67,68] In contrast to SHF, where numerous studies in many thousands of patients have generated a rich evidence base to direct therapy, there is essentially only one large, multicenter trial in DHF. This is remarkable given the high prevalence, substantial morbidity, and significant mortality of DHF.[53,68–70] This is particularly regrettable for older women who bear the brunt of DHF.

Considering the storied journey to definitive, evidence-based therapy for SHF during the past three decades (recall the seemingly paradoxical failure of inotropes and success of beta-blockers), one should expect a number of surprising reversals during the journey toward evidence-based therapy for DHF. Several large trials are now in progress.

General approach

The approach to the patient with heart failure and a normal EF should begin with a search for a primary etiology. Most such patients will be found to have hypertension as their main underlying condition.[20] Screening for CHD with a noninvasive stress test or coronary angiography should be considered, especially in patients with chest pain and/or 'flash pulmonary edema', to exclude severe CHD.[20] When found, manifest ischemia should be treated, including invasively if indicated,[20] since ischemia is a therapeutic target in its own right and also strongly impairs diastolic relaxation. A small but important number of patients will be found to have hypertrophic cardiomyopathy,[71,72] with or without dynamic obstruction, undiagnosed valvular disease, or rarely amyloid heart disease.[73]

Control of hypertension may be the single most important treatment strategy for DHF.[74] Chronic hypertension causes LV hypertrophy (LVH) and fibrosis which impair diastolic chamber compliance. Acute hypertension significantly impairs diastolic relaxation. In addition, meta-analyses indicate that therapy of chronic, mild systolic hypertension in the elderly is a potent means of preventing the development of heart failure, and it is likely that a major proportion of cases prevented are due to DHF (Table 28.2).[74–78] ALLHAT showed that the diuretic chlorthalidone was at least as effective for prevention of CHF as other antihypertensive medications.[79]

Loss of atrial contraction is deleterious to LV filling, and atrial fibrillation with fast ventricular rate is a common precipitant to decompensated DHF. Therefore, sinus rhythm should be maintained.[20] Achieving and maintaining sinus rhythm can be difficult in the elderly where the rate of atrial fibrillation is high. When sinus rhythm cannot be maintained, a more modest goal of rate control should be pursued.

Management goals in women with DHF include relief of symptoms, improvement in functional capacity and quality of life, prevention of acute exacerbations and related hospital admissions, and prolongation of survival. A systematic approach should comprise several elements: diagnosis and staging of disease, search for reversible etiology, judicious use of medications, patient education, enhancement of self-management skills, coordination of care across disciplines, and effective followup. Every heart failure patient should have a scale, weigh regularly, and know what steps to take if weight increases beyond pre-specified ranges. Diuretic adjustments can be performed by nurses over the telephone, and in some cases by patients themselves. There must be easy access to health-care providers so that problems can be addressed early to avoid decompensation with periodic telephone calls, frequent follow-up appointments, and monitoring programs utilizing telephone and the internet.[20,80]

There is now undisputed evidence of the efficacy of a multidisciplinary approach to care in reducing acute exacerbations leading to rehospitalization,

Table 28.2 Effect of antihypertensive therapy on incident heart failure

Trial	n	Age range (years)	Risk reduction
European Working Party	840	>60	22%
INDANA Group	884	60–79	32%
Swedish Trial	1627	70–84	51%
SHEP	4736	≥60	55%
Syst-Eur	4695	≥60	36%
STONE	1632	60–79	68%

Adapted from reference 11.

improving quality of life, reducing total costs, and increasing survival.[81–84] Notably, many of these studies included significant numbers of female patients with normal EF.[82] Women with heart failure often have severe deconditioning and severe exercise intolerance and they should be encouraged to undertake regular moderate physical activity.

Pharmacological therapy (see also Chapter 39)

Despite the fact that numerous randomized, controlled trials have shown a marked decrease in development of heart failure in patients treated for systolic hypertension (Table 28.2),[75–78] community surveys consistently show undertreatment of hypertension. Thus, adequate treatment of systemic hypertension is a potent means for prevention of DHF.

Diuretics

Diuretics are indispensable for rapid relief of pulmonary congestion and peripheral edema and are necessary in most patients with moderate to severe heart failure to mitigate volume overload. However, they may accelerate activation of the renin–angiotensin system and cause renal insufficiency and electrolyte disturbances. Therefore, the lowest dose capable of maintaining euvolemia should be utilized. Although some patients with mild DHF can be treated effectively with a thiazide diuretic for some time, usually a loop diuretic will eventually be required in order to maintain euvolemia.

Most patients with heart failure have an intrinsic 'diuretic threshold' below which minimal diuresis occurs, even when repeated doses are administered. Thus, multiple daily doses are not usually necessary and are inconvenient, particularly in older women in whom they can exacerbate urinary incontinence.[54] Usually, a single morning oral dose somewhat above the diuretic threshold will provide effective control of salt and fluid retention. Nonsteroidal anti-inflammatory medications, frequently used in older patients, can cause relative diuretic resistance and should be discontinued if possible. During active diuresis, careful monitoring and replacement of electrolytes, particularly potassium and magnesium, are important; fluid restriction may be needed to avoid or alleviate hyponatremia.[85]

Digoxin

Since most inotropes enhance early diastolic relaxation, digoxin might theoretically have a similar effect. Indeed, in the the Digitalis Investigation Group Trial (DIG), which included a subset of elderly patients with preserved systolic function, results were similar regardless of EF, with symptomatic improvement and prevention of hospitalizations but no difference in overall mortality compared with placebo.[86] This suggests that digoxin could play a role in adjunctive therapy to help relieve symptoms in this disorder. However, a recent retrospective analysis of the DIG trial showed that among patients with SHF, digoxin therapy was associated with increased risk of death from any cause in women. There were relatively few events in patients with DHF to evaluate the potential detrimental effect of digitalis in women with DHF.[87]

Angiotensin-converting enzyme inhibitors

ACE inhibitors and angiotensin-receptor blockers (ARBs) are attractive as therapy for patients with DHF. They are the cornerstone of systolic heart failure therapy where they reduce mortality and hospital admissions, and improve exercise tolerance and symptoms. As discussed above, patients with DHF also appear to have neuroendocrine activation, increased LV filling pressure and decreased stroke volume similar to those with systolic failure.[25,26,39] ACE inhibition reduces blood pressure and LVH and improves LV relaxation as well as aortic distensibility.[88–92]

Aronow et al. showed in a group of New York Heart Association class III heart failure patients and presumed diastolic dysfunction (EF >50%) that enalapril significantly improved functional class, exercise duration, EF, diastolic filling, and LV mass.[93] In an observational study of 1402 patients admitted to 10 community hospitals, ACE inhibitor use in DHF patients was associated with substantially reduced all-cause mortality (odds ratio 0.61) and CHF death (odds ratio 0.55).[94,95] The European trial PEP-CHF is assessing the effect of the ACE inhibitor perindopril in elderly (age >70 years) heart failure patients with an LVEF ≥40% on death, heart failure admission, quality of life, and 6-minute walk distance.[96]

Angiotensin-receptor blockers

In a blinded, randomized, controlled, cross-over trial of 20 elderly patients with diastolic dysfunction and an exaggerated blood pressure response to exercise, the ARB losartan substantially improved exercise capacity and quality of life.[97] The much anticipated, recently reported CHARM-Preserved trial assessed the effect of candesartan on death and hospital admission in heart failure patients with EF >40%.[98] This study included a substantial number of women (n = 1200+) and elderly. Over a median follow-up of 36 months, cardiovascular death did not differ from placebo; however, fewer patients in the candesartan group than in the placebo group (230 vs 279, p = 0.017) were admitted to the hospital for new episodes of CHF. The I-PRESERVE trial is assessing the effect of the ARB irbesartan compared with placebo and is recruiting a larger number of DHF patients and using more specific inclusion criteria.

Calcium channel antagonists

Calcium channel antagonists have often been suggested for DHF. In hypertrophic cardiomyopathy, a disorder in which diastolic dysfunction is common, verapamil appears to improve symptoms and objec-

tively measured exercise capacity.[99–102] In laboratory animal models calcium antagonists, particularly dihydropyridines, prevent ischemia-induced increases in LV diastolic stiffness[103] and improve diastolic performance in pacing-induced heart failure.[104–106] However, negative inotropic calcium antagonists significantly impair early relaxation.[106–110] Negative inotropic calcium antagonists have in general shown a tendency toward adverse outcome in patients with SHF.[106] However, Setaro et al. examined 22 men (mean age 65) with clinical heart failure despite EF >45% in a randomized, double-blind, placebo-controlled cross-over trial of verapamil.[111] There was a 33% improvement in exercise time and significant improvements in clinicoradiographic heart failure scoring and peak filling rate.

β-Adrenergic antagonists

β-Adrenergic antagonists have also been successful as therapy for hypertrophic obstructive cardiomyopathy.[112] In addition, they substantially improve mortality in SHF patients. Furthermore, they reduce blood pressure, assist in the regression of ventricular hypertrophy, and increase the ischemic threshold, all of hypothetical importance in DHF.[28,30,34,113,114] However, Cheng et al. and others have shown that early diastolic relaxation is impaired by β-adrenergic blockade.[115,116] Delineating the role of beta-blockers in DHF will require well-designed clinical trials.

Aldosterone antagonists

The addition of low-dose spironolactone (12.5–50 mg daily) to standard therapy has been shown to reduce mortality by 30% in patients with severe SHF.[117] Aldosterone antagonism has numerous potential benefits in patients with DHF, including LV remodeling, reversal of myocardial fibrosis, and improved LV diastolic function and vascular function.[118–120] However, few data are presently available regarding aldosterone antagonism in DHF. In one small study, low-dose spironolactone was well tolerated and appeared to improve exercise capacity and quality of life in older women with isolated DHF.[121] Notably, spironolactone is much better tolerated in women, who have lower rates of mastodynia than men.[117] Spironolactone and eplerenone are both contraindicated in patients with advanced renal dysfunction or pre-existing hyperkalemia. Delineation of the role of this potentially promising strategy will have to await results of clinical trials.[53]

References

1. Schocken DD. Epidemiology and risk factors for heart failure in the elderly. In: Rich MW (ed). Philadelphia: WB Saunders Company, 2000: 407–18.

2. Kitzman DW, Gardin JM, Gottdiener JS, et al. Importance of heart failure with preserved systolic function in patients > or = 65 years of age. CHS Research Group. Cardiovascular Health Study. *Am J Cardiol* 2001; **87**:413–19.

3. Gottdiener JS, Arnold AM, Aurigemma GP, et al. Predictors of congestive heart failure in the elderly: the Cardiovascular Health Study. *J Am Coll Cardiol* 2000; **35**:1628–37.

4. Senni M, Tribouilloy CM, Rodeheffer RJ, et al. Congestive heart failure in the community: a study of all incident cases in Olmsted County, Minnesota, in 1991. *Circulation* 1998; **98**:2282–9.

5. Ramachandran S, Vasan RS, Larson MG, et al. Congestive heart failure in subjects with normal versus reduced left ventricular ejection fraction. *J Am Coll Cardiol* 1999; **33**:1948–55.

6. Gottdiener JS, McClelland R, Marshall RJ, et al. Outcome of congestive heart failure in elderly persons: influence of left ventricular systolic function. The Cardiovascular Health Study. *Ann Intern Med* 2002; **137**:631–9.

7. Devereux RB, Roman MJ, Liu JE, et al. Congestive heart failure despite normal left ventricular systolic function in a population-based sample: the Strong Heart Study. *Am J Cardiol* 2000; **86**:1090–6.

8. Kupari M, Lindroos M, Iivanainen AM, Heikkila J, Tilvis R. Congestive heart failure in old age: prevalence, mechanisms and 4-year prognosis in the Helsinki Ageing Study. *J Intern Med* 1997; **241**:387–94.

9. Havranek EP, Masoudi FA, Westfall KA, Wolfe P, Ordin DL, Krumholz HM. Spectrum of heart failure in older patients: results from the National Heart Failure project. *Am Heart J* 2002; **143**:412–17.

10. Masoudi FA, Havranek EP, Smith G, et al. Gender, age, and heart failure with preserved left ventricular systolic function. *J Am Coll Cardiol* 2003; **41**:217–23.

11. Rich MW, Kitzman DW. Heart failure in octogenarians: a fundamentally different disease. *Am J Geriatr Cardiol* 2000; **9** (Suppl 5):97–104.

12. Samuel RS, Hausdorff JM, Wei JY. Congestive heart failure with preserved systolic function: is it a woman's disease? *Womens Health Issue* 1999; **9**:219–22.

13. Bella JN, Palmieri V, Kitzman DW, et al. Gender difference in diastolic function in hypertension (the HyperGEN study). *Am J Cardiol* 2002; **89**:1052–6.

14. Gerdts E, Zabalgoitia M, Bjornstad H, Svendsen TL, Devereux RB. Gender differences in systolic left ventricular function in hypertensive patients with electrocardiographic left ventricular hypertrophy (the LIFE study). *Am J Cardiol* 2001; **87**:980–3.

15. Kane GC, Hauser MF, Behrenbeck TR, Miller TD, Gibbons RJ, Christian TF. Impact of gender on rest Tc-99m sestamibi-gated left ventricular ejection fraction. *Am J Cardiol* 2002; **89**:1238–41.

16. Bella JN, Wachtell K, Palmieri V, et al. Relation of left ventricular geometry and function to systemic hemodynamics in hypertension: the LIFE Study. Losartan Intervention For Endpoint Reduction in Hypertension Study. *J Hypertens* 2001; **19**:127–34.

17. Douglas PS, Katz SE, Weinberg EO, Chen MH, Bishop SP, Lorell BH. Hypertrophic remodeling: gender differences in the early response to left ventricular pressure overload. *J Am Coll Cardiol* 1998; **32**:1118–25.

18. Aurigemma GP, Silver KH, McLaughlin M, Mauser J, Gaasch WH. Impact of chamber geometry and gender on left ventricular systolic function in patients >60 years of age with aortic stenosis. *Am J Cardiol* 1994; **74**:794–8.

19. Aurigemma GP, Gaasch WH, McLaughlin M, McGinn R, Sweeney A, Meyer TE. Reduced left ventricular systolic pump performance and depressed myocardial contractile function in patients >65 years of age with normal ejection fraction and a high relative wall thickness. *Am J Cardiol* 1995; **76**:702–5.

20. Mendes LA, Davidoff R, Cupples LA, Ryan TJ, Jacobs

AK. Congestive heart failure in patients with coronary artery disease: the gender paradox. *Am Heart J* 1997; **134** (2 Pt 1):207–12.

21. Freshour JR, Chase SE, Vikstrom KL. Gender differences in cardiac ACE expression are normalized in androgen-deprived male mice. *Am J Physiol Heart Circ Physiol* 2002; **283**:H1997–2003.

22. Ogawa T, Spina RJ, Martin WH, Kohrt WM, Schechtman KB. Effect of aging, sex, and physical training on cardiovacular responses to exercise. *Circulation* 1992; **86**:494–503.

23. Spina RJ, Ogawa T, Miller TR, Kohrt WM, Ehsani AA. Effect of exercise training on left ventricular performance in older women free of cardiopulmonary disease. *Am J Cardiol* 1993; **71**:99–104.

24. Sullivan M, Cobb FR, Knight JD, Higginbotham MB. Stroke volume increases by similar mechanisms in men and women. *Am J Cardiol* 1991; **67**:1405–12.

25. Kitzman DW, Little WC, Brubaker PH, et al. Pathophysiological characterization of isolated diastolic heart failure in comparison to systolic heart failure. *JAMA* 2002; **288**:2144–50.

26. Kitzman DW, Higginbotham MB, Cobb FR, Sheikh KH, Sullivan M. Exercise intolerance in patients with heart failure and preserved left ventricular systolic function: failure of the Frank–Starling mechanism. *J Am Coll Cardiol* 1991; **17**:1065–72.

27. Hundley WG, Kitzman DW, Morgan TM, et al. Cardiac cycle dependent changes in aortic area and aortic distensibility are reduced in older patients with isolated diastolic heart failure and correlate with exercise intolerance. *J Am Coll Cardiol* 2001; **38**:796–802.

28. Little WC. Enhanced load dependence of relaxation in heart failure: clinical implications. *Circulation* 1992; **85**:2326–8.

29. Gelpi RJ. Changes in diastolic cardiac function in developing and stable perinephritic hypertension in conscious dogs. *Circ Res* 1991; **68**:555–67.

30. Shannon RP, Komamura K, Gelpi RJ, Vatner SF. Altered load: an important component of impaired diastolic function in hypertension and heart failure. In: Lorell BH, Grossman W (eds). *Diastolic Relaxation of the Heart*. Norwell, MA: Kluwer Academic Publishers, 1994: 177–85.

31. Little WC, Braunwald E. Assessment of cardiac performance. In: Braunwald E (ed.). *Heart Disease*. Philadelphia: WB Saunders Company, 1999: 479–502.

32. Hoit BD, Walsh RA. Diastolic dysfunction in hypertensive heart disease. In: Gaasch WH, LeWinter MM (eds). *Left Ventricular Diastolic Dysfunction and Heart Failure*. Philadelphia: Lea & Febiger, 1994: 354–72.

33. Little WC, Ohno M, Kitzman DW, Thomas JD, Cheng CP. Determination of left ventricular chamber stiffness from the time for deceleration of early left ventricular filling. *Circulation* 1995; **92**:1933–9.

34. Iriarte M, Murga N, Morillas M, Salcedo A, Etxebeste J. Congestive heart failure from left ventricular diastolic dysfunction in systemic hypertension. *Am J Cardiol* 1993; **71**:308–12.

35. Iriarte MM, Perez OJ, Sagastagoitia D, Molinero E, Murga N. Congestive heart failure due to hypertensive ventricular diastolic dysfunction. *Am J Cardiol* 1995; **76**:43D–7D.

36. Cohen-Solal A, Desnos M, Delahaye F, Emeriau JP, Hanania G. A national survey of heart failure in French hospitals. The Myocardiopathy and Heart Failure Working Group of the French Society of Cardiology, the National College of General Hospital Cardiologists and the French Geriatrics Society. *Eur Heart J* 2000; **21**:763–9.

37. Kramer K, Kirkman P, Kitzman DW, Little WC. Flash pulmonary edema: association with hypertension, reocurrence despite coronary revascularization. *Am Heart J* 2000; **140**:451–5.

38. Gandhi SK, Powers JE, Fowle KM, et al. The pathogenesis of acute pulmonary edema associated with hypertension. *N Engl J Med* 2000; **344**:17–22.

39. Clarkson PBM, Wheeldon NM, MacFadyen RJ, Pringle SD, MacDonald TM. Effects of brain natriuretic peptide on exercise hemodynamics and neurohormones in isolated diatsolic heart failure. *Circulation* 1996; **93**:2037–42.

40. Bella JN, Palmieri V, Liu JE, et al. Relationship between left ventricular diastolic relaxation and systolic function in hypertension: The Hypertension Genetic Epidemiology Network (HyperGEN) study. *Hypertension* 2001; **38**:424–8.

41. Arnett D, Hong Y, Bella J, Oberman A, et al. Sibling correlation of left ventricular mass and geometry in hypertensive African Americans and whites: The HyperGEN Study. *Am J Hypertens* 2001; **14**:1226–30.

42. Tang W, Arnett DK, Devereux RB, Atwood L, Kitzman DW, Rao DC. Linkage of left ventricular diastolic peak filling velocity to chromosome 5 in hypertensive African Americans: the HyperGEN echocardiography study. *Am J Hypertens* 2002; **15** (7 Pt 1):621–7.

43. Vikstrom KL, Leinwand LA. The molecular genetic basis of familial hypertrophic cardiomyopathy. *Heart Fail* 1995; **11**:5–14.

44. Webster KA, Bishopric NH. Molecular aspects and gene therapy prospects for diastolic failure. *Cardiol Clin* 2000; **18**:621–35.

45. Ghali JK, Kadakia S, Cooper R, Liao Y. Bedside diagnosis of preserved versus impaired left ventricular systolic function in heart failure. *Am J Cardiol* 1991; **67**:1002–6.

46. Nagueh SF, Middleton KJ, Kopelen HA, Zoghbi WA, Quinones MA. Doppler tissue imaging: a noninvasive technique for evaluation of left ventricular relaxation and estimation of filling pressures. *J Am Coll Cardiol* 1997; **30**:1527–33.

47. European Study Group on Diastolic Heart Failure. How to diagnose diastolic heart failure. *Eur Heart J* 1998; **19**:990–1003.

48. Vasan RS, Levy D. Defining diastolic heart failure: a call for standardized diagnostic criteria. *Circulation* 2000; **101**:2118–21.

49. Zile MR, Gaasch WH, Carroll JD, et al. Heart failure with a normal ejection fraction: is measurement of diastolic function necessary to make the diagnosis of diastolic heart failure? *Circulation* 2001; **104**:779–82.

50. Zile MR, Baicu CF, Gaasch WH. Diastolic heart failure – abnormalities in active relaxation and passive stiffness of the left ventricle. *N Engl J Med* 2004; **350**:1953–9.

51. Zile MR, Brutsaert DL. New concepts in diastolic dysfunction and diastolic heart failure: Part I: diagnosis, prognosis, and measurements of diastolic function. *Circulation* 2002; **105**:1387–93.

52. Zile MR, Brutsaert DL. New concepts in diastolic dysfunction and diastolic heart failure: Part II: causal mechanisms and treatment. *Circulation* 2002; **105**:1503–8.

53. Redfield MM. Understanding 'diastolic' heart failure. *N Engl J Med* 2004; **350**:1930–1.

54. Kitzman DW. Heart failure and cardiomyopathy. In: Abrams WB, Beers MH, Berkow B (eds). *The Merck Manual of Geriatrics*. Whitehouse Station, NJ: Merck Research Laboratories, 2000: 900–14.

55. Redfield MM, Rodeheffer RJ, Jacobsen SJ, Mahoney DW, Bailey KR, Burnett JC Jr. Plasma brain natriuretic peptide concentration: impact of age and gender. *J Am Coll Cardiol* 2002; **40**:976–82.

56. Davis KM, Fish LC, Minaker KL, Elahi D. Atrial natriuretic peptide levels in the elderly: differentiating normal aging changes from disease. *J Gerontol* 1996; **51**:M95–101.

57. Pernenkil R, Vinson JM, Shah AS, Beckham V, Wittenberg C, Rich MW. Course and prognosis in patients ≥70 years of age with congestive heart failure and normal versus abnormal left ventricular ejection fraction. *Am J Cardiol* 1997; **79**:216–19.

58. Vinson JM, Rich MW, Sperry JC, Shah AS, McNamara T. Early readmission of elderly patients with congestive heart failure. *J Am Geriatr Soc* 1990; **38**:1290–5.

59. Rich MW, Vinson JM, Sperry JC, et al. Prevention of readmission in elderly patients with congestive heart failure: results of a prospective, randomized pilot study. *J Gen Intern Med* 1993; **8**:585–90.

60. Kitzman DW. Heart failure in the elderly: systolic and diastolic dysfunction. *Am J Geriatr Cardiol* 1995; **5**:20–6.

61. Schocken DD, Arrieta MI, Leaverton PE, Ross EA. Prevalence and mortality rate of congestive heart failure in the United States. *J Am Coll Cardiol* 1992; **20**:301–6.

62. Senni M, Tribouilloy CM, Rodeheffer RJ, et al. Congestive heart failure in the community: trends in incidence and survival in a 10-year period. *Arch Intern Med* 1999; **159**:29–34.

63. Taffet GE, Teasdale TA, Bleyer AJ, Kutka NJ, Luchi RJ. Survival of elderly men with congestive heart failure. *Age Ageing* 1992; **21**:49–55.

64. Aronow WS, Ahn C, Kronzon I. Prognosis of congestive heart failure in elderly patients with normal versus abnormal left ventricular systolic function associated with coronary artery disease. *Am J Cardiol* 1990; **66**:1257–9.

65. Opasich C, Tavazzi L, Lucci D, et al. Comparison of one-year outcome in women versus men with chronic congestive heart failure. *Am J Cardiol* 2000; **86**:353–7.

66. Krumholz HM, Chen YT, Vaccarino V, et al. Correlates and impact on outcomes of worsening renal function in patients > or =65 years of age with heart failure. *Am J Cardiol* 2000; **85**:1110–13.

67. Kitzman DW. Therapy for diastolic heart failure: on the road from myths to multicenter trials. *J Card Fail* 2001; **7**:229–31.

68. Vasan RS, Benjamin EJ. Diastolic heart failure – no time to relax. *N Engl J Med* 2001; **344**:56–9.

69. Tresch DD, McGough MF. Heart failure with normal systolic function: a common disorder in older people. *J Am Geriatr Soc* 1995; **43**:1035–42.

70. Dauterman K, Massie BM, Gheorghiade M. Heart failure associated with preserved systolic function: a common and costly clinical entity. *Am Heart J* 1998; **135** (6 Pt 2):S310–17.

71. Lewis JF, Maron BJ. Clinical and morphologic expression of hypertrophic cardiomyopathy in patients ≥65 years of age. *Am J Cardiol* 1994; **73**:1105–11.

72. Lewis JF, Maron BJ. Elderly patients with hypertrophic cardiomyopathy: a subset with distinctive left ventricular morphology and progressive clinical course late in life. *J Am Coll Cardiol* 1989; **13**:36–45.

73. Olson LJ, Gertz MA, Edwards WD, et al. Senile

cardiac amyloidosis with myocardial dysfunction. Diagnosis by endomyocardial biopsy and immuno-histochemistry. *N Engl J Med* 1987; **317**:738–42.

74. Moser M, Hebert PR. Prevention of disease progression, left ventricular hypertrophy and congestive heart failure in hypertension treatment trials. *J Am Coll Cardiol* 1996; **27**:1214–18.

75. Amery A, Birkenhager W, Brixko P, et al. Mortality and morbidity results from the European Working Party on High Blood Pressure in the Elderly Trial. *Lancet* 1985; **1**:1349–54.

76. Dahlof B, Lindholm L, Hannson L, Schersten B, Ekbom T, Wester PO. Morbidity and mortality in the Swedish Trial in Old Patients with Hypertension (STOP-Hypertension). *Lancet* 1991; **338**:1281–5.

77. Stassen JA, Fagard R, Thijs L, et al. Randomised double-blind comparison of placebo and active treatment for older patients with isolated systolic hypertension. *Lancet* 1997; **350**:757–64.

78. Gong LS, Zhang W, Zhu Y. Shanghai Trial of Nifedipine in the Elderly (STONE). *J Hypertension* 2001; **14**:1237–45.

79. Major outcomes in high-risk hypertensive patients randomized to angiotensin-converting enzyme inhibitor or calcium channel blocker vs diuretic: the Antihypertensive and Lipid-Lowering Treatment to Prevent Heart Attack Trial (ALLHAT). *JAMA* 2002; **288**:2981–97.

80. Kitzman DW. Diastolic dysfunction in the elderly; genesis and diagnostic and therapeutic implications. In: Kovacs SJ (ed.). *Cardiology Clinics of North America – Diastolic Function.* Philadelphia: WB Saunders, 2000: 597–617.

81. Stewart S, Marley JE, Horowitz JD. Effects of a multidisciplinary, home-based intervention on unplanned readmissions and survival among patients with chronic congestive heart failure: a randomised controlled study. *Lancet* 1999; **354**:1077–83.

82. Rich MW, Beckham V, Wittenberg C, Leven CL, Freedland KE, Carney R. A multidisciplinary intervention to prevent the readmission of elderly patients with congestive heart failure. *N Engl J Med* 1995; **333**:1190–5.

83. Stewart S, Vanderheyden M, Pearson S, Horowitz JD. Prolonged beneficial effects of a home-based intervention on unplanned readmissions and mortality among patients with congestive heart failure. *Arch Intern Med* 1999; **159**:257–61.

84. Tsuyuki RT, McKelvie RS, Arnold JM, et al. Acute precipitants of congestive heart failure exacerbations. *Arch Intern Med* 2001; **161**:2337–42.

85. Leier CV, Dei Cas L, Metra M. Clinical relevance and management of the major electrolyte abnormalities in congestive heart failure: hyponatremia, hypokalemia, and hypomagnesemia. *Am Heart J* 1994; **128**:564–74.

86. Digoxin Investigators Group. The effect of digoxin on mortality and morbidity in patients with heart failure. *N Engl J Med* 1997; **336**:525–33.

87. Rathore SS, Wang Y, Krumholz HM. Sex-based differences in the effect of digoxin for the treatment of heart failure. *N Engl J Med* 2002; **347**:1403–11.

88. Lorell BH, Grossman W. Cardiac hypertrophy: the consequences for diastole. *J Am Coll Cardiol* 1987; **9**:1189–93.

89. Lorell BH. Cardiac renin–angiotensin system in cardiac hypertophy and failure. In: Lorell BH, Grossman W (eds). *Diastolic Relaxation of the Heart*, 2nd edn. Norwell, MA: Kluwer Academic Publishers, 1996: 91–9.

90. Oren S, Grossman E, Frohlich ED. Reduction in left ventricular mass in patients with systemic hypertension treated with enalapril, lisinopril, or fosenopril. *Am J Cardiol* 1996; **77**:93–6.

91. Friedrich SP, Lorell BH, Douglas PS, et al. Intracardiac ACE inhibition improves diastolic distensibility in patients with left ventricular hypertophy due to aortic stenosis. *Circulation* 1992; **86** (Suppl I):I-119.

92. Lakatta E. Cardiovascular aging research: the next horizons. *J Am Geriatr Soc* 1999; **47**:613–25.

93. Aronow WS, Kronzon I. Effect of enalapril on congestive heart failure treated with diuretics in elderly patients with prior myocardial infarction and normal left ventricular ejection fraction. *Am J Cardiol* 1993; **71**:602–4.

94. Philbin EF, Rocco TA. Use of angiotensin-converting enzyme inhibitors in heart failure with preserved left ventricular systolic function. *Am Heart J* 1997; **134**:188–95.

95. Philbin EF, Rocco TA Jr, Lindenmuth NW, Ulrich K, Jenkins PL. Clinical outcomes in heart failure: report from a community hospital-based registry. *Am J Med* 1999; **107**:549–55.

96. Cleland JG, Tendera M, Adamus J, et al. Perindopril for elderly people with chronic heart failure: the PEP-CHF study. The PEP investigators. *Eur J Heart Fail* 1999; **1**:211–17.

97. Abraham TP, Kon ND, Nomeir AM, Cordell AR, Kitzman DW. Accuracy of transesophageal echocardiography in preoperative determination of aortic anulus size during valve replacement. *J Am Soc Echocardiogr* 1997; **10**:149–54.

98. Yusuf S, Pfeffer MA, Swedberg K, et al. Effects of candesartan in patients with chronic heart failure and

preserved left-ventricular ejection fraction: the CHARM-Preserved Trial. *Lancet* 2003; **362**:777–81.

99. Vandenberg VF, Rath LS, Stuhlmuller P, Melton H, Skorton DJ. Estimation of left ventricular cavity area with on-line, semiautomated echocardiographic edge detection system. *Circulation* 1992; **86**:159–66.

100. Bonow RO, Leon MB, Rosing DR, et al. Effects of verapamil and propranolol on left ventricular systolic function and diastolic filling in patients with coronary artery disease: radionuclide angiographic studies at rest and during exercise. *Circulation* 1981; **65**:1337–50.

101. Bonow RO, Dilsizian V, Rosing DR, Maron BJ, Bacharach SL, Green MV. Verapamil-induced improvement in left ventricular diastolic filling and increased exercise tolerance in patients with hypertrophic cardiomyopathy: short- and long-term effects. *Circulation* 1985; **72**:853–64.

102. Udelson J, Bonow RO. Left ventricular diastolic function and calcium channel blockers in hypertrophic cardiomyopathy. In: Gaasch WH (ed). *Left Ventricular Diastolic Dysfunction and Heart Failure.* Malvern, PA: Lea & Febiger, 1996: 465–89.

103. Serizawa T, Shin-Ichi M, Nagai Y, et al. Diastolic abnormalities in low-flow and pacing tachycardia-induced ischemia in isolated rat hearts – modification by calcium antagonists. In: Lorell BH, Grossman W (eds). *Diastolic Relaxation of the Heart.* Norwell, MA: Kluwer Academic Publishers, 1996: 266–74.

104. Cheng CP, Pettersson K, Little WC. Effects of felodipine on left ventricular systolic and diastolic performance in congestive heart failure. *J Pharmacol Exp Ther* 1994; **271**:1409–17.

105. Cheng CP, Noda T, Ohno M, Little WC. Differential effects of enalaprilat and felodipine on diastolic function during exercise in dogs with congestive heart failure. *Circulation* 1993; **88**:I-294.

106. Little WC, Cheng CP, Elvelin L, Nordlander M. Vascular selective calcium entry blockers in the treatment of cardiovascular disorders: focus on felodipine. *Cardiovasc Drugs Ther* 1995; **9**:657–63.

107. Ten Cate FJ, Serruys PW, Mey S, Roelandt JR. Effects of short-term administration of verapamil on left ventricular filling dynamics measured by a combined hemodynamic–ultrasonic technique in patients with hypertrophic cardiomyopathy. *Circulation* 1983; **68**:1274–9.

108. Hess OM, Murakami T, Krayenbuehl HP. Does verapamil improve left ventricular relaxation in patients with myocardial hypertrophy? *Circulation* 1996; **74**:530–43.

109. Brutsaert DL, Rademakers F, Sys SU, Gillebert TC, Housmans PR. Analysis of relaxation in the evalua-

tion of ventricular function of the heart. *Prog Cardiovasc Dis* 1985; **28**:143–63.

110. Brutsaert DL, Sys SU, Gillebert TC. Diastolic failure: pathophysiology and therapeutic implications. *J Am Coll Cardiol* 1993; **22**:318–25.

111. Setaro JF, Zaret BL, Schulman DS, Black HR. Usefulness of verapamil for congestive heart failure associated with abnormal left ventricular diastolic filling and normal left ventricular systolic performance. *Am J Cardiol* 1990; **66**:981–6.

112. Sasayama S, Asanoi H, Ishizaka S, Kihara Y. Diastolic dysfunction in experimental heart failure. In: Lorell BH, Grossman W (eds). *Diastolic Relaxation of the Heart.* Norwell, MA: Kluwer Academic Publishers, 1994: 195–202.

113. Copeland JL, Consitt LA, Tremblay MS. Hormonal responses to endurance and resistance exercise in females aged 19–69 years. *J Gerontol A Biol Sci Med Sci* 2002; **57**:B158–65.

114. Udelson J, Bonow RO. Left ventricular diastolic function and calcium channel blockers in hypertrophic cardiomyopathy. In: Gaasch WH, LeWinter MM (eds). *Left Ventricular Diastolic Dysfunction and Heart Failure.* Philadelphia: Lea & Febiger, 1994: 462–89.

115. Cheng CP, Igarashi Y, Little WC. Mechanism of augmented rate of left ventricle filling during exercise. *Circ Res* 1992; **70**:9–19.

116. Cheng CP, Noda T, Nozawa T, Little WC. Effect of heart failure on the mechanism of exercise induced augmentation of mitral valve flow. *Circ Res* 1993; **72**:795–806.

117. Pitt B, Zannad F, Remme WJ, et al. The effect of spironolactone on morbidity and mortality in patients with severe heart failure. *N Engl J Med* 1999; **341**:709–17.

118. Pitt B, Reichek N, Willenbrock R, et al. Effects of eplerenone, enalapril, and eplerenone/enalapril in patients with essential hypertension and left ventricular hypertrophy: the 4E-left ventricular hypertrophy study. *Circulation* 2003; **108**:1831–8.

119. Rajagopalan S, Pitt B. Aldosterone as a target in congestive heart failure. *Med Clin North Am* 2003; **87**:441–57.

120. Zannad F, Alla F, Dousset B, Perez A, Pitt B. Limitation of excessive extracellular matrix turnover may contribute to survival benefit of spironolactone therapy in patients with congestive heart failure: insights from the randomized aldactone evaluation study (RALES). Rales Investigators. *Circulation* 2000; **102**:2700–6.

121. Daniel KR, Wells GL, Fray B, Stewart KP, Kitzman DW. The effect of spironolactone on exercise tolerance and quality of life in elderly women with diastolic heart failure. *Am J Geriatr Cardiol* 2003; **12**:131.

29

Heart failure in women

Ileana L. Piña and Shadi Daoud

Introduction

Cardiovascular disease (CVD) is the leading cause of death in women, responsible for more deaths each year than all other causes combined. As treatment options have broadened and long-term survival improved, more women are living with chronic cardiovascular conditions which can ultimately lead to end-stage heart disease, i.e. heart failure.

More than half of all patients in the US with heart failure are women. Among persons older than 70 years, the incidence of congestive heart failure (HF) in women is higher than in men[1-3] with the largest increase in prevalence occurring in the 65–74-year-old age group[4] (Fig. 29.1).

The incidence of heart failure in women, however, has declined in the past 40 years, perhaps due to better blood pressure control or perhaps due to a reduction in rheumatic heart disease. The incidence in men during the same period has remained unchanged. In spite of a decline in the rates of heart failure death for both women and men, as noted in Fig. 29.2, 50% of patients who were diagnosed in the 1990s had died in 5 years.[5]

This chapter will review heart failure gender differences in several areas, including risk factors, source of data on women with heart failure, pathophysiology in the development of heart failure, survival, and any gender differences in response to therapy.

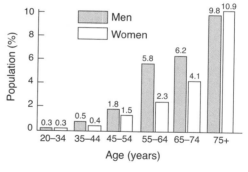

Figure 29.1
Prevalence of congestive heart failure by sex and age according to National Health and Nutrition Examination Survey, 1999–2002. Note the near doubling of the prevalence in women from the 55–64 age group to the 65–74 group with a further increase in the over 75 age group. Many of the women in the over 75 group may have heart failure with preserved systolic function. Source: Centers for Disease Control and Prevention/National Center for Health Statistics and National Heart, Lung, and Blood Institute. From reference 4.

Gender differences in risk factors

Hypertension is a stronger risk factor for the development of HF in women than in men. In the

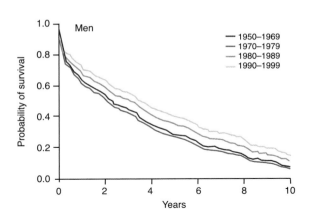

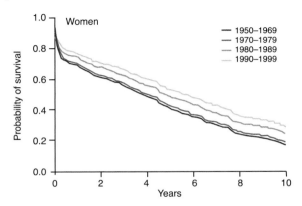

Figure 29.2
Age-adjusted survival after the onset of heart failure for men (a) and for women (b). The graph is divided into time periods from the Framingham database. The age-adjusted survival after the onset of heart failure improved over time. The 5-year mortality rate in men dropped from 70% in the years 1950–1969 to 59% in the years 1990–1999 and that in women in the same time period decreased from 57% to 45%. Reproduced from reference 5 with permission.

Framingham Study, hypertension conferred a two-fold excess risk of developing heart failure in men and a threefold risk in women.[6] This observation has been duplicated in more recent studies and may be due to a gender-based difference in cardiac response to pressure overload (see below).

The incidence of heart failure is five times higher in patients who have had a myocardial infarction (MI) compared with those who have not and survivors of an MI are at increased risk for heart failure as they grow older. Although the incidence of MI is lower in women than in men, women who sustain a MI are more likely to develop heart failure, 46% compared with 22%, respectively.[4]

In addition, diabetes mellitus is a more potent risk factor in women than in men for the development of CHD, and diabetes increases the risk of death following an acute MI. Several studies[7–9] have shown that diabetes mellitus is a stronger risk factor for the development of heart failure in women, with or without an ischemic etiology, as well. Risk factors also co-exist more often in diabetics. In the SAVE trial, the diabetic patients were more likely to have concomitant hypertension and more likely to have heart failure after 2 years of follow-up.[10]

Who are the women with heart failure?

Information on the women with heart failure can be derived from various sources:

- Large epidemiologic studies
- Health plans
- Registries – usually derived from clinical trials or procedures
- Clinical trials
- Heart specialty clinics

Each of these sources has its unique perspective and its positive and negative aspects. Epidemiologic studies examine a large population with its natural history and do not usually provide an active intervention. Health plans today collect data on their constituency primarily to identify the healthier segment of their population and to control rising costs. They rely primarily on the coding for diagnosis and do not verify the patient presentations. Registries derived from clinical trials provide information on the natural course of a focused disease process in a population that for multiple reasons did not enter the parent trial. The population tends to be more homogeneous than those of epidemiologic data or those of health plans. Clinical trials, on the other hand, examine focused populations that fit specific entry criteria and are therefore more uniform but may not be generalized to the population at large with the disease process. Specialty clinics, by their very nature, concentrate strongly on a certain disease or syndrome and attract patients who are more ill and have been referred to the clinics for careful follow-up.

The Framingham data are an example of a large epidemiologic group which report that the prevalence of heart failure in women is less than that of men until their 80s, when the prevalence in women surpasses that of men.[4] A more recent report by Levy et al. finds that, over a 40-year period, the incidence of heart failure has decreased in women but remains unchanged in men. The authors speculate that the decrease in incidence may be due to better recognition of hypertension as a risk factor for heart failure and better pharmacologic therapy development in the same time period. Another plausible explanation may be the near eradication of rheumatic fever and subsequent rheumatic heart disease in the US, which in the 1950s was a significant cause of heart failure, particularly in women.[11,12]

Health plans such as the Henry Ford Hospital Health System report that the prevalence of heart failure increased in both women and men in the late 1990s. Of the patients with heart failure, 53% are women and 54% of those are African-American. Women with heart failure are older than the men. Over a 5-year period, the women had a better survival than the men overall. The data do not distinguish between ischemic and nonischemic etiologies.[13]

Registries are often a byproduct of large trials giving a distinct view of the population being described which was not randomized into the parent trial. The SOLVD (Studies of Left Ventricular Dysfunction) Registry contained 1640 women. The women with heart failure in the Registry were more likely to have a dilated than an ischemic cardiomyopathy, and to have hypertension or valvular disease as an etiology. More women were also diabetic.[14,15]

The clinical trials have not enrolled a significant number of women, since there appear to be more women with heart failure in health plans and in epidemiologic databases than are included in trials. Table 29.1[7,10,16–32] depicts the number and percentage of women in clinical trials dedicated to heart failure. To date, the CHARM trial has included the largest

Table 29.1 The number of women in heart failure trials

Study	Number of patients	Number of women	Percentage of women
CONSENSUS-I[18]	253	75	30
SOLVD-T[7]	2569	504	23
SOLVD-P[19]	4228	476	31
ELITE-I[21]	722	240	31
ELITE-II[22]	3152	966	30
MERIT-HF[23]	3991	451	23
CIBIS II[24]	2647	515	20
COPERNICUS[25]	2287	465	28
Val HEFT[26]	5010	1002	20
RALES[27]	1663	446	27
SAVE[10]	2231	390	28
TRACE[28]	1749	501	22
CHARM[29]	7599	243	32
SCD HeFT[30]	2521	580	23
DIG[31]	6800	1520	22.4
Total	47 422	10 907	23

Adapted from reference 32.

percentage of women at 32%.[29] This difference may be due to the CHARM-Preserved trial, which had 40% women with heart failure and preserved systolic function.[33] There is consistency, however, across clinical trials in that women who enter are more symptomatic and more likely to have a higher NYHA class, more hypertension, and a higher ejection fraction. Whether the women are diagnosed later or whether symptoms develop in a different way from men is purely speculative.

Heart specialty clinics associated with heart failure programs offer a different view on the number of women attending outpatient services. Adams et al. examined the patient demographics in their Heart Failure Clinic and found that the women were older than the men but had a history of hypertension similar to that of the men.[34] The men, however, were more likely to have an ischemic etiology for heart failure and more likely to have had coronary artery bypass graft surgery. In contrast to the men, the women had higher ejection fractions but were nonetheless more symptomatic, particularly with edema. It is therefore, not surprising that there were more women with NYHA

Table 29.2 Differences in characteristics between women and men in several heart failure trials and in a specialty heart failure clinic

Parameter	SOLVD[7,19]	FIRST[36]	MERIT[23]	CIBIS-II[24]	Heart failure clinic[34]
n (% women)	6271 (26)	471 (24)	898 (22.5)	2647 (19)	557 (32)
Age	Older	Older	Older	Older	Younger
Ischemia	Less	Less	Less	Less	Less
EF	Same	Same	Same	Same	Higher
Diabetes	More	Same	More	More	More
Hypertension	More	More	More	More	More
HR	Higher	Higher	Higher	Same	–
Race	↑AA	↑AA	–	–	↑AA
Mortality	Higher	Lower in IDC	Lower	Lower in nonIDC	Lower in nonIDC

EF, ejection fraction; HR, hazard ratio; AA, African American; IDC, ischemic cardiomyopathy.
Reproduced from reference 32 with permission.

class IV compared with men (40% vs 25%, respectively).

In summary, all the above-mentioned sources provide important information about women with heart failure. There is a consistency in several factors relating to women with heart failure. These include: a greater proportion with hypertension and diabetes, a more advanced set of symptoms on presentation (in spite of higher ejection fractions), and less ischemic etiology (Table 29.2).[7,19,32,34–36]

Gender differences in pathophysiology (see also Chapter 28)

Physiology

The syndrome of heart failure is initiated by an injury or a maladaptive repair process of the myocardium which results in altered molecular and cellular activities. These changes ultimately cause either relaxation or contraction abnormalities, or both. The end result is a combination of neurohormonal and circulatory changes which are responsible for the syndrome of heart failure. This process includes activation of the renin–angiotensin–aldosterone system, upregulation of the sympathetic nervous system and the release of inflammatory mediators such as interleukin (IL)-1, IL-6, and tumor necrosis factor-α (TNF-α).

A growing body of basic and clinical data points to fundamental gender-related differences in the nature and extent of myocardial hypertrophy and adaptation, which might account for the survival advantage of women with dilated cardiomyopathy. Early studies of spontaneously hypertensive rats suggested that the adverse influence of hypertrophy on cardiac function was greater in male than female rats.[37] Gender differences in upregulation of left ventricular (LV) angiotensin-converting enzyme (ACE) activity during pressure overload hypertrophy have been reported.[38] Importantly, gender has been found to influence the nature of LV adaptation in patients with aortic stenosis with women more likely to have well preserved systolic function and less ventricular dilatation and hypertrophy than their male counterparts.[39] A similar situation exists with regard to hypertension, with women more likely have LV hypertrophy (LVH).[40]

Etiology (see also Chapters 28 and 31)

Women have more heart failure related to hypertension and valvular heart disease and are less likely to have an ischemic etiology than men.[41,42] In addition, women are more sensitive to cardiac toxins such as ethanol and may have specific immune risk factors such as seen peripartum.[43,44] Women with heart failure are also more likely to be diabetic. In all patients, diabetes disproportionately increases the risk for heart failure; however, this is even more common in young women.[45] Although CHD plays a stronger role in men, women are at a higher risk than men for heart failure development following MI.[45]

Women present with heart failure later in life and are more likely to have preserved systolic function. This prevalence increases with age. Overall, LVH, hypertension, older age, and being female are all independent contributors to the likelihood of developing heart failure with preserved systolic function.[46]

Remodeling

There is strong laboratory and clinical research evidence for gender differences in cardiac function and adaptation to injury and stress.[37,47–49] In animals, Weinberg et al. observed less contractile reserve in male rats in response to identical degrees of LVH and systolic wall stress. Myocytes from male rats were found to have less expression of sarcoplasmic reticulum Ca^{2+}-adenosine triphosphate (SERCA-2) and increased expression of β-myosin than myocytes from female rats.[38] Pfeffer et al. have shown in spontaneously hypertensive rats that LVH reduces cardiac performance in males to a lesser degree than in females.[37]

In humans, women tend to have preserved or even supernormal ejection fractions with smaller but thicker-walled chambers in response to hypertension and aortic stenosis.[50–53]

Carroll et al. first reported the importance of sex-associated differences in LV function when they showed that women with aortic stenosis tended to have more preserved LV function than men with the same degree of aortic stenosis.[50]

Mendes et al. studied the LV pressure–volume relationship in patients referred for cardiac catheterization. When patients were stratified according to LV end-diastolic pressure, women had significantly lower end-diastolic volume than men.[54] Women tend to develop a pattern of concentric hypertrophy whereas men develop an eccentric pattern.[55]

Cell death

Gender differences influence the aging process of the heart. Cell death occurs by apoptosis, necrosis, or a combination of both. These processes contribute to the evolution of heart failure. Women appear to be more protected from necrotic and apoptotic death signals.[56] The myocardium in women may be less vulnerable to the aging process. Olivetti et al. found that aging in men is associated with myocyte death and reactive hypertrophy; however, this was not found in women, who have a constant number of myocytes throughout their life.[49]

Hormonal influences

Data from experimental animals, epidemiologic surveys, and clinical investigations suggest that the circulating and tissue levels of the renin–angiotensin system are affected by gender. Oral estrogen upregulates angiotensinogen but downregulates renin, ACE and angiotensin-1 receptor. The net effect is similar to the effects of angiotensin receptor blockers (ARBs) and ACE inhibitors.[57] Estrogen can be synthesized locally by myocytes from both females and males. Since more estrogen is produced in females, it is postulated that estrogen, by signaling through the adult myocyte estrogen receptor, may explain the gender differences.[58]

Estrogen can play a role by phosphorylating insulin-like growth factor 1 (IGF-1) receptors, which can confer protection through stimulation of nitric oxide and other pathways.[59–61] Other pathophysiologic differences have also been noted. Aronson et al. found that women have an attenuated sympathetic activation and an attenuated parasympathetic withdrawal when they studied heart rate variability in patients with nonischemic heart failure.[62]

Gender differences in survival

Discrepancies exist in the early literature regarding gender-based differences in survival in patients with heart failure. Several studies revealed a better prognosis for women than for men with symptomatic HF. In the Framingham database,[45,63] the prognosis for women after the diagnosis of heart failure was better than for men (despite an older age at presentation) with a median survival of 3.2 years compared with 1.7 years. The short median survivals are reflective of the fact that patients were enrolled between 1948 and 1988, well before the widespread use of ACE inhibitors and beta-blockers for the treatment of heart failure. In the early days of Framingham, echocardiographic estimation of LV function was not obtained, and thus the heart failure population undoubtedly represents a heterogeneous array of differing physiologic causes of heart failure.

In distinction to the early Framingham data, the SOLVD Trial Registry reported a worse outcome in women than men presenting with symptomatic heart failure (22% vs 17%, respectively).[15] Event-free survival was worse in women, with an odds ratio of death or heart failure hospital admission for men compared with women of 0.67 (p <0.001). Women were older than men at study entry, but had an equivalent abnormality of ventricular function.

These seemingly disparate results may reflect the inclusion of patients with heart failure with preserved LV systolic function in the Framingham cohort and the probable inclusion of a greater percentage of women with coronary heart disease in the SOLVD registry prior to the extensive use of ACE inhibitors.

Although some of this gender-based survival advantage has been ascribed to the lesser prevalence of CHD in women, mortality has been shown to be lower for women with heart failure in several large clinical trials following adjustment for differences in baseline variables. In the MERIT-HF study, the relative risk for total mortality in the placebo arm was significantly lower for women as compared with men (RR 0.63) regardless of heart failure etiology.[64]

The etiology of heart failure, however, does seem to impact the survival of women. The Flolan International Randomized Survival Trial (FIRST), a trial of advanced heart failure patients randomized to either epoprostenol or placebo, enrolled 359 men and 112 women.[36] After adjustment for important variables, significant gender-based differences in survival were noted. Among patients with a nonischemic etiology of heart failure, the relative risk of death for men versus women was 3.08, whereas among those with ischemic heart disease the relative risk of death for men versus women was a modest and statistically insignificant 1.64.

Further confirmation of this observation was made by Adams and colleagues at the University of North Carolina, where a database has been in existence since 1984.[34] A study of 557 patients (380 men and 177 women) with symptomatic heart failure, predominantly nonischemic in origin (68%), and severe LV dysfunction with a mean LV ejection fraction (LVEF) of 25%, revealed a better survival in women compared with men when heart failure was due to a nonischemic cause but not in women with an ischemic cause. With a follow-up of 2.4 years, the risk of death was similar for the subset of women and men with ischemic heart disease as the primary cause of heart failure.

Ghali et al. have reported the findings from the BEST trial, which randomized class III and IV heart failure patients to either placebo or bucindolol.[64] The trial as a whole failed to meet its hypothesis of reduction in mortality. The women were younger, had greater both left and right ventricular EFs, lower plasma norepinephrine and more non-ischemic disease. However, the women with ischemic disease had a worse outcome than the men. In the women, CHD and LVEF were stronger predictors of mortality. The authors concluded that the survival benefit in women existed only in the nonischemic group.

These observations underline the need for trials that prospectively plan to analyze women separately and that include enough women to make definitive statements. It is also a reminder that women can have CHD as a cause of heart failure and that risk factors cannot be ignored in women and should be addressed as vigorously as in men.[65]

Treatment of established heart failure (see also Chapter 39)

ACE inhibitors

No ACE inhibitor heart failure trial to date has prospectively planned to review the results in women. We are therefore left with retrospective analyses of a small percentage of women in ACE inhibitor trials. The first trial to demonstrate a survival benefit with the use of ACE inhibitors in

Table 29.3 Effects of ACE inhibitors on women compared with men as reflected in heart failure trials

Study name	RR analysis					
	Total n	Male n	Female n	RR male (95% CI)	RR female (95% CI)	RRR (95% CI)
CONSENSUS	253	179	74	0.61 (0.44–0.85)	1.14 (0.68–1.90)	1.86 (1.01–3.42)
SAVE	2231	1841	390	0.80 (0.68–0.95)	0.99 (0.67–1.47)	1.24 (0.80–1.90)
SMILE	1556	1128	428	0.61 (0.39–0.96)	0.74 (0.47–1.18)	1.22 (0.64–2.32)
SOLVD-Prevention	4228	3752	476	0.90 (0.77–1.05)	1.15 (0.74–1.78)	1.27 (0.80–2.02)
SOLVD-Treatment	2569	2065	504	0.89 (0.80–0.99)	0.86 (0.67–1.09)	0.97 (0.74–1.26)
TRACE	1749	1248	501	0.79 (0.68–0.91)	0.90 (0.74–1.11)	1.15 (0.90–1.48)
Random effects pooled estimate		10213	2373	0.82 (0.74–0.90)	0.92 (0.81–1.04)	1.15 (0.99–1.33)

ACE, angiotensin-converting enzyme; CI, confidence interval; RR, relative risk; RRR, ratio of relative risk. Adapted from reference 68.

heart failure was the CONSENSUS trial, reported in 1987.[18] Women comprised 23% of the 253 patients with NYHA class IV heart failure who were enrolled. While the men enjoyed a 51% reduction in 6-month mortality, women achieved only a nonsignificant 6% reduction.[66] The small sample size, and therefore the small number of events in women, without a doubt contributed to this apparent discrepancy in survival benefit. In addition, one cannot ignore that many women may have had heart failure with preserved systolic function and inherently had a better survival probability.

The SAVE trial enrolled 390 women with a low LVEF following MI and suggested that ACE inhibitors may be less effective in women than men with heart failure.[10] Although the mortality risk reduction was 22% in men compared with 2% in women, risk reduction in women and men was similar (21% vs 19%) after adjustment for baseline variables.

An early meta-analysis of ACE inhibitor trials[67] found significant reductions in mortality and the combined endpoints of all-cause mortality and hospitalizations for heart failure for men only. The apparent lack of benefit for women in this analysis most likely once again reflects the small number of women in these trials. Shekelle et al. synthesized data from 12 of the largest randomized trials of ACE inhibitors and beta-blockers and analyzed the results to test differences by gender, race and co-morbidities.[68] The ACE inhibitor trials reviewed included

SAVE, SOLVD treatment, SOLVD prevention, SMILE, TRACE, and CONSENSUS.[7,10,18,19,28,69] Table 29.3 illustrates that although the risk reduction (RR) is better for men, the random pooled data showed some benefit in women, although less so than for men. Studies that reported a hazard ratio (HR) yielded values of 0.76 in men and 0.84 in women. This difference only approached statistical significance, p = 0.07. If the treatment and prevention studies are divided, the women have a more attenuated effect of ACE inhibition but the RR is better in the treatment than in the prevention trials. Therefore, there are no convincing data to suggest that women do not benefit from ACE inhibition, particularly when overt symptoms are present; however, the effect may be less than in men. ACE inhibitors, nonetheless, should be administered to women similarly to men with heart failure.

Beta-blockers

The Cardiac Insufficiency Bisoprolol Study (CIBIS II) was the first large-scale randomized, double-blind, placebo-controlled European study to show a reduction in all-cause mortality rates with the addition of the beta-1 selective antagonist bisoprolol to standard treatment with ACE inhibitors and diuretics. The study enrolled 2647 patients with NYHA class III–IV heart failure and a LVEF of ≤35%.[24]

Of the total study population, 515 were women. As is often seen, the women were older than the men by approximately 5 years.[70] They had a higher NYHA score, with 21% versus 16% in class IV. Despite being sicker at baseline, women had a lower mortality after an average follow-up of 1.3 years. The rates of sudden death, fatal MI, unknown cause of death, and all-cause hospital admissions did not differ between women and men. The number of women with non-ischemic cardiomyopathy may have had a better survival in parallel to the observations made above.

MERIT-HF was a randomized, placebo-controlled study of metoprolol controlled-release/extended-release in 3991 patients with NYHA class II–IV heart failure due to LV systolic dysfunction.[23] Women constituted 23% of the patients enrolled. Compared with the men, the women were older, were more often in NYHA class III and IV, less often were classified as previous or current smokers, and had similar LVEFs.[64] They had a higher prevalence of hypertension and diabetes mellitus and a lower prevalence of CHD and prior MI. Overall, treatment with extended-release metoprolol led to a 21% decrease in the combined endpoint of all-cause hospitalization and all-cause mortality in women, but did not lead to a significant reduction in mortality when viewed as separate endpoints. There was a 29% decrease in cardiovascular hospitalizations and a 42% decrease in hospitalizations due to worsening heart failure. In the subset of women with severe heart failure, there was a 44% reduction in the combined endpoint, a 57% reduction in cardiovascular hospitalization, and a 72% reduction in hospitalization due to worsening heart failure. In contrast to women, actively treated men had a significant but less robust reduction in all-cause hospitalization rates. A significant reduction in all-cause mortality was seen in actively treated men.

Although there was no significant survival advantage demonstrated in women randomized to beta-blocker treatment in the MERIT-HF trial, this may be due to the relatively small number of women enrolled and the small number of deaths in women which totaled 64. The meta-analysis of Shekelle et al. confirms that in pooling the four most important beta-blocker trials in heart failure (i.e. COPERNICUS, MERIT-HF, US Carvedilol Trials, and CIBIS II), the RRs for women and men are similar (0.63 vs 0.66); therefore women seem to enjoy the same benefit from beta-blockade as men. In summary, the beta-blocker trials confirm the observations made by single centers and databases that women present with more advanced symptoms and fewer have CHD, although the co-morbidities of hypertension and diabetes are more frequent.[68]

Angiotensin II receptor blockers

Although ACE inhibitors continue to be the first recommendation for patients with heart failure, women have been reported to have more side effects, such as cough. In the SOLVD trial, the women had a higher rate of adverse events both at first dosing and at rechallenge.[35,71,72] In addition, in African-American women, the incidence of angioedema is also greater. There are no known explanations for these observations.

Given these observations, alternative agents have to be considered for women with intolerable cough or with angioedema. Although the combination of hydralazine and isosorbide dinitrate was shown to improve survival versus placebo in heart failure, all subjects in the VHeFT trials were men.[16,17] To date, there are few data on women using this vasodilator combination. The angiotensin II receptor blockers (ARBs) are now being recommended as alternative therapy for patients who are intolerant of ACE inhibitors. The Val-HeFT trial studied the ARB valsartan versus placebo in combination with background therapy which consisted mostly of ACE inhibitors, beta-blockers, digoxin, and diuretics in 5010 patients (20% of whom were women) with class II–IV heart failure due to LV systolic dysfunction.[26] Although overall mortality was similar in the two groups, there was a 13.2% reduction in the combined endpoint of morbidity and mortality. A similar benefit was seen in women and men. In a small percentage of patients, the mortality and morbidity was significant; these patients were not on an ACE inhibitor for a variety of reasons. This group drove the results of the reduction in hospitalizations. This study gives an initial glance at alternative therapy, although the analysis is retrospective.

The CHARM trial, which was a combination of three distinct studies plus the combined studies as a fourth, addressed ACE intolerance directly with the Alternative trial.[29,73] This study enrolled 2028 patients, 32% women, which is the largest number of women thus far enrolled in a heart failure clinical trial. It is not surprising to note the larger percentage of women with 'intolerance' to ACE inhibitors, given the observations in the SOLVD trial. The overall benefit was significantly greater with candesartan compared with placebo for cardiovascular death and heart failure hospitalizations. The number of hospitalizations was also reduced. The incidence of angioedema was extremely low with only one patient of 39 with previous angioedema developing angioedema with candesartan. The Added arm of the CHARM trial enrolled 2548 patients, 22% of whom were women.[74]

This study showed a HR of 0.85 for the combined endpoint. However, the data have not been divided by gender. Overall, in the CHARM program, the women with heart failure were older than the men (mean age of 68 vs 65 years), and were more likely to have a hypertensive etiology for their heart failure (21% vs 9%) and were less likely to be treated with beta-blockers (57% vs 52%). At baseline, women also had more symptoms and clinical evidence of systemic and pulmonary vascular congestion, despite a higher LVEF (43% vs 37%).[75]

In summary, women who develop cough or angioedema with an ACE inhibitor can be administered at least two proven ARBs, i.e. candesartan or valsartan.

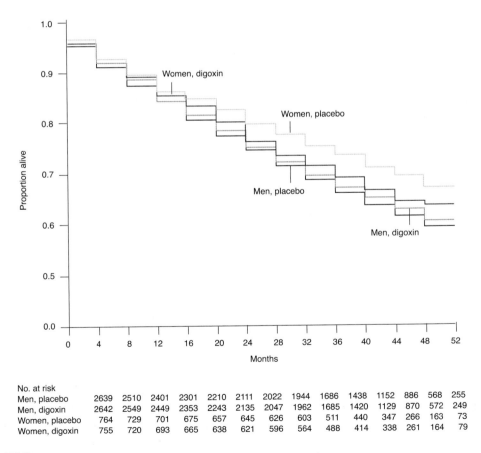

Figure 29.3
Kaplan–Meier survival estimates for men and women in the Digitalis Investigation Group (DIG) trial randomized to digoxin or placebo. Reproduced from reference 78.

Aldosterone inhibitors

The RALES trial enrolled 1663 patients with class IV heart failure;[27] 27% were women. The women appeared to have the same benefit of relative risk reduction in mortality as the men, although the confidence intervals were wider due to the smaller number of women. No other formal analysis of the RALES trial according to gender has been published. A new aldosterone inhibitor, eplerenone, was studied in a population of patients with MI.[76] Of 6642 patients studied, 29% were women. The women enjoyed an equal benefit from the administration of eplerenone versus placebo in the endpoint of death from any cause. Therefore, although the data are limited, there is no reason to withhold aldosterone inhibitors from women with heart failure who fit the entry criteria for either of the two trials discussed above.

Digoxin

The Digitalis Investigation Group trial reported that treatment with digoxin did not decrease overall mortality in patients with heart failure due to depressed LV systolic function.[31] The trial did find a modest reduction in hospitalizations. An analysis post hoc by gender showed that the women assigned to digoxin had a higher mortality than those assigned to placebo (33% vs 28.9%)[77,78] (Fig. 29.3). The digoxin serum levels, however, were higher in the women than in the men and may represent a smaller muscle mass. The study concluded that serum digoxin levels should be kept below 1.0 ng/ml and that higher levels may be detrimental. The possibility of keeping digoxin levels even lower in women has been suggested by others.

Peripartum cardiomyopathy

Peripartum cardiomyopathy (PPCM) as an etiology of heart failure is unique to women and is discussed in Chapter 24. Therefore it will not be discussed further here.

Summary

In summary, heart failure in women is a real entity, complex in presentation with more advanced disease, although ejection fractions are higher than in men. The myth that women with heart failure fare better than men in survival needs to be reassessed, since data are accumulating that CHD as an etiology for heart failure in women is a deadly disease. In addition, new therapies have to be prospectively tested in women, with sufficient power analysis to make definitive statements regarding the benefits of therapy and applicability to women. Failure to do this would be a disservice to a female population that is under-represented in clinical trials.

References

1. Redfield MM, Jacobsen SJ, Burnett JC Jr, Mahoney DW, Bailey KR, Rodeheffer RJ. Burden of systolic and diastolic ventricular dysfunction in the community: appreciating the scope of the heart failure epidemic. *JAMA* 2003; **289**:194–202.
2. Senni M, Tribouilloy CM, Rodeheffer RJ, et al. Congestive heart failure in the community: a study of all incident cases in Olmsted County, Minnesota, in 1991. *Circulation* 1998; **98**:2282–9.
3. Senni M, Tribouilloy CM, Rodeheffer RJ, et al. Congestive heart failure in the community: trends in incidence and survival in a 10–year period. *Arch Intern Med* 1999; **159**:29–34.
4. American Heart Association. *Heart Disease and Stroke Statistics – 2003*. American Heart Association, 2003.
5. Levy D, Kenchaiah S, Larson MG, et al. Long-term trends in the incidence of and survival with heart failure. *N Engl J Med* 2002; **347**:1397–1402.

6. Levy D, Larson MG, Vasan RS, Kannel WB, Ho KK. The progression from hypertension to congestive heart failure. *JAMA* 1996; **275**:1557–62.

7. Effect of enalapril on survival in patients with reduced left ventricular ejection fractions and congestive heart failure. The SOLVD Investigators. *N Engl J Med* 1991; **325**:293–302.

8. Ho KK, Pinsky JL, Kannel WB, Levy D. The epidemiology of heart failure: the Framingham Study. *J Am Coll Cardiol* 1993; **22** (4 Suppl A):6A–13A.

9. Kannel WB. Epidemiological aspects of heart failure. *Cardiol Clin* 1989; **7**:1–9.

10. Pfeffer MA, Braunwald E, Moye LA, et al. Effect of captopril on mortality and morbidity in patients with left ventricular dysfunction after myocardial infarction. Results of the survival and ventricular enlargement trial. The SAVE Investigators. *N Engl J Med* 1992; **327**:669–77.

11. Schaffer WL, Galloway JM, Roman MJ, et al. Prevalence and correlates of rheumatic heart disease in American Indians (the Strong Heart Study). *Am J Cardiol* 2003; **91**:1379–82.

12. Kaplan EL. T. Duckett Jones Memorial Lecture. Global assessment of rheumatic fever and rheumatic heart disease at the close of the century. Influences and dynamics of populations and pathogens: a failure to realize prevention? *Circulation* 1993; **88** (4 Pt 1):1964–72.

13. McCullough PA, Philbin EF, Spertus JA, Kaatz S, Sandberg KR, Weaver WD. Confirmation of a heart failure epidemic: findings from the Resource Utilization Among Congestive Heart Failure (REACH) study. *J Am Coll Cardiol* 2002; **39**:60–9.

14. Bangdiwala SI, Weiner DH, Bourassa MG, Friesinger GC, Ghali JK, Yusuf S. Studies of Left Ventricular Dysfunction (SOLVD) Registry: rationale, design, methods and description of baseline characteristics. *Am J Cardiol* 1992; **70**:347–53.

15. Bourassa MG, Gurne O, Bangdiwala SI, et al. Natural history and patterns of current practice in heart failure. The Studies of Left Ventricular Dysfunction (SOLVD) Investigators. *J Am Coll Cardiol* 1993; **22** (4 Suppl A):14A–19A.

16. Cohn JN, Archibald DG, Ziesche S, et al. Effect of vasodilator therapy on mortality in chronic congestive heart failure. Results of a Veterans Administration Cooperative Study. *N Engl J Med* 1986; **314**:1547–52.

17. Cohn JN, Johnson G, Ziesche S, et al. A comparison of enalapril with hydralazine-isosorbide dinitrate in the treatment of chronic congestive heart failure. *N Engl J Med* 1991; **325**:303–10.

18. Effects of enalapril on mortality in severe congestive heart failure. Results of the Cooperative North Scandinavian Enalapril Survival Study (CONSENSUS). The CONSENSUS Trial Study Group. *N Engl J Med* 1987; **316**:1429–35.

19. Effect of enalapril on mortality and the development of heart failure in asymptomatic patients with reduced left ventricular ejection fractions. The SOLVD Investigators. *N Engl J Med* 1992; **327**:685–91.

20. Pitt B, Segal R, Martinez FA, et al. Randomised trial of losartan versus captopril in patients over 65 with heart failure (Evaluation of Losartan in the Elderly Study, ELITE). *Lancet* 1997; **349**:747–52.

21. Pitt B, Poole-Wilson PA, Segal R, et al. Effect of losartan compared with captopril on mortality in patients with symptomatic heart failure: randomised trial – the Losartan Heart Failure Survival Study ELITE II. *Lancet* 2000; **255**:1582–7.

22. Costill DL, Fink WJ, Flynn MJPK. Muscle fiber composition and enzyme activities in elite female distance runners. *Int J Sport Med* 1987; **8** (Suppl 2):103–6.

23. Hjalmarson A, Goldstein S, Fagerberg B, et al. Effects of controlled-release metoprolol on total mortality, hospitalizations, and well-being in patients with heart failure: the Metoprolol CR/XL Randomized Intervention Trial in congestive heart failure (MERIT-HF). MERIT-HF Study Group. *JAMA* 2000; **283**:1295–302.

24. The Cardiac Insufficiency Bisoprolol Study II (CIBIS-II): a randomised trial. *Lancet* 1999; **353**:9–13.

25. Packer M, Fowler MB, Roecker EB, et al. Effect of carvedilol on the morbidity of patients with severe chronic heart failure: results of the carvedilol prospective randomized cumulative survival (COPERNICUS) study. *Circulation* 2002; **106**:2194–9.

26. Cohn JN, Tognoni G. A randomized trial of the angiotensin-receptor blocker valsartan in chronic heart failure. *N Engl J Med* 2001; **345**:1667–75.

27. Pitt B, Zannad F, Remme WJ, et al. The effect of spironolactone on morbidity and mortality in patients with severe heart failure. Randomized Aldactone Evaluation Study Investigators. *N Engl J Med* 1999; **341**:709–17.

28. The TRAndolapril Cardiac Evaluation (TRACE) study: rationale, design, and baseline characteristics of the screened population. The Trace Study Group. *Am J Cardiol* 1994; **73**:44C–50C.

29. Pfeffer MA, Swedberg K, Granger CB, et al. Effects of candesartan on mortality and morbidity in patients with chronic heart failure: the CHARM-Overall programme. *Lancet* 2003; **362**:759–66.

30. Klein H, Auricchio A, Reek S, Geller C. New primary prevention trials of sudden cardiac death in patients with left ventricular dysfunction: SCD-HEFT and MADIT-II. *Am J Cardiol* 1999; **83**:91D–97D.

31. The effect of digoxin on mortality and morbidity in patients with heart failure. The Digitalis Investigation Group. *N Engl J Med* 1997; **336**:525–33.

32. Jessup M, Pina IL. Is it important to examine gender differences in the epidemiology and outcome of severe heart failure? *J Thorac Cardiovasc Surg* 2004; **127**:1247–52.

33. Yusuf S, Pfeffer MA, Swedberg K, et al. Effects of candesartan in patients with chronic heart failure and preserved left-ventricular ejection fraction: the CHARM-Preserved Trial. *Lancet* 2003; **362**: 777–81.

34. Adams KF Jr, Dunlap SH, Sueta CA, et al. Relation between gender, etiology and survival in patients with symptomatic heart failure. *J Am Coll Cardiol* 1996; **28**:1781–8.

35. Johnstone D, Limacher M, Rousseau M, et al. Clinical characteristics of patients in studies of left ventricular dysfunction (SOLVD). *Am J Cardiol* 1992; **70**:894–900.

36. Califf RM, Adams KF, McKenna WJ, et al. A randomized controlled trial of epoprostenol therapy for severe congestive heart failure: The Flolan International Randomized Survival Trial (FIRST). *Am Heart J* 1997; **134**:44–54.

37. Pfeffer JM, Pfeffer MA, Fletcher P, Fishbein MC, Braunwald E. Favorable effects of therapy on cardiac performance in spontaneously hypertensive rats. *Am J Physiol* 1982; **242**:H776–H784.

38. Weinberg EO, Thienelt CD, Katz SE, et al. Gender differences in molecular remodeling in pressure overload hypertrophy. *J Am Coll Cardiol* 1999; **34**:264–73.

39. Carroll JD, Carroll EP, Feldman T, et al. Sex-associated differences in left ventricular function in aortic stenosis of the elderly. *Circulation* 1992; **86**:1099–107.

40. Devereux RB, Pickering TG, Alderman MH, Chien S, Borer JS, Laragh JH. Left ventricular hypertrophy in hypertension. Prevalence and relationship to pathophysiologic variables. *Hypertension* 1987; **9** (2 Pt 2):II53–60.

41. Opasich C, Tavazzi L, Lucci D, et al. Comparison of one-year outcome in women versus men with chronic congestive heart failure. *Am J Cardiol* 2000; **86**:353–7.

42. Halm MA, Penque S. Heart failure in women. *Prog Cardiovasc Nurs* 2000; **15**:121–33.

43. Mehta NJ, Mehta RN, Khan IA. Peripartum cardiomyopathy: clinical and therapeutic aspects. *Angiology* 2001; **52**:759–62.

44. Fernandez-Sola J, Nicolas-Arfelis JM. Gender differences in alcoholic cardiomyopathy. *J Gend Specif Med* 2002; **5**:41–7.

45. Ho KK, Anderson KM, Kannel WB, Grossman W, Levy D. Survival after the onset of congestive heart failure in Framingham Heart Study subjects. *Circulation* 1993; **88**:107–15.

46. Silber DH. Heart failure in women. *Curr Womens Health Rep* 2003; **3**:104–9.

47. Scheuer J, Malhotra A, Schaible TF, Capasso J. Effects of gonadectomy and hormonal replacement on rat hearts. *Circ Res* 1987; **61**:12–19.

48. Buttrick P, Scheuer J. Sex-associated differences in left ventricular function in aortic stenosis of the elderly. *Circulation* 1992; **86**:1336–8.

49. Olivetti G, Giordano G, Corradi D, et al. Gender differences and aging: effects on the human heart. *J Am Coll Cardiol* 1995; **26**:1068–79.

50. Carroll JD, Carroll EP, Feldman T, Ward DM, Lang RM, McGaughey D, et al. Sex-associated differences in left ventricular function in aortic stenosis of the elderly. *Circulation* 1992; **86**:1099–107.

51. Aurigemma GP, Gaasch WH. Gender differences in older patients with pressure-overload hypertrophy of the left ventricle. *Cardiology* 1995; **86**:310–17.

52. Aurigemma GP, Silver KH, McLaughlin M, Mauser J, Gaasch WH. Impact of chamber geometry and gender on left ventricular systolic function in patients > 60 years of age with aortic stenosis. *Am J Cardiol* 1994; **74**:794–8.

53. Douglas PS, Otto CM, Mickel MC, Labovitz A, Reid CL, Davis KB. Gender differences in left ventricle geometry and function in patients undergoing balloon dilatation of the aortic valve for isolated aortic stenosis. NHLBI Balloon Valvuloplasty Registry. *Br Heart J* 1995; **73**:548–54.

54. Mendes LA, Davidoff R, Cupples LA, Ryan TJ, Jacobs AK. Congestive heart failure in patients with coronary artery disease: the gender paradox. *Am Heart J* 1997; **134** (2 Pt 1):207–12.

55. Krumholz HM, Larson M, Levy D. Sex differences in cardiac adaptation to isolated systolic hypertension. *Am J Cardiol* 1993; **72**:310–13.

56. Guerra S, Leri A, Wang X, et al. Myocyte death in the failing human heart is gender dependent. *Circ Res* 1999; **85**:856–66.

57. Fischer M, Baessler A, Schunkert H. Renin angiotensin system and gender differences in the cardiovascular system. *Cardiovasc Res* 2002; **53**:672–7.

58. Grohe C, Kahlert S, Lobbert K, Vetter H. Expression of oestrogen receptor alpha and beta in rat heart: role of local oestrogen synthesis. *J Endocrinol* 1998; **156**:R1–7.

59. Richards RG, DiAugustine RP, Petrusz P, Clark GC,

Sebastian J. Estradiol stimulates tyrosine phosphorylation of the insulin-like growth factor-1 receptor and insulin receptor substrate-1 in the uterus. *Proc Natl Acad Sci USA* 1996; **93**:12002–7.

60. Tsukahara H, Gordienko DV, Tonshoff B, Gelato MC, Goligorsky MS. Direct demonstration of insulin-like growth factor-I-induced nitric oxide production by endothelial cells. *Kidney Int* 1994; **45**:598–604.

61. Huang A, Sun D, Koller A, Kaley G. Gender difference in myogenic tone of rat arterioles is due to estrogen-induced, enhanced release of NO. *Am J Physiol* 1997; **272**:H1804–9.

62. Aronson D, Burger AJ. Gender-related differences in modulation of heart rate in patients with congestive heart failure. *J Cardiovasc Electrophysiol* 2000; **11**:1071–7.

63. McKee PA, Castelli WP, McNamara PM, Kannel WB. The natural history of congestive heart failure: the Framingham study. *N Engl J Med* 1971; **285**:1441–6.

64. Ghali JK, Pina IL, Gottlieb SS, Deedwania PC, Wikstrand JC. Metoprolol CR/XL in female patients with heart failure: analysis of the experience in Metoprolol Extended-Release Randomized Intervention Trial in Heart Failure (MERIT-HF). *Circulation* 2002; **105**:1585–91.

65. Pina IL. A better survival for women with heart failure? It's not so simple. *J Am Coll Cardiol* 2003; **42**:2135–8.

66. Petrie MC, Dawson NF, Murdoch DR, Davie AP, McMurray JJ. Failure of women's hearts. *Circulation* 1999; **99**:2334–41.

67. Garg R, Yusuf S. Overview of randomized trials of angiotensin-converting enzyme inhibitors on mortality and morbidity in patients with heart failure. Collaborative Group on ACE Inhibitor Trials. *JAMA* 1995; **273**:1450–6.

68. Shekelle PG, Rich MW, Morton SC, et al. Efficacy of angiotensin-converting enzyme inhibitors and beta-blockers in the management of left ventricular systolic dysfunction according to race, gender, and diabetic status: a meta-analysis of major clinical trials. *J Am Coll Cardiol* 2003; **41**:1529–38.

69. Ambrosioni E, Borghi C, Magnani B. The effect of the angiotensin-converting-enzyme inhibitor zofenopril on mortality and morbidity after anterior myocardial infarction. The Survival of Myocardial Infarction Long-Term Evaluation (SMILE) Study Investigators. *N Engl J Med* 1995; **332**:80–5.

70. Simon T, Mary-Krause M, Funck-Brentano C, Jaillon P. Sex differences in the prognosis of congestive heart failure: results from the Cardiac Insufficiency Bisoprolol Study (CIBIS II). *Circulation* 2001; **103**:375–80.

71. Kostis JB, Shelton B, Gosselin G, et al. Adverse effects of enalapril in the Studies of Left Ventricular Dysfunction (SOLVD). SOLVD Investigators. *Am Heart J* 1996; **131**:350–5.

72. Limacher MCYS. Gender differences in presentation, morbidity and mortality in the Studies of Left Ventricular Dysfunction (SOLVD): a preliminary report. In: Wenger NK (ed.). *Cardiovascular Health and Disease in Women*. Greenwich, CT: Le Jacq Communications, 1993: 345–8.

73. Granger CB, McMurray JJ, Yusuf S, et al. Effects of candesartan in patients with chronic heart failure and reduced left-ventricular systolic function intolerant to angiotensin-converting-enzyme inhibitors: the CHARM-Alternative trial. *Lancet* 2003; **362**:772–6.

74. McMurray JJ, Ostergren J, Swedberg K, et al. Effects of candesartan in patients with chronic heart failure and reduced left-ventricular systolic function taking angiotensin-converting-enzyme inhibitors: the CHARM- Added trial. *Lancet* 2003; **362**:767–71.

75. McMurray J, Ostergren J, Pfeffer M, et al. Clinical features and contemporary management of patients with low and preserved ejection fraction heart failure: baseline characteristics of patients in the Candesartan in Heart failure-Assessment of Reduction in Mortality and morbidity (CHARM) programme. *Eur J Heart Fail* 2003; **5**:261–70.

76. Pitt B, Williams G, Remme W, et al. The EPHESUS trial: eplerenone in patients with heart failure due to systolic dysfunction complicating acute myocardial infarction. Eplerenone Post-AMI Heart Failure Efficacy and Survival Study. *Cardiovasc Drugs Ther* 2001; **15**:79–87.

77. Eichhorn EJ, Gheorghiade M. Digoxin – new perspective on an old drug. *N Engl J Med* 2002; **347**:1394–5.

78. Rathore SS, Wang Y, Krumholz HM. Sex-based differences in the effect of digoxin for the treatment of heart failure. *N Engl J Med* 2002; **347**:1403–11.

30
Cardiac transplantation

Sharon A. Hunt

Heart transplantation has become a mature and widely adopted clinical field over the past 20 years; its maturity was preceded by several decades of preclinical and preliminary clinical work. This work involved diverse disciplines including immunology, pathology, pharmacology, and infectious disease in addition to cardiology and cardiac surgery. While donor availability kept pace with demand for the decade of the 1980s, it became clear in the 1990s that a plateau in donor numbers had been reached and that plateau remains today, making recipient selection and donor distribution and matching very important societal as well as medical issues. This chapter addresses the basic issues involved in recipient selection and postoperative management, describes the results to be expected currently, and examines gender-specific results and issues.

Recipient selection

Transplantation of the heart began as, and remains, the most 'radical' form of therapy for end-stage heart disease. The morbidity and mortality and need for ongoing care associated with the procedure as well as the fact, alluded to above, that donor organs are a scarce societal resource, make selection of appropriate recipients an important medical and ethical issue. Criteria to assure that recipient selection meets these goals were first codified in a consensus form in the American College of Cardiology Bethesda Conference in 1993[1] and have changed little since that time. These criteria are summarized in Box 30.1.

Data on the demographics of patients undergoing heart transplantation have been accrued in an international registry since 1982 and are published annually in the *Journal of Heart and Lung Transplantation*. This registry has been sponsored by the International Society for Heart and Lung

---

Box 30.1 Cardiac recipient selection criteria

1. End-stage heart disease not remediable by more conservative means
2. Absence of:
   a. Advanced age
   b. Severe peripheral or cerebrovascular disease
   c. Irreversible dysfunction of another organ (kidney, liver, lung), unless being considered for multi-organ transplantation
   d. History of malignancy with probability of recurrence
   e. Inability to comply with complex medical regimen
   f. Irreversible pulmonary hypertension (>4 Wood units)
   g. Active systemic infection

Transplantation (ISHLT) and, since 1999, has been administered jointly in the US with the federally contracted United Network for Organ Sharing (UNOS). Reporting of data is mandatory in the US, but voluntary in other countries. In this database, which now includes >62 000 transplant recipients,[2] the underlying type of heart disease leading to the need for transplant is approximately evenly divided between coronary heart disease (CHD) and primary myocardial disease; this pattern has changed little over the two decades of reporting. The gender of transplant recipients has always been predominantly male, overall ~80% male, and the percentage has changed little over the years. This predominance of males most likely relates to the fact that women develop end-stage heart disease later in life when they are considered to be too old for transplant candidacy.

Donor selection

Appropriate cardiac donors are individuals who have been declared brain dead (with death from a variety of causes including violent death and subarachnoid hemorrhage), who have normal hearts, and whose families consent to donation. In the earlier days of transplantation, donors were almost without exception less than 30 years of age, but in more recent history the average donor age has climbed in concert with the increased demand, with the most recent registry report documenting donor age listing about 10% of donors >50. Such 'loosening' of donor criteria is accompanied by more rigorous documentation of the normalcy of the heart in question, often requiring coronary arteriography to be performed on the older potential donor heart, to assure its freedom from significant coronary artery disease.

Many states in the US give their citizens the option to state their willingness (or unwillingness) to donate organs on their drivers' licenses, but in the current legal climate the donor's family's wishes will generally over-ride this statement, especially when the family is unwilling to donate. Several other countries have passed 'presumed consent' laws which allow the use of organs from brain-dead individuals unless a family specifically objects, and these countries have higher donor retrieval rates than the US.

The gender of cardiac donors is also predominantly male, averaging around 65% in recent years. Since approximately 50% of donors die of trauma, it can be speculated that the male preponderance of donors could be related to a stronger tendency to be involved in violence in the male gender.

Donor distribution

The donor organ distribution system in the US is federally supervised through contract with the independent organization UNOS, which in turn creates and updates the rules for organ distribution with input from a wide variety of constituencies including transplant physicians and surgeons, donor families, ethicists, and others. Currently, medical donor/recipient matching requires only ABO blood type compatibility and general body size matching. Prioritization otherwise is given according to severity of illness, length of time on the waiting list, and geographic distance between donor and recipient. A 'transport' or 'ischemic' time of 3 hours is considered maximum for a donated heart.

Surgical technique

Virtually all heart transplantation currently places the donor heart in the orthotopic, or anatomically normal, position after excision of the diseased recipient heart. In the classical procedure, excision and re-anastamosis involve incision at the mid-atrial level and across the great vessels just above the semilunar valves. A more recent variation on this technique, known as the bicaval technique, makes the venous anastamoses at the level of the superior and inferior vena cavae instead of the mid-atrial level. This technique is thought to result in more normal right atrial geometry and, in turn, fewer atrial arrhythmias and less tricuspid regurgitation.[3]

Atypical physiology

The transplanted heart is surgically denervated; thus, the donor sinoatrial node does not have autonomic neural input, although it responds to circulating catecholamines. Because of this denervated state, the heart cannot respond acutely to increased demand, such as commencing exercise, with an increase in heart rate. Instead, it relies on the intrinsic Frank-Starling mechanism to increase stroke volume in response to increased venous return. This mechanism turns out to be remarkably efficient and transplant patients are quite capable of carrying out normal activities and vigorous exercise, even though (on average) their measured peak exercise oxygen consumption is below normal.[4]

Immunosuppression

Suppression of the normal immune reaction which rejects a foreign tissue is necessary to maintain the integrity of an organ allograft. The pharmacologic means to accomplish this immunosuppression are in a constant state of evolution, seemingly a more rapid evolution with each passing year. All currently used regimens are nonspecific, however, providing general hyporeactivity to foreign antigens rather than donor-specific hyporeactivity. For this reason, all current regimens lead to an unwanted susceptibility to infections and malignant complications in the recipient.

Most cardiac transplant centers currently introduce immunosuppression with a three-drug regimen commencing immediately at the time of transplant. Most include a calcineurin inhibitor (cyclosporine or tacrolimus), an inhibitor of T cell proliferation or differentiation (azathioprine or mycophenolate mofetil or sirolimus), and at least a short course of corticosteroids. Many also include a period of 'induction' therapy with polyclonal (anti-thymocyte preparations) or monoclonal (mouse CD3 monoclonal antibodies such as Orthoclone OKT3) anti-T cell antibodies in the perioperative period to decrease the frequency or severity of early post-transplant rejection. Most recently introduced have been monoclonal antibodies (daclizumab and basiliximab), which block the interleukin-2 receptor and may provide prevention of allograft rejection without additional global immunosuppression.[5] The 'tapering' or adjustment of the immunosuppressive regimen after the perioperative period is a process which is highly individualized for each patient and determined by the patient's rejection history and tolerance to and complications from the drugs or modalities used.

Cardiac allograft vasculopathy

The development of a chronologically premature and anatomically quite diffuse and often rapidly progressive obliterative pattern of coronary artery disease, a vascular disease which is limited to the allograft, is currently the major complication limiting truly long-term survival in cardiac transplant recipients. Its etiology is likely complex and is thought to involve an interplay of immunologic (HL-A and other mismatches), infectious (cytomegalovirus (CMV) and others), and more usual (lipid status, diabetes, etc.) factors.

Some angiographic evidence of this disease is present by 1 year post-transplant in 10% of patients and 50% have some evidence by 5 years. In recent years, the use of intravascular ultrasound has provided earlier and more sensitive diagnosis of the intimal thickening that characterizes the disease and the technique has provided a surrogate end-point for clinical trials of newer immunosuppressive agents designed to evaluate changes in the incidence of the disease consequent to changed immunosuppression.[6]

Since transplant recipients generally have a persistent state of both afferent and efferent denervation, they are usually not capable of experiencing the subjective sensation of angina pectoris. Ischemic sequelae in these patients can include arrhythmias leading to sudden death as well as ischemic left ventricular dysfunction leading to the clinical syndrome of heart failure. The very diffuseness of the disease makes the use of standard revascularization with percutaneous or surgical interventions palliative at best. The prognosis once graft vasculopathy has led to clinical events is poor, with one study finding only 18–20% survival in heart transplant recipients after an ischemic clinical event. No drug or agent has been shown to reverse this disease and the only definitive therapy available is retransplantation. The overall survival rates reported after retransplantation late after a first transplant are slightly inferior

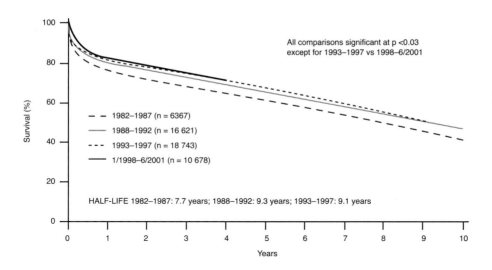

Figure 30.1 Actuarial survival curves from the International Society for Heart and Lung Transplantation (ISHLT) Registry. Reproduced from reference 2 with permission from Elsevier.

to those after the first transplant, and the use of scarce donor hearts for this purpose is a somewhat contentious issue in the transplant community.

Overall results

As noted above, the Registry of the ISHLT is updated annually. Reports indicate a plateau of approximately 2500 heart transplants annually in the US and 4000 worldwide over the last decade. One-year survival rates are currently around 80%, with 5- and 10-year survival rates of 66% and 47%, respectively (Fig. 30.1). Patient half-life (i.e. time to 50% survival) is 9.3 years based on registry data between 1982 and 2001.[2] There are no differences in survival between male and female recipients. Approximately 40% of patients are rehospitalized during the first post-transplant year, often for treatment of rejection or infection. By the second post-transplant year only 20% require rehospitalization. The vast majority report good functional status after transplantation, although in the US less than 40% return to work. This fact is no doubt a result of the usual linkage between insurability and employability in the US health-care system.

Specific gender issues related to heart transplantation

Gender matching/mismatching between donor and recipient – does it matter?

A small difference in graft survival (which is identical with patient survival in the field of heart transplantation) has been repeatedly documented in male recipients of female hearts,[7,8] but no statistical difference according to donor gender was demonstrable in female recipients. There is no apparent correlation of this difference in survival with the proportion of patients treated for rejection episodes.[7] One study showed that male recipients of female allografts have a greater degree of coronary arterial intimal hyperplasia detected by intravascular ultrasound at 1 year post-transplant,[9] suggesting that more aggressive graft vasculopathy may account for the worse survival.

Pregnancy and childbearing (see also Chapters 22 and 24)

It is estimated that 1 of every 20 women of childbearing age with a functioning organ transplant will become pregnant. Several medical issues are intuitively raised when a female heart transplant recipient considers the possibility of childbearing. The first is the possible teratogenicity of the drugs she takes which are required to prevent rejection of her cardiac allograft. The second is the physiologic changes of pregnancy and whether the transplanted heart will be able to cope with them and, if not, whether that poses unacceptable risks to either mother or fetus. The third, and perhaps less intuitive, concern is whether the tremendous hormonal changes inherent in the state of pregnancy will affect the immunologic 'balance' between the donor and recipient. The 'news' on all of these strictly medical issues is good and favors the woman's safety and child's normalcy should the woman choose to become pregnant. The choice to bear a child that she might well not live to raise to adulthood is clearly a non-medical one, but one that at least has to be acknowledged by the involved health-care professionals.

Despite concern about these issues, the outcomes, both for mother and fetus, have been excellent. These outcomes have been followed since 1991 in the National Transplantation Pregnancy Registry based in Philadelphia and the most recent update was published in 2002.[10] This is a voluntary registry and can be accessed through the internet at www.tju.edu/ntpr. Children of heart transplant recipients (n = 52 in the most recent report, which also includes outcomes on >7000 mothers with renal transplants) have no reported pattern of or excess incidence of birth defects and the mothers have no excess incidence of miscarriage, and no excess incidence of rejection. It should be noted that the majority of these data have been accrued in patients receiving azathioprine and cyclosporine; there are relatively few data so far regarding mycophenolate, tacrolimus, or sirolimus in pregnancy. Most babies are somewhat premature (average gestational age 34 weeks) and somewhat small for gestational age, but appear to grow and develop normally. The incidence of pre-eclampsia is high, but the cardiac allograft generally tolerates the hemodynamic stresses of pregnancy well. Pregnant heart transplant recipients should be considered high risk and their course managed by a team including high-risk obstetric consultants and transplant cardiologists.[11] The most common alteration in immunosuppressive therapy during pregnancy involved 40% of patients needing to increase cyclosporine dose because of decreasing cyclosporine blood levels during pregnancy.[12] All of the immunosuppressive agents are present in breast milk and there is a consensus that mothers should avoid breastfeeding for this reason.

References

1. Hunt SA (Chair). Cardiac Transplantation: Bethesda Conference 24, November 5–6, 1992. *J Am Coll Cardiol* 1993; **22**:1–64.
2. Hertz MI, Mohacsi PH, Taylor DO, et al. The registry of the International Society for Heart and Lung Transplantation: introduction to the twentieth annual reports – 2003. *J Heart Lung Transplant* 2003; **22**:610–15.
3. Dreyfus G, Jebara V, Mihaileaun S, Carpentier AF. Total orthotopic heart transplantation: an alternative to standard technique. *Ann Thorac Surg* 1991; **52**:1181–4.
4. Osada N, Chaitman BR, Donohue TJ, Wolford TL, Stelken AM, Miller LW. Long-term cardiopulmonary exercise performance after heart transplantation. *Am J Cardiol* 1997; **79**:451–6.
5. Beniaminovitz A, Itescu S, Lietz K, et al. Prevention of rejection in cardiac transplantation by blockade of the interleukin-2 receptor with a monoclonal antibody. *N Engl J Med* 2000; **342**:613–19.
6. Kobashigawa JA. First-year intravascular ultrasound results as a surrogate marker for outcomes after heart transplantation. *J Heart Lung Transplant* 2003; **22**: 711–14.
7. Zeier M, Hohler B, Opelz G, Ritz E. The effect of donor gender on graft survival. *J Am Soc Nephrol* 2002; **13**:2570–6.
8. Taylor DO, Edwards LB, Mohacsi PJ, et al. The registry of the International Society for Heart and Lung Transplantation: twentieth official adult heart transplant report – 2003. *J Heart Lung Transplant* 2003; **22**:616–24.
9. Mehra MR, Stapleton DD, Ventura HO, et al.

Influence of donor and recipient gender on cardiac allograft vasculopathy. An intravascular ultrasound study. *Circulation* 1994; **90** (5 Pt 2):II78–82.

10. Armenti VT, Radomski JS, Moritz MJ, et al. Report from the national transplantation pregnancy registry (NTPR): outcomes of pregnancy after transplantation. In: Cecka JM, Terasaki PI (eds). *Clinical Transplants*, 2nd edn. Los Angeles, CA: UCLA Tissue Typing Laboratory, 2002: 121–30.

11. Alston PK, Kuller JA, McMahon MJ, Pregnancy in transplant recipients. *Obstet Gynecol Surv* 2001; **56**:289–95.

12. Wagoner LE, Taylor DO, Olsen SL, et al. Immunosuppressive therapy, management, and outcome of heart transplant recipients during pregnancy. *J Heart Lung Transplant* 1993; **12**:993–9.

Part 4
Other Cardiovascular Diseases

31
Hypertension

Andrew P. Miller, Vera A. Bittner and Suzanne Oparil

Introduction

Over 64 million Americans suffer from cardiovascular disease (CVD), and women comprise 54% of these.[1] CVD is the leading killer of women, accounting for 1 in 2.5 deaths in women, which markedly eclipses breast cancer at 1 in 30.[1] Furthermore, trends in women's mortality have shown a worrisome plateau in the number of deaths attributable to CVD despite improving diagnostic and therapeutic tools.[1] This trend may be related to increases in the prevalence of several cardiovascular risk factors, including obesity and type 2 diabetes mellitus, coupled with stagnation of improvements in hypertension control, smoking prevention/cessation, and dyslipidemia treatment since 1990.[2] Of these, hypertension is the most common modifiable risk factor in women.

Sexual dimorphism in hypertension

Hypertension is defined as blood pressure (BP) ≥140 mmHg systolic and/or ≥90 mmHg diastolic. According to the National Health and Nutrition Examination Survey (NHANES), the prevalence of hypertension in the US population tracks remarkably closely with the prevalence of CVD[1] (Fig. 31.1). Interestingly, there is a striking age-dependent sexual

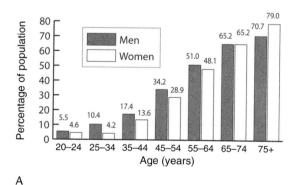

A

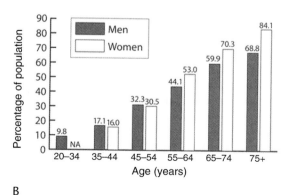

B

Figure 31.1
(A) Prevalence of cardiovascular diseases in Americans aged 20 and older by age and sex (NHANES III, 1988–94). (B) Prevalence of high blood pressure in Americans aged 20 and older by age and sex (NHANES IV, 1999–2000). From reference 1 with permission of the American Heart Association.

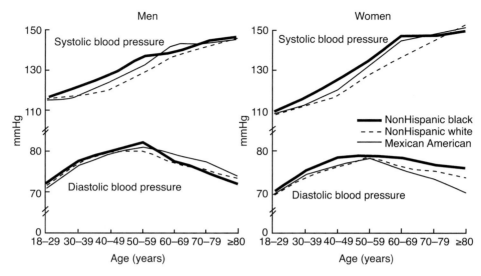

Figure 31.2
Mean systolic and diastolic blood pressures by age and race/ethnicity for men and women (NHANES III, 1988–1991). Reproduced with permission from reference 3.

dimorphism in the prevalence of both CVD and hypertension. Women have lower systolic BP levels than men during early adulthood, while the opposite is true after the sixth decade of life. Diastolic BP tends to be slightly lower in women than men regardless of age (Fig. 31.2).[3-5] Similarly, in early adulthood, hypertension is less common among women than men. However, after the fifth decade of life, the incidence of hypertension increases more rapidly in women than men, with the prevalence of hypertension in women equal to or exceeding that in men during the sixth decade of life. The highest prevalence rates of hypertension are observed in elderly black women, with hypertension occurring in more than 75% of women older than 75 years of age.[6]

Awareness, treatment, and control of high blood pressure in women (see also Chapter 2)

Women are more likely than men to know that they have hypertension and to have it treated; however, they are less likely to have it controlled.[7] In NHANES 1999–2000, approximately 71% of hypertensive

black and white women were aware of their high BP in contrast to just 66% of hypertensive men in these ethnic groups. Overall, 62% of hypertensive women, but only 54% of men were being treated with antihypertensive medications. The higher antihypertensive treatment rates in women have been attributed to increased numbers of physician contacts because of visits for reproductive health and childcare, as well as a lower probability of employment outside the home. However, despite higher treatment rates, only 48% of treated women and 30% of all women had their BP controlled (<140/90 mmHg) compared with 60% and 33% of treated and all men, respectively (Fig. 31.3).

The greatest burden of hypertension in the US in absolute numbers falls on the elderly. Compared with only 7.5 million persons aged 25–44 years, an estimated 18.5 million persons over age 65 are hypertensive[8] (Fig. 31.4). Numbers of hypertensives who are treated but have inadequate BP control or are unaware of their condition are disproportionately greater in the elderly than in the middle-aged and younger age groups. Systolic hypertension, in particular, is highly prevalent in the elderly, since systolic BP increases throughout the entire lifespan in the

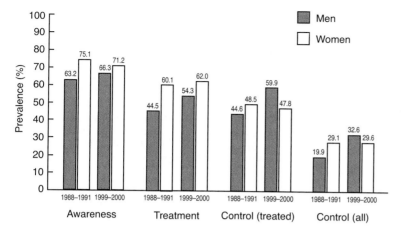

Figure 31.3
Awareness, treatment, and control of blood pressure for men/women in the United States, 1988–2000. Adapted with permission from reference 7.

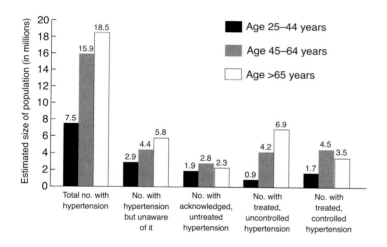

Figure 31.4
Numbers of Americans classified by hypertension category in each age group (NHANES III, 1988–1991). Reproduced with permission from reference 8.

population as a whole, while diastolic BP tends to fall after age 60. The prevalence of isolated systolic hypertension (systolic BP ≥140 mmHg and diastolic BP ≤90 mmHg) increased from 52% in younger (age 25–44) persons unaware of their diagnosis to 90% of similarly undiagnosed persons >65 years in NHANES III (Table 31.1). Data from the Framingham Heart Study indicate that the residual lifetime risk of hypertension for normotensive men and women aged 55–65 in the cohort is 90%, indicating a huge public health burden and need for frequent monitoring of BP levels as patients advance in years.[9] More than half of the 55-year-old participants and two-thirds of the 65-year-old participants

developed hypertension within 10 years. In this report, lifetime risk for hypertension was similar in the two sexes.

Observational data from the Women's Health Initiative (WHI) underscore the gravity of the hypertension problem in menopausal women.[10] The WHI, best known for its findings on the effects of hormone replacement therapy (HRT) on breast cancer and CVD, provides valuable data on the largest multiethnic, best characterized cohort of menopausal women ever studied. WHI collected data on risk factors for CVD, including BP, as well as for other common conditions, including breast cancer, colorectal cancer, and osteoporosis from 98 705

Table 31.1. Blood pressure (BP) in subjects with uncontrolled hypertension according to age (NHANES III)

Age (years)	Mean BP (mmHg)	Unaware SBP ≥140 mmHg and DBP <90 mmHg (%)	Mean BP (mmHg)	Aware untreated SBP ≥140 mmHg and DBP <90 mmHg (%)	Mean BP (mmHg)	Treated uncontrolled SBP ≥140 mmHg and DBP <90 mmHg (%)
25–44	138/91	52	141/94	25	147/95	29
45–64	148/86	70	152/89	54	150/87	66
≥65	153/77	90	160/81	82	159/78	88

DBP, diastolic BP; SBP, systolic BP. Data from reference 8.

women aged 50–79 years. Baseline characteristics of the cohort are shown in Table 31.2.

The prevalence of hypertension in women enrolled in WHI was 38% (34 339 women). An additional 4% of the cohort reported a history of hypertension but had normal screening BPs while not on medication. Among the hypertensives, only 36% (12 383) were controlled while 64% (22 096) were on treatment. Normal diastolic BP with elevated systolic BP was found in 17% (15 821) of the cohort at baseline. Prevalence rates were directly related to age (Fig. 31.5) and varied markedly with race/ethnicity (Fig. 31.6). Other major determinants of hypertension prevalence included alcohol consumption (46% in nondrinkers, 32% in moderate drinkers, and 36% in heavier drinkers), physical activity (45% in those with no moderate or strenuous activity vs 31% in those with ≥4 sessions/week) and body weight (48% in those with body mass index (BMI) >27.3 vs 29% in those with BMI <27.3). History of CVD and concomitant CVD risk factors were associated with marked increases in hypertension prevalence.

Treatment rates did not change with age but did vary with race/ethnicity and were highest among black women (Figs 31.5 and 31.6). As might be predicted, current users of HRT were more likely than never users to be on antihypertensive drug treatment (odds ratio (OR) 1.26, 95% confidence interval (CI) 1.2–1.3), supporting the widely held concept that HRT users are generally more health conscious and adherent to medical recommendations than nonusers. Despite comparable treatment rates in the three decades, BP control rates were inversely related to age (Fig. 31.5). Whether this is related to biological determinants of responsiveness

Table 31.2 Baseline characteristics of the Women's Health Initiative (WHI)

Characteristic	%
Age	
50–59 years	40
60–69 years	40
70–79 years	20
Race/ethnicity	
White	84
Black	9
Hispanic	3
Other	4
Education	
College degree or higher	40
Income	
Family income >$50 000	36
CV risk factors	
Current smoker	7
Overweight	46
Current HRT user	42

CV, cardiovascular; HRT, hormone replacement therapy. Data from reference 10.

to antihypertensive treatment, e.g. increased stiffness and increased pulse wave velocity in conduit vessels of older women, or to the possibility that older women may not be treated as aggressively as younger ones, remains to be determined from future studies.

Analysis of antihypertensive drug treatment patterns revealed that the majority of women were treated with a single drug (Fig. 31.7). Monotherapy with diuretics achieved the highest control rates (63%), while control was intermediate with beta-blockers (57%) or angiotensin-converting enzyme

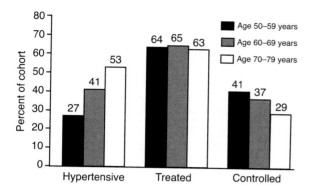

Figure 31.5
Prevalence of hypertension in women and treatment status by age at baseline in the Women's Health Initiative (WHI). Adapted with permission from reference 10.

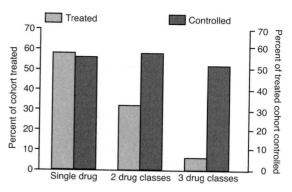

Figure 31.7
Antihypertensive drug treatment patterns at baseline in the Women's Health Initiative (WHI). Adapted with permission from reference 10.

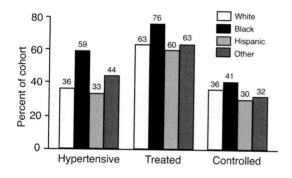

Figure 31.6
Prevalence of hypertension in women and treatment status by race/ethnicity in the Women's Health Initiative (WHI). Adapted with permission from reference 10.

(ACE) inhibitors (56%) and lowest on calcium channel blockers (CCBs) (50%). Adding drugs from different therapeutic classes did not improve control rates. Whether this is related to underdosing of individual drugs, to inappropriate choices of combinations, or to true resistance to antihypertensive treatment is uncertain. CCBs, the favorite class of antihypertensive agents, were used as monotherapy in 16% and either as monotherapy or in combination

in 34% of participants. Diuretics and beta-blockers, which were recommended by JNC 6 as first-line therapy for hypertension, were used as monotherapy less often (diuretics 14%; beta-blockers 9% of participants). Diuretics were used more often than any other drug class in combination. The presence of co-morbid conditions influenced drug choices: (1) beta-blockers were used more often in women with a history of MI, (2) combination therapy was more common in women with a history of CVD, and (3) CCBs were used more frequently in combination with other drugs in diabetics than in nondiabetics.

While the randomized trials of HRT have not confirmed a cardioprotective role for menopausal hormone therapy, they have provided important data specific to women and CVD. Like the WHI, data from the Heart and Estrogen/progestin Replacement Study (HERS) have demonstrated underutilization of proven treatment strategies in women, including the use of antihypertensive agents.[11,12] A looming crisis exists, with the burgeoning public health problems of obesity, diabetes, and hypertension increasing in prevalence and the use of interventions for these stagnating. Future research on intervention utilization, such as the American Heart Association's 'Get With The Guidelines Program', is urgently needed.[13] In the interim, evidence-based guidelines for CVD prevention for women have begun to address this problem.[14]

Menopause and blood pressure

The effect of menopause on BP is controversial. Longitudinal studies such as Framingham have not documented a rise in BP with menopause, while cross-sectional studies have found significantly higher systolic and diastolic BP in postmenopausal versus premenopausal women.[4] In NHANES III and the Canadian Heart Health Surveys (CHHS), the rate of rise in systolic BP tends to steepen in post-menopausal compared with premenopausal women until the sixth decade, when the rate of increase tends to slow.[15] Staessen et al. reported that, even after adjustment for age and BMI, postmenopausal women are more than twice as likely to have hypertension as premenopausal women.[16] In a prospective study of conventional and ambulatory BP levels in pre-, peri-, and postmenopausal women, the postmenopausal women had higher systolic BP (4–5 mmHg) than the pre- and perimenopausal controls.[17] The increase in systolic BP per decade was 5 mmHg greater in the peri- and postmenopausal women than in the premenopausal group. Thus, there is evidence that at least part of the rise in BP (particularly systolic BP) seen later in life in women is due to menopause. A menopause-related increase in BP has been attributed to a variety of factors, including estrogen withdrawal, overproduction of pituitary hormones, weight gain, or a combination of these and other yet undefined neurohumoral influences.[5]

Menopausal hormone therapy and blood pressure (see also Chapter 26)

Results of studies evaluating the effects of hormone replacement therapy (HRT) on BP have been inconsistent. The WHI found a 1 mmHg increase from baseline in systolic BP among 8506 menopausal women randomized to conjugated equine estrogen and medroxyprogesterone acetate compared with a placebo group at 1 year of follow-up.[18] This difference persisted throughout the 5.6 years of follow-up. There was no difference in diastolic BP between treatment groups. Further, in the WHI, cross-sectional

analysis of almost 100 000 women aged 50–79 years indicated that current hormone use was associated with a 25% greater likelihood of having hypertension compared with past use or no prior use.[10]

Smaller observational and interventional studies have found different results. The Baltimore Longitudinal Study on Aging (BLSA) followed 226 normotensive, menopausal women for an average of 5.7 years.[19] Women receiving HRT had a significantly smaller increase in systolic BP over time than nonusers, but diastolic BP was not affected by hormone therapy. The Postmenopausal Estrogen/Progestin Interventions (PEPI) trial followed 596 normotensive menopausal women, aged 45–64 years for an average of 3 years. HRT had no significant effect on systolic or diastolic BP.[20] Smaller studies have used 24-hour ambulatory monitoring to evaluate the effects of HRT on BP in normotensive and hypertensive women. While overall results are inconsistent, several of the studies suggest that HRT improves or restores the normal night-time reduction ('dipping') in BP that may be diminished in menopausal women. Such an effect would tend to reduce total BP load and thereby reduce target organ damage.[5]

Overall, HRT-related changes in BP are likely to be modest and should not preclude hormone use in normotensive or hypertensive women. However, HRT does not appear to reduce BP significantly, and should not be prescribed for that indication. All hypertensive women treated with HRT should have their BP monitored closely at first and then at 6-month intervals.

Oral contraceptives and blood pressure

Many women taking oral contraceptives experience a small but detectable increase in BP, and a small percentage experience the onset of frank hypertension, which resolves with withdrawal of oral contraceptive therapy. This is true even with modern preparations that contain only 30 µg estrogen. The Nurses' Health Study found that current users of oral contraceptives had a significantly increased (relative risk (RR) 1.8; 95% CI, 1.5–2.3) risk of hypertension compared with never users.[21] Absolute risk was small (only 41.5 cases of hypertension per 10 000 person-years could be attributed to oral contraceptive use) and risk decreased quickly with cessation of contraceptive use (past users had only a slightly increased (RR, 1.2; CI, 1.0–1.4) risk compared with never users). Controlled prospective studies have demonstrated a return of BP to pretreatment levels within 3 months of discontinuing oral contraceptives, indicating that their BP effect is readily reversible.

Oral contraceptives occasionally appear to precipitate accelerated, or malignant, hypertension. Genetic characteristics such as family history of hypertension, as well as environmental characteristics, including pre-existing pregnancy-induced hypertension, occult renal disease, obesity, middle age (>35 years) and duration of oral contraceptive use, increase susceptibility to oral contraceptive-induced hypertension. Contraceptive-induced hypertension appears to be related to the progesterogenic, not the estrogenic, potency of the preparation.[21] The risk of hypertension is greater among users of monophasic combination oral contraceptives than among users of biphasic or triphasic combinations, perhaps because the total dose of progestin is greater with the monophasic preparations.

The diagnosis of oral contraceptive-induced hypertension is made by documenting the onset of hypertension de novo during contraceptive therapy and the resolution of the hypertension on drug withdrawal. Regular monitoring of BP throughout contraceptive therapy is recommended, and it has been suggested that contraceptive prescriptions be limited to 6 months to ensure at least semi-annual re-evaluations. Withdrawal of the offending contraceptive agent is generally desirable in cases of contraceptive-induced hypertension, but such therapy may have to be continued in some women (e.g. if other contraceptive methods are not suitable) and combined with antihypertensive therapy.

Outcomes of antihypertensive trials in women

There is a strong evidence base for the use of antihypertensive treatment in the prevention of CVD in women. A subgroup meta-analysis of individual patient data according to sex based on seven older randomized controlled trials from the INDANA (Individual Data Analysis of Antihypertensive) intervention database showed significant treatment benefits for women (Fig. 31.8).[22] Significant reductions in stroke (total and fatal)

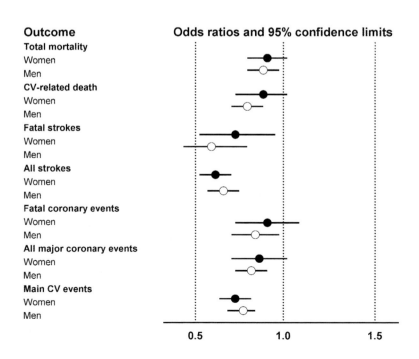

Figure 31.8
Data from the Individual Data Analysis of Antihypertensive (INDANA) intervention database showing significant treatment benefits for women. CV, cardiovascular. Reproduced with permission from reference 22.

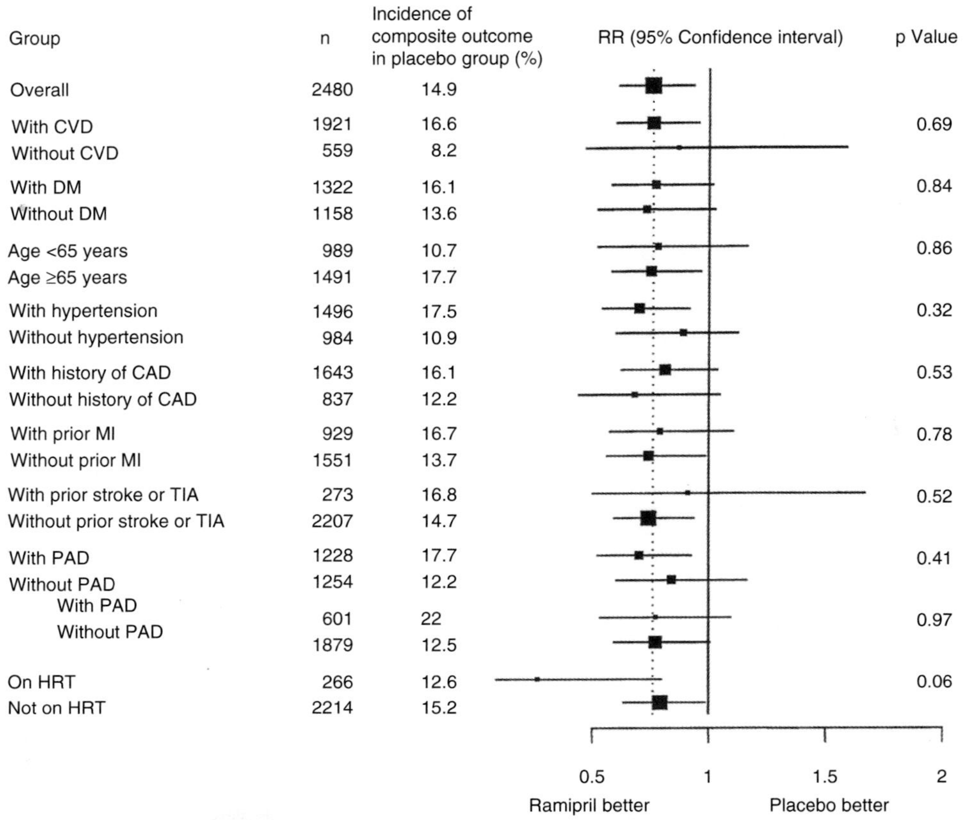

Group	n	Incidence of composite outcome in placebo group (%)	RR (95% Confidence interval)	p Value
Overall	2480	14.9		
With CVD	1921	16.6		0.69
Without CVD	559	8.2		
With DM	1322	16.1		0.84
Without DM	1158	13.6		
Age <65 years	989	10.7		0.86
Age ≥65 years	1491	17.7		
With hypertension	1496	17.5		0.32
Without hypertension	984	10.9		
With history of CAD	1643	16.1		0.53
Without history of CAD	837	12.2		
With prior MI	929	16.7		0.78
Without prior MI	1551	13.7		
With prior stroke or TIA	273	16.8		0.52
Without prior stroke or TIA	2207	14.7		
With PAD	1228	17.7		0.41
Without PAD	1254	12.2		
With PAD	601	22		0.97
Without PAD	1879	12.5		
On HRT	266	12.6		0.06
Not on HRT	2214	15.2		

0.5   1   1.5   2

Ramipril better   Placebo better

Figure 31.9
The effects of ramipril on primary study outcomes in key subgroups of women. RR, relative risk; CVD, cardiovascular disease; DM, diabetes mellitus; CAD, coronary artery disease; PAD, peripheral arterial disease; HRT, hormone replacement therapy. Reproduced with permission from reference 26.

and major cardiovascular events were seen in women randomized to thiazide diuretic or beta-blocker treatment compared with placebo. Expressed as relative risk, treatment benefits did not differ between the sexes. Absolute risk reduction, in contrast, is dependent on untreated risk, and while untreated risk for stroke was similar in both sexes, untreated risk for coronary events was greater in men. Therefore, absolute risk reduction for coronary events was less in women and did not attain statistical significance. Similarly, a placebo-controlled trial of CCB treatment showed treatment benefits for both sexes, although men were at higher risk than women.[23,24]

More recent trials that evaluated the newer classes of antihypertensive agents and included larger proportions of older, higher risk women showed even greater benefit. The Heart Outcomes Prevention Evaluation (HOPE) study evaluated the effects of long-term ACE inhibitor (ramipril) use on CVD outcomes in women and men aged >54 years with documented vascular disease or with diabetes and an additional cardiovascular risk factor.[25] At the time of enrollment, approximately half of the participants had controlled hypertension. Ramipril treatment of the 2480 female participants was associated with a 23% reduction in the composite end-point of myocardial infarction (MI), stroke, or cardiovascular death with a number needed to treat (NNT) to prevent one event of 27.[26] Importantly, relative risk reduction for cardiovascular death alone was 38% in women. Event reductions for women were similar to those for men (Fig. 31.9).

The Losartan Intervention For Endpoint reduction in hypertension (LIFE) study randomized 9193 persons, 4963 of whom were women, to an antihypertensive treatment regimen based on either the angiotensin receptor blocker (ARB) losartan or the beta-blocker atenolol.[27] Participants were older (aged 55–80), higher risk hypertensives with left ventricular hypertrophy by electrocardiographic criteria. Despite nearly equal BP reductions in the two groups, participants randomized to losartan had a 13% reduction in the composite endpoint of MI, stroke or cardiovascular death and 25% reductions in stroke and new onset diabetes. Subgroup analysis indicated that the benefit of losartan compared with atenolol treatment was greater in women than in men and in older (>70 years) than in younger persons (Fig. 31.10).

The Antihypertensive and Lipid Lowering to Prevent Heart Attack Trial (ALLHAT), the largest outcome study of antihypertensive treatment ever conducted, enrolled 42 448 high-risk (age 55 and over, with at least one additional CVD risk factor) hypertensive persons, 19 865 of whom were women.[28] ALLHAT tested the hypothesis that the combined incidence of fatal coronary heart disease (CHD) and nonfatal MI is lower in hypertensive persons randomized to a representative of one of the newer classes of antihypertensive agents (the CCB amlodipine, the ACE inhibitor lisinopril or the alpha-blocker doxazosin) than in those randomized to a thiazide-like diuretic (chlorthalidone) as first-line therapy. The alpha-blocker arm of ALLHAT was stopped early because of an excess of heart failure and major CVD events and the extreme improbability of finding benefit with alpha-blocker treatment compared with the diuretic.[29,30] The main result of ALLHAT was that there was no difference between treatments in the primary (coronary) endpoint or in all-cause mortality.[31] There was a higher rate of heart failure with the CCB than with the diuretic, and rates of stroke, heart failure, and combined CVD were higher with the ACE inhibitor than with the diuretic. Treatment effects were similar in women and men. Because the diuretic was superior to newer classes of antihypertensive drugs in preventing a variety of CVD outcomes, and because diuretics are less costly, the

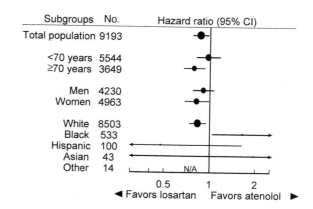

Figure 31.10
Age, gender, and race/ethnicity subgroup analysis from the Losartan Intervention For Endpoint reduction in hypertension (LIFE) study. Reproduced with permission from reference 27.

ALLHAT investigators concluded that thiazide-type diuretics should be preferred for first-line antihypertensive therapy and that a diuretic should be included in all multi-drug antihypertensive regimens, if possible. These observations, coupled with the additional benefits of thiazide-type diuretics discussed later in this chapter, provide a strong basis for use of these agents in high-risk older women with hypertension.

Although these active control trials do not provide information about absolute benefit derived from any particular antihypertensive treatment, they do suggest that women and men respond similarly to treatment with various antihypertensive drug classes. The totality of evidence from randomized controlled outcome trials indicates that the sex of the patient should not play a role in decisions about whether or not to treat high BP.

Choice of antihypertensive therapy for women

Thresholds for instituting antihypertensive treatment, BP goals, and choices of antihypertensive drugs are generally the same for women as for men and are outlined in Table 31.3.[32] In a clinical advisory statement, the National High Blood Pressure

Table 31.3 Classification and management of blood pressure (BP) for adults aged 18 years or older

BP classification	Systolic BP (mmHg)*		Diastolic BP (mmHg)*	Lifestyle modification	Initial drug therapy without compelling indication	Initial drug therapy with compelling indications†
Normal	<120	and	<80	Encourage	–	–
Prehypertension	120–139	or	80–89	Yes	No antihypertensive drug indicated	Drugs for the compelling indications‡
Stage 1 hypertension	140–159	or	90–99	Yes	Thiazide-type diuretics for most; may consider ACE inhibitor, ARB, beta-blocker, CCB, or combination	Drug(s) for the compelling indications; other antihypertensive drugs (diuretics, ACE inhibitor, ARB, beta-blocker, CCB) as needed
Stage 2 hypertension	≥160	or	≥100	Yes	Two-drug combination for most (usually thiazide-type diuretics and ACE inhibitor or ARB or beta-blocker or CCB)§	Drug(s) for the compelling indications; other antihypertensive drugs (diuretics, ACE inhibitor, ARB, beta-blocker, CCB) as needed

ACE, angiotensin-converting enzyme; ARB, angiotensin-receptor blocker; CCB, calcium channel blocker.
*Treatment determined by highest BP category.
†Heart failure: diuretic, beta-blocker, ACE inhibitor, ARB, aldosterone antagonist; post-myocardial infarction: beta-blocker, ACE inhibitor, aldosterone antagonist; high coronary disease risk: diuretic, beta-blocker, ACE inhibitor, CCB; diabetes: diuretic, beta-blocker, ACE inhibitor, ARB, CCB; chronic kidney disease: ACE inhibitor, ARB; recurrent stroke prevention: diuretic, ACE inhibitor.
‡Treat patients with chronic kidney disease or diabetes to BP goal of <130/80 mmHg.
§Initial combined therapy should be used cautiously in those at risk for orthostatic hypotension.
From reference 32 with permission.

Education Program has identified systolic BP as the 'principal clinical endpoint' for the management (both treatment threshold and BP goals) of hypertension.[33] Current guidelines also suggest lifestyle modification and specific drug therapy, including certain drug classes for compelling indications, for women with hypertension.[32]

Lifestyle modification is indicated in all persons with clinical hypertension or with BP in the 'prehypertension' range because of its potential for preventing CVD outcomes and the progression to higher BPs and for increasing pharmacologic treatment efficacy. The National High Blood Pressure Education Program Coordinating Committee has made specific recommendations for prevention of hypertension by modifying lifestyle[34] and these recommendations have been supported by AHA guidelines.[14] Specifically, all women should be encouraged to obtain an optimal BP of <120/80 mmHg via lifestyle approaches. Of the lifestyle interventions, aerobic exercise and weight

loss are the most efficacious in reducing BP and related CVD risk factors such as dyslipidemia.[35,36]

Important determinants of the aggressiveness of antihypertensive treatment are, in addition to the extent of BP elevation, the presence of co-morbid conditions. These factors play a role in determining an individual's risk of sustaining a CVD event or death from CVD over time. Persons with multiple risk factors or target organ damage (e.g. renal insufficiency, proteinuria or heart failure) should be treated to a lower goal and often require combination therapy, with special consideration given to newer agents with proven benefits beyond BP-lowering.

With the exception that older persons are generally at higher risk and merit particularly aggressive treatment, there are no age- or gender-specific recommendations for BP management. The BP-lowering effect of antihypertensive drugs is generally similar in both sexes, but some special issues may dictate treatment choices for women. ACE inhibitors and ARBs are contraindicated for women who are or intend to become pregnant because of the risk of fetal developmental abnormalities. Beta-blockers tend to be less effective in women than men,[37] while diuretics have added value in older women because of their association with decreased bone loss and reduced risk of hip fracture.[38] Further, some antihypertensive drugs have gender-specific adverse effect profiles. For example, in the Treatment Of Mild Hypertension Study (TOMHS), in which 902 women and men received nonpharmacologic treatment plus treatment with a drug chosen at random from each class of antihypertensive agent then available, women reported twice as many side effects as men.[39]

Biochemical responses to drugs may also be gender-dependent. While men are more likely to develop gout, women are more likely to develop hyponatremia and hypokalemia associated with diuretic therapy.[40] Women develop cough related to ACE inhibitor therapy three times more often than men.[41] Minoxidil-induced hirsutism and lower extremity edema induced by CCBs are much more common in women than in men. Further, there is evidence that sexual dysfunction related to antihypertensive therapy may be a problem in women as well as in men, and is most often associated with centrally acting agents, beta-blockers, and thiazide diuretics, while ARB therapy may improve these symptoms.[42–44]

Conclusions

Hypertension is the most common modifiable risk factor for CVD in women and its modification offers significant hope for tackling this public health crisis. Currently, hypertension is underappreciated and often undertreated in the United States. Evidence-based guidelines recommend lifestyle interventions for all women with 'prehypertension' or with clinical disease and pharmacotherapy for those with BP >140/90 mmHg.[14] The treatment threshold is even lower for those with target organ damage or diabetes. Largely based on evidence from ALLHAT, thiazide-type diuretics should be first-line agents, but multidrug therapy is usually required to obtain BP control, and additional agents should be aggressively employed.

References

1. American Heart Association. *2004 Heart and Stroke Statistical Update*. Dallas, TX: American Heart Association, 2003.
2. Cooper R, Cutler J, Desvigne-Nickens P, et al. Trends and disparities in coronary heart disease, stroke, and other cardiovascular diseases in the United States: findings of the national conference on cardiovascular disease prevention. *Circulation* 2000; **102**:3137–47.
3. Burt VL, Whelton P, Roccella EJ, et al. Prevalence of hypertension in the US adult population: results from the Third National Health and Nutrition Examination Survey, 1988–91. *Hypertension* 1995; **25**:305–13.
4. Rosenthal T, Oparil S. Hypertension in women. *J Hum Hypertens* 2000; **14**:691–704.
5. Calhoun D, Oparil S. Gender and blood pressure. In: Izzo JL, Black HR (eds). *Hypertension Primer*, 3rd edn. Baltimore, MD: Lippincott, Williams & Wilkins, 2003: 253–7.
6. Wolz M, Cutler J, Roccella EJ, et al. Statement from the National High Blood Pressure Education Program: prevalence of hypertension. *Am J Hypertens* 2000; **13**:103–4.
7. Hajjar I, Kotchen TA. Trends in prevalence, awareness, treatment and control of hypertension in the United States, 1988–2000. *JAMA* 2003; **290**:199–206.
8. Hyman DJ, Pavlik VN. Characteristics of patients with uncontrolled hypertension in the United States. *N Engl J Med* 2001; **345**: 479–86.
9. Vasan RS, Beiser A, Seshadri S, et al. Residual lifetime risk for developing hypertension in middle-aged women and men: The Framingham Heart Study. *JAMA* 2002; **287**:1003–10.
10. Wassertheil-Smoller S, Anderson G, Psaty BM, et al. Hypertension and its treatment in postmenopausal women: baseline data from the Women's Health Initiative. *Hypertension* 2000; **36**:780–9.
11. Vittinghoff E, Shlipak MG, Varosy PD, et al. Risk factors and secondary prevention in women with heart disease: the Heart and Estrogen/progestin Replacement Study. *Ann Intern Med* 2003; **138**:81–9.

12. Miller AP, Oparil S. Secondary prevention of coronary heart disease in women: a call to action. *Ann Intern Med* 2003; **138**:150–1.

13. AHA Get With The Guidelines (GWTG) web page: http://www.americanheart.org/presenter.jhtml?identifier=1165.

14. Mosca L, Appel LJ, Benjamin EJ, et al. Evidence-based guidelines for cardiovascular disease prevention in women. *Circulation* 2004; **109**:672–93.

15. Joffres MR, Hamet P, MacLean DR, et al. Distribution of blood pressure and hypertension in Canada and the United States. *Am J Hypertens* 2001; **14**:1099–105.

16. Staessen JA, Celis H, Fagard R. The epidemiology of the association between hypertension and menopause. *J Hum Hypertens* 1998; **12**:587–92.

17. Staessen JA, Ginocchio G, Thijs L, Fagard R. Conventional and ambulatory blood pressure and menopause in a prospective population study. *J Hum Hypertens* 1997; **11**:507–14.

18. Manson JE, Hsia J, Johnson KC, et al. Estrogen plus progestin and the risk of coronary heart disease. *N Engl J Med* 2003; **349**:523–34.

19. Scuteri A, Bos AJ, Brant LJ, Talbot L, Lakatta EG, Fleg JL. Hormone replacement therapy and longitudinal changes in blood pressure in postmenopausal women. *Ann Intern Med* 2001; **135**:229–38.

20. The Writing Group for the PEPI Trial. Effects of estrogen or estrogen/progestin regimens on heart disease risk factors in postmenopausal women: the Postmenopausal Estrogen/Progestin Interventions (PEPI) Trial. *JAMA* 1995; **273**:199–208.

21. Chasan-Taber L, Willett WC, Manson JE, et al. Prospective study of oral contraceptives and hypertension among women in the United States. *Circulation* 1996; **94**:483–9.

22. Gueyffier F, Boutitie F, Boissel J-P, et al. Effect of antihypertensive drug treatment on cardiovascular outcomes in women and men: a meta-analysis of individual patient data from randomized, controlled trials. The INDANA Investigators. *Ann Intern Med* 1997; **126**:761–7.

23. Staessen JA, Fagard R, Thijs L, et al. Randomised double-blind comparison of placebo and active treatment for older patients with isolated systolic hypertension. *Lancet* 1997; **350**:757–64.

24. Staessen JA, Fagard R, Thijs L, et al. Subgroup and per-protocol analysis of the randomized European trial on isolated systolic hypertension in the elderly. *Arch Intern Med* 1998; **158**:1681–91.

25. Yusuf S, Sleight P, Dagenais G, et al. Effects of an angiotensin-converting-enzyme inhibitor, ramipril, on cardiovascular events in high-risk patients. *N Engl J Med* 2000; **342**:145–53.

26. Lonn E, Roccaforte R, Yi Q, et al. Effect of long-term therapy with ramipril in high-risk women. *J Am Coll Cardiol* 2002; **40**:693–702.

27. Dahlöf B, Devereux RB, Kjeldsen SE, et al. Cardiovascular morbidity and mortality in the Losartan Intervention For Endpoint reduction in hypertension study (LIFE): a randomised trial against atenolol. *Lancet* 2002; **359**:995–1003.

28. Davis BR, Cuttler JA, Gordon DJ, et al. Rationale and design for the Antihypertensive and Lipid-Lowering Treatment to Prevent Heart Attack Trial (ALLHAT): ALLHAT Research Group. *Am J Hypertens* 1996; **9**:342–60.

29. The ALLHAT Officers and Coordinators for the ALLHAT Collaborative Research Group. Major cardiovascular events in hypertensive patients randomized to doxazosin vs chlorthalidone: the Antihypertensive and Lipid-Lowering Treatment to Prevent Heart Attack Trial (ALLHAT). *JAMA* 2000; **283**:1967–75.

30. Davis BR, Cutler JA, Furberg CD, et al. Relationship of antihypertensive treatment regimens and change in blood pressure to risk for heart failure in hypertensive patients randomly assigned to doxazosin or chlorthalidone: further analyses from the Antihypertensive and Lipid-Lowering Treatment to Prevent Heart Attack Trial. *Ann Intern Med* 2002; **137**:313–20.

31. The ALLHAT Officers and Coordinators for the ALLHAT Collaborative Research Group. Major outcomes in high-risk hypertensive patients randomized to angiotensin-converting enzyme inhibitor or calcium channel blocker versus diuretic: the Antihypertensive and Lipid-Lowering Treatment to Prevent Heart Attack Trial (ALLHAT). *JAMA* 2002; **288**:2981–97.

32. Chobanian AV, Bakris GL, Black HR, et al. The seventh report of the Joint National Committee on prevention, detection, evaluation, and treatment of high blood pressure: The JNC 7 report. *JAMA* 2003; **289**:2560–72.

33. Izzo JL, Levy D, Black HR. Clinical advisor statement: importance of systolic blood pressure in older Americans. *Hypertension* 2000; **35**:1021–4.

34. Whelton PK, He J, Appel LJ, et al. Primary prevention of hypertension: clinical and public health advisory from The National High Blood Pressure Education Program. *JAMA* 2002; **288**:1882–8.

35. Stevens VJ, Obarzanek E, Cook NR, et al. Long-term weight loss and changes in blood pressure: results of the Trials of Hypertension Prevention, phase II. *Ann Intern Med* 2001; **134**:1–11.

36. Whelton SP, Chin A, Xin X, He J. Effect of aerobic exercise on blood pressure: a meta-analysis of randomized, controlled trials. *Ann Intern Med* 2002; **136**:493–503.

37. Lewis CE. Characteristics and treatment of hypertension in women: a review of the literature. *Am J Med Sci* 1996; **11**:193–9.

38. Cauley JA, Cummings SR, Seeley DG, et al. Effects of thiazide diuretic therapy on bone mass, fractures, and falls: the Study of Osteoporotic Fractures Research Group. *Ann Intern Med* 1993; **118**:666–73.

39. Lewis CE, Grandits GA, Flack J, et al. Efficacy and tolerance of antihypertensive treatment in men and women with stage 1 diastolic hypertension. *Arch Intern Med* 1996; **156**:377–85

40. August P, Oparil S. Hypertension in women. In: Oparil S, Weber M (eds). *Hypertension*. Philadelphia, PA: WB Saunders, 1999: 546–50.

41. Os I, Bratland B, Dahlof B, et al. Female sex as an important determinant of lisinopril induced cough. *Lancet* 1992; **339**:372.

42. Wassertheil-Smoller S, Blaufox MD, Oberman A, et al. Effect of antihypertensives on sexual function and quality of life: the TAIM study. *Ann Intern Med* 1991; **114**:613–20.

43. Grimm RH, Grandits GA, Prineas RF. Long-term effects on sexual function of five antihypertensive drugs and nutritional hygienic treatment of hypertensive men and women: Treatment of Mild Hypertensive Study (TOMHS). *Hypertension* 1997; **27**:8–14.

44. Fogari R, Preti P, Zoppi A, et al. Effect of valsartan and atenolol on sexual behavior in hypertensive postmenopausal women. *Am J Hypertens* 2004; **17**:77–81.

32

Women and congenital heart disease

Craig S. Broberg, Steve M. Yentis, Philip J. Steer and
Michael A. Gatzoulis

Introduction

Women with congenital heart disease make up an
ever-increasing fraction of any adult cardiology
practice for several reasons. First, congenital problems
are increasing in prevalence. Though estimates vary
considerably, current prevalence is 0.8%.
Approximately 1600 patients with moderate to severe
forms of congenital heart abnormalities in the UK
enter adulthood each year,[1] a conservative estimate
according to the European Society of Cardiology.[2]
Second, diagnostic tools are more sophisticated and
widely available, meaning that diagnoses are made
earlier with better sensitivity and accuracy. Third,
improved medical and surgical therapeutic options
allow more patients to reach adulthood. Of children
with congenital lesions, 77–90% will survive into
maturity.[3,4] Fourth, even though the above reasons
apply equally to both genders, the female patients with
congenital heart disease seek medical attention far
more frequently because of pregnancy. Occasionally
previously undiagnosed lesions are first discovered
during antenatal visits. In high-risk pregnancy clinics
in North America the majority of heart disease
encountered will be congenital,[5] although in developing countries rheumatic heart disease is still more
common.[6]

Many women with congenital heart defects have
difficulty obtaining adequate care for their complex
problems, because of both poor insurance coverage
(notably in the United States) and the lack of
adequately trained providers. Treatment of congenital lesions with or without pregnancy can also be
expensive.[7] For all these reasons, there is a tremendous need for proper education about congenital
heart disease and its complexities, but a shortage of
providers. Worldwide health task forces have been
formed to address the need.

This chapter will highlight the key issues that
women with congenital heart defects face. Although
pregnancy is addressed in detail elsewhere in this
book, it is a major issue for women with congenital
heart disease, and thus will also be addressed as
appropriate here. The chapter will first review
incidence data, followed by recommendations about
contraception. Then pregnancy will be considered,
both in terms of management issues and maternal
and fetal risks. Thereafter, the chapter will focus on
specific congenital lesions and how they affect
women in particular. Finally, it will highlight the
importance of women as caregivers for affected
children.

Incidence of congenital heart disease in women

Overall, women and men have a similar incidence of
congenital heart disease with few differences. Mitral

valve prolapse is more common in women. Slightly more patients with atrial septal defects (ASD) are female.[8] An Egyptian survey found a slight female predominance in patent ductus arteriosus (PDA) and AV septal defects.[9] Primary pulmonary hypertension is also more common in women, and in the classic patient cohort with Eisenmenger syndrome reported in 1958 there were four times as many women as men.[10] Although more contemporary studies do not find such a radical gender difference in this group, females still tend to predominate.

Other lesions are less common in women, including pulmonic stenosis (PS),[9] transposition of the great arteries (TGA), and coarctation of the aorta.[11] Men with bicuspid aortic valve outnumber women by as much as 4 to 1.[4] Ventricular septal defect (VSD), hypertrophic obstructive cardiomyopathy (HOCM), and tetralogy of Fallot (TOF) tend to affect men and women equally. Marfan's syndrome, an autosomal dominant mutation, is also gender neutral. Lesions such as Ebstein's anomaly of the tricuspid valve, tricuspid atresia, double inlet ventricle, truncus arteriosus, and anomalous pulmonary venous return are rarer and always reported in small numbers, but no gender differences are suspected.

Contraception

In the past, paternalistic providers made contraception decisions for patients, even sometimes coercing sterilization. Today's caregiver should educate and enable the patient to reach her own conclusions about the appropriateness of pregnancy and methods of contraception. This is best done well before conception so that any necessary investigations or procedures can be expedited, even when lack of overt symptoms would not necessarily warrant the same intervention in a man. Since pregnant women should not be exposed to ionizing radiation such as catheterization, and since coronary artery bypass graft surgery in pregnancy is high risk, pre-emptive action before pregnancy will often be key to a healthy newborn and mother. For this reason, women of reproductive age ought to be encouraged to seek attention from trained professionals well before considering conception.

Discussions about contraception should therefore begin in early adolescence. Despite this, information is not always conveyed, and 6 of 35 women with congenital heart disease in one study had an unplanned pregnancy.[12] It is important that an appropriate method suits the patient's own life situation. However, no form of contraception is flawless. The ill-named 'natural' methods are faulty because they rely on unnatural timing. Hormone therapy requires regular compliance and increases the risk of thromboembolic events, which is already greater in this patient group. Many patients with congenital heart defects using oral contraception do so incorrectly.[12] Barrier methods must be conveniently on hand, and even when used properly have a known failure rate.

Intrauterine contraceptive devices (IUCD) have a good success rate but can increase the risk of endocarditis. The recent introduction of an IUCD carrying slow release progestogen (Mirena) has been an important advance. The pregnancy rate associated with it is similar to that of sterilization; the amount of menstrual bleeding is substantially reduced thereby lowering the risk of anemia; and suppression of the endometrium greatly reduces the incidence of infectious complications, and thus endocarditis (although antibiotic prophylaxis at insertion is probably wise). Fertility is restored on removal, and coil change is necessary only every 5 years.

Current recommendations are as follows. Hormonal contraception should be avoided in cyanotic patients because of associated thromboembolic risk. IUCDs should be discouraged in patients with high risk of endocarditis, but the use of the Mirena may be acceptable. Barrier methods should be encouraged. Tubal occlusion (with clips) should be offered only to patients with high risk of pregnancy-related complications such as those with Eisenmenger syndrome, but there is still a 1 in 200 pregnancy rate.[13]

Pregnancy – management (see also Chapter 22)

General considerations

As opposed to nonrheumatic acquired forms of heart disease, which tend to affect older women, congenital heart disease plays a significant physiologic role during a patient's childbearing years. Thanks to advances in cardiac surgery and fertility medicine, more women with congenital heart defects are surviving with better chances of conception. Even those once considered infertile, such as patients with Turner's syndrome, can use ovum donation successfully. Pregnancy presents some of the most difficult issues in the field of congenital heart disease. The strains of pregnancy on the mother, both psychosocial and physiologic, can be both life-altering and life-threatening.

There is little written about the ideal obstetric and anesthetic management of congenital heart disease patients. Because of the risks involved, the pregnant patient with congenital heart disease deserves a highly specialized team approach to her labor and delivery whenever possible. This ought to include cardiologists, obstetricians, midwives, anesthetists, intensivists, and neonatologists who have experience with this group and the nature of problems that may arise. They should work closely in decision-making with both patient and partner.

The team approach should start with a general assessment of the patient's risk,[14] which should be conveyed clearly to the patient. Risk assessment is also important for planning a safe labor and delivery. An assessment of symptom limitation such as New York Heart Association (NYHA) classification should be made and factored into this plan. Although most congenital heart disease patients can be expected to do well (apart from those with Eisenmenger syndrome), it is very important to monitor the patient for obstetric complications such as pre-eclampsia, which can be especially dangerous when superimposed on underlying cardiac disease.

Considerations during pregnancy

The cardiovascular changes that occur with pregnancy are well recognized. As the fetus develops, maternal blood volume increases by 30–50%. Both stroke volume and heart rate contribute to a 50% increase in cardiac output, and systemic resistance drops to compensate for the higher flow. Thus, any right-to-left shunt increases because of reductions in systemic vascular resistance. Hypoxia can worsen because the fetus takes increasing amounts of oxygen from the

bloodstream and because maternal functional residual capacity and thus gas exchange is reduced. For all of the above reasons, stenotic or cyanotic lesions (right-to-left shunt), where effective cardiac output is limited, are not well tolerated. In contrast, regurgitant lesions or volume overload (left-to-right shunt) pose less difficulty, although increased blood volume may precipitate congestive heart failure. Patients should be seen frequently and monitored for the development of heart failure, arrhythmias, pre-eclampsia, and poor fetal growth. Often medications need to be switched to those felt to be safe during pregnancy. Warfarin (early on) and angiotensin-converting enzyme (ACE) inhibitors are particularly contraindicated because of teratogenicity.[15]

In the final trimester bed rest is often recommended, especially for patients with cyanotic and obstructive lesions. Anti-thrombotic prophylaxis should be used in most cases. Patients should be warned to avoid lying flat on their backs because of aortocaval compression, which can impair venous return and produce catastrophic effects on cardiovascular function. In fact most women in late pregnancy avoid this position themselves. Patients with congenital heart lesions should be warned not to allow medical staff to lie them flat, for example, for vaginal examination or assessment of the fetus, and to remind all concerned that aortocaval compression can occur even in the semi-sitting and semi-lateral positions.

Labor and delivery

The cardiovascular stress of labor can be intense. Inadequate oxygen delivery for the reasons listed above can be worsened by regional analgesia/ anesthesia unless steps are taken to avoid it, either by using low-dose epidural techniques or by careful titration of anesthesia and use of vasoconstrictors. Maternal oximetry coupled with serial scanning of the fetus can be useful in determining optimal timing of delivery. Peripartum monitoring should be instituted as appropriate and would normally include ECG and pulse oximetry as well as blood pressure (BP). Intra-arterial BP monitoring may be required in patients with labile cardiovascular status or in those with aortic conditions (Marfan's or coarctation). Placement of a central venous or pulmonary artery catheter may be required in severe conditions, particularly if pulmonary edema is present. However, placement of such lines is not straightforward given increased subcutaneous tissue fluid, breast enlargement, and the difficulty that pregnant patients with congenital lesions have in lying head down.

Decisions about method of delivery should be made by obstetricians and anesthetists who have experience and understanding of the issues faced. Traditionally, elective cesarean section under general anesthesia has been recommended in women with congenital heart problems to avoid the risks associated with labor, especially pushing in the second stage. Cesarean deliveries reported in the recent literature are usually done for obstetric rather than cardiovascular reasons.[16] More recently, there has been a trend towards vaginal delivery with low-dose epidural analgesia with limited or no pushing and elective vacuum assistance.[16] Low-dose epidural analgesia is remarkably stable cardiovascularly, reduces stress on the heart, allows elective assisted vaginal delivery, and permits slow extension for anesthesia if required.[17] For cesarean section, regional or general anesthesia may be used. The choice probably has little impact on outcome if both are done with precision. Oxytocin may result in calamitous drops in BP and induce severe tachycardia.[18] Therefore, avoidance altogether is preferable (though there is a risk of bleeding). It is also possible that patients with congenital defects have uterine malformations that pose difficulty for the obstetrician.[19]

Postpartum

Because many patients, especially those with cyanosis, will have complications in the week after delivery, thorough monitoring must continue through the high-risk postpartum period. Risk is due to dramatic changes in venous return, blood loss, and the thrombogenic milieu. Most deaths in Eisenmenger patients, for example, occur in the first or second week after delivery. Extra care should be taken to detect bleeding, since reduced venous return may be poorly tolerated. Fluid balance should also be controlled. Good analgesia in the postoperative

period with either epidural or spinal opioids will reduce the adverse cardiovascular effects of pain such as tachycardia and hypertension.

Pregnancy – specific risks (see also Chapter 22)

Problems with risk assessment

Even with adequate preparation, the patient's informed decision about childbirth is often difficult and soul-searching. She must consider the risks to both herself and the unborn baby. She also needs to consider long-term risks such as whether the child will have a similar heart defect or whether she will be present and capable during her child's upbringing. Unfortunately, accurate data for risk assessment are often elusive. Because of the rarity of many conditions, reports have low numbers. Wide discrepancies between studies reflect the variability of data as well as the inherent morphologic and hemodynamic spectra in the lesions themselves. Referral and recall bias are often a problem. Despite these shortcomings, the literature does shed some light on the issues. Current studies are listed uniformly (Tables 32.1 and 32.2), which, although considerable heterogeneity exists, can offer approximate risks to guide decision-making. In general, the literature confirms the expectation that there is increased risk with increased anatomic complexity, cyanosis, and severity of obstructive lesions.

Maternal mortality

Cardiac disease remains the leading cause of maternal death in the UK.[20] Data on maternal morbidity and mortality with congenital heart disease are listed in Table 32.1. However, many of these studies were compiled from patient questionnaires retrospectively; thus they may underestimate true maternal mortality (and are thus not shown in such circumstances). The lack of complete data is readily apparent. Overall, the risk of maternal death is approximately 1/100–1/1000, depending greatly on which studies/conditions are included. This is higher

Table 32.1 Data on maternal outcome in congenital heart disease

Reference	Congenital heart disease lesion	Mothers	Pregnancies	Maternal deaths	CV complications*
All congenital heart disease combined					
Shime, 1987[21]	All congenital heart disease	74	144	1 (1.35%)	18 (13%)
Siu, 2001†[5]	All congenital heart disease	445	445	1 (0.22%)	36 (8%)
Avila, 2003[6]	All congenital heart disease	191	191	7 (3.66%)	44 (23%)
	Combined data	710	780	9 (1.27%)	98 (13%)
Shime, 1987[21]	All acyanotic	50	101	0	6 (6%)
Intracardiac shunts					
Whittemore, 1982[19]	PDA	42	105		1 (1%)
Whittemore, 1982[19]	VSD	50	98		8 (8%)
Whittemore, 1982[19]	ASD	36	66		4 (6%)
	Combined data	128	269		13 (5%)
Obstructive lesions					
Beachesne, 2001[34]	Coarctation	50	118	1 (2%)	0
Whittemore, 1982[19]	Any left-sided obstruction	27	59		8 (14%)
Lao, 1993[13]	AS	13	25	0	2 (8%)
Lao, 1993[13]	AS (literature summary)	65	106	7 (11%)	
Whittemore, 1982[19]	PS	24	46		5 (11%)
Cyanotic conditions					
Shime, 1987[21]	All cyanotic	24	43	1 (4%)	8 (19%)
Presbitero, 1994[23]	All cyanotic	44	96	1 (2%)	14 (15%)
	Combined data	68	139	2 (3%)	22 (16%)
Connolly, 1997[36]	PA all	15	26	0	2 (8%)
Neumeyer, 1997[37]	PA all	15	41		
Whittemore, 1982[19]	PA (cyanotic)	22	42		2 (5%)
Presbitero, 1994[23]	PA (TOF, cyanotic)	21	46	1 (5%)	8 (17%)
Neumeyer, 1997[37]	PA (cyanotic)	9	26		3 (12%)
	Combined data	52	114	1 (2%)	13 (11%)
Shime, 1987[21]	Eisenmenger syndrome	9	19	1 (11%)	8 (42%)
Avila, 1995[39]	Eisenmenger syndrome	12	13	3 (25%)	3 (23%)
Avila, 2003[6]	Eisenmenger syndrome	21	21	6 (29%)	
	Combined data	42	53	10 (24%)	
Other lesions					
Neumeyer, 1997[37]	PA (acyanotic)	7	15	1 (14%)	5 (33%)
Connolly, 1999‡[43]	CC-TGA	22	61	0	6 (10%)
Therrien, 1999[62]	CC-TGA	19	45	0	5 (11%)
	Combined data	41	106	0	11 (10%)
Presbitero, 1994[23]	CC-TGA + VSD/PS (cyanotic)	5	10		1 (10%)
Lao, 1994[40]	D-TGA (Mustard/Rastelli)	4	7	0	3 (43%)
Clarkson, 1994[41]	D-TGA (Mustard repair)	9	15	0	0
	Combined data	13	22	0	1 (5%)
Cannobbio, 1996[46]	Fontan repair	21	33		2 (6%)
Presbitero, 1994[23]	TA, single vent (cyanotic)	10	26		2 (8%)
Connolly, 1994[44]	Ebstein's anomaly	44	111	0	0
Presbitero, 1994[23]	Ebstein's + ASD (cyanotic)	8	14		3 (21%)
Rossiter, 1995[47]	Marfan's syndrome	21	45		5 (11%)

CV, cardiovascular; PDA, patent ductus arteriosus; VSD, ventricular septal defect; ASD, atrial septal defect; AS, aortic stenosis; PS, pulmonic stenosis; PA, pulmonic atresia; TOF, tetralogy of Fallot; CC-TGA, congenitally corrected transposition of the great arteries; D-TGA, dextrorotatory transposition of the great arteries; TA, tricuspid atresia.

*Cardiovascular complications (expressed as a per cent of pregnancies) include arrhythmia, treatment for congestive heart failure, syncope, need for cardiac surgery, endocarditis, significant bleeding, or cerebral vascular event. It does not include pre-eclampsia, hypertension, or isolated deterioration of NYHA class.

†Siu did not report explicitly the number of mothers, 445 is used here for calculations.

‡Five of the six maternal complications occurred in the same patient, who carried 12 pregnancies.

Table 32.2 Data on fetal outcome in congenital heart disease

Reference	Congenital heart disease lesion	Pregnancy	TAB	Live births*	Fetal loss	Premature†	CHD
All congenital heart disease combined							
Whittemore, 1982[19]	All congenital heart disease	482	41	367 (83%)	74 (17%)		60 (16%)
Shime, 1987[21]	All congenital heart disease	144	37	81 (76%)	26 (24%)	14 (17%)	
Siu, 2002[27]	All congenital heart disease	194		183 (94%)	11 (6%)		15 (8%)
Avila, 2003[6]	All congenital heart disease	191	8	159 (87%)	24 (13%)	31 (19%)	11 (7%)
	Combined data	1011	86	790 (85%)	135 (15%)		
Shime, 1987[21]	All acyanotic	101	25	61 (80%)	15 (20%)	6 (10%)	
Intracardiac shunts							
Whittemore, 1982[19]	PDA	105	1	83 (80%)	21 (20%)		9 (11%)
Whittemore, 1982[19]	VSD	98	6	78 (85%)	14 (15%)		17 (22%)
Whittemore, 1982[19]	ASD	66	1	52 (80%)	13 (20%)		3 (6%)
	Combined data	269	8	213 (82%)	48 (18%)		29 (14%)
Obstructive lesions							
Beauchesne, 2001‡[34]	Coarctation	118	0	105 (89%)	13 (11%)	4 (4%)	4 (4%)
Whittemore, 1982[19]	Any left-sided obstruction	59	5	46 (85%)	8 (15%)		12 (26%)
Lao, 1993[13]	AS	25	5	20 (100%)	0	0	1 (5%)
Lao, 1993[13]	AS (literature summary)	106	24?§	79		4 (5%)	
Whittemore, 1982[19]	PS	46	4	36 (86%)	6 (14%)		7 (19%)
Cyanotic conditions							
Shime, 1987[21]	All cyanotic	43	12	20 (65%)	11 (35%)	8 (40%)	
Presbitero, 1994[23]	All cyanotic	96		41 (43%)	55 (57%)	15 (37%)	2 (5%)
	Combined data	139	12	61 (48%)	66 (52%)		
Connolly, 1997[36]	PA all	26	6	10 (50%)	10 (50%)	4 (40%)	0
Neumeyer, 1997[37]	PA all	41	3	23 (61%)	15 (39%)	0	2 (9%)
Whittemore, 1982[19]	PA (cyanotic)	42	13	21 (72%)	8 (28%)	8 (38%)	3 (14%)
Presbitero, 1994[23]	PA (TOF, cyanotic)	46	0	15 (33%)	31 (67%)	9 (60%)	
Neumeyer, 1997[37]	PA (cyanotic)	26	3	8 (35%)	15 (65%)	1 (13%)	
	Combined data	114	16	44 (45%)	54 (55%)		
Shime, 1987[21]	Eisenmenger syndrome	19	5	8 (57%)	6 (43%)	6 (75%)	
Avila, 2003[6]	Eisenmenger syndrome	21		11 (52%)	10 (48%)		
Avila, 1995[39]	Eisenmenger syndrome	13	0	7 (54%)	6 (46%)	4 (57%)	1 (14%)
	Combined data	53	5	26 (54%)	22 (46%)		
Other lesions							
Neumeyer, 1997[37]	PA (acyanotic)	15	0	12 (80%)	3 (20%)	0	1 (8%)
Connolly, 1999[43]	CC-TGA	61	0	50 (82%)	11 (18%)	1 (2%)	0
Therrien, 1999[62]	CC-TGA	45	6	27 (69%)	12 (31%)	5 (19%)	1 (4%)
	Combined data	106	6	77 (77%)	23 (23%)	6 (8%)	1 (1%)
Presbitero, 1994[23]	CC-TGA + VSD/PS (cyanotic)	10	0	6 (60%)	4 (40%)	2 (33%)	
Lao, 1994[40]	D-TGA (Mustard/Rastelli)	7	1	6 (100%)	0	3 (50%)	
Clarkson, 1994[41]	D-TGA (Mustard repair)	15	0	12 (80%)	3 (20%)		0
	Combined data	22	1	18 (86%)	3 (14%)		
Cannobbio, 1996[46]	Fontan repair	33	5	15 (54%)	13 (46%)	1 (7%)	1 (7%)
Presbitero, 1994[23]	TA, single vent (cyanotic)	26	0	8 (31%)	18 (69%)	3 (38%)	
Connolly, 1994[44]	Ebstein's anomaly	111		85 (77%)	26 (23%)		
Presbitero, 1994[23]	Ebstein's + ASD (cyanotic)	14	0	12 (86%)	2 (14%)	1 (8%)	
Rossiter, 1995[47]	Marfan's syndrome	45	10	26 (74%)	9 (26%)	1 (4%)	

TAB, therapeutic abortion; PDA, patent ductus arteriosus; VSD, ventricular septal defect; ASD, atrial septal defect; AS, aortic stenosis; PS, pulmonic stenosis; PA, pulmonic atresia; TOF, tetralogy of Fallot; CC-TGA, congenitally corrected transposition of the great arteries; D-TGA, dextrorotatory transposition of the great arteries; TA, tricuspid atresia.

*Live births exclude all miscarriages, stillbirths, and neonatal deaths, and implies hospital discharge of the infant, and are expressed as a percentage of non-aborted pregnancies.

†Prematurity is defined differently in various studies; therefore data were not combined. Number here is as reported by the study.

§Therapeutic and spontaneous abortions reported together.

than for the general population, 1/10 000. In a Brazilian series of 191 pregnant patients with congenital heart defects the maternal mortality rate was 3.6%, but nearly all deaths were in those with Eisenmenger syndrome.[6] By far the greatest mortality in any series is found in women with cyanosis, pulmonary hypertension, or both (Eisenmenger syndrome).

Maternal morbidity

Heart failure

Many patients who are asymptomatic before conception develop classic symptoms of heart failure while pregnant. Several publications have demonstrated deterioration in NYHA class during gestation.[21,22] Typically this reverses to baseline following delivery. Congestive heart failure will require hospitalization for intravenous diuretics.[23] Cardiovascular complications (listed in Table 32.1) include hospitalization for heart failure but not NYHA deterioration alone because of its subjectivity. In general, patients with good functional class at the start of pregnancy tend to have fewer complications than those starting with compromised function.[19] Heart failure can lead to poor fetal growth and prematurity.

Endocarditis

Bacteremia during labor and delivery is not uncommon, and turbulent flow makes one susceptible to bacterial endocarditis, sometimes with fatal consequences. In a series of 44 cyanotic pregnant patients, two patients developed bacterial endocarditis following labor, and one died.[23] The American Heart Association does not currently recommend the routine use of prophylactic antibiotics during labor, but some high-risk centers practice otherwise.[23] Thus, although proven benefit does not exist, the use of intravenous antibiotic prophylaxis seems reasonable in high-risk patients such as those with known valvular abnormalities or those undergoing cesarean or operative vaginal delivery (forceps, ventouse).

Thromboembolic disease

For all women, thromboembolism is six times more common during gestation. Since cyanotic congenital heart disease is also an independent risk factor for thrombosis, pregnancy creates additional risk for these patients. Those with mechanical valves who require anticoagulation place themselves and the fetus at particular risk during pregnancy, and management decisions must weigh the risks and benefits of warfarin versus heparin. Most specialized centers tend to recommend unfractionated heparin during the first trimester when embryopathy due to warfarin is greatest. Thereafter, warfarin conveys good cover against valve thrombosis but crosses the placenta and is associated with neonatal cerebral hemorrhage. Thus heparin is usually reinstated at 36 weeks' gestation or earlier if premature delivery is anticipated. The risk of thromboembolic disease is greater following cesarean section and is thought to be increased further after general anesthesia; however, for patients on anticoagulants, even at prophylactic doses, care needs to be taken over the timing of regional anesthesia, to minimize the risk of neuraxial hematoma.[24]

Arrhythmias

Atrial arrhythmias are common in pregnancy,[20] especially in patients with atrial surgical scars or atrial enlargement from lesions such as Ebstein's, valvular regurgitation, or left-to-right shunts. In practice, arrhythmias are poorly tolerated when the patient is pregnant because of the likely drop in cardiac output.[25] Management of rhythm abnormalities during pregnancy can be challenging, since antiarrhythmic drugs cannot always be used.[25] Antiarrhythmics that are safe during gestation are listed in Table 32.3. As a general rule they should be avoided unless the arrhythmia is significantly worrisome. For ventricular tachycardia, lidocaine is probably the drug of choice. For atrial arrhythmias, adenosine is safe,[26] as well as atrioventricular node blocking agents such as calcium channel blockers. Beta-blockers are reasonably safe although there is an association with intrauterine growth restriction. In our experience, this risk is very small, and most patients should be monitored for growth restriction anyway. Direct

Table 32.3 Cardiac drug safety in pregnancy

Relatively safe	Unstudied, probably safe	Unsafe
Digoxin	Sotalol	ACE inhibitors
Procainamide	Mexilitine	Warfarin
Flecainide*		Amiodarone†
Calcium channel blockers		Phenytoin
Beta-blockers		
Heparin		
Lidocaine		
Quinidine		
Adenosine		

ACE, angiotensin-converting enzyme.
*May cause fetal hyperbilirubinemia.
†Can be used in special circumstances with specialized consultation.

Table 32.4 Neonatal complications and rate by maternal congenital heart disease lesion

Lesion	Pregnancies	Complications (%)
PDA/VSD/ASD	142	17 (12)
Coarctation	51	7 (14)
AS/BAV	73	17 (23)
PS	58	10 (17)
Cyanotic	4	2 (50)
TOF/DORV	53	11 (21)
Single ventricle	5	4 (80)
D-TGA	25	3 (12)
CC-TGA	6	0
Pulmonary hypertension	3	1 (33)
Ebstein's anomaly	12	4 (33)
Marfan's syndrome	10	5 (50)

PDA, patent ductus arteriosus; VSD, ventricular septal defect; ASD, atrial septal defect; AS, aortic stenosis; BAV, bicuspid aortic valve; PS, pulmonic stenosis; TOF, tetralogy of Fallot; DORV, double outlet right ventricle; D-TGA, dextrorotatory transposition of the great arteries; CC-TGA, congenitally corrected transposition of the great arteries.
Modified from reference 5.

current (DC) cardioversion can usually be performed safely in a pregnant patient, although there are isolated reports of adverse outcome. During delivery, use of ephedrine to counter the hypotensive effects of regional analgesia/anesthesia may provoke arrhythmias in susceptible patients. Therefore purer vasoconstrictors such as phenylephrine may be more suitable. After delivery a lactating mother can safely use most cardiovascular drugs, including warfarin and heparin. Anti-arrhythmic drugs and atrioventricular node blocking agents are excreted in breast milk, however, so it is important to continue close monitoring of the baby's heart rate.

Fetal mortality

Reported data on fetal morbidity and mortality are listed in Table 32.2. Fetal loss calculations shown in the table include stillbirth and neonatal death but exclude therapeutic termination, yet over a third of such terminations are performed because of perceived cardiovascular risk. Overall there is a much higher chance of fetal loss in these patients than in the general population, although immense variations in data exist. Mortality ranges from 6%[27] to 24%.[21] Again, lesions such as cyanosis and obstruction, where cardiac output may be limited, have the worst fetal survival. Hemoglobin level and oxygen saturation have been demonstrated as significant predictors of adverse events (both maternal and fetal).[23]

Fetal morbidity

Prematurity or poor fetal growth

By far the most common complication in the fetus is growth restriction. Risk of any complication from a recent large Canadian series following 445 pregnancies is shown in Table 32.4, and the majority of these were prematurity or low birth weight.[5] Poor fetal growth often necessitates early delivery. Particularly in mothers with cyanotic or stenotic lesions, the restriction or lack of adequate rise in cardiac output can slow fetal growth and sometimes necessitate early delivery. There is ample evidence showing how intrauterine growth restriction increases the risk for multiple health challenges throughout that child's life, including diabetes and hyperlipidemia.[28]

Congenital heart defects in offspring

The potential for heart lesions in the offspring must be considered before conception. There is large variation in reported risk of transmission from a woman with congenital heart disease. Generally

Table 32.5 Risk of congenital heart disease recurrence in offspring

Lesion	Risk of transmission (%)			
	Mother affected	Father affected	One sibling affected	Two siblings affected
PDA	4.1	2.5	3	10
VSD	9.5–15.6	2	3	10
ASD	4.6–11	1.5	2.5	8
AVSD	13.9			
Coarctation	4.1			6
AS	15–17.9	3	2	6
PS	6.5	2	2	6
TOF	2.6	1.5	2.5	8
TGA				5
Marfan's syndrome	50	50		

PDA, patent ductus arteriosus; VSD, ventricular septal defect; ASD, atrial septal defect; AVSD, atrioventricular septal defect; AS, aortic stenosis; PS, pulmonic stenosis; TOF, tetralogy of Fallot; TGA, transposition of the great arteries (either form). Modified from references 29 and 30.

accepted risks from various lesions depending on which family member is affected are shown in Table 32.5.[29] Overall the chance is 3–6%, although one large series reported an incidence as high as 16.3%.[19] If two prior children have a heart defect, the risk of a third affected child is 5–10%.[30] There is some suggestion that women with congenital heart lesions are more likely to have affected children than men with heart defects.[31,32] This does not hold for all conditions nor in all studies, and in some reports, the opposite is true.[33] When both parents have a congenital heart problem one would expect a higher risk of transmission, but this has not been demonstrated in the literature. Congenital syndromes (Marfan's, Noonan's, etc.) have up to a 50% risk of transmission.

Premature loss of a parent

When considering the life of the newborn, it is worth recognizing that many women with congenital lesions, corrected or uncorrected, have a limited prognosis, depending of course on the type and severity of their condition. Although life expectancy cannot be predicted accurately on an individual basis, there will certainly be children born to patients with congenital lesions who will tragically lose a parent prematurely. This is an important consideration that should be addressed when planning a family.

Specific diagnoses considered

Left-to-right shunts

Generally ASD, VSD, and PDA are well tolerated until volume overload leads to pulmonary hypertension and reversed or bi-directional shunt (Eisenmenger syndrome). This primarily depends on defect size. It is more common in PDA than VSD, and is rare in ASD. Lesions may not be discovered until much later in life, especially an ASD, yet there still may be low pulmonary vascular resistance and hence suitability for closure. The general concerns in this group are atrial arrhythmias from atrial enlargement, stroke from thromboemboli, and eventual pulmonary vascular disease leading to reversed shunt.

Pregnancy tends to be well tolerated in a previously asymptomatic woman without pulmonary hypertension, with no maternal mortality and fetal loss that is similar to the normal population.[19] This is because left-to-right shunting stays relatively constant from the combination of increased cardiac output and reduced afterload.[4] Lesions should be closed electively after delivery if the shunt is large enough. ASDs and PDAs can most often be closed percutaneously.

Atrioventricular defects are another type of left-to-right shunt. They range from simple ostium primum ASD with an abnormal left atrioventricular valve (often, though erroneously, called a 'cleft mitral valve') to complete septal defect with a common valve orifice. These are often associated with Down syndrome. Generally, morbidity relates to the severity of the defect. There is little published about the effects of pregnancy in such lesions, although physiologically they behave similarly to other intra-cardiac shunts. When uncorrected, they lead to Eisenmenger syndrome usually by early adult life.

Stenotic lesions

Coarctation of the aorta

Patients are often first found to have coarctation of the aorta incidentally during work-up for other problems. Eighty-five percent will have a bicuspid aortic valve, and cerebral aneurysms and VSD are relatively common. The need for repair is mostly dependent on the pressure gradient across the coarctation. Concerns after repair are recoarctation, aortic aneurysm, and hypertension. The latter increases the risk of dissection. Patients should routinely be checked for delay between the radial and femoral pulses and a difference between right arm and leg blood pressures. Often patients will need to undergo a second release (surgical or percutaneous) in their lifetime. Even in those with adequate repair, hypertension can develop and should be treated aggressively, as there is still a risk of dissection or rupture later in life. Hypertension is more common in women with significant gradients across the coarctation (58% vs 11%),[34] for which beta-blockers are the treatment of choice.

During pregnancy, complete control of proximal hypertension may be counterproductive as it leads to lower body hypotension, thus compromising placental flow. In a recent series there was one maternal death reported out of 50 pregnant patients.[34] The live birth rate was 90%. There did not seem to be a difference in patients who had prior repair of coarctation versus those without. Pregnant patients should be encouraged to decrease activity level significantly to avoid blood pressure rises. Beta-blockers, although associated with intrauterine growth restriction generally, are still preferred and used widely. Fetuses should be monitored for growth restriction regardless of what pharmacologic option is used. If anesthe-sia is required, steps should be taken to minimize the hypertensive response to tracheal intubation, for example, with opioid drugs.

Aortic stenosis from bicuspid aortic valve

Although much more common in men, bicuspid aortic valve has a high enough prevalence that it affects 0.2–0.4% of all women.[4] It is not uncommon for aortic stenosis (AS) to be mild or missed during childhood. Most often it manifests itself as AS. Alternatively patients may present with aortic insufficiency (AI) or bacterial endocarditis. There is a tendency for coexistent coarctation of the aorta, which should be sought. When symptoms develop (CHF, syncope, angina or a reduction in exercise tolerance), aortic valve surgery should be offered. Some patients will have undergone surgical repair by the time they are adults. More frequently this is being done using the Ross procedure, where the native pulmonary valve is inserted into the aortic position and an autograft is placed in the pulmonic position. These patients should be followed for pulmonic autograft valve dysfunction as well as neo-aortic dilation with or without AI.

Although still considered relatively high risk,[4] congenital AS during pregnancy usually leads to a satisfactory outcome, depending on severity and the presence of symptoms.[13] In one series, two patients with symptomatic severe AS did poorly whereas one asymptomatic patient with severe AS did well. It is important to appreciate that the nonpregnant gradient across the valve may double during pregnancy merely as a result of physiologic changes. Apparent worsening of the gradient during pregnancy should not necessarily cause alarm. On the other hand absence of such an increase can be falsely reassuring since it may herald cardiac failure. A better indication of severity is valve area. AI is less risky than AS during pregnancy since the fixed obstruction in the latter is less tolerant of increases in cardiac output. Anticipated pregnancy may be an indication for AS surgery, even in an asymptomatic patient.

Pulmonic stenosis

Pulmonic stenosis (PS) can occur in isolation but is often associated with other congenital lesions such as

ASD or PR. It is common in patients with Noonan's syndrome. Unless the stenosis is severe, patients rarely experience symptoms. However, mild gradients can worsen as flow increases with pregnancy.[4] The strain on the right ventricle in severe stenosis can precipitate right heart failure or arrhythmias. Catheter-based intervention is the treatment of choice, including balloon dilation and deployment of the recently developed percutaneous valve. Patients with Noonan's syndrome may have associated problems such as restrictive cardiomyopathy, bleeding disorders or difficulty with tracheal intubation. Noonan's syndrome is also more likely to be passed on to offspring.

Cyanotic conditions

Cyanosis is the result of a number of lesions where mixing of oxygenated and deoxygenated blood can occur. Erythrocytosis develops to maintain tissue oxygen delivery. Patients will usually exhibit clubbing and can develop symptoms of hyperviscosity including head, muscle, and joint aches, which become worse as hemoglobin rises. In the past, regular venosection was performed to alleviate such symptoms, although now this is discouraged as iron deficiency may lead to microcytosis and poor red blood cell flexibility. Patients can be prone to gallstones, renal dysfunction, and gout. Daily allopurinol is often warranted. Patients still menstruate, but patterns are definitely different to those without cyanosis.[35]

Pregnancy in cyanotic heart disease has traditionally been considered high risk for both maternal and fetal death.[6] Erythrocytosis coupled with an increased thrombotic tendency during pregnancy can be problematic. When patients with Eisenmenger syndrome are excluded, maternal mortality may not be so grave. In 24 pregnant women with cyanosis a single death occurred from coagulopathy in a patient with Eisenmenger syndrome.[21] In another study involving 43 cyanotic mothers without Eisenmenger syndrome, there was only one death (due to endocarditis) in a woman with TOF.[23] Still, fetal deaths in both studies were high (35% and 57%, respectively). Predictors of fetal mortality were baseline hemoglobin levels and oxygen saturation in the mother.

Tetralogy of Fallot

TOF is the most common cyanotic form of congenital heart disease. The vast majority of patients will have had a complete repair by the time they reach adulthood and for the most part will have a good prognosis without cyanosis. This of course is dependent on cardiac and pulmonary artery morphology. There is a later risk of ventricular arrhythmia, residual shunt, right ventricular (RV) dysfunction, and pulmonary valve dysfunction (stenosis or regurgitation) that is often dependent on the morphology of the RVOT and the type of repair employed. Very occasionally, patients may be at risk for pulmonary hypertension due to palliative arterial shunts (Blalock–Taussig, Waterston, or Potts) performed prior to repair.

There are surprisingly very few data on pregnancy and TOF, but it is generally felt that pregnancy can be safe for both mother and fetus especially after successful repair. The exception is cyanotic patients, where one maternal death in 21 women has been reported.[23]

Pulmonary atresia

Complex pulmonary atresia (PA) is vastly different in those with or without a VSD. Patients with an intact septum do very poorly and rarely survive to maturity.[11] In contrast, patients with a VSD develop aortopulmonary collaterals to maintain pulmonary blood flow. If the right ventricle and pulmonary arteries are of reasonable size, they may be repaired in childhood with a conduit from the right ventricle to the pulmonary artery. As adults, conduit obstruction is the norm, requiring replacement. Patients should also be watched for ventricular arrhythmias, or cyanosis from residual collaterals.

Miscarriage rates in these patients are high[36] and, in at least one series, so are maternal complications.[37] Interestingly, this study concluded that previous repair decreased chances of miscarriage but increased maternal morbidity. Many of these patients have Di George syndrome, associated with a 50% recurrence risk in the offspring.

Eisenmenger syndrome

Eisenmenger syndrome is defined as pulmonary hypertension secondary to left-to-right shunt, which then leads to bi-directional or reversed shunt and cyanosis.[10] Patients with this condition can live fairly normal lives for decades despite their cyanotic condition. In fact, their prognosis is better than for patients with primary pulmonary hypertension. Like any cyanotic patient, symptoms related to high hemoglobin levels may include headaches, myalgias, arthralgias, and general fatigue. There is a small but finite risk of stroke due to venous emboli in these patients, and thus care should be taken when using intravenous lines. Usually patients die of pulmonary hemorrhage due to thrombotic infarct, or of congestive heart failure.

There is little doubt about the high risk to both mother and fetus in pregnant patients with this combination. While systemic vascular resistance falls to compensate for the increased cardiac output, pulmonic resistance does not, leading to more right-to-left shunting, cyanosis, and heart failure. Added to this is the risk of thromboembolic disease that is inherent in Eisenmenger syndrome. Some reports show a maternal mortality of nearly 50%,[38] although this may be lower when series are combined (Table 32.1). Most deaths occur in the first 7 days after delivery. A Brazilian group treated 12 women aggressively through 13 pregnancies with oxygen, heparin, antibiotics, and bed rest.[39] Despite this, 3 of 12 mothers died and only 7 of 13 babies survived. Eisenmenger syndrome remains one of the few conditions for which pregnancy is always contraindicated.

Other conditions

Transposition of the great arteries

In D-TGA (dextro-rotatory transposition of the great arteries), there is discordance between the ventricles and arteries only, such that survival is not possible without a large septal defect (created by catheter intervention at birth if necessary). This is followed by a corrective procedure, either an 'atrial switch' (Mustard or Senning procedures done until the 1980s) or an arterial switch (patients just now reaching childbearing age). Women with an atrial switch will often develop atrial arrhythmias as well as leak or obstruction of the atrial baffles. The right ventricle will eventually fail under the systemic load, but often not until the fifth or sixth decade. Patients with arterial switch have a systemic left ventricle, which is favorable. They should be followed for problems with proximal coronary artery obstruction, since repair involves replacement of the coronary ostia.

There are only two small series involving a total of 13 patients with atrial switch operations undergoing pregnancy.[40,41] No maternal deaths were reported, there were three maternal complications, and 86% of nonaborted pregnancies were discharged home. In patients with arterial switch, little is known about their ability to cope with pregnancy, but major difficulties are not anticipated.

Congenitally corrected transposition of the great arteries

When there is also discordance between the atria and ventricles, such that venous blood travels from right atrium to left ventricle then to pulmonary artery, it is known as congenitally corrected transposition (CC-TGA), or L-TGA. This may be unrecognized until well into adulthood. Other frequent associations include dextrocardia, VSD, pulmonary stenosis, Ebstein's anomaly (the tricuspid valve is the systemic atrioventricular valve), and complete heart block. They remain at risk for systemic RV failure later in life. Otherwise outcome is determined most by associated lesions and the status of the right ventricle.

Generally, pregnancy is well tolerated in these patients.[42] There is a published series of 22 pregnant women with CC-TGA, most of who had other associated anomalies but were not cyanotic.[43] Seven unsuccessful pregnancies occurred in women in whom the diagnosis had not yet been made. There was no maternal mortality, and an 83% pregnancy success rate. Generally stress and strain through pregnancy should be minimized so as to decrease the risk of systemic ventricular failure.

Ebstein's anomaly of the tricuspid valve

In this defect the septal insertion of the tricuspid valve is displaced towards the right ventricular apex, resulting in severe regurgitation, right atrial enlarge-ment, and impaired RV volume and function. Although the lesion is uncommon, it is sometimes not detected until adulthood. Half the patients will also have an ASD and a quarter will have an accessory conduction pathway (Wolff–Parkinson–White syndrome). Surgical attempts to repair the valve are often unsuccessful. In severe lesions the RV volume is small and nearly nonfunctional, which leads to cyanosis via shunting through an ASD. In this instance an aorto-pulmonary shunt combined with valve surgery may be necessary to improve pulmonary circulation and systemic cardiac output.

For the majority of patients, pregnancy is well tolerated with a small increased risk of atrial arrhythmias,[44] though fetal loss can be high. In the cyanotic form, pregnancy is associated with more maternal complications (three out of eight patients).[23] Fetal mortality was 14% in this study.

Fontan

The Fontan operation shunts blood directly from the venous system to the pulmonary circulation, and is therefore a palliative technique for patients with a single ventricle, such as tricuspid atresia or double inlet ventricles. Usually this is performed in child-hood or early adolescence. These patients have diffi-culty increasing cardiac output to meet demands because of the limited venous flow reserve. The adult with a Fontan may face a number of problems includ-ing atrial arrhythmias, right atrial dilatation, clot formation, collateral shunts, and residual cyanosis. Problems related to elevated venous pressure include hepatomegaly, cirrhosis, ascites, and protein-losing enteropathy (PLE). Ten-year survival is 60–80%,[4] and significantly less if PLE develops. Adult patients with a prior classic Fontan, where blood transverses the right atrium to the pulmonary artery, may benefit from transition to total cavopulmonary connection (TCPC), with a Glenn shunt (superior vena cava to pulmonary artery) and a lateral tunnel Fontan (inferior vena cava to pulmonary artery). This avoids some of the problems of atrial arrhythmias and right atrial thrombus. However, since access to the right atrium will not be possible afterwards, it is worth-while to offer patients an electrophysiologic study

beforehand with the aim of ablating common rhythm pathways.

Menstruation has been studied in 72 patients with Fontan circulation, 70% of whom had normal menses,[45] 30% had amenorrhea, including many who had normal cycles before the creation of the Fontan. It is not clear what factors were associated with amenorrhea in these women.

Fontan patients have difficulty raising cardiac output during pregnancy. While this leads to cardio-vascular complications in 10–20% of the mothers, it has more drastic consequences for the fetus. In one series, there was no maternal mortality in 21 patients, but nearly half of the babies did not survive.[46] In another series of Fontan patients with cyanosis, only 31% resulted in live births and 38% were preterm.[23]

Marfan's syndrome

Women with Marfan's syndrome face a number of challenges in adult life. The biggest threat is aortic dilation and rupture, a potentially fatal complica-tion. Therefore, keen observation and careful timing of aortic root surgery are of paramount importance. All affected women should be on beta-blocker therapy even if normotensive. Even after reparative surgery, the remaining segments of the native aorta and aortic valve may well require a second operation. Endocarditis of affected valves is not uncommon.

The overall maternal mortality rate from pregnancy is 4%, with 21% failed pregnancies.[4] In a series of 21 pregnant patients (45 pregnancies) there were three who showed dilation of the aortic root during pregnancy.[47] Patients need to plan childbearing around expected surgery, as many will have significant aortic dilation before or during their childbearing years. Large shearing forces may increase risk of aortic rupture across the aorta; both severe hypotension and hyper-tension should therefore be avoided. Cardiostability is particularly important should anesthesia for cesarean section be required. The condition is autosomal dominant, thus there is a 50% transmission rate.

Mitral valve prolapse

Prolapse of the mitral valve leaflets with myxoma-tous change (usually valvular thickening) is found commonly in young women. It can be a completely benign incidental finding not associated with any morbidity. Diagnosis is made by the coexistence of both auscultatory and echocardiographic features rather than either alone.

There are two clinical concerns in patients with mitral valve prolapse (MVP). The first is the risk of infective endocarditis, which can be prevented by prophylactic antibiotics when appropriate[15] such as before dental work. The second is the development of significant mitral insufficiency. Indications for mitral valve surgery depend on the severity of regurgitation and associated findings. An experienced surgeon can often repair the valve, avoiding the need for replacement. Patients with MVP may develop palpitations from ventricular ectopic beats or sustained supraventricular rhythms. When necessary these are treated with beta-blockers. Sudden death has been reported,[48] though it is not certain whether MVP is simply an incidental finding in such cases.

During pregnancy, MVP patients do well, as demonstrated in several small series.[49,50] In some cases prolapse was improved,[51] presumably from LV volume changes that occur during pregnancy. There are case reports of thromboembolic events during pregnancy, including cerebrovascular events,[52,53] but these are felt to be rare.

Hypertrophic obstructive cardiomyopathy

Severe congenital LV hypertrophy (LVH) can sometimes produce a septal bulge that dynamically obstructs outflow of the left ventricle during systole. The anterior leaflet of the mitral valve can be pulled towards the septum resulting in mitral regurgitation. The condition is worse when the LV filling volume is low. In general the outcome of the condition is related to the degree of obstruction present,[54] which may need to be measured both at rest and during stress. Patients are at risk for atrial fibrillation as well as ventricular arrhythmias and sudden death. Generally, patients have good long-term survival.[55] Treatment options traditionally have included beta-blockers, pacing, and surgical myomectomy.[56] Recently, a catheter-based alcohol ablation of the first septal perforator has been perfected.[57] Good improvement in selected patients has been reported

from this minimally invasive procedure, with the most common complication being AV nodal block requiring pacemaker implantation.

Two maternal deaths in 100 pregnant patients have been reported, where both patients were felt to be high risk before pregnancy.[58] Usually pregnant patients do quite well, in theory because of the increased volume of the left ventricle and hence less obstruction. In another series of 127 patients with 271 pregnancies, patients continued to experience symptoms but there were no major clinical events and only three fetal losses.[59] Still, pulmonary edema during pregnancy has been reported elsewhere.[60,61]

Women as parents of affected children

It is worth remembering that even a woman without congenital heart disease has a 1% chance of having a child with a congenital heart defect. Here she will play an additional role, educating herself about the condition, making important decisions, becoming her child's advocate, scheduling the child's clinic visits and diagnostic tests, supporting the child through surgery, and then educating the child about the problem. Having a child with a heart defect can involve a huge commitment of time and financial resources. Although optimally both mother and father will equally take part in the care of an affected child, the traditional role of the mother as the primary caregiver cannot be overlooked. Such women also must consider the risk of having a second child with a similar defect (Table 32.5).

A number of patient/family support networks exist to offer assistance to parents of children with heart disease. Online resources can be found easily. Some more prominent sites that focus on support for parents include:

- http://tchin.org/support/index.htm
- http://www.tchin.org/family/c_4parents1.htm
- http://www.csun.edu/~hcmth011/heart/
- http://www.pediheart.org/parents/index.html

In the UK, http://www.guch.org.uk/ is mostly geared towards adult patients themselves.

Conclusions

Women with congenital heart disease represent a vast range of problems, from those wholly unaware of their illness through most of their lives, to those with severe problems who have had previous heart surgeries and may still face debilitating symptoms, limited prognosis, and difficult decisions. Despite many of the problems highlighted in this chapter, the majority of women with congenital heart problems are able to lead normal healthy lives, including having healthy children of their own.

Because of their growing prevalence it is incumbent upon the provider to recognize the various issues that these women face, which become particularly important during childbearing, and know when to refer the patient to a tertiary center with congenital heart disease experience. Particularly during pregnancy, a multidisciplinary approach involving a specialized cardiologist, high-risk obstetrician and anesthetist, who jointly develop a clear plan for pregnancy and the peripartum, is required to minimize risks and optimize maternal and fetal outcomes.

References

1. Wren C, O'Sullivan JJ. Survival with congenital heart disease and need for follow up in adult life. *Heart* 2001; **85**:438–43.
2. Deanfield J, Thaulow E, Warnes C, et al. Management of grown up congenital heart disease. *Eur Heart J* 2003; **24**:1035–84.
3. Samanek M, Voriskova M. Congenital heart disease among 815,569 children born between 1980 and 1990 and their 15-year survival: a prospective Bohemia survival study. *Pediatr Cardiol* 1999; **20**:411–17.
4. Colman JM, Sermer M, Seaward PG, Siu SC. Congenital heart disease in pregnancy. *Cardiol Rev* 2000; **8**:166–73.
5. Siu SC, Sermer M, Colman JM, et al. Prospective multicenter study of pregnancy outcomes in women with heart disease. *Circulation* 2001; **104**:515–21.
6. Avila WS, Rossi EG, Ramires JA, et al. Pregnancy in patients with heart disease: experience with 1000 cases. *Clin Cardiol* 2003; **26**:135–42.
7. Smith M, Cooper GM, Clutton-Brock TH, et al. Five cases of severe cardiac disease in pregnancy: outcomes and costs. *Int J Obstet Anesth* 2001; **10**:58–63.
8. Perloff JK, Child JS. *Congenital Heart Disease in Adults*, 2nd edn. Philadelphia: WB Saunders, 1998.
9. Bassili A, Mokhtar SA, Dabous NI, Zaher SR, Mokhtar MM, Zaki A. Congenital heart disease among school children in Alexandria, Egypt: an overview on prevalence and relative frequencies. *J Trop Pediatr* 2000; **46**:357–62.
10. Wood P. The Eisenmenger syndrome or pulmonary hypertension with reversed central shunt. *BMJ* 1958; **2**:701–9,755–62.
11. Redington A, Shore D, Oldershaw P. *Congenital Heart Disease in Adults: A Practical Guide.* London: WB Saunders, 1994.
12. Leonard H, O'Sullivan JJ, Hunter S. Family planning requirements in the adult congenital heart disease clinic. *Heart* 1996; **76**:60–2.
13. Lao TT, Sermer M, MaGee L, Farine D, Colman JM. Congenital aortic stenosis and pregnancy – a reappraisal. *Am J Obstet Gynecol* 1993; **169**:540–5.
14. Connolly HM, Warnes C. Pregnancy and contraception. In: Gatzoulis MA, Webb G, Daubeney PEF (eds). *Diagnosis and Management of Adult Congenital Heart Disease*, 1st edn. Philadelphia: Churchill Livingstone, 2003:135–44.
15. Bonow RO, Carabello B, de Leon AC Jr, et al. Guidelines for the management of patients with valvular heart disease: executive summary. A report of the American College of Cardiology/American Heart Association Task Force on Practice Guidelines (Committee on Management of Patients with Valvular Heart Disease). *Circulation* 1998; **98**:1949–84.
16. Lewis DP, Dob DP, Yentis SM. UK registry of high-risk obstetric anaesthesia: arrhythmias, cardiomyopathy, aortic stenosis, transposition of the great arteries and Marfan's syndrome. *Int J Obstet Anesth* 2003; **12**:28–34.
17. Suntharalinam G, Dob DP, Yentis SM. Obstetric epidural analgesia in aortic stenosis: a low-dose technique for labour and instrumental delivery. *Int J Obstet Anesth* 2001; **10**:129–34.
18. Bolton TJ, Randall K, Yentis SM. Effect of the

Confidential Enquiries into Maternal Deaths on the use of Syntocinon at Caesarean section in the UK. *Anaesthesia* 2003; **58**:277–9.

19. Whittemore R, Hobbins JC, Engle MA. Pregnancy and its outcome in women with and without surgical treatment of congenital heart disease. *Am J Cardiol* 1982; **50**:641–51.

20. Lewis G. *Why Mothers Die. Report on Confidential Enquiries into Maternal Deaths in the United Kingdom.* London: Royal College of Obstetrics and Gynaecology, 2004.

21. Shime J, Mocarski EJ, Hastings D, Webb GD, McLaughlin PR. Congenital heart disease in pregnancy: short- and long-term implications. *Am J Obstet Gynecol* 1987; **156**:313–22.

22. Siu SC, Colman JM. Heart disease and pregnancy. *Heart* 2001; **85**:710–15.

23. Presbitero P, Somerville J, Stone S, Aruta E, Spiegelhalter D, Rabajoli F. Pregnancy in cyanotic congenital heart disease. Outcome of mother and fetus. *Circulation* 1994; **89**:2673–6.

24. Horlocker TT, Wedel DJ, Benzon H, et al. Regional anesthesia in the anticoagulated patient: defining the risks (the second ASRA Consensus Conference on Neuraxial Anesthesia and Anticoagulation). *Reg Anesth Pain Med* 2003; **28**:172–97.

25. Rotmensch HH, Rotmensch S, Elkayam U, Frishman W. Management of cardiac arrhythmias during pregnancy. Current concepts. *Drugs* 1987; **33**:623–33.

26. Leffler S, Johnson DR. Adenosine use in pregnancy: lack of effect on fetal heart rate. *Am J Emerg Med* 1992; **10**:548–9.

27. Siu SC, Colman JM, Sorensen S, et al. Adverse neonatal and cardiac outcomes are more common in pregnant women with cardiac disease. *Circulation* 2002; **105**:2179–84.

28. Barker DJ. Fetal origins of cardiovascular disease. *Ann Med* 1999; **31** (Suppl 1):3–6.

29. Lupton M, Oteng-Ntim E, Ayida G, Steer PJ. Cardiac disease in pregnancy. *Curr Opin Obstet Gynecol* 2002; **14**:137–43.

30. Nora JJ, Nora AH. Familial risk of congenital heart defect. *Am J Med Genet* 1988; **29**:231, 233.

31. Burn J, Brennan P, Little J, et al. Recurrence risks in offspring of adults with major heart defects: results from first cohort of British collaborative study. *Lancet* 1998; **351**:311–16.

32. Nora JJ, Nora AH. Maternal transmission of congenital heart diseases: new recurrence risk figures and the questions of cytoplasmic inheritance and vulnerability to teratogens. *Am J Cardiol* 1987; **59**:459–63.

33. Driscoll DJ, Michels VV, Gersony WM, et al.

Occurrence risk for congenital heart defects in relatives of patients with aortic stenosis, pulmonary stenosis, or ventricular septal defect. *Circulation* 1993; **87**(2 Suppl):I114–20.

34. Beauchesne LM, Connolly HM, Ammash NM, Warnes CA. Coarctation of the aorta: outcome of pregnancy. *J Am Coll Cardiol* 2001; **38**:1728–33.

35. Canobbio MM, Rapkin AJ, Perloff JK, Lin A, Child JS. Menstrual patterns in women with congenital heart disease. *Pediatr Cardiol* 1995; **16**:12–15.

36. Connolly HM, Warnes CA. Outcome of pregnancy in patients with complex pulmonic valve atresia. *Am J Cardiol* 1997; **79**:519–21.

37. Neumayer U, Somerville J. Outcome of pregnancies in patients with complex pulmonary atresia. *Heart* 1997; **78**:16–21.

38. Yentis SM, Steer PJ, Plaat F. Eisenmenger's syndrome in pregnancy: maternal and fetal mortality in the 1990s. *Br J Obstet Gynaecol* 1998; **105**:921–2.

39. Avila WS, Grinberg M, Snitcowsky R, et al. Maternal and fetal outcome in pregnant women with Eisenmenger's syndrome. *Eur Heart J* 1995; **16**:460–4.

40. Lao TT, Sermer M, Colman JM. Pregnancy following surgical correction for transposition of the great arteries. *Obstet Gynecol* 1994; **83** (5 Pt 1):665–8.

41. Clarkson PM, Wilson NJ, Neutze JM, North RA, Calder AL, Barratt-Boyes BG. Outcome of pregnancy after the Mustard operation for transposition of the great arteries with intact ventricular septum. *J Am Coll Cardiol* 1994; **24**:190–3.

42. Yarrow S, Russell R. Transposition of the great vessels: a series of three cases with a review of the literature. *Int J Obstet Anesth* 2000; **9**:179–85.

43. Connolly HM, Grogan M, Warnes CA. Pregnancy among women with congenitally corrected transposition of great arteries. *J Am Coll Cardiol* 1999; **33**:1692–5.

44. Connolly HM, Warnes CA. Ebstein's anomaly: outcome of pregnancy. *J Am Coll Cardiol* 1994; **23**:1194–8.

45. Canobbio MM, Mair DD, Rapkin AJ, Perloff JK, George BL. Menstrual patterns in females after the Fontan repair. *Am J Cardiol* 1990; **66**:238–40.

46. Canobbio MM, Mair DD, van der Velde M, Koos BJ. Pregnancy outcomes after the Fontan repair. *J Am Coll Cardiol* 1996; **28**:763–7.

47. Rossiter JP, Repke JT, Morales AJ, Murphy EA, Pyeritz RE. A prospective longitudinal evaluation of pregnancy in the Marfan syndrome. *Am J Obstet Gynecol* 1995; **173**:1599–606.

48. Corrado D, Basso C, Nava A, Rossi L, Thiene G. Sudden death in young people with apparently isolated mitral valve prolapse. *G Ital Cardiol* 1997; **27**:1097–105.

49. Chia YT, Yeoh SC, Viegas OA, Lim M, Ratnam SS. Maternal congenital heart disease and pregnancy outcome. *J Obstet Gynaecol Res* 1996; **22**:185–91.

50. Jana N, Vasishta K, Khunnu B, Dhall GI, Grover A. Pregnancy in association with mitral valve prolapse. *Asia Oceania J Obstet Gynaecol* 1993; **19**:61–5.

51. Rayburn WF, LeMire MS, Bird JL, Buda AJ. Mitral valve prolapse. Echocardiographic changes during pregnancy. *J Reprod Med* 1987; **32**:185–7.

52. Artal R, Greenspoon JS, Rutherford S. Transient ischemic attack: a complication of mitral valve prolapse in pregnancy. *Obstet Gynecol* 1988; **71** (6 Pt 2):1028–30.

53. Bergh PA, Hollander D, Gregori CA, Breen JL. Mitral valve prolapse and thromboembolic disease in pregnancy: a case report. *Int J Gynaecol Obstet* 1988; **27**:133–7.

54. Maron MS, Olivotto I, Betocchi S, et al. Effect of left ventricular outflow tract obstruction on clinical outcome in hypertrophic cardiomyopathy. *N Engl J Med* 2003; **348**:295–303.

55. Maron BJ, Casey SA, Hauser RG, Aeppli DM. Clinical course of hypertrophic cardiomyopathy with survival to advanced age. *J Am Coll Cardiol* 2003; **42**:882–8.

56. Maron BJ. Hypertrophic cardiomyopathy: a systematic review. *JAMA* 2002; **287**:1308–20.

57. Seggewiss H. Current status of alcohol septal ablation for patients with hypertrophic cardiomyopathy. *Curr Cardiol Rep* 2001; **3**:160–6.

58. Autore C, Conte MR, Piccininno M, et al. Risk associated with pregnancy in hypertrophic cardiomyopathy. *J Am Coll Cardiol* 2002; **40**:1864–9.

59. Thaman R, Varnava A, Hamid MS, et al. Pregnancy related complications in women with hypertrophic cardiomyopathy. *Heart* 2003; **89**:752–6.

60. Tessler MJ, Hudson R, Naugler-Colville M, Biehl DR. Pulmonary oedema in two parturients with hypertrophic obstructive cardiomyopathy (HOCM). *Can J Anaesth* 1990; **37** (4 Pt 1):469–73.

61. Oakley GD, McGarry K, Limb DG, Oakley CM. Management of pregnancy in patients with hypertrophic cardiomyopathy. *BMJ* 1979; **1**:1749–50.

62. Therrien J, Barnes I, Somerville J. Outcome of pregnancy in patients with congenitally corrected transposition of the great arteries. *Am J Cardiol* 1999; **84**:820–4.

33
Acquired valvular heart disease*

Delphine Détaint, Maurice Enriquez-Sarano and A. Jamil Tajik

Introduction

Over the past 25 years there have been marked changes in the demographics, clinical presentation, etiology, and treatment of acquired valvular heart diseases.[1] In western countries, with the decline of rheumatic fever and with the aging population, degenerative valve disease has become the main etiology. However, this shift in etiology is limited to industrialized countries, as rheumatic heart disease remains the most frequent etiology of valvular heart disease in developing countries.

In several forms of valvular heart disease gender distributions have changed in parallel to these changes in etiology. Indeed men predominate in degenerative valvular diseases which share a common pattern with atherosclerosis. Conversely other forms of valvular disease may affect women predominantly or even exclusively. In addition to these epidemiologic disparities, women face specific issues related to their smaller size, to unequal age at diagnosis, to different sensitivity to genetic-related diseases, to economic considerations and to pregnancy. These overt differences affect the outcome of women presenting with valvular heart disease. Indeed women, because they encounter specific problems, require special attention and their sex-related issues should be taken into account in the management of valvular heart disease.

Thus, to improve the management of women and to eliminate the gap in outcomes that exists in valvular heart disease between genders, this chapter describes and discusses the specific issues encountered by women in the major types of acquired valve disease.

Rheumatic fever and rheumatic heart disease

Rheumatic fever (RF) is an inflammatory disease which involves immunological cross-reactivity between streptococcal components and host antigens.[2,3] Acute RF may involve different organ systems such as the heart (carditis, pericarditis), joints, central nervous system, and skin. Following the initial episode and an asymptomatic latent period of 16 ± 5 years,[4] RF may lead to rheumatic heart disease, which constitutes the severity of the disease.

The incidence of rheumatic fever and the prevalence of rheumatic heart disease show marked variations from country to country. In the western world, the prevalence of rheumatic valvular heart disease has drastically decreased. However, rheumatic valve disease remains a major public health problem worldwide with an estimated 12 million people affected by acute RF and its cardiac complications.[5] Table 33.1 shows the death rates from acute RF and

Table 33.1 Worldwide mortality of rheumatic heart disease and rheumatic fever

WHO regions	Mortality of rheumatic heart disease (per 100 000)		Mortality of acute rheumatic fever (per 100 000)	
	Women	Men	Women	Men
Africa	15*		35*	
America	0.7–1.67	0.2–0.79	0–0.10	0–0.07
Eastern Mediterranean	2–9.8	0.7–7.64	0–0.7	0–0.48
Europe	1.29–2.77	0.9–2.05	0–0.23	0–0.11
Southeast Asia	1	0.64	0.08	0.02
Western Pacific	1.24–2.99	0.69–1.52	0.002	0.002

From World Health Organization, September 2003 (http//www.cvdinfobase.ca).
*No gender data available.

from rheumatic heart disease according to data from the World Health Organization (WHO). As previously reported,[6] mortality is slightly higher in women than in men, whatever the geographic origin, but it is unclear whether this female predominance is due to a higher incidence or females are more severely affected, as suggested by a higher incidence of mitral valve repair for acute carditis in women.[7] Eradication of RF should be based on primary and secondary prevention programs. However, the lack of good quality prevalence surveys and the economic status of most developing countries may limit prevention campaign efficiency.[8]

Mitral stenosis (see also Chapter 22)

The most common etiology of mitral stenosis (MS) by far is rheumatic heart disease that causes thickening of the mitral valve leaflets with fusion of the commissures. Therefore the incidence of MS is highly dependent on the geographic origin. In industrialized nations, MS is currently the least frequent valvular disease, representing only 9.5% of native valve disease in a recent European prospective survey.[9] Regardless of the geographic origin, there is a uniform sex distribution characterized by a strong female predominance (over 70% of patients with MS are women in all large published series[10–14]). The pathogenic mechanisms underlying the female predominance remain

unknown. Although recent progress has been made in understanding the genetic susceptibility to rheumatic heart diseases,[15,16] further studies are needed to investigate these gender disparities.

The clinical presentation and management of women presenting with MS differ from country to country. In developing countries women presenting with MS are younger (mean age about 30 years in published series from India and Tunisia[11,12]), compared with western countries where women are older (mean age 49 years in a study from Western Europe[14]) and where symptoms often occur in the fifth to seventh decades of life. Rheumatic MS is a progressive disease but the latent period between acute RF and symptomatic MS is variable and related to the magnitude of the severity of preceding episodes of RF. Indeed in certain developing countries the ineffective use of antibiotics or increased virulence of the streptococcus causes a more severe primary affront that shortens the latent period.

Over time, the progressive valve narrowing is associated with a gradual loss of orifice area, resulting in an increase in transmitral pressure gradient leading to increased pulmonary pressures and poor clinical exercise tolerance. As such, any situation that increases cardiac output can precipitate symptoms even in patients with mild stenosis.[17] Figure 33.1 shows the effect of exercise on the transmitral pressure gradient.

Increased left atrial and pulmonary pressures commonly lead to dyspnea and may lead to hemoptysis and pulmonary edema. In some cases, the initial

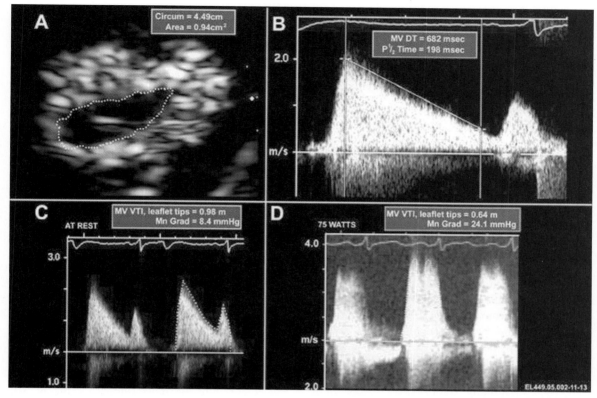

Figure 33.1
Rheumatic mitral stenosis in a 34-year-old woman. Mitral valve area was quantified at 0.94 cm² by planimetry (A) and at 1.12 cm² by pressure half time (B). The mean gradient at rest was 8 mmHg (C) and increased with exercise stress to 24 mmHg (D).

manifestation of MS is the onset of atrial fibrillation or an embolic event. However, age at diagnosis deeply influences the clinical presentation. In women of childbearing age the first symptoms often occur during pregnancy. Indeed increased cardiac output, increased heart rate, and subsequent reduced diastolic time lead to increased flow in a shorter time through a fixed orifice, which is poorly tolerated and may require emergent intervention with balloon valvuloplasty.[18,19] The most hazardous time is late pregnancy, labor, and the early puerperium when these changes are maximal.[20] Older patients, particularly elderly women with less activity, may complain of fewer symptoms. In these sedentary patients further investigations such as hemodynamic exercise testing with Doppler echocardiography may be

needed to evaluate their functional capacity and their exercise tolerance.[21]

Classically the physical examination of a patient with MS consists of a loud first sound, an opening snap, and a diastolic rumble. Doppler echocardiography is the current gold standard for diagnosis, for quantification of severity, and for determination of suitability of mitral commissurotomy and/or repair. Two-dimensional echocardiography is important in identifying the morphology of the mitral leaflet and the subvalvular apparatus, which are essential in deciding the type and timing of intervention. Patients with mobile noncalcified leaflets, no commissural calcification, and little subvalvular fusion are excellent candidates for percutaneous or surgical commissurotomy.[21,22] Importantly young patients have a far better anatomic condition than older patients who may present with severe alteration of subvalvular apparatus, thickened leaflets, and calcification.[23] With regard to the impact of gender on anatomy, men are more likely to present with unfavorable valve anatomy with extensive calcification.[10] Doppler echocardiography can be used to assess the severity of the obstruction, allowing calculation of the mitral valve area and the mean transmitral gradient. A valve area <1.5 cm^2 and a resting mean gradient >10 mmHg indicate hemodynamically severe MS and an area <1.0 cm^2 defines critical MS.[24]

Patients presenting with symptoms or MS complications such as atrial fibrillation, thrombo-embolism, pulmonary hypertension, or moderate to severe MS (mitral valve area <1.5 cm^2) should be considered for interventional therapy.[21] However, age, echocardiographic features, clinical presentation, and economic considerations influence patient management and choice of procedure (surgical commissurotomy, percutaneous mitral balloon valvulotomy (PMBV) or mitral valve replacement).[21,23,25] In selected patients, particularly in younger patients with a pliable valve, PMBV is an accepted alternative to surgical approaches[11] and similar good results are observed in female and male patients.[14,26] In older women and men, less favorable anatomy for PMBV (presence of calcification), and decreased interest in deferring surgery (over 70 years) may lead to the consideration of valve replacement.[23,27]

MS is the most common valvular lesion in women of childbearing age.[28] The hemodynamic changes associated with normal pregnancy may be poorly tolerated (see above). Therefore ideally patients with known MS should receive definitive treatment before pregnancy. When first symptoms occur during pregnancy and evaluation reveals MS, the management of pregnant women includes restricted activity and judicious use of diuretics. Throughout pregnancy the increase in maternal blood volume contributes to worsening symptoms. If symptoms progress, beta-blockers may be given in addition to diuretic therapy to optimize diastolic filling.[21,29] For patients with severe MS who remain symptomatic despite medical therapy, the PMBV procedure has changed the prognosis.[20,30,31] Indeed, with limited fluoroscopy exposure and echocardiographic guidance, this procedure avoids surgery during pregnancy.[21]

Of note, the nonrheumatic causes of MS are rare ($<4.5\%$[4]). MS may result from degenerative causes (entrapment of mitral leaflets in heavy calcification), which is more common in women; and from congenital MS, where the prevalence in women and men is equally distributed.[32] Uncommonly, MS may be associated with inflammatory disease, such as lupus and rheumatoid arthritis.

Mitral regurgitation

There is a wide array of disease processes that lead to organic mitral regurgitation (MR). Organic MR can be due to a primary disease of the valve apparatus or can be related to a systemic disease involving the mitral valve. In mitral regurgitation, the impact of gender on clinical presentation, on left ventricular (LV) and atrial remodeling, and on outcome remains unclear. Furthermore, several gender discrepancies between benign and severe MR are observed and need to be clarified.

With the decrease of rheumatic heart disease, distribution in etiology has changed over time. Degenerative MR is currently the most common cause of MR (61.3%[9]) and includes the mitral valve prolapse syndrome (discussed later), flail leaflet, and degenerative MR without prolapse (valve sclerosis or annular calcification). Rheumatic disease, ischemic MR and endocarditis represent other less frequent etiologies of MR; their prevalence rates in the recent European Heart Survey were 14.2%, 7.3%, and 3.5%, respectively.[9] The gender distribution has changed in parallel to the changes in the etiologic spectrum. Severe MR predominates in men (60% vs 40%) and MR increases with aging of the population (from 0.6% under 50 years old to 5.6% over 70 years old).[33] Uncommonly, MR can be due to systemic disease such as systemic lupus erythematosus (90% in women[34]).

In organic MR, the abnormal coaptation of the mitral leaflets creates a regurgitant orifice, which results in a regurgitant volume entering into the left atrium. Tolerance of MR and occurrence of symptoms are determined by its severity, its cause, its rapidity of development and by the compliance of the left atrium and left ventricle. In acute severe MR, the sudden volume overload markedly increases left atrial pressure and leads to pulmonary congestion and edema. In chronic MR the natural history is characterized by an initial compensated phase lasting many years followed by progressive LV dysfunction that leads to poor outcome.[35–37]

In chronic MR, the clinical presentation is similar in women and men and is characterized by a prolonged asymptomatic phase. Later as LV function deteriorates, patients may develop dyspnea, orthopnea, and paroxysmal nocturnal dyspnea. Clinically, a holosystolic murmur is the hallmark of mitral regurgitation and the intensity of murmur has good correlation with the severity of MR.[38] In patients with organic MR, a grade 1–2 intensity murmur is indicative of mild-moderate MR, while a grade ≥4 intensity murmur is strongly indicative of severe (regurgitant volume ≥50 ml) MR. Of note, there is a wide range of MR severity for a grade 3/6 intensity murmur. An inferolaterally displaced hyperdynamic apex impulse and presence of an S3 gallop are also indicative of severe MR. 2D-Echocardiography is essential in assessing the morphology of the mitral valve apparatus (leaflets, commissures, annulus, chordae, papillary muscles) and a systematic evaluation of these structures helps define the mechanism of MR. Moreover Doppler echocardiography characterizes MR severity, which is essential for prognostic evaluation.[21,39] The American Society of Echocardiography (ASE) Task Force recommends the combined use of several parameters to assess MR degree, as semi-quantification by color Doppler has technical and hemodynamic limitations, and as measurement of regurgitant flow rate and effective regurgitant orifice by Pisa and by quantitative Doppler has been previously validated.[39–44] Finally, Doppler echocardiography can evaluate the impact of MR on LV and atrial size and function and on hemodynamics, which are essential in deciding the necessity and the timing of surgery.[21]

Surgical correction of nonischemic MR should be performed before the development of LV dysfunction. According to the American College of Cardiology/American Heart Association (ACC/AHA) guidelines,[21] the current class 1 indication for surgical correction is severe MR with either notable symptoms or overt LV dysfunction (ejection fraction (EF) <60% or end systolic diameter >45 mm). In selected asymptomatic patients with severe MR (low surgical risk, repairable valves), a strategy of early surgery may improve outcome.[42,45,46]

Importantly the current management of patients does not take indexed cavity dimensions into account. Nevertheless, recent data from our institution identified that elderly women, with at least moderate MR, despite lower absolute LV cavity size, displayed higher indexed cavity diameters.[47] Thus, further studies are needed to confirm whether the management of women may improve with the use of body surface area-adjusted parameters (regurgitant volume, effective regurgitant orifice, LV and LA dimensions). In published studies from our institution no difference was observed between women and men in the progression of MR and LV remodeling.[48] Several surgical series have reported similar operative mortality and similar long-term postoperative outcomes for MR in both sexes.[49–52] The type of procedure, mitral repair versus mitral valve replacement, is important in the timing of surgery. The choice of valve repair versus replacement depends on the cause of the MR, the anatomy of the mitral valve, and the surgeon. When feasible, repair compared with replacement improves LV function and survival.[53–55]

Mitral valve prolapse

In western countries, mitral valve prolapse (MVP) refers to the systolic billowing of one or both mitral leaflets into the left atrium and represents the most common cause of chronic mitral regurgitation.[10,56] MVP differs in some ways from the other causes of MR and may occur alone or in association with other connective tissue disorders such as Marfan's syndrome. Histologically, MVP is characterized by a myxomatous degeneration of the mitral valve resulting in thickened leaflets and chordae. The mechanisms accompanying the myxomatous valvular degeneration are still uncertain, but seem related to extracellular matrix remodeling.[57] The estimated prevalence of MVP – defined by 2D-echocardiographic criteria – ranges from 0.6 to 2.4% of the population.[58,59] In general, MVP is more common in females; however, in community-based studies, age and gender were similar in patients and subjects without MVP. Several studies[56,60–65] support the hypothesis of a familial form of MVP with an autosomal pattern of inheritance in which young age and female gender seem to influence MVP gene expression.

MVP is clinically diagnosed by a typical mid-systolic click and late systolic murmur. The echocardiographic criteria have been reviewed recently and are more rigorous than the initial diagnostic criteria, explaining the prevalence discrepancies between prior and current studies.[58,66,67] There are a wide variety of clinical features associated with MVP. In particular, some atypical complaints (palpitations, atypical chest pain, anxiety, and fatigue) have been associated with MVP and have been related to autonomic and neuroendocrine dysfunction.[68,69]

With regard to outcome, the natural history of MVP is widely heterogeneous and subsets of patients display high morbidity and even excess mortality.[70] Patients can be classified in low-, medium- and high-risk groups according to a combination of clinical and echocardiographic parameters.[70] Importantly, the risk factors for outcome are mainly related to MR severity and its consequences (low ejection fraction, atrial fibrillation, enlarged left atrium). Notably, female gender may be protective against adverse events since women more often have MVP without much MR. Management of MR should be similar in both genders. Antibiotic prophylaxis is advised for patients presenting with click and systolic murmur of MR or for patients with evidence of MVP and MR.[21] When systemic atypical symptoms are present, especially in young women, beta-blocker therapy is recommended.

Pregnancy is tolerated well in women with MVP, as both increased blood volume and decreased peripheral resistance help to improve valve function. Indeed, increased LV size may reduce MVP. In rare cases in which surgery is required during pregnancy because of sudden worsening of the regurgitant lesion, such as ruptured chordae, valve repair is preferred to avoid the need for anticoagulation.[21]

Aortic stenosis

Aortic stenosis (AS) is the most frequent valvular heart disease and is characterized by progressive LV outflow obstruction due to decreased orifice area. The most common causes of AS are congenital, rheumatic, and degenerative. Although male gender predominates in adults with symptomatic AS, age, etiology, and stage of the disease may influence the gender distribution. Women, because of their smaller size and older age at diagnosis, encounter specific issues, which affect outcome.

Acquired aortic stenosis

Acquired AS may be degenerative or rheumatic in origin. Rheumatic AS is undoubtedly in regression in western countries and is associated with a male predominance. Rheumatic AS is characterized by commissural fusion leading to a fixed narrowed orifice. Conversely, in 'degenerative' AS, increased valve rigidity and calcification,[71] without commissural fusion result in a dynamic valvular stenosis[72] (Fig. 33.2). 'Degenerative' AS is a frequent disease and has become the main etiology as a result of the decline of rheumatic fever and the aging of the population.[73,74] Indeed, the Cardiovascular Health Study[71,75,76] reported a prevalence of 2% for AS and 26% for aortic sclerosis in the ≥65-year-old population. However, rather than being merely consequences of aging, the development of these degenerative lesions is an active inflammatory process, which shares many similarities with the development of atherosclerosis. These include extracellular matrix remodeling, fibrosis, deposition of lipoproteins, infiltration of inflammatory cells and calcification.[77] Several clinical risk factors for coronary heart disease (CHD) are also associated with calcific AS including male sex, smoking, hypertension, older age, hypercholesterolemia, and diabetes.[71,78-80] Consequently, the predominance of men is very marked in patients with AS and parallels the clinical features of atherosclerosis.[24,71,75,76] Nevertheless in subgroups of older patients (>75 years), women are more likely than men to present with aortic valve stenosis.[71,81,82] In the Helsinki aging study (501 patients, aged 75–86) moderate and severe AS were more frequent in women (8.8% vs 3.6% in men).[82] This discrepancy occurs because of the longer life expectancy of women, allowing more time for them to develop severe AS. Consequently at the time of diagnosis and valve replacement, women are older.[83,84]

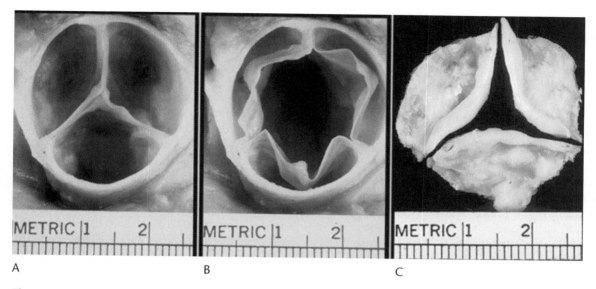

Figure 33.2
Macroscopic lesion of degenerative aortic stenosis (C): thickened cusps, calcification, valve opening limitation, and a reduced orifice compared with a normal aortic valve (A and B).

In both sexes, some patients may be completely asymptomatic and have a murmur detected on physical examination, while others may present with the classic triad of exertional symptoms of dyspnea, angina and syncope. Notably sedentary elderly women may present with fewer symptoms. 2D/Doppler echocardiography is the modality of choice for diagnosing AS, quantifying its severity, and assessing LV and LA remodeling. LV adaptation to AS has been reported to be different in women and men. For the same aortic valve area, women have been suggested to develop a greater degree of LV hypertrophy and higher preoperative LV ejection fraction.[83,85–89] However, a recent study showed that the normalization by body surface area weakens and even eliminates the differences between women and men in LV geometry.[84,90] These contrasting data emphasize the importance of accounting for body size in women with AS. Therefore, as recommended by ACC/AHA guidelines, some consideration of body size should be included in any estimation of valve area. Severe AS is diagnosed when the valve area is <0.6 cm²/m²or <1.0 cm² and when the mean transvalvular gradient is ≥50 mmHg.[21,91]

Natural history studies have demonstrated a marked increase in mortality after the development of symptoms.[92–94] Therefore, prompt replacement of the aortic valve is recommended when patients present with any symptom of angina, syncope or dyspnea.[21] In asymptomatic patients with severe AS, the outcome may vary widely and management decisions are more controversial. Nevertheless possible subgroups of patients at high risk have been suggested on the basis of a rapid increase in aortic jet velocity over time and marked valvular calcification;[75,93,95] such patients require early aortic valve replacement even if asymptomatic.[25,96] Severe pulmonary hypertension may occur in patients with severe AS and is associated with a dismal prognosis with nonoperative management. Therefore patients with severe pulmonary hypertension, despite higher risk of surgery, should be considered for early aortic valve replacement.[97]

Women, because of their smaller size and older age, may be at higher operative risk and should receive special attention. Women compared with men tend to have a small aortic annulus, leading to implantation of a smaller valve prosthesis. These smaller prostheses are more likely to have a larger transprosthetic gradient and to create a prosthesis–patient mismatch associated with poor prognosis.[98–101] To prevent this mismatch, an aortic root enlargement should be performed, allowing the use of a larger prosthesis.[102] After aortic valve replacement, women and men have a similar prognosis.[83,103] However, operative mortality is higher in women compared with men in the subgroups of octogenarians and in patients undergoing concomitant coronary artery bypass surgery.[104,105] Currently the only treatment for severe aortic valve stenosis is the standard aortic valve replacement (AVR) using cardiopulmonary bypass. Recently a catheter-based approach for AVR has been introduced for very high-risk patients. In patients with mild-moderate AS, promising experimental and clinical data focusing on the pathophysiology suggest the use of statin agents for reduction of the progression of AS. These observational studies pave the way to investigate further medical treatment in 'degenerative' AS.[106–109]

Aortic stenosis and bicuspid aortic valve (see also Chapter 22)

Congenital bicuspid aortic valve is the most common congenital valvular malformation, with an incidence in the general population of 1.0–2%.[110–112] Men are affected three to four times more frequently than women.[113] However, both sexes share identical clinical presentations and the development of AS in patients with bicuspid valves[114] is similar in women and men.

The most common cause of AS in pregnant women in western countries is congenital bicuspid aortic valve disease. Pregnancy is often well tolerated because of the physiologic increase of intravascular volume.[115] However, severe AS (>50 mmHg and valve area <1 cm^2) may increase maternal and fetal risk during pregnancy and should be managed before conception. Labor and delivery are hazardous because hypovolemia due to anesthesia and hemorrhage may hinder adequate cardiac output.[21] Therefore in the rare case of severe symptomatic AS, balloon dilatation has been proposed as a palliative procedure.[116,117]

Aortic regurgitation (see also Chapter 22)

Isolated aortic regurgitation (AR) represents about 10% of native valve disease.[9] AR can either result from intrinsic valvular abnormalities or aortic root diseases (dilatation of the aortic root and sinuses). As with AS, AR also principally affects men, whatever the causal disease.[113,118] In the Framingham population-based study, AR of ≥ trace on color Doppler echocardiography was present in 13% of men and 8.5% of women.[33] However, women with AR have a worse prognosis than men. To understand and overcome these differences it is important to highlight the gender-specific issues encountered by women with AR.

All forms of AR result in a varying severity of regurgitant volume leading to an increase in LV end-diastolic volume and in wall stress. In chronic AR, the heart responds with a compensatory hypertrophy (eccentric type) that tends to return wall stress to normal, although wall stress remains elevated in severe AR.[119] Therefore patients with chronic AR, despite a progressive LV dilatation, remain asymptomatic for many years.[120]

The clinical features of severe AR are related to the high volume ejection of blood with rapid fall of pressure in diastole, with widened pulse pressure, and bounding and collapsing peripheral pulses. On cardiac auscultation, a holodiastolic murmur is the hallmark of AR. The intensity of the murmur correlates well with the degree of aortic regurgitation and murmur intensity greater than grade 2 carries a high probability of severe regurgitation.[38]

A number of tests can help to document the presence and assess the severity of chronic aortic regurgitation. 2D/Doppler echocardiography is useful to confirm the diagnosis, to assess the etiology and the severity of AR, and evaluate LV dimension, LV function, and aortic root size.[21]

In both sexes, occurrence of symptoms (NYHA class from II to IV) corresponds to the transition to a decompensated stage, and is associated with an increased mortality rate.[121,122] In asymptomatic patients, measurement of LV size and function is useful to detect this transition and provides important prognostic information.[120,123–125]

Therefore in both sexes, the indications for aortic valve replacement are the development of symptoms

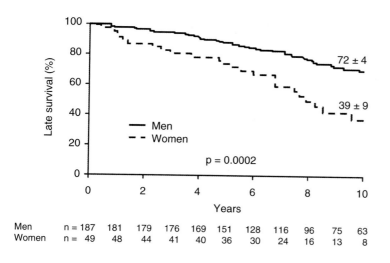

Figure 33.3
Late survival in women (dashed line) and men (solid line) after aortic valve replacement for severe chronic AR. Reproduced from reference 126 with permission.

or progressive LV dilatation and dysfunction.[21,25] The current thresholds reported in the ACC/AHA guidelines are EF <50%, end-systolic dimension >55 mm and end-diastolic dimension >75 mm. Although it is recommended to consider lower thresholds for patients of small stature, there is no guideline for the specific management of women with AR. Nevertheless, the outcome after aortic valve replacement is remarkably different for women and men.

Women exhibit a significant excess of late mortality (10-year survival 72 ± 4% vs 39 ± 9%[126]) (Fig. 33.3). A study from our institution showed that women compared with men underwent aortic valve replacement at a later stage. In women the indication for surgery was mainly triggered by the development of symptoms. Indeed, because of their smaller size, they almost never reached the unadjusted LV diameter (diastolic diameter ≥80 mm or systolic diameter ≥55 mm[120]) as a surgical indication. Therefore the use of a body surface area-corrected value of LV systolic diameter (threshold ≥25 mm/m²) is helpful for the management of AR, particularly in women.[121,126]

During pregnancy AR can usually be managed medically with a combination of diuretics and vasodilators. Surgery should be considered only for the control of refractory class III or IV symptoms.[21,127]

Aortic root disease

Among patients with aortic root disease, such as Marfan's syndrome or aortic dilatation, the valvular regurgitation may be less important in the decision-making process.[21] A population-based cohort study reported that the incidence rate of thoracic aorta dilatation was currently 10.4 per 100 000 person-years.[128] Women are usually older than men when diagnosed with aortic aneurysms and incur a higher rate of aortic rupture (5 years after diagnosis, 33% vs 9% in men).[128] Although the size of the aorta in patients with aortic aneurysms is identical in women and men, this higher rate of rupture raises the question whether aortic dimension should be normalized to body size. The excess rate of aortic rupture in women was also suggested in a series of patients having undergone aortic valve replacement for AR.[129] This excess rate may be one of the reasons for the excess mortality observed in women after surgery for AR. Furthermore, special attention should be brought to women with Marfan's syndrome. Marfan's syndrome is the most common heritable disorder, with a prevalence of 1 in 10 000 births in the United States.[130,131] Both sexes are affected,[132] but women are at high risk of aortic dissection during pregnancy.[133–135] Dissection and rupture are most likely to occur during the third trimester or at the time of delivery. Enlargement of the aortic root >4.0 cm constitutes a high-risk group and women with enlargement ≥5.0 cm should be considered for aortic repair before conception. The use of prophylactic beta-blockade is strongly recommended throughout pregnancy and optimal hemodynamic control should be performed during labor and delivery.[21]

Valvular heart disease induced by drugs (see also Chapter 35)

The fight against obesity has led many patients and physicians to adopt an aggressive strategy. Accordingly, appetite-suppressing or anorectic drugs have been prescribed to obese patients, mainly women. Fenfluramine and phentermine are anorexic agents which, when used in combination, are associated with a higher prevalence of cardiac valvular insufficiency.[136] The initial report involved only 24 women who had taken both drugs and who developed multivalvular disease involving the mitral, aortic, and tricuspid valves.[137] These data were further confirmed in larger series.[136,138,139] With regard to the pathogenesis, the anorexic drugs augment serotonergic activity, which has the potential to stimulate fibrogenesis. Macroscopically, the leaflets are thickened by a thick layer of amorphous material, the chordae tendinae are shortened but no commissural fusion is observed. Although the appetite suppressant-related valvular heart diseases are established disorders, several issues of clinical relevance remain uncertain. The relationship between dose and duration of exposure and incidence of valvular abnormalities is controversial.[138,140] The cessation of drugs seems to be associated with stabilization and improvement of lesions but larger series with longer follow-up are needed to confirm the reversibility. These drugs have been withdrawn from the market by the US Food and Drug Administration (FDA).

In addition, valvular disease has been also reported after exposure to serotonin-like drugs such as ergotamine and methysergide.[141,142] These drug-induced valvular diseases share a common patho-physiology with increased serotonergic activity and result in identical echocardiographic features.

Prosthetic heart valves and women (see also Chapter 22)

Women with prosthetic heart valves face special problems related to the type of valve (mechanical, bioprosthetic or homograft). For young women who wish to become pregnant it is essential to implant the optimal prosthesis associated with the lowest health risk. Women with mechanical valves are at risk of thromboembolic events and are exposed to the lifelong risk of anticoagulation.[143] During pregnancy, the rate of complications including maternal thromboembolic events and fetal loss with warfarin therapy is high.[144] Therefore, bioprosthetic or homograft valves have been preferred in childbearing women,[145] even though bioprosthetic valves are not as durable as mechanical valves. In a recent review of young women with prosthetic valves, 10-year valve survival was greater with a mechanical valve than a bioprosthetic valve, but mechanical valves may be associated with reduced patient survival.[146] With regard to valve loss, pregnancy does not increase the failure of mechanical or homograft valves and does not accelerate the deterioration of bioprosthetic valves. For elderly women, particularly octogenarian patients, the choice of a bioprosthesis is the best because their life expectancy may be shorter than the bioprosthesis durability.[147] However, when elderly women present with a small aortic annulus, it is advisable to use a stentless aortic prosthesis, which provides a larger orifice for a same annulus size[148] or to enlarge the aorta with a patch.

Conclusions

The presentation of valvular heart disease in women is markedly related to age, geographic origin, and type of disease. Indeed, elderly women in western countries are mainly affected by degenerative etiologies, whereas rheumatic heart disease continues to be the most important cause affecting the younger women in developing countries. This chapter has identified the sex-related issues encountered by women with valvular heart disease in these different situations. Thus, understanding female-specific issues in prevalence, clinical presentation, and physiopathology helps to develop an optimal gender-specific management plan to improve outcome in women.

References

1. Edwards WD. The changing spectrum of valvular heart disease pathology. In: Braunwald E (ed.). *Harrison's Advances in Cardiology*. New York: McGraw-Hill, 2003: 317–23.

2. Guedez Y, Kotby A, El-Demellawy M, et al. HLA class II associations with rheumatic heart disease are more evident and consistent among clinically homogeneous patients. *Circulation* 1999; **99**:2784–90.

3. Figueroa F, Gonzalez M, Carrion F, et al. Restriction in the usage of variable beta regions in T-cells infiltrating valvular tissue from rheumatic heart disease patients. *J Autoimmun* 2002; **19**:233–40.

4. Horstkotte D, Niehues R, Strauer BE. Pathomorphological aspects, aetiology and natural history of acquired mitral valve stenosis. *Eur Heart J* 1991; **12** (Suppl B):55–60.

5. Strategy for controlling rheumatic fever/rheumatic heart disease, with emphasis on primary prevention: memorandum from a joint WHO/ISFC meeting. *Bull World Health Organ* 1995; **73**:583–7.

6. Douglas PS. Rheumatic heart disease and other valvular disorders in women. *Cardiovasc Clin* 1989; **19**:259–65.

7. Stollerman G. Acute rheumatic fever and its management. In: Hurst JW (ed.). *The Heart*, 5th edn. New York: McGraw-Hill, 1982: 854–63.

8. Steer AC, Carapetis JR, Nolan TM, Shann F. Systematic review of rheumatic heart disease prevalence in children in developing countries: the role of environmental factors. *J Paediatr Child Health* 2002; **38**:229–34.

9. Iung B, Baron G, Butchart EG, et al. A prospective survey of patients with valvular heart disease in Europe: The Euro Heart Survey on Valvular Heart Disease. *Eur Heart J* 2003; **24**:1231–43.

10. Olson LJ, Subramanian R, Ackermann DM, Orszulak TA, Edwards WD. Surgical pathology of the mitral valve: a study of 712 cases spanning 21 years. *Mayo Clin Proc* 1987; **62**:22–34.

11. Ben Farhat M, Ayari M, Maatouk F, et al. Percutaneous balloon versus surgical closed and open mitral commissurotomy: seven-year follow-up results of a randomized trial. *Circulation* 1998; **97**:245–50.

12. Arora R, Kalra GS, Murty GS, et al. Percutaneous transatrial mitral commissurotomy: immediate and intermediate results. *J Am Coll Cardiol* 1994; **23**:1327–32.

13. Multicenter experience with balloon mitral commissurotomy. NHLBI Balloon Valvuloplasty Registry Report on immediate and 30-day follow-up results. The National Heart, Lung, and Blood Institute Balloon Valvuloplasty Registry Participants. *Circulation* 1992; **85**:448–61.

14. Iung B, Garbarz E, Michaud P, et al. Late results of percutaneous mitral commissurotomy in a series of 1024 patients. Analysis of late clinical deterioration: frequency, anatomic findings, and predictive factors. *Circulation* 1999; **99**:3272–8.

15. Carlquist JF, Ward RH, Meyer KJ, Husebye D, Feolo M, Anderson JL. Immune response factors in rheumatic heart disease: meta-analysis of HLA-DR associations and evaluation of additional class II alleles. *J Am Coll Cardiol* 1995; **26**:452–7.

16. Zabriskie JB. T-cells and T-cell clones in rheumatic fever valvulitis. Getting to the heart of the matter? *Circulation* 1995; **92**:281–2.

17. Messika-Zeitoun D, Fung Yiu S, Cormier B, et al. Sequential assessment of mitral valve area during diastole using colour M-mode flow convergence analysis: new insights into mitral stenosis physiology. *Eur Heart J* 2003; **24**:1244–53.

18. Gupta A, Lokhandwala YY, Satoskar PR, Salvi VS. Balloon mitral valvotomy in pregnancy: maternal and fetal outcomes. *J Am Coll Surg* 1998; **187**:409–15.

19. de Souza JA, Martinez EE Jr, Ambrose JA, et al. Percutaneous balloon mitral valvuloplasty in comparison with open mitral valve commissurotomy for mitral stenosis during pregnancy. *J Am Coll Cardiol* 2001; **37**:900–3.

20. Iung B, Cormier B, Elias J, et al. Usefulness of percutaneous balloon commissurotomy for mitral stenosis during pregnancy. *Am J Cardiol* 1994; **73**:398–400.

21. Bonow RO, Carabello B, de Leon AC Jr, et al. Guidelines for the management of patients with valvular heart disease: executive summary. A report of the American College of Cardiology/American Heart Association Task Force on Practice Guidelines (Committee on Management of Patients with Valvular Heart Disease). *Circulation* 1998; **98**: 1949–84.

22. Cannan CR, Nishimura RA, Reeder GS, et al. Echocardiographic assessment of commissural calcium: a simple predictor of outcome after percutaneous mitral balloon valvotomy. *J Am Coll Cardiol* 1997; **29**:175–80.

23. Iung B, Vahanian A. The long-term outcome of balloon valvuloplasty for mitral stenosis. *Curr Cardiol Rep* 2002; **4**:118–24.

24. Braunwald E. *Heart Disease: A Textbook of Cardiovascular Medicine*, 5th edn. Philadelphia: Saunders, 1997.

25. Iung B, Gohlke-Barwolf C, Tornos P, et al. Recommendations on the management of the asymptomatic patient with valvular heart disease. *Eur Heart J* 2002; **23**:1252–66.

26. Iung B, Garbarz E, Doutrelant L, et al. Late results of percutaneous mitral commissurotomy for calcific mitral stenosis. *Am J Cardiol* 2000; **85**:1308–14.

27. Iung B, Cormier B, Farah B, et al. Percutaneous mitral commissurotomy in the elderly. *Eur Heart J* 1995; **16**:1092–9.

28. McFaul PB, Dornan JC, Lamki H, Boyle D. Pregnancy complicated by maternal heart disease. A review of 519 women. *Br J Obstet Gynaecol* 1988; **95**:861–7.

29. al Kasab SM, Sabag T, al Zaibag M, et al. Beta-adrenergic receptor blockade in the management of pregnant women with mitral stenosis. *Am J Obstet Gynecol* 1990; **163**:37–40.

30. Ben Farhat M, Gamra H, Betbout F, et al. Percutaneous balloon mitral commissurotomy during pregnancy. *Heart* 1997; **77**:564–7.

31. Mangione JA, Lourenco RM, dos Santos ES, et al. Long-term follow-up of pregnant women after percutaneous mitral valvuloplasty. *Catheter Cardiovasc Interv* 2000; **50**:413–17.

32. Osterberger LE, Goldstein S, Khaja F, Lakier JB. Functional mitral stenosis in patients with massive mitral annular calcification. *Circulation* 1981; **64**:472–6.

33. Singh J, Evans J, Levy D, et al. Prevalence and clinical determinants of mitral, tricuspid and aortic regurgitation. *Am J Cardiol* 1999; **83**:897–902.

34. Bulkley BH, Roberts WC. The heart in systemic lupus erythematosus and the changes induced in it by corticosteroid therapy. A study of 36 necropsy patients. *Am J Med* 1975; **58**:243–64.

35. Gaudron P, Eilles C, Kugler I, Ertl G. Progressive left ventricular dysfunction and remodeling after myocardial infarction. Potential mechanisms and early predictors. *Circulation* 1993; **87**:755–63.

36. Ling H, Enriquez-Sarano M, Seward J, et al. Clinical outcome of mitral regurgitation due to flail leaflets. *N Engl J Med* 1996; **335**:1417–23.

37. Enriquez-Sarano M, Tajik A, Schaff H, et al. Echocardiographic prediction of left ventricular function after correction of mitral regurgitation: results and clinical implications. *J Am Coll Cardiol* 1994; **24**:1536–43.

38. Desjardins VA, Enriquez-Sarano M, Tajik AJ, Bailey KR, Seward JB. Intensity of murmurs correlates with severity of valvular regurgitation. *Am J Med* 1996; **100**:149–56.

39. Zoghbi WA, Enriquez-Sarano M, Foster E, et al. Recommendations for evaluation of the severity of native valvular regurgitation with two-dimensional and Doppler echocardiography. *Am J Echocardiog* 2003; **16**:777–802.

40. Dujardin K, Enriquez-Sarano M, Bailey K, Nishimura R, Seward J, Tajik A. Grading of mitral regurgitation by quantitative Doppler echocardiography – calibration by left ventricular angiography in routine clinical practice. *Circulation* 1997; **96**:3409–15.

41. Enriquez-Sarano M, Bailey K, Seward J, Tajik A, Krohn M, Mays J. Quantitative Doppler assessment of valvular regurgitation. *Circulation* 1993; **87**:841–8.

42. Enriquez-Sarano M, Miller FJ, Hayes S, Bailey K, Tajik A, Seward J. Effective mitral regurgitant orifice area: clinical use and pitfalls of the proximal isovelocity surface area method. *J Am Coll Cardiol* 1995; **25**:703–9.

43. Rokey R, Sterling L, Zoghbi W, et al. Determination of regurgitant fraction in isolated mitral or aortic regurgitation by pulsed Doppler two-dimensional echocardiography. *J Am Coll Cardiol* 1986; **7**:1273–8.

44. Enriquez-Sarano M, Seward J, Bailey K, Tajik A. Effective regurgitant orifice area: a noninvasive doppler development of an old hemodynamic concept. *J Am Coll Cardiol* 1994; **23**:443–51.

45. Mohty D, Orszulak TA, Schaff HV, Avierinos JF, Tajik JA, Enriquez-Sarano M. Very long-term survival and durability of mitral valve repair for mitral valve prolapse. *Circulation* 2001; **104**:I1–I7.

46. Ling L, Enriquez-Sarano M, Seward J, et al. Early surgery in patients with mitral regurgitation due to partial flail leaflet: a long-term outcome study. *Circulation* 1997; **96**:1819–25.

47. Avierinos JF, Enriquez-Sarano M. Sex-dependent disparities between local and tertiary care centers in the presentation and management of patients with mitral valve prolapse. *Circulation* 2003; **108** (Suppl): Abstract.

48. Enriquez-Sarano M, Basmadjian A, Rossi A, Bailey K, Seward J, Tajik A. Progression of mitral regurgitation: a prospective Doppler echocardiographic study. *J Am Coll Cardiol* 1999; **34**:1137–44.

49. Cosgrove DM, Chavez AM, Lytle BW, et al. Results of mitral valve reconstruction. *Circulation* 1986; **74**:I82–7.

50. Cohn LH, Couper GS, Kinchla NM, Collins JJ Jr. Decreased operative risk of surgical treatment of mitral regurgitation with or without coronary artery disease. *J Am Coll Cardiol* 1990; **16**:1575–8.

51. Cohn LH, Couper GS, Aranki SF, Rizzo RJ, Adams DH, Collins JJ Jr. The long-term results of mitral valve reconstruction for the 'floppy' valve. *J Card Surg* 1994; **9**:278–81.

52. Dahlberg PS, Orszulak TA, Mullany CJ, Daly RC, Enriquez-Sarano M, Schaff HV. Late outcome of mitral valve surgery for patients with coronary artery disease. *Ann Thorac Surg* 2003; **76**:1539–48; discussion 1547–8.

53. Mohty D, Enriquez-Sarano M. The long-term outcome of mitral valve repair for mitral valve prolapse. *Curr Cardiol Rep* 2002; **4**:104–10.

54. Tribouilloy C, Enriquez-Sarano M, Schaff H, et al. Impact of preoperative symptoms on survival after surgical correction of organic mitral regurgitation: rationale for optimizing surgical indications. *Circulation* 1999; **99**:400–5.

55. Enriquez-Sarano M, Schaff H, Orszulak T, Tajik A, Bailey K, Frye R. Valve repair improves the outcome of surgery for mitral regurgitation. *Circulation* 1995; **91**:1264–5.

56. Devereux RB. Mitral valve prolapse. *J Am Med Womens Assoc* 1994; **49**:192–7.

57. Rabkin E, Aikawa M, Stone JR, Fukumoto Y, Libby P, Schoen FJ. Activated interstitial myofibroblasts express catabolic enzymes and mediate matrix remodeling in myxomatous heart valves. *Circulation* 2001; **104**:2525–32.

58. Freed LA, Levy D, Levine RA, et al. Prevalence and clinical outcome of mitral-valve prolapse. *N Engl J Med* 1999; **341**:1–7.

59. Flack JM, Kvasnicka JH, Gardin JM, Gidding SS, Manolio TA, Jacobs DR Jr. Anthropometric and physiologic correlates of mitral valve prolapse in a biethnic cohort of young adults: the CARDIA study. *Am Heart J* 1999; **138**:486–92.

60. Chen WW, Chan FL, Wong PH, Chow JS. Familial occurrence of mitral valve prolapse: is this related to the straight back syndrome? *Br Heart J* 1983; **50**:97–100.

61. Devereux RB, Brown WT, Kramer-Fox R, Sachs I. Inheritance of mitral valve prolapse: effect of age and sex on gene expression. *Ann Intern Med* 1982; **97**:826–32.

62. Devereux RB, Kramer-Fox R, Shear MK, Kligfield P, Pini R, Savage DD. Diagnosis and classification of severity of mitral valve prolapse: methodologic, biologic, and prognostic considerations. *Am Heart J* 1987; **113**:1265–80.

63. Strahan NV, Murphy EA, Fortuin NJ, Come PC, Humphries JO. Inheritance of the mitral valve prolapse syndrome. Discussion of a three-dimensional penetrance model. *Am J Med* 1983; **74**:967–72.

64. Weiss AN, Mimbs JW, Ludbrook PA, Sobel BE. Echocardiographic detection of mitral valve prolapse. Exclusion of false positive diagnosis and determination of inheritance. *Circulation* 1975; **52**:1091–6.

65. Devereux RB, Kramer-Fox R. Gender differences in mitral valve prolapse. *Cardiovasc Clin* 1989; **19**: 243–58.

66. DeMaria AN, King JF, Bogren HG, Lies JE, Mason DT. The variable spectrum of echocardiographic manifestations of the mitral valve prolapse syndrome. *Circulation* 1974; **50**:33–41.

67. Levine RA, Stathogiannis E, Newell JB, Harrigan P, Weyman AE. Reconsideration of echocardiographic standards for mitral valve prolapse: lack of association between leaflet displacement isolated to the apical four chamber view and independent echocardiographic evidence of abnormality. *J Am Coll Cardiol* 1988; **11**:1010–19.

68. Gaffney FA, Karlsson ES, Campbell W, et al. Autonomic dysfunction in women with mitral valve prolapse syndrome. *Circulation* 1979; **59**:894–901.

69. Boudoulas H, Kolibash AJ Jr, Baker P, King BD, Wooley CF. Mitral valve prolapse and the mitral valve prolapse syndrome: a diagnostic classification and pathogenesis of symptoms. *Am Heart J* 1989; **118**:796–818.

70. Avierinos JF, Gersh BJ, Melton LJ 3rd, et al. Natural history of asymptomatic mitral valve prolapse in the community. *Circulation* 2002; **106**:1355–61.

71. Stewart BF, Siscovick D, Lind BK, et al. Clinical factors associated with calcific aortic valve disease. Cardiovascular Health Study. *J Am Coll Cardiol* 1997; **29**:630–4.

72. Shively BK, Charlton GA, Crawford MH, Chaney RK. Flow dependence of valve area in aortic stenosis:

relation to valve morphology. *J Am Coll Cardiol* 1998; **31**:654–60.

73. Otto CM, O'Brien KD. Why is there discordance between calcific aortic stenosis and coronary artery disease? *Heart* 2001; **85**:601–2.

74. Iung B. Interface between valve disease and ischaemic heart disease. *Heart* 2000; **84**:347–52.

75. Otto CM, Lind BK, Kitzman DW, Gersh BJ, Siscovick DS. Association of aortic-valve sclerosis with cardiovascular mortality and morbidity in the elderly. *N Engl J Med* 1999; **341**:142–7.

76. Branch KR, O'Brien KD, Otto CM. Aortic valve sclerosis as a marker of active atherosclerosis. *Curr Cardiol Rep* 2002; **4**:111–17.

77. Otto CM, Kuusisto J, Reichenbach DD, Gown AM, O'Brien KD. Characterization of the early lesion of 'degenerative' valvular aortic stenosis. Histological and immunohistochemical studies. *Circulation* 1994; **90**:844–53.

78. Mohler ER, Sheridan MJ, Nichols R, Harvey WP, Waller BF. Development and progression of aortic valve stenosis: atherosclerosis risk factors – a causal relationship? A clinical morphologic study. *Clin Cardiol* 1991; **14**:995–9.

79. Aronow WS, Schwartz KS, Koenigsberg M. Correlation of serum lipids, calcium and phosphorus, diabetes mellitus, aortic valve stenosis and history of systemic hypertension with presence or absence of mitral anular calcium in persons older than 62 years in a long-term health care facility. *Am J Cardiol* 1987; **59**:381–2.

80. Peltier M, Trojette F, Sarano ME, Grigioni F, Slama MA, Tribouilloy CM. Relation between cardiovascular risk factors and nonrheumatic severe calcific aortic stenosis among patients with a three-cuspid aortic valve. *Am J Cardiol* 2003; **91**:97–9.

81. Boon A, Cheriex E, Lodder J, Kessels F. Cardiac valve calcification: characteristics of patients with calcification of the mitral annulus or aortic valve. *Heart* 1997; **78**:472–4.

82. Iivanainen AM, Lindroos M, Tilvis R, Heikkila J, Kupari M. Natural history of aortic valve stenosis of varying severity in the elderly. *Am J Cardiol* 1996; **78**:97–101.

83. Morris JJ, Schaff HV, Mullany CJ, Morris PB, Frye RL, Orszulak TA. Gender differences in left ventricular functional response to aortic valve replacement. *Circulation* 1994; **90**:II183–9.

84. Milavetz DL, Hayes SN, Weston SA, Seward JB, Mullany CJ, Roger VL. Sex differences in left ventricular geometry in aortic stenosis: impact on outcome. *Chest* 2000; **117**:1094–9.

85. Carroll JD, Carroll EP, Feldman T, et al. Sex-associated differences in left ventricular function in aortic stenosis of the elderly. *Circulation* 1992; **86**:1099–107.

86. Favero L, Giordan M, Tarantini G, et al. Gender differences in left ventricular function in patients with isolated aortic stenosis. *J Heart Valve Dis* 2003; **12**:313–18.

87. Kostkiewicz M, Tracz W, Olszowska M, Podolec P, Drop D. Left ventricular geometry and function in patients with aortic stenosis: gender differences. *Int J Cardiol* 1999; **71**:57–61.

88. Legget ME, Kuusisto J, Healy NL, Fujioka M, Schwaegler RG, Otto CM. Gender differences in left ventricular function at rest and with exercise in asymptomatic aortic stenosis. *Am Heart J* 1996; **131**:94–100.

89. Rohde LE, Zhi G, Aranki SF, Beckel NE, Lee RT, Reimold SC. Gender-associated differences in left ventricular geometry in patients with aortic valve disease and effect of distinct overload subsets. *Am J Cardiol* 1997; **80**:475–80.

90. Bech-Hanssen O, Wallentin I, Houltz E, Beckman Suurkula M, Larsson S, Caidahl K. Gender differences in patients with severe aortic stenosis: impact on preoperative left ventricular geometry and function, as well as early postoperative morbidity and mortality. *Eur J Cardiothorac Surg* 1999; **15**:24–30.

91. Rahimtoola SH. Perspective on valvular heart disease: an update. *J Am Coll Cardiol* 1989; **14**:1–23.

92. Horstkotte D, Loogen F. The natural history of aortic valve stenosis. *Eur Heart J* 1988; **9** (Suppl E):57–64.

93. Rosenhek R, Binder T, Porenta G, et al. Predictors of outcome in severe, asymptomatic aortic stenosis. *N Engl J Med* 2000; **343**:611–17.

94. Ross J Jr, Braunwald E. Aortic stenosis. *Circulation* 1968; **38**:61–7.

95. Roger VL, Tajik AJ, Bailey KR, Oh JK, Taylor CL, Seward JB. Progression of aortic stenosis in adults: new appraisal using Doppler echocardiography. *Am Heart J* 1990; **119**:331–8.

96. Pellikka PA, Nishimura RA, Bailey KR, Tajik AJ. The natural history of adults with asymptomatic, hemodynamically significant aortic stenosis. *J Am Coll Cardiol* 1990; **15**:1012–17.

97. Malouf JF, Enriquez-Sarano M, Pellikka PA, et al. Severe pulmonary hypertension in patients with severe aortic valve stenosis: clinical profile and prognostic implications. *J Am Coll Cardiol* 2002; **40**:789–95.

98. Rao V, Jamieson WR, Ivanov J, Armstrong S, David TE. Prosthesis-patient mismatch affects survival after aortic valve replacement. *Circulation* 2000; **102**:III5–9.

99. Pibarot P, Dumesnil JG. Hemodynamic and clinical impact of prosthesis-patient mismatch in the aortic valve position and its prevention. *J Am Coll Cardiol* 2000; **36**:1131–41.

100. Pibarot P, Dumesnil JG, Lemieux M, Cartier P, Metras J, Durand LG. Impact of prosthesis-patient mismatch on hemodynamic and symptomatic status, morbidity and mortality after aortic valve replacement with a bioprosthetic heart valve. *J Heart Valve Dis* 1998; **7**:211–18.

101. Blais C, Dumesnil JG, Baillot R, Simard S, Doyle D, Pibarot P. Impact of valve prosthesis-patient mismatch on short-term mortality after aortic valve replacement. *Circulation* 2003; **108**:983–8.

102. Sommers KE, David TE. Aortic valve replacement with patch enlargement of the aortic annulus. *Ann Thorac Surg* 1997; **63**:1608–12.

103. Buttrick P, Scheuer J. Sex-associated differences in left ventricular function in aortic stenosis of the elderly. *Circulation* 1992; **86**:1336–8.

104. Aranki SF, Rizzo RJ, Couper GS, et al. Aortic valve replacement in the elderly. Effect of gender and coronary artery disease on operative mortality. *Circulation* 1993; **88**:II17–23.

105. Gehlot A, Mullany CJ, Ilstrup D, et al. Aortic valve replacement in patients aged eighty years and older: early and long-term results. *J Thorac Cardiovasc Surg* 1996; **111**:1026–36.

106. Bellamy MF, Pellikka PA, Klarich KW, Tajik AJ, Enriquez-Sarano M. Association of cholesterol levels, hydroxymethylglutaryl coenzyme-A reductase inhibitor treatment, and progression of aortic stenosis in the community. *J Am Coll Cardiol* 2002; **40**: 1723–30.

107. Novaro GM, Tiong IY, Pearce GL, Lauer MS, Sprecher DL, Griffin BP. Effect of hydroxymethylglutaryl coenzyme a reductase inhibitors on the progression of calcific aortic stenosis. *Circulation* 2001; **104**:2205–9.

108. Shavelle DM, Takasu J, Budoff MJ, Mao S, Zhao XQ, O'Brien KD. HMG CoA reductase inhibitor (statin) and aortic valve calcium. *Lancet* 2002; **359**:1125–6.

109. Rajamannan NM, Subramaniam M, Springett M, et al. Atorvastatin inhibits hypercholesterolemia-induced cellular proliferation and bone matrix production in the rabbit aortic valve. *Circulation* 2002; **105**:2660–5.

110. Roberts WC. The congenitally bicuspid aortic valve. A study of 85 autopsy cases. *Am J Cardiol* 1970; **26**:72–83.

111. Davies MJ, Treasure T, Parker DJ. Demographic characteristics of patients undergoing aortic valve replacement for stenosis: relation to valve morphology. *Heart* 1996; **75**:174–8.

112. Beppu S, Suzuki S, Matsuda H, Ohmori F, Nagata S, Miyatake K. Rapidity of progression of aortic stenosis in patients with congenital bicuspid aortic valves. *Am J Cardiol* 1993; **71**:322–7.

113. Olson LJ, Edwards WD, Tajik AJ. Aortic valve stenosis: etiology, pathophysiology, evaluation, and management. *Curr Probl Cardiol* 1987; **12**:455–508.

114. Chan KL, Ghani M, Woodend K, Burwash IG. Case-controlled study to assess risk factors for aortic stenosis in congenitally bicuspid aortic valve. *Am J Cardiol* 2001; **88**:690–3.

115. Lao TT, Sermer M, MaGee L, Farine D, Colman JM. Congenital aortic stenosis and pregnancy – a reappraisal. *Am J Obstet Gynecol* 1993; **169**:540–5.

116. Lao TT, Adelman AG, Sermer M, Colman JM. Balloon valvuloplasty for congenital aortic stenosis in pregnancy. *Br J Obstet Gynaecol* 1993; **100**:1141–2.

117. Banning AP, Pearson JF, Hall RJ. Role of balloon dilatation of the aortic valve in pregnant patients with severe aortic stenosis. *Br Heart J* 1993; **70**:544–5.

118. Smith HJ, Neutze JM, Roche AH, Agnew TM, Barratt-Boyes BG. The natural history of rheumatic aortic regurgitation and the indications for surgery. *Br Heart J* 1976; **38**:147–54.

119. Wisenbaugh T, Booth D, DeMaria A, Nissen S, Waters J. Relationship of contractile state to ejection performance in patients with chronic aortic valve disease. *Circulation* 1986; **73**:47–53.

120. Bonow R, Lakatos E, Maron B, Epstein S. Serial long-term assessment of the natural history of asymptomatic patients with chronic aortic regurgitation and normal left ventricular systolic function. *Circulation* 1991; **84**:1625–35.

121. Dujardin KS, Enriquez-Sarano M, Schaff HV, Bailey KR, Seward JB, Tajik AJ. Mortality and morbidity of aortic regurgitation in clinical practice. A long-term follow-up study. *Circulation* 1999; **99**:1851–7.

122. Klodas E, Enriquez-Sarano M, Tajik AJ, Mullany CJ, Bailey KR, Seward JB. Optimizing timing of surgical correction in patients with severe aortic regurgitation: role of symptoms. *J Am Coll Cardiol* 1997; **30**:746–52.

123. Borer J, Hochreiter C, Herrold E, et al. Prediction of indication for valve replacement among asymptomatic or minimally symptomatic patients with chronic aortic regurgitation and normal left ventricular performance. *Circulation* 1998; **97**:525–34.

124. Chaliki HP, Mohty D, Avierinos JF, et al. Outcomes after aortic valve replacement in patients with severe aortic regurgitation and markedly reduced left ventricular function. *Circulation* 2002; **106**:2687–93.

125. Klodas E, Enriquez-Sarano M, Tajik AJ, Mullany CJ, Bailey KR, Seward JB. Aortic regurgitation complicated by extreme left ventricular dilation: long-term outcome after surgical correction. *J Am Coll Cardiol* 1996; **27**:670–7.

126. Klodas E, Enriquez-Sarano M, Tajik AJ, Mullany CJ, Bailey KR, Seward JB. Surgery for aortic regurgitation in women. Contrasting indications and outcomes compared with men. *Circulation* 1996; **94**:2472–8.

127. Sheikh F, Rangwala S, DeSimone C, Smith HS, O'Leary AM. Management of the parturient with severe aortic incompetence. *J Cardiothorac Vasc Anesth* 1995; **9**:575–7.

128. Clouse WD, Hallett JW Jr, Schaff HV, Gayari MM, Ilstrup DM, Melton LJ 3rd. Improved prognosis of thoracic aortic aneurysms: a population-based study. *JAMA* 1998; **280**:1926–9.

129. McDonald ML, Smedira NG, Blackstone EH, Grimm RA, Lytle BW, Cosgrove DM. Reduced survival in women after valve surgery for aortic regurgitation: effect of aortic enlargement and late aortic rupture. *J Thorac Cardiovasc Surg* 2000; **119**:1205–12.

130. Kouchoukos NT, Dougenis D. Surgery of the thoracic aorta. *N Engl J Med* 1997; **336**:1876–88.

131. Baumgartner WA, Cameron DE, Redmond JM, Greene PS, Gott VL. Operative management of Marfan syndrome: the Johns Hopkins experience. *Ann Thorac Surg* 1999; **67**:1859–60; discussion 1868–70.

132. Gott VL, Greene PS, Alejo DE, et al. Replacement of the aortic root in patients with Marfan's syndrome. *N Engl J Med* 1999; **340**:1307–13.

133. Pedowitz P, Perell A. Aneurysms complicated by pregnancy. I. Aneurysms of the aorta and its major branches. *Am J Obstet Gynecol* 1957; **73**:720–35.

134. Pyeritz RE. Maternal and fetal complications of pregnancy in the Marfan syndrome. *Am J Med* 1981; **71**:784–90.

135. Rossiter JP, Repke JT, Morales AJ, Murphy EA, Pyeritz RE. A prospective longitudinal evaluation of pregnancy in the Marfan syndrome. *Am J Obstet Gynecol* 1995; **173**:1599–606.

136. Khan MA, Herzog CA, St Peter JV, et al. The prevalence of cardiac valvular insufficiency assessed by transthoracic echocardiography in obese patients treated with appetite-suppressant drugs. *N Engl J Med* 1998; **339**:713–18.

137. Connolly HM, Crary JL, McGoon MD, et al. Valvular heart disease associated with fenfluramine-phentermine. *N Engl J Med* 1997; **337**:581–8.

138. Jick H, Vasilakis C, Weinrauch LA, Meier CR, Jick SS, Derby LE. A population-based study of appetite-suppressant drugs and the risk of cardiac-valve regurgitation. *N Engl J Med* 1998; **339**:719–24.

139. Gardin JM, Schumacher D, Constantine G, Davis KD, Leung C, Reid CL. Valvular abnormalities and cardiovascular status following exposure to dexfenfluramine or phentermine/fenfluramine. *JAMA* 2000; **283**:1703–9.

140. Burger AJ, Sherman HB, Charlamb MJ, et al. Low prevalence of valvular heart disease in 226 phentermine-fenfluramine protocol subjects prospectively followed for up to 30 months. *J Am Coll Cardiol* 1999; **34**:1153–8.

141. Pritchett AM, Morrison JF, Edwards WD, Schaff HV, Connolly HM, Espinosa RE. Valvular heart disease in patients taking pergolide. *Mayo Clin Proc* 2002; **77**:1280–6.

142. Redfield MM, Nicholson WJ, Edwards WD, Tajik AJ. Valve disease associated with ergot alkaloid use: echocardiographic and pathologic correlations. *Ann Intern Med* 1992; **117**:50–2.

143. Cannegieter SC, Rosendaal FR, Briet E. Thromboembolic and bleeding complications in patients with mechanical heart valve prostheses. *Circulation* 1994; **89**:635–41.

144. Reimold SC, Rutherford JD. Clinical practice. Valvular heart disease in pregnancy. *N Engl J Med* 2003; **349**:52–9.

145. Hanania G, Thomas D, Michel PL, et al. Pregnancy and prosthetic heart valves: a French cooperative retrospective study of 155 cases. *Eur Heart J* 1994; **15**:1651–8.

146. North RA, Sadler L, Stewart AW, McCowan LM, Kerr AR, White HD. Long-term survival and valve-related complications in young women with cardiac valve replacements. *Circulation* 1999; **99**:2669–76.

147. Kvidal P, Bergstrom R, Malm T, Stahle E. Long-term follow-up of morbidity and mortality after aortic valve replacement with a mechanical valve prosthesis. *Eur Heart J* 2000; **21**:1099–111.

148. David TE, Puschmann R, Ivanov J, et al. Aortic valve replacement with stentless and stented porcine valves: a case-match study. *J Thorac Cardiovasc Surg* 1998; **116**:236–41.

34

Severe pulmonary hypertension

Michael J. Landzberg

Current state of diagnosis

The ramifications of medical and legal discussions surrounding modern use of anorexigens,[1] coupled with increasing pathophysiologic understanding and availability of pharmacotherapies directed at vascular inflammation,[2] have all helped to reposition severe pulmonary hypertension into a greater center of awareness for caregivers and patients. Whereas the classification of 'primary' (or, unknown etiology) pulmonary hypertension (PPH) comprised a relatively small percentage of the extensive incidence of pulmonary hypertensive disorders, a newer classification of 'pulmonary arteriolar hypertension' (PAH), either of a familial or sporadic, nonfamilial nature, has expanded the clinical entity to include various disorders sharing common pathophysiologic and anatomic features of vascular inflammation. Similarities among these syndromes have been sufficient to allow and to promote increase in standardized study populations for testing of mechanisms of disease and application of therapeutics.

Epidemiologic associations (see also Chapters 22, 35 and 37)

Multicenter national and international registries established from 1981 to the present[3,4] have assisted in the clarification of the prevalence and incidence of PPH (1–2 per million and 1–2/million/year, respectively), identification of associated occurrences, risks, or triggers (Box 34.1), and untreated survival of patients affected by severe pulmonary hypertension (PHT). Association (typically >2:1) with female gender remains unexplained, and persists for PAH associated with many other triggers (Box 34.2). A peak in PAH incidence during the second to fourth decades of life tracks most women's childbearing years. An increased awareness of PAH during the hemodynamic changes and stress of pregnancy, coupled with the noted increased incidence of pulmonary hypertension in women has suggested an association of PAH with pregnancy as well as with hormonal contraception use. Severely, if not prohibitively, worsened outcomes during pregnancy and, in particular, during the immediate postpartum period are recognized, and are discussed below. The association between PAH and pregnancy or oral contraception use is debated, and, for the greatest part, has recently been refuted, suggesting that hormonal differences alone may not explain the noted gender-based variations in incidence of disease.[5] Alternative causative or associative mechanisms have been suggested, including recognized gender-based increased autoantibody effects leading to development of PAH, as well as linkage of the presence of BMPR2 mutation (see below) with increased female births. These factors are unlikely to be sole causative mechanisms, as they occur frequently in nonaffected individuals, thus suggesting additional genetic or environmental modifiers. Likewise, additional associative environmental triggers appear more common in women, including use of cooking oil contaminated with L-tryptophan, use of certain described petroleum-based solvents, as well as anorexigenic agent use. These multiple risks appear to be cumulative in an as yet poorly defined manner, contributing to the increased female gender predominance of PAH.

Additional associated conditions with higher prevalence of PAH in the affected population have led to increased awareness of PAH (e.g. scleroderma, especially of the limited skin involvement type, with estimated prevalence of PHT of 12–14%; HIV, with estimated cumulative incidence of 0.5%; and portal hypertension, with estimated prevalence of 0.25–2%).[6–8] The tremendous differences in therapy and outcomes for patients with severe PHT associated with valvular or cardiomyopathic heart disease, or proximal or distal chronic thromboembolic disease mandate a thorough search for 'secondary' etiologies, as outlined.

Analyses of epidemiologic databases associated with patients with PPH have suggested similar untreated survival of patients with severe PHT, nearly universally regardless of etiology (with median survival between 2.8 and 3.4 years for the affected adult patient). Correlation of survival with variables relating to right ventricular (RV) function (typically assessed by hemodynamic measure of systemic cardiac output/mixed venous oxygen saturation and right atrial pressure) and physical capacity (typically measured by 6-minute walking capacity), emphasizes the delicate balance and direct relationships between pulmonary afterload, cardiac function, physical capacity, and survival (Fig. 34.1).[9] The improved survival outcomes seen in persons with severe PAH associated with Eisenmenger syndrome, or shunt-related PHT with associated cyanosis (10–20-year survival >80%),[10] suggest potential for improved response to increased pulmonary afterload when it is shared between right and left heart muscle.[1]

Symptoms and diagnosis

Persons with PHT typically come to attention either due to symptoms (dyspnea, chest fullness or pain,

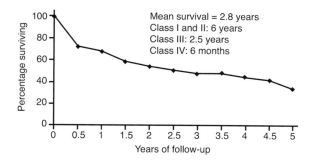

Figure 34.1
Untreated survival with severe pulmonary arteriolar hypertension (PAH). Adapted from reference 9.

bloating, volume retention, palpitations or syncope), incidentally during evaluation for other disease, or more recently, during family screening for PHT or in patients with identified risks or triggers. Typically, diagnosis may be suggested by evidence on cardiac examination of RV failure (volume retention, elevated jugular venous column, prominence of RV impulse with third heart sound) and increased afterload (loud pulmonary component of the second heart sound), but is strengthened by echocardiography, with estimates of RV and pulmonary artery (PA) pressures frequently ascertained by measure of Doppler-based tricuspid velocities. In general, systolic PA pressures >50 mm (or half systemic levels) or <36 mm (or one-third systemic levels) tend to define or exclude diagnosis of PHT, with intermediate values frequently requiring increased assessment. Echocardiography is at best able to estimate pressures and diastolic cardiac function (relative stiffness and impedance to filling), but does reliably assess systolic ventricular function.

Due to the high prevalence of diastolic cardiac abnormalities, the limitations inherent in echocardiographic measure, as well as the additional anatomic and functional etiologies of PHT not accurately defined and measured by such methods, confirmatory and diagnostic testing rely on hemodynamic assessment at cardiopulmonary catheterization. Typically, such approaches include measure of right- and left-sided pressures, flow, and resistance (assisting in diagnosis and prognostic assessment), limited angiography as indicated, as well as maneu-

vers to test reactivity of flow and resistance to acute administration of pulmonary vasodilator agents (typically inhalation of nitric oxide (NO) with or without oxygen, inhalation or intravenous administration of specific prostanoids, or intravenous administration of acetylcholine or adenosine). Catheterization is suggested to be carried out in regional specialty centers where such is done with increased frequency, potentially decreasing associated risk and improving reliability of diagnosis and testing. In general, catheter-based measure of mean PA pressure >25 mm (or systolic pressure > one-third to one-half systemic levels) or <36 mm (or one-third systemic levels) defines PHT. Exercise-induced PHT remains less well defined, but is suggested when mean PA pressure rises to >30 mmHg upon exertion. Response to acute administration of pulmonary vasodilator therapy (seen in 10–20% of tested patients, potentially reflecting a subset of patients with an earlier, or less lethal phase of disease) has classically, yet in uncontrolled study, been described as ≥20% decrease in systolic PA pressure with stability or improvement in pulmonary blood flow. Vasoresponsiveness was initially felt to correlate with improved functional and survival outcomes (>80% 5-year survival) in response to therapy with calcium channel blocker therapy.[11] Recent study has suggested lesser correlation of percent reduction in PA pressure with long-term responsiveness to calcium channel blocker therapy, and has led to the suggestion of adding an absolute drop of mean PA pressure to ≤35 mmHg to be classified as a 'responder', with improved correlation with improvement upon use of calcium channel blocker therapy.[12] In the past, acute vasodilator responsiveness was critical to choice of therapy and determination of outcome, and still carries importance for both aspects of care. Nonetheless, the long-term benefits on PA pressure, functional capacity or survival (albeit less than that seen with calcium channel blockers in 'responsive' patients) that have been documented with newer agents (prostanoids, endothelin antagonists) administered to patients who do not demonstrate acute vasodilator responsiveness (see below) raise new hope for such patients.

Definition of alternative triggers, and elimination of additional treatable etiologies for PHT mandate additional patient testing, typically including chest

X-ray, pulmonary function assessment (with spirometry, volumes, and measure of diffusion capacity – shown to correlate with patient outcome); high-resolution chest CT scan, typically with angiography and pulmonary embolism protocol; serologic testing (collagen vascular screening, liver and renal function, complete blood count and assessment, HIV testing when appropriate); abdominal ultrasound with or without flow assessment in the portal veins or liver–spleen scintigraphy when appropriate; sleep testing as appropriate (although nearly always indicated due to overlap in presenting symptomatology); and tuberculosis (TB) testing when indicated. Disease-specific therapies, including oxygen administration, positive airway ventilation, alternative organ therapy or transplantation, surgical pulmonary endarterectomy,[13] or balloon pulmonary angioplasty[14,15] may be indicated as primary therapy, based on the results of such testing.

Functional capacity, as assessed by exercise testing, with formal measure of 6-minute walking capacity (typically used due to ease and patient functional restriction) or cardiopulmonary exercise testing with measure of maximal oxygen consumption,[16] has become routine as a prognostic tool, both for initial survival prediction and for response to therapy. Subjective assessment of functional capacity using NYHA or WHO functional scales has correlated with both untreated and treated outcomes and has also been used to define tested populations in a randomized controlled study of medical therapy. Improved outcomes for less functionally limited patients has led to recommendation to treat less severely ill patients with functional class ≥2 (dyspneic with at least moderate activity).[17] Dyspnea scales have been utilized in randomized controlled trials, although their individual additive prognostic potential remains undefined.

Serologic testing of biomarkers, including troponins and measure of natriuretic peptides, remains under investigation, but appears promising as regards markers of disease severity.

Current state of therapy

Calcium channel blockers were the first widely accepted therapeutic agents causing a change in outcome for patients with PAH. Their use was modeled on the 'vasoconstrictor' model of pulmonary arteriolar hypertension, envisioning pathology to be due to a disorder and disregulation of small pulmonary arteries, characterized by lamellar intimal fibrosis, medial hypertrophy, and neovascular plexiform lesions. To date, no randomized trial exists testing effect and risk of calcium channel blockade, although nifedipine has remained the prototype therapy for the small percentage of patients (5–15%) who are 'responders' to acute administration of vasodilator agents during cardiopulmonary catheterization. Given that clinical effect typically requires drug doses 5–10 times those commonly used for systemic hypertension therapy and that such dosage requirements are unpredictable and may be accompanied by considerable adversity, dose-response testing is typically performed with indwelling PA pressure monitoring to identify eventual effective target dosage. Most centers will recommend achieving this goal dosage in graded fashion, to allow adversity to be minimized as the systemic vasculature accommodates to drug effect. As suggested above, more recent uncontrolled databases suggest that calcium channel blocker use may be even less effective than previously thought, and may require a change to a more stringent definition of 'acute vasodilator responsiveness' to better define the population where this class of medication will be effective. Calcium channel blocker therapy is generally felt to be contraindicated in those patients presenting with substantial right atrial (RA) pressure elevation or marked decrease in cardiac output.

The use of what is considered 'conventional' PAH therapy, including warfarin, oxygen, oral inotropy with digoxin, and diuretics, is controversial. Benefit of warfarin has been extrapolated from subset analyses of retrospective single-center studies, and is based on pathologic data from lung biopsies and postmortem examinations, confirming in situ thrombosis within the pulmonary vasculature. Warfarin is generally advised, with an ill-defined, though typically suggested, goal for target INR of 2.0–3.0, dependent upon individual patient risk of bleeding. Recent multicenter randomized controlled trials (RCTs) of other therapeutic agents for PAH have noted use of oral anticoagulants at time of inclusion in 51–86% of enrolled patients (see below).

Long-term digoxin administration for patients with right heart dysfunction due to PAH has not been studied. Its use has been declining, with digoxin administration at time of inclusion in recent multicenter RCTs of other therapy between 18 and 53%. Diuretic therapy may assist in volume control, is likewise unstudied in the chronic state, and its use has been documented in 49–70% of patients during recent multicenter RCTs of other therapies for PAH. Use of oxygen, other than that defined for appropriate patients with chronic lung disease and hypoxemia, is unsupported.

Over the past decade, the 'vasoconstriction' monolayer model of PPH has fallen away to the current vascular wall inflammation paradigm, with therapies reflecting this change in pathobiologic thought. For the majority of affected patients, modern treatment, however indirectly, centers on mediators of chemotaxis, cellular proliferation and differentiation, and regulation of vasoactive peptides and growth factors. These mediators currently include prostanoids (intravenous, inhaled, oral), endothelin antagonists, nitroso-compounds and phosphodiesterase inhibitors.

The earliest multicenter randomized clinical trials focused on the use of the intravenous prostanoid, epoprostenol, or Flolan®. An epoprostenol + conventional therapy treated group showed improved survival and exercise tolerance, increased cardiac output, and decreased pulmonary vascular resistance when compared with controls using conventional therapy alone.[18] These results have been confirmed both in patients with PPH and in patients with PAH associated with scleroderma, with longer-term benefit shown in multiple subsequent studies (Fig. 34.2).[19] However, the personal and financial costs of Flolan use are protean, with need for continuous administration via a commercially available personal pump attached via tubing to a centrally placed indwelling catheter and daily personal admixture of drug. Common drug side effects include flushing, headache, peculiar jaw pain with the first bite of each meal, bony and muscular pain, local and systemic infection, nausea, diarrhea, hypotension, tachyphylaxis, and potential for rebound – worsened, if not threatening, PHT upon drug withdrawal. Typical dosing begins at 0.5–2.0 ng/kg/min, with adjustments based upon

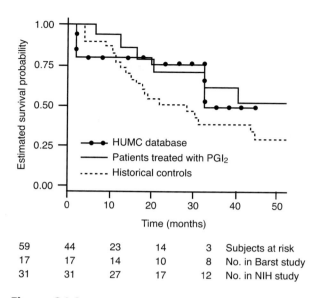

Figure 34.2
Survival in severe pulmonary arteriolar hypertension (PAH): treatment with Flolan®. HUMC, Harbor-UCLA Medical Center. Adapted from reference 19.

effect and tachyphylaxis, typically every 3–10 days. Eventual 'plateauing' of dose may occur, without need for dosage augmentation. Periodic invasive hemodynamic assessment is required to ensure adequacy of dosage, as well as avoidance of overdosage. This medication is currently Food and Drug Administration (FDA)-approved for PAH patients who are in functional class (FC) III–IV. Pharmaceutical cost may be in the range US$75–150 000, yearly. Drug benefit is modest, including improved walking within 6 minutes of more than 20–30 meters, and extension of survival to 63% at 3 years. Predictors of survival at start of therapy have included functional class (poor prognosis if initially <250 m), cardiac index, mean RA pressure (poor prognosis if ≥12 mmHg), and mean PA pressure, with predictors of survival after 1 year of therapy including improvement in cardiac index and decrease in RA pressure.

Recent multicenter randomized clinical trials, outlined below, have placed prostanoids and endothelin antagonists into a positive spotlight, and include the following:

The *Treprostinil® (SQ prostanoid: Remodulin®; tricyclic benzidine analog of prostacyclin) study.*[20] This was a 12-week double-blind randomized, therapeutic trial, ending in 2001, with enrollment based on baseline 6-minute walk capacity (mean 327 meters). Right heart catheterization was required. Study drug was started at 2 ng/kg/min, with weekly dosage increases, with endpoints measured at 12 weeks, including 6-minute walk and hemodynamic parameters. The study was followed by an optional open-label study; 470 patients were enrolled, 81% were women, 271 with PPH, 90 with connective tissue disease, 109 with congenital heart disease, with a mean age of 44 years at enrollment. Functional capacity was notably WHO FC II (12%), III (81%), IV (7%). At trial end, there was only a 10-meter difference in 6-minute walk distance between the study groups. However, this difference increased as final tolerated drug dosage increased, with 36.1 ± 10 m difference between groups when study drug dosage was >13.8 ng/kg/min. Benefits persisted at 18 months of therapy, with the most common side effect being infusion site pain. This medication is currently FDA-approved for patients with PAH and FC III or IV, and has benefits of being a more stable compound, requiring a smaller mechanical pump, and a nonintravenous administration. Local injection site pain has been frequent, although various strategies have been designed to reduce such pain. Financial cost per year has been estimated at US $93 000.[21]

The *Beraprost® (oral prostacyclin analog) ALPHA-BET trial.*[22] This was a 12-week double-blind randomization, therapeutic trial, with enrollment based on baseline 6-minute walk (mean 373 meters). Right heart catheterization was required. Study drug was started at 20 µg p.o. q.i.d., with weekly dosage increases, with maximal dose of 120 µg q.i.d. (mean 80 µg q.i.d.), with endpoints measured at 12 weeks, including 6-minute walk and hemodynamic parameters and Borg dyspnea index. One hundred and thirty patients were enrolled, 62% were women, 63 with PPH, 13 with connective tissue disease, 24 with congenital heart disease, 21 with portal hypertension, nine with HIV, and with mean age at enrollment of 45 years. Functional capacity at enrollment was FC II (50%), III (50%), IV (0%). At trial end, there was nearly a 30-meter difference in 6-minute walk distance between the study groups. This difference

was more pronounced in patients with PPH than in those with other recognized triggers of PAH. Continued drug benefit after 1 year of therapy was lost in subsequent trial, with no current or expected FDA approval for this agent.[23]

The *Iloprost® (inhaled prostacyclin analog) AIR trial.*[24] This was a 12-week double-blind randomization, therapeutic trial, with enrollment based on baseline 6-minute walk (mean 323 meters). Right heart catheterization was required. Study drug was started at 2.5–5.0 µg inhaled 6–9 times daily with overnight 'breaks', with dosage adjustments over the first 8 days, with endpoints measured at 12 weeks as a 'combined endpoint' defined as 10% improvement of 6 minute walk + improved WHO FC, hemodynamic parameters, Borg dyspnea scale, and quality of life scale. Two hundred and three patients were enrolled, 67% were women, 102 with PPH, 35 with connective tissue disease, 57 with chronic thromboembolic PHT, nine anorexigen-related PHT, with mean age at enrollment of 51 years, and functional capacity at enrollment of FC II (0%), III (59%), IV (41%). At trial end, there was a 36-meter difference in 6-minute walk distance between the study groups (Fig. 34.3). This difference was more pronounced in patients with PPH than in those with other recognized triggers of PAH. To date, the FDA has not addressed drug approval, although a similar phase III US trial is not anticipated.

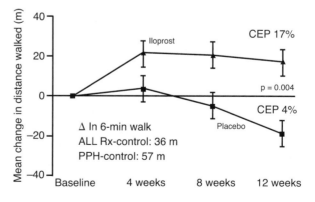

Figure 34.3
Functional capacity in severe pulmonary arteriolar hypertension (PAH): treatment with Iloprost®. Adapted from reference 24.

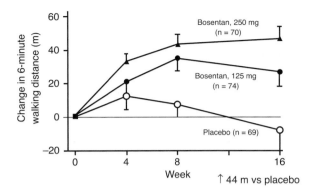

Figure 34.4
Functional capacity in severe pulmonary arteriolar hypertension (PAH): treatment with bosentan. Adapted from reference 25.

Bosentan (Tracleer®: combined endothelin a and b receptor antagonist): BREATHE Study.[25] This was a 16-week double-blind randomization, therapeutic trial, with enrollment based on baseline 6-minute walk (mean 335 meters). Right heart catheterization was required. Study drug was started at 62.5 mg b.i.d. for 4 weeks with two arms of dosage increase to either 125 or 250 mg p.o. b.i.d. for 12 weeks, with endpoints measured at 16 weeks, including 6-minute walk and hemodynamic parameters, Borg dyspnea scale, and WHO functional class. The trial was followed by an optional open-label study: 213 patients were enrolled, 79% were women, 151 with PPH, 62 with connective tissue disease, with mean age at enrollment of 48 years, with functional capacity at enrollment of FC II (0%), III (92%), IV (8%). At trial end, there was a 44-meter difference in 6-minute walk distance between the study groups (Fig. 34.4). Benefits have persisted during long-term follow-up, with the most common side effect being liver function test (LFT) abnormalities (mandating monthly LFT checks), and mild dilutional anemia. The FDA has approved bosentan use in patients with PAH in FC III or IV. Cost per year is currently US $36 000.[26]

Similar trials utilizing (a) *sole endothelin A antagonists*, and (b) *sildenafil*, are underway, and remain to be completed or interpreted.

Prescription of current intravenous and nonparenteral therapies for PAH in the US focuses on FDA-approved therapies, administered to patients in particular WHO FCs in which the approved medications were tested: e.g. Flolan® for FC IV patients, and bosentan and treprostinil for patients in FC III. If patients do not respond to initial diagnostic acute vasodilator challenge our recommendations for therapy include:

- WHO FC II:
  - US: bosentan (tested in FC III patients), or remodulin
  - elsewhere: also short-term beraprost or long-term iloprost
- WHO FC III:
  - US: bosentan, or remodulin
  - elsewhere: also short-term beraprost or iloprost
- WHO FC IV:
  - US: Flolan® (consideration of bosentan, if lag time tolerable)
  - elsewhere: iloprost
  - AVOID: beraprost/treprostinil due to lag in response time.

Patients without improvement to <FC III by several months of therapy, those initiating in FC IV, or those persisting with elevated RA pressure or low systemic cardiac output, are typically referred for consideration of organ transplantation (single lung/double lung/heart-lung depending on institutional availability and success).[27] Worsening of FC, new symptoms of neurohormonal activation, or decrement in 6-minute walk time >10% baseline with worsening dyspnea typically prompt a full reassessment for potential causes of deterioration, or to alter therapy.

Therapy designed to support RV contractile function, decrease muscular remodeling, decrease neurohormonal activation, decrease 'inflammation', or even reduce alveolar hypoxia (with agents such as beta-blockade, brain natriuretic peptide, angiotensin-converting enzyme (ACE) inhibitors or angiotensin receptor blockade, and spironolactone), as shown to be of assistance in left ventricular (LV) failure syndromes with increased afterload, have not been effectively trialed in patients with PAH. Effects of exercise training, stress reduction, nutritional support, and therapy of sleep abnormalities have yet to be scientifically examined. How to, and when best to, combine or transition therapies, as well as elucidation of markers of responsiveness to such therapies, are topics of current investigation. Use of implanted continuous hemodynamic recording devices of RA, RV or PA pressures have been described, and while their use remains intriguing, clinical benefit from such procedures remains to be examined.

General patient recommendations to practice (1) safe airline travel (most commercial airlines pressurize to an equivalent of 1800–2400 m, with hypobaric hypoxia typically seen at 1500–2000 m), with frequent rests and concomitant oxygen use; (2) budgeting of energy to personal goals; (3) excellent skin, dental, and overall infection risk reduction strategies to minimize increased tissue demand scenarios; (4) episodic laboratory checks (autoimmune associations, renal and hepatic function, complete blood count) to minimize high-risk additional body demands; (5) vigilance regarding use of even simple, over-the-counter agents with potential for renal or hepatic function alterations; and (6) overall educated consumerism, are typically encouraged.

New paradigms?

There is increasing evidence for genetically inherited abnormalities in endothelial cell apoptosis and growth potential, with links of familial and sporadic PPH to transforming growth factor-β (TGF-β) superfamily bone morphogenetic protein receptor BMPR2 (as well as angiopoietin-1, its specific endothelial cell receptor, BMPR1, and ALK 1, encoding a BMPR receptor). Currently, assays for mutations in these genes are not sufficiently standardized to allow for clinical family guidance, although there is speculation that specific defects may correlate with more robust PAH phenotypes and improved definitions of susceptibility to PAH.[28–30]

Increasing data suggest that the hallmark lesion of PPH/PAH, the plexiform lesion, is a response phenomenon to local hypoxia or inflammation, and represents a tumor-like proliferation of endothelial cells (monoclonal in PPH, polyclonal in secondary forms of PAH). To date, the functional significance of these lesions and their components, and the temporal control of vascular growth remain elusive.[31]

Markers of cellular inflammation, matrix stimulation, and cellular growth, as well as platelet and coagulant activity, can now be studied in circulation and in situ, with alterations of fractalkine, RANTES (Regulated on Activation, Normal T Expressed and Secreted), interleukin (IL) 1-β, IL-6, soluble intercellular cell adhesion molecule (sICAM), soluble vascular cell adhesion molecule (sVCAM), sP-selectin, S-electin, von Willebrand factors, as well as serotonin, plasminogen activator inhibitor (PAI), fibrinopeptide A (fpA), and thrombomodulin, noted in biopsy samples and circulation of patients with PAH. To date, there remains need to further characterize as well as correlate changes in these factors with disease severity or progression.[32,33]

Endothelial cell (EC) activation abnormalities have been at the heart of modern understanding and therapies for PAH. Successful use of chronic NO has been demonstrated, although randomized clinical trials of such therapies remain to be orchestrated. Abnormalities in vascular endothelial growth factor (VEGF) have been described in patients with PAH, although where these abnormalities lie in the activation of the overall inflammation/constriction scheme, and the effect of modulators of these factors remain unknown.

The role of serotonin as a trigger for development of PAH was highlighted by the fen-Phen epidemic, with direct action on PA smooth muscle cell 5-hydroxy-tryptamine (5-HT)-2A and 5-HT-1B receptors (↓ cAMP), as well as via direct cellular entry to trigger proliferation (phosphorylation of guanosine 5'-triphosphate (GTP)-ase activating protein).[34] A unified theory of serotonin activation remains to be clearly defined, though trials of serotonin receptor blockers and serotonin transporters have been suggested. Other abnormalities in smooth muscle (sM) cell components in patients with PAH may include dysfunctional voltage-dependent potassium channels, which can be altered with anorexigenic agents including aminorex, dexfenfluramine, and phentermine (Kv 1.5 and Kv 2.1). Similar to changes in EC, where sM abnormalities lie in the activation of the overall inflammation/constriction scheme of PAH, and the effect of modulators of these factors, remain unknown.

Increased extracellular matrix production is a hallmark of PAH, with abnormalities of serine elastase, causing elevation in basic fibroblast growth factor (bFGF) leading to changes in matrix metalloproteinase (MMP) production of tenascin and phophorylation of growth factor receptors and sM cell proliferation.[35] Where such abnormalities in matrix activation lie in the overall inflammation/constriction scheme of PAH, and the effect of modulators of these factors also remain unknown.

General considerations (see also Chapter 22)

The risk of pregnancy-related death for women with PAH is substantial, with mortality in the modern era anecdotally similar to that previously reported as 30–50%, despite use of modern pulmonary vasoactive agents.[36] For women who present during pregnancy, maternal and fetal risk of termination may be equally substantial, if not greater, depending upon timing of presentation. Warfarin-based teratogenic risk may be substantial at doses typically used in PAH therapy, although it is less clearly defined. Any such patient maintaining pregnancy is advised to do so only in regional centers of such expertise, with access to all levels of supportive and heroic maternal and fetal care. Reliable and educated contraception remains a hallmark of appropriate care, though the appropriateness and effectiveness of individual therapies (in particular, hormonal contraception) remain untested in this population. Tubal ligation, similar to any noncardiopulmonary surgery, in patients with PAH, may carry substantial morbid and mortal risk, and should not be undertaken without consideration of alternatives.

Summary

We have begun to better understand the genetic, inflammatory, growth, and apoptosis bases supporting the mechanisms underlying the development and sustenance of PAH. Gender-based differences in occurrence and effect of PAH require further study. Translation of this understanding to improving markers to define current state, progression, disease untreated prognosis, potential for regulation and control of disease, and responsiveness to therapy, may be within closer reach. Similarly, study of mechanisms of RV acute and chronic decompensation, as well as study of innovative techniques to support the right ventricle during afterload manipulation, can be practically undertaken, and will likely lead to new therapies and practice paradigms in the practical future. In addition, understanding of the multiple triggers combining to cause PA hypertension, with targeting of therapies frequently derived from nonstandard modalities, will lead to increasingly novel approaches with improvement in life quality and quantity for patients affected with PAH, as well as secondary forms of pulmonary hypertension. These therapies have proven to be costly, though they have already added greatly to life quality and quantity for those affected.

References

1. Rich S, Rubin L, Walker AM, Scheewiess S, Abenheim L. Anorexigens and pulmonary hypertension in the United States: results from the Surveillance of North American Pulmonary Hypertension. *Chest* 2000; **117**: 870–4.

2. Newman JH, Fanburg BL, Archer SL, et al. Pulmonary arterial hypertension. Future directions. Report of a National Heart, Lung and Blood Institute/Office of Rare Diseases Workshop. *Circulation* 2004; **109**: 2947–52.

3. Rich S, Dantzker DR, Ayres SM, et al. Primary pulmonary hypertension: a national prospective study. *Ann Intern Med* 1987; **107**:216–23.

4. The International Primary Pulmonary Hypertension Study Group. The international primary pulmonary hypertension study (IPPHS). *Chest* 1994; **105**:37S–41S.

5. Abenheim L, Moride Y, Brenot F, et al. Appetite-suppressant drugs and the risk of primary pulmonary hypertension. International Primary Pulmonary

Hypertension Study Group. *N Engl J Med* 1996; **335**: 609–16.

6. Yamane K, Ihn H, Asano Y, et al. Clinical and laboratory features of scleroderma patients with pulmonary hypertension. *Rheumatology* 2000; **39**:1269–71.

7. Speich R, Jenni R, Opravil M, Pfab M, Russi EW. Primary pulmonary hypertension in HIV infection. *Chest* 1991; **100**:128–71.

8. Hadengue A, Benhayoun M, Lebrec D, Benhamou JP. Portal hypertension complication portal hypertension. Prevalence and relation to splanchnic hemodynamics. *Gastroenterology* 1991; **100**:520–8.

9. D'Alonzo GG, Barst RJ, Ayres SM, et al. Survival in patients with primary pulmonary hypertension: results from a natural prospective registry. *Ann Intern Med* 1991; **115**:343–9.

10. Oya H, Nagaya N, Uematsu M, et al. Poor prognosis and related factors in adults with Eisenmenger syndrome. *Am Heart J* 2002; **143**:739–44.

11. Rich S, Kaufmann E, Levy PS. The effect of high doses of calcium-channel blockers on survival in primary pulmonary hypertension. *N Engl J Med* 1992; **327**:76–81.

12. Sitbon O, Humbert M, Ioos V, Simmoneau G. Who does benefit from calcium-channel blocker therapy in primary pulmonary hypertension? *Am J Respir Crit Care Med* 2003; **167**:A440.

13. Moser KM, Auger WR, Fedullo PF. Chronic major-vessel thromboembolic pulmonary hypertension. *Circulation* 1990; **81**:1735–43.

14. Kreutzer J, Landzberg MJ, Preminger TJ, et al. Isolated peripheral pulmonary artery stenoses in the adult. *Circulation* 1996; **93**:1417–23.

15. Feinstein JA, Goldhaber SZ, Lock JE, et al. Balloon pulmonary angioplasty for treatment of chronic thromboembolic pulmonary hypertension. *Circulation* 2001; **103**:10–13.

16. Wensel R, Optiz CF, Anker SD, et al. Assessment of survival in patients with primary pulmonary hypertension: importance of cardiopulmonary exercise testing. *Circulation* 2002; **106**:319–24.

17. McLaughlin VV, Presberg KW, Doyle RL, et al. Prognosis of pulmonary arterial hypertension: ACCP evidence-based clinical practice guidelines. *Chest* 2004; **126**:78S–92S.

18. Barst RJ, Rubin LJ, Long WA, et al for the Primary Pulmonary Hypertension Study Group. A comparison of continuous intravenous epoprostenol (prostacyclin) with conventional therapy for primary pulmonary hypertension. *N Engl J Med* 1996; **334**:296–301.

19. Shapiro SM, Oudiz RF, Cao T, et al. Primary pulmonary hypertension: improved long-term effects and survival with continuous intravenous epoprostenol infusion. *J Am Coll Cardiol* 1997; **30**:343–9.

20. Simonneau G, Barst RJ, Galie N, et al. Continuous subcutaneous infusion of treprostinil, a prostacyclin analogue, in patients with pulmonary arterial hypertension: a double-blind, randomized, placebo-controlled trial. *Am J Respir Crit Care Med* 2002; **165**: 800–4.

21. *Medical Letter* 2002; **1139** (September 16):80–2.

22. Galie N, Humbert M, Vachiery JL, et al. Effects of beraprost sodium, an oral prostacylcin analogue, in patients with pulmonary arterial hypertension: a randomized double-blind, placebo-controlled trial. *J Am Coll Cardiol* 2002; **39**:1496–502.

23. Barst RJ, McGoon M, McLaughlin V, et al. Beraprost therapy for pulmonary arterial hypertension. *J Am Coll Cardiol* 2003; **41**:2119–25.

24. Olschewski H, Simonneau G, Galie N, et al. Inhaled iloprost in severe pulmonary hypertension. *N Engl J Med* 2002; **347**:322–9.

25. Rubin LJ, Badesch DB, Barst RJ, et al. Bosentan therapy for pulmonary arterial hypertension. *N Engl J Med* 2002; **346**:896–903 [erratum: *N Engl J Med* 2002; **346**:1258].

26. *Medical Letter* 2002; **1127** (April 1):30–2.

27. McLaughlin VV, Shillington A, Rich S. Survival in primary pulmonary hypertension: the impact of epoprostenol therapy. *Circulation* 2002; **106**:1477–82.

28. Du L, Sullivan CC, Chu D, et al. Signalling molecules in nonfamilial pulmonary hypertension. *N Engl J Med* 2003; **348**:500–9.

29. Newman JH, Wheeler L, Lane KB, et al. Mutation in the gene for bone morphogenetic protein receptor II as a cause of pulmonary hypertension in a large kindred. *N Engl J Med* 2001; **345**:319–24.

30. Trembath RC, Thomson JR, Machado RD, et al. Clinical and molecular genetic features of pulmonary hypertension in patients with hereditary hemorrhagic telangiectasia. *N Engl J Med* 2001; **345**:325–34.

31. Lee SD, Shroyer KR, Markham NE, et al. Monoclonal endothelial cell proliferation is present in primary but not secondary pulmonary hypertension. *J Clin Invest* 1998; **101**:927–34.

32. Dorfmuller P, Zarka V, Durand-Gasselin I, et al. Chemokine RANTES in severe pulmonary arterial hypertension. *Am J Respir Crit Care Med* 2002; **165**: 534–9.

33. Welsh CH, Hassell KL, Badesch DB, et al. Coagulation and fibrinolytic profiles in patients with severe pulmonary hypertension. *Chest* 1996; **110**:710–17.

34. McLean MR, Herve P, Eddahibi S, Adnot S.

5–hydroxytryptamine and the pulmonary circulation: receptors, transporters, and relevance to pulmonary arterial hypertension. *Br J Pharmacol* 2000; **131**: 161–8.

35. Cowan KN, Jones PL, Rabinovitch M, et al. Elastase and matrix metalloproteinase inhibitors induce regression, and tenascin antisense prevents regression of vascular disease. *J Clin Invest* 2000; **105**:21–34.

36. Weiss BM, Zemp L, Seifert B, Hess OM. Outcome of pulmonary vascular disease in pregnancy. A systematic overview from 1978–1996. *J Am Coll Cardiol* 1998; **31**:1650–7.

35

Anorectic drugs and their cardiopulmonary effects

Sangeeta B. Shah and Neil J. Weissman

Introduction

In spite of society's preoccupation with weight loss, the epidemic of obesity is continuing to increase. The 1999–2000 National Health and Nutrition Examination Survey (NHANES) estimated that 64% of US adults are either overweight or obese, an increase of 8% in just 6 years (Fig. 35.1). Furthermore, more of the overweight subjects are becoming obese. The prevalence of obesity has doubled during this same period from 15% to 30.5%. Women predominate among the obese population. The NHANES 1999–2000 data report a greater percentage of obesity among women (33%) than men (28%). While there was no difference in obesity and overweight based on race among men, nonHispanic black women have the highest rate of obesity in women. The prevalence of overweight or obesity in nonHispanic black women over 40 years old is greater than 80%![1]

Obesity is a matter of considerable public health importance and needs to be treated effectively. Obese patients have a higher rate of cardiovascular disease (CVD), diabetes, obstructive sleep apnea, some cancers, osteoarthritis, and psychological disorders. Overweight is defined as a body mass index (BMI) of 25–29.9 kg/m² and obesity is defined as a BMI of at least 30 kg/m². The National Institutes of Health (NIH) recommends weight loss for all obese individuals and for overweight individuals with two or more risk factors for obesity-related diseases listed above. Currently, pharmacologic treatment of obesity is approved for individuals with a BMI of ≥27 with obesity-related disease or a BMI of ≥30, even in the absence of an obesity-related disease.[2]

Of the 59 million obese adults in the US, at least 10% of women and 3% of men report use of medication for weight loss.[3] For these reasons, it is important to understand the mechanisms and cardiopulmonary effects of weight loss agents. This chapter will review

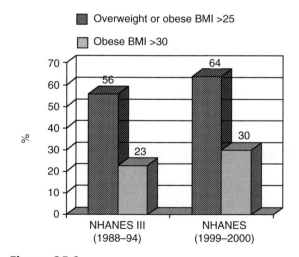

Figure 35.1
Age-adjusted prevalence of overweight and obese individuals among US adults aged 20 years and older. BMI, body mass index. Source: http://www.cdc.gov/nchs/products/pubs/pubd/hestats/obese/obse99figs1and2.htm#fig%202.

Table 35.1 Appetite suppressants

Noradrenergic	Serotonergic	Combination noradrenergic and serotonergic	Lipase inhibitor
Benzphetamine (Didrex)	Fenfluramine (Pondimin)*	Sibutramine (Meridia)	Orlistat (Xenical)
Diethylpropion (Tenuate, Tenuate Dospan, Tepanil Ten-Tab)	Dexfenfluramine (Redux)*		
Phendimetrazine (Adipost, Bontril, Melfiat, Obezine, Phendiet, Plegine, Prelu-2, PT 105)			
Mazindol (Mazanor, Sanorex)			
Phentermine (Ionamin, Fastin, Pro-fast, Teramine, Zantyrl)			
Contraindications: hypertension, advanced cardiovascular disease, hyperthyroidism, glaucoma, known hypersensitivity to appetite suppressants, history of drug abuse, epilepsy	Contraindications	Contraindications: severe hypertension, CHD, CHF, arrhythmias, stroke, glaucoma, hepatic/renal dysfunction, known hypersensitivity	Contraindications: chronic malabsorption syndrome or cholestasis
Potential drug interactions: MAOI, SSRI, other appetite suppressants, asthma drugs, CNS stimulants, TCA	Potential drug interactions	Potential drug interactions: MAOI, other serotonergic drugs, CNS stimulants, other appetite suppressants	Potential drug interactions: cyclosporine

MAOI, monoamine oxidase inhibitor; SSRI, selective serotonin reuptake inhibitors; TCA, tricyclic antidepressants.
[Source: www.pdr.net].
*No longer on the market.

the anorectic drugs used over the last 20 years, their association with pulmonary hypertension and valvular heart disease and recommendations for patients who have taken such anorectic drugs.

Pharmacotherapy

As the prevalence of obesity increases, the market for anorectic drugs is increasing in both women and men. A phenomenal $321 million was spent in the US in 1 year (1999) on prescription medications for the treatment of obesity.[4] In addition, more than $5.1 million was spent on herbal therapies.[5] As is evident from their increasing prevalence of obesity and prescription use, women are the leading users of anorectic drugs. The use of these agents was greatest between 1994 and 1996, with the use of the combina-

tion of fenfluramine and phentermine (fen-phen). Monthly prescriptions of phentermine and fenfluramine were estimated at approximately 11 million in 1996.[6] Anorectic medications are divided into two major groups: (1) the reduction of intake by decreasing appetite or increasing satiety and (2) reduction of nutrient absorption (Table 35.1).

Reduction of intake

These appetite suppressants act on neurotransmitters and are grouped into two classes: noradrenergic and serotonergic.

Noradrenergic anorectic drugs

One of the first and most familiar noradrenergic drugs introduced in 1959 was phentermine.[7] Other noradrenergic drugs approved in the US include benzphetamine, diethlypropion, phendimetrazine, and mazindol.[8] Noradrenergic agents produce appetite suppression but the exact mechanism of action is not known. The Food and Drug Administration (FDA) recommends appetite suppressants for the treatment of obesity only for 'a few weeks', while patients learn new ways to eat and exercise. Noradrenergic drugs are contraindicated in individuals with advanced atherosclerosis, CVD, moderate to severe hypertension, hyperthyroidism, glaucoma, and known hypersensitivity to sympathomimetics agents. Additionally, co-administration with selective serotonin reuptake inhibitors (SSRIs) is not established and not recommended in the product labeling.[9]

Serotonergic drugs

In 1973 fenfluramine (Pondimin) became available as an appetite suppressant and more than two decades later, in 1996 dexfenfluramine (Redux) was approved by the FDA.[10] The rationale for the use of these agents is that serotonin suppresses appetite. Fenfluramine and dexfenfluramine increase serotonin concentrations in the brain by inhibiting reuptake and simultaneously stimulating release of serotonin. Fenfluramine was inconsistent in its effect on weight loss and showed disappointing weight gain at 1 year when compared with the behavioral control group.[11] Dexfenfluramine, the d-isomer of fenfluramine, was the active form of the racemic mixture and had greater potency. It reduced daily energy intake by 10–15% and maintained significant weight loss at 1 year, with the most weight loss occurring in the first 6 months. The FDA approved dexfenfluramine for treatment up to 1 year.[12] In 1997, both of these agents were withdrawn from the market because of their association with valvular heart disease and pulmonary hypertension.[13] SSRIs such as fluoxetine and sertraline initially illustrated weight loss, but failed to show long-term efficacy. There is no evidence of an association between valvular disease and the SSRIs.[14]

Combination noradrenergic and serotonergic

In an effort to reduce side effects of the anorectic drugs, and produce consistent and significant weight loss, Weintraub in 1992 published results of dramatic weight loss, maintained up to 4 years, with the combination of the noradrenergic agent, phentermine, and the serotonergic agent, fenfluramine (fen-phen).[15] Although the FDA approved each drug individually, combination therapy was an 'off-label' use. It was during the peak use of this famous fen-phen combination that fenfluramine was removed from the market. On November 24, 1997, soon after the withdrawal of fenfluramine and dexfenfluramine, another combination drug, sibutramine (Meridia), was introduced to the market.[16] Sibutramine not only inhibits reuptake of both serotonin and norepinephrine, but also weakly inhibits dopamine uptake. Sibutramine, in combination with diet management, achieves weight loss of 5–8% and can be taken for up to 2 years. The most common side effects of sibutramine include dry mouth, headache, constipation, insomnia, tachycardia, and elevation of blood pressure. It can be used with caution in patients with controlled hypertension, but is contraindicated in patients with uncontrolled hypertension, coronary heart disease, congestive heart failure, arrhythmias or stroke. Sibutramine results in an average heart rate increase of 3–4 beats/min and an average increase in blood pressure of 2 mmHg.[17] In March 2002, Public Citizen, a national consumer organization, petitioned the FDA to ban sibutramine. They claimed that sibutramine resulted in 29 deaths in the US and that an additional 143 patients developed cardiac arrhythmias. There was concern that the paradoxical increase in blood pressure and heart rate with weight loss may aggravate obesity-related co-morbidities.[18] This created international concern since by 2002 nearly 8.5 million individuals worldwide were taking sibutramine. Once the data were reviewed, the fatality numbers were lower than one would expect in a similarly ill obese population. It was determined that the overall risk/benefit ratio was favorable and the drug was not removed from the market.[19] In a study performed by Bach et al., sibutramine demonstrated no association with valvular disease. This may be because, unlike fenfluramine and dexfenfluramine, sibutramine does not induce serotonin release.[20]

Reduction of nutrient absorption

Orlistat (Xenical), introduced in April 1999, reduces nutrient absorption by binding to gastrointestinal lipases in the gut lumen and preventing hydrolysis of the dietary fats. It effectively blocks absorption of approximately 30% of ingested fat calories, resulting in an average weight loss of 9% in the individual taking the drug for 1 year. However, there is also a high rate of discontinuation secondary to the side effects of flatulence, fecal urgency and incontinence, steatorrhea, and increased frequency of defecation. No cardiovascular side effects or contraindications have been reported. One potential drug interaction is a change in anticoagulation levels with the use of warfarin, since orlistat inhibits absorption of vitamins.[21]

Herbal supplements

Herbal supplements, which are not regulated by the FDA, are widely available to the public. Not only are the data on herbal supplements based on poorly designed trials, but also the supplements have variable amounts of active ingredients that could result in life-threatening adverse events. Some agents which promote weight loss are chitosan, conjugated linoleic acid, *Garcinia cambogia*, chromium picolinate, and ephedra alkaloids. Ephedra alkaloid, an adrenergic agent, is often combined with caffeine. Serious cardiovascular and neurologic events, such as hypertension, myocardial infarction (MI), sudden death, arrhythmias, stroke and seizures, have been reported.[5] It is crucial to be aware of products containing herbal supplements and to check for drug–drug interactions. At this time the NIH does not endorse the use of any herbal supplement for the treatment of obesity and after the withdrawal of phenylpropanolamine in 2000, there is no over-the-counter approved appetite suppressant.[22]

Other potential anorectic drugs

There have been several clinical trials investigating the use of bupropion (Wellbutrin), topiramate (Topamax), and metformin (Glucophage) for the treatment of obesity. Bupropion, generally used for the treatment of depression or smoking addiction, has a chemical structure similar to diethylpropion, a noradrenergic anorectic drug. It is a weak inhibitor of the reuptake of dopamine, serotonin, and norepinephrine and results in weight loss. Although the overall incidence is very low, bupropion has been associated with an increased incidence of hypertension for which close monitoring is recommended.[23] A study at the Veterans Administration Medical Center showed a weight loss of 5%, 7.2%, and 10.1% at the end of 24 weeks for placebo, bupropion SR 300 mg/day, and 400 mg/day, respectively, with sustained weight loss at 48 weeks.[24] Weight loss is also observed in patients taking the antiepileptic, topiramate. The mechanism of weight loss with topiramate is most likely reduced caloric intake. The initial safety and efficacy studies showed a 5–10% weight reduction compared with placebo. However, there was a high rate of withdrawal from the study, with the most frequent complaints being paresthesia, somnolence, and difficulty with memory and concentration. All events were dose-related and usually resolved spontaneously with discontinuation of the drug.[25] There are no known significant cardiovascular side effects from topiramate.[26] Metformin (Glucophage) is used for the treatment of type 2 diabetes mellitus by decreasing hepatic glucose production, decreasing intestinal absorption, and improving insulin sensitivity. Most recently the Diabetes Prevention Program Research Group randomized nondiabetic, obese individuals with elevated fasting blood sugars (95–125 mg/dl) and post-load blood glucose (140–199 mg/dl) to placebo, metformin, or lifestyle modification for a mean of 2.8 years. The weight loss was modest in the metformin group (2 kg). More importantly, compared with placebo, there was a reduction in the incidence of diabetes of 31% in the metformin group. The benefit appears to be greatest in those with metabolic syndrome. Metformin has a low incidence of cardiovascular side effects; however, it is contraindicated in patients with congestive heart failure requiring pharmacologic treatment.[27] Ongoing studies will continue to evaluate the efficacy and long-term safety of these drugs for the treatment of obesity.

Another interesting drug is leptin, a cytokine-like protein made in the adipose tissue and transported into the brain where it inhibits food intake by altering the expression of hypothalamic neurotransmitters. Leptin raises the hope that a normally occurring hormone could result in weight loss without adverse effects. Leptin works effectively in individuals with hyperphagia as a result of low leptin levels. However, studies in obese individuals with high leptin levels (leptin insensitive) have been disappointing. To achieve effective weight loss, it may be necessary to overcome the leptin insensitivity by developing agents that act distal to leptin action.[28]

Pulmonary hypertension (see also Chapter 34)

Pulmonary hypertension is defined as a mean pulmonary artery pressure exceeding 25 mmHg at rest or 30 mmHg with exercise. The incidence of primary pulmonary hypertension is 2 per 1 million with the mean age of occurrence of 35 years and a predominance in women (2.4:1 ratio).[29] Today it is known that some anorectic drugs contribute to the risk of developing pulmonary hypertension but the exact mechanism for these drugs remains elusive.

The first epidemiologic evidence suggesting an association between appetite suppressants and pulmonary hypertension came in the 1960s from Western Europe. Aminorex fumarate (Menocil), introduced in Austria, Germany, and Switzerland in 1965, has chemical properties similar to epinephrine and amphetamines. Prior to 1965, it was noted that the prevalence of primary pulmonary hypertension in the area was 0.87%. However by 1967, the prevalence had increased to 13.5%. This 10-fold increase in incidence led to the withdrawal of aminorex fumarate from the market in 1972. Unfortunately, the morbidity and mortality from this drug was monumental. The number of women who developed drug-induced pulmonary hypertension outnumbered the men 4:1 and sadly only 50% of the women prescribed the drug suffered from obesity. The mortality rate from aminorex-induced pulmonary hypertension was approximately 50%.[30]

In 1993, a national referral center for pulmonary hypertension in France retrospectively reviewed their population of primary pulmonary hypertension from 1988 to 1992. Of the 73 patients with pulmonary hypertension, 15 patients had taken fenfluramine for a minimum of 3 months. All subjects were women and it was concluded that 20% of patients with primary pulmonary hypertension had exposure to fenfluramine derivatives. They noted that the survival in this group of patients was no different from the survival of those with other forms of primary pulmonary hypertension.[31]

A landmark study from the International Primary Pulmonary Hypertension Study Group (IPPHS) published in 1996 was a prospective case-control study conducted in France, Belgium, the UK, and the Netherlands. The study sought to investigate the causative roles of suspected risk factors, especially anorectic drugs, in primary pulmonary hypertension. The following appetite suppressants were analyzed: derivatives of fenfluramine (fenfluramine and dexfenfluramine), mazindol, fenproporex, amphetamine-like anorexic drugs (diethylpropion), chobenzorex, and phenmetrazine. Ninety-five eligible patients with primary pulmonary hypertension were recruited from 1992 to 1994 at the time of right heart catheterization. Four matched controls for each patient with primary pulmonary hypertension were recruited for a total of 355 control patients. Among the patients with primary pulmonary hypertension, the incidence in women outnumbered men 2.3:1. The odds ratio of pulmonary hypertension secondary to the use of appetite suppressants was 6.3 with a 95% confidence interval (CI) of 3.0–13.2. Women who have primary pulmonary hypertension are almost eight times more likely to have taken anorectic drugs. Interestingly, the odds ratio increases dramatically when the duration of exposure was greater than 3 months to 23.1 (95% CI 6.9–77.7), implying that duration of treatment may increase the risk of pulmonary hypertension. Both dexfenfluramine and fenfluramine were primarily used in both groups. The IPPHS group was able to suggest strongly a causal relationship between anorectic drugs and pulmonary hypertension. They boldly state that the absolute risk of pulmonary hypertension for obese patients on appetite suppressants for longer than 3 months would be more than 30 times higher than nonusers.[32] The FDA approved dexfenfluramine 2 months prior to the publication of the IPPHS results. The labeling of dexfenfluramine was modified and, based on the risk:benefit ratio, the use was acceptable in appropriate patients.[10]

A year later, the first case implicating combination therapy of fenfluramine and phentermine as a cause of pulmonary hypertension was reported in the US. After only 23 days of treatment, an obese (BMI 32 kg/m^2) 29-year-old woman developed symptoms of pulmonary hypertension with shortness of breath. Although symptoms initially improved with discontinuation of the drug, she returned with symptoms of shortness of breath and right heart failure and died several months later.[33]

Possible mechanisms

The mechanism by which fenfluramine, dexfenfluramine, and aminorex increase the risk of pulmonary hypertension is unknown. However, many avenues of investigation are seeking to delineate the mechanism in the hope of avoiding this fatal complication with new drug formulations.

Serotonergic hypothesis

Serotonin (5-HT) promotes pulmonary smooth muscle cell proliferation, which can result in potent pulmonary vasoconstriction in susceptible individuals. Anorectic drugs increase serum serotonin levels by inhibition of serotonin reuptake and release of serotonin from receptors and nerve endings. This increased serotonin has been implicated as the cause of anorectic-induced pulmonary hypertension.[34] However, this theory does not provide a complete explanation for several reasons. (1) Pathological levels of serotonin occur in patients with carcinoid who fail to develop pulmonary hypertension. (2) Serotonin levels are not consistently elevated in patients taking these anorectic drugs. In fact, chronic use of fen-phen lowered plasma serotonin levels in some patients.[35] (3) Despite similar increases in serotonin levels, SSRIs used as antidepressants are not associated with a higher incidence of pulmonary hypertension.[14] In attempts to reconcile these inconsistencies in the serotonin hypothesis, investigators have focused on the serotonin transporter (5-HTT) and its role in the development of pulmonary hypertension. 5-HTT is abundantly located in the smooth muscle cells (SMC) of the pulmonary vasculature. In addition to its involvement in the uptake and inactivation of serotonin, 5-HTT also mediates the proliferation of

SMC. Studies have shown an overexpression of 5-HTT in pulmonary artery SMC from patients with pulmonary hypertension. The anorectic drug attaches to the transporter resulting in inhibition of reuptake of serotonin at one site and in proliferation of SMCs of the pulmonary vasculature at another. In addition, there may be genetic predisposition to anorexigen-induced pulmonary hypertension.[36] Research has shown heterogeneity of the promoter region of the 5-HTT. The L-allele of the promoter region results in a two to three times higher level of 5-HTT transcription than the S-allele. Preliminary studies show that the L/L genotype occurs in 60–70% of individuals with pulmonary hypertension as compared with only 20–30% of a control population.[37]

Epidemiologic studies now strongly suggest an increased incidence of pulmonary hypertension associated with the anorectic drugs fenfluramine, dexfenfluramine, and aminorex. However, the exact mechanism remains unclear. Anorectic drugs may result in pulmonary hypertension secondary to elevated circulating serotonin levels, substrate-induced activation of 5-HTT, increased expression of 5-HTT, a genetic predisposition, and/or inhibition of ion channels.

Clinical treatment for anorectic drug-induced pulmonary hypertension

All patients with a history of appetite suppressant use should be questioned about symptoms of pulmonary hypertension, type of drug used, and duration of treatment. No diagnostic evaluation is recommended unless the patient has symptoms or abnormal physical findings. Treatment of patients with anorectic drug-induced pulmonary hypertension is the same as patients with primary pulmonary hypertension: anticoagulation, supplemental oxygen, diuretics, and vasodilators.[38] Although regression with discontinuation of the anorectic drug is occasionally seen, the prognosis of these individuals is truly unknown. Some feel that the prognosis is based on histopathology since the cases display a wide range of pathologic grades from grade 1 – medial hypertrophy to grade 4 – plexogenic arteriopathy.[33] Others have conducted a retrospective study showing no survival difference between the fenfluramine-induced pulmonary hypertension and primary pulmonary hypertension (PPH).[31] However, recent analysis of the NIH Registry of PPH, produced very alarming results. The survival at 36 months in patients with fenfluramine-induced pulmonary hypertension was 18% compared with 46% in the non-diet pill group with pulmonary hypertension.[39]

Appetite suppressants and valvular heart disease (see also Chapter 33)

Originally, the only two drugs associated with valvular heart disease were ergotamine and methysergide. The overall prevalence of valvulopathy from exposure to either one of these drugs is very small since its use is limited. However, the implication of valvulopathy from appetite suppressants created a national scare because of the potential consequences for over 5 million individuals. This potential side effect led to the withdrawal of fenfluramine and dexfenfluramine from the market and to numerous investigations to determine the association of these agents and valvular heart disease. This topic is fundamentally important to women's health since women are more likely to use appetite suppressants, as evidenced by the fact that 80–90% of patients receiving a prescription for these agents or involved in these clinical studies were women.

The initial MeritCare/Mayo report

Beginning in 1994, the sonographers and physicians at MeritCare Center in Fargo, ND noticed an uncanny increase in the incidence of valvular regurgitation in obese women taking the combination of fenfluramine and phentermine. This observation prompted the physicians to contact the Mayo Clinic who, unaware of any association of anorectic drugs with valvular regurgitation, evaluated the cases from MeritCare and additional cases from their center. In the summer of 1997, these investigators published a report of 24 patients (18 from MeritCare) in whom valvular regurgitation was associated with the use of combination fenfluramine and phentermine. The patients were women between the ages of 30 and 63, who presented with either cardiovascular symptoms or a new murmur after taking fen-phen for 1–28 months. All 24 patients were women and all had echocardiograms revealing morphologically abnormal left and/or right-sided cardiac valves: thickening and restricted motion of the mitral, aortic and tricuspid (especially the septal and anterior leaflets) valve(s) resulting in lack of coaptation. These morphological abnormalities led to various degrees of regurgitation of the mitral, tricuspid and aortic valves. Most of the women had aortic regurgitation (79%) and mitral regurgitation (92%) (Fig. 35.2). The most troublesome observation was that five women developed severe regurgitation requiring surgery and valve replacement and eight women

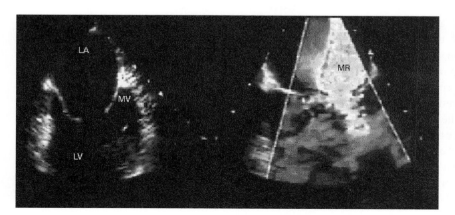

Figure 35.2
Intraoperative transesophageal echocardiography. Thickened mitral valve (MV) during diastole (left) and severe mitral regurgitation (MR) (right). LA, left atrium; LV, left ventricle.

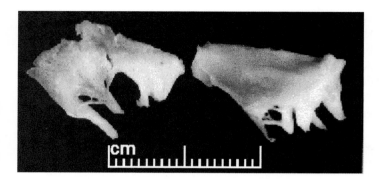

Figure 35.3
Excised mitral valve. Glistening white leaflets and chordae with mild to moderate irregular diffuse thickening. Reproduced from reference 40 with permission.

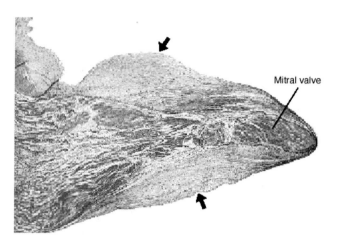

Mitral valve

Figure 35.4
Histology of mitral valve. Intact valve architecture with 'stuck-on' plaques (arrows). Reproduced from reference 40 with permission.

developed pulmonary hypertension with right ventricular systolic pressures >50 mmHg, mostly due to the severity of valvular regurgitation. The gross and histologic findings were similar to carcinoid-induced valvular disease, suggesting a serotonin-mediated mechanism. Gross pathology of the women who underwent surgery showed glistening white, thickened leaflets with chordal thickening (Fig. 35.3). Microscopically, the diseased valves revealed proliferative myofibroblasts in an abundant extracellular matrix creating a 'stuck-on' appearance of plaques on the leaflet[40] (Fig. 35.4). Interestingly, a few years later, a detailed examination of the Fargo patients discovered that some of these patients may have had reasons other than the consumption of fen-phen for valvular disease: two of 18 patients had a history of rheumatic fever and ergotamine use, an additional four had murmurs prior to the use of fen-phen, and most used

concomitant SSRIs, which may have a synergistic effect with fen-phen.[41]

FDA case definition and prevalence data

Because of the high sensitivity of Doppler echocardiography, it was very important to determine the amount of regurgitation that should be considered abnormal. The FDA used several epidemiologic studies to sort out the true 'background' prevalence of valvular regurgitation. Using CARDIA, an epidemiologic study of 4000 healthy adults between the ages of 23 and 35 years and other data (Framingham Heart Study, Cardiovascular Health Study and others), the FDA case definition of significant regurgitation was defined as the presence of at least moderate mitral regurgitation or at least mild aortic regurgitation. This degree of regurgitation is expected in <5% of young, healthy adults.[42,43]

Subsequently, several hundred patients with appetite suppressant-related valvular disease were reported to the FDA MedWatch program. By September 1997, 21 patients treated with anorectic drugs required valvular surgery, of whom three died. Five centers which performed echocardiograms on patients who had taken dexfenfluramine and fenfluramine alone or in combination with phentermine found a prevalence of valvulopathy (using the FDA definition) from 28.7 to 38.3%. Most subjects were women (87%) with a mean age of 48 years and median duration of drug exposure of 14 months.[13] This significant prevalence of valvulopathy in a group of young and middle-aged women raised serious public health concerns about the safety of anorectic drugs. On September 15, 1997 the FDA announced the withdrawal of fenfluramine and its isomer, dexfenfluramine, from the market.

The uncertainty (1997–1998)

In an effort to better define the association between appetite suppressants and valvular heart disease, three studies examined this relationship and were published in September 1998 in the *New England Journal of Medicine*. Using the General Practice Research Database in the UK, Jick et al. evaluated the risk of newly diagnosed valvular disease in users of fenfluramine, dexfenfluramine, and phentermine compared with obese patients not using these drugs.[44] In the case group of individuals, 87% of patients were women with an average age of 43 years. This group was composed of 6532 dexfenfluramine users, 2371 fenfluramine users, and 862 phentermine users. The control population was composed of obese subjects matched for age, sex, and weight. Of the 11 newly diagnosed cases of valve disease, five used dexfenfluramine and six used fenfluramine. No cases of valvulopathy occurred among the obese control population or those taking phentermine alone. These data supported the fact that obesity by itself does not cause a higher prevalence of valvular regurgitation. The 5-year cumulative incidence of valvular disease in individuals who

had taken fenfluramine or its derivative for less than 4 months was 7.1 per 10 000 subjects. An important observation was that duration of ≥4 months of treatment dramatically increased the 5-year cumulative incidence to 35 per 10 000 subjects. Nevertheless, the prevalence of valvular disease secondary to appetite suppressants in this study was approximately 0.1%, drastically different from the initial reports of up to 38%.

In the same *Journal* issue, Khan et al. reported a cross-sectional, case-controlled investigation to evaluate the prevalence and severity of valve regurgitation in obese patients on anorectic drugs.[45] They enrolled 233 patients who had previously enrolled in pharmacologic appetite suppressant studies (87% women) and compared them to 233 obese controls matched for age, sex, BMI, and height. Echocardiography was performed on all subjects and was read in a blinded fashion. Compared with the control group, a significant number of patients who had taken an appetite suppressant developed a valvulopathy (22.7% vs 1.3%); the most common valvular dysfunction was aortic regurgitation. The prevalence was higher in the patients taking fen-phen (25.2%) and dex-fen (22.6%) than patients taking dexfenfluramine alone (12.8%).

A third study performed by Weissman et al. was a modification of an ongoing randomized, double-blind, placebo-controlled trial comparing dexfenfluramine, sustained-release dexfenfluramine, and placebo.[46] When dexfenfluramine was withdrawn from the market, the study was discontinued and echocardiographic examinations were performed within 1 month. A total of 1072 echocardiograms were performed in 366 patients in the dexfenfluramine group, 352 patients in the slow-release dexfenfluramine group, and 354 patients in the placebo group. The majority of subjects were female (80%) and the average duration of treatment was 72 days. Analysis using the FDA criteria for significant regurgitation illustrated no significant difference among the three groups. Aortic regurgitation of mild or greater was present in 5.0% of the dexfenfluramine (dex) group, 5.8% of the dexfenfluramine slow-release (dex SR) group, 5.4% in the combined (dex and dex SR) treatment group, and 3.6% of the placebo group. Mitral regurgitation of moderate or greater occurred in 1.7% of the dex group, 1.8% of the dex SR group, 1.8% of the combined treatment group, and 1.2% of the placebo group. There was no increase in the prevalence of pulmonary hypertension or right-sided valve disease. The lower prevalence of valvular disease in this study may be due to the short duration, less than 3 months, of treatment in these patients.

All these studies were case-controlled without sequential echocardiographic data in the same patient. In another attempt to determine the risk of valvulopathy in individual patients who had taken appetite suppressants, Wee et al. searched their database for patients who had taken appetite suppressants for at least 14 days and had an echocardiogram performed previous to treatment.[47] They were able to compare before and after therapy echocardiograms on a total of 46 patients. The 2.6% risk of developing a new or worsening valvular disease in patients on anorectic drugs was also significantly lower than previously believed. Ironically, two patients with baseline regurgitation had regression of their regurgitation after taking appetite suppressants.

Resolving the uncertainty (1999–present)

Although all these studies utilized different study designs, by the end of 1999, research seemed to support the association of valvular disease with appetite suppressants, but many issues remained unresolved including the true prevalence of association, influence of duration of treatment or combination therapy, and natural history.

True prevalence

The true prevalence of disease will never be delineated since a prospective trial comparing echocardiograms pre- and post-treatment cannot be performed now that the drug has been withdrawn from the market. However, if the trials with controls are evaluated, the overall prevalence of valvulopathy in individuals taking anorectic drugs is 6–15% with the prevalence of valvulopathy in the controls of 3–6%.[43–46] Therefore, the incremental increase in prevalence of aortic and/or mitral regurgitation, in

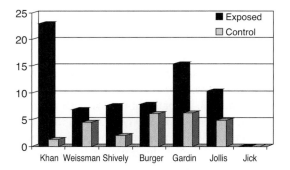

Figure 35.5
Prevalence of aortic regurgitation and mitral regurgitation. Data taken from references 44–46, 48–52.

patients taking appetite suppressants, FDA criteria regurgitation, is approximately 4–9% above background rates of regurgitation (Fig. 35.5).

Influence of duration of treatment

There is strong evidence that the incidence of valvular regurgitation increases with prolonged duration of anorectic drug use. In an initial study it was 7.4 times higher if the individual took appetite suppressants for ≥4 months.[44] In a multicenter, reader-blinded controlled design to determine the effect of duration of fenfluramine and phentermine treatment on prevalence of valvular disease, 1137 obese patients who had taken fen-phen for varying lengths of time and 672 control patients who had never taken the drug combination were enrolled.[48] The treatment group was predominantly middle-aged (mean 46 years) women (85%) who consumed the combination fen-phen for a mean duration of 11.2 months. There was a significant increased incidence of aortic regurgitation, primarily mild, in 8.8% of the treatment group compared with 3.6% of the control patients (p <0.001). The subjects treated for <6 months had a 3.6% prevalence of aortic regurgitation while those treated for >2 years had a prevalence of 17.4%; this is a fivefold increase in the prevalence of 'significant' aortic regurgitation. The consensus is that there is an increase in the prevalence of appetite suppressant-associated valvulopathy with increased duration of treatment, especially >6–9 months.

The relationship between daily dose of appetite suppressant and valvulopathy is not clear since few studies have addressed this issue. Burger et al. performed a substudy analysis of their original study and showed no difference in valvular regurgitation between low dose (less than three tablets) of phen-fen (maximum of 15 mg of phentermine and 20 mg of fenfluramine/day) and high dose (three or more tablets) of fen-phen (maximum of 45 mg of phentermine and 60 mg of fenfluramine/day).[49] However, this was a relatively small retrospective analysis.

Influence of combination therapy

It is postulated that the combination of phentermine and fenfluramine or dexfenfluramine produces an adverse synergistic effect. Some have suggested that phentermine is a monoamine oxidase inhibitor that further increases serotonin levels.[50] Khan et al. showed that combination therapy increased the risk of developing valvular regurgitation with an odds ratio of 12.7 with the use of dexfenfluramine, 24.5 with the use of dexfenfluramine and phentermine, and 26.3 with the use of fenfluramine and phentermine.[45] To address this issue, Gardin et al. performed a multicenter, reader-blinded, controlled study comparing the occurrence of valvular regurgitation in patients taking dexfenfluramine, fen-phen, and untreated controls.[51] Once again, the population was primarily middle-aged (47 years) women (74%) who were prescribed dexfenfluramine for a mean of 6.0 months and fen-phen for a mean of 11.9 months. The prevalence of aortic regurgitation, predominantly mild, was increased in the treatment group with a more pronounced increase with combination therapy; prevalence was 8.9% in the dexfenfluramine group, 13.7% in the fen-phen group, and 4.1% in the untreated group. However, the data from these two studies are confounded by the fact that the duration of treatment in each of the groups was different. Of note, patients who took anorexigens for no more than 3 months showed no increase in significant aortic regurgitation.

Natural history

Fortunately, valvulopathy secondary to appetite suppressants is likely to stabilize or regress in the majority of patients with time.[52–54] Also, latent valvular disease is unlikely to develop in an individual who does not have regurgitation soon after discontinuation of the drug.[53] To assess the natural history, follow-up echocardiograms at 1 year were performed on several cohorts.[53,54] The original and follow-up echocardiograms were evaluated side-by-side with no knowledge of treatment group or which echocardiogram was the initial and which was the follow-up. These studies showed that there was no progression or development of mitral or aortic regurgitation. In fact, there was a statistically significant decrease in aortic regurgitation in the treatment (fen-phen or dexfenfluramine) groups as compared with the untreated group. In all studies, the vast majority of patients (>80%) had no change in regurgitation severity but among those that demonstrated a change, appetite suppressant users were more likely to show regression.

Possible mechanisms of valve injury

Echocardiograms of appetite suppressant patients may demonstrate aortic or mitral regurgitation, with aortic regurgitation being more common. Initial cases reported various degrees of thickening and restricted motion of the mitral, aortic, and tricuspid leaflets and shortening of the chordal apparatus of the mitral valve. Subsequent studies have not shown this to be a consistent finding. The histology of the early cases showed irregular leaflet thickening with fibromyxoid plaques and central myxoid degeneration.[55] The echocardiographic and histologic features appeared similar to those seen with carcinoid disease and ergotamine use.

The true mechanism of appetite suppressant-induced valvulopathy is not known. One leading theory is the serotoninergic mechanism. Both fenfluramine and dexfenfluramine promote the release and prevent the reuptake of serotonin. Since the valvular pathology is similar to carcinoid disease and ergotamine use and because there is an increased concentration of serotonin metabolite receptors on the valve leaflets, the increased serotonin becomes a plausible explanation.[56] However, controversy remains, since circulating levels of serotonin and urinary metabolites of serotonin are actually lower in appetite suppressant users.[35]

Management of patients exposed to appetite suppressants

Physicians caring for patients with history of appetite suppressant use should follow the American College of Cardiology (ACC) guidelines on valvular heart disease and the specific recommendations for patients who have taken appetite suppressants. All patients must discontinue fenfluramine or its derivative and should undergo cardiac history and physical examination. If the patient has cardiac symptoms, murmur, or a body habitus that precludes proper auscultation, then an echocardiogram with Doppler study should be performed. Routine echocardiogram in all patients with a history of appetite suppressant use is not recommended. If valvular disease is present, then prophylaxis for bacterial endocarditis should be prescribed[57] (Table 35.2).

Table 35.2 ACC guidelines for patients who have used anorectic drugs: fenfluramine and or dexfenfluramine with or without phentermine

Indication	Class
Discontinuation of the anorectic drug(s)	I
Cardiac physical exam	I
Echocardiogram in patients with murmur, symptoms, associated physical findings or inadequate cardiac auscultation secondary to body habitus	I
Repeat physical exam in 6–8 months in those without murmur	IIa
Echocardiogram in all patients prior to dental procedures in the absence of symptoms, heart murmur or associated cardiac findings	IIb
Echocardiogram in all patients	III

Class I, useful/recommended; class II, conflicting evidence/controversial; class III, not useful/not recommended.

Conclusion

More women than men use appetite suppressants, which is why women were predominantly affected by pulmonary hypertension and valvular regurgitation caused by fenfluramine and dexfenfluramine. However, only a small percentage of appetite suppressant users (4–9%) actually develop valvular regurgitation, and when they do it is more likely to be milder degrees of aortic or mitral regurgitation. Furthermore, now that these agents are no longer available, the important issue is that there is no latent development or evidence of progression once the drug is withdrawn.

References

1. Flegal KM, Carroll MD, Ogden CL, Johnson CL. Prevalence and trends in obesity among US adults 1999–2000. *JAMA* 2002; **288**:1723–7.
2. NHLBI Expert Panel in the Identification, Evaluation, and Treatment of Overweight and Obesity in Adults. Clinical guidelines on the identification, evaluation, and treatment of overweight and obesity in adults: the evidence report. *Obes Res* 1998; **6** (Suppl 2):51S-2909S.
3. Khan LK, Serdula MK, Bowman BA, Williamson DF. Use of prescription weight loss pills among US adults in 1996–1998. *Ann Intern Med* 2001; **134**:282–6.
4. Wilhelm C. Growing the market for antiobesity drugs. *Chemical Market Reporter* 2000: FR23–24.
5. Roerig JL, Mitchell JE, de Zwaan M. The eating disorders medicine cabinet revisited: a clinician's guide to appetite suppressants and diuretics. *Int J Eat Disord* 2003; **33**:443–57.
6. Connolly HM, McGoon M. Obesity drugs and the heart. *Curr Prob Cardiol* 1999; **24**:745–92.
7. Phentermine. http://www.fda.gov/cder/da/da.htm [accessed December 6, 2003].
8. Drug information: appetite suppressants, sympathomimetics (systemic). http://www.nlm.nih.gov/medlineplus/druginfo/uspdi/202069.html [accessed August 10, 2003].
9. Phentermine. http://www.pdr.net/ [accessed December 6, 2003].
10. Fenfluramine and dexfenfluramine. http://www.fda.gov/cder/da/da.htm [accessed December 6, 2003].

11. Douglas JG, Gough J, Preston PG, et al. Long-term efficacy of fenfluramine in treatment of obesity. *Lancet* 1983; 1:384–6.

12. McTavish D, Heel RC. Dexfenfluramine: a review of its pharmacological properties and therapeutic potential in obesity. *Drugs* 1992; 43:713–33.

13. Cardiac valvulopathy associated with exposure to fenfluramine or dexfenfluramine: US Department of Health and Human Services interim public health recommendations, November 1997. *MMWR Morb Mortal Wkly Rep* 1997; 46:1061–6.

14. Mast ST, Gersing KR, Anstrom KJ, et al. Association between selective serotonin-reuptake inhibitor therapy and heart valve regurgitation. *Am J Cardiol* 2001; 87:989–93.

15. Weintraub M. Long-term weight control study: conclusions. *Clin Pharmacol Ther* 1992; 51:642–6.

16. Sibutramine. http://www.fda.gov/cder/da/da.htm [accessed December 6, 2003].

17. Sibutramine hydrochloride monohydrate. http://www.pdr.net/ [accessed December 6, 2003].

18. Petition to the FDA to ban the diet drug sibutramine (Meridia) (HRG Publication #1613). http://www.citizen.org/publications/print_release.cfm>ID=7160 [accessed October 14, 2003].

19. Abbott Laboratories reassures patients of the efficacy and safety of Meridia (sibutramine) and denounces public citizen's petition to the US FDA as incorrect and misleading. March 20, 2002. http:// www.abbott.com/news/press_release.cfm ?id=353 [accessed December 6, 2003].

20. Bach DS, Rissanen AM, Mendel CM, et al. Absence of cardiac valve dysfunction in obese patients treated with sibutramine. *Obes Res* 1999; 7:363–9.

21. Heck AM, Yanovski JA, Calis KA. Orlistat, a new lipase inhibitor for the management of obesity. *Pharmacotherapy* 2000; 20:270–9.

22. Kernan WN, Viscoli CM, Brass LM, et al. Phenylpropanolamine and the risk of hemorrhagic stroke. *N Engl J Med* 2000; 343:1826–32.

23. Bupropion Sustained Release Tablets. http://www.pdr.net [accessed December 6, 2003].

24. Anderson JW, Greenway FL, Fujioka K, et al. Bupropion SR enhances weight loss: a 48 week double blinded, placebo-controlled trial. *Obes Res* 2002; 10:633–41.

25. Bray GA, Hollander P, Klein S, et al. A 6–month randomized, placebo-controlled, dose ranging trial of topiramate for weight loss in obesity. *Obes Res* 2003; 11:722–33.

26. Topiramate tablets. http://www.pdr.net [accessed December 6, 2003].

27. Diabetes Prevention Program Research Group. Reduction in the incidence of type 2 diabetes with lifestyle intervention or metformin. *N Engl J Med* 2002; 346:393–403.

28. Proietto J, Thornburn AW. The therapeutic potential of leptin. *Expert Opin Investig Drugs* 2003; 12:373–8.

29. Rubin LJ, Barst RJ, Kaiser LR, et al. Primary pulmonary hypertension. *Chest* 1993; 104:236–50.

30. Gurtner HP. Aminorex and pulmonary hypertension: a review. *Cor Vasa* 1985; 27:160–71.

31. Brenot F, Herve P, Petitpretz P, Parent F, Duroux P, Simmonneau G. Primary pulmonary hypertension and fenfluramine use. *Br Heart J* 1993; 70:537–41.

32. Abenhaim L, Moride Y, Brenot F, et al. Appetite-suppressant drugs and the risk of primary pulmonary hypertension. *N Engl J Med* 1996; 335:609–16.

33. Mark EJ, Patalas ED, Chang HT, et al. Fatal pulmonary hypertension associated with short-term use of fenfluramine and phentermine. *N Engl J Med* 1997; 337:602–6.

34. Herve P, Launay JM, Scrobohaci ML, et al. Increased plasma serotonin in primary pulmonary hypertension. *Am J Med* 1995; 99:249–54.

35. Rothman RB, Redmon B, Raatz SK, et al. Chronic treatment with phentermine combined with fenfluramine lowers plasma serotonin. *Am J Cardiol* 2000; 85:913–16.

36. Rothman RB, Ayestas MA, Dersch CM, Baumann MH. Aminorex, fenfluramine, and chlorphentermine are serotonin transporter substrates: implication for primary pulmonary hypertension. *Circulation* 1999; 100:869–75.

37. Eddahibi S, Adnot S. Anorexigen-induced pulmonary hypertension and the serotonin hypothesis: lessons for the future in pathogenesis. *Respir Res* 2002; 3:9–12.

38. Rich S. Primary pulmonary hypertension. *Curr Treat Options Cardiovasc Med* 2000; 2:135–40.

39. Rich S, Shillington A, McLaughlin. Comparison of survival in patients with pulmonary hypertension associated with fenfluramine to patients with primary pulmonary hypertension. *Am J Cardiol* 2003; 92:1366–8.

40. Connolly HM, Crary JL, McGoon MD, et al. Valvular heart disease associated with fenfluramine-phentermine. *N Engl J Med* 1997; 337:581–8.

41. Kimmel SE, Keane MG, Crary JL, et al. Detailed examination of fenfluramine-phentermine users with valve abnormalities identified in Fargo, North Dakota. *Am J Cardiol* 1999; 84:304–8.

42. Klein AL, Burstow DJ, Tajik AJ, et al. Age-related prevalence of valvular regurgitation in normal subjects: a comprehensive color flow examination of 118 volunteers. *J Am Soc Echocardiogr* 1990; 3:54–63.

43. Reid CL, Gardin JM, Yunis C, Kurosaki T, Flack JM. Prevalence and clinic correlated of aortic and mitral regurgitation in a young adult population: the CARDIA Study [Abstract]. *Circulation* 1994; **90**:1519.

44. Jick, H, Vasilakis C, Weinrauch LA, Meier CR, Jick SS, Derby L. A population-based study of appetite suppressant drugs and the risk of cardiac-valve regurgitation. *N Engl J Med* 1998; **339**:719–24.

45. Khan MA, Herzog CA, St Peter JV, et al. The prevalence of cardiac valvular insufficiency assessed by transthoracic echocardiography in obese patients treated with appetite-suppressant drugs. *N Engl J Med* 1998; **339**:713–18.

46. Weissman NJ, Tighe JF, Gottdiener JS, Gwynne JT. An assessment of heart-valve abnormalities in obese patients taking dexfenfluramine, sustained-release dexfenfluramine, or placebo. *N Engl J Med* 1998; **339**:725–32.

47. Wee CC, Phillips RS, Aurigemma G, et al. Risk of valvular heart disease among users of fenfluramine and dexfenfluramine who underwent echocardiography before use of medication. *Ann Intern Med* 1998; **129**:870–4.

48. Jollis JG, Landolfo CK, Kisslo J, et al. Fenfluramine and phentermine and cardiovascular findings: effect of treatment duration on prevalence of valve abnormalities. *Circulation* 2000; **101**:2071–7.

49. Burger AJ, Sherman HB, Charlamb MJ, et al. Low prevalence of valvular heart disease in 226 phentermine-fenfluramine protocol subjects prospectively followed for up to 30 months. *J Am Coll Cardiol* 1999; **34**:1153–8.

50. Wellman PJ, Maher TJ. Synergistic interactions between fenfluramine and phentermine. *Int J Obes* 1999; **23**:723–32.

51. Gardin JM, Schumacher D, Constantine G, Davis K, Leung C, Reid CL. Valvular abnormalities and cardiovascular status following exposure to dexfenfluramine or phentermine/fenfluramine. *JAMA* 2000; **283**:1703–9.

52. Shively BK, Roldan CA, Gill EA, Najarian T, Loar SB. Prevalence and determinants of valvulopathy in patients treated with fexfenfluramine. *Circulation* 1999; **100**:2161–7.

53. Weissman, NJ, Panza JA, Tighe JF, Gwynne JT. Natural history of valvular regurgitation 1 year after discontinuation of dexfenfluramine therapy: a randomized, double-blind, placebo-controlled trial. *Ann Intern Med* 2001; **134**:267–73.

54. Gardin JM, Weissman NJ, Leung C, et al. Clinical and echocardiographic follow-up of patients previously treated with dexfenfluramine or phentermine/fenfluramine. *JAMA* 2001; **286**:2011–14.

55. Steffee CH, Singh HK, Chitwood WR. Histologic changes in three explanted native cardiac valves following use of fenfluramines. *Cardiovasc Pathol* 1999; **8**:245–53.

56. Rothman RB, Baumann MH, Savage JE, et al. Evidence for possible involvement of 5–HT$_{2B}$ receptors in the cardiac valvulopathy associated with fenfluramine and other serotonergic medications. *Circulation* 2000; **102**:2836–41.

57. Bonow RO, Carabello B, de Leon AC, et al. Guidelines for the management of patients with valvular heart disease: a report of the American College of Cardiology/American Heart Association tasks force on practice guidelines. *J Am Coll Cardiol* 1998; **32**:1486–582.

36

Women, their hearts and their strokes

Bartłomiej Piechowski-Józwiak and Julien Bogousslavsky

Introduction

Stroke and coronary heart disease (CHD) are leading causes of death in the adult population.[1] These two disease entities share common risk factors such as hypertension, tobacco use, and increased body mass index (BMI).[2–4] The burden of cardiovascular disease (CVD) is extremely high, as almost 20% of women in the United States have CVD. Approximately 40% of deaths in women are due to CVD, compared with only 3% of deaths in women due to breast cancer.[5] However, only a minority of women consider CVD to impose an important risk to their well-being. At the same time, two-thirds of women consider breast cancer as a major threat to their lives.[6] In the United States in 1998 there were more than 500 000 deaths in women due to CVD compared with 41 000 deaths from breast cancer.[5]

Epidemiology of stroke

Although stroke may seem to be a uniform disorder, there are important differences between the sexes in demographics, stroke risk factors, subtypes of stroke, management, and outcomes. According to a recently published review of population-based studies, the age-standardized prevalence of stroke in men >65 years of age ranged from 58.8 to 92.6/1000 population, while in women in the same age group the prevalence of stroke was lower with a range from 32.2 to 61.2/1000 population.[7] When taking into account crude data from different studies that used different age ranges, stroke prevalence rates in men in developed countries ranged from 5.0 (95% confidence interval (CI) 4.2–5.8) to 9.6 (6.9–12.3) per 1000 population.[8,9] In women the crude prevalence ranged from 3.2 to 9.7 per 1000 population.[10,11] These differences are more evident when considering individual studies. In the Rotterdam study, the crude stroke prevalence was 5.0 (4.2–5.8) in men and 4.3 (3.7–4.9) per 1000 population in women, and in the L'Aquila study it was 9.6/1000 (6.9–12.3) for men and 5.5/1000 (3.6–7.3) population in women.[8,9] Regarding the age of onset of stroke in different studies, women were older, with the mean age ranging from 74.6 to 75.5 years, compared with the age range of 68.8–73.2 years reported for men.[12–14] Stroke incidence increases with increasing age.[15] In men aged 65–69 years first-ever stroke incidence was 4.5/1000 person-years, and increased to 15.3/1000 person-years in those aged 80–84 years. In women aged 65–69 years stroke incidence was 4.6/1000 person-years and rose to 13.5/1000 person-years in women aged 80–84 years.[16] In men aged 80–84 years the incidence rate was 18.3/1000 population, and increased to 33/1000 population for those over 90 years of age. In women these rates were 16.8/1000 population, and 28.5/1000 population, respectively. The difference in stroke incidence between the elderly men and women is less

Table 36.1 Distribution of stroke risk factors among female vs male patients

Reference/patients	Hypertension	Atrial fibrillation	Diabetes mellitus	Smoking	Alcohol
Arboix et al.[24] n = 2000; 48%*	55 vs 50%†	30 vs 18%†	Not reported	1 vs 21%†	0.1 vs 5%†
Di Carlo et al.[13] n = 4499; 50%	51 vs 47%†	21 vs 15%†	21 vs 21%	18 vs 57%†	21 vs 48%†
Glader et al.[14] n = 20761; 49%	48 vs 46%	21 vs 17%	20 vs 22%	12 vs 15%	Not reported
Holroyd-Leduc et al.[25] n = 44832; 50%	34 vs 30%†	13 vs 10%†	19 vs 20%†	Not reported	Not reported
Roquer et al.[12] n = 1581; 48%	65 vs 53%†	31 vs 19%†	28 vs 27%	5 vs 52%†	3 vs 25%†
Worall BB et al.[26] n = 1087; 53%	88 vs 80%	Not reported	45 vs 32%	48 vs 78%	1 vs 5%
LSR n = 4200; 39%	50 vs 48%	13 vs 9%	12 vs 16%	21 vs 51%	Not reported

LSR, Lausanne Stroke Registry.
*Number of cases, % of women in the studied sample.
†Statistical significance (where available).

evident, as it was 22.1/1000 population in men over the age of 80 years and 21.2/1000 population in women.[17] Similar results were demonstrated in another population, where the incidence of first-ever stroke was 15.3/1000 person-years in men 80–84 years of age, and 13.5/1000 person-years in women.[16] In favor of the hypothesis of an increased stroke incidence in elderly women is the higher proportion of women older than 80 years with stroke when compared with younger (<80 years) female stroke patients (61% vs 48%).[17] The increased stroke incidence in elderly women, their increased longevity by about 10 years,[1] and shorter life expectancy in men may in part explain the equal absolute lifetime risk of stroke for those aged 55 years that was shown to be 21% for both sexes. Indirectly, the comparable frequency of ischemic strokes between men and women >25 years of age may also add to accepting the same lifetime risk of stroke in both sexes.[18,19] However, the burden of stroke in women seems greater than in men, as they live longer than men, and their life expectancy is expected to increase in the next 15 years to a mean of 85–90 years in developed countries, thus imposing a real threat of a stroke epidemic.[1]

substantially between the sexes. The frequency of risk factors among stroke patients varies considerably in different studies depending on the study design and the size of the studied population. The frequency of hypertension ranges from 34% to 88% in women, and 3% to 80% in men; atrial fibrillation from 13% to 31% in women, and from 9% to 19% in men; diabetes mellitus from 12% to 45% in women, and from 16% to 32% in men; cigarette smoking from 1% to 48% in women, and from 15% to 78% in men; alcohol abuse from to 0.1% to 21% in women, and from 5% to 48% in men.[12–14,24–26] In our hospital-based register (Lausanne Stroke Registry) collecting first-ever ischemic strokes,[27] hypertension was more frequent in female than male stroke patients (50% vs 48%), as was atrial fibrillation (13% vs 9%) (Table 36.1).[12–14,24–26] When analyzing the predictive value of different variables for stroke, congestive heart failure and atrial fibrillation were independently associated with female gender with the odds of 1.76 (95% CI 1.0–2.84) and 1.5 (1.2–1.9), respectively.[24] In general terms, hypertension and atrial fibrillation are more common in female stroke patients, while cigarette use, alcohol intake and peripheral arterial disease (not shown in the table) are more common in male patients.

Stroke risk factors

Women have the same key risk factors for stroke as men: cigarette smoking, hypertension, diabetes, and cardiac disorders.[20–23] However, the risk of stroke from some of these risk factors and their prevalence differ

Cardiac disorders and stroke

Cardiac conditions associated with an increased risk of cerebral ischemic complications may be stratified by the anatomic structure of the heart that is

Table 36.2 Sources of cardiogenic embolism. After reference 28.

Type	High-risk sources	Low-risk sources
Valvular	Mechanical prosthetic valves Left heart endocarditis	Mitral valve prolapse Mitral annulus calcification Mitral stenosis Aortic stenosis Fibroelastoma
Atrial	Atrial fibrillation Left atrial thrombus Atrial myxoma Sick sinus syndrome	Left atrial turbulence Patent foramen ovale Atrial septal aneurysm Atrial flutter
Ventricular	Myocardial infarction (<4 weeks) Left ventricular thrombus Dilated cardiomyopathy Akinetic left ventricular segment Left ventricular myxoma	Congestive heart failure Hypokinetic left ventricular segment Myocardial infarction (>4 weeks)

involved in the disease process (i.e. atria, valves, ventricles), or according to the risk of stroke they carry (i.e. high and low risk) (Table 36.2).[28] There are many possible risk factors for cardioembolic stroke (Fig. 36.1). Here we concentrate on the most frequent and most widely studied disorders such as atrial fibrillation, heart failure, and CHD, including myocardial infarction (MI). The mechanism of stroke in atrial fibrillation is probably related to local, intra-atrial stasis of blood (especially in the left atrial

appendage) that allows for thrombus formation that can embolize to an extracranial or intracranial cerebral artery. In MI the presumed basis of cerebral embolism is formation of a mural thrombus. However, other mechanisms such as atrial fibrillation or left ventricular dysfunction should also be considered. Thrombus formation is more frequent in anterior than inferior MI. Most often embolic complications of acute MI appear from the first to seventh day from onset. In heart failure, formation of emboligenic material is probably due to sluggish blood flow in a poorly contracting left ventricle, endothelial and epicardial dysfunction, and venous stasis, and the risk of embolism is probably inversely related to the ventricular ejection fraction.[29]

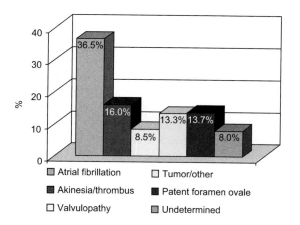

Figure 36.1
Presumed causes of cardiogenic strokes in the Lausanne Stroke Registry (1982–1998).

Atrial fibrillation (see also Chapter 37)

When considering the relation between cardiac disorders and stroke, some differences can be observed between women and men. The incidence of atrial fibrillation increases with age from 0.5/1000 person-years for those aged 50 years or less, to 16.9/1000 person-years by age 85.[30] In the Framingham cohort the prevalence of atrial fibrillation increased from 5/1000 population for patients in their sixth decade to 88/1000 population in octogenarians. Atrial fibrillation was more prevalent in men than women (men-to-women ratio of 1.7). In this cohort the incidence of stroke attributed to nonvalvular atrial fibrillation was 4.8 times greater when compared with the incidence of stroke in the general population without atrial fibrillation.[31] In another population-based study atrial fibrillation was shown to increase the risk of stroke 2.1-fold.[30] The risk of stroke in patients with nonvalvular atrial fibrillation is approximately 5% per year. When considering different age groups, the risk of stroke attributable to atrial fibrillation increases significantly with increasing age from 1.5% for those aged 50–59 years to 23.5% for octogenarians.[31] Additionally when comparing the age of onset of atrial fibrillation, women are significantly older than men (65.4 ± 0.7 vs 60.5 ± 0.6; p <0.001) and a tendency to an increased frequency of stroke is observed.[32] Atrial fibrillation in patients with rheumatic heart disease is now less common due to the introduction of effective antimicrobial regimens to decrease recurrent rheumatic fever. It is important to mention data from the Framingham Study which clearly show that coexistence of atrial fibrillation and a history of rheumatic heart disease increases the risk of stroke 17-fold.[33] History of rheumatic heart disease is also significantly more frequent in female than in male stroke patients (6.4% vs 3.5%).[24]

Heart failure (see also Chapter 29)

The prevalence of heart failure displays a similar pattern to that of stroke, as it increases with age from 8/1000 population for patients aged 50–59 years to 91/1000 population in octogenarians. Heart failure increased the incidence of stroke 4.3-fold, compared with the general population.[31] It is more frequently present in female (from 6% to 7%) than in male stroke patients (from 3% to 5%) (p <0.001).[24,25] The risk of stroke attributable to heart failure rises from 2.3% in the sixth decade to 6% in the ninth decade of life.[31] Women with heart failure have a significantly greater incidence of all thromboembolic complications (cerebral, pulmonary, and peripheral) when compared with men (2.4 vs 1.8/100 patient-years).

Irrespective of gender, cerebral embolism is the prevailing embolic complication of heart failure. However, the frequency of nonfatal cerebral embolic events is lower in women than in men (58% vs 68%).[29]

Coronary heart disease and myocardial infarction (see also Chapter 18)

Prevalence of CHD rises with increasing age as is the case with heart failure and atrial fibrillation. In subjects 50–59 years of age, CHD was present in 66/1000 population and in those aged 80–89 years it was 270/1000 population. The history of CHD increased stroke incidence twofold according to the Framingham cohort results. However, with increasing age the influence of CHD and heart failure on stroke risk decreased, and only atrial fibrillation remained an important risk factor for stroke in octogenarians.[31] Hospital-based registries show that CHD was more prevalent among male stroke patients with a frequency ranging from 15% to 18%. In women the frequency was lower and ranged from 10% to 15% (p <0.001).[24,25] Acute MI is one manifestation of CHD and sometimes its initial presentation. The frequency of stroke related to acute coronary syndromes varies between different studies depending on the design and sample size from 0.6% (n = 10 948) to 2.4% (n=740).[34,35] The risk of stroke was the highest during the first 5 days after acute MI, with more than 50% of strokes occurring in this period.[36] A positive correlation was demonstrated between the patient's age and the frequency of post-MI stroke and/or transient ischemic attack. The frequency of stroke complicating the acute MI in patients younger than 59 years ranged from 0.4% to 0.8%, while for those older than 70 years it was higher, from 1.4% to 1.6%.[36,37] No clear-cut correlation between gender and stroke incidence/prevalence was demonstrated.

In clinical practice, overlapping of risk factors is often encountered. In patients with atrial fibrillation, both heart failure and CHD may also be present. In patients with atrial fibrillation and co-existent heart failure, the relative risk of stroke in women was significantly greater than in men (2.8 vs 1.7). In patients with atrial fibrillation and CHD, the stroke risk was also significantly higher in women than in men (4.9 vs 2.3). It is important to highlight an almost twofold higher risk of stroke in women with atrial fibrillation and co-existing CHD compared with those with atrial fibrillation and heart failure (4.9 vs 2.8).[31] In patients with post-MI heart failure, ejection fraction below 28% was shown to increase the risk of stroke 1.86-fold (95% CI 1.15–3.04), and every absolute decrease of 5% in ejection fraction yielded an 18% increase of stroke risk. However, no differences in stroke risk between genders were demonstrated.[38]

Cardiogenic stroke

Does the fact that some epidemiological data speak in favor of an increased frequency of stroke in women with heart disease compared with men translate directly into increased frequency of cardiogenic stroke? To go further with our discussion we have to define a cardiogenic stroke, as different studies used different definitions of cardiogenic stroke. The most useful and straightforward seems the definition that classifies strokes as cardiogenic based on the presence of cerebral or cerebellar symptoms, detection of an ischemic lesion >1.5 cm with neuroimaging, finding a cardiac source of emboli, and excluding other possible stroke mechanisms.[28] Population-based data (Rochester Epidemiology Project) show that cardiogenic embolism is the most frequent determined cause of first-ever stroke in women, with an age-adjusted incidence rate of 37 (95% CI 29–45) per 100 000 population. The second in frequency is lacunar stroke, with an incidence of 22 (15–29) per 100 000 population. The least frequent cause of stroke in women is stenosis of large extra- or intra-cranial arteries, with an age-adjusted incidence rate of 12 (7–17) per 100 000 population. In men, the most frequent determined cause of stroke is arterial stenosis, with an incidence rate of 47 (34–61) per 100 000 population. The second most frequent cause of stroke in men is cardiac embolism, with an incidence of 42 (30–55) per 100 000 population. The absolute difference of the incidence of cardiogenic strokes between the sexes in this study should be interpreted with

caution as the incidence of cardiogenic stroke in women was approximately 20% lower than the incidence in men, while the incidence of all strokes was 40% higher in men than in women (173 (148–199) vs 124 (109–140)).[39] Other studies demonstrated that cardioembolic stroke was more frequent in women (range 22–30%) when compared with men (range 13–22%), and was either the first or the second most frequent cause of stroke in women.[12,24,40] In our stroke register, cardiogenic stroke was also more frequent in women than in men (23% vs 20%), and women with presumed cardiogenic stroke were older than men (68 vs 65 years). These data point toward a linkage between female sex, increased age, and increased frequency of cardioembolic strokes.

Stroke-related disability

The burden of stroke is related mainly to stroke outcome and stroke-related disability. In this section we address the question whether there are differences between the sexes, and if there is any relation between stroke outcome and the presence of cardiac disease in female stroke patients. Among stroke survivors up to three-quarters are left with some degree of disability.[11,41,42] In the Multicenter Multinational Hospital-Based Registry female sex was an independent factor that increased the odds of being disabled (odds ratio (OR) 1.4; 95% CI 1.1–1.8), and handicapped (OR 1.5; 95% CI 1.1–1.9) at 3 months post-stroke. However, the baseline characteristics of patients were different, as women had significantly more disability (defined as pre-stroke modified Rankin score 2–5) before the index stroke compared with men (32% vs 23%).[13] Another study on first-ever strokes demonstrated that women had odds of 1.87 (95% CI 1.5–2.35) for being more disabled (modified Rankin score 3–5) compared with men (p <0.001).[12]

Why should women be more disabled than men? Is there a correlation between female gender, clinical symptomatology, anatomical lesion, stroke etiology and outcome? In the Multicenter Multinational Hospital-Based Registry women, compared with men, had significantly more frequent aphasia (35% vs 30%), paralysis (42% vs 36%), and coma (10% vs

7%). At the same time they had more partial anterior circulation infarcts compared with men (32% vs 28%; p = 0.029).[13] Data from another hospital-based study also showed that aphasia was significantly more frequent in women (29%) compared with men (22%), as well as visual deficits (17% vs 14%).[12] Another group reported similar findings with more female stroke patients being aphasic than male patients (37% vs 28%), and after controlling for stroke mechanism, an excess of aphasia in women with cardioembolic strokes was demonstrated.[43] The presence of visual deficits (i.e. hemianopia), Wernicke's aphasia, and partial involvement of anterior circulation territories (posterior division of middle cerebral artery, anterior cerebral artery, multiple territories) were linked with a potential cardiac source of brain embolism.[44] Higher frequency of aphasia, visual deficits, paralysis, and consciousness abnormalities in women may be the consequence of the greater severity of stroke in women than in men, which indeed seems to be a fact, as stroke severity assessed with the Canadian Stroke Scale was significantly higher in women than in men (6.6 vs 7.4).[12]

Short-term case fatality (in-hospital, 28- or 30-day) is reported to be either equal for both sexes or slightly higher in women (range 11–17%) than in men (range 11–13%). Long-term case fatality was reported to be either equal for both sexes or lower in women, with odds of dying during the first year post-stroke of 0.94 (95% CI 0.89–0.98).[12–14,24,25]

Summary

Stroke jeopardizes life and well-being of both women and men. Yet women live longer than men, and their lifespan will increase even more; thus a stroke epidemic in women should be previewed. Women, compared with men, have a predilection for cardioembolic strokes. The burden of cardioembolic stroke in women is high as they are elderly at stroke onset and have more stroke-related disability and handicap than men. These factors should enhance a global effort to increase both public awareness of the importance of cerebrovascular disease in women and the introduction of effective stroke preventive strategies.

References

1. Murray CJ, Lopez AD. Mortality by cause for eight regions of the world: Global Burden of Disease Study. *Lancet* 1997; **349**:1269–76.

2. Colditz GA, Bonita R, Stampfer MJ, Willet W, Rosner B, Speizer IE. Cigarette smoking and risk of stroke in middle-aged women. *N Engl J Med* 1988; **18**:937–41.

3. MacMahon S, Peto R, Cutler J, et al. Blood pressure, stroke, and coronary heart disease, part 1: prolonged differences in blood pressure: prospective observational studies corrected for the regression dilution bias. *Lancet* 1990; **335**:765–74.

4. Robertson TL, Kato H, Gordon T, et al. Epidemiologic studies of coronary heart disease and stroke in Japanese men living in Japan, Hawaii and California: coronary heart disease risk factors in Japan and Hawaii. *Am J Cardiol* 1997; **39**:244–9.

5. American Heart Association. *2002 Heart and stroke statistical update.* Dallas, TX: American Heart Association, 2001.

6. Robertson RM. Women and cardiovascular disease: the risk of misperception and the need for action. *Circulation* 2001; **103**:2318–20.

7. Feigin V, Lawes C, Bennett DA, Anderson CS. Stroke epidemiology: a review of population-based studies of incidence, prevalence, and case-fatality in the late 20th century. *Lancet Neurology* 2003; **2**:43–53.

8. Bots ML, Looman SJ, Koudstaal PJ, Hofman A, Hoes AW, Grobbee DE. Prevalence of stroke in the general population: the Rotterdam study. *Stroke* 1996; **27**:1499–501.

9. Prencipe M, Ferretti C, Casini AR, Santini M, Giubilei F, Culasso F. Stroke, disability, and dementia: results of a population survey. *Stroke* 1997; **28**:531–6.

10. Mittelmark MB, Psaty BM, Rautaharju PM, et al. Prevalence of cardiovascular disease among older adults: the cardiovascular health study. *Am J Epidemiol* 1993; **137**:311–17.

11. Bonita R, Solomon N, Broad JB. Prevalence of stroke and stroke-related disability: estimates from the Auckland stroke studies. *Stroke* 1997; **28**:1898–902.

12. Roquer J, Campello AR, Gomis M. Sex differences in first-ever acute stroke. *Stroke* 2003; **34**:1581–5.

13. Di Carlo A, Lamassa M, Baldereschi M, et al. Sex differences in the clinical presentation, resource use, and 3-month outcome of acute stroke in Europe: data from a multicenter multinational hospital-based registry. *Stroke* 2003; **34**:1114–19.

14. Glader EL, Stegmayr B, Norrving B, et al. Sex differences in management and outcome after stroke. A Swedish national perspective. *Stroke* 2003; **34**:1970–5.

15. Marini C, Triggiani L, Cimini N, et al. Proportion of older people in the community as a predictor of increasing stroke incidence. *Neuroepidemiology* 2001; **20**:91–5.

16. Di Carlo A, Baldereschi M, Gandolfo C, et al. Stroke in an elderly population: incidence and impact on survival and daily function. The Italian Longitudinal Study on Aging. *Cerebrovasc Dis* 2003; **16**:141–50.

17. Marini C, Baldassarre M, Russo T, et al. Burden of first-ever ischemic stroke in the oldest old. Evidence from a population-based study. *Neurology* 2004; **62**:77–81.

18. Hollander M, Koudstaal PJ, Bots ML, Grobbee DE, Hofman A, Breteler MM. Incidence, risk, and case fatality of first ever stroke in the elderly population. The Rotterdam Study. *J Neurol Neurosurg Psychiatry* 2003; **74**:317–21.

19. Zhang LF, Yang J, Hong Z, et al. Proportion of different subtypes of stroke in China. *Stroke* 2003; **34**:2091–6.

20. Njolstad I, Arnesen E, Lund-Larsen PG. Body height, cardiovascular risk factors, and risk of stroke in middle-aged men and women. A 14-year follow-up of the Finnmark Study. *Circulation* 1996; **94**:2877–82.

21. Lindenstrom E, Boysen G, Nyobe J. Lifestyle factors and risk of cerebrovascular disease in women: the Copenhagen City Heart Study. *Stroke* 1993; **24**:1468–72.

22. Shinton R, Beevers G. Meta-analysis of relation between cigarette smoking and stroke. *BMJ* 1989; **298**:789–94.

23. Boysen G, Nyobe J, Appleyard M, et al. Stroke incidence and risk factors for stroke in Copenhagen, Denmark. *Stroke* 1988; **19**:1345–53.

24. Arboix A, Oliveres M, Garcia-Eroles L, Maragall C, Massons J, Targa C. Acute cerebrovascular disease in women. *Eur Neurol* 2001; **45**:199–205.

25. Holroyd-Leduc JM, Kapral MK, Austin PC, Tu JV. Sex differences and similarities in the management and outcome of stroke patients. *Stroke* 2000; **31**:1833–7.

26. Worall BB, Johnston KC, Kongable G, Hung E, Richardson D, Goerlick PB, for the AAASPS

Investigators. Stroke risk factor profiles in American women. An interim report from the African-American Antiplatelet Stroke Prevention Study. *Stroke* 2002; **33**:913–19.

27. Bogousslavsky J, Van Melle G, Regli F. The Lausanne Stroke Registry: analysis of 1000 consecutive patients with first stroke. *Stroke* 1988; **19**:1083–92.

28. Adams HP Jr, Bendixen BH, Kappelle LJ, et al. Classification of subtype of acute ischemic stroke. Definitions for use in a multicenter clinical trial. TOAST. Trial of Org 10172 in Acute Stroke Treatment. *Stroke* 1993; **24**:35–41.

29. Dries DL, Rosenberg YD, Waclawiw MA, Domanski MJ. Ejection fraction and risk of thromboembolic events in patients with systolic dysfunction and sinus rhythm: evidence for gender differences in the studies of left ventricular dysfunction trials. *J Am Coll Cardiol* 1997; **29**:1074–80.

30. Krahn AD, Manfreda J, Tate RB, Mathewson FA, Cuddy TE. The natural history of atrial fibrillation: incidence, risk factors, and prognosis in the Manitoba Follow-Up Study. *Am J Med* 1995; **98**:476–84.

31. Wolf PA, Abbott RD, Kannel WB. Atrial fibrillation as an independent risk factor for stroke: the Framingham Study. *Stroke* 1991; **22**:983–8.

32. Humphries KH, Kerr CR, Connolly SJ, et al. New-onset atrial fibrillation: sex differences in presentation, treatment, and outcome. *Circulation* 2001; **103**:2365–70.

33. Wolf PA, Dawber TR, Thomas HE Jr, Kannel WB. Epidemiologic assessment of atrial fibrillation and risk of stroke: the Framingham Study. *Neurology* 1978; **28**:973–7.

34. Mahaffey KW, Harrington RA, Simoons ML, et al. Stroke in patients with acute coronary syndromes: incidence and outcomes in the platelet glycoprotein IIb/IIIa in unstable angina. Receptor suppression using integrilin therapy (PURSUIT) trial. The PURSUIT Investigators. *Circulation* 1999; **99**:2371–7.

35. Komrad MS, Coffey CE, Coffey KS, McKinnis R, Massey EW, Califf RM. Myocardial infarction and stroke. *Neurology* 1984; **34**:1403–9.

36. Mooe T, Eriksson P, Stegmayr B. Ischemic stroke after acute myocardial infarction. A population-based study. *Stroke* 1997; **28**:762–7.

37. Behar S, Tanne D, Abinader E, et al. Cerebrovascular accident complicating acute myocardial infarction: incidence, clinical significance and short- and long-term mortality rates. The SPRINT Study Group. *Am J Med* 1991; **91**:45–50.

38. Loh E, Sutton MS, Wun CC, et al. Ventricular dysfunction and the risk of stroke after myocardial infarction. *N Engl J Med* 1997; **336**:251–7.

39. Petty GW, Brown RD, Whisnant JP, Sicks JD, O'Fallon WM, Wiebers DO. Ischemic stroke subtypes. A population-based study of incidence and risk factors. *Stroke* 1999; **30**:2513–16.

40. Grau AJ, Weimar C, Buggle F, et al. Risk factors, outcome, and treatment in subtypes of ischemic stroke: the German stroke data bank. *Stroke* 2001; **32**:2559–66.

41. Geddes JM, Fear J, Tennant A, Pickering A, Hillman M, Chamberlain MA. Prevalence of self reported stroke in a population in northern England. *J Epidemiol Community Health* 1996; **50**:140–3.

42. O'Mahony PG, Thomason RG, Dobson R, Rodgers H, James OF. The prevalence of stroke and associated disability. *J Public Health Med* 1999; **21**:166–71.

43. Hier DB, Yoon WB, Mohr JP, Price TR, Wolf PA. Gender and aphasia in the Stroke Data Bank. *Brain Lang* 1994; **47**:155–67.

44. Bogousslavsky J, Cachin C, Regli F, Despland PA, Van Melle G, Kappenberger L. Cardiac sources of embolism and cerebral infarction – clinical consequences and vascular concomitants: the Lausanne Stroke Registry. *Neurology* 1991; **41**:855–9.

37

Arrhythmia and arrhythmia management

Richard H. Hongo and Melvin M. Scheinman

Introduction

Studies assessing the gender differences in arrhythmias have been distinctly limited, relative to the importance of this topic. Notwithstanding, differences in the clinical presentation and manifestations of a variety of arrhythmias have been observed, and these differences have impacted the management of women with arrhythmias. At the same time, established treatments such as radiofrequency catheter ablation and implantable cardioverter defibrillators have been found to be equally efficacious in women as in men. Fortunately, there is growing interest in this topic of late, and with a better understanding of the etiology of these differences, further advances in the management of women with arrhythmias may follow.

Gender differences in electrocardiographic parameters

Heart rate

A higher heart rate in women was first reported by Bazett in 1920.[1] In a population-based study of 5116 healthy young adults, Liu et al.[2] subsequently estimated this increase in heart rate in women to be between 3 and 5 beats/min on average. A report of a

shorter sinus node recovery time in women compared with men (1135 ± 214 ms vs 1215 ± 297 ms, p <0.05) has suggested an intrinsic difference in sinus node function.[3] In apparent support of this, Burke et al.[4] found that after double autonomic blockade (propranolol and atropine) of the sinus

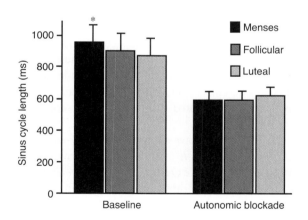

Figure 37.1
Menstrual phase versus sinus cycle length in women. The sinus cycle length was significantly longer (p <0.03) during the menstrual phase than during the follicular or luteal phase. After autonomic blockade with propranolol 0.2 mg/kg and atropine 0.04 mg/kg these differences were no longer present. Reproduced from reference 5 with permission.

node, women still had a shorter sinus cycle length (faster heart rate) when compared with men (594 ± 57 ms vs 645 ± 41 ms, p <0.0001). Covariance analysis, however, found that gender did not have a significant effect on heart rate, and maximal exercise capacity was instead the most significant predictor of sinus cycle length. Whether there is an intrinsic gender difference in sinus node function is debatable. Burke et al.[5] also observed that the average heart rate during the menstrual phase was increased, compared with both follicular and luteal phases, and that these differences disappeared with double autonomic blockade, thus supporting a hormonal influence on heart rate gender difference (Fig. 37.1).

Rate-corrected QT interval

A longer rate-corrected QT interval in women was also recognized by Bazett,[1] and has since been confirmed by others.[6,7] In a North American population-based study of 14 379 children and adults, Rautaharju et al.[8] demonstrated that the difference in rate-corrected QT interval emerged after a sudden drop in rate-corrected QT interval (20 ms) in boys that coincided with puberty and with a sudden surge in androgen levels (Fig. 37.2). On the other hand, rate-corrected QT interval in women appeared relatively unaffected by expected changes in hormonal balance, such as during menopause. These observations strongly suggest that the gender difference in rate-corrected QT interval is, in fact, caused by androgen-mediated shortening of rate-corrected QT interval in men.

Animal studies have supported the rate-corrected QT shortening effects of androgens, but have found estrogen to influence QT prolongation as well. Liu et al.[9] observed significantly lower potassium current densities (I_{Kr} and I_{Kl}) in female rabbit ventricular tissue compared with the male. In oophorectomized rabbits, Drici et al.[10] found that administration of dihydrotestosterone (DHT) and estradiol resulted in down-regulation of potassium channels (I_{sK} and H_{K2}) in ventricular tissue, more prominently with estradiol; those treated with DHT were more refractory to quinidine-induced QT prolongation. In oophorectomized rabbits, Hara et al.[11] demonstrated that ventricular repolarization was significantly length-

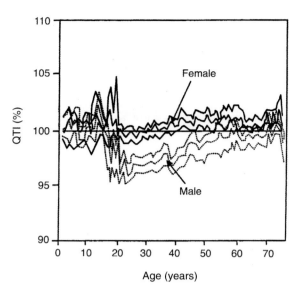

Figure 37.2
Heart rate-corrected QT interval expressed as QT index by age in 14 379 children and adults from birth to 75 years. Mean values of the QT index (QTI = (QT/QTp) × 100) with 95% confidence intervals calculated for each age subinterval of 1 year for men and women using the formula QTp = 656/(1 + 0.01 HR). A distinct decrease in rate-corrected QT values in men following puberty is followed by a linear increase through a major part of adult life. The slight nonsignificant age trend present in women at reproductive age disappears after inclusion of a correction term for QRS duration. Reproduced from reference 8 with permission.

ened with estradiol while shortened with DHT. Maximum action potential prolongation was seen in the estradiol group with administration of E4031 (I_{Kr} blocker), which also resulted in induction of early afterdepolarizations (EADs). Similarly, Pham et al.[12] demonstrated marked action potential prolongation and induction of EADs in estradiol-treated oophorectomized rabbits with dofetilide (I_{Kr} blocker) administration (Fig. 37.3). In this particular study, gender difference in baseline action potential duration persisted in castrated rabbits, suggesting that extragonadal factors may influence ventricular repolarization in addition to estrogen.

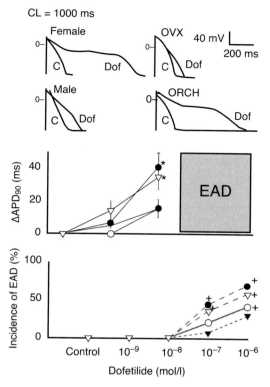

Figure 37.3
Effects of dofetilide on APD (action potential duration) and EAD (early afterdepolarizations) incidence at CL = 1000 ms. Top, representative action potentials; C indicates control; Dof, 10^{-6} mol/l dofetilide; OVX, oophorectomized rabbit; ORCH, orchiectomized rabbit. Middle, relationship of ΔAPD_{90} to increasing dofetilide concentrations. Bottom, incidence of EADs induced by dofetilide. n = 12, 10, 13, and 16 for female (●), male (○), OVX (▼), and ORCH (▽), respectively. *p <0.05 vs OVX and control male; +p <0.05 vs respective predrug control. Reproduced from reference 12 with permission.

The effect of estrogen on QT prolongation in women has not yet been elucidated by clinical studies. In a study of 3103 women from the Atherosclerosis Risk in Communities cohort, Carnethon et al.[13] did find a small (6.6 ms) but statistically significant (p <0.01) increase in corrected QT interval in women who used estrogen replacement therapy compared with never-users. The clinical significance of this small difference, however, is unclear. Rodriguez et al.[14] found that ibutilide-induced QT prolongation was most pronounced during menses and ovulation as compared with the luteal phase of the menstrual cycle. They found, however, that the progesterone and the progesterone-to-estradiol ratio, not estradiol or testosterone, inversely correlated with ibutilide-induced corrected QT prolongation, suggesting that progesterone may have a major role in determining rate-corrected QT interval in women. Whereas in men androgens appear to protect against rate-corrected QT prolongation, in women a more complex interplay of estrogen and progesterone may determine the risk of rate-corrected QT prolongation.

Gender differences in clinical arrhythmias

Supraventricular tachycardias

There are distinct gender differences in the distribution of certain supraventricular tachycardias (Table 37.1). Inappropriate sinus tachycardia is predominantly (approximately 90%) seen in women.[15–17] In 623 consecutive patients referred for catheter ablation of supraventricular tachycardia, Rodriguez et al.[18] found that arrhythmia due to an accessory pathway was twice as common in men as in women, and conversely, atrioventricular (AV) nodal re-entry tachycardia was twice as common in women (Table 37.2). Calkins et al.[19] found a similar distribution among 873 consecutive patients, with women representing 42% and 70% of accessory pathways and AV nodal re-entry tachycardias, respectively. A shorter refractory period has been observed for the AV node slow pathway in women[20] that may represent a wider tachycardia zone and larger window of opportunity for induction of AV nodal re-entry tachycardia. Women who present with Wolff–Parkinson–White syndrome have a better prognosis with less aborted sudden death due to the progression of atrial fibrillation to ventricular fibrillation.[18,21] The mean age of symptom onset in patients with accessory pathway-mediated tachycardia has been found to be 3 years younger in women.[22]

Table 37.1 Gender differences in frequency of clinical arrhythmias

Arrhythmia	More common in men	More common in women
Bradyarrhythmias	High-degree AV block* Carotid sinus syndrome*	Sinus node dysfunction*
Supraventricular tachyarrhythmias	Atrial fibrillation WPW syndrome	AVNRT Inappropriate sinus tachycardia
Ventricular tachyarrhythmias	Ischemic VT/VF Brugada syndrome† SUDS‡ Left fascicular VT§ Sudden cardiac death	Nonischemic VT/VF Congenital LQT syndrome Acquired LQT syndrome RVOT-VT§

*Bjerregaard P. Mean 24 hour heart rate, minimal heart rate and pauses in healthy subjects 40–79 years of age. *Eur Heart J* 1983; **4**:44–51, and Manolio TA, Furberg CD, Rautaharju PM, et al. Cardiac arrhythmias on 24-h ambulatory electrocardiography in older women and men: The Cardiovascular Health Study. *J Am Coll Cardiol* 1994; **23**:916–25.
†Brugada J, Brugada P, Brugada R. The syndrome of right bundle branch block ST segment elevation in V1 to V3 and sudden death. The Brugada syndrome. *Europace* 1999; **1**:156–66.
‡Nadamanee K, Veerakul G, Nimmannit S, et al. Arrhythmogenic marker for the sudden unexplained death syndrome in Thai men. *Circulation* 1997; **96**:2595–600.
§Nakagawa M, Takahashi N, Nobe S, et al. Gender differences in various types of idiopathic ventricular tachycardia. *J Cardiovasc Electrophysiol* 2002; **13**:633–8.
AV, atrioventricular; AVNRT, atrioventricular nodal re-entry tachycardia; WPW, Wolff–Parkinson–White; VT, ventricular tachycardia; VF, ventricular fibrillation; LQT, long QT; SUDS, sudden unexplained death syndrome; RVOT, right ventricular outflow tract. Adapted from Linde C. Women and arrhythmia. *Pacing Clin Electrophysiol* 2000; **23**:1553, with permission.

Table 37.2 Gender of patients with supraventricular tachycardias

Type of arrhythmia	Male	Female	Sex ratio (M/F)
Accessory pathways	273	136	2.00
AV nodal tachycardias	52	113	0.46
Atrial tachycardias	23	26	0.88

AV, atrioventricular. Reproduced from reference 7 with permission from Excerpta Medica.

The menstrual cycle appears to influence supraventricular tachycardias. Rosano et al.[23] observed significantly more episodes on day 28 compared with days 7, 14, and 21, and the number of episodes correlated directly with serum progesterone levels and inversely with estradiol levels. Myerburg et al.[24] observed that in women with perimenstrual clustering of spontaneous supraventricular tachycardia episodes, inducibility during electrophysiology study was highest when performed either in the premenstrual phase or at the onset of menses. They recommended scheduling of electrophysiologic procedures during times of low estrogen levels (premenstrual and off estrogen replacement) in order to facilitate inducibility of tachycardia.

Despite concerns about a higher degree of difficulty in performing catheter ablation within a smaller female heart, success and complication rates of supraventricular tachycardia ablation appear to be equal between genders.[20,25] In a study of 894 consecutive patients presenting for either accessory pathway or AV nodal re-entry tachycardia ablation, Dagres et al.[25] found ablation success to be 93% and 95% in men and women, respectively, and rates of major procedural complications were 1.1% for both men and women. Women compared with men, however, were more symptomatic, received more antiarrhythmic drugs before ablation (1.6 ± 1.2 vs 1.3 ± 1.1, p <0.001), and were referred for ablation later after onset of symptoms (185 ± 143 vs 157 ± 144 months, p <0.001). The delay to ablative therapy is difficult to explain, but there are likely many factors ranging from unique concerns of radiation exposure in women to the tendency of supraventricular tachycardia to mimic symptoms of anxiety. Lessmeier et al.[26] found that in patients with unrecognized supraventricular tachycardia, women were more likely to have symptoms attributed to panic disorder than men (65% vs 32%, respectively; p <0.04).

Atrial fibrillation

In the Framingham Heart Study,[27,28] men were found to have a 1.5-fold higher risk for developing atrial fibrillation when compared with women. In the Coronary Artery Surgery Study Registry,[29] men with coronary disease had an even higher 5.4-fold risk for developing atrial fibrillation. Atrial fibrillation after cardiothoracic surgery is also more common in men.[30] Despite a higher prevalence of atrial fibrillation in men in any given age group, because there are close to twice as many women >75 years old as men, the absolute number of women with atrial fibrillation is equal to, if not more than (53%) that of men.[31] In the Framingham cohort, atrial fibrillation in men was associated with myocardial infarction (MI), whereas in women it was associated with congestive heart failure and valvular heart disease.[27,28]

Women with atrial fibrillation appear to have a lower survival rate than their male counterparts. Multivariate analysis of the Framingham data found the odds of death in patients with atrial fibrillation to be increased 1.9-fold in women compared with 1.5-fold in men.[27] Atrial fibrillation in women may also be more difficult to manage because of more symptoms, longer durations of episodes, and higher heart rates during arrhythmia.[32] Recurrence of atrial fibrillation after cardioversion is more common in women,[33] and there is evidence to suggest that risk of embolic stroke related to atrial fibrillation may be higher in women.[34] In addition, many of the anti-arrhythmic agents used to treat atrial fibrillation are associated with more proarrhythmia in women.

Drug-induced torsade de pointes (see also Chapter 39)

Torsade de pointes is a characteristic polymorphic ventricular tachycardia that occurs in the setting of QT prolongation. In a survey of 93 articles, Makkar et al.[35] found that women made up 70% of 332 identified cases of anti-arrhythmic drug-induced

Table 37.3 Prevalence of women among cases of torsade de pointes, by drug

| Drug | n | Female prevalence | |
		%	95% CI
Quinidine	108	60	50–70
Procainamide	39	49	32–66
Disopyramide	49	86	72–94
Amiodarone	28	68	47–85
Sotalol	21	76	52–92

CI, confidence interval. Adapted from reference 35 with permission.

torsade de pointes, and that most cases were with corrected QT interval >500 ms (Table 37.3). The risk of torsade de pointes appears especially high in anti-arrhythmic agents that block the rapid component of the delayed rectifier potassium current (I_{Kr}) such as sotalol and dofetilide. In a database compiled from 22 clinical trials, Lehmann et al.[36] found that among 3135 subjects, the occurrence of drug-induced torsade de pointes with d,l-sotalol was 4.1% in women, compared with 1.9% in men (p <0.001). Other risk factors for proarrhythmia included sustained ventricular arrhythmia, congestive heart failure, a sotalol dose >320 mg/day, and a serum creatinine >1.4 mg/dl. After adjusting for these risk factors, women were found to have a 3-fold greater odds of developing torsade de pointes than men. There was also a 3.2-fold greater odds of women developing torsade de pointes with dofetilide, but the risk of mortality was not different between genders.[37]

Female predominance in drug-induced torsade de pointes, however, is not confined to anti-arrhythmic agents. In a survey of 129 articles, Bednar et al.[38] identified 189 cases of nonanti-arrhythmic drug-induced torsade de pointes, and found that women comprised 67.2% of cases. The most commonly involved drugs included terfenadine, haloperidol, and erythromycin (Table 37.4). The reasons for this observed increase in proarrhythmia in women is not entirely understood, but it is likely related to hormonal influences that may prolong and destabilize ventricular repolarization in women, and to a protective effect of androgens in men. These findings underscore the importance of close monitoring when administering drug therapy in women, particularly with agents known to prolong the QT interval.

Table 37.4 Distribution of drug use in cited cases of torsade de pointes

Drug	Distribution (%) of drug use of total cases of TdP cited	Distribution (%) of female gender among cases of TdP cited
Terfenadine	14.3	59.3
Haloperidol	13.2	62.5
Erythromycin	11.6	68.2
Pentamidine	9.5	33.3
Astemizole	9.0	94.1
Thioridazine	6.9	76.9
Cisapride	4.8	77.8
Probucol	4.2	100.0
Clarithromycin	4.2	75.0
Ketanserin	3.7	42.9
Terodiline	3.7	85.7
Halofantrine	3.2	66.7

TdP, torsade de pointes. Adapted from reference 38 with permission from Excerpta Medica, Inc.

Congenital long QT syndromes

In a study by Locati et al.[39] of patients in the International Long QT Syndrome Registry, 70% of probands and 58% of affected family members were women. However, the study found men to have more fatal first events (32% vs 19%, p <0.05) and to be at higher risk for first events before puberty, both in probands and in family members (Fig. 37.4). The risk of a first event occurring after age 15, on the other hand, was higher in women for both probands and family members, with a hazard ratio of 1.87 and 3.25, respectively. Clinically, this would suggest that discontinuation of therapy later on in life would be reasonable to consider in men yet to experience their first episode, especially in the setting of shortening of the corrected QT interval. Women, however, have a continued risk for first events and, generally speaking, should be maintained on therapy for life.

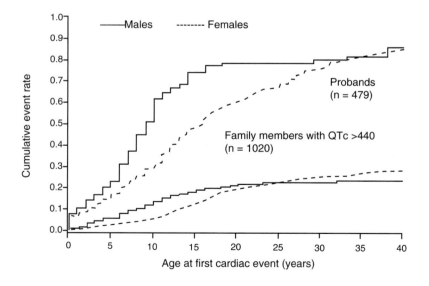

Figure 37.4
Cumulative age-related probability of event from birth to time of first event by Kaplan–Meier life-table analysis in affected LQTS patients (QTc >440 ms) referred to LQTS registry in 479 probands (366 with cardiac events) and 1020 affected family members (230 with cardiac events, 21 family members excluded for missing data) in males (solid lines) and females (dashed lines). Probability of first events by age 15 years was higher in males than females among probands (74% vs 51%, p <0.0001) and among family members (20% vs 16%, p <0.01), whereas it was similar by sex by age 40 years in both groups. Reproduced from reference 39 with permission.

In a more recent study of the same registry, Zareba et al.[40] evaluated recurrent events by genotype, and found that in children <15 years of age, LQT1 females had a significantly lower risk of recurrent cardiac events compared with LQT1 males (hazard ratio 0.58, p = 0.005). In those older than age 15, LQT1 and LQT2 females had significantly higher risks of recurrent events compared with their male counterparts (hazard ratio 3.35, p = 0.007; hazard ratio 3.71, p = 0.010, respectively). The lethality of cardiac events was higher in both LQT1 and LQT2 men (5% and 6%) compared with LQT1 and LQT2 women (2% for both), but was highest in LQT3 men and women (19% and 18%) without gender difference.

Sudden cardiac death and ventricular tachycardias

Analysis of the Framingham data by Kannel et al.[41] indicates that the incidence of sudden cardiac death (SCD) in women of all age groups appears to be less than half that of men. The incidence of SCD in women, in fact, lagged by more than 10 years behind men and appeared to be related to the delay in onset of CHD in women. The presence of CHD, however, did not completely explain the lower incidence of SCD in women in that 63% of SCD in women was in the absence of CHD, compared with only 44% in men. The Framingham data also suggest[42] that risk factors for SCD differ between genders. Whereas left ventricular hypertrophy, total cholesterol, smoking and body weight were risk factors for SCD in men, reduced vital capacity, increased hematocrit, and hyperglycemia were risk factors in women. However, in a more recent study of 121 701 women from the Nurses' Health Study cohort, Albert et al.[43] found that of those who suffered SCD, 94% had previously reported at least one, and 73% had reported at least two traditional CHD risk factors. While a prior history of MI conferred a 4.1 relative risk of SCD, smoking, hypertension, diabetes, and family history were also associated with increased relative risks between 1.6 and 4.1. These data suggest that traditional CHD risk factors indeed predict SCD in women, and modification of these risk factors in women should not be neglected.

Assessment of SCD risk in women is difficult. Ventricular premature beats and nonsustained ventricular tachycardia have not been found to predict SCD in women.[44,45] Numerous studies[46–49] have reported ventricular tachyarrhythmias less likely to be induced during electrophysiology study in women. One retrospective analysis of 355 consecutive cardiac arrest survivors by Albert et al.[50] did find that when corrections were made for the presence of CHD, the rates of noninducibility were similar between women and men (22.2% vs 23.5%). Women, however, had less CHD (45% vs 80%, p <0.0001) and higher ejection fraction (0.46 ± 0.18 vs 0.41 ± 0.18, p <0.05), and whereas low ejection fraction (<0.40) was the most powerful predictor of total and cardiac mortality in men, presence of CHD was the only predictor in women. Nonetheless, the utility of electrophysiologic testing in assessing SCD risk in women remains undetermined.

The role of implantable cardioverter defibrillators in the treatment of SCD in women appears undiminished. In a retrospective analysis of 213 men and 55 women survivors of cardiac arrest who subsequently received an implantable cardioverter defibrillator, Kudenchuk et al.[51] found that even though women had a better baseline ejection fraction, had less underlying structural heart disease, and were younger, there remained a substantial 37% arrhythmia recurrence resulting in device therapy after 2 years (vs 52% in men, p = 0.11). Complication rates for defibrillator implantation were similar between genders.

Management of arrhythmia during pregnancy (see also Chapter 22)

General considerations

Palpitations and premature atrial and ventricular complexes have been found to be increased during pregnancy in women without heart disease, and to be essentially benign without need of treatment.[52] Although smaller studies[53–56] have observed supraventricular tachycardia to be more common with pregnancy, it is unclear if a true increase in

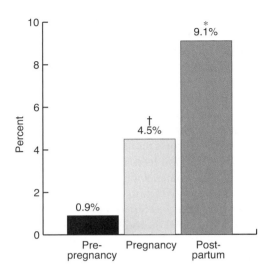

Figure 37.5
Percentage of LQTS probands with multiple cardiac events before, during, and after pregnancy. Multiple cardiac events were significantly more common among probands during the postpartum interval. The pregnancy interval was not associated with a significant increase in multiple events. *p = 0.01 vs the pregnancy interval; †p = 0.10 vs the pre-pregnancy interval. Reproduced from reference 61 with permission.

incidence exists. In a retrospective study of 60 women with supraventricular tachycardia, Tawam et al.[57] reported an increased risk of onset or exacerbation of supraventricular tachycardia during pregnancy (relative risk 5.1, p <0.001). In contrast, a larger retrospective study of 207 women by Lee et al.[58] observed only 3.9% of women to have a first-onset supraventricular tachycardia during pregnancy. Both studies, however, found symptoms of supraventricular tachycardia to be increased during pregnancy.

There have been a few case reports[59,60] of new-onset ventricular tachycardia during pregnancy, mostly in the setting of no structural heart disease. Brodsky et al.[59] observed these episodes to occur in the setting of physical and emotional stress, and postulated that the ventricular tachycardia was catecholaminergic and

responsive to beta-blocker therapy. In analyzing the International Long QT Syndrome Registry, Rashba et al.[61] reported that among patients with long QT syndrome, there was an increase in the risk of cardiac events (death, aborted cardiac arrest, syncope) during the postpartum period, but not during pregnancy itself (Fig. 37.5). Although the increase in events only after pregnancy is not well understood, a possible protective effect of increased heart rate during pregnancy has been postulated. Treatment with beta-blockers was found to significantly decrease the risk of cardiac events (odds ratio 0.023; 95% CI 0.001–0.44; p = 0.01).

Fortunately, most arrhythmias during pregnancy occur in the setting of a structurally normal heart, and are well tolerated. When symptoms are brief and only mildly symptomatic, reassurance and observation are preferred over drug therapy. In recommending rest, a left lateral decubitus position is recommended. Lying directly supine can lead to compression of the inferior vena cava by the gravid uterus and can result in decreased cardiac output.[62] As previously mentioned, however, symptoms of some arrhythmias appear to be enhanced during pregnancy and further treatment may become necessary. Women of childbearing age should be encouraged to undergo cure of arrhythmia by catheter ablation prior to becoming pregnant.

Symptomatic bradyarrhythmia during pregnancy is rare. Uterine compression of the inferior vena cava resulting in a reflex sinus bradycardia has been reported.[62] Patients with unrecognized congenital AV node disease may present with advanced heart block during pregnancy. Temporary pacing can be considered for symptomatic advanced heart block, and is recommended for asymptomatic complete heart block prior to labor and delivery.[63] Permanent pacemaker implantation can be safely performed with endovascular lead positioning guided by limited fluoroscopy. Procedures should be performed with maximal radiation shield protection for the fetus, and if possible, delayed until after 8 weeks' gestation when the risk of radiation is considerably lessened because of completed organogenesis. There are reports of successful permanent pacemaker implantation without the use of fluoroscopy, utilizing instead either transthoracic or transesophageal echocardiography to guide lead positioning.[64]

Anti-arrhythmic drug therapy

The decision to administer any drug during pregnancy is made after weighing benefit against potential risk, the main concern being fetal teratogenesis. The most vulnerable period for the fetus is during the first 8 weeks after fertilization prior to completion of organogenesis.[65] Most of the anti-arrhythmic drugs appear to be relatively safe during pregnancy, and other than a few exceptions, fall into the US Food and Drug Administration (FDA) category C (risk suggested by animal studies unconfirmed by human studies, or lack of controlled studies).[66]

The three most notable exceptions are phenytoin, amiodarone, and atenolol, all FDA category D (risk indicated by human studies) agents. Phenytoin, mostly utilized as an anticonvulsant, has some anti-arrhythmic activity (Vaughan Williams class IB) and is occasionally used to treat arrhythmias. Phenytoin has been associated with serious fetal abnormalities and should not be used during pregnancy. Amiodarone (class III) has been reported to cause hypothyroidism, growth retardation, and premature delivery[67] and should only be used in the setting of life-threatening ventricular tachyarrhythmias.[68] Beta-blockers (class II) have been safely used during pregnancy for years and are generally considered to be safe. Several studies,[69,70] however, have reported growth retardation to be associated with atenolol administration during pregnancy, mostly with first-trimester use, and thus it is probably advisable to avoid beta-blockers, if possible, during the first trimester.

Vagal maneuvers should be considered first in the acute treatment of supraventricular tachycardias during pregnancy, as successful termination may obviate the need to administer drugs. Intravenous adenosine (endogenous nucleoside) transiently blocks AV node conduction with a half-life of <2 seconds, and is the drug of choice in terminating re-entry supraventricular tachycardias. Adenosine, in boluses of 6–18 mg, has been administered safely[71–74] without deleterious effect on monitored fetal heart rate. Intravenous verapamil should be avoided because of reports of maternal and fetal bradycardia, heart block, hypotension, and depressed contractions.[75] If pre-exitation is evident or the etiology of

wide-complex tachycardia is unclear, intravenous procainamide can be given safely.[76]

Digoxin has the longest safety record in the chronic treatment of supraventricular tachycardia during pregnancy,[67,77] but unfortunately is not especially effective. Metoprolol, a cardioselective beta-blocker, has not been associated with growth retardation and is a reasonable first choice agent.[78] When possible, beta-blocker therapy should be delayed till after the first trimester. Propafenone and flecainide (class IC) appear safe and can be used appropriately.[67] Serum drug levels may need to be monitored as many factors influence therapeutic dosing of drugs during pregnancy including increased intravascular volume, reduced plasma protein concentration, increased renal blood flow, increased hepatic metabolism, and altered gastrointestinal absorption.[79] Successful radiofrequency ablation using echocardiography-guided catheter manipulation has been reported.[80]

Treatment of stable ventricular tachycardia in the setting of cardiomyopathy can start with intravenous lidocaine, which has limited efficacy but is quite safe. Intravenous procainamide is more likely to be effective and has also been found to be safe during pregnancy.[76] If the ventricular tachycardia is idiopathic (occurs without associated structural heart disease), intravenous beta-blockers should be considered. Intravenous adenosine may be effective if a right or left ventricular outflow tract focus is suspected. Amiodarone should be avoided during the first trimester, and only be considered for life-threatening arrhythmias. Although use of sotalol appears safe during pregnancy,[81] because of concerns for torsade de pointes, especially in the postpartum period, corrected QT interval should be followed closely during initiation of therapy and with any increase in dose.

Cardioversion and defibrillator implantation

When dealing with an episode of tachyarrhythmia during pregnancy, one must remember the importance of a stable blood pressure for the well-being of the fetus, and assessment and treatment should therefore be prompt. Any unstable tachyarrhythmia should be treated with external cardioversion without hesitation. Direct current shocks of up to 400 J have been used during pregnancy without significant complication.[82–84] The safety of the procedure appears to be a function of the small amount of energy that reaches the fetus and the high fibrillation threshold of a small fetal heart.[85] Isolated instances of transient fetal distress have been observed,[85,86] however, and fetal monitoring during the procedure is preferred. If either the mother or fetus is threatened, emergent cesarean section should be considered.

Internal shocks from previously implanted cardioverter defibrillators also appear safe during pregnancy, based on a report from Natale et al.[87] Of 44 women studied, 42 had nonpectoral devices, and the majority of lead systems were epicardial. The total number of shocks during pregnancy ranged from 0 to 11, and averaged 0.66 ± 1.9 shocks per patient. There were no adverse fetal outcomes as a result of the shocks. Contractions were not found to precipitate arrhythmias or myopotentials that might trigger defibrillator discharge. It would appear that a woman with a previously implanted defibrillator can safely undergo pregnancy from an arrhythmic standpoint. There has been one reported case of successful implantation of a defibrillator during pregnancy.[88]

Anticoagulation

The need for anticoagulation for arrhythmia during pregnancy is unusual, and is essentially confined to women with atrial fibrillation who are also at high risk for embolic complications. Factors that increase this risk are a history of previous transient ischemic attack or stroke, mitral stenosis, hypertension, diabetes, age above 65 years, coronary disease, and congestive heart failure.[89] Most of these risk factors are rarely found in pregnant women, and atrial fibrillation is often isolated in this population without need of anticoagulation. If, however, atrial fibrillation is associated with any of these risk factors, or if there is a pre-existing need for anticoagulation (such as mechanical prosthetic valve), anticoagulation must be considered.

Warfarin crosses the placenta and first-trimester exposure can result in severe embryopathy. Less frequently, central nervous system abnormalities and fetal bleeding have been reported with exposure beyond the first trimester.[90] Thus, warfarin should be avoided, especially during the first trimester, and only used thereafter under extenuating circumstances.

Heparin, on the other hand, does not cross the placenta and is the preferred agent for anticoagulation during pregnancy. Heparin can be administered subcutaneously as twice-daily injections starting with a total daily dose of 35 000 U, adjusted to an activated partial thromboplastin time >1.5 times normal range. Heparin-binding proteins increase in the third trimester and the need for increasing doses should be anticipated. Alternatively, low-molecular-weight heparin (LMWH) can be given subcutaneously as 100 anti-Xa U/kg twice-daily injections, adjusted to anti-Xa levels between 0.5 and 1.0 U/ml drawn 4–6 hours after injections. Heparin and LMWH should be discontinued 12 hours before labor induction. Warfarin can be restarted after delivery even if the mother plans to nurse. Studies have shown that warfarin will not cause an anticoagulant effect in breastfed infants.[91,92] Either heparin or LMWH therapy should be reinstituted postpartum until warfarin levels are therapeutic.

Anticoagulation of patients with mechanical heart valves is a separate, more complex issue. Heparin failure resulting in thromboembolic complication has been reported in patients with mechanical heart valves.[93–95] LMWH has also been associated with complications in these patients (FDA and Aventis advisory warning). In women with mechanical heart valves, warfarin may need to be reconsidered for treatment during the second and third trimesters, and perhaps even during the first trimester if maternal risk is assessed greater than fetal risk. The American Heart Association and American College of Cardiology scientific statement[96] outlines three potential options of therapy, which are, (1) heparin or LMWH throughout pregnancy, (2) warfarin throughout pregnancy, (3) heparin or LMWH during the first trimester followed by switch to warfarin in the second trimester. If heparin or LMWH is used in women with mechanical heart valves, they should be given in adequate doses and followed closely with at least twice-weekly blood level checks. If warfarin is used, a switch back to heparin or LMWH at 38 weeks' gestation is recommended to avoid bleeding complications during delivery, and labor induction should be planned at 40 weeks' gestation.

References

1. Bazett HC. An analysis of the time-relations of electrocardiograms. *Heart* 1920; **7**:353–70.
2. Liu K, Ballew C, Jacobs DR Jr, et al. Ethnic differences in blood pressure, pulse rate, and related characteristics in young adults. The CARDIA study. *Hypertension* 1989; **14**:218–26.
3. Teneja T, Mahnert BW, Passman R, Goldberger J, Kadish A. Effects of sex and age on electrocardiographic and cardiac electrophysiological properties in adults. *Pacing Clin Electrophysiol* 2001; **24**:16–21.
4. Burke JH, Goldberger JJ, Ehlert FA, Kruse JT, Parker MA, Kadish AH. Gender differences in heart rate before and after autonomic blockade: evidence against an intrinsic gender effect. *Am J Med* 1996; **100**:537–43.
5. Burke JH, Ehlert FA, Kruse JT, Parker MA, Goldberger JJ, Kadish AH. Gender-specific differences in the QT interval and the effect of autonomic tone and menstrual cycle in healthy adults. *Am J Cardiol* 1997; **79**:178–81.
6. Stramba-Badiale M, Locati EH, Martinelli A, Courville J, Schwartz PJ. Gender and the relationship between ventricular repolarisation and cardiac cycle length during 24–h Holter recordings. *Eur Heart J* 1997; **18**:1000–6.
7. Merri M, Benhorin J, Alberti M, Locati E, Moss AJ. Electrocardiographic quantification of ventricular repolarization. *Circulation* 1989; **80**:1301–8.
8. Rautaharju PM, Zhou SH, Wong S, et al. Sex differences in the evolution of the electrocardiographic QT interval with age. *Can J Cardiol* 1992; **8**:690–5.
9. Liu XK, Katchman A, Drici MD, et al. Gender difference in the cycle length-dependent QT and potassium currents in rabbits. *J Pharmacol Exp Ther* 1998; **285**:672–9.
10. Drici MD, Burklow TR, Haridasse V, Glazer RI, Woosley RL. Sex hormones prolong the QT interval and downregulate potassium channel expression in the rabbit heart. *Circulation* 1996; **94**:1471–4.
11. Hara M, Danilo P, Rosen MR. Effects of gonadal steroids on ventricular repolarisation and the response to E4031. *J Pharmacol Exp Ther* 1998; **285**:1068–72.
12. Pham TV, Sosunov EA, Gainullin RZ, Danilo P, Rosen MR. Impact of sex and gonadal steroids on prolongation of ventricular repolarization and arrhythmias induced by I_K-blocking drugs. *Circulation* 2001; **103**:2207–12.
13. Carnethon MR, Anthony MS, Cascio WE, et al. A prospective evaluation of the risk of QT prolongation with hormone replacement therapy: the atherosclerosis risk in communities study. *Ann Epidemiol* 2003; **13**:530–6.
14. Rodriguez I, Kilborn MJ, Liu X-K, Pezzullo JC, Woosley RL. Drug-induced QT prolongation in women during the menstrual cycle. *JAMA* 2001; **285**:1322–6.
15. Krahn AD, Yee R, Klein GJ, Morillo C. Inappropriate sinus tachycardia: evaluation and therapy. *J Cardiovasc Electrophysiol* 1995; **6**:1124–8.
16. Lee RJ, Shinbane JS. Inappropriate sinus tachycardia. Diagnosis and treatment. *Cardiol Clin* 1997; **15**:599–605.
17. Morillo CA, Klein GJ, Thakur RK, Li H, Zardini M, Yee R. Mechanism of 'inappropriate' sinus tachycardia: role of sympathovagal balance. *Circulation* 1994; **90**:873–7.
18. Rodriguez LM, de Chillou C, Metzger J, et al. Age at onset and gender of patients with different types of supraventricular tachycardias. *Am J Cardiol* 1992; **70**:1213–15.
19. Calkins H, Yong P, Miller JM, et al. Catheter ablation of accessory pathways, atrioventricular nodal reentrant tachycardia, and the atrioventricular junction. *Circulation* 1999; **99**:262–70.
20. Insulander P, Kenneback G, Straat E, Jensen-Urstad M, Vallin H. Differences in dual AV nodal properties between men and women. *Eur Heart J* 1999; **20**:568 (abstract).
21. Timmermans C, Smeets JL, Rodriguez LM, Vrouchos G, van den Dool A, Wellens HJ. Aborted sudden death in the Wolff–Parkinson–White syndrome. *Am J Cardiol* 1995; **76**:492–4.
22. Tada H, Oral H, Greenstein R, et al. Analysis of age of onset of accessory pathway-mediated tachycardia in men and women. *Am J Cardiol* 2002; **89**:470–1.
23. Rosano GM, Leonardo F, Sarrel PM, Beale CM, De Luca F, Collins P. Cyclical variation in paroxysmal supraventricular tachycardia in women, *Lancet* 1996; **347**:786–8.
24. Myerburg RJ, Cox MM, Interian A Jr, et al. Cycling of inducibility of paroxysmal supraventricular tachycardia in women and its implications for timing of electrophysiologic procedures. *Am J Cardiol* 1999; **83**:1049–54.
25. Dagres N, Clague JR, Breithardt G, Borggrefe M.

Significant gender-related differences in radiofrequency catheter ablation therapy. *J Am Coll Cardiol* 2003; **42**:1103–7.

26. Lessmeier TJ, Gamperling D, Johnson-Liddon V, et al. Unrecognized paroxysmal supraventricular tachycardia. *Arch Intern Med* 1997; **157**:537–43.

27. Benjamin EJ, Levy D, Vaziri SM, D'Agostino RB, Belanger AJ, Wolf PA. Independent risk factors for atrial fibrillation in a population-based cohort. The Framingham Heart Study. *JAMA* 1994; **271**:840–4.

28. Benjamin EJ, Wolf PA, D'Agostino RB, Silvershatz H, Kannel WB, Levy D. Impact of atrial fibrillation on the risk of death: the Framingham Heart Study. *Circulation* 1998; **98**:946–52.

29. Cameron A, Schwartz MJ, Kronmal RA, Kosinski AS. Prevalence and significance of atrial fibrillation in coronary artery disease (CASS Registry). *Am J Cardiol* 1988; **61**:714–17.

30. Cooklin M, Gold MR. Implications and treatment of atrial fibrillation after cardiothoracic surgery. *Curr Opin Cardiol* 1998; **13**:20–7.

31. Feinberg WM, Blackshear JL, Laupacis A, Kronmol R, Hart RG. Prevalence, age distribution, and gender of patients with atrial fibrillation. Analysis and implications. *Arch Intern Med* 1995; **155**:469–73.

32. Hnatkova K, Walstare JEP, Murgatroyd FD. Age and gender influences on rate and duration of paroxysmal atrial fibrillation. *Pacing Clin Electrophysiol* 1998; **21**:2455–8.

33. Suttorp MJ, Kingma JH, Koomen EM, van't Hof A, Tijssen JG, Lie KI. Recurrence of paroxysmal atrial fibrillation or flutter after successful cardioversion in patients with normal left ventricular function. *Am J Cardiol* 1993; **71**:710–13.

34. Cabin HS, Clubb KS, Hall C, Perlmutter RA, Feinstein AR. Risk of systemic embolization of atrial fibrillation without mitral stenosis. *Am J Cardiol* 1990; **65**:1112–16.

35. Makkar RR, Fromm BS, Steinman RT. Female gender as a risk factor for torsades de pointes associated with cardiovascular drugs. *JAMA* 1993; **270**:2590–7.

36. Lehmann MH, Hardy S, Archibald D, Quart B, MacNeil DJ. Sex difference in risk of torsade de pointes with d,l-sotalol. *Circulation* 1996; **94**:2535–41.

37. Torp-Pedersen C, Moller M, Bloch-Thomsen PE, et al. for the Danish Investigations of Arrhythmia & Mortality on Dofetilide Study Group. Dofetilide in patients with congestive heart failure and left ventricular dysfunction. *N Engl J Med* 1999; **34**:857–65.

38. Bednar MM, Harrigan EP, Ruskin JN. Torsades de pointes associated with nonarrhythmic drugs and

observations on gender and QTc. *Am J Cardiol* 2002; **89**:1316–19.

39. Locati EH, Zareba W, Moss AJ, et al. Age- and sex-related differences in clinical manifestations in patients with congenital long-QT syndrome: findings from the International LQTS Registry. *Circulation* 1998; **97**:2237–44.

40. Zareba W, Moss AJ, Locati EH, et al. Modulating effects of age and gender on the clinical course of long QT syndrome by genotype. *J Am Coll Cardiol* 2003; **42**:103–9.

41. Kannel WB, Wilson PWF, D'Agostino RB, Cobb J. Sudden coronary death in women. *Am Heart J* 1998; **136**:205–12.

42. Kannel WB, Schatzkin A. Sudden death: lessons from subsets of population studies. *J Am Coll Cardiol* 1985; **5**:141B–9B.

43. Albert CM, Chae CU, Grodstein F, et al. Prospective study of sudden cardiac death among women in the United States. *Circulation* 2003; **107**:2096–101.

44. Cupples LA, Gagnon DR, Kannel WB. Long and short term risk of sudden coronary death. *Circulation* 1992; **85**:I11–18.

45. Dittrich H, Gilpin E, Nicod P. Acute myocardial infarction in women: influence of gender on mortality and prognostic variables. *Am J Cardiol* 1988; **62**:1–7.

46. Schoenfeld MH, McGovern B, Garan H, Kelly E, Grant G, Ruskin JN. Determinants of the outcome of electrophysiology study in patients with ventricular tachyarrhythmias. *J Am Coll Cardiol* 1985; **6**:298–306.

47. Freedman RA, Swerdlow CD, Soderholm-Difatte V, Mason JW. Clinical predictors of arrhythmia inducibility in survivors of cardiac arrest: importance of gender and prior myocardial infarction. *J Am Coll Cardiol* 1988; **12**:973–8.

48. Vaitkus PT, Kindwall E, Miller JM, Marchlinski FE, Buxton AE, Josephson ME. Influence of gender on inducibility of ventricular arrhythmias in survivors of cardiac arrest with coronary artery disease. *Am J Cardiol* 1991; **67**:537–9.

49. Buxton AE, Hafley GE, Lehmann MH, et al. Prediction of sustained ventricular tachycardia inducible by programmed stimulation in patients with coronary artery disease: utility of clinical variables. *Circulation* 1999; **99**:1843–50.

50. Albert CM, McGovern BA, Newell JB, Ruskin JN. Sex differences in cardiac arrest survivors. *Circulation* 1996; **93**:1170–6.

51. Kudenchuk PJ, Bardy GH, Poole JE, et al. Malignant sustained ventricular tachyarrhythmias in women; characteristics and outcome of treatment with an

implantable cardioverter defibrillator. *J Cardiovasc Electrophysiol* 1997; **8**:2–10.

52. Shotan A, Ostrzega E, Mehra A, Johnson JV, Elkayam U. Incidence of arrhythmia in normal pregnancy and relation to palpitations, dizziness, and syncope. *Am J Cardiol* 1997; **79**:1061–4.

53. Widerhorn J, Widerhorn AL, Rahimtoola SH, Elkayam U. WPW syndrome during pregnancy: increased incidence of supraventricular arrhythmias. *Am Heart J* 1992; **123**:796–8.

54. Mendelson DL. Disorder of the heart beat during pregnancy. *Am J Obstet Gynecol* 1956; **72**:1268–301.

55. Szekely P, Snaith L. Paroxysmal tachycardia in pregnancy. *Br Heart J* 1953; **15**:195–8.

56. Gleicher N, Meller J, Sandler RZ, Sullum S. Wolff–Parkinson–White syndrome in pregnancy. *Obstet Gynecol* 1981; **58**:748–52.

57. Tawam M, Levine J, Mendelson M, Goldberger J, Dyer A, Kadish A. Effect of pregnancy on paroxysmal supraventricular tachycardia. *Am J Cardiol* 1993; **72**:838–40.

58. Lee SH, Chen SA, Wu TJ, et al. Effects of pregnancy on first onset and symptoms of paroxysmal supraventricular tachycardia. *Am J Cardiol* 1995; **76**:675–8.

59. Brodsky M, Doria R, Allen B, Sato D, Thomas G, Sada M. New-onset ventricular tachycardia during pregnancy. *Am Heart J* 1992; **123**:933–41.

60. Russell RO Jr. Paroxysmal ventricular tachycardia associated with pregnancy. *Ala J Med Sci* 1969; **6**:111–20.

61. Rashba EJ, Zareba W, Moss AJ, et al. Influence of pregnancy on the risk for cardiac events in patients with hereditary long QT syndrome. LQTS Investigators. *Circulation* 1998; **97**:451–6.

62. McAnulty JH, Morton MJ, Ueland K. The heart and pregnancy. *Curr Probl Cardiol* 1988; **13**:589–665.

63. Dalvi BV, Chaudhuri A, Kulkarni HL, Kale PA. Therapeutic guidelines for congenital complete heart block presenting in pregnancy. *Obstet Gynecol* 1992; **79**:802–4.

64. Antonelli D, Bloch L, Rosenfeld T. Implantation of permanent dual chamber pacemaker in a pregnant woman by transesophageal echocardiographic guidance. *Pacing Clin Electrophysiol* 1999; **22**:534–5.

65. Cunningham FG, MacDonald PC, Leveno KJ, Gant NF, Gilstrap LC. *Williams Obstetrics*, 19th edn. Norwalk, CT: Appleton & Lange, 1993: 166–8.

66. *Physicians' Desk Reference*, 57th edn. Montvale, NJ: Medical Economics, 2003.

67. Cox JL, Gardner MJ. Treatment of cardiac arrhythmias during pregnancy. *Prog Cardiovasc Dis* 1993; **36**:137–78.

68. Wilderhorn J, Bhandari AK, Bughi S, Rahimtoola SH, Elkayam U. Fetal and neonatal adverse effects profile of amiodarone treatment during pregnancy. *Am Heart J* 1991; **122**:1162–6.

69. Butters L, Kennedy S, Rubin PC. Atenolol in essential hypertension during pregnancy. *BMJ* 1990; **301**:587–9.

70. Lip GY, Beevers M, Churchill D, Shaffer LM, Beevers DG. Effect of atenolol on birth weight. *Am J Cardiol* 1997; **79**:1436–8.

71. Alfridi I, Moise KJ, Rokey R. Termination of supraventricular tachycardia with intravenous adenosine in a pregnant woman with Wolff–Parkinson–White syndrome. *Obstet Gynecol* 1992; **80**:481–3.

72. Mason BA, Ricci-Goodman J, Koos BJ. Adenosine in the treatment of maternal paroxysmal supraventricular tachycardia. *Obstet Gynecol* 1992; **80**:478–80.

73. Leffler S, Johnson DR. Adenosine use in pregnancy: lack of effect on fetal heart rate. *Am J Emerg Med* 1992; **10**:548–9.

74. Elkayam U, Goodwin TM. Safety and efficacy of intravenous adenosine therapy for supraventricular tachycardia during pregnancy-results of a national survey. *J Am Coll Cardiol* 1994; **23**:91A (abstract).

75. Kleinman CS, Copel JA, Weinstein EM, Santulli TV, Hobbins JC. Treatment of fetal supraventricular tachyarrhythmias. *J Clin Ultrasound* 1985; **13**:265–73.

76. Allen NM, Page RL. Administration of procainamide during pregnancy. *Clin Pharm* 1993; **12**:58–60.

77. Rotmensch HH, Elkayam U, Frishman W. Antiarrhythmic drug therapy during pregnancy. *Ann Intern Med* 1983; **98**:487–97.

78. Frishman WH, Chesner M. Beta-adrenergic blockers in pregnancy. *Am Heart J* 1988; **115**:147–52.

79. Page RL. Treatment of arrhythmias during pregnancy. *Am Heart J* 1995; **130**:871–6.

80. Lee MS, Evans SJ, Blumberg S, Bodenheimer MM, Roth SL. Echocardiographically guided electrophysiologic testing in pregnancy. *J Am Soc Echocardiogr* 1994; **7**:182–6.

81. Mason JW. A comparison of seven antiarrhythmic drugs in patients with ventricular tachyarrhythmias. Electrophysiologic Study versus Electrocardiographic Monitoring Investigators. *N Engl J Med* 1993; **329**:452–8.

82. Ogburn PL, Schmidt G, Linman J, Cefalo RC. Paroxysmal tachycardia and cardioversion during pregnancy. *J Reprod Med* 1992; **27**:359–66.

83. Curry JJ, Quintana FJ. Myocardial infarction with ventricular fibrillation during pregnancy treated by direct current defibrillation with fetal survival. *Chest* 1970; **58**:82–4.

84. Klepper I. Cardioversion in late pregnancy. *Anaesthesia* 1981; **36**:611–16.

85. DeSilva RA, Graboys TB, Podrid PJ, Lown B. Cardioversion and defibrillation. *Am Heart J* 1980; **100**:881–95.

86. Finlay AY, Edmonds V. D.C. cardioversion in pregnancy. *Br J Clin Pract* 1979; **33**:88–94.

87. Natale A, Davidson T, Geiger MJ, Newby K. Implantable cardioverter-defibrillators and pregnancy: a safe combination? *Circulation* 1997; **96**:2808–12.

88. Wydra D, Ciach K, Matkowski S, Sawicki S, Emerich J. Cardiac arrest and implantation of a cardioverter-defibrillator in a pregnant woman. *Ginekol Pol* 2003; **74**:545–8.

89. The Stroke Prevention in Atrial Fibrillation Investigators. Predictors of thromboembolism in atrial fibrillation: I. Clinical feature of patients at risk. *Ann Intern Med* 1992; **116**:1–5.

90. Hall JG, Pauli RM, Wilson KM. Maternal and fetal sequelae of anticoagulation during pregnancy. *Am J Med* 1980; **68**:12–40.

91. McKenna R, Cole ER, Vasan U. Is warfarin sodium contraindicated in the lactating mother? *J Pediatr* 1983; **103**:325–7.

92. Lao TT, de Swiet M, Letsky SE, Walters BN. Prophylaxis of thromboembolism in pregnancy: an alternative. *Br J Obstet Gynaecol* 1985; **92**:202–6.

93. Altman R, Rouvier J, Gurfinkel E, et al. Comparison of two levels of anticoagulant therapy in patients with substitute heart valves. *J Thorac Cardiovasc Surg* 1991; **101**:427–31.

94. Sbarouni E, Oakley CM. Outcome of pregnancy in women with valve prostheses. *Br Heart J* 1994; **71**:196–201.

95. Hanania G. Management of anticoagulants during pregnancy. *Heart* 2001; **86**:125–6.

96. Hirsh J, Fuster V, Ansell J, Halperin JL. American Heart Association/American College of Cardiology foundation guide to warfarin therapy. *J Am Coll Cardiol* 2003; **41**:1633–52.

38

Peripheral arterial disease in women

Janet T. Powell and Tamsin Ribbons

The umbrella of cardiovascular disease (CVD) covers diseases of the heart, the cardiac and cerebral circulations, the great vessels, the abdominal aorta, and its distal branches. Peripheral arterial disease (PAD), atherosclerotic-thrombotic disease of the abdominal aorta and its distal branches (including abdominal aortic aneurysm, AAA), can be considered as the Cinderella of CVD, often neglected in favor of coronary heart disease and stroke. The reasons for this apparent lack of interest in PAD are diverse, but prominent among them is the fact that PAD is rarely fatal, although this does not apply to AAA. Nevertheless, PAD is a cause of considerable morbidity and decreasing quality of life in the elderly population. PAD is also the unwanted herald of future cardiovascular events and for this reason there is increased interested in the detection of both symptomatic and asymptomatic disease.[1] The symptom most commonly reported is intermittent claudication, although some patients first present with ulceration, rest pain, or gangrene. The environmental and genetic risk factors that contribute to the development of PAD and AAA appear to be rather different from those for other forms of CVD. Smoking is particularly important: less than 10% of the patients with symptomatic PAD or AAA have never smoked.[2,3] Hypertriglyceridemia has been another factor particularly associated with the development and progression of PAD.[4,5]

Apart from the occlusive form of atherosclero-thrombotic disease of the abdominal aorta and its distal branches, the atherosclerotic abdominal aorta may dilate to form an AAA. Again this disorder is strongly associated with smoking, which has been the only consistent risk factor for AAA in population studies. Although femoral and popliteal aneurysms also may occur, these are very rare in women. AAA is the herald of future cardiovascular death.[6] Both PAD and AAA are discussed in this chapter.

Prevalence of PAD in women

Many early epidemiologic studies used the Rose questionnaire[7] to detect the presence of intermittent claudication. In more recent studies focusing on PAD more sensitive questionnaires, such as the Edinburgh artery questionnaire, have been used. These have been supplemented by objective measurements, particularly the ankle/brachial systolic pressure index (ABI) to provide estimates of asymptomatic disease. Many of the earlier studies were conducted in men only and from these one could have been led to believe that PAD was a disease of men, rather than a disease of smokers.

In 1991 Fowkes et al.[8] reported on the prevalence of both asymptomatic and symptomatic disease in 2720 subjects from the general population of Lothian, Scotland: the Edinburgh Artery Study. The principal finding of this study was that 4.5% of the population aged 55–74 years had intermittent claudication and a further 8.0% had findings that indicated the presence of asymptomatic disease. Although relatively more men than women had an ABI of <0.8 (the cut-off point chosen for the presence of asymptomatic disease), this did not achieve statistical significance. In summary, even using a sensitive and relatively specific questionnaire, the prevalence of both symptomatic and asymptomatic disease was similar in women and men. More recent European studies have been conducted in Rotterdam and Limburg.[9,10] These both used different criteria for the presence of asymptomatic PAD, using an ABI of <0.9 and <0.95, respectively. Therefore, unsurprisingly the Rotterdam study, conducted among the general population aged 55 years and older, showed a higher prevalence of asymptomatic PAD than the Edinburgh study. The prevalence of asymptomatic PAD in Rotterdam was 20.9% in women and 16.9% in men, with symptoms being reported by 2.2% of men and 1.2% of women.[9] The Limburg study included younger subjects (from 45 to 74 years), resulting in a lower prevalence of PAD, 6.9%, but with a similar prevalence in women and men.[10] There was some evidence from the Limburg study that the symptomatic PAD was more severe in men than women.

The findings for asymptomatic PAD in the United States are similar. In the Cardiovascular Health Study, ABI was measured in 5201 persons aged over 65 years recruited from a stratified random sample of Medicare recipients taken from communities in four states.[9] A similar percentage of women (11.4%) and men (13.8%) had an ABI <0.9 (the cut-off point chosen for the detection of PAD in this study). There was a very strong association of reduced ABI (<0.9) with increasing age (p <0.0001), but no association with gender. The earlier California study of Criqui et al.[11] found that the prevalence of intermittent claudication was 1.7% in women and 2.2% in men.

The accumulating evidence shows that where thresholds of ABI or ankle pressure are used to determine the prevalence of PAD, the prevalence in women and men is similar. The lack of uniform definitions of asymptomatic PAD, as assessed by ABI, hampers reliable estimates of the prevalence in women. The detection of symptomatic disease remains questionnaire-based or determined from hospital case records and the true incidence may be difficult to determine. However, the Rotterdam Study showed that symptomatic PAD (intermittent claudication using the Rose questionnaire) was two

to three times more common in men than women. There are several reasons that might underlie this important observation, including previous differences in smoking habit and stoicism. Exercise improves walking distance. Therefore it is possible that the exercise involved in performing routine household chores, which continues after retirement, may attenuate the severity of PAD in women. Nevertheless, there are preliminary indications that both asymptomatic and symptomatic PAD has a greater impact on women than men, with decreased physical functioning, more bodily pain, and greater mood disturbance than in men.[12] These effects are progressive and indicate that medical therapy for PAD in women should address these issues.

Over and above all these considerations, it must be remembered that PAD and ABI are markers of future cardiovascular death.[13] The management of PAD in women should be directed both at alleviating symptoms and preventing future cardiovascular events. Recent data from the large trials of hormone replacement therapy (HRT) have indicated that HRT is not a treatment to prevent cardiovascular morbidity and mortality.[14,15]

Prevalence of AAA in women and men

The majority of AAA have no symptoms before impending rupture. The prevalence of AAA has been determined by ultrasonographic screening of asymptomatic populations over the age of 60 years. The definition of AAA, like the definition of asymptomatic PAD, is variable, but many studies have based their definition of AAA on a minimum anterior-posterior diameter of 3.0 cm. This was the definition used by the Chichester screening program, which showed the prevalence of AAA to be 1.4% in women and 4.8% in men.[16] This threefold difference in prevalence has been confirmed in several other smaller studies. While the prevalence of AAA in women might be low, there is clear evidence that in women the risk of AAA rupture is higher and that AAA rupture at smaller diameters than in men.[17,18] Small AAA (<5.5 cm diameter) have a very low annual risk of rupture, about 1% per annum.

However, the risk of rupture for small AAA is up to fourfold higher for women than men. In a study which included AAA that enlarged to beyond 5.5 cm in diameter, the mean diameter preceding rupture was 5.0 cm in women versus 6.0 cm in men.[17] So AAA is less common among women, but when present it is likely to be more dangerous than in men.

Anatomic factors associated with the development of PAD in women

There may be anatomic factors that predispose to sex-specific differences in the development of PAD and AAA. There is clear evidence that the diameter of the abdominal aorta and femoral arteries is smaller in women.[19,20] In addition, the age-dependent increase in arterial diameter appears to be less marked in women than in men. This contributes to the low prevalence of AAA in women and potentially could aggravate the symptoms of occlusive PAD. In addition to these matters of size, there are other gender-specific differences in the development of disease. Atherosclerotic femoral artery aneurysms appear to be found in men only, probably related to arterial anatomy at the level of the inguinal ligament. Popliteal artery aneurysms and popliteal artery entrapment syndrome both have a very strong male predominance and may be exacerbated by trauma from repetitive vigorous physical exercise. Historically there was a high prevalence of popliteal aneurysms among cavalry officers. Beyond this, aneurysmal disease progresses in a different manner in women, the aneurysm having a shorter, but wider neck than in men.[21] In addition, severe angulation of the neck or arteries at the distal end of the aneurysm is seen more commonly in women. Both of these considerations impact on treatment options: AAA in women are less likely to be suitable for endovascular repair.[21]

The small aorta syndrome is observed exclusively in women.[22] This is a syndrome confined to women of small stature, who present with intermittent claudication or rest pain at an early age, often premenopausal women between the ages of 40 and 55 years. These women are heavy smokers and usually have hypercholesterolemia or other lipid abnormalities. Angiography demonstrates a narrow infrarenal aorta, narrow iliac and common femoral arteries, and a straight course of the iliac arteries, with atherosclerotic lesions involving principally the aorto-iliac segment. The mean diameter of the distal aorta is about 12 mm and the diameter of the iliac arteries about 7 mm, significantly smaller than in other women. Among these patients there is a high incidence of single bifurcating lumbar arteries at the fourth and fifth lumbar vertebrae. Therefore, it has been suggested that the aortic hypoplasia results from embryonic overfusion of the dorsal aortas.

The smoking habits of women (see also Chapter 5)

Smoking is the major risk factor for PAD and AAA. Although tobacco was introduced into England by Sir Walter Raleigh in the late sixteenth century, it was not until after the industrial revolution that cigarettes were available for mass marketing. Among British men, the popularity of cigarette smoking increased sharply between 1900 and 1940.[23] The percentage of British men who smoked decreased from a peak of around 70% in 1945 to 40% in 1980 to less than 30% today. The story for women is very different. In the UK, women did not smoke in large numbers until after World War II. Cigarette consumption among women increased sharply between 1945 and 1975, at which time about 40% of all women over the age of 16 years smoked. Today, smoking is more common among women than men, with a third of all women still smoking. This is likely to underlie the trend of an ever increasing proportion of women presenting for vascular surgery. It is worrying that smoking is so common among teenage women.

It has been difficult to establish any clear relationship between the extent of tobacco exposure and the severity of either PAD or AAA. To obtain information about this and other risk factors a case-control study of smokers was established at Charing Cross Hospital, London in 1988.[24,25] The cases were consecutive referrals to the Vascular Surgical Service, the presence of PAD being confirmed by an ABI of ≤0.8 and an AAA as a maximum anterior-posterior aortic diameter of ≥3.0 cm. Controls were patients in other outpatient departments of the hospital (mainly orthopedics, dermatology, and urology). While there was a clear association between risk of developing PAD and previous smoking history (pack-years) and depth of inhalation in men, there was no such association observed in women. In contrast, women smokers with PAD had much higher serum cholesterol and lipoprotein(a) concentrations than women smokers without PAD. A similar situation has been observed for the development of AAA in women; hypercholesterolemia appears to be a significant risk factor, whereas in men the evidence is inconsistent.

Although women smokers develop PAD or AAA in large numbers, they almost never suffer from Buerger's disease – a diffuse inflammatory disease of the distal artery, vein and nerve, restricted to younger male smokers. On another positive note, with sufficient commitment women can be persuaded to stop smoking after cardiovascular events. A recent study has shown that, with cognitive behavioral intervention, there was almost a 50% success rate for smoking cessation in older women who had been in hospital for management of CVD.[26]

Diabetes and PAD in women
(see also Chapter 3)

Diabetes is the endocrine disorder most commonly associated with the development of PAD. On average, one in seven patients referred to vascular surgeons with PAD are women; some 20% or more of the women have diabetes. In a study of the prevalence of intermittent claudication in Finland, the age-adjusted prevalence of PAD was 5.7 times higher in diabetic women than in diabetic men.[27] The prevalence of asymptomatic PAD (ABI <0.8) after at least 25 years of diabetes is reported as being 30% in women compared with only 11% in men.[28]

Outcomes of surgical intervention in women

Although several single-center studies have indicated that female gender was associated with worse outcome following conventional open repair of AAA, population data do not support this prejudice.[29,30] There was no difference in 30-day mortality for women and men. However, the late survival of women who have survived AAA repair is substantially less than that for an age/sex-matched population, a phenomenon not observed in men.[30] There may be sociological explanations for this phenomenon. Whereas often wives act as the carers for men who return home from AAA repair, many of the women may be living alone. An increasing number of peripheral arterial reconstructions (bypass surgery) is performed in women. Despite often being older than men, with a high proportion of diabetics, there is no difference in morbidity or mortality following infra-inguinal reconstructions for limb salvage. A large study has shown that primary graft patency after 5 years was 65% in women and 61% in men.[31] This same study showed that the 30-day mortality was 3.5% in women and 2.9% in men. Although wound infection appeared to be more common in women, this could be related to the underlying high prevalence of diabetes (53%) in women.

Summary

Sexual equality is being accomplished. The total prevalence of PAD is similar in women and men. However, far fewer women than men complain of intermittent claudication. This difference could result from past differences in smoking habit or other factors. In contrast, AAA remains largely a disease of men. With smoking now being more prevalent among women than men, in the future PAD could lose its status as a disease of men and the prevalence of AAA in women might increase. Gender does not influence postoperative morbidity and mortality for either condition. Both PAD and AAA are degenerative diseases with increasing prevalence in later life. The dream that HRT might alleviate the burden of disease has been rudely shattered. The recommended treatments for PAD and AAA are the same in women and men.

References

1. Newman AB, Siscovick DS, Manolio TA, et al. Ankle-arm index as a marker of atherosclerosis in the Cardiovascular Health Study. *Circulation* 1993; **88**:837–45.

2. Fowkes FGR. Epidemiology of atherosclerotic arterial disease in the lower limbs. *Eur J Vasc Surg* 1988; **2**: 283–91.

3. Powell JT, Greenhalgh RM. Changing the smoking habit and its influence on the managements of vascular disease. *Acta Chir Scand* 1990; **555**:99–103.

4. Greenhalgh RM, Lewis B, Rosengarten DS, et al. Serum lipids and lipoproteins in peripheral vascular disease. *Lancet* 1971; **ii**: 947–50.

5. Smith I, Franks PJ, Greenhalgh RM, et al. The influence of hypertriglyceridaemia and smoking cessation on the progression of peripheral arterial disease and the onset of critical ischaemia. *Eur J Vasc Surg* 1996; **11**:402–8.

6. Brady AR, Thompson SG, Fowkes FGR, Powell JT. Aortic aneurysm diameter and risk of cardiovascular mortality. *Arterioscler Thromb Vasc Biol* 2001; **21**:1203–7.

7. Smith GD, Shipley MJ, Rose G. Intermittent claudication, heart disease risk factors and mortality: the Whitehall Study. *Circulation* 1990; **82**:1925–31.

8. Fowkes FGR, Housley E, Cawood EHH, et al. Edinburgh Artery Study: prevalence of asymptomatic and symptomatic PAD in the general population. *Int J Epidemiol* 1991; **20**:384–92.

9. Meijer WT, Hoes AW, Rutgers D, et al. Peripheral arterial disease in the elderly. The Rotterdam Study. *Arterioscler Thromb Vasc Biol* 1998; **18**:185–92.

10. Hooi JD, Stoffers HE, Kester AD, et al. Risk factors and cardiovascular diseases associated with asymptomatic peripheral arterial occlusive disease. The Limburg PAOD study. *Scand J Prim Health Care* 1998; **16**:177–82.

11. Criqui MH, Fronek A, Barrett-Connor E, et al. The prevalence of peripheral arterial disease in a defined population. *Circulation* 1985; **71**:510–15.

12. Oka RK, Szuba A, Giacomini JC, Cooke JP. Gender differences in perception of PAD: a pilot study. *Vasc Med* 2003; **8**:89–94.

13. Newman AB, Shemanski L, Manolio TA, et al. The ankle-arm index as a predictor of cardiovascular disease and mortality in the Cardiovascular Health Study. The Cardiovascular Health Study Group. *Arterioscler Thromb Vasc Biol* 1999; **19**:538–45.

14. Grady D, Herrington D, Bittner V, et al. Cardiovascular outcomes during 6.8 years of hormone therapy: the estrogen/progestin replacement study follow-up (HERS II). *JAMA* 2002; **288**:49–57.

15. Hsia J, Criqui MH, Rodabough RJ, Langer RD, et al. Women's Health Initiative Investigators. Estrogen plus progestin and the risk of peripheral arterial disease: the Women's Health Initiative. *Circulation* 2004; **109**:620–6.

16. Scott RA, Ashton HA, Kay DN. Abdominal aortic aneurysm in 4237 screened patients: prevalence, development and management over 6 years. *Br J Surg* 1991; **78**:1122–5.

17. Brown LC, Powell JT. Risk factors for aneurysm rupture in patients kept under ultrasound surveillance. UK Small Aneurysm Trial Participants. *Ann Surg* 1999; **230**:289–96.

18. UK Small Aneurysm Trial Participants. Long-term outcomes of immediate repair compared with surveillance for small abdominal aortic aneurysm. *N Engl J Med* 2002; **346**:1445–52.

19. Schnyder G, Sawhney N, Whisenant B, Tsimikas S, Turi ZG. Common femoral artery anatomy is influenced by demographics and comorbidity: implications for cardiac and peripheral invasive studies. *Catheter Cardiovasc Interv* 2001; **53**:289–95.

20. Singh K, Bonaa KH, Jacobsen BK, et al. Prevalence and risk factors for abdominal aortic aneurysms in a population-based study. The Tromso Study. *Am J Epidemiol* 2001; **154**:236–44.

21. Velazquez OC, Larson RA, Baum RA, et al. Gender-related differences in infrarenal aortic aneurysm morphologic features: issues relevant to Ancure and Talent endografts. *J Vasc Surg* 2001; **33**:S77–S84.

22. Caes F, Cham B, Van den Brande P, Welch W. Small artery syndrome in women. *Surg Gynaecol Obstet* 1985; **161**:165–70.

23. Kiryluk S, Wald N. Trends in cigarette smoking habits in the United Kingdom 1905–1985. In: Wald N, Froggatt P (eds). *Nicotine, Smoking and the Low Tar Programme.* Oxford: Oxford University Press, 1989: 53–69.

24. Franks PJ, Edwards RJ, Greenhalgh RM, Powell JT. Risk factors for abdominal aortic aneurysm in smokers. *Eur J Vasc Endovasc Surg* 1996; **11**: 487–92.

25. Powell JT, Edwards RJ, Worrell PC, et al. Risk factors for peripheral arterial disease in smokers: a case-control study. *Atherosclerosis* 1997; **129**:41–8.

26. Froelicher ESSN, Houston Miller N, Christopherson DJ, et al. High rates of smoking cessation in women hospitalised with cardiovascular disease. *Circulation* 2004; **109**:587–93.

27. Reuanen A, Takkunen H, Aromaa A. Prevalence of intermittent claudication and its effect upon mortality. *Acta Med Scand* 1982; **211**:249–56.

28. Orchard TJ, Dorman JS, Maser RE, et al. Prevalence and complications in IDDM by sex and duration. Pittsburgh Epidemiology of Diabetes Complications Study II. *Diabetes* 1990; **39**:1116–24.

29. Brady AR, Fowkes FGR, Greenhalgh RM, et al. Risk factors for post-operative death following elective surgical repair of abdominal aortic aneurysm: results from the UK Small Aneurysm Trial. *Br J Surg* 2000; **87**:742–9.

30. Norman PE, Semmens JB, Lawrence-Brown MM, Holman CD. Long term relative survival after surgery for abdominal aortic aneurysm in Western Australia: population based study. *BMJ* 1998; **317**:852–6.

31. Roddy SP, Darling C, Maharaj D, et al. Gender-related differences in outcome: an analysis of 5880 infrainguinal arterial reconstructions. *J Vasc Surg* 2002; **37**:399–402.

Part 5
Related Issues

39

Gender and cardiovascular medications

Janice B. Schwartz

Introduction

While there is increasing evidence to support diet and exercise interventions to both prevent and improve cardiovascular health, most therapeutic cardiac interventions are pharmacologic. The net effect following drug administration in vivo depends on the sum of a number of processes summarized as pharmacokinetics (that determine drug concentrations in the body) and pharmacodynamic (that determine the physiologic response, or effects, to drug concentrations). An understanding of these processes is key to optimizing medication therapy for all patients. However, it is also clear that responses to pharmacologic agents may differ between the sexes. This has been demonstrated in the recent past with cardiovascular toxicity from combined antihistamine and antibiotic use in younger women;[1] rhabdomyolysis with an HMG Co-A reductase inhibitor primarily in older, smaller women;[2] with dexfenfluramine valvular toxicity in women of all ages, with ephedra-containing dietary agents;[3] and with troglitazone, cisapride,[4] dofetilide[5] and mibefradil[6] toxicity more commonly in women than men; with increased bleeding complications with warfarin anticoagulation for atrial fibrillation, with thrombolytic agents and intravenous (i.v.) IIbIIIa agents in women after myocardial infarction (MI),[7,8] and with less certain benefit for digoxin[9] or beta-blockade in women compared with men with heart failure.[10-12] It is therefore important to review both the principles of pharmacokinetics and pharmacodynamics and how they relate to the design of therapeutic regimens as well as sex-related differences in both pharmacokinetics and pharmacodynamics to improve drug selection and modifications in dosing regimens for women compared with men.

Principles of pharmacokinetics

Pharmacokinetics has been summarized as 'what the body does to the drug'. Pharmacokinetic processes determine the appearance, distribution throughout tissues, and elimination of drug from the body. The major pharmacokinetic parameters are volume of distribution, bioavailability, and clearance. Sex differences in these parameters are summarized in Table 39.1.

Volume of distribution

Volume of distribution terms relate amount of drug in the body to measured concentrations. The 'central' volume of distribution of a drug is most often determined during preclinical evaluation of a drug by rapid administration of an i.v. dose by bolus or infusion of a known amount of drug followed by

Table 39.1 Summary of sex differences in bioavailability, distribution volumes, and drug clearance

Parameter	Men > women	Men = women	Women > men
Bioavailability			
Oral			X[13–18]
Transdermal		X[19,20]	
Distribution volume*			
Water-soluble, nonlipophilic	X[21]		
Lipophilic			X[22–24]
Drug clearance			
Renal glomerular filtration	X		
Renal tubular secretion	x	X	
Renal tubular reabsorption	x	X	
Enzymatic – Phase I oxidation			
CYP1A	X		
CYP2C9		X	
CYP2C19		X	
CYP2D6	X		
CYP2E1	X		
CYP3A		x	X
Phase II conjugative			
Glucuronidation	X		
Sulfation	X		
Catechol-o-methyltransferase	X		
Dihydropyridine dehydrogenase	X		
N-Acetyltransferase		X	
Thiopurine methyltransferase	X		
UDP-glucuronosyl transferase	X		
Transporter: P-glycoprotein			X

*In general, total volumes are greater in men due to greater body size. The smaller x notations represent the presence of lesser data to support the difference.

measurement of the concentration immediately following drug administration:

$$\text{volume of distribution} = \frac{\text{drug dose}}{\text{concentration}}$$

This initial or 'central' volume of distribution does not represent a 'real' volume but the volume if the drug were immediately and equally distributed throughout the circulation and highly perfused organs such as the heart, liver, and kidney. It is often expressed in units of volume per kilogram body weight. The volume of distribution defines the loading dose of a drug as can be seen by its definition:

$$\text{loading dose} = \text{desired concentration} \times \text{volume of drug distribution}$$

Later phases occur with drug distribution into less highly perfused tissues such as muscle, viscera, skin,

and fat. The volume of distribution at steady-state estimates total body distribution when these processes have reached equilibrium. Modified loading regimens with infusions or multiple doses are often used for drugs with large steady-state volume of distributions to avoid higher than desired initial concentrations in the circulation and more rapidly perfused tissues.

Sex effects on volume of distribution (see Table 39.1)

Women, on average, are smaller than men at all ages. Intravascular volumes, organ volumes, and muscle volume are usually smaller than in men. A smaller distribution volume for a drug results in a higher drug concentration after a dose compared with concentrations in a larger person given the same dose. A widely recognized consequence is the higher alcohol concentrations found in women compared with men after consumption of equal amounts of alcohol. During clinical care, the impact of a reduced volume of drug distribution will be most evident when a loading or intravenous bolus dose of a medication is given and for those drugs that have narrow toxic to therapeutic ratios. Weight adjustment for loading doses of the cardiovascular drugs digoxin, lidocaine and other type I anti-arrhythmic drugs, type III anti-arrhythmic drugs, aminoglycoside antibiotics, chemotherapy regimens, and for unfractionated heparin are standard. The increased risk of intracranial bleeding in older patients, usually women, can be reduced by use of weight-based dosing of heparin.[25] There are more women at older ages than men and body size and volumes decrease after age 65 years, further underscoring the need to adjust dosages for body weight in older female patients. The difference in body weight is thought by some to be the most important gender difference that affects drug concentrations.[26,27]

Women have a greater percentage of body fat compared with men at all ages, but this difference decreases at older ages.[22] Steady-state distribution volumes will be higher for lipophilic drugs such as the benzodiazepines and may contribute to the prolonged effect of such drugs in women compared with men (later release from fat reservoirs of drug).

Clinical implications:
- *Loading doses of medications will generally be lower in women compared with men*
- *Doses will be lowest in older women*
- *Weight-based loading regimens are recommended*
- *Lipid-soluble drugs may have greater distribution volumes in women and may reside in the body for longer than in men.*

Bioavailability

Bioavailability is the fraction (F) of drug that reaches the circulation after administration. Intravascular (i.v.) administration of a drug results in a bioavailability of 1 or 100%. Bioavailability for other routes of drug administration (oral, nasal, inhaled, buccal, intramuscular, subcutaneous, topical, etc.) is

estimated by comparing the area under the curve (AUC) of drug concentration versus time after extravascular administration divided by the AUC of drug concentration versus time data after i.v. dosage (AUC extravascular/AUC intravascular) expressed as a fraction of one or a percentage. Bioavailability determines dose adjustments for different drug administration routes. After oral drug administration, absorption usually occurs in the intestine where metabolism and active transport back into the lumen can affect systemic bioavailability. The primary drug-metabolizing enzyme found in the intestinal villi is cytochrome P450 (CYP)3A; the drug transporter P-glycoprotein is found adjacent.

Interactions with nutrients and dietary factors are most common for lower bioavailable drugs undergoing CYP3A metabolism. Grapefruit juice has a direct inhibitory effect on gut CYP3A that is at least partly irreversible, and has been reported to increase bioavailability of a number of CYP3A substrates including amiodarone, buspirone, dihydropyridines (felodipine, nifedipine), verapamil, terfenadine, ethinylestradiol, midazolam, saquinavir, cyclosporin A, several HMG Co-A reductase inhibitor medications (lovastatin, simvastatin, not fluvastatin), and sildenafil. Seville orange juice and pomelos have also been reported to interact with bowel CYP3A while regular orange juice, sweet oranges, and tangerines do not.[28–33] Cranberry juice has more recently been reported to prolong anticoagulation times when co-administered with warfarin; although enzymatic inhibition of metabolism has been postulated, the mechanism has not been elucidated nor has the location of the effect (gut vs liver).

Sex effects on bioavailability (see Table 39.1)

Investigations using oral midazolam (trade name, Versed®) as a probe of intestinal CYP3A show higher bioavailability in women compared with men with greater inhibition of clarithromycin on intestinal metabolism in women compared with men.[13] Oral bioavailability of verapamil, a mixed CYP3A and P-glycoprotein substrate,[14,15] is also greater in women compared with men, as is bioavailability of aspirin.[16] The data are not completely uniform, with bioavailability of traditionally formulated oral cyclosporine reported to be lower in women compared with men. A newer formulation (as Neoral®) appears to have improved bioavailability with less sex differences (as Sandimmune®),[34] and bioavailability of tacrolimus, another CYP3A substrate, is relatively low without sex differences.[35]

Nonoral routes of drug administration

Greater subcutaneous lipid in women compared with men could be hypothesized to affect transdermal drug delivery but equal availability of transdermal clonidine in hypertensive women and men has been reported.[19] In vitro data with skin from women and men also showed similar absorption with fentanyl and sufentanil.[36] No data are available on nitrates. Less delivery of inhaled aerosol drugs such as ribavirin and cyclosporine has been reported in women compared with men.[37,38] The clinical relevance of these observations is not known.

Clearance

Drugs are eliminated from the body either by metabolism (enzymatic biotransformation in the liver, intestine, or bloodstream) or by excretion (renal or biliary). Total body drug clearance is the net rate of removal of drug from the body described as a unit of volume cleared of drug per unit time (i.e. ml/min). In experimental preparations, this is corrected for amount of metabolizing enzyme or microsome or protein. Descriptions of human drug clearance rates and investigations of sex, age, or race differences often report clearance in volume cleared per unit time per kg body weight or per body surface area of 1.73 m². This again underscores the principle that consideration of size should be incorporated into chronic dosage choices as well as for loading doses of medications.

Steady-state drug concentrations are determined by drug clearance; thus clearance defines the drug dosing rate per unit time to maintain a stable drug concentration. Drug clearance is often considered as renal, hepatic, and nonrenal nonhepatic.

Renal clearance

The kidney is the major organ of drug excretion of either parent drug compounds or metabolites resulting from biotransformation of parent drug. There are three renal processes of drug clearance: glomerular filtration, tubular secretion, and tubular reabsorption.

Glomerular filtration

Although glomerular filtration is proportional to body weight, there may also be a weight-independent sex difference in glomerular filtration rate (GFR). In addition, men produce more creatinine than women due to larger muscle mass. Thus, algorithms to estimate creatinine clearance or glomerular filtration often include sex and weight or more recently, sex and race as variables.[39,40] Examination of two methods for estimation of renal filtration suggest a sex difference of 15–25% at all ages as well as an age-dependent decrease:

$$\text{creatinine clearance} = (140 - \text{age (yr)} \times \text{weight(kg)})/(\text{creatinine} \times 72)$$

multiplied by 0.85 for women.[39]

$$\text{glomerular filtration} = 186.3 \times (\text{creat})^{-1.154} \times (\text{age})^{-0.203} \times 1.212 \text{ (if black)} \times 0.742 \text{ (if female)}^{40,41}$$

Table 39.2 illustrates the effects of sex, age, body size, race, and serum creatinine on estimates of creatinine clearance and glomerular filtration. Using definitions of renal function from the National Kidney Foundation 2001 guidelines (available at http://www.kidney.org), a white woman of average weight and over the age of 65 years with a serum creatinine of 1 will have a glomerular filtration rate classified as Stage 3 renal function or moderate renal failure (see Table 39.2). Thus, serum creatinine may be normal when glomerular filtration is significantly reduced. In the older woman with an elevation of serum creatinine, severe renal impairment may be present. Investigations of patient groups confirm lower renal clearances of drugs with narrow therapeutic to toxic ratios such as digoxin[42] and aminoglycosides[43] in women compared with men. It has been postulated that the poorer overall outcomes of

Table 39.2 Estimated renal clearance by age, sex, and race

Age (years)		Cr = 1						Cr = 1.2						Cr = 1.5				
		35	45	55	65	75	85	35	45	55	65	75	85	35	45	55	65	75
White	CrCL	119	109	100	87	71	55	99	83	76	65	53	41	79	66	61	52	42
men*	GFR	91	86	82	80	77	75	73	70	67	65	63	61	57	54	52	50	49
White	CrCL	80	75	72	61	50	39	66	55	51	44	36	28	53	44	41	35	29
women	GFR	67	64	61	59	57	56	54	52	50	48	47	45	42	40	38	37	36
Black	CrCL	117	107	98	81	69	55	98	78	71	60	49	39	78	72	65	54	46
men	GFR	110	104	100	97	94	91	89	84	81	78	76	74	69	65	63	61	59
Black	CrCL	90	88	79	68	56	40	75	62	56	49	40	29	66	61	55	46	39
women	GFR	81	77	74	72	70	68	66	63	60	58	56	55	51	48	46	45	44

Data present average estimated creatinine clearance (CrCL) in ml/min using the Cockcroft and Gault method[39] based on average weight per age for women and men (source: NHANES[44]) and glomerular filtration rate (GFR)[40,41] for serum creatinine of 1 mg/dl (Cr = 1), 1.2 mg/dl (Cr = 1.2), and 1.5 mg/dl (Cr = 1.5). Darkly shaded areas indicate glomerular filtration rate estimates <60 ml/min/1.73 m² classified as moderate decreases in GFR or stage 3 chronic renal disease.
*All groups exclude Hispanics.

women with heart failure who received digoxin compared with men may have been due to the higher digoxin concentrations in these women.[9,45] For drugs undergoing renal filtration, algorithms for estimation of renal clearance should be used to estimate drug dosages – especially for drugs with low therapeutic to toxic ratios and/or adverse effects related to concentrations (note: online calculators for creatinine clearance and glomerular filtration rate (GFR) and definitions of renal function by GFR are available at http://www.kidney.org). These algorithms are not accurate during periods of clinical instability. Currently, other markers of renal function such as cystatin C are being evaluated that may be sex-independent and may reflect changes in renal function more rapidly.[46–48]

Renal tubular secretion and reabsorption

Renal tubular secretion is detected in vivo when renal clearance of a substance exceeds clearance rates by filtration. Secretion is an active process with separate processes for acids and bases that efficiently eliminate protein-bound drugs. Tubular reabsorption is detected when urinary excretion of a compound is less than filtration rates. For most drugs, reabsorption is passive and can be affected by urine flow and by changes in pH. Both processes slow with age (about 7% per decade), but sex differences in trans-

porters have not been described in humans. Nonetheless, there are data to suggest that secretion is higher in men compared with women and that inhibitors of renal secretion have greater effects in men compared with women.[49]

Clinical implications:
- *Renal clearance cannot accurately be estimated by serum creatinine alone*
- *Renal clearance should be estimated using algorithms that include adjustments for sex, age, serum creatinine, weight, and race*
- *Initial dosages of renally-cleared medications should be based on estimates of renal clearance*
- *Estimates of renal clearance may not be accurate during conditions associated with rapid changes in renal function.*

Hepatic and intestinal enzymatic drug clearance

The rate and extent of hepatic drug metabolism is influenced by hepatic and extrahepatic factors. Hepatic blood flow determines the delivery rate of drug to the liver and enzyme type, numbers, affinity, and activity rate determine hepatic biotransformation rates. Metabolic biotransformation usually converts drugs to more polar or water-soluble metabolites to facilitate excretion. Administered drugs may also be 'prodrugs' that are biotransformed into biologically active compounds; drugs may also be metabolized to toxic metabolites. Drug metabolism pathways are classified as phase I reactions (i.e. oxidation, reduction, and hydrolysis that usually remove groups from the drug) or phase II, conjugation reactions (i.e. acetylation, glucuronidation, sulfation, and methylation that add groups to the drug) that may occur in any sequence. The following information is presented within the context of the metabolic enzyme involved to provide a framework for anticipating metabolic drug interactions and potential impact of genetics on drug metabolism.

Oxidative drug metabolism

The cytochrome P450 (CYP) superfamily of heme-containing microsomal enzymes is responsible for the majority of phase I metabolism of drugs, environmental chemicals, a number of hormones, foods, and toxins. CYP isoforms are categorized by their amino acid sequences. Sequences with over 40% homology are classed in the same family identified by an Arabic number. Within the family, sequences with over 55% homology are considered in the same subfamily identified with a letter. Within subfamilies, different forms are further designated with an Arabic numeral. Human CYP protein content is largely from eight to ten isoforms from three major groups – CYP1, CYP2, and CYP3.

It is estimated that 50–55% of therapeutic medications are biotransformed by CYP3A enzymes. CYP3A proteins comprise about 25% of the protein in the liver and are also found and are the dominant form in the intestine. The CYP3A forms found in adult humans are 3A4 or 3A5 that differ in metabolic characteristics and distributions between races and 3A7 that is found in neonates.[50–54] Although genetic polymorphisms have been identified, no distinct slow or rapid metabolizer phenotypes for this enzyme have been clinically identified.

CYP3A4 is the enzyme for which faster clearance of a number of substrates (such as alfentanil, cyclosporine, diazepam, erythromycin, methylprednisolone, midazolam, nifedipine, tirilazad, verapamil), has been reported in women compared with men.[55–59] CYP3A4 expression has recently been reported to be greater in liver tissues from women

compared with men with correlations between pregnane X receptor (PRX) expression and mRNA for CYP3A4.[60] Estrogen receptor element sequences are also present in the 5'-untranslated region that may influence the expression of the enzyme.[61]

The majority of data suggest sex differences in i.v. clearance of CYP3A substrates of mild to modest size that are influenced by concomitant medications and alternative routes of drug metabolism. Midazolam is currently considered the purest CYP3A substrate and most studies with midazolam detect both sex- and age-related decreases in clearance.[62–67] There appears to be faster i.v. clearance in women compared with men in the order of 20–40%. Intravenous midazolam is used for conscious sedation. While initial bolus doses may be somewhat smaller on average in women compared with men because of smaller body size, repeated dosing may need to be more frequent or infusion dosing may need to be higher (when considered as mg/kg) to maintain equivalent anesthesia in women compared with men.[51]

Conclusions regarding sex differences in orally administered CYP3A substrates are less uniform. In patients receiving oral nifedipine or verapamil, faster clearance in women compared with men has been reported.[56,68] These comparisons showing faster clearance in women compared with men are for data corrected for body weight (i.e. presented as clearance in ml/min/kg). Clinically, faster clearance in women may be masked by smaller body weight resulting in similar drug concentrations when female and male patients are given the same chronic oral doses of CYP3A substrates. In contrast, cyclosporine is cleared faster in women than men after renal transplantation and also has a greater volume of distribution in women compared with men and lower bioavailability, suggesting that higher cyclosporine doses may be required in female transplant patients.[59]

CYP3A metabolizes many beta-blockers (except atenolol, propranolol), calcium channel blockers (dihydropyridines, verapamil, diltiazem), lidocaine, quinidine, amiodarone, many HMG Co-A reductase inhibitors (excluding fluvastatin), most benzodiazepines, estrogens, astemizole, carbamazepine, cisapride, clarithromycin, cortisol, erythromycin, itraconazole, ketoconazole, nefazodone, sertraline, tamoxifen, terfenadine and troglitazone among others (for information on CYP pathway of metabolism by drug see reference 51).

Multiple isoforms of CYP2 are found in humans. CYP2D6 is estimated to be responsible for metabolism of 25% of phase I-metabolized drugs. The CYP2D6 enzyme has multiple genetic polymorphisms that produce distinct phenotypes of ultra-rapid, rapid, slow and ultra-slow drug clearance. Drugs metabolized by this pathway include encainide, metoprolol, warfarin, debrisoquine, dextromethorphan, dehydroepiandrosterone (DHEA), mexiletine, propafenone, propranolol, the selective serotonin reuptake inhibitor paroxetine, most tricyclic antidepressants, and the neuroleptics, haloperidol and resperidone. Because the opiate codeine requires activation of the parent compound to the active moiety by CYP2D6, clinical efficacy may be determined by the genotype; i.e. slow and ultra-slow metabolizers may have no or lesser responses. CYP2C accounts for another 20% of phase I drug metabolism. CYP2C9 metabolizes fluvastatin, losartan, phenytoin, s-warfarin (the active enantiomer), and many nonsteroidal anti-inflammatory drugs (NSAIDs). CYP2C19 metabolizes the proton pump inhibitors lansoprazole, omeprazole, and pantoprazole. CYP1A2 accounts for metabolism of about 5% of drugs undergoing oxidative phase I metabolism. CYP1A demonstrates genetic polymorphisms with the extensive metabolizer phenotype being more prevalent. Acetaminophen, caffeine, nicotine, tacrine, and theophylline are metabolized via CYP1. For these enzymes, clearance has been reported to be either faster in men compared with women (CYP2D6, CYP1A, CYP2E1) or the same in women and men (CYP2C9 and CYP2C19).[69] (See Table 39.1).

Alterations in CYP-mediated drug clearance

CYP-mediated clearance rates vary markedly in human populations. Contributing factors include genetics, differing environmental exposures, enzyme induction or inhibition, multiple pathways for metabolism of a number of compounds, and other factors not fully elucidated. There are data that support the concept of hormonal regulation of drug clearance including the effects of estrogen or oral contraceptive administration to decrease clearance of CYP1A2 substrates such as caffeine[70] and ropinirole,[71] and inhibitory effects of oral contraceptives on CYP2C19 clearance rates.[72] There have also been variably detected changes in drug clearance during the menstrual cycle in women.[73–78] Recently, it has been shown that a number of xenobiotics can activate PXR.[79] Interactions between PXR and genomic effects of estrogens occur and may provide a potential mechanism for sex-dependent regulation of CYP3A activity.

Cardiovascular disease presents, on average, later in life in women than men. Decreases in clearance due to aging have been shown for many CYP substrates, and for those undergoing biotransformation by CYP3A pathways, in particular. In patient groups, effects of disease, gender, smoking or alcohol consumption and other environmental factors have had larger effects on drug clearance than age.[56,68] The influence of herbs and nutritional supplements has become recognized as another source of variability due to either enzyme induction or inhibition.[80] St. John's wort induces CYP3A and can lead to clinically significant decreases in concentrations of immunosuppressants and decreased antihypertensive effects of medications metabolized by CYP3A.[81–83]

Clinical implications:
- *Enzymatic hepatic and intestinal drug clearance is more variable than renal clearance*
- *Sex differences in enzymatic and intestinal drug clearance exist*
- *Co-medications, smoking, drinking, disease states, and dietary intake or supplements may influence clearance by CYP pathways*
- *Increasing age may also decrease clearance by CYP pathways.*

Metabolism by phase II enzymes

Phase II metabolism includes conjugative reactions of glucuronidation (morphine, diazepam), sulfation (methyldopa), acetylation (procainamide), methylation, and glutathione conjugation. Drugs that are metabolized solely by conjugation are, in general, cleared faster by men than women.[84,85] Cardiovascular medications undergoing glucuronidation include propranolol,[86,87] labetalol[88] (cleared by combined processes), and the immunosuppressant drug mycophenolic acid.[89] Faster clearance in men compared with women has also been reported for catechol-o-methyltransferase (COMT) that metabolizes the neurotransmitters norepinephrine, epinephrine and dopamine, and levo-dopamine; for dihydropyrimidine dehydrogenase (metabolizes fluorouracil); UDP-glucuronosyl transferase (metabolizes clofibric acid, ibuprofen); and thiopurine methyltransferase (metabolizes mercaptopurine, thioguanine, partial metabolism of azathioprine).

Drug transporters

A focus on investigations of drug transporters in the liver and bowel has been more recent than the study of metabolic enzymes. The human multidrug-efflux transporter P-glycoprotein is found in the liver and intestine. P-glycoprotein content has been reported to be higher in liver tissue of men than women[90] but phenotyping with fexofenadine, a model P-glycoprotein substrate, did not demonstrate sex differences in clearance.[91] Recently, CYP3A metabolism (and not P-glycoprotein transport into the gut lumen) has been identified as the major determinant of presystemic intestinal first-pass metabolism of verapamil, a mixed CYP3A and P-glycoprotein substrate, that has been used as an in vitro marker of P-glycoprotein transport and activity.[83] Digoxin, although renally eliminated, undergoes enterohepatic recycling and is a P-glycoprotein substrate that is also used as an in vitro marker of P-glycoprotein transport. The clinical relevance of P-glycoprotein and its genetic polymorphisms to digoxin clearance in vivo is less clear.

Elimination half-lives

The terminal elimination half-life (t 1/2) describes the time it takes for the amount of drug in the body to decrease by half after drug distribution has occurred throughout the body. It is dependent on volume of distribution and clearance:

$$\text{t } 1/2 = 0.693 \times \frac{\text{volume of distribution}}{\text{clearance}}$$

The half-life defines the time to reach steady-state during both drug initiation and after drug discontinuation. Approximately 90% of steady-state is reached after 3.3 half-lives.

For a summary of pharmacokinetic differences between the sexes see Table 39.1.

Sex-specific pharmacokinetic considerations in women: hormones, oral contraceptives, and pregnancy (see also Chapters 22 and 26)

Neither estradiol nor estriol affects GFR, or tubular reabsorption.[92] In most studies of menopausal women receiving estrogen therapy, no effect on CYP3A-mediated drug clearance has been reported.[55,62] Combined estrogen and progesterone hormone therapy in older women has not been sufficiently studied to allow conclusions to be drawn. Similarly, although black cohosh has not been reported to interact with any drugs or to influence laboratory tests, this has not been rigorously studied.[93]

Oral contraceptives are one of the most widely prescribed class of drugs in the world and the most commonly prescribed medication in young women. The most frequently prescribed are composed of both an estrogen (ethinyl estradiol most commonly) and one of a number of progestins. Both the estrogens and progestins undergo intestinal absorption and metabolism, hepatic metabolism, and enterohepatic recycling. Metabolism is via oxidation by the cytochrome P450 enzymes (CYP) including the 3A isozyme (see above). Drug interactions can either increase the clearance of the oral contraceptive leading to lower concentrations, and potentially failure of contraception; or, decrease the clearance of the oral contraceptive leading to increased concentrations of the drugs with potential side effects. Oral contraceptives can increase or decrease concentrations of co-administered medications and concomitant medications can alter both concentrations and effects of oral contraceptives. Reported interactions are summarized in Tables 39.3 and 39.4. Further discussion of oral contraceptives can be found in Chapter 26.

Clinical considerations:
- *When initiating or discontinuing a drug in a woman on oral contraceptives, drug interactions and alterations in contraceptive efficacy should be considered*
- *When initiating or discontinuing oral contraceptives in a woman receiving other medications, effects on medication concentrations and efficacy should be considered*

Table 39.3 Drug interactions that alter oral contraceptive concentrations and effects[94-100]

Decreased drug effect or concentrations	Increased drug effect or concentrations

Mechanism: increased drug clearance
  Anticonvulsants: phenytoin, primidone and
  carbamazepine
  Antituberculous: rifampin*
Mechanism: inhibited enterohepatic recirculation
  Antibiotics: penicillin, ampicillin, tetracyclines,
  cephalosporins
	Mechanism: decreased drug clearance
	  Antifungals*: ketoconazole, fluconazole, itraconazole
	  griseofulvin
	  Anticoagulant: warfarin

*Most potent.

Table 39.4 Changes in effects or concentrations of medications co-administered with oral contraceptives[94-100]

Decreased effect or concentrations	Increased effect or concentrations

Mechanism: increased drug clearance
  Benzodiazepines (lorazepam, temazepam, and
  oxazepam; related to estrogen dose)
  Clofibric acid
  Cyclosporine
  Phenytoin
  Rifampin
 	
Mechanism unknown
  Warfarin
	Mechanism: decreased drug clearance
	  Antidepressants: imipramine, amitryptyline
	  Caffeine
	  Corticosteroids (prednisone, prednisolone)
	  Selegiline
	  Theophylline

- *In general, menopausal hormone therapy has not been associated with altered pharmacokinetics or pharmacodynamics of other medications.*

Pregnancy (see also Chapter 22)

Most drugs currently marketed in the United States carry statements in their labeling that warn that adequate and well-controlled studies have not been performed in pregnant women. Nonetheless, it is well recognized that maternal physiologic changes occur during gestation that have the potential to affect the pharmacokinetics of medications.[101] These changes include increased intravascular and total volumes that can, on average, increase drug distribution volume and lower peak drug concentrations unless dosing is corrected for body weight. Increases in cardiac output with changes in blood flow distribution favoring uterine and renal blood flow with relative decreases in hepatic blood flow that can change renal and/or enzymatic drug clearance are also seen. In addition, decreased drug binding to plasma proteins may be seen.[102] For hepatically or enzymatically cleared drugs, changes associated with pregnancy cannot always be predicted. A consistent finding has been lower plasma concentrations of most anticonvulsants drugs (phenytoin, carbamazepine) during pregnancy. In addition, for several CYP3A substrates (nifedipine, methadone), and CYP1A substrates (theophylline), and for citalopram (mixed CYP2C19, 2D6, and 3A4 metabolism) increased clearance has been reported during pregnancy.

Clinical considerations:
- *Drug distribution volumes are, on average, larger during pregnancy; dosage corrections for total weight should be considered*
- *Glomerular filtration rate is increased during pregnancy and adjustments of dosages for renal clearance should be made*
- *Upward adjustments in anticonvulsant medications may be needed during pregnancy and measurement of drug concentrations is recommended.*

Pharmacodynamics

The Institute of Medicine Report[26] concluded that although there are very limited data on sex differences in pharmacodynamics, these differences may be *more important* than pharmacokinetic changes. The evidence for sex/gender differences in physiology, receptors, prevalence, and responses to pharmacologic therapy are strongest in two major areas: the central nervous system and the cardiovascular system. Aspects of sex differences in presentation and physiology of cardiovascular diseases are reviewed in the preceding disease-specific sections and depression is discussed in Chapter 41. Sex differences in pharmacologic responses to specific cardiovascular medications are discussed below.

Sex differences in responses to pharmacologic therapy

Arrhythmias (see also Chapter 37)

Basal QT intervals corrected for heart rate are the same in boys and girls and become longer after puberty in women compared with men, while at older ages the sex-related differences decrease in magnitude.[103] Gender differences in the rate-corrected QT interval are present even in adults with inherited cardiac ion channel mutations.[104] While gender-related differences in QT intervals alone do not increase the risk for torsade de pointes arrhythmias, gender is a risk factor for an increased incidence of torsade de pointes during administration of drugs which produce QT prolongation.[1,4,105–107] Torsade de pointes occurs more frequently in women than in men with both drugs that have minor effects to prolong the QT interval (antihistamines) and drugs with a primary action to prolong cardiac repolarization (type I-C anti-arrhythmic drugs quinidine, disopyramide, dofetilide, amiodarone, bepridil, prenylamine, and sotalol). The data suggest that both pharmacokinetic interactions to increase drug concentrations and pharmacodynamic factors showing increased sensitivity to QT-prolonging effects in women play a role.[5,108]

Clinical correlates:
- *Women are more likely to develop clinically important QT prolongation and torsade de pointes arrhythmias with drugs that prolong the QT interval*
- *QT-prolonging properties of drugs should be reviewed prior to administration to women*
- *QTc intervals should be monitored in women receiving anti-arrhythmic or other drugs that prolong cardiac repolarization and QT intervals*
- *Drugs with QT-prolonging effects should not be co-administered in women unless careful monitoring is performed*
- *Use of equally efficacious drugs which do not produce prolongation of the QT interval should be favored over drugs which produce even mild QT-prolonging effects in women*
- *Inhibitors of CYP3A metabolism may increase concentrations of drugs leading to greater increases in QT intervals.*

Heart failure (see also Chapters 28 and 29)

Digitalis
A post hoc analysis of the Digitalis Investigation (DIG) trial of 6800 patients found that the rate of cardiovascular deaths and deaths from worsening heart failure were reduced in men taking digoxin, but were increased in women taking digoxin.[9] Hospitalization rates were reduced in women taking digoxin but not to the same extent as in men. Digoxin concentration data were not routinely collected, but were higher in the women than in the men in the small numbers in whom it was measured.

Beta-blockers

Relatively small numbers of women were enrolled in individual trials. Both the metoprolol for the treatment of congestive heart failure (MERIT-HF) trial[10] and the Carvedilol Prospective Randomized Cumulative Survival (COPERNICUS) trial found survival benefits in men but not women.[12,109] In contrast, a post hoc analysis of the Cardiac Insufficiency Bisoprolol Study (CIBIS II) adjusted for the older age of the women enrolled, found greater benefit in women compared with men.[110] A recent meta-analysis of beta-blocker trials for heart failure reached the conclusion that the beneficial effects of beta-blockade in dilated heart failure extend to women with clinically stable severe heart failure after adjustment for age and risk factor differences between women and men.[111]

ACE inhibitors

Several meta-analyses of the published randomized trials of ACE inhibitors for heart failure have appeared.[112,113] The meta-analyses from about 13 000 patients show confidence intervals for benefit to include 1.0 for women (0.71–1.02) and for patients over 75 years of age (0.74–1.22).

The incidence of ACE inhibitor-induced cough varies, with reports ranging from 5% to 39%[114–116] and cough is a major reason for medication discontinuation. The frequency of cough with ACE inhibitors is higher in women and nonsmokers.[114,117,118]

Diuretics

The incidence of hyponatremia as well as hypokalemia appears to be higher in women compared with men treated with diuretics, with hyponatremia being more common in the elderly. This appears to be true for thiazide and nonthiazide diuretics.[119]

Anticoagulants

No gender differences have been confirmed for the metabolism of the currently available antithrombotic drugs. Despite the lack of sex differences in overall metabolism, lighter body weight and older age (on average) at time of presentation for therapy may lead to increased sensitivity to antithrombotic drugs in women. Bleeding risk appears higher with use of anticoagulant and thrombolytic agents in older patients[120,121] and women compared with men, especially older women.[7,8] Increased risk for intracranial hemorrhage with thrombolytic therapy may be related in part to lack of weight correction of dosing, but increased bleeding and cardiac rupture have also been seen in older women when dosages were corrected for weight and/or creatinine clearance.[13,122,123] An underlying pharmacodynamic mechanism is also suggested by increased risk of intracranial bleeding during chronic oral warfarin administration for atrial fibrillation in patients over 75 years of age, more often women than men, when drug doses were titrated to a target effect.[121] Although there are currently no algorithms that individualize dosing of heparins or thrombolytics other than for weight,[124] adjustment of heparin dosing regimens on the basis of multiple factors that include gender may result in safer and more efficacious regimens.[125]

Factors that influence the response to warfarin include the presence of other drugs, diet, and acute and chronic illnesses. Gender effects have not usually been found when data are controlled for age and weight. However, because women are usually of smaller size than men and may be older than men when receiving warfarin for nonvalve-related cardiovascular indications, warfarin dose requirements may be lower in women, especially older women. The American Geriatrics Society (AGS) guidelines suggest initiation at estimated maintenance doses (or 2.5 mg/day) and no more than 5 mg/day (see http://www.americangeriatrics.org/products/positionpapers/).

Vitamin K plays a role in bone metabolism, and warfarin antagonizes vitamin K. In analyses of women receiving chronic oral anticoagulation compared with nonanticoagulated cohorts, increased risk of osteoporosis and higher rates of vertebral and rib fractures were associated with oral anticoagulation for more than 12 months.[126] Shorter exposures may also confer osteoporosis risk in some individuals. Administration of unfractionated heparin for more than 3–6 months has also been associated with increased rates of bone mineral loss.[127] It is anticipated that osteoporosis may also be a consequence of long-term low-molecular-weight heparin administration. Measures to prevent osteoporosis should accompany long-term anticoagulation with warfarin and be considered during use of heparin or low-molecular-weight heparin for more than 3 months.

Clinical correlate:
- *Osteoporosis is a risk of chronic anticoagulation and routine administration of calcium and vitamin D should accompany chronic anticoagulation and additional pharmacologic measures should be considered if osteoporosis is present (hormones, bisphosphonates, calcitonin).*

Lipid-lowering drugs (see also Chapter 4)

Statins

The vast majority of lipid-lowering medications prescribed worldwide are the HMG-CoA reductase inhibitors or 'statin' drugs. Common adverse effects include elevation of serum hepatic transaminases and myopathy. Risk of myopathy is higher when co-administered with gemfibrozil or if CYP3A-metabolized statins (atorvastatin, lovastatin, simvastatin) are co-administered with drugs such as erythromycin, cyclosporine, or the antifungal azoles that are also metabolized via CYP3A (see above). Additional risk factors include advanced age (>80 years and in women more than men), small body frame and frailty, multisystem disease (chronic renal insufficiency, especially due to diabetes), and multiple medications. It is clear that the older woman with cardiovascular disease will be at higher risk for statin-induced myopathy. Therapy should be initiated at a low dose and monitored closely, recognizing that myopathy may not be accompanied by rises in muscle enzymes, especially in older women.

Clinical correlate:
- *Older women may be at increased risk for myopathy and should be closely monitored and co-administration of HMG Co-A reductase inhibitors and gemfibrozil should be avoided if possible.*

Vitamins

During evaluation of extended-release niacin (Niaspan), women given the same dose as men had greater low-density lipoprotein (LDL) cholesterol response but also experienced more side effects, especially at higher doses.[128] Conclusions were 'that use of lower dosages of niacin may be desirable in women'. At least one large, randomized, blinded study performed exclusively in menopausal women with coronary disease failed to demonstrate benefit of antioxidants and vitamins but suggested adverse effects.[129]

NSAIDs

Arthritis is more common in women and use of NSAIDs by prescription or over the counter is frequent. It has become recognized that administration of both cyclo-oxygenase II selective and non-selective NSAIDs can lead to loss of antihypertensive control. Hyperkalemia may also occur with NSAID administration, especially if co-administered with ACE inhibitors, angiotensin receptor blocking drugs, or aldosterone antagonists. Very rare adverse renal effects of NSAID therapy include nephritic syndrome and papillary necrosis. Acute interstitial nephritis can develop at any time during therapy and usually occurs in combination with minimal-change glomerulonephritis. The exact risk factors for NSAID-related nephrotic syndrome have not been identified, but it seems that it occurs more frequently in women and the elderly.[130]

Clinical correlate:
- *NSAID use is common in women and the elderly and monitoring to avoid adverse interactions, especially hyperkalemia, with ACE inhibitors, ARBs, or aldosterone antagonists is necessary.*

Summary

There are sex differences in both the pharmacokinetics and pharmacodynamics of drugs. Recent analyses of data from bioequivalence trials submitted to the Center for Drug Evaluation and Research (CDER), Food and Drug Administration (FDA), found statistically significant sex differences in about 28% of the data sets and that differences in drug exposure could be greater than 50%.[131] A portion of the differences may be due to differences in body size. However, 'usual dosing instructions for adult women and men do not take into account weight differences'.[131] Adjustment for only weight, however, will not avoid all sex-related differences in toxicity and other factors must be considered. It is also important to consider concomitant medications, disease states, age, diet, and nutraceutical intake and estimates of renal or enzymatic drug clearance when initiating a medication regimen. It is also key to evaluate responses to guide either dose titration or dose reduction in the clinical setting. Women have been under-represented in clinical trials of cardiovascular

therapies; yet the data suggest they may benefit less than men for many of the current cardiovascular interventions. Data also suggest that women have more adverse effects from cardiovascular drug therapy. Recommendations to improve cardiovascular drug therapy for women with cardiovascular disease include individualization of drug selection as well as drug dosage. At this point in time, it is also important that the clinician, educator, and researcher recognize that optimal pharmacological therapy for the woman with cardiovascular disease remains an area of uncertainty and in critical need of further investigation.

References

1. Woosley R, Chen Y, Freiman J, Gillis R. Mechanism of the cardiotoxic actions of terfenadine. *JAMA* 1993; **269**:1532–6.
2. FDA. CDER. Report No.: http: www.fda.gov/cder/foi/label2001/207S6lbl.pdf.
3. Haller C, Benowitz N. Adverse cardiovascular and central nervous system events associated with dietary supplements containing ephedra alkaloids. *N Engl J Med* 2000; **343**:1833–8.
4. Wysowski D, Bacsanyi J. Cisapride and fatal arrhythmia. *N Engl J Med* 1996; **335**:290–1.
5. Torp-Pedersen C, Moller M, Bloch-Thomsen P, et al. Dofetilide in patients with congestive heart failure and left ventricular dysfunction. Danish Investigations of Arrhythmia and Mortality on Dofetilide Study Group. *N Engl J Med* 1999; **341**:857–65.
6. SoRelle R. Withdrawal of posicor from market. *Circulation* 1998; **98**:831–2.
7. Gurwitz J, Gore J, Goldberg R, et al. Risk for intracranial hemorrhage after tissue plasminogen activator treatment for acute myocardial infarction. Participants in the National Registry of Myocardial Infarction 2. *Ann Intern Med* 1998; **129**:597–604.
8. Brass LM, Lichtman JH, Wang Y, Gurwitz JH, Radford MJ, Krumholz HM. Intracranial hemorrhage associated with thrombolytic therapy for elderly patients with acute myocardial infarction: results from the Cooperative Cardiovascular Project. *Stroke* 2000; **31**:1802–11.
9. Rathore S, Wang Y, Krumholz H. Sex-based differences in the effect of digoxin for the treatment of heart failure. *N Engl J Med* 2002; **347**:1403–11.

10. Group M-HS. Effect of metoprolol CR/XL in chronic heart failure: Metoprolol CR/XL. Randomized Intervention Trial in Congestive Heart Failure (MERIT-HF). *Lancet* 1999; **353**:2001–6.
11. Packer M, Fowler BM, Cohn JN, et al. The effect of carvedilol on morbidity and mortality in patients with chronic heart failure. US Carvedilol Heart Failure Study Group. *N Engl J Med* 1996; **334**:1349–55.
12. Packer M, Fowler MB, Roecker EB, et al., for the Carvedilol Prospective Randomized Cumulative Survival (COPERNICUS) Study Group. Effect of carvedilol on the morbidity of patients with severe chronic heart failure: results of the Carvedilol Prospective Randomized Cumulative Survival (COPERNICUS) study. *Circulation* 2002; **106**:2194–9.
13. Gorski J, Jones D, Haehner-Daniels B, Hamman M, O'Mara E, Hall S. The contribution of intestinal and hepatic CYP3A to the interaction between midazolam and clarithromycin. *Clin Pharmacol Ther* 1998; **64**:133–43.
14. Krecic-Shepard M, Barnas C, Slimko J, Jones M, Schwartz J. Gender-specific effects on verapamil pharmacokinetics and pharmacodynamics in humans. *J Clin Pharmacol* 2000; **40**:219–30.
15. Kates R, Keefe D, Schwartz J, Harapat S, Kirsten E, Harrison D. Verapamil disposition kinetics in chronic atrial fibrillation. *Clin Pharmacol Ther* 1981; **30**:44–51.
16. Ho P, Triggs E, Bourne D, Heazlewood V. The effects of age and sex on the disposition of acetylsalicyclic acid and its metabolites. *Br J Clin Pharmacol* 1985; **19**:675–84.

17. Frezza M, di Padova C, Pozzato G, Terpin M, Baraona E, Lieber C. High blood alcohol levels in women: the role of gastric alcohol dehydrogenase activity and first pass metabolism. *N Engl J Med* 1990; **322**:95–9.

18. Seitz H, Egerer G, Simanowski V, et al. Human gastric alcohol dehydrogenase activity: effect of age sex, and alcoholism. *Gut* 1993; **34**:1433–7.

19. Dias V, Tendler B, Oparil S, Reilly P, Snarr P, White W. Clinical experience with transdermal clonidine in African-American and Hispanic-American patients with hypertension: evaluation from a 12-week prospective, open label clinical trial in community-based clinics. *Am J Ther* 1999; **6**:19–24.

20. Van Horn L, Ballew C, Liu K, et al. Diet, body size, and plasma lipids-lipoproteins in young adults: differences by race and sex. The Coronary Artery Risk Development in Young Adults (CARDIA) Study. *Am J Epidemiol* 1991; **133**:9–23.

21. Kristjansson F. Disposition of alprazolam in human volunteers. Differences between genders. *Acta Pharm Nord* 1991; **3**:249–50.

22. Vahl N, Moller N, Lauritzen T, Christiansen J, Jorgensen JOL. Metabolic effects and pharmacokinetics of a growth hormone pulse in healthy adults: relation to age, sex, and body composition. *J Clin Endocrinol Metab* 1998; **82**:3612–18.

23. Greenblatt D, Wright C. Clinical pharmacokinetics of alprazolam: therapeutic implications. *Clin Pharmacokinet* 1993; **24**:453–71.

24. Kirkwood C, Moore A, Hayes P, DeVane C, Pelonero A. Influence of menstrual cycle and gender on alprazolam pharmacokinetics. *Clin Pharmacol Ther* 1991; **50**:404–9.

25. Van de Werf F. ASSENT-3: implications for future trial design and clinical practice. *Eur Heart J* 2002; **23**:911–12.

26. Wizeman T, Pardue M-L. *Exploring the Biological Contributions to Human Health. Does Sex Matter?* Report No. ASBN 0–309–07281–6. Washington, DC: Institute of Medicine, 2001.

27. Beierle I, Meibohm B, Derendorf H. Gender differences in pharmacokinetics and pharmacodynamics. *Int J Clin Pharmacol Ther* 1999; **37**:529–47.

28. Fuhr U. Drug interactions with grapefruit juice. Extent, probable mechanism, and clinical relevance. *Drug Safety* 1998; **18**:251–72.

29. Spence JD. Drug interactions with grapefruit: whose responsibility is it to warn the public? *Clin Pharmacol Ther* 1997; **61**:395–400.

30. Bailey DG, Arnold JMO, Munoz C, Spence JD. Grapefruit juice-felodipine interaction: mechanism,

31. Kupferschmidt HH, Ha HR, Ziegler WH, Meier PJ, Krahenbuhl S. Interaction between grapefruit juice and midazolam in humans. *Clin Pharmacol Ther* 1995; **58**:20–8.

32. Lown KS, Bailey DG, Fontana RJ, et al. Grapefruit juice increases felodipine oral availability in humans by decreasing intestinal CYP3A protein expression. *J Clin Invest* 1997; **99**:2545–53.

33. Anon. Drug interactions with grapefruit juice. *Medical Letter* 2004; **46**:2–3.

34. Valantine H. Neoral use in the cardiac transplant recipient. *Transplant Proc* 2000; **32**:27S-44S.

35. Fitzsimmons W, Bekersky D, Dressler D, Raye K, Hodosh E, Mekki Q. Demographic considerations in tacrolimus pharmacokinetics. *Transplant Proc* 1998; **30**:1359–64.

36. Roy S, Flynn G. Transdermal delivery of narcotic analgesics: pH, anatomical, and subject influences on cutaneous permeability of fentanyl and sufentanil. *Pharm Res* 1990; **7**:842–7.

37. Rohatagi S, Calic F, Harding N, et al. Pharmacokinetics, pharmacodynamics, and safety of inhaled cyclosporin A (ADI628) after single and repeated administration in healthy male and female subjects and asthmatic patients. *J Clin Pharmacol* 2000; **40**:1211–26.

38. Knight V, Yu C, Gilbert B, et al. Estimating the dosage of ribavirin aerosol according to age and other variables. *J Infect Dis* 1988; **158**:443–7.

39. Cockcroft DW, Gault MH. Prediction of creatinine clearance from serum creatinine. *Nephron* 1976; **16**:31–41.

40. Levey A, Bosch J, Lewis J, Greene T, Rogers N, Roth D. A more accurate method to estimate glomerular filtration rate from serum creatinine: a new prediction equation. *Ann Intern Med* 1999; **130**:461–70.

41. Manjunath G, Sarnak M, Levey A. Prediction equations to estimate glomerular filtration rate: an update. *Curr Opin Nephrol Hypertens* 2001; **10**:785–92.

42. Yukawa E, Mine H, Higuchi S, Aoyama T. Digoxin population pharmacokinetics from routine clinical data: role of patient characteristics for estimating dosing regimens. *J Pharm Pharmacol* 1992; **44**:761–5.

43. Ducharme M, Slaughter R, Edwards D. Vancomycin pharmacokinetics in a patient population: effect of age, gender, and body weight. *Ther Drug Monit* 1994; **16**:513–18.

44. National Center for Health Statistics: National Health and Nutrition Examination Survey (NHANES).

Anthropomorphic reference data, United States, 1988–1994. Available at www.cdc.gov.nchs

45. Eichhorn E, Gheorghiade M. Digoxin – new perspective on an old drug. *N Engl J Med* 2002; **347**:1394–5.

46. Johnston N, Jernberg T, Lindahl B, et al. Biochemical indicators of cardiac and renal function in a healthy elderly population. *Clin Biochem* 2004; **37**:210–16.

47. Dharnidharka V, Kwon C, Stevens G. Serum Cystatin C is superior to serum creatinine as a marker of kidney function: a meta-analysis. *Am J Kidney Dis* 2002; **40**:221–6.

48. Delanaye P, Lambermont B, Chapelle J-P, Gielen J, Gerard P, Rorive G. Plasmatic cystatin C for the estimation of glomerular filtration rate in intensive care units. *Intensive Care Med* 2004; **30**:980–3.

49. Gaudry S, Sitar D, Smyth D, McKenzie J, Aoki F. Gender and age as factors in the inhibition of renal clearance of amantadine by quinine and quinidine. *Clin Pharmacol Ther* 1993; **54**:23–7.

50. Evans W, Relling M. Pharmacogenomics: translating functional genomics into rational therapeutics. *Science* 1999; **286**:487–91.

51. Rendic S. Summary of information on human CYP enzymes: human P450 metabolism data. *Drug Metab Rev* 2002; **34**:83–448.

52. Weinshilboum R. Inheritance and drug response. *N Engl J Med* 2003; **348**:529–37.

53. Wandel C, Witte J, Hall J, Stein CM, Wood A, Wilkinson G. CYP3A activity in African American and European American men: population differences and functional effect of the CYP3A4*1B5'-promoter region polymorphism. *Clin Pharmacol Ther* 2000; **68**:82–91.

54. Kuehl P, Zhang J, Lin Y, et al. Sequence diversity in CYP3A promoters and characterization of the genetic basis of polymorphic CYP3A5 expression. *Nat Genet* 2001; **27**:383–91.

55. Krecic-Shepard ME, Barnas C, Slimko J, Gorski J, Wainer I, Schwartz JB. *In vivo* comparison of putative probes of CYP3A4/5 activity: erythromycin, dextromethorphan, and verapamil. *Clin Pharmacol Ther* 1999; **66**:40–50.

56. Krecic-Shepard M, Park K, Barnas C, Slimko J, Kerwin D, Schwartz J. Race and sex influence clearance of nifedipine: results of a population study. *Clin Pharmacol Ther* 2000; **68**:130–42.

57. Lew K, Ludwig E, Milad M, et al. Gender-based effects on methylprednisolone pharmacokinetics and pharmacodynamics. *Clin Pharmacol Ther* 1993; **54**: 402–14.

58. Hunt C, Westerkam W, Stave G. Effect of age and gender on the activity of human hepatic CYP3A. *Biochem Pharmacol* 1992; **44**:275–83.

59. Kahan B, Kramer W, Wideman C, et al. Demographic factors affecting the pharmacokinetics of cyclosporine estimated by radioimmunoassay. *Transplantation* 1986; **41**:459–64.

60. Wolbold R, Klein K, Burk O, et al. Sex is a major determinant of CYP3A4 expression in human liver. *Hepatology* 2003; **38**:978–88.

61. Guengerich F. Cytochrome P-450 3A4: regulation and role in drug metabolism. *Annu Rev Pharmacol Toxicol* 1999; **39**:1–17.

62. Gorski J, Wang Z, Haehner-Daniels B, Wrighton S, Hall S. The effect of hormone replacement therapy on CYP3A activity. *Clin Pharmacol Ther* 2000; **68**:412–17.

63. Greenblatt D, Abernethy D, Locniskar A, Harmatz J, Limjuco R, Shader R. Effect of age, gender, and obesity on midazolam kinetics. *Anesthesiology* 1984; **61**:27–35.

64. Holazo A, Winkler M, Patel I. Effects of age, gender and oral contraceptives on intramuscular midazolam pharmacokinetics. *J Clin Pharmacol* 1988; **28**:1040–5.

65. Smith M, Heazlewood V, Eadie M, Brophy T, Tyrer J. Pharmacokinetics of midazolam in the aged. *Eur J Clin Pharmacol* 1984; **26**:381–8.

66. Platten H, Schweizer E, Dilger K, Mikus G, Klotz U. Pharmacokinetics and the pharmacodynamic action of midazolam in young and elderly patients undergoing tooth extraction. *Clin Pharmacol Ther* 1998; **63**:552–60.

67. Nishiyama T, Matsukawa T, Hanaoka K. The effects of age and gender on the optimal premedication dose of intramuscular midazolam. *Anesth Analg* 1998; **86**:1103–8.

68. Kang D, Verotta D, Krecic-Shepard ME, Modi NM, Gupta SK, Schwartz JB. Population analyses of sustained-release verapamil in patients: effects of sex, race, and smoking. *Clin Pharmacol Ther* 2003; **73**:31–40.

69. Schwartz J. The influence of sex on pharmacokinetics. *Clin Pharmacokinet* 2003; **42**:4–10.

70. Kalow W, Tang B. Use of caffeine metabolite ratios to explore CYP1A2 and xanthine oxidase ratios. *Clin Pharmacol Ther* 1991; **50**:508–19.

71. Kaye C, Nicholls B. Clinical pharmacokinetics of ropinirole. *Clin Pharmacokinet* 2000; **39**:243–54.

72. Tamminga A, Wemer J, Oosterhuis B, et al. CYP2D6 and CYP2C19 activity in a large population of Dutch healthy volunteers: indications for oral contraceptive-related gender differences. *Eur J Clin Pharmacol* 1999; **55**:177–84.

73. Kashuba A, Bertino J, Kearns G, et al. Quantitation of three-month intraindividual variability and influence of sex and menstrual cycle phase on CYP1A2, N-

acetyltransferease-2, and xanthine oxidase activity determined with caffeine phenotyping. *Clin Pharmacol Ther* 1998; **63**:540–51.

74. Kharasch E, Russell M, Garton K, Lentz G, Bowdle T, Cox K. Assessment of cytochrome P450 3A4 activity during the menstrual cycle using alfentanil as a noninvasive probe. *Anesthesiology* 1997; **87**:26–35.

75. Ròdriguez I, Killborn M, Liu X, Pezzullo J, Woosley R. Drug-induced QT prolongation in women during the menstrual cycle. *JAMA* 2001; **285**:1322–6.

76. Bruguerolle B, Toumi M, Faraj F, Vervloet D, Razzouk H. Influence of the menstrual cycle on theophylline pharmacokinetics in asthmatics. *Eur J Clin Pharmacol* 1990; **39**:59–61.

77. Sweeting J. Does the time of the month affect the function of the gut. *Gastroenterology* 1992; **102**: 1084–5.

78. Jochemsen R, Van Der Graaff M, Boeijinga J, Breimer D. Influence of sex, menstrual cycle and oral contraception on the disposition of nitrazepam. *Br J Clin Pharmacol* 1982; **13**:319–24.

79. Kliewer SA. The nuclear pregnane X receptor regulates xenobiotic detoxification. *J Nutr* 2003; **133**:2444S–7S.

80. Ioannides C. Pharmacokinetic interactions between herbal remedies and medicinal drugs. *Xenobiotica* 2002; **32**:451–78.

81. Risk of drug interactions with St. John's wort and indinavir and other drugs. In: www.fda.gov/cderdrugadvisory/stjwort.htm. Ed: FDA Public Health Advisory, 2000.

82. Ernst E, Rand J, Barnes J, Stevinson C. Adverse effects profile of the herbal antidepressant St. John's wort. *Eur J Clin Pharmacol* 1998; **54**:589–94.

83. Tannergren C, Engman H, Knurson L, Hedeland H, Bondesson U, Lennernas H. St. John's wort decreases the bioavailability of R- and S-verapamil through induction of the first pass metabolism. *Clin Pharamcol Ther* 2004; **75**:298–309.

84. Divoll M, Greenblatt D, Harmatz J, Shader R. Effect of age and gender on disposition of temazepam. *J Pharm Sci* 1981; **70**:1104–7.

85. Greenblatt D, Divoll M, Harmatz J, Shader R. Oxazepam kinetics: effects of age and sex. *J Pharmacol Exp Ther* 1980; **215**:86–91.

86. Walle T, Walle U, Cowart T, Conradi E. Pathway-selective sex differences in the metabolic clearance of propranolol in human subjects. *Clin Pharmacol Ther* 1989; **46**:257–63.

87. Walle T, Byington R, Furberg C, McIntypre K, Vokonos P. Biologic determinants of propranolol disposition. Results from 1308 patients in the beta-blocker heart attack trial. *Clin Pharmacol Ther* 1985; **38**:509–18.

88. Johnson J, Akers W, Herring V, Wolfe M, Sullivan J. Gender differences in labetalol kinetics: importance of determining stereoisomer kinetics for racemic drugs. *Pharmacotherapy* 2000; **20**:622–8.

89. Morissette P, Albert C, Busque S, St-Louis G, Vinet B. In vivo higher glucuronidation of mycophenolic acid in male than in female recipients of a cadaveric kidney allograft and under immunosuppressive therapy with mycophenolate mofetil. *Ther Drug Monit* 2001; **23**:520–5.

90. Schuetz E, Furuya K, Schuetz J. Interindividual variation in expression of P-glycoprotein in normal human liver and secondary hepatic neoplasms. *J Pharmacol Exp Ther* 1995; **275**:1011–18.

91. Kim R, Leake B, Choo E, et al. Identification of functionally variant MDR1 alleles among European Americans and African Americans. *Clin Pharmacol Ther* 2001; **70**:189–99.

92. Christy N, Shaver J. Estrogens and the kidney. *Kidney Int* 1974; **6**:366–76.

93. Anon. Questions and answers about black cohosh and the symptoms of menopause. In: *NIH Office of Dietary Supplements and National Center for Complementary and Alternative Medicine*, 2004. Available at http://ods.od.nih.gov/factsheets/blackcohosh.html

94. Fazio A. Oral contraceptive drug interactions: important considerations. *South Med J* 1991; **84**:997–1002.

95. Back D, Orme M. Pharmacokinetic drug interactions with oral contraceptives. *Clin Pharmacokinet* 1990; **18**:472–84.

96. Crawford P, Chadwick D, Martin C, Tjia J, Back D, Orme M. The interaction of phenytoin and carbamazepine with combined oral contraceptive steroids. *Br J Clin Pharmacol* 1990; **30**:892–6.

97. Shapiro B, Agrawal A, Pampori N. Gender differences in drug metabolism regulated by growth hormone. *Int J Biochem Cell Biol* 1995; **27**:9–20.

98. Teichmann A. Influence of oral contraceptives on drug therapy. *Am J Obstet Gynecol* 1990; **163**:2208–13.

99. Rasmussen B, Brosen K. Determination of urinary metabolites of caffeine, for the assessment of cytochrome 4501A2, xanthine oxidase, and N-acetyltransferase activity in humans. *Ther Drug Monit* 1996; **18**:254–62.

100. Weisberg E. Interactions between oral contraceptives and antifungals/antibacterials. Is contraceptive failure the result? *Clin Pharmacokinet* 1999; **36**:309–13.

101. Loebstein R, Lalkin A, Koren G. Pharmacokinetic changes during pregnancy and their clinical relevance. *Clin Pharmacokinet* 1997; **33**:328–43.

102. Gleichmann W, Bachmann G, Dengler H, Dudeck J. Effects of hormonal contraceptives and pregnancy on serum protein pattern. *Eur J Clin Pharmacol* 1973; **5**:218–25.

103. Rautaharju P, Zhou S, Wong S, et al. Sex differences in the evolution of the electrocardiographic QT interval with age. *Can J Cardiol* 1992; **8**:690–5.

104. Lehmann M, Timothy K, Frankovich D, et al. Age-gender influence on the rate-corrected QT intervals in the QT-heart rate relation in families with genotypically characterized long QT syndrome. *J Am Coll Cardiol* 1997; **29**:93–9.

105. Makkar R, Fromm B, Steinman R, Meissner M, Lehmann M. Female gender as a risk factor for torsade de pointes associated with cardiovascular drugs. *JAMA* 1993; **270**:2590–7.

106. Drici M, Knollman B, Wang W, Woosley R. Cardiac actions of erythromycin: influence of female sex. *Am Heart J* 1998; **131**:1184–91.

107. Lehmann MH, Hardy S, Archibald D, et al. Sex difference in risk of torsade de pointes with d,l-sotalol. *Circulation* 1996; **94**:2535–41.

108. Benton R, Sale M, Flockhart D, Woosley R, Greater quinidine-induced QTc interval prolongation in women. *Clin Pharmacol Ther* 2000; **67**:413–18.

109. Packer M, Coats AJ, Fowler MB, et al. Effect of carvedilol on survival in severe chronic heart failure. *N Engl J Med* 2001; **344**:1651–8.

110. Simon T, Mary-Krause M, Funck-Brentano C, Jaillon P. Sex differences in the prognosis of congestive heart failure. Results from the Cardiac Insufficiency Bisoprolol Study (CIBIS II). *Circulation* 2001; **103**:375–80.

111. Ghali JK, Pina IL, Gottlieb SS, Deedwania PC, Wikstrand JC, on Behalf of the MERIT-HF Study Group. Metoprolol CR/XL in Female Patients With Heart Failure: analysis of the experience in Metoprolol Extended-Release Randomized Intervention Trial in Heart Failure (MERIT-HF). *Circulation* 2002; **105**:1585–91.

112. Garg R, Yusuf S. Overview of randomized trials of angiotensin converting enzyme inhibitors on mortality and morbidity in heart failure. Collaborative Group on ACE Inhibitor Trials. *JAMA* 1995; **273**:1450–6.

113. Flather M, Yusuf S, Kober L, et al. for the ACE-Inhibitor Myoardial Infarction Collaborative Group. Long-term ACE-inhibitor therapy in patients with heart failure or left-ventricular dysfunction: a systematic overview of data from individual patients. *Lancet* 2000; **355**:1575–81.

114. Israeli Z, Hall W. Cough and angioneurotic edema associated with angiotensin-converting enzyme inhibitor therapy. A review of the literature and pathophysiology. *Ann Intern Med* 1992; **117**: 234–42.

115. Sebastian J, McKinney W, Kaufman J, Young M. Angiotensin-converting enzyme inhibitors and cough: prevalence in an outpatient medical clinic population. *Chest* 1991; **99**:36–9.

116. Simon S, Black H, Moser M, Berland W. Cough and ACE inhibitors. *Arch Intern Med* 1992; **152**:1698–700.

117. Os I, Bratland B, Dahlöf B, Gisholt K, Syvertsen J, Tretli S. Female sex as an important determinant of lisinopril-induced cough. *Lancet* 1992; **339**:372.

118. Lee S, Kim H, Choi C, et al. Clinical characteristics and angiotensin converting enzyme gene polymorphism in the susceptibility to angiotensin converting enzyme inhibitor-induced cough. *Korean Circ J* 1996; **26**:1099–106.

119. Chapman M, Hanrahan R, McEwen J, Marley J. Hyponatraemia and hypokalemia due to indapamide. *Med J Aust* 2002; **176**:219–21.

120. Hart RG, Boop BS, Anderson DC. Oral anticoagulants and intracranial hemorrhage. Facts and hypotheses. *Stroke* 1995; **26**:1471–7.

121. Morley J, Marinchak R, Rials SJ, Kowey P. Atrial fibrillation, anticoagulation, and stroke. *Am J Cardiol* 1996; **77**:38A–44A.

122. Becker RC, Hochman JS, Cannon CP, et al. Fatal cardiac rupture among patients treated with thrombolytic agents and adjunctive thrombin antagonists: observations from the Thrombolysis and Thrombin Inhibition in Myocardial Infarction 9 Study. *J Am Coll Cardiol* 1999; **33**:479–87.

123. Van de Werf F, Barron H, Armstrong P, et al. Incidence and predictors of bleeding events after fibrinolytic therapy with fibrin-specific agents. *Eur Heart J* 2001; **22**:2253–61.

124. Lee M, Wali A, Menon V, et al. The determinants of activated partial thromboplastin time, relation of activated partial thromboplastin time to clinical outcomes, and optimal dosing regimens for heparin treated patients with acute coronary syndromes: a review of GUSTO-IIb. *J Thromb Thrombolysis* 2002; **14**:91–101.

125. Menon V, Berkowitz S, Antman E, Fuchs R, Hochman J. New heparin dosing recommendations for patients with acute coronary syndromes. *Am J Med* 2001; **110**:641–50.

126. Caraballo P, Heit J, Atkinson E, et al. Long-term use of oral anticoagulants and the risk of fracture. *Arch Intern Med* 1999; **159**:1750–6.

127. Hirsh J. Heparin. *N Engl J Med* 1991; **324**:1565–74.

128. Goldberg A. Clinical trial experience with extended-release niacin (Niaspan): dose-escalation study. *Am J Cardiol* 1998; **82**:35–8.

129. Waters D, Alderman E, Hsia J, et al. Effects of hormone replacement therapy and antioxidant vitamin supplements on coronary atherosclerosis in postmenopausal women. A randomized controlled trial. *JAMA* 2002; **288**:2432–40.

130. Porile J, Bakris G, Garella S. Acute interstitial nephritis with glomerulopathy due to nonsteroidal anti-inflammatory agents: a review of its clinical spectrum and effects of steroid therapy. *J Clin Pharmacol* 1990; **30**:468–75.

131. Chen M-L, Lee S-C, Ng M-J, Schuirmann D, Lesko L, Williams R. Pharmacokinetic analysis of bioequivalence trials: implications for sex-related issues in clinical pharmacology and biopharmaceutics. *Clin Pharmacol Ther* 2000; **68**:510–21.

40

Social stress, strain, and heart disease in women

Kristina Orth-Gomér, Margaret A. Chesney and David E. Anderson

Introduction

The prevalence of cardiovascular disease (CVD) among women and men, and its position as the leading cause of death, underscores the need for a comprehensive risk factor profile to direct prevention efforts. The knowledge of the female risk profile is unsatisfactory, largely because most research on risk factors and prediction of CVD has been conducted in men.[1,2] What is known about traditional risk factors in women is based on such population-based longitudinal studies as the Framingham Study, the Gothenburg Study, and the MONICA study.[3–5] The Framingham Study, for example, generated a risk equation for women that includes age, systolic blood pressure, cholesterol, high-density lipoprotein (HDL), glucose intolerance, cigarette smoking, and electrocardiogram (ECG) evidence of myocardial hypertrophy. The Framingham women who were aged between 60 and 64 years and at highest risk, i.e. in the upper 10% of the risk factor distribution, had a 12% probability of developing coronary heart disease (CHD) during a 6-year follow-up; the comparable probability for men was 20%.[6] These small probabilities indicate the lack of specificity in the prediction of CHD risk, in particular for women but also for men. It is also evident that the traditional risk factors incorporated in the equations explain only a portion of the risk, and that other risk factors must contribute as well. These less well-established factors include social, psychological, and behavioral variables, the role of

which has been less extensively studied in women than in men.[7] The purpose of this chapter is to highlight the relative importance of psychosocial, as compared with traditional factors, in understanding CVD among women.

One of the reasons that psychosocial factors are not included in traditional risk factor equations is the lack of models demonstrating mechanisms by which these factors exert increased risk. In the first section of this chapter, a model is proposed linking social strain, depressed mood, health behavior, and increased CVD risk. In addition, the hypothesis that psychosocial factors might contribute to the development of sodium-sensitive forms of hypertension via an inhibited breathing mechanism is discussed. In the second section, data are presented from two major Swedish studies that provide a 'test' of the proposed model. Finally, the implications for further research and risk factor reduction among women are discussed.

Model of social strain and CVD risk

Social isolation and cardiovascular outcomes: relevance for women?

Social isolation, low levels of social support, and limited social networks have been associated with numerous adverse health outcomes, including CHD.

In a 5-year prospective study of patients with CHD, being unmarried or living without a confidant was associated with a threefold increase in mortality compared with being married or having a confidant.[8] This relationship was independent of the standard risk factors. Living alone was also found to be associated with recurrent heart disease in another prospective study of patients with pre-existing heart disease.[9] It is important to note that the percentage of women in each of these studies was small (18% and 19%, respectively), precluding an analysis by gender.

In another prospective study of postmyocardial infarction (MI) patients, having fewer sources of emotional support was associated with 6-month mortality among women and men.[10] This relationship was independent of the severity of MI, of co-morbidity, and of the standard risk factors such as smoking and hypertension. Specifically, there was a clear linear association between the number of sources of support and the percentage of postMI subjects who died during the 6 months of follow-up. These studies suggest that lack of social support, lack of social contacts, and particularly social isolation create social strain and lead to behavioral and physiological response patterns, the long-term effects of which may be harmful and cause heart disease.

Other studies have suggested that having social ties does not always confer protection from social strain. Population-based studies, which have used quantitative measures of social networks, have almost invariably shown that social ties are health-promoting in men.[11] In women, however, the findings are contradictory. Specifically, in North Karelia, a northeastern region of Finland, and in Evans County, Georgia, no association was observed between the number of social ties and cardiovascular risk in women.[12,13] It is possible that, to the extent that social ties increase the number of roles, there might also be an associated increase in social strain. Perhaps, in North Karelia and Georgia, increases in strain associated with more social ties may 'offset' the benefit of increased social support that these ties may deliver. The model proposed in Fig. 40.1 is based on a review of the existing literature that documents significant relationships between social strain, depressed mood, health behaviors and increased CVD risk.

With strain we understand social and psychological influences in the environment, which may cause

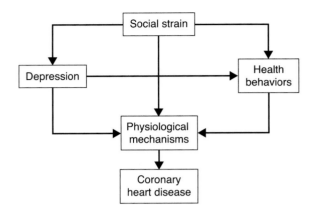

Figure 40.1
Relationship between social strain and coronary heart disease.

unhealthy reactions. With stress we understand physiological and psychological responses to strain, which may affect health in a negative way.

Women's multiple roles and social strain

Women's lives are often characterized by multiple social roles, including spouse, manager in the home, worker, and caregiver for the family members. There is the possibility that these relationships, although providing a number of potentially beneficial contacts, also increase the likelihood of conflicting demands, and a high total workload. The effects of these demands on health-related factors are documented by studies showing harmful neuroendocrine reactions in women with a total work overload.[14]

In considering psychosocial risk factors for women, the number of social contacts cannot be considered as a measure of social support. More specifically, it cannot be assumed that the absence of contacts will be associated with adverse health outcomes, nor that the presence of many contacts is protective. Research contrasting the health outcomes for men and single women supports this point. Specifically, Mortiz and Satariano[15] found that women who lived with a spouse had a higher odds ratio (2.02) of being diagnosed with more advanced breast cancer than did women living alone. The investigators in this study concluded, 'The presence of a spouse may detract from the attention a woman pays to her own health'.

Thus, for women, marriage may be associated with increased strain and does not provide the protection against adverse health effects that has been observed in samples consisting primarily of men. The above studies demonstrate that, in the context of women's lives, social relationships are not a proxy for social support. Marriage, rather than being the buffer against adverse health effects that it can be for men, appears to have some detrimental effects for women. In summary, in studies of women, it is important to test measures of social strain or low social support that take into account the female subjects' perceptions of both strain and support.

Social strain, depressed mood, and CVD (see also Chapter 41)

One of the pathways by which social strain affects CVD risk is through depressed mood. Low levels of social support are associated with depression.[16–18] On the basis of studies examining the relationship between social support and depression, Palinkas et al. wrote, 'At any age the deterioration of social networks is a risk factor for depression'.[19] In a population-based survey of over 1600 adults aged 65 years or older, the research team found that depressive symptoms were associated with a smaller network size, greater distance to primary support, and less participation in community organizations. The association between social strain and depressed mood is reciprocal, with each factor influencing the other. Thus, while social strain may influence depression, longitudinal research indicates that depressive symptoms can also predict a decline in social relationships over time.[20] Depressive mood may affect social networks in a number of ways, including reducing a person's capacity to become involved with others in their social network, discouraging members of a social support system from providing support, and diminishing a person's perception of the adequacy of the support they are receiving.[19]

Depression is associated with increased risk for MI as well as other cardiac events.[21–23] This association was noted in the 1980s by Kaplan[24] and others but was overlooked for many years, while attention was focused on coronary-prone behavior. In 1987, Booth-Kewley and Friedman[25] published a meta-analysis of psychosocial predictors of CHD and pointed out that among variables including type A behavior and anxiety, depression had the strongest association with CHD. Recently, new studies have provided compelling evidence regarding the importance of depression in CHD risk. In a longitudinal study, Frasure-Smith and her colleagues[26] found that depressed postMI patients had a fivefold greater risk of mortality 6 months after MI compared with nondepressed postMI patients. At the time that these findings were published, results from the Recurrent Coronary Prevention Project, showing depression to be an independent predictor of mortality and recurrence of clinical cardiac events, were presented by Powell and her associates.[27] It has been argued that depression may be more important as a CHD risk factor for women than for men. Noting both the higher postMI mortality rate among women than men and the twofold greater prevalence of depression among women with CHD than men, Freedland and Carney argued that depression may explain the observed sex difference in mortality rates associated with MI.[28] The specific mechanisms by which depression increases CHD risk remain to be determined. A number of factors associated with decreased central nervous system serotonergic functioning, including increased norepinephrine and weaker parasympathetic function, have been observed in depressed patients and proposed as possible pathways linking depression to heart disease risk.

Social strain and health behaviors

Significant relationships between social strain and adverse health behaviors provide another pathway by which social strain may influence CHD risk. Decreases in social ties lead to increases in health-damaging behaviors, according to Broman.[29] The inverse has also been confirmed. That is, increases in the number of social ties predict increases in positive health behaviors. Focusing on exercise, for example,

King and her associates reported that being either separated or divorced places people at increased risk for failing to adhere to exercise regimens.[30] Conversely, beginning and maintaining exercise is significantly related to high levels of social support.[31,32] Depression may mediate some of the association between social strain and health behavior. For example, major disruptions in social ties, such as divorce, are associated with depressive symptoms, which in turn are associated with adverse health behaviors including smoking and alcohol consumption.[29]

The model presented thus far describes significant relationships between social isolation, depressive symptoms and adverse health behaviors. Consistent with this is a study of a community sample which demonstrated that, among women, working full time, marital conflict, negative life events, and a history of depression are associated with current cigarette smoking.[33] History of depression and the presence of marital conflict were also associated with alcohol use in this sample. Apart from its relationship with social strain variables, such as marital conflict, depressed mood is significantly related to such adverse health behaviors as current smoking,[34] and difficulty in adherence to postMI regimens, including diet, exercise, medications, and smoking cessation.[35] Among postMI women, depressed mood predicts poorer adherence to weight loss and exercise recommendations, two key aspects of cardiac rehabilitation.[36]

Physiological mechanisms – social strain and cardiovascular reactivity

New research with female primates is providing important insights into the mechanisms by which social strain may increase cardiovascular risk among females. Using a primate model, Shively and her colleagues demonstrated that monkeys who have socially subordinate positions in social living groups are more often the targets of aggression, are more vigilant, and spend more time alone than their socially dominant counterparts.[37,38] Physiological characteristics of these subordinate monkeys indicate that they are experiencing social stress and that this stress causes impaired ovarian function.[39]

To test the specific effects of social isolation, Shively and her associates conducted a study[38] comparing coronary artery atherosclerosis in singly housed and socially housed female monkeys. In both conditions, the monkeys were fed an atherogenic diet for 2 years. After the 2 years, singly housed monkeys had four times more coronary artery atherosclerosis than the socially housed monkeys. It was also possible to examine the extent of coronary artery atherosclerosis within the socially housed monkeys. Socially dominant monkeys in the socially housed group had the least coronary atherosclerosis. The extent of coronary atherosclerosis of the socially housed subordinate monkeys fell between that seen for the dominant monkeys and the singly housed monkeys. Shively concluded that 'the results of these experiments suggest that psychosocial stress exerts an effect on CHD risk. Part of this effect appears to be mediated by ovarian function'. While research on the effects of impaired premenopausal ovarian function on subsequent CHD is difficult to carry out, there is evidence from one study that irregular menstrual cycles elevate risk of CHD in women.[40] Thus, this animal research provides evidence that one mechanism by which social strain in general, and social isolation in particular, exerts its influence on CHD is impaired ovarian function.

Physiological mechanisms – interactions of stress and salt intake

Another area in which animal models have been informative regarding cardiovascular regulation in humans is that of the interactions of stress and high dietary sodium intake in blood pressure regulation. Epidemiological studies of humans have consistently found that the prevalence of hypertension in a society is a positive function of dietary sodium intake.[41] However, within a society, only a substantial minority of individuals is salt-sensitive, suggesting that genetic or other environmental factors mediate this association. Previous experimental studies have found that laboratory animals are resistant to the effects of salt loading on blood pressure unless they have been conditioned to remain vigilant in anticipation of the onset of a stressful task. Under those conditions, breathing frequency slows as the onset of the task approaches and levels of blood carbon dioxide rise, that transiently acidify, and then expand the plasma volume.[42] Animals that repeatedly engage in this inhibited breathing pattern become susceptible to the hypertensive effects of high salt intake over periods of days.[43]

This mechanism may also contribute to blood pressure elevation in humans, particularly women. It is well established that humans differ significantly in breathing pattern, with some breathing more rapidly and maintaining lower levels of carbon dioxide in blood and expired air, while others breathe more slowly and maintain higher levels of carbon dioxide.[44] Rapid breathing and hypocapnia are typically associated with anxiety, while slower breathing and hypercapnia are typically associated with an absence of emotional arousal. Hypercapnic breathing is also accompanied by increased cerebral blood flow, which could enhance vigilance during stress. When this inhibited breathing pattern is elicited in humans, a cascade of physiological changes can be observed that could potentiate sodium retention and hypertension. Several studies have produced findings in accord with this hypothesis. In one recent study, women who reported that they had been under high stress for the past month were characterized by slower breathing and higher blood carbon dioxide than women who reported less stress.[45] This is consistent with the view that they were maintaining a vigilant orientation to the environment. A similar, but less significant, trend was observed in men. In another study, voluntary and sustained inhibited breathing by humans during 30-minute performance sessions using a feedback procedure elicited decreases in plasma pH, together with decreases in renal sodium excretion and increases in natriuretic compounds that are produced by expansion of plasma volume.[46] Thus, the stress-induced suppression of breathing might be accompanied by increased circulating fluid volume even in persons on a normal salt diet, and thereby increase susceptibility to the hypertensive effects of a high sodium diet. Support for this view was obtained in a study that showed that blood pressure of older humans with high carbon dioxide was more sensitive to the hypertensive effects of a high salt diet than in those whose carbon dioxide levels were lower.[47] A similar finding was reported for humans with low

resting plasma pH.[48] From these observations, it can be suggested that social stresses that create an emotionally quiescent but vigilant state of mind provide the conditions for sodium sensitivity of blood pressure in humans, as well as laboratory animals.

Swedish research on social strain and CVD

A series of important research studies have yielded insights into the association between social support and CHD. In particular, these studies provide an excellent test of the model.

In the Swedish Survey of living conditions, which examined a representative sample of the entire Swedish population, 17 400 women and men were interviewed about quantitative aspects of their social networks and then followed for a 6-year period. In both women and men there was an excess cardiovascular mortality risk in those with few contacts. Controlling for standard risk factors, there was an excess CVD mortality of 50% in the lower compared with the middle and upper third of the social network index. Thus, it seems that both women and men in the Swedish population benefit from having a crucial number of social contacts. However, there was no beneficial effect of an increased number of contacts. In fact older women, who had the largest number of contacts, also had the highest CVD mortality.[49]

In an attempt to understand these relationships, we asked whether the function of the contacts could be more important than the number of available persons in the network or the frequency of interaction with network members. We wanted to know whether these contacts were mostly supportive or whether they were perhaps demanding and stressful. Few studies, however, have made the link between functional measures of social support and prospective prediction of cardiovascular endpoints.

In men, functional aspects of social support in relation to CHD have included:

- Emotional support or attachment, usually provided by close friends or family members

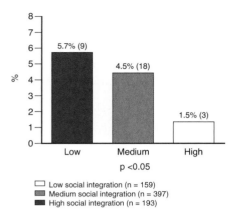

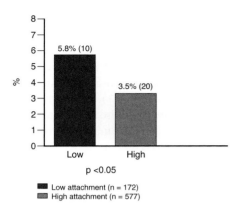

Figure 40.2
Six-year incidence of myocardial infarction by social integration (749 men, 50 years of age). Odds ratio for coronary heart disease in men with low social integration: 3.8 (95% CI: 1.1–13.9).

Figure 40.3
Six-year incidence of myocardial infarction by attachment (749 men, 50 years of age). Odds ratio for coronary heart disease in men with low attachment: 3.1 (95% CI: 1.3–7.6).

• Tangible support, meaning practical help
• Appraisal support, meaning good advice, and help properly to recognize and cope with problems and difficulties
• Belongingness, meaning the need to belong to groups of people with whom one shares interests and values.[50]

The latter three functions are usually provided by the extended social network, whereas emotional support is typically found within family and close friends.

In the studies of 50-year-old men born in Gothenburg (men born in 1913, 1923 and 1933), these aspects of social support have been evaluated in relation to other CHD risk factors. As the Gothenburg studies have been respected for their representativity, methodological accuracy and conclusiveness, it was particularly useful to examine this study group in terms of socially supportive functions and determine to what extent these would predict the incidence of MI in previously healthy men.

The strongest effect was seen for lack of social integration, i.e. the functions provided by the extended network that give guidance, advice, practical help, and belongingness (Fig. 40.2). It is perhaps not surprising that these functions were highly correlated with social class, so that men at higher occupa-

tional levels had more efficient support and were better socially integrated.

The other important aspect of social support, the very close emotional relationships that provide comfort, trust, and love and enhance self-esteem, were marginally predictive of MI in these men. However, a smaller group of men (23%), who lacked this kind of support, also had an increase in MI risk, although not as strong as for lack of social integration (Fig. 40.3).

Social support in women

In women, the picture is not as clear and unambiguous as in men, as was discussed earlier in this chapter. In the Swedish Survey of living conditions, women were as much in need as men of a *basic* number of contacts for their survival.[49] This is similar to the previously cited study from Alameda County, where women who lacked social ties had an excess mortality risk, which was even slightly higher than that of men.[51] However, as previously discussed, there is evidence that additional social ties can add to women's roles and increase workload and strain. The Stockholm Study of Female Coronary Risk provided an excellent opportunity to disentangle the role of strain and the role of support in women's lives and their significance for cardiovascular health. The study is a population-based case–control study of all women aged 65 years and below, who were hospitalized for an acute CHD event within a 3-year time period. Thus, the patient group represents all women with a known diagnosis of CHD in the greater Stockholm area. Age-matched healthy control subjects were obtained from the census register of the county, so they were representative of women in the same age group of the general population.

In Sweden practically all women are employed outside the home. There is even formal legislation requiring every citizen, woman or man, to work and to provide an income for herself or himself. Under these circumstances it is not surprising that only two homemakers were identified among the 600 women who were included in the study. That employment outside the home really means an additional workload has been elegantly described by Frankenhäuser and co-workers.[52] In their studies of female and male employees in large companies, they estimated the total number of hours per week spent on paid work and on work at home for the service of the family.

Full-time employed women and men without children both spent a total average of 60 work hours per week; women with children increased their total workload to as much as 90 hours/week with three children. Men in the same situation increased their total workload to 70 hours per week (Fig. 40.4). The cardiovascular health effects of chronically increased workload in women are not yet known, but psychosomatic symptoms have been found to be related to multiple stressors, both at work and at home, in Swedish women, but not in Swedish men.[53]

When the Stockholm women characterized their social supports using the functional measures also used in Gothenburg men, the effects were generally weaker for women than for men. Only the scale describing social integration, which was also the best predictor for men, showed a significant, but small, difference between cases and controls. This difference disappeared, however, after adjustment for standard risk factors including blood pressure, cholesterol, high-density lipoprotein (HDL), body mass index, smoking, exercise and education (Fig. 40.5). This failure of social strain to maintain its effects when controlling for standard risk factors

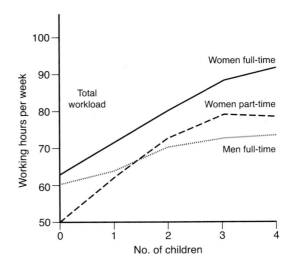

Figure 40.4
Total workload for women and men in relation to number of children in the family.

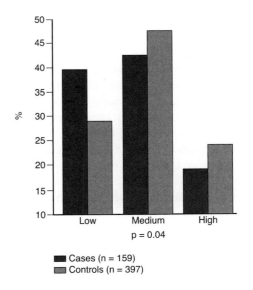

Figure 40.5
Social integration and coronary heart disease (CHD) in women. Odds ratio for CHD in women with low social integration: 1.65 (95% CI: 1.16–2.35).

supports the model that one of the pathways by which strain increases risk is through other factors, including health behaviors.

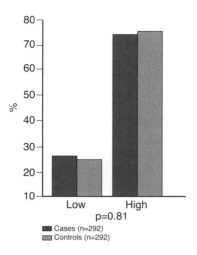

Figure 40.6
Attachment and coronary heart disease (CHD) in women. Odds ratio for CHD in women with low attachment: 1.06 (95% CI: 0.72–1.55).

The scale describing lack of attachment, which predicted CHD in men, showed absolutely no difference between women with and without heart disease (Fig. 40.6). In contrast, in the Gothenburg men, lack of social integration remained significant after controlling for standard risk factors. In fact, lack of social support and smoking were equally strong and independent risk factors in the multivariate analysis.

Social ties, social strain, and multiple roles

Because of these contradictory patterns when examining the social network structure and its function, a semistructured interview procedure was used to explore not just the concept of support, but also the concept of strain from the social sphere. The general goal of the interview was to describe all possible sources of stress and strain in women. The concept and methodology to assess family strain were similar to those used by Karasek and Theorell for work strain, i.e., both demand and control dimensions were considered.[54] The interview was structured to describe both the work and family career of these women, specifically addressing employment, marriage, divorce and separation, childbirth and the rearing of children, as well as caring responsibilities for elderly and other relatives. The general methodology of the interview procedure is described elsewhere.[55] Here, it is sufficient to point out that the interview questions were aimed at concrete and 'objective' events, that would not be affected by disease and ill health.

In Figure 40.7, the sources of strain from different life domains are compared in women with CHD and in healthy women. Consistent with the model proposed at the beginning of this chapter, a significant association was observed between strain and CHD. Most pronounced are the excess strain scores for CHD women, concerning strain from the present job and strain from having too little time for relaxation, for leisure, and for personal growth and development. This is also in accordance with the results from other measures of work demand and decision latitude at work. Thus, in women with CHD, there was lack of opportunity for growth and development, both at work and in leisure time. When the job strain variables were combined into the demand, control model, proposed by Karasek and Theorell,[54] the odds ratio of CHD for the highest versus the lowest quartile of job strain was 2.5 and highly significant. The effect persisted after adjustment for multivariate traditional confounders, thus confirming the results from the interview using a standardized well-validated job strain measure. In the absence of similar, well-validated family strain measures, we have to rely on semistructured interview data, obtained according to the same concept of demand and control as for job strain.

Family strain

Women with CHD had both more children and more separations than healthy controls and the proportion of women without children was larger in healthy women (14%) than in women with CHD (10%). Women with CHD also reported more strain from problems with children, but above all more problems associated with their spouse relationships. In particular, the separations caused these women to report stress and strain when interviewed. As these were assessments made in women who were already ill, it is of course possible that their perception of

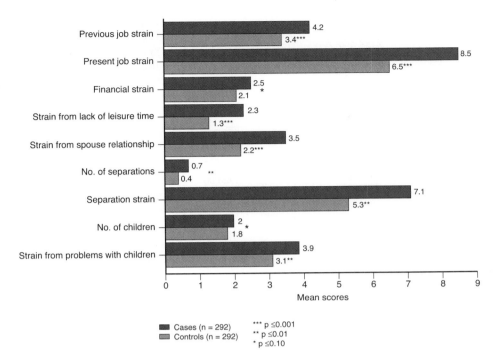

Figure 40.7
Psychosocial strain and coronary heart disease in women.

family strain was compromised by the knowledge of their heart disease. It is unlikely, however, that the women with a history of CHD would consciously blame their heart disease on family problems. When asked this question directly, most of them blamed it on their own unhealthy lifestyle, e.g., smoking and lack of exercise. It is also unlikely that many of the women could have had a direct contamination of their disease on family life. Most of the women had their first clinical signs of CVD less than a year before examination. Their mean age at interview was 56 years, so most of them were already beyond the reproductive and child-rearing ages.

Social strain, depressed mood, and CHD
(see also Chapter 41)

In this context, it is also interesting to note that women with heart disease had significantly more depressive symptoms than healthy women.

Depressive symptoms were measured by means of a nine-item questionnaire derived from Pearlin et al.[56] The original scale consisted of 10 questions but in this study the question about sexual activity was excluded in an effort to reduce the number of potentially threatening items. The shorter version thus included nine questions with yes/no options. The 'yes' answers were summarized with a low value indicating a low degree of depressive feelings. The scale includes questions on mood, sleeping problems, appetite, interest in normal activities, crying, feelings about the future, and energy. Some examples of questions are: Do you feel bored or do you have little interest in doing things? Do you feel downhearted or blue? Do you feel hopeless about the future? Women with CHD had almost twice as many symptoms of depression, 3.7 (± 2.7), compared with 2.0 (± 2.2) in healthy women.

Prospective evidence has recently confirmed these early findings. The Stockholm women with CHD were followed longitudinally and their rate of recurrent clinical events, which required hospitalization,

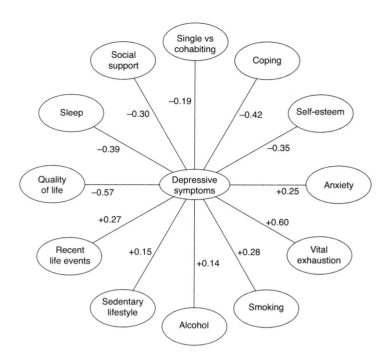

Figure 40.8
Factors associated with depressive symptoms in women with coronary heart disease.

was monitored. These events included cardiac death, acute MI, and surgical revascularization (coronary artery bypass graft surgery and percutaneous coronary angioplasty).[57] Within a 5-year follow-up period, recurrent events occurred in 81 of 292 women.

The opportunity to follow the patients was scientifically useful, because we were able to examine whether the social influences, as suggested in cross-sectional analyses, were prospectively confirmed. Among the clinical cardiac factors, a previous history of acute MI was the most significant prognostic marker. Women who had symptoms of angina pectoris, but no definite myocardial damage, had a much better prognosis. Furthermore, the presence of clinically manifest diabetes, and a low HDL cholesterol value (below 18 mg/dl), were statistically significant, and independent predictors of poor prognosis. It was interesting that the social factors were almost as important prognostically as the biological markers. Thus, both depression and vital exhaustion were associated with poor prognosis and increased mortality. The worst outcome was in women who were both depressed and socially isolated.[57]

Such symptoms are likely to be to some extent caused by the heart condition itself. In the Stockholm women with CHD, however, depression and social isolation were also linked to the experience of severe stress, in particular in the context of the spousal relationship.

Among women who were both working outside the home, and either married or otherwise cohabiting, we calculated the 5-year risk of a recurrent event due to stress from various sources. Women with marital stress were at greater risk than women with stress at work. Both the risk of being depressed and that of having a new heart attack almost tripled in women under marital stress.[58,59] In many previous studies, depression and depressive symptoms have been found to increase mortality risk, in both female and male patients. Studies from North America and Europe all point in the same direction; that is, depressed cardiac patients run a greater risk of dying, and this is not solely due to more advanced heart disease.[60]

In the clinical setting, it is crucial to diagnose and treat the mood disturbance. Clinical experience and trials of selective serotonin reuptake inhibitors

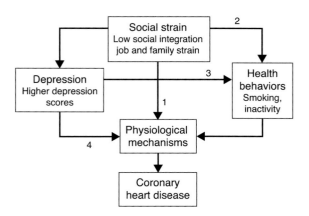

Figure 40.9
Modified model of social strain, depression, and
health behaviors.

confirm that these drugs are safe to use, and that they
are effective against depression in cardiac patients.
Whether they improve the cardiac prognosis is not
yet clear, nor is it clear whether psychological treatment of the depressive disorder is beneficial for the
heart. In recent pioneering controlled trials, treatment with individual and group-based psychotherapy was found to decrease cardiac recurrences in
men but not in women.[61]

Why women did not benefit can only be a subject
of speculation. One possibility is that the therapy did
not sufficiently address the causes of depressive
symptoms, such as stress and strain at work and at
home. In Swedish women, who are frequently
employed outside the home, pilot data support the
notion that a group-based, psychosocial educational
program aiming at increased social support, and
improved coping and mastery of stress, may be
beneficial for the heart. In a pilot study with female
CHD patients living in the south of Stockholm, the
2-year rehospitalization rate was reduced to half in
those who received the psychosocial program. Those
women spontaneously expressed increases in

personal security, trust, and better social support, as
an outcome of the intervention.[62]

Implications for future research

Social strain, depression, and adverse health behaviors are risk factors in their own right and closely
linked to each other. This creates implications for
interventions and for future research. To be effective
in intervening on one factor, such as smoking, one
must consider the psychosocial context that is associated with this behavior, including distress (depression) and social strain variables. This means that
prevention efforts need to be multidimensional.
However, if such multidimensional intervention
efforts are effective, the chances for successful interventions may be multiplied, since different pathways
are being acted upon at the same time.[63]

There is clearly a need for secondary prevention
and rehabilitation in women with CHD. In view of
the data discussed above, it seems inevitable to
develop intervention programs that are tailored
specifically for women. These need to address
adverse health behaviors, but also to focus on factors
that cause social strain as well as depressive reactions.
Doing so may not only decrease the risk of recurrent
events in women with CHD, but also increase their
quality of life in general terms.

Furthermore, future research on behavioral and
psychosocial risk factors for CHD in women has to
take into account the complex and multidimensional
patterns. Clearly, the standard epidemiological
models are unsatisfactory in this respect. Further
development of tools to study interactive patterns and
pathways are strongly needed. Most urgent, perhaps,
is the need for population-based longitudinal studies,
which are able prospectively to test the hypotheses that
have emerged from studies like the Stockholm Female
Coronary Risk Study. With such studies to confirm
the results, the basis for psychosocial preventive
actions will be considerably strengthened.

References

1. Wenger NK, Speroff L, Packard B. Cardiovascular health and disease in women. *N Engl J Med* 1993; **329**:247–56.

2. Eaker ED, Chesebro JH, Sacks F, Wenger NK, Whisnant JP. Cardiovascular disease in women. *Circulation* 1993; **88**:1999–2009.

3. Eaker ED, Pinsky J, Castelli WP. Myocardial infarction and coronary death among women: psychosocial predictors from a 20-year follow-up of women in the Framingham Study. *Am J Epidemiol* 1992; **135**:854–64.

4. Johansson S. Female myocardial infarction in Göteborg. Thesis: University of Göteborg, 1983.

5. Tunstall-Pedoe H, Kuulasmaa K, Amouyel P, Arveiler D, Rajakangas A-M, Pajak A. Myocardial infarction and coronary deaths in the World Health Organization MONICA project. *Circulation* 1994; **90**:583–612.

6. Andersson KM, Wilson PWF, Odell PM, Kannel WB. An updated coronary risk profile. A statement for health professionals. *Circulation* 1991; **83**:356–62.

7. LaCroix AZ. Psychosocial factors and risk of coronary heart disease in women: an epidemiologic perspective. *Fertil Steril* 1994; **62**:133S–9S.

8. Williams RB. Hostility, depression and CHD: a common biological mechanism? Paper presented at the Third International Congress of Behavioral Medicine, Amsterdam, The Netherlands, 1994.

9. Case RB, Moss AM, Case N, McDermot M, Eberly S. Living alone after myocardial infarction. *JAMA* 1992; **26**:515–19.

10. Berkman LF, Orth-Gomér K. Prevention of cardiovascular morbidity and mortality. Role of social relations. In: Orth-Gomér K, Schneiderman N (eds). *Behavioral Medicine Approaches to Cardiovascular Disease Prevention*. Hillsdale: Lawrence Erlbaum Associates, 1996: 1–315.

11. House JS, Landis KR, Umberson D. Social relationships and health. *Science* 1988; **241**:540–5.

12. Kaplan GA, Salonen JT, Cohen RD, Brand RJ, Syme SL, Puska P. Social connections and mortality from all causes and from cardiovascular disease: prospective evidence from Eastern Finland. *Am J Epidemiol* 1988; **128**:370–80.

13. Schoenbach VR, Kaplan BH, Fredman L, Kleinbaum DG. Social ties and mortality in Evans county, Georgia. *Am J Epidemiol* 1986; **123**:577–91.

14. Frankenhäuser M (ed). *Kvinnligt, Manligt, Stressigt*. Höganäs: Förlags AB Wiken, 1993.

15. Moriz DJ, Satariano WA. Factors predicting stage of breast cancer at diagnosis in middle aged and elderly women. The role of living arrangements. *J Clin Epidemiol* 1993; **46**:443–54.

16. Monroe SM, Bromet EJ, Connell MM, Steiner SC. Social support, life events and depressive symptoms: a 1-year prospective study. *J Consult Clin Psychol* 1986; **54**:424–31.

17. George LK, Blazer DG, Hughes DC, Fowler N. Social support and the outcome of major depression. *Br J Psychiatry* 1989; **154**:478–85.

18. Henderson S. Social relationships adversity and neurosis: an analysis of prospective observations. *Br J Psychiatry* 1981; **138**:391–8.

19. Palinkas LA, Wingard DL, Barrett-Connor E. The biocultural contest of social networks and depression among the elderly. *Soc Sci Med* 1990; **30**:441–7.

20. Cerhan JR, Wallace RB. Predictors of decline in social relationships in the rural elderly. *Am J Epidemiol* 1993; **137**:870–80.

21. Carney RM, Freedland KE, Eisen SA, Rich MW, Jaffe AS. Major depression and medication adherence in elderly patients with coronary artery disease. *Health Psychol* 1995; **14**:88–90.

22. Barefoot JC, Schroll M. Symptoms of depression, acute myocardial infarction and total mortality in a community sample. *Circulation* 1996; **93**:1976–80.

23. Frasure-Smith N, Lespérance F, Talajic M. Depression and 18–month prognosis after myocardial infarction. *Circulation* 1995; **91**: 999–1005.

24. Kaplan G. Psychosocial aspects of chronic illness: direct and indirect association with ischemic heart disease mortality. In: Kaplan R and Crique M (eds). *Behavioral Epidemiology and Disease Prevention*. New York: Plenum, 1985: 237–69.

25. Booth-Kewley S, Friedman HS. Psychological predictors of heart disease: a quantitative review. *Psychol Bull* 1987; **101**:343–62.

26. Frasure-Smith N, Lespérance F, Talajic M. Depression following myocardial infarction. *JAMA* 1993; **270**:1819–25.

27. Powell L, Shaker L, Jones B, Vaccarino L, Thoresen C, Pattillo J. Psychosocial predictors of mortality in 83 women with premature acute myocardial infarction. *Psychosom Med* 1993; **55**:426–33.

28. Freedland KE, Carney RM. Depression as a risk factor for coronary heart disease. Paper presented at the Third International Congress of Behavioral Medicine, Amsterdam, The Netherlands, 1994.

29. Broman CL. Social relationships and health-related behavior. *J Behav Med* 1993; **16**:335–50.

30. King AC, Taylor CB, Haskell WL. Smoking in older women: is being female a 'risk factor' for continued cigarette use? *Arch Intern Med* 1990; **150**:1841–6.

31. King AC, Young DR, Oka RK, Haskell WL. Effects of exercise format and intensity on two-year health outcomes in the aging adult. *Gerontologist* 1992; **32**:190 (abstract).

32. Dishman RK, Sallis JF, Orenstein DR. The determinants of physical activity and exercise. *Public Health Rep* 1985; **100**:158–71.

33. Cohen S, Schwartz JE, Bromet EJ, Parkinson DK. Mental health, stress, and poor health behaviors in two community samples. *Prev Med* 1991; **20**:306–15.

34. Franks P, Campbell TL, Shields CG. Social relationships and health: the relative roles of family functioning and social support. *Soc Sci Med* 1992; **34**:779–88.

35. Conn VS, Taylor SG, Wiman P. Anxiety, depression, quality of life, and self-care among survivors of myocardial infraction. *Issues Ment Health Nurs* 1991; **12**:321–31.

36. Finnegan DL, Suler JR. Psychological factors associated with maintenance of improved health behaviors in postcoronary patients. *J Psychol* 1985; **119**:87–94.

37. Shively CA, Kaplan JR, Adams MR. Effects of ovariectomy, social instability and social status on female *Macaca fascicularis* social behavior. *Physiol Behav* 1986; **36**:1147–53.

38. Shively CA, Clarkson TB, Kaplan JR. Social deprivation and coronary artery atherosclerosis in female cynomologus monkeys. *Atherosclerosis* 1989; **77**:69–76.

39. Shively CA, Watson SL, Williams JK, Adams MR. Social stress, reproductive hormones, and coronary heart disease risk in primates. In: Orth-Gomér K, Chesney M, Wenger NK (eds). *Women, Stress & Heart Disease*. New York: Lawrence Erlbaum, 1996: 205–17.

40. La Vechia C, Decarli A, Franceschi S, Gentile A, Negri E, Parazzini F. Menstrual and reproductive factors and the risk of myocardial infarction in women under fifty-five years of age. *Am J Obstet Gynecol* 1987; **157**:1108–12.

41. Muntzel M, Drueke T. A comprehensive review of the salt and blood pressure relationship. *Am J Hypertens* 1992; **5**:1S–42S.

42. Anderson DE, Fedorova OV, French AW. Preavoidance hypercapnia and decreased hematocrit in micropigs. *Physiol Behav* 1996; **59**:857–61.

43. Anderson DE. Behavior analysis and the search for the origins of hypertension. *J Exp Anal Behav* 1994; **61**:255–61.

44. Grossman P. Respiration, stress and cardiovascular function. *Psychophysiology* 1983; **20**:284–99.

45. Anderson DE, Chesney MA. Gender-specific association of perceived stress and inhibited breathing pattern. *Int J Behav Med* 2002; **9**:216–27.

46. Anderson DE, Bagrov AY, Austin JL. Inhibited breathing decreases renal sodium excretion. *Psychosom Med* 1995; **57**:373–80.

47. Anderson DE, Dhokalia A, Parsons DJ, Bagrov AY. End tidal CO_2 association with blood pressure response to sodium loading in older adults. *J Hypertens* 1996; **14**:1073–9.

48. Sharma AM, Cetto C, Schorr U, Spies KP, Distler A. Renal acid-base excretion in normotensive salt-sensitive humans. *Hypertension* 1993; **22**:884–90.

49. Orth-Gomér K, Johnsson JV. Social network interaction and mortality. A six year follow-up study of a random sample of the Swedish population. *J Chronic Dis* 1987; **40**:949–57.

50. Cohen S, Syme SL (eds). *Social Support and Health*. New York: Academic Press, 1985.

51. Berkman LF, Syme SL. Social networks, host resistance, and mortality: a nine-year follow-up study of Alameda County residents. *Am J Epidemiol* 1979; **109**:186–204.

52. Frankenhäuser M, Lundberg U, Chesney M (eds). *Women, Work and Health*. New York: Plenum Press, 1991.

53. Hall E. Women's work: an inquiry into the health effects of invisible and visible labor. Thesis: Karolinska Institute, Stockholm, 1990.

54. Karasek R, Theorell T (eds). *Healthy Work*. New York: Basic Books, 1990.

55. Moser V, Blom M. Källor till Social Stress hos Kvinnor med Kjärtsjukdom. Stress Research Report. Stockholm: National Institute for Psychosocial Factors and Health, 1995.

56. Pearlin LI, Menaghan EG, Lieberman MA, Mullan JT. The stress process. *J Health Soc Behav* 1981; **22**: 337–56.

57. Horsten M, Mittleman MA, Wamala SP, Schenck-Gustafsson K, Orth-Gomér K. Depressive symptoms and lack of social integration in relation to prognosis of CHD in middle-aged women. The Stockholm Female Coronary Risk Study. *Eur Heart J* 2000; **21**:1043–5.

58. Orth-Gomér K, Wamala SP, Horsten M, Schenck-Gustafsson K, Schneiderman N, Mittleman MA. Marital stress worsens prognosis in women with coronary heart disease. The Stockholm Female Coronary Risk Study. *JAMA* 2000; **284**:3008–14.

59. Balog P, Janszky I, Leineweber C, Blom M, Wamala SP, Orth-Gomér K. Depressive symptoms in relation to marital and work stress in women with and

without coronary heart disease. The Stockholm Female Coronary Risk Study. *J Psychosom Res* 2003; **54**:113–19.

60. De Backer G, Ambrosioni E, Borch-Johnsen K, et al. European Guidelines on cardiovascular disease prevention in clinical practice: third joint task force of European and other societies on cardiovascular disease prevention in clinical practice (constituted by representatives of eight societies and by invited experts). *Eur J Cardiovasc Prev Rehabil* 2003; **10**:S1–10.

61. Berkman LF, Blumenthal J, Burg M, et al. Enhancing recovery in coronary heart disease patients investiga-tors (ENRICHD). Effects of treating depression and low perceived social support on clinical events after myocardial infarction: the Enhancing Recovery In Coronary Heart Disease patients (ENRICHD) Randomized Trial. *JAMA* 2003; **289**:3106–16.

62. Orth-Gomér K, et al. Friskare kvinnohjärtan [Healthier female hearts – new study provides hope for the future. *Medicinsk Vetenskap Karolinska Institute* 2000; **3**:12–16.

63. Orth-Gomér K, Schneiderman N (eds). *Behavioral Medicine Approaches to Cardiovascular Disease Prevention*. Hillsdale: Lawrence Erlbaum, 1996.

41
Depression and heart disease

Viola Vaccarino

Introduction

The cardiovascular system has long been considered vulnerable to the effects of psychosocial stress.[1,2] Although several psychosocial factors have been linked to the pathogenesis of coronary heart disease (CHD),[3] this field of research has been challenged by the fact that it requires a multidisciplinary approach, as well as because the exposure (i.e. 'stress' or other psychosocial characteristics) is often difficult to define in a rigorous way.

Depression is probably the psychosocial factor most consistently associated with increased cardiovascular risk.[4] In part, this is because the definition and measurement of depression are better established than other psychosocial factors. Depression is a psychiatric diagnosis; therefore it can be assessed clinically. In addition, numerous validated scales are available for the measurement of depressive symptoms. Research on the role of depression on the pathophysiology or outcome of CHD is particularly relevant to women, because of the high prevalence of this condition among women. Effective treatments are available for depression, making it an attractive target for intervention.

The burden of depression in women

Major depression is a highly prevalent condition, particularly in women. Worldwide, the Global Burden of Disease Study estimated that major depression was the fourth leading cause of disability in 1990[5] and predicted that it would be the second leading cause by the year 2020, surpassed only by CHD, making depression and CHD the two projected most disabling health problems worldwide.[6]

As defined by the *Diagnostic and Statistical Manual of Mental Disorders*, 4th edition (DSM-IV),[7] major depressive disorder is characterized by depressed mood or loss of interest in nearly all activities for at least 2 weeks accompanied by at least four of the following symptoms: appetite or weight change, insomnia or hypersomnia, psychomotor agitation or retardation, fatigue or loss of energy, feelings of worthlessness or inappropriate guilt, diminished ability to think or concentrate, and recurrent thoughts of death. In addition, these symptoms must cause clinically significant distress or impairment in important areas of functioning.

The National Comorbidity Survey Replication (NCS-R) has produced up-to-date population estimates of the prevalence of major depression.[8] This population-based survey used the World Health Organization's Composite International Diagnostic Interview (CIDI) instrument, which provides a diagnosis of major depressive disorder according to DSM-IV. The prevalence of lifetime major depression was 16.2% in both women and men combined, and was about 70% higher in women than in men. The overall 12-month prevalence was 6.6% and was 40% higher in women than in men. These figures translate to national population projections of 33–35 million US adults with lifetime major depression and

13–14 million with 12-month prevalence of the disorder, many of whom are women. These recent figures confirm previous estimates of a relatively high population prevalence of major depression, with considerably higher prevalence rates in women than in men.[9,10] Prospective studies have also demonstrated higher incidence rates of depression in women compared with men, with female to male incidence rate ratios varying from 1.6 to 3.4.[11]

Depression is an even greater problem among patients with CHD. Prevalence rates of current major depression or moderate/severe depressive symptoms are reported between 12% and 30% in most series, including patients with acute myocardial infarction (MI),[12–14] heart failure,[15–17] unstable angina,[18] patients undergoing cardiac catheterization[19] and coronary bypass surgery,[20–22] as well as patients with stable CHD in the outpatient setting.[23] Most series of cardiac patients report rates of major depression of at least 20%, suggesting that the typical cardiologist doing rounds in a 25-bed hospital unit sees about five patients with this disorder. An even greater proportion of cardiac patients have a minor form of depression, i.e., they have depressive symptoms but not quite to the level of meeting the criteria for major depressive disorder.[12,15,16,18–20,24] As discussed below, minor depression is also important to recognize. Again, women with CHD are more vulnerable to depression than men,[13,14,24] with prevalence rates that are 1.5–2.0 times higher than their male counterparts.[13,24,25]

The female preponderance in depression rates begins during mid-puberty and continues in adult age with no evidence of a decline in older age groups. In fact, the majority of studies have found that higher rates of depression in women are maintained throughout the lifespan, with no attenuation of the sex gap in older age.[26,27]

It is not entirely clear why women are more vulnerable to depression than men. This phenomenon is true not only in the US but is found across a variety of cultural settings.[11] For example, cross-national studies found that, while the absolute lifetime and point prevalence rates of depression varied across centers, such rates were consistently higher among women, with women-to-men ratios on average 2 to 1.[28,29] Possible ascertainment bias has often been suggested as an explanation for sex differences in depression rates, for example the fact that women may have a higher tendency than men to seek medical attention or to recall past affective states, or the fact that the ascertainment of depression may more strongly favor the expression of 'female' symptoms, such as sadness. However, there is little scientific basis to suggest that these factors explain sex differences in the prevalence of depression.[11] There is also no consistent evidence in favor of sex differences in genetic susceptibility for depression,[30] or that hormonal status per se plays a role.[31,32]

Another potential explanation which has received attention in recent years is a dysregulation of the hypothalamus–pituitary–adrenal (HPA) axis, possibly due to exposure to early trauma.[33,34] Childhood sexual abuse in particular, which is distinctly more common in girls,[35,36] is associated with adult-onset depression as well as with sustained abnormalities in the HPA axis in adult life characterized by higher response to stressful stimuli.[33,34] Conservative estimates of childhood sexual abuse range between 7–19% of women and 3–7% of men, and as much as 35% of the sex difference in adult depression can be explained by differences in exposure to childhood sexual abuse.[11,35] In addition, the female HPA axis may be more susceptible to stress-induced dysregulation, which may also contribute to higher vulnerability to depression in adulthood. This effect may be in part due to estrogen, which has been shown to elevate cortisol levels after stress.[37,38]

Gender roles may also contribute to the higher risk of depression in women, since they may predispose to psychosocial stressors such as poverty, low educational status, and lack of decisional control which may in turn increase the risk for depression. That this may be true is suggested by the observation that sex differences in depression are less pronounced in societies where the traditional female role is valued similarly to that of men.[39] In addition, accounting for differences in social roles and inequities in workload reduces substantially the sex ratio in depression rates.[28,40]

Depression and CHD

Observational studies have provided strong evidence of the association between clinical depression (or depressive symptoms) and CHD endpoints, both among individuals initially free of CHD,[41-53] and cardiac patients,[13,24,54-58] with few exceptions.[59,60] Several aspects of this literature support the validity of the relationship between depression and CHD risk. The first is the consistency of the findings, as pointed out by several reviews.[3,61-66] The second is the large effect size associated with depression after adjustment for potential confounders, ranging from about 1.5 to 6 times. The third is the robustness of the relationship, i.e. an increased risk is found despite different measurement scales for depression, ranging from DSM-based clinical criteria for major depressive episode, to a host of different symptom-based scales. The fourth is the presence of a dose–response relationship between the number of depressive symptoms, or severity of depression, and cardiovascular risk.[12,41,43,44] The fifth is the persistence of the relationship for long-term follow-up (10 years and longer), even after a single determination of depression status.[47,50,54]

Depression and CHD incidence

Two recent meta-analyses of depression as a predictor of CHD have reported overall adjusted relative risks of 2.69 for clinical depression,[66] 1.49 for depressive mood,[66] and 1.64 for a combination of the two.[4,66]

Of the studies that have reported results stratified by sex, some found that depression was a stronger predictor of cardiovascular events among women,[60,67,68] while in others the effect was more marked in men.[46,69] The majority of the studies, however, found significantly elevated and fairly comparable relative risks in women and in men.[45,52,70-72] In older women, depression also predicts all-cause mortality,[48,49,52] and in a study of middle-aged women, recurrent major depressive episodes were associated with a twofold increased risk of carotid plaques assessed by B-mode ultrasound.[73]

Depression and prognosis of CHD

Patients with major depression or elevated level of depressive symptoms have remarkably higher morbidity and mortality rates after acute MI, often three to four times higher, than patients without depression[12-14,24,55,56] even after controlling for clinical predictors of mortality. Similarly elevated risks attributable to depression are found in other cardiac patient groups, including patients undergoing coronary artery bypass surgery,[20-22] patients with heart failure,[15] and patients with unstable angina.[18] Depression appears to be at least as strong a prognostic factor as traditional risk indicators such as low ejection fraction or other indicators of left ventricular dysfunction,[13,18,20] history of previous MI,[13] number of diseased vessels and electrocardiographic evidence of ischemia.[18] Similar to that found in community studies, depressed mood in cardiac patients predicts mortality also in the absence of a clinical diagnosis of depression. Indeed, higher levels of depressive symptoms measured by self-rating questionnaires show a clear dose–response relationship with mortality: the higher the level of depressive symptoms, the higher the mortality risk.[12]

Depression not only predicts higher mortality but also poor functional status of cardiac patients. In stable outpatients with CHD, depression predicts worse symptomatic status, lower physical function, and worse overall quality of life.[23,74] Interestingly, traditional prognostic indicators, such as low ejection fraction or presence of wall motion abnormalities, are not useful predictors of these outcomes.[23] A strong relationship between depression and worse functional status/quality of life is also found in patients with heart failure,[16,17] as well as patients undergoing coronary artery bypass surgery, among whom depressive symptoms predict lower functional gains after the procedure,[75] hospital readmissions and failure to return to work.[22]

Studies of the impact of depression on outcomes in cardiac patients have not usually shown results stratified by sex, perhaps due to the relatively small number of women included in several of these studies. In a cohort of coronary artery bypass surgery patients, however, the effect of depression on cardiac events did not differ between women and men.[20] Similarly, in a prospective study of MI patients, an elevated level of depressive symptoms was significantly related to cardiac mortality in both sexes, with an odds ratio of 3.29 in women and 3.05 in men.[24] These data indicate that women and men with CHD are similarly susceptible to the adverse effects of depression on prognosis.

Sex, depression, and prognosis after MI
(see also Chapter 18)

Once women develop MI they appear to lose much of their protection compared with men and experience more complications and higher mortality, a difference that is particularly seen among younger women.[76–79] In part, this observation is attributable to the higher prevalence of pre-existing diseases and risk factors in women compared with men, but in many studies the sex-related outcome differences remain unexplained. Given that women have substantially higher rates of depression compared with men, and that this condition is more common in young and middle-aged persons,[8] it is possible that depression plays a role in explaining the worse outcomes of women after MI compared with men. However, this issue has not been thoroughly evaluated. Frasure-Smith et al.[24] have found that adjustment for depression in the regression models explained 68% of the higher odds of death and 38% of the higher odds of recurrent MI in women compared with men, suggesting that the higher rate of depression in women was indeed a major determinant in women's poorer outcomes. However their study, which included 283 women and 613 men, was under-powered to detect significant sex differences in outcomes, and therefore these results remain inconclusive.

Biological mechanisms

Despite the considerable epidemiological evidence favoring a role of depression in CHD, this association is still questioned.[63,65,80] Several studies have failed to control completely for physical illness,[63] which may act as a confounder. In addition, pathways linking depression to CHD may include noncausal relationships due to presence of depressive symptoms in persons with pre-existing CHD, or common antecedents in depression and CHD (Fig. 41.1). In addition, the exact mechanisms through which depression increases CHD risk have not been

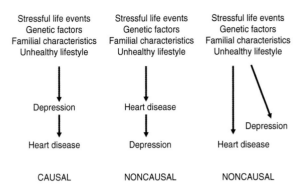

Figure 41.1
Three possible pathways linking depression to coronary heart disease: causal and noncausal associations.

clarified. For example, it is not clearly established whether this effect occurs solely by adversely influencing health behaviors (such as physical inactivity, decreased adherence to medications, and poor self-care) or rather by directly or indirectly affecting the cardiovascular system. Nonetheless, the relationship between depression and CHD makes biological sense through a number of possible pathophysiological pathways, as described below, lending support to the notion that depression is etiologically linked to CHD.

Neurohormonal effects

Many of the hypothesized adverse effects of depression on the cardiovascular system are thought to occur because of sustained dysregulation of the HPA axis and the autonomic nervous system, leading to a number of neurohormonal abnormalities. The first is HPA axis hyperactivity, which has been clearly documented in untreated patients with major depression in a number of ways, including elevations of corticotropin-releasing factor (CRF) in cerebrospinal fluid, blunting of corticotropin response after CRF administration, nonsuppression of cortisol secretion following dexamethasone administration, hypercortisolemia, and postmortem findings of an increased number of CRF neurons in the hypothalamus of depressed patients.[62,81–84] Studies have also

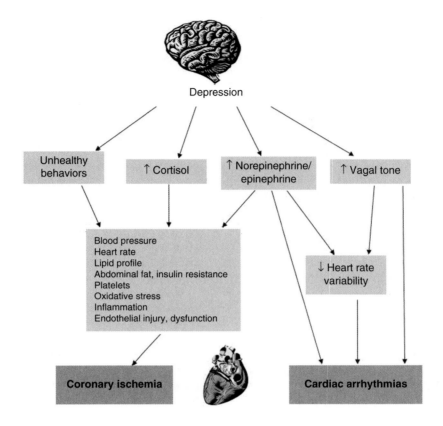

Figure 41.2
Major pathophysiological pathways linking depression to coronary heart disease.

shown that severe early life stress such as childhood abuse, which is a risk factor for depression, is associated with sustained abnormalities in the HPA response to stress which can be observed in adult life long after the stressor had subsided.[33,34,85] In a study of adult women, these abnormalities were particularly evident in women with a history of both major depression and childhood abuse.[34]

The second key neuroendocrine abnormality in major depression is hyperactivity of the sympathoadrenal system (SNS). Hypersecretion of norepinephrine (NE) has been documented by elevated NE and NE metabolite concentrations in plasma and urine,[25,86–88] and treatment with tricyclic antidepressants decreases plasma and urinary levels of NE and NE metabolites.[89,90]

Activation of the HPA axis and the SNS can lead to increased CHD risk through a variety of mecha-

nisms, for example, adverse effects on inflammation and oxidative stress, as well as blood pressure, heart rate, insulin resistance, and platelet activity. Each of these mechanisms will be discussed in this chapter. Direct signs of adverse cardiovascular effects due to neuro-adrenergic activation include the fact that elevated morning plasma cortisol levels correlate with coronary atherosclerosis in young and middle-aged individuals,[91] that administration of steroid hormones may induce injury of the intima,[92,93] and that the effect of stress on coronary plaque area[94] and on endothelial injury[95] is abolished by beta-adrenergic blockade in cynomolgus monkeys.

The two broad pathophysiological pathways through which depression might increase CHD risk include higher susceptibility to myocardial ischemia and higher risk for cardiac arrhythmias and sudden death (Fig. 41.2).

Myocardial ischemia

Depression may increase susceptibility to myocardial ischemia because of the direct effects of HPA and SNS activation on the heart and the coronary arteries, or through changes in established CHD risk factors and/or hemostatic/inflammatory factors as described later in this chapter. A direct effect of depressive mood on triggering ischemia has been suggested by the study of Gullette et al.,[96] in which self-reported feelings of sadness were associated with an almost threefold higher risk of myocardial ischemia detected by ambulatory ECG monitoring in patients with CHD. This observation mimics the effects of mental stress on the induction of myocardial ischemia in patients with CHD,[97–99] and may be due to increased oxygen demands on the heart (in part due to an increase in blood pressure and heart rate) as well as a possible stress-related coronary vasoconstriction.[3]

Heart rate and heart rate variability

Normotensive depressed patients with increased plasma NE concentrations,[88,100] but also without,[101] have greater heart rates at rest, after orthostasis and after exercise, compared with controls. Elevated resting heart rate, in turn, has been related to increased cardiovascular mortality in community samples[102] and in cardiac patients.[103]

The hyperactivity of the sympathetic system in depression described above, coupled with impaired vagal tone, could lead to excess CHD deaths by affecting heart rate variability (HRV) and increasing the risk for lethal ventricular arrhythmias. HRV is a measure of the beat-to-beat heart rate fluctuations/periodicities over time. These periodicities can be identified through spectral analysis of the heart rate, in which the power spectrum is integrated over four discrete frequency bands: ultra low frequency, very low frequency, low frequency, and high frequency.[104] HRV is thought to express the modulation of the sympathetic and parasympathetic activity on the heart. The low-frequency power is a marker of sympathetic tone, while the high-frequency power is a marker of vagal modulation on the heart.[105] Reduced HRV is thought to result from autonomic

imbalance, involving either increased sympathetic or decreased parasympathetic tone, although the latter may predominate.[62]

Depression is associated with reduced HRV, both in patients with CHD,[106–108] and in community subjects,[109] and one uncontrolled study reported normalization of reduced HRV in depressed patients after successful treatment of depression.[110] In turn, decreased HRV is a strong and consistent predictor of outcome after myocardial infarction[111–114] as well as a predictor of CHD endpoints in healthy populations, including all-cause mortality[115–117] and CHD incidence and mortality.[118] Lower HRV has also been related to sudden cardiac death.[119] Both low-frequency power[115] and high-frequency power[118] have been associated with risk of CHD and total mortality.

Decreased HRV is thought to increase CHD mortality by predisposing to ventricular arrhythmias. In animal models, vagal output is protective against ventricular fibrillation during myocardial ischemia,[120–122] and during electrical induction of ventricular fibrillation.[123,124] High sympathetic tone, on the other hand, lowers the threshold for ventricular fibrillation in animal models,[123,125] and in humans, increased NE levels have been associated with ventricular arrhythmias.[126]

Conventional CHD risk factors and metabolic syndrome

Higher cortisol and catecholamine levels may increase the risk for cardiovascular disease by adversely affecting CHD risk factors, particularly those associated with the metabolic syndrome. A role of the sympathoadrenal system in the etiology of hypertension has long been suspected.[127] More recently, several if not all the components of the metabolic syndrome have been linked with adrenocortical and autonomic disturbances.[128–132] For example, the relationship between neurohormonal abnormalities induced by stress or depression, visceral fat and insulin resistance is now well-established,[133–137] and psychosocial factors explain a large portion of the association between adrenocortical/autonomic disturbances and metabolic syndrome.[132,138]

Possible pathophysiological mechanisms linking depression, neurohormonal activation, and metabolic syndrome risk factors include glucocorticoid-mediated accumulation of central adipose tissue; direct metabolic effects of cortisol and catecholamines on glucose and lipid metabolism; activation of the renin–angiotensin system which, through the type 1 angiotensin II receptor (AT1), in turn increases blood pressure and induces production of reactive oxygen species and inflammatory mediators; and, finally, catecholamine-mediated induction of cytokines in the adipose tissue and other tissues.[139,140] Recent evidence suggests that innate immunity and inflammation play a significant role in the development of insulin resistance and predict the development of diabetes.[141,142] For example, higher production of reactive oxygen species and inflammatory cytokines in the setting of increased abdominal fat depots may induce insulin resistance, possibly through phosphorylation of the insulin receptor.[139] Therefore, the link between depression, neurohormonal abnormalities, and the metabolic syndrome may be due to the effects of depression on inflammation and oxidative stress (as described in the next section). In addition to systemic inflammatory effects and cytokine production, however, the neurohumoral stimulation may cause secretion of other factors in the adipose tissue. Recently it has been recognized that the adipose tissue is an active secretory organ that elaborates a variety of molecules known as adipocytokines. Of these, inflammatory cytokines such as interleukin-6 (IL-6) and tumor necrosis factor-α (TNF-α), have an established role in atherogenesis.[143] Others, in particular leptin and adiponectin, are of significance due to their emerging role in CHD. Plasma leptin, which is elevated in obesity and other insulin-resistant states, is predictive of CHD events independent of traditional risk factors, body mass index, and C-reactive protein.[144] In contrast, plasma adiponectin, which is reduced in obesity and diabetes, has anti-atherogenic properties in mice models[145] and in humans.[146]

Inflammation and oxidative stress

Several lines of basic and clinical research indicate that inflammation and oxidative stress play a central role in the initiation and progression of atherosclerosis.[143,147–149] Inflammation and oxidative stress are thought to mediate all stages of this disease, from initiation through progression and, ultimately, its thrombotic complications leading to acute coronary syndromes. Oxidative stress and inflammation are linked phenomena in the pathophysiology of atherosclerosis. For example, reactive oxygen species can induce activation of redox-sensitive genes which, in turn, lead to increased expression of pro-inflammatory cytokines and activation of monocytes and other inflammatory cells.[148] The latter, in turn, leads to production of reactive oxygen species and more cytokines. These processes amplify inflammation and endothelial damage and predispose to plaque rupture and thrombotic effects.[143] Indeed, serum markers of inflammation and oxidative stress predict the incidence of cardiovascular disease[150–155] as well as a worse prognosis following acute coronary syndromes.[156–160]

Many studies have shown an association between depression and elevated levels of acute phase proteins, such as C-reactive protein, and inflammatory cytokines, such as IL-6, in patients with and without CHD[161–166] as well as in community samples of younger[167] and older[168,169] adults. Inflammatory markers may be reduced by antidepressant treatment,[170,171] and correlate with recency of the depressive episode.[167] It is generally assumed that these effects are true for both women and men, and studies usually have not stratified by sex, in part also due to the small sample of many studies. However, in a recent analysis of the Third National Nutrition and Examination Survey (NHANES-III),[167] history of a major depressive episode was a stronger risk factor for elevated C-reactive protein in the men than in women. In men, the more recent the depressive episode, the higher was the probability of having elevated C-reactive protein, while in women a similar relationship was less clear-cut (Fig. 41.3).[167] It should be noted that the women had higher levels of C-reactive protein in the absence of depression, perhaps because of the pro-inflammatory effects of estrogen in this pre-menopausal sample.[172] Because of these higher values in the absence of depression, it may be more difficult to detect an increase due to depression in women than in men.

A growing literature also suggests that depression and other forms of chronic psychological stress may

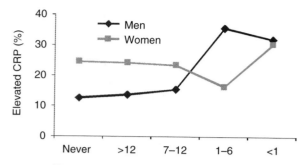

Figure 41.3
Prevalence of elevated C-reactive protein (CRP)
(≥0.22 mg/dl) according to sex and presence or
recency of history of major depressive episode in
6149 adults aged 17 to 39 years in the Third
National Health and Nutrition Survey (NHANES-III).
Depression was assessed by using the Diagnostic
Interview Schedule. CRP was measured with a
latex-enhanced Behring Nephelometer Analyzer
System. p Value for trend, men: p = 0.004;
women: p = 0.85. Modified from reference 167.

increase oxidative stress. Animals exposed to psychological stress have increased release of superoxide from neutrophils[173] and develop higher levels of 8-hydroxy-deoxyguanosine (8-OH-dG) in liver DNA, a marker of oxidative damage.[174] Experimentally stressed pigs have higher levels of circulating catecholamines which correlate with cardiac lesions, and treatment with antioxidants has been shown to have a protective effect.[175] In human studies, female workers with increased subjective workload were found to have higher levels of peripheral 8-OH-dG,[176] and lipid peroxide levels are lower in subjects who practice transcendental meditation than in those who do not.[177] Data specific for depression have shown that plasma antioxidant capacity is reduced in major depression patients.[178,179] In other studies, nitrite content was reduced in the polymorphonuclear leucocytes of depressed patients compared with controls, although the activity of antioxidant enzymes (superoxide dismutase, catalase, and glutathione peroxidase) did not differ.[180] The effect of depression on oxidative stress is also demonstrated by the finding that depressed

patients have markedly reduced endothelial function measured by means of flow-mediated vasodilation in the brachial artery,[181] a phenomenon that is dependent on nitric oxide (NO) production in the endothelium.[182]

A high inflammatory and oxidant state in depression probably contributes to worsening of depression or the neuroendocrine abnormalities associated with depression. For example, it is well established that pro-inflammatory cytokines exert potent enhancing effects on the HPA axis,[183] thereby exacerbating neurohormonal abnormalities in depression. NO is a putative neurotransmitter,[184] and a modulator of HPA axis function.[185] In addition, tetrahydrobiopterin, a cofactor in the synthesis of NO, is also an essential cofactor in the biosynthesis of neurotransmitters such as noradrenaline, serotonin, and dopamine, involved in the pathogenesis of depressive disorders.[186]

The effects of depression on oxidative state and inflammation are likely to be due to HPA and SNS activation. For example, sustained elevation of epinephrine levels, due to either cardiac sympathetic nerve stimulation[187] or myocardial ischemia and reperfusion,[188] positively correlates with enhanced generation of hydroxyl radicals. One possible mechanism is the auto-oxidation of catecholamines,[189] resulting in the formation of cyclized o-quinone and o-semiquinones which, when oxidized, produce superoxide. Another potential mechanism is SNS-mediated activation of the renin–angiotensin system, which in turn leads to activation of the AT1 receptor,[190,191] a major pathway leading to production and release of reactive oxygen species.[148] Sympathetic nervous system activation and catecholamine release can also increase systemic IL-6 concentrations, presumably through β_2-adrenergic receptors.[183] In addition, cortisol has been shown to inhibit nitric oxide synthase (NOS) activity, by inhibiting the induction of NOS by lipopolysaccharide and interferon gamma[192] but also increasing gene expression of guanosine triphosphate (GTP) cyclohydrolase, a rate-limiting enzyme in the formation of tetrahydrobiopterin.[193] There is also evidence of a role of the NO system in cortisol-induced hypertension in humans,[194] although the specific enzyme systems and neurohumoral stimuli mediating these effects have not been clarified.

Platelet activation and thrombogenesis

Catecholamines, in particular epinephrine, are potent platelet activators,[195] and heightened platelet activity has been consistently found in depression.[196–198] Platelet activation contributes to early atherosclerosis, to plaque growth as well as to acute occlusion (resulting in acute coronary syndromes), the latter due to acute thrombus formation on pre-existing plaques and acute vasoconstriction by releasing thromboxane A2 and serotonin.[195] Thrombogenic factors released by platelets (platelet factor 4 and beta-thromboglobulin) have been shown to be elevated in patients with either MI or unstable angina,[199–203] giving further support to the pathophysiological role of platelets in acute coronary syndromes.

Stress exposure (see also Chapter 40)

As mentioned above, environmental stressors are known to be important risk factors for major depression. Since exposure to stress in itself is thought to be a risk factor for CHD, the effect of depression on the vascular system could be due to stress exposure (Fig. 41.1). Data from animal studies support the idea that stress, acting through increased sympathoadrenal activity, has several effects on cardiovascular function which in animal models include endothelial injury, accelerated atherosclerosis, and impaired endothelial responsivity.[1]

As in depression, stress exposure results in HPA axis and SNS activation,[204,205] which, if severe, can result in a chronic dysregulation of these systems.[34] In many instances, a distinction between depression and chronic stress may be an artificial one, as there is ample evidence for their inter-relationship, coexistence, and synchronistic effects.[33, 34]

Behavioral factors

In addition to the direct pathophysiological effects described above, depression has been associated with unhealthy lifestyle behaviors that could influence CHD risk and therefore mediate the relationship between depression and CHD. These mainly include smoking[206,207] and decreased adherence with medica-

tions.[208,209] Behaviors and depression may also share genetic/familial influences. For example, the relationship between smoking and major depression results solely from genes that predispose to both conditions.[210] The association between depression and CHD, however, usually persists after behaviors are controlled for,[61] indicating that the latter only play a partial role in the increased CHD risk associated with depression.

Treating depression in cardiac patients

Although results of individual trials have been mixed, meta-analyses of psychosocial interventions in cardiac patients have reported improvement in psychosocial distress and CHD risk factors,[211] as well as morbidity and mortality.[211,212] In the recently published Enhancing Recovery in Coronary Heart Disease (ENRICHD) trial, however, cognitive behavioral therapy for the treatment of depression and social isolation was ineffective in reducing death and nonfatal MI as well as a number of secondary cardiovascular endpoints.[213] An unexpected finding however, which might have played a role in the negative results, was that both the intervention and the usual care group substantially improved in their depression and social support ratings over the follow-up, although the intervention group improved more. In addition, a substantial proportion of patients in both arms received drug treatment for depression, which, at the end of the follow-up, was prescribed to 28% of the intervention and 21% of the usual care arm. These findings prompted the investigators to perform post hoc analyses to determine the impact of pharmacological treatment of depression on their findings. The results were quite surprising. First, exclusion of patients using antidepressants did not change the results (the relative risk comparing the intervention to the usual care group remained very close to one). Second, when patients using antidepressants were compared with those not using antidepressants in the two arms combined, use of selective serotonin reuptake inhibitors (SSRI), as well as any antidepressant use, were associated with a significantly lower risk for the main study endpoint (death or MI), with a relative risk of 0.57 and 0.63, respectively.[214] Total deaths were similarly reduced. Although these non-randomized post-hoc analyses should be taken with caution, they suggest that pharmacological treatment of depression may be more beneficial in CHD patients than psychotherapy approaches, particularly the use of SSRI medications which, in addition to being effective in improving mood, also have anti-platelet effects.

The safety of the SSRI sertraline in depressed patients with acute coronary syndromes has been demonstrated by another recent randomized trial, the Sertraline Antidepressant Heart Attack Randomized Trial (SADHART).[215] The main end-point of this safety trial was left ventricular ejection fraction, which remained unaffected by the treatment both in the overall sample as well as among patients who had reduced ejection fraction from the start. It is noteworthy that the incidence of cardiovascular events, which were evaluated as secondary endpoints, was reduced by SSRI treatment. For example, the risk of death was reduced by 61%, the risk of MI and heart failure each by 30%, and the risk of any cardiovascular event by 23%. Because of the limited sample size (369 patients) however, none of these relative risks were significantly different from one. Overall, the SADHART results indicate that SSRI use is safe in CHD patients with major depression and they suggest, as the ENRICHD trial, that their use may be associated with better cardiovascular outcomes. A larger clinical trial of SSRI use in CHD patients with clinical endpoints is needed. However, the data available so far do indicate that women with CHD should be evaluated for the presence of depression and referred or treated for depression as needed. Indeed, this approach has been included in recently published guidelines for CVD prevention in women.[216]

Conclusions

Evidence from epidemiological studies indicates that depression is a risk factor for new cardiovascular events in individuals initially free of CHD, as well as for recurrent events and mortality among cardiac patients. There is a host of possible pathophysiological mechanisms supporting the link between depressive mood and increased susceptibility to atherosclerosis and its complications. The impact of depression on cardiac outcomes may be particularly substantial for women, who suffer higher rates of depression than men. Depression is relatively easy to recognize and screen for by the attentive clinician. Given the high prevalence of depression in the US population, particularly among women, early recognition and treatment of depression could substantially reduce the burden of CVD and related disability, in addition to improving the emotional well-being of the affected patients. While the most effective treatment of depression for cardiovascular risk reduction awaits confirmation, SSRI medications are safe in the cardiac patient and should be considered in patients who are clinically depressed.

References

1. Kaplan JR, Petterson K, Manuck SB, Olsson G. The role of sympathoadrenal medullary activation in the initiation and progression of atherosclerosis. *Circulation* 1991; **84** (Suppl V):V123–V32.

2. Chrousos GP, Gold PW. The concepts of stress and stress system disorders: overview of physical and behavioral homeostasis. *JAMA* 1992; **267**:1244–52.

3. Rozanski A, Blumenthal JA, Kaplan J. Impact of psychological factors on the pathogenesis of cardiovascular disease and implications for therapy. *Circulation* 1999; **99**:2192–217.

4. Wulsin LR, Singal BM. Do depressive symptoms increase the risk for the onset of coronary disease? A systematic quantitative review. *Psychosom Med* 2003; **65**:201–10.

5. Murray CJL, Lopez AD. Global mortality, disability, and the contribution of risk factors: Global Burden of Disease Study. *Lancet* 1997; **349**:1436–42.

6. Murray CJ, Lopez AD. Alternative projections of mortality and disability by cause 1990–2020: Global Burden of Disease Study. *Lancet* 1997; **349**:1498–504.

7. American Psychiatric Association. *Diagnostic and*

Statistical Manual of Mental Disorders, 4th edn, Text revision. Washington, DC: American Psychiatric Association, 2000.

8. Kessler RC, Berglund P, Demler O, et al. The epidemiology of major depressive disorder: results from the National Comorbidity Survey Replication (NCS-R). *JAMA* 2003; **289**:3095–105.

9. Weissman MM, Leaf PJ, Tischler GL, et al. Affective disorders in five United States communities. *Psychol Med* 1988; **18**:141–53.

10. Kessler RC, McGonagle KA, Zhao S, et al. Lifetime and 12-month prevalence of DSM-III-R psychiatric disorders in the United States. *Arch Gen Psychiatry* 1994; **51**:8–19.

11. Kuehner C. Gender differences in unipolar depression: an update of epidemiological findings and possible explanations. *Acta Psychiatr Scand* 2003; **108**:163–74.

12. Lesperance F, Frasure-Smith N, Talajic M, Bourassa M. Five-year risk of cardiac mortality in relation to initial severity and one-year changes in depression symptoms after myocardial infarction. *Circulation* 2002; **105**:1049–53.

13. Frasure-Smith N, Lesperance F, Talajic M. Depression following myocardial infarction. *JAMA* 1993; **270**:1819–25.

14. Frasure-Smith N, Lesperance F, Talajic M. Depression and 18-month prognosis after myocardial infarction. *Circulation* 1995; **91**:999–1005.

15. Jiang W, Alexander J, Christopher E, et al. Relationship of depression to increased risk of mortality and rehospitalization in patients with congestive heart failure. *Arch Intern Med* 2001; **161**:1849–56.

16. Vaccarino V, Kasl SV, Abramson J, Krumholz HM. Depressive symptoms and risk of functional decline and death in patients with heart failure. *J Am Coll Cardiol* 2001; **38**:199–205.

17. Rumsfeld JS, Havranek E, Masoudi FA, et al. Depressive symptoms are the strongest predictors of short-term declines in health status in patients with heart failure. *J Am Coll Cardiol* 2003; **42**:1811–17.

18. Lesperance F, Frasure-Smith N, Juneau M, Theroux P. Depression and 1-year prognosis in unstable angina. *Arch Intern Med* 2000; **160**:1354–60.

19. Hance M, Carney RM, Freedland KE, Skala J. Depression in patients with coronary heart disease: a 12-month follow-up. *Gen Hosp Psychiatry* 1996; **18**:61–5.

20. Connerney I, Shapiro PA, McLaughlin JS, Bagiella E, Sloan R. Relation between depression after coronary artery bypass surgery and 12-month outcome: a prospective study. *Lancet* 2001; **358**:1766–71.

21. Blumenthal JA, Lett HS, Babyak MA, et al. Depression as a risk factor for mortality after coronary artery bypass surgery. *Lancet* 2003; **362**:604–9.

22. Burg MM, Benedetto MC, Rosenberg R, Soufer R. Presurgical depression predicts medical morbidity 6 months after coronary artery bypass graft surgery. *Psychosom Med* 2003; **65**:111–18.

23. Ruo B, Rumsfeld JS, Hlatky MA, Liu H, Browner WS, Whooley MA. Depressive symptoms and health-related quality of life: The Heart and Soul Study. *JAMA* 2003; **290**:215–21.

24. Frasure-Smith N, Lesperance F, Juneau M, Talajic M, Bourassa MG. Gender, depression and one-year prognosis after myocardial infarction. *Psychosom Med* 1999; **61**:26–37.

25. Lake CR, Pickar D, Ziegler MG, Lipper S, Slater S, Murphy DL. High plasma NE levels in patients with major affective disorder. *Am J Psychiatry* 1982; **139**:1315–18.

26. Beekman AT, Copeland JR, Prince MJ. Review of community prevalence of depression in later life. *Br J Psychiatry* 1999; **174**:307–11.

27. Copeland JR, Beekman AT, Dewey ME, et al. Depression in Europe. Geographical distribution among older people. *Br J Psychiatry* 1999; **174**:312–21.

28. Maier W, Gansicke M, Gater R, Rezaki M, Tiemens B, Florenzano Urzua R. Gender differences in the prevalence of depression: a survey in primary care. *J Affect Dis* 1999; **53**:241–52.

29. Weissman MM, Bland RC, Canino GJ, et al. Cross-national epidemiology of major depression and bipolar disorder. *JAMA* 1996; **276**:293–9.

30. Sullivan PF, Neale MC, Kendler KS. Genetic epidemiology of major depression: review and meta-analysis. *Am J Psychiatry* 2000; **157**:1552–62.

31. Hankin BL, Abramson LY. Development of gender differences in depression: an elaborated cognitive vulnerability-transactional stress theory. *Psychol Bull* 2001; **127**:773–96.

32. Beck CT. Predictors of post-partum depression: an update. *Nurs Res* 2001; **50**:275–85.

33. Weiss EL, Longhurst JG, Mazure CM. Childhood sexual abuse as a risk factor for depression in women: psychosocial and neurobiological correlates. *Am J Psychiatry* 1999; **156**:816–28.

34. Heim C, Newport DJ, Heit S, et al. Pituitary-adrenal and autonomic responses to stress in women after sexual and physical abuse in childhood. *JAMA* 2000; **284**:592–7.

35. Cutler SE, Nolen-Hoeksema S. Accounting for sex differences in depression through female victimization: childhood sexual abuse. *Sex Roles* 1991; **24**:425–38.

36. Paolucci EO, Genuis ML, Violato C. A meta-analysis of the published research on the effects of child sexual abuse. *J Psychol* 2001; **135**:17–36.

37. Young EA. Sex differences and the HPA axis: implications for psychiatric disease. *J Gend Specif Med* 1998; **1**:21–7.

38. Kirschbaum C, Schommer N, Federenko I, et al. Short-term estradiol treatment enhances pituitary-adrenal axis and sympathetic responses to psychosocial stress in healthy young men. *J Clin Endocrinol Metab* 1996; **81**:3639–43.

39. Piccinelli M, Wilkinson G. Gender differences in depression. Critical review. *Br J Psychiatry* 2000; **177**:486–92.

40. Nolen-Hoeksema S, Larson J, Grayson C. Explaining the gender difference in depressive symptoms. *J Pers Soc Psychol* 1999; **77**:1061–72.

41. Anda R, Williamson D, Jones D, et al. Depressed affect, hopelessness, and the risk of ischemic heart disease in a cohort of US adults. *Epidemiology* 1993; **4**:285–94.

42. Aaroma A, Raitasalo R, Reunanen A, et al. Depression and cardiovascular diseases. *Acta Psychiatr Scand* 1994; **377**(Suppl):77–82.

43. Everson SA, Goldberg DE, Kaplan GA, et al. Hopelessness and risk of mortality and incidence of myocardial infarction and cancer. *Psychosom Med* 1996; **58**:113–21.

44. Pratt LA, Ford DE, Crum RM, Armenian HK, Gallo JJ, Eaton WW. Depression, psychotropic medication, and risk of myocardial infarction: prospective data from the Baltimore ECA follow-up. *Circulation* 1996; **94**:3123–9.

45. Barefoot J, Schroll M. Symptoms of depression, acute myocardial infarction, and total mortality in a community sample. *Circulation* 1996; **93**:1976–80.

46. Hippisley-Cox J, Fielding K, Pringle M. Depression as a risk factor for ischemic heart disease in men: population based case-control study. *BMJ* 1998; **316**:1714–19.

47. Ford DE, Mead LA, Chang PP, Cooper-Patrick L, Wang N, Klag MJ. Depression is a risk factor for coronary artery disease in men. *Arch Intern Med* 1998; **158**:1422–6.

48. Fredman L, Magaziner J, Hebel JR, Hawkes W, Zimmerman SI. Depressive symptoms and 6-year mortality among elderly community-dwelling women. *Epidemiology* 1999; **10**:54–9.

49. Whooley MA, Browner WS. Association between depressive symptoms and mortality in older women. *Arch Intern Med* 1998; **158**:2129–35.

50. Everson SA, Roberts RE, Goldberg DE, Kaplan GA.

Depressive symptoms and increased risk of stroke mortality over a 29-year period. *Arch Intern Med* 1998; **158**:1133–8.

51. Murphy JM, Monson RR, Olivier DC, Sobol AM, Leighton AH. Affective disorders and mortality: a general population study. *Arch Gen Psychiatry* 1987; **44**:473–80.

52. Ariyo AA, Haan M, Tangen CM, et al. Depressive symptoms and risks of coronary heart disease and mortality in elderly Americans. Cardiovascular Health Study Collaborative Research Group. *Circulation* 2000; **102**:1773–9.

53. Sesso HD, Kawachi I, Vokonas PS, Sparrow D. Depression and the risk of coronary heart disease in the normative aging study. *Am J Cardiol* 1998; **82**:851–6.

54. Barefoot JC, Helms MJ, Mark DB. Depression and long-term mortality risk in patients with coronary artery disease. *Am J Cardiol* 1996; **78**:613–17.

55. Ahern DK, Gorkin L, Anderson JL, et al. Biobehavioral variables and mortality or cardiac arrest in the Cardiac Arrhythmia Pilot Study (CAPS). *Am J Cardiol* 1990; **66**:59–62.

56. Carney RM, Rich MW, Freedland KE, et al. Major depressive disorder predicts cardiac events in patients with coronary artery disease. *Psychosom Med* 1988; **50**:627–33.

57. Silverstone PH. Depression and outcome in acute myocardial infarction. *BMJ* 1987; **294**:219–20.

58. Denollet J, Brutsaert DL. Personality, disease severity, and risk of long-term cardiac events in patients with a decreased ejection fraction after myocardial infarction. *Circulation* 1998; **97**:167–73.

59. Vogt T, Pope C, Mullooly J, Hollis J. Mental health status as a predictor of morbidity and mortality: a 15-year follow-up of members of a health maintenance organization. *Am J Public Health* 1994; **84**:227–31.

60. Wassertheil-Smoller S, Applegate WB, Berge K, et al. Changes in depression as a precursor of cardiovascular events. SHEP Cooperative Research Group (Systolic Hypertension in the Elderly). *Arch Intern Med* 1996; **156**:553–61.

61. Glassman AH, Shapiro PA. Depression and the course of coronary artery disease. *Am J Psychiatry* 1998; **155**:4–11.

62. Musselman DL, Evans DL, Nemeroff CB. The relationship of depression to cardiovascular disease. *Arch Gen Psychiatry* 1998; **55**:580–92.

63. Wulsin LR, Vaillant GE, Wells VE. A systematic review of the mortality of depression. *Psychosom Med* 1999; **61**:6–17.

64. Barrett-Barrick C. Sad, glad, or mad hearts?

Epidemiological evidence for a causal relationship between mood disorders and coronary artery disease. *J Affect Dis* 1999; **53**:193–201.

65. Hemingway H, Marmot M. Psychosocial factors in the aetiology and prognosis of coronary heart disease: systematic review of prospective cohort studies. *BMJ* 1999; **318**:1460–7.

66. Rugulies R. Depression as a predictor for coronary heart disease. A review and meta-analysis. *Am J Prev Med* 2002; **23**:51–61.

67. Mendes de Leon CF, Krumholz HM, Seeman TS, et al. Depression and risk of coronary heart disease in elderly men and women: New Haven EPESE, 1982–1991. Established Populations for the Epidemiologic Studies of the Elderly. *Arch Intern Med* 1998; **158**:2341–8.

68. Williams SA, Kasl SV, Heiat A, Abramson JL, Krumholz HM, Vaccarino V. Depression and risk of heart failure among the elderly: a prospective community-based study. *Psychosom Med* 2002; **64**:6–12.

69. Penninx BW, Guralnik JM, Mendes de Leon CF, et al. Cardiovascular events and mortality in newly and chronically depressed persons >70 years of age. *Am J Cardiol* 1998; **81**:988–94.

70. Aromaa A, Raitasalo R, Reunanen A, et al. Depression and cardiovascular diseases. *Acta Psychiatr Scand Suppl* 1994; **377**:77–82.

71. Ferketich AK, Schwartzbaum JA, Frid DJ, Moeschberger ML. Depression as an antecedent to heart disease among men and women in the NHANES I study. *Arch Intern Med* 2000; **160**:1261–8.

72. Penninx BW, Beekman AT, Honig A, et al. Depression and cardiac mortality: results from a community-based longitudinal study. *Arch Gen Psychiatry* 2001; **58**:221–7.

73. Jones DJ, Bromberger JT, Sutton-Tyrrell K, Matthews KA. Lifetime history of depression and carotid atherosclerosis in middle-aged women. *Arch Gen Psychiatry* 2003; **60**:153–60.

74. Spertus JA, McDonell M, Woodman CL, Fihn SD. Association between depression and worse disease-specific functional status in outpatients with coronary artery disease. *Am Heart J* 2000; **140**:105–10.

75. Mallik S, Krumholz HM, Lin Z, et al. Patients with depressive symptoms have lower health status benefits after coronary artery bypass surgery. *Circulation* 2005; **111**:271–7.

76. Vaccarino V, Krumholz HM, Yarzebski J, Gore JM, Goldberg RJ. Sex differences in 2-year mortality after hospital discharge for myocardial infarction. *Ann Intern Med* 2001; **134**:173–81.

77. Vaccarino V, Parsons L, Every NR, Barron HV, Krumholz HM. Sex-based differences in early mortality after myocardial infarction. *N Engl J Med* 1999; **341**:217–25.

78. MacIntyre K, Stewart S, Capewell S, et al. Gender and survival: a population-based study of 201,114 men and women following a first acute myocardial infarction. *J Am Coll Cardiol* 2001; **38**:729–35.

79. Mukamal KJ, Muller JE, Maclure M, Sherwood JB, Mittleman MA. Evaluation of sex-related differences in survival after hospitalization for acute myocardial infarction. *Am J Cardiol* 2001; **88**:768–71.

80. Whooley MA. Depression and medical illness. *Ann Epidemiol* 1999; **9**:281–2.

81. Rubin RT, Poland RE, Lesser IM, Winston RA, Blodgett AL. Neuroendocrine aspects of primary endogenous depression. I. Cortisol secretory dynamics in patients and matched controls. *Arch Gen Psychiat* 1987; **44**:328–36.

82. Nemeroff CB, Widerlov E, Bissette G, et al. Elevated concentrations of CSF corticotropin-releasing factor-like immunoreactivity in depressed patients. *Science* 1984; **226**:1342–4.

83. Risch SC, Lewine RJ, Kalin NH, et al. Limbic-hypothalamic-pituitary-adrenal axis activity and ventricular-to-brain ratio studies in affective illness and schizophrenia. *Neuropsychopharmacology* 1992; **6**:95–100.

84. Raadsheer FC, Hoogendijk WJG, Stam FC, Tilders FJH, Swaab DF. Increased numbers of corticotropin-releasing hormone expressing neurons in the hypothalamic paraventricular nucleus of depressed patients. *Neuroendocrinology* 1994; **60**:436–44.

85. Francis DD, Caldji C, Champagne F, Plotsky PM, Meaney MJ. The role of corticotropin-releasing factor – norepinephrine systems in mediating the effects of early experience on the development of behavioral and endocrine responses to stress. *Biol Psychiatry* 1999; **46**:1153–66.

86. Wyatt RJ, Portnoy B, Kupfer DJ, Synder F, Engelman K. Resting plasma catecholamine concentrations in patients with depression and anxiety. *Arch Gen Psychiatry* 1971; **24**:65–70.

87. Roy A, Pickar D, DeJong J, Karoum F, Linnoila M. Norepinephrine and its metabolites in cerebrospinal fluid, plasma, and urine: relationship to hypothalamic-pituitary-adrenal axis function in depression. *Arch Gen Psychiatry* 1988; **45**:849–57.

88. Veith RC, Lewis L, Linares OA, et al. Sympathetic nervous system activity in major depression: basal and desipramine-induced alterations in plasma norepinephrine kinetics. *Arch Gen Psychiatry* 1994; **51**:411–22.

89. Charney DS, Menkes DB, Henninger GR. Receptor sensitivity and the mechanism of action of antidepressant treatment. *Arch Gen Psychiatry* 1981; **38**:1160–80.

90. Golden RN, Markey SP, Risby ED, Rudorfer MV, Cowdry RW, Potter WZ. Antidepressants reduce whole-body norepinephrine turnover while enhancing 6-hydroxymelatonin output. *Arch Gen Psychiatry* 1988; **45**:150–4.

91. Troxler RG, Sprague EA, Albanese RA, Fuchs R, Thompson AJ. The association of elevated plasma cortisol and early atherosclerosis as demonstrated by coronary angiography. *Atherosclerosis* 1977; **26**: 151–62.

92. Kemper JW, Baggenstoss AH, Slocumb CH. The relationship of therapy with cortisone to the incidence of vascular lesions in rheumatoid arthritis. *Ann Intern Med* 1957; **46**:831–51.

93. Nahas GG, Brunson JG, King WM, Cavert HM. Functional and morphologic changes in heart lung preparations following administration of adrenal hormones. *Am J Clin Pathol* 1958; **34**:717–29.

94. Kaplan JR, Manuck SB, Adams MR, Weingand KW, Clarkson TB. Inhibition of coronary atherosclerosis by propranolol in behaviorally predisposed monkeys fed an atherogenic diet. *Circulation* 1987; **76**:1364–72.

95. Skantze HB, Kaplan J, Pettersson K, et al. Psychosocial stress causes endothelial injury in cynomolgus monkeys via [beta]1–adrenoceptor activation. *Atherosclerosis* 1998; **136**:153–61.

96. Gullette EC, Blumenthal JA, Babyak M, et al. Effect of mental stress on myocardial ischemia during daily life. *JAMA* 1997; **277**:1521–6.

97. Rozanski A, Bairey CN, Krantz DS, et al. Mental stress and the induction of silent myocardial ischemia in patients with coronary artery disease. *N Engl J Med* 1988; **318**:1005–12.

98. Jain D, Burg M, Soufer R, Zaret BL. Prognostic implications of mental stress-induced silent left ventricular dysfunction in patients with stable angina pectoris. *Am J Cardiol* 1995; **76**:31–5.

99. Sheps DS, McMahon RP, Becker L, et al. Mental stress-induced ischemia and all-cause mortality in patients with coronary artery disease: results from the Psychophysiological Investigations of Myocardial Ischemia study. *Circulation* 2002; **105**:1780–4.

100. Lechin F, van der Dijs B, Orozco B, et al. Plasma neurotransmitters, blood pressure, and heart rate during supine-resting, orthostasis, and moderate exercise conditions in major depressed patients. *Biol Psychiatry* 1995; **38**:166–73.

101. Carney RM, Freedland KE, Veith RC, et al. Major depression, heart rate, and plasma norepinephrine in patients with coronary heart disease. *Biol Psychiatry* 1999; **45**:458–63.

102. Kannel WB, Kannel C, Paffenbarger RS Jr, Cupples PH, Cupples LA. Heart rate and cardiovascular mortality: The Framingham Study. *Am Heart J* 1987; **113**:1489–94.

103. Hjalmarson A, Gilpin EA, Kjekshus J, Schieman G, Nicod P, Henning H. Influence of heart rate on mortality after acute myocardial infarction. *Am J Cardiol* 1990; **65**:547–53.

104. Bigger JT, Steinman RC, Rolnitzky LM, Fleiss JL, Albrecht P, Cohen RJ. Power-law behavior of RR-interval variability in healthy middle-aged persons, patients with recent acute myocardial infarction, and patients with heart transplant. *Circulation* 1996; **93**:2142–51.

105. Akselrod S, Gordon D, Ubel FA, Shannon DC, Barger AC, Cohen RJ. Power spectrum analysis of heart rate fluctuation: a quantitative probe of beat-to-beat cardiovascular control. *Science* 1981; **213**:220–2.

106. Krittayaphong R, Cascio W, Light K, et al. Heart rate variability in patients with coronary artery disease: differences in patients with higher and lower depression scores. *Psychosom Med* 1997; **59**:231–5.

107. Carney R, Saunders R, Freedland K, Stein P, Rich M, Jaffe A. Association of depression with reduced heart rate variability in coronary artery disease. *Am J Cardiol* 1995; **76**:562–4.

108. Carney RM, Blumenthal JA, Stein PK, et al. Depression, heart rate variability and acute myocardial infarction. *Circulation* 2001; **104**:2024–8.

109. Hordsten M, Ericson M, Perski A, Wamala S, Schenk-Gustafsson K, Orth-Gomer K. Psychosocial factors and heart rate variability in healthy women. *Psychosom Med* 1999; **61**:49–57.

110. Balogh S, Fitzpatrick DF, Hendricks SE, Paige SR. Increases in heart rate variability with successful treatment in patients with major depressive disorder. *Psychopharmacol Bull* 1993; **29**:201–6.

111. Bigger J, Fleiss J, Steinman R, Rolnitsky L, Kleiger R, Rottman J. Frequency domain measures of heart period variability and mortality after myocardial infarction. *Circulation* 1992; **85**:164–71.

112. Kleiger RE, Miller JP, Bigger JT, Moss AJ (The Multicenter Post-Infarction Research Group). Decreased heart rate variability and its association with increased mortality after acute myocardial infarction. *Am J Cardiol* 1987; **59**:256–62.

113. Lampert R, Ickovics J, Viscoli C, Horwitz R, Lee W. Inter-relationship between effect on heart rate variability and effect on outcome by beta-blockers in

the Beta Blocker Heart Attack Trial (BHAT). *Circulation* 1998; **98**:I-80 (abstract).

114. Zuanetti G, Neilson JMM, Latini R, Santoro E, Maggioni AP, Ewing DJ. Prognostic significance of heart rate variability in post-myocardial infarction patients in the fibrinolytic era. *Circulation* 1996; **94**:432–6.

115. Tsuji H, Larson MG, Venditti FJ, et al. Impact of reduced heart rate variability on risk for cardiac events: The Framingham Heart Study. *Circulation* 1996; **94**:2850–5.

116. Huikuri HV, Makikallio TH, Airaksinen J, et al. Power-law relationship of heart rate variability as a predictor of mortality in the elderly. *Circulation* 1998; **97**:2031–6.

117. Dekker JM, Schouten EG, Klootwijk P, Pool J, Swenne CA, Kromhout D. Heart rate variability from short electrocardiographic recordings predicts mortality from all causes in middle-aged and elderly men. The Zutphen Study. *Am J Epidemiol* 1997; **145**:899–908.

118. Liao D, Cai J, Rosamond WD, et al. Cardiac autonomic function and incident coronary heart disease: a population-based case-cohort study. The ARIC Study. Atherosclerosis Risk in Communities Study. *Am J Epidemiol* 1997; **145**:696–706.

119. Martin GJ, Magid NM, Myers G, et al. Heart rate variability and sudden cardiac death secondary to coronary artery disease during ambulatory electrocardiographic monitoring. *Am J Cardiol* 1987; **60**:86–9.

120. Meyers R, Pearlman A, Hyman R, et al. Beneficial effects of vagal stimulation and bradycardia during experimental acute myocardial ischemia. *Circulation* 1974; **49**:943–7.

121. Hull SJ, Evans A, Vanoli E, et al. Variability before and after myocardial infarction in conscious dogs at high and low risk of sudden death. *J Am Coll Cardiol* 1990; **16**:978–85.

122. Hull SS, Vanoli E, Adamson PB, Verrier RL, Foreman RD, Schwartz PJ. Exercise training confers anticipatory protection from sudden death during acute myocardial ischemia. *Circulation* 1994; **89**:548–52.

123. Kolman BS, Verrier RL, Lown B. The effect of vagus nerve stimulation upon vulnerability of the canine ventricle. *Circulation* 1975; **52**:578–85.

124. Kent KM, Smith ER, Redwood DR, Epstein SE. Electrical stability of acutely ischemic myocardium: influences to heart rate and vagal stimulation. *Circulation* 1973; **47**:291–8.

125. Han J, Garcia de Jalon P, Moe GK. Adrenergic effects on ventricular vulnerability. *Circ Res* 1964; **14**:516–24.

126. Meredith IT, Broughton A, Jennings GL, Esler MD. Evidence of a selective increase in cardiac sympathetic activity in patients with sustained ventricular arrhythmias. *N Engl J Med* 1991; **325**:618–24.

127. Goldstein DS. Plasma catecholamines and essential hypertension: an analytical review. *Hypertension* 1983; **5**:86–99.

128. Bjorntorp P, Holm G, Rosmond R. Hypothalamic arousal, insulin resistance and type 2 diabetes mellitus. *Diabetic Med* 1999; **16**:373–83.

129. Reaven GM, Lithell H, Landsberg L. Hypertension and associated metabolic abnormalities: the role of insulin resistance and the sympathoadrenal system. *N Engl J Med* 1996; **334**:374–81.

130. Liao D, Sloan R, Cascio W, et al. Multiple metabolic syndrome is associated with lower heart rate variability. The Atherosclerosis Risk in Communities Study. *Diabetes Care* 1998; **21**:2116–22.

131. Phillips DIW, Barker DJP, Fall CHD, et al. Elevated plasma cortisol concentrations: a link between low birth weight and the insulin resistance syndrome? *J Clin Endocrinol Metab* 1998; **83**:757–60.

132. Brunner EJ, Hemingway H, Walker BR, et al. Adrenocortical, autonomic, and inflammatory causes of the metabolic syndrome: nested case-control study. *Circulation* 2002; **106**:2659–65.

133. Weber-Hamann B, Hentschel F, Kniest A, et al. Hypercortisolemic depression is associated with increased intra-abdominal fat. *Psychosom Med* 2002; **64**:274–7.

134. Epel EE, Moyer AE, Martin CD, et al. Stress-induced cortisol, mood, and fat distribution in men. *Obes Res* 1999; **7**:9–15.

135. Esler M, Rumantir M, Wiesner G, Kaye D, Hastings J, Lambert G. Sympathetic nervous system and insulin resistance: from obesity to diabetes. *Am J Hypertens* 2001; **14** (11 Pt 2):304S–9S.

136. Raikkonen K, Hautanen A, Keltikangas-Jarvinen L. Association of stress and depression with regional fat distribution in healthy middle-aged men. *J Behav Med* 1994; **17**:605–16.

137. Raikkonen K, Matthews KA, Kuller LH. Anthropometric and psychosocial determinants of visceral obesity in healthy postmenopausal women. *Int J Obes Relat Metab Disord* 1999; **23**:775–82.

138. Raikkonen K, Matthews KA, Kuller LH, Reiber C, Bunker CH. Anger, hostility, and visceral adipose tissue in healthy postmenopausal women. *Metabolism* 1999; **48**:1146–51.

139. Black PH. The inflammatory response is an integral part of the stress response: implications for atherosclerosis, insulin resistance, type II diabetes and metabolic syndrome X. *Brain Behav Immun* 2003; **17**:350–64.

140. Rosmond R. Stress induced disturbances of the HPA axis: a pathway to type 2 diabetes? *Med Sci Monit* 2003; **9**:RA35–9.

141. Schmidt MI, Duncan BB, Sharrett AR, et al. Markers of inflammation and prediction of diabetes mellitus in adults (Atherosclerosis Risk in Communities study): a cohort study. *Lancet* 1999; **353**:1649–52.

142. Pradhan AD, Manson JE, Rifai N, Buring JE, Ridker PM. C-Reactive protein, interleukin 6, and risk of developing type 2 diabetes mellitus. *JAMA* 2001; **286**:327–34.

143. Libby P. Inflammation in atherosclerosis. *Nature* 2002; **420**:868–74.

144. Wallace AM, McMahon AD, Packard CJ, et al. Plasma leptin and the risk of cardiovascular disease in the West of Scotland Coronary Prevention Study (WOSCOPS). *Circulation* 2001; **104**:3052–6.

145. Okamoto Y, Kihara S, Ouchi N, et al. Adiponectin reduces atherosclerosis in apolipoprotein E-deficient mice. *Circulation* 2002; **106**:2767–70.

146. Kumada M, Kihara S, Sumitsuji S, et al. Association of hypoadiponectinemia with coronary artery disease in men. *Arterioscler Thromb Vasc Biol* 2003; **23**:85–9.

147. Libby P, Ridker PM, Maseri A. Inflammation and atherosclerosis. *Circulation* 2002; **105**:1135–43.

148. Nickening G, Harrison DG. The AT1–type angiotensin receptor in oxidative stress and atherogenesis. Part I: Oxidative stress and atherogenesis. *Circulation* 2002; **105**:393–6.

149. Griendling KK, FitzGerald GA. Oxidative stress and cardiovascular injury: Part II: animal and human studies. *Circulation* 2003; **108**:2034–40.

150. Ridker PM. Inflammation, infection, and cardiovascular risk. How good is the evidence? *Circulation* 1998; **97**:1671–4.

151. Ridker PM. Evaluating novel cardiovascular risk factors: can we better predict heart attacks? *Ann Intern Med* 1999; **130**:933–7.

152. Libby PL, Ridker PM. Novel inflammatory markers of coronary risk. Theory versus practice. *Circulation* 1999; **100**:1148–50.

153. Zhang R, Brennan ML, Fu X, et al. Association between myeloperoxidase levels and risk of coronary artery disease. *JAMA* 2001; **286**:2136–42.

154. Brennan ML, Hazen SL. Emerging role of myeloperoxidase and oxidant stress markers in cardiovascular risk assessment. *Curr Opin Lipidol* 2003; **14**:353–9.

155. Shishehbor MH, Aviles RJ, Brennan M-L, et al. Association of nitrotyrosine levels with cardiovascular disease and modulation by statin therapy. *JAMA* 2003; **289**:1675–80.

156. Guillen I, Blanes M, Gomez-Lechon MJ, Castell JV. Cytokine signaling during myocardial infarction: sequential appearance of IL-1 beta and IL-6. *Am J Physiol* 1995; **269**:R229–35.

157. Biasucci L, Vitelli A, Liuzzo G, et al. Elevated levels of interleukin-6 in unstable angina. *Circulation* 1996; **94**:874–7.

158. Buffon A, Biasucci LM, Liuzzo G, D'Onofrio G, Crea F, Maseri A. Widespread coronary inflammation in unstable angina. *N Engl J Med* 2002; **347**:5–12.

159. Lindmark E, Diderholm E, Wallentin L, Siegbahn A. Relationship between interleukin 6 and mortality in patients with unstable coronary artery disease: effects of an early invasive or noninvasive strategy. *JAMA* 2001; **286**:2107–13.

160. Brennan M-L, Penn MS, Van Lente F, et al. Prognostic value of myeloperoxidase in patients with chest pain. *N Engl J Med* 2003; **349**:1595–604.

161. Maes M, Scharpe S, Meltzer HY, et al. Relationships between interleukin-6 activity, acute phase proteins, and function of the hypothalamic-pituitary-adrenal axis in severe depression. *Psychiatry Res* 1993; **49**:11–27.

162. Maes M, Meltzer HY, Buckley P, Bosmans E. Plasma-soluble interleukin-2 and transferrin receptor in schizophrenia and major depression. *Eur Arch Psychiatry Clin Neurosci* 1995; **244**:325–9.

163. Kop WJ, Gottdiener JS, Tangen CM, et al. Inflammation and coagulation factors in persons >65 years of age with symptoms of depression but without evidence of myocardial ischemia. *Am J Cardiol* 2002; **89**:419–24.

164. Lesperance F, Frasure-Smith N, Theroux P, Irwin M. The association between major depression and levels of soluble intercellular adhesion molecule 1, interleukin-6, and C-reactive protein in patients with recent acute coronary syndromes. *Am J Psychiatry* 2004; **161**:271–7.

165. Sluzewska A, Rybakowski L, Bosmans E, et al. Indicators of immune activation in major depression. *Psychiatry Res* 1996; **64**:161–7.

166. Berk M, Wadee AA, Kuschke RH, O'Neill-Kerr A. Acute-phase proteins in major depression. *J Psychosom Res* 1997; **43**:529–34.

167. Danner M, Kasl SV, Vaccarino V. Association between major depressive episode and elevated C-reactive protein. *Psychosom Med* 2003; **65**:347–56.

168. Dentino AN, Pieper CF, Rao KMK, et al. Association of interleukin-6 and other biological variables with depression in older people living in the community. *J Am Geriatr Soc* 1999; **47**:6–11.

169. Penninx BWJH, Kritchevsky SB, Yaffe K, et al.

Inflammatory markers and depressed mood in older persons: results from the health, aging and body composition study. *Biol Psychiatry* 2003; **54**:566–72.

170. Lanquillon S, Krieg JC, Bening-Abu-Shach U, Vedder H. Cytokine production and treatment response in major depressive disorder. *Neuropsychopharmacology* 2000; **22**:370–9.

171. Hornig M, Goodman DBP, Kamoun M, Amsterdam JD. Positive and negative acute phase proteins in affective subtypes. *J Affect Dis* 1998; **49**:9–18.

172. Cushman M, Legault C, Barrett-Connor E, et al. Effect of postmenopausal hormones on inflammation-sensitive proteins: the Postmenopausal Estrogen/Progestin Interventions (PEPI) Study. *Circulation* 1999; **100**:717–22.

173. Kang D-H, McCarthy DO. The effect of psychological stress on neutrophil superoxide release. *Res Nursing Health* 1994; **17**:363–70.

174. Adachi S, Kawamura K, Takemoto K. Oxidative damage of nuclear DNA in liver of rats exposed to psychological stress. *Cancer Res* 1993; **53**:4153–5.

175. Haggendal J, Jonsson L, Johansson G, Bjurstrom S, Carlsten J, Thoren-Tolling K. Catecholamine-induced free radicals in myocardial cell necrosis on experimental stress in pigs. *Acta Physiol Scand* 1987; **131**:447–52.

176. Irie M, Asami S, Nagata S, Masakazu M, Kasai H. Relationship between perceived workload, stress and oxidative DNA damage. *Int Arch Occup Environ Health* 2001; **74**:153–7.

177. Schneider RH, Nidich SI, Salerno JW, et al. Lower lipid peroxide levels in practitioners of the Transcendental Meditation Program. *Psychosom Med* 1998; **60**:38–41.

178. Maes M, Stevens W, De Clerck L, et al. Neutrophil chemotaxis, phagocytosis and superoxide relapse in depressed illness. *Biol Psychiatry* 1992; **31**:1220–4.

179. Peets M, Murphy B, Shay J, Horrobin D. Depletion of omega-3–fatty acid levels in red blood cell membranes of depressive patients. *Biol Psychiatry* 1998; **43**:315–19.

180. Srivastava N, Barthwal MK, Dalal PK, et al. A study on nitric oxide, beta-adrenergic receptors and antioxidant status in the polymorphonuclear leukocytes from the patients of depression. *J Affect Dis* 2002; **72**:45–52.

181. Rajagopalan S, Brook R, Rubenfire M, Pitt E, Young E. Abnormal brachial artery flow-mediated vasodilation in young adults with major depression. *Am J Cardiol* 2001; **88**:196–8.

182. Abrams J. Role of endothelial dysfunction in coronary artery disease. *Am J Cardiol* 1997; **79**:2–9.

183. Chrousos GP. The hypothalamic-pituitary-adrenal axis and immune-mediated inflammation. *N Engl J Med* 1995; **332**:1351–62.

184. Snyder SH, Dawson TM. Nitric oxide and related substances as neural messengers. In: Bloom FE, Kupfer DJ (eds). *Psychopharmacology: The Fourth Generation of Progress*. New York: Raven Press, 1995: 609–18.

185. Van Amsterdam JG, Opperhuizen A. Nitric oxide and biopterin in depression and stress. *Psychiatry Res* 1999; **85**:33–8.

186. Abou-Saleh MT, Anderson DN, Collins J, et al. The role of pterins in depression and the effects of antidepressive therapy. *Biol Psychiatry* 1995; **38**:458–63.

187. Obata T, Yamanaka Y. Cardiac microdialysis of salicylic acid to detect hydroxyl radical generation associated with sympathetic nerve stimulation. *Neurosci Lett* 1996; **211**:216–18.

188. Obata T, Yamanaka Y. Prazosin attenuates hydroxyl radical generation in the rat myocardium. *Eur J Pharmacol* 1999; **379**:161–6.

189. Dhalla N, Temsah RM, Netticadan T. Role of oxidative stress in cardiovascular disease. *J Hypertension* 2000; **18**:655–73.

190. Nickening G, Harrison DG. The AT1-type angiotensin receptor in oxidative stress and atherogenesis. Part II: AT1 receptor regulation. *Circulation* 2002; **105**:530–6.

191. Aguilera G, Kiss A, Luo X. Increased expression of type 1 angiotensin II receptors in the hypothalamic paraventricular nucleus following stress and glucocorticoid administration. *J Neuroendocrinol* 1995; **7**:775–83.

192. Di Rosa M, Radomski M, Carnuccio R, Moncada S. Glucocorticoids inhibit the induction of nitric oxide synthase in macrophages. *Biochem Biophys Res Commun* 1990; **172**:1246–52.

193. Serova L, Nankova B, Rivkin M, Kvetnansky R, Sabban EL. Glucocorticoids elevate GTP cyclohydrolase I mRNA levels in vivo and in PCI2 cells. *Mol Brain Res* 1997; **48**:251–8.

194. Kelly JJ, Tam SH, Williamson PM, Lawson J, Whitworth JA. The nitric oxide system and cortisol-induced hypertension in humans. *Clin Exp Pharmacol Physiol* 1998; **25**:945–6.

195. Markovitz JH, Matthews KA. Platelets and coronary heart disease: potential psychophysiologic mechanisms. *Psychosom Med* 1991; **53**:643–68.

196. Musselman DL, Tomer A, Manatunga AK, et al. Exaggerated platelet reactivity in major depression. *Am J Psychiatry* 1996; **153**:1313–17.

197. McAdams C, Leonard BE. Changes in platelet aggre-

gatory responses to collagen and 5-hydroxytrypta-mine. *Int Clin Psychopharmacol* 1992; **7**:81–5.

198. Laghrissi-Thode F, Wagner WR, Pollock BG, Johnson PC, Finkel MS. Elevated factor 4 and beta-thromboglobulin plasma levels in depressed patients with ischemic heart disease. *Biol Psychiatry* 1997; **42**:290–5.

199. van Hulsteijn H, Kolff J, Briet E, van der Laarse A, Bertina R. Fibrinopeptide A and beta thromboglobulin in patients with angina pectoris and acute myocardial infarction. *Am Heart J* 1984; **107**:39–45.

200. Nichols AB, Owen J, Kaplan KL, Sciacca RR, Nossel HL. Fibrinopeptide A, platelet factor 4, and beta-thromboglobulin levels in coronary heart disease. *Blood* 1982; **60**:650–4.

201. Rasi V, Ikkala E, Torstila I. Plasma beta-thromboglobulin in acute myocardial infarction. *Thromb Res* 1982; **25**:203–12.

202. Sobel M, Salzman EW, Davies GC, et al. Circulating platelet products in unstable angina pectoris. *Circulation* 1981; **63**:300–6.

203. de Boer AC, Turpie AGG, Butt RW, Johnston RV, Genton E. Platelet release and thromboxane synthesis in symptomatic coronary artery disease. *Circulation* 1982; **66**:327–33.

204. Bremner JD, Krystal JH, Southwick SM, Charney DS. Noradrenergic mechanisms in stress and anxiety: I. Preclinical studies. *Synapse* 1996; **23**:28–38.

205. Bremner JD, Krystal JH, Southwick SM, Charney DS. Noradrenergic mechanisms in stress and anxiety: II. Clinical studies. *Synapse* 1996; **23**:39–51.

206. Glassman AH, Helzer JE, Covey LS, et al. Smoking, smoking cessation and major depression. *JAMA* 1990; **264**:1546–9.

207. Anda RF, Williamson DF, Escobedo LG, Mast EE, Giovino GA, Remington PL. Depression and the dynamics of smoking; a national perspective. *JAMA* 1990; **264**:1541–5.

208. Carney RM, Freedland KE, Eisen SA, Rich MW, Jaffe AS. Major depression and medication adherence in elderly patients with coronary artery disease. *Health Psychol* 1995; **14**:88–90.

209. Zigelstein RC, Bush DE, Fauerbach JA. Depression, adherence behavior, and coronary disease outcomes. *Arch Intern Med* 1998; **158**:808–9.

210. Kendler KS, Neale MC, Maclean CJ, Heath AC, Eavens LJ, Kessler RC. Smoking and major depression: a causal analysis. *Arch Gen Psychiatry* 1993; **50**:36–43.

211. Linden W, Stossel C, Maurice J. Psychological interventions for patients with coronary artery disease. *Arch Intern Med* 1996; **156**:745–52.

212. Dusseldorp E, van Elderen T, Maes S, Meulman J, Kraaij V. A meta-analysis of psychoeducational programs for coronary heart disease patients. *Health Psychol* 1999; **18**:506–19.

213. Writing Committee for the ENRICHD Investigators. Effects of treating depression and low level social support on clinical events after myocardial infarction: The Enhancing Recovery in Coronary Heart Disease (ENRICHD) patients randomized trial. *JAMA* 2003; **289**:3106–16.

214. The ENRICHD Investigators. Enhancing Recovery in Coronary Heart Disease (ENRICHD): baseline characteristics. *Am J Cardiol* 2001; **88**:316–22.

215. Glassman AH, O'Connor CM, Califf RM, et al. Sertraline treatment of major depression in patients with acute MI or unstable angina. *JAMA* 2002; **288**:701–9.

216. Mosca L, Appel LJ, Benjamin EJ, et al. Evidence-based guidelines for cardiovascular disease prevention in women. *Circulation* 2004; **109**:672–93.

42

Clinical trial evidence for women's cardiovascular health: what we know and what we must learn

Nanette K. Wenger

Introduction

That women and men have different lifespans, different patterns of illness, that they differ in metabolism and in disease processes, and that they respond differently to therapies was highlighted in the landmark 2001 Institute of Medicine report 'Exploring the Biological Contribution to Human Health. Does Sex Matter?'[1] The report posited that the ascertainment of sex-based differences in disease components, pathogenesis, diagnostic modalities, preventive approaches, and therapeutic interventions is pivotal for clinicians to appreciate how women and men react differently to diseases and to drugs. The report recommended the analysis and presentation of sex-based differences in clinical research and further urged that journal editors encourage researchers to report the results of sex-specific analyses. Examples offered include that women have a greater risk of developing life-threatening ventricular arrhythmias with a variety of potassium channel blocking drugs; and that women recover language ability more rapidly than men after a left hemisphere stroke. The report further advocated that clinicians incorporate these sex-based differences in responses in preventive, diagnostic, and therapeutic strategies.

Although cardiovascular disease (CVD) is the leading killer of women in the United States, clinical decisions for preventive, diagnostic, and therapeutic medical care have historically been based on evidence from clinical trials performed predominately or exclusively in men. Clinical trials provide the most reliable research evidence of the benefits and risks of an intervention. In a review of sex representation in clinical trials (1966–1998) males outnumbered females 3.66 to 1 in heart disease trials.[2] This chapter displays selected overviews and several examples of the relevance of sex-based analyses of cardiovascular clinical trials to clinical decision-making and health-care policy for women.

Diligent efforts are needed to change the paradigm of clinical practice to improve the heart health of women; the major challenge is expanding the knowledge base. As noted, until recently women have been excluded from many clinical research studies, and current participation remains suboptimal. In particular, few data are available for women of racial and ethnic minorities. As well, the recently available sex-specific epidemiologic data often remain incomplete, particularly in regard to information for subsets of women. The sex-specific clinical outcome data that have only recently become available are equally incomplete, with limited information deriving from these subsets of women. Analyses of existing databases may reverse prior missed opportunities.

The US Food and Drug Administration (FDA) and clinical trials

Beginning in 1993, the US Food and Drug Administration (FDA) provided guidance to industry to include sufficient women as participants in clinical drug trials such that significant differences in drug safety and efficacy could be detected, and advised that analyses of sex differences were to be presented in New Drug Applications (NDAs). Although participation of women in phase 3 clinical trials increased from 44% to 56% between 1992 and 2000, this increase included trials for clinical issues that involved solely women.

In 1998, the guidance was updated to a regulation, where the FDA required separate presentation of safety and efficacy data for women and men in the NDAs and mandated tabulation of study participants by sex. Nonetheless, these regulations lacked specific criteria for the numbers of women needed and specific requirements for data analysis. As subsequently noted by an oversight group, one-third of current NDAs did not fulfill this requirement. Moreover, until very recent years there was no FDA system to track women in clinical trials, no procedures regarding the requirements for NDA presentation of sex differences for drug side effects, and no information mandated about dosage adjustment based on sex that reflected issues such as body weight; body fat distribution; differential drug absorption, metabolism or excretion; and resultant drug concentrations. Also noted was a failure to address inclusion of women in early-phase clinical pharmacologic trials, to identify the stages of the menstrual cycle regarding hormonal variability or the notation of menopausal status when appropriate. The reason that sex-based differences in drug response require more broad exploration is that of the ten prescription drugs withdrawn from the US market since 1997, eight caused more adverse events in women than in men.

In 2001 the General Accounting Office (GAO) of the US Government[3] challenged the FDA for failure to enforce industry adherence to these 1998 regulations for reporting data on sex differences in NDAs. More than one-third of all drugs approved by the FDA between 1998 and 2000 failed to provide information on sex-related responses in their NDAs; 22% of these reports did not present separate efficacy data for women and men, and 17% omitted sex-based safety data. The GAO suggested that this information, although available, was not included in the reporting. The GAO defined a compelling need for the FDA to monitor the inclusion of women in all stages of pharmacologic research, as well as to improve the oversight of the analyses and presentation of data related to sex differences in clinical trials. Emphasized was that the initial small-scale safety trials involved women as only 22% of participants, even for those drugs where the later stage clinical trials included sufficient numbers of women for safety and efficacy determinations.

In response to this GAO report, the FDA has implemented management systems to improve review of sex-specific data. The FDA Office of Women's Health has created a clinical trials demographic data base.

US National Heart, Lung, and Blood Institute (NHLBI) and cardiovascular clinical trials

The sex-based differences in CVD are a compelling basis for inclusion of women in clinical trials of cardiovascular problems. NHLBI data from 1965 to 1998 show that 215 769 women and 183 005 men were included in such trials, with a resultant percentage of 54% women. However, when single sex trials were excluded, only 38% of the participants in NHLBI cardiovascular trials were women. Over time there has been increased representation of women in clinical trials addressing coronary heart disease (CHD), but no change in participation of women in clinical trials of hypertension, of arrhythmia, or of heart failure (Fig. 42.1).[4] The representation of women in NHLBI-supported clinical trials of hypertension has remained substantial, ranging from 40 to 50%. Similarly, women and men were equally represented in NHLBI-supported clinical trials involving statin therapy. By contrast, women constituted fewer than 20% of participants in trials of heart failure and of anti-arrhythmic therapies.

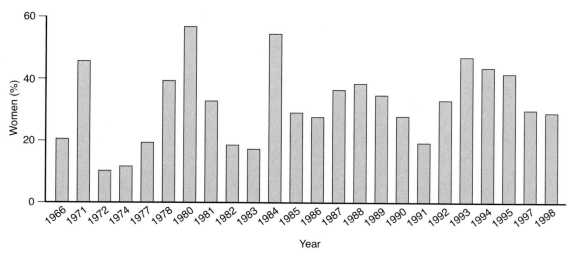

Figure 42.1
Percentages of women among enrollees in cardiovascular trials involving men and women, according to the year in which the trial was started. Years are shown for trials for which data on sex were available. Single-sex trials are not included. Reproduced from reference 4 with permission.

Since 1990 the US National Institutes of Health (NIH) has mandated the inclusion of women in all NIH-sponsored research, and since 1994 has required the analysis of outcomes by sex. Despite these advances, specific data for women are not uniformly evident in the published research findings.

A December 2002 report, monitoring the adherence of the NIH policy of inclusion of women and minorities as clinical research subjects identified that, when female-only and male-only studies were excluded, there was equal representation of women and men in all NIH extramural studies, 50.2% versus 49.3%.[5]

The Cochrane Reviews

In an analysis of Cochrane Reviews related to the treatment of CVD that examined eight systematic reviews by the heart group, three by the hypertension group, and 19 by the peripheral vascular diseases group, a total of 196 studies were evaluated for sex-based analyses. Women comprised 27% of the pooled population of the total 258 clinical trials. Of 196 clinical trials that included both women and men, only one-third examined the outcomes by sex; however, among trials that supplied sex-based analyses, 20% reported significant differences in cardiovascular-related outcomes between women and men.

The conclusion of the authors was that there were insufficient large-scale clinical trials or meta-analyses concerning CVD in women to determine if their medical treatment should differ from that for men. The recommendation was that all clinical trials relating to the management of CVD should enroll significantly more female participants, and that sex-based analysis should be performed and published as currently mandated for NIH-sponsored research by the NIH Revitalization Act of 1993. Finally, the authors suggested that the Cochrane Library would be more useful for the evidence-based health care of women if the systematic reviews included all available sex-based information in their analyses.[6]

Agency for Healthcare Research and Quality (AHRQ) review

A systematic review of research on the diagnosis and treatment of CHD in women, conducted for the

Agency for Healthcare Research and Quality (AHRQ),[7] concluded that much of the evidence supporting contemporary recommendations for prevention, testing, and treatment of CHD in women is extrapolated from studies conducted predominantly in middle-aged men. In general, there was no evidence to address differences in the accuracy of diagnostic tests, the strength of risk factors, the effects of treatment, and the prognostic value of markers for ischemia in women of different races or ethnicity. The only evidence regarding ethnicity differences suggested that African American women may benefit more from treatment of hypertension than white women. Fair evidence suggested that the accuracy of exercise electrocardiography (ECG) and exercise thallium testing for CHD in women is low; the accuracy of exercise echocardiography, based on limited data, appeared to be higher. There was weak evidence that the absence of coronary calcification may be useful to exclude CHD in both women and men.

There was fair to good evidence that beta-blockers, aspirin, and angiotensin-converting enzyme (ACE) inhibitors reduced the risk for coronary events in women known to have heart disease, and good evidence that nitrates do not reduce such risk. There was fair evidence that glycoprotein IIb/IIIa inhibitor drugs given to women undergoing percutaneous coronary intervention (PCI) decreased the risk of CHD events and the need for revascularization, but this treatment increased mortality in women with acute coronary syndromes. The latter was the only evidence of possible interaction by sex in that men treated with the IIb/IIIa platelet inhibitor drugs for acute coronary syndromes had better outcomes. There was weak evidence regarding the efficacy of major treatments for CHD in women including calcium channel blocking drugs, heparin, ticlopidine, clopidogrel, coronary artery bypass graft surgery, PCI, and coronary stenting.

Despite fair to good evidence that hyperlipidemia, diabetes, and hyperhomocysteinemia are risk factors for CHD in women, only weak evidence links most risk factors to coronary risk in women because most of such studies were observational and few good quality systematic reviews have been accomplished. Risk factors appeared to impart comparable risk for the sexes with the possible exception of age, diabetes, and certain lipoproteins conferring excess risk for women. Fair to good evidence suggests that smoking cessation after myocardial infarction (MI) and treatment of hypertension and of hyperlipidemia lowered the risk for CHD events in women, without evidence available for the effectiveness of other interventions to modify coronary risk in women.

There was weak evidence that women were less likely than men to undergo diagnostic testing and treatment for CHD, but that women were more likely than their male peers to be treated for hypertension. Differences in the utilization of tests or treatments may reflect differences in physician perception of the severity and prognosis of CHD between the sexes, differences in physician perception of the risks and efficacies of diagnostic and therapeutic procedures between the sexes, differences in the severity of the disease or of comorbidities between the sexes or may represent overuse of such tests or treatments for men.

A subsequent report of systematic reviews of evidence on selected topics regarding the diagnosis and treatment of CHD in women, again performed for the AHRQ,[8] suggested that the accuracy of exercise myocardial perfusion imaging for the diagnosis of CHD is low, but does not differ clinically in women and men; with little difference in the diagnostic accuracy of exercise myocardial perfusion imaging and exercise echocardiography in women. The accuracy of exercise myocardial perfusion imaging for the diagnosis of CHD in women was similar whether thallium or sestamibi was used as the imaging agent.

Regarding the efficacy of lipid-lowering for CHD risk reduction in women, treatment with lipid-lowering therapy in women with established CHD reduced CHD mortality by 26%, nonfatal MI by 36%, and major CHD events by 21%. There was insufficient evidence that lipid-lowering reduced rates of revascularization procedures and no evidence of reduction in total mortality risk. Insufficient evidence of lipid-lowering benefit was available for women without CHD.

Summary estimates for the risk for CHD mortality due to diabetes in white women and men were similar to those for all ethnicities combined. The difference in CHD outcomes between diabetic women and men was progressively attenuated with adjustment for major cardiovascular risk factors.

This may reflect that women with diabetes have more risk factors and more severe risk factor abnormalities than women without diabetes, a difference not present in men with and without diabetes.

Finally, women with acute coronary syndromes were older and more likely to have diabetes and hypertension than men. Elevated troponin levels similarly increased the risk of death for both sexes but were associated with a greater increase in risk of nonfatal MI for women.[8]

Clinical trials of menopausal hormone therapy and CVD (see also Chapter 26)

Despite biologically plausible mechanisms for menopausal hormone benefit in the prevention of CVD, and in particular CHD in women; observational studies initially suggesting substantial benefit,[9] and intermediate outcome trials also defining that surrogate markers of coronary risk were improved with hormone therapy;[10] randomized clinical trial data have displayed lack of cardiovascular benefit and increased risk with hormone therapy.[11] The results from these single-sex randomized clinical trials of hormone therapy dramatically changed the evidence for the preventive health benefits of menopausal hormone therapy, drastically changed clinical practice patterns, and culminated in revised national and international clinical practice guidelines and recommendations of regulatory agencies.[12]

The Women's Health Initiative Hormone Trial was the pivotal study addressing menopausal hormone therapy for the primary prevention of CVD. About 25 000 women were randomized to conjugated equine estrogen plus medroxyprogesterone acetate daily versus placebo if they had an intact uterus and conjugated equine estrogen versus placebo for women after hysterectomy. The estrogen/progestin arm was terminated prematurely in 2002 owing to an excess risk of invasive breast cancer and an unfavorable global risk score. Specifically, harms were identified for CHD, stroke, venous thrombo-embolism, and invasive breast cancer.[13] Subsequent analyses also identified that hormone therapy did not forestall dementia, but rather entailed a small increased risk of

dementia and mild cognitive impairment.[14,15] The estrogen-only arm was terminated prematurely in 2004 because of an increased risk of stroke and a lack of coronary benefit.[16]

The pivotal secondary prevention trial was the Heart and Estrogen/progestin Replacement Study (HERS)[17] and its follow-up in HERS II.[18] HERS randomized 2763 women with established CHD to conjugated equine estrogen plus medroxyprogesterone acetate daily versus placebo. At trial end, there was no difference in the primary outcome of CHD mortality and nonfatal MI; however, there was a suggestion of early harm and potential late benefit. Follow-up of 93% of the surviving cohort in an open-label observational study (HERS II) for a total duration of 6.8 years, failed to show benefit in any primary or secondary cardiovascular outcome. Of concern were the harms of increased venous thromboembolism and increased risk for gallbladder disease requiring surgical intervention. The Women's Estrogen for Stroke Trial (WEST) directed attention to cerebrovascular disease and showed no cerebrovascular benefit but rather harm from estradiol therapy.[19] Comparable data for lack of menopausal hormone cardiovascular benefit and potential harms derived from the Papworth HRT Atherosclerosis Study (PHASE), the Women's Angiographic Vitamin and Estrogen (WAVE) trial, the Women's Estrogen-progestin Lipid-Lowering Hormone Atherosclerosis Regression Trial (WELL-HART), and the oEStrogen in the Prevention of ReInfarction Trial (ESPRIT).[20–23]

Clinical trials of therapies for acute MI[24] (see also Chapters 17 and 18)

CHD claims the lives of over 250 000 US women annually. In 1975 women comprised 30% of US patients with acute MI, with this percentage increasing to 43% by 1995. Analysis of 593 randomized controlled clinical trials of acute coronary syndromes between 1966 and 2000[24] showed that women constituted only 20% of the study population between 1966 and 1990. This percentage increased to 25% for the years 1991–2000; and analysis of the subset enrolled after 1995 and published after that year showed

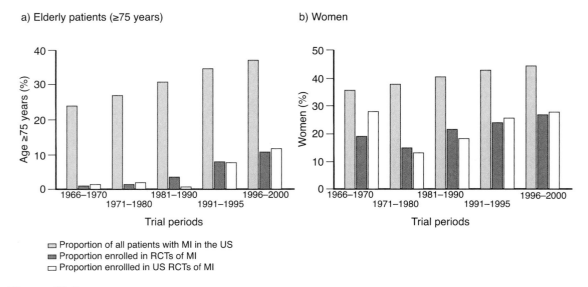

a) Elderly patients (≥75 years)

b) Women

Trial periods

Trial periods

▱ Proportion of all patients with MI in the US
▰ Proportion enrolled in RCTs of MI
▱ Proportion enrollled in US RCTs of MI

Figure 42.2
Representation of elderly patients and women in randomized trials of myocardial infarction (MI). The lightest gray bars are based on the Worcester Heart Attack Study. RCTs, randomized controlled trials. Reproduced from reference 24 with permission.

27–29% participation for women. Of concern are the adverse consequences of CHD, in that women characteristically have increased complications of MI including heart failure, shock, and ventricular rupture.

Most mega-trials of CHD therapies were conducted in patients with acute MI and most were studies of thrombolytic therapy. Figure 42.2 displays the percentage of women recruited in such trials, in addition to the percentage of elderly participants, defined as those older than 75 years of age. Exclusion of elderly patients from clinical trials doubly disadvantages women owing to the predominance of their coronary events at elderly age.[24]

Gruppo Italiano per lo Studio della Sporavvivenza nell'Infarto Miocardico (GISSI)-1, comparing streptokinase versus placebo, enrolled 11 712 patients, 2310 of whom were women. The female mortality was double that for men. One-year survival benefit with streptokinase was evident only for men and for patients younger than 65 years of age. GISSI-2 compared tPA (tissue plasminogen activator) versus streptokinase and heparin versus no heparin; 23% of the 20 891 participants were women. There was comparable sex-based benefit with both drugs, but

increased mortality was described for women. An excess risk of hemorrhagic stroke occurred in women, even after adjustment for risk factors.[25]

ISIS-2 randomized 17 187 patients, 23% women, to streptokinase, aspirin alone, or combined therapy compared with placebo. Greater benefit occurred with combination therapy. The absolute decrease in mortality was greatest in the high-risk patients: women, the elderly, those with anterior infarction, and those with prior infarction, among others. Nonetheless, there was a substantial excess of mortality in women compared with men.

Streptokinase was compared with tPA and with APSAC in ISIS-3, as was aspirin plus heparin versus aspirin alone. Twenty-seven per cent of the 41 299 patients randomized were women. Although there was similar benefit of all three lytic agents, no sex-specific data were presented.

Global Use of Strategies to Open Occluded Arteries (GUSTO)-1 compared streptokinase with tPA or both plus heparin. Twenty-five per cent of the 41 021 randomized patients were women. Survival benefit was greater with tPA plus heparin, but sex-specific data were not provided.

In GUSTO-3 reteplase (recombinant plasminogen activator) was compared with alteplase (tPA). Twenty-seven per cent of the 15 059 patients were women. Although there was comparable benefit of both drugs, no sex-specific data were provided. There was an increased stroke risk in participants older than 75 years of age.

TIMI IIIB assessed the effect of tPA compared with an early invasive strategy in patients with unstable angina and nonQ wave MI; 34% of the 1473 patients were women. Thrombolysis was not beneficial and possibly harmful; there was no difference between the early invasive and conservative strategies. Again no sex-specific data were provided.

Finally, in GUSTO-V, comparison was undertaken between reteplase and half-dose reteplase plus a glycoprotein IIb/IIIa inhibitor. Twenty-five per cent of the 16 588 patients were women. There was comparable outcome of both therapies, but again no sex-specific data were provided; as in GUSTO-3, there was an excess of intracranial hemorrhage in patients older than 75 years of age; again sex-specific information was absent.

Opportunities exist for deriving additional information about contemporary interventions for acute MI in women. Sex-specific analyses from this compendium of mega-trials, designed to explore a variety of therapeutic issues, are needed. First, why is the mortality greater for women? Second, why is there less benefit and increased intracranial hemorrhage and stroke with thrombolysis in the population older than age 75 – does this reflect sex-specific issues? Third, were there sex differences in the delay to arrival at hospital, in concomitant therapies, and in co-morbid illnesses in these cohorts?

Clinical trials in acute coronary syndromes (see also Chapters 17 and 18)

The GUSTO IIB trial[26] enrolled 12 142 patients, 3662 of them women. Women displayed major differences in baseline characteristics in that they were older and more likely to have diabetes, hypertension, prior heart failure, and cerebrovascular disease. GUSTO also defined major sex-based differences in the clinical presentation of acute coronary syndromes. Women were more likely than men to have unstable angina than acute MI; among the women with MI, fewer had ST elevation MI. Women with unstable angina had a better prognosis than their male peers. Women uniformly had greater mortality and an excess of in-hospital complications, although the outcomes were similar after adjustment for age and baseline characteristics. This simply means that women fare poorly not specifically because of their sex, but rather because of their older age and greater prevalence of co-morbidities.

Two European trials, FRISC II[27] and RITA 3,[28] addressing the invasive management for acute coronary syndromes, randomized patients to early invasive compared with noninvasive strategies. In general, the women were older and had less severe angiographic coronary disease than the men. Although the early invasive strategy improved the composite outcomes in men, women had a nonsignificant increase in adverse outcomes of MI or death. By contrast, the US trial TACTICS TIMI-18[29] showed equal favorable outcomes for women and men with an early invasive approach. This difference between trials likely reflects the increased procedural risk for women, including an increased risk of bleeding with invasive strategies, such that only those studies that enrolled higher-risk status women, more specifically women with elevated troponin levels, had sufficient benefit of the early invasive intervention to over-ride the procedural risk.

Although exercise testing is often considered less reliable for the diagnosis and prognosis of CHD in women than in men, exercise testing in women with acute coronary syndromes provided particular benefit.[30] In the FRISC study group, exercise testing on day 5–8 best predicted subsequent cardiac events, and proved a better predictor for women than any of the clinical variables tested.

Clinical trials of PCI compared with medical therapy (see also Chapter 19)

In the initial trials of PCI that antedated the use of coronary stents, of glycoprotein IIb/IIIa platelet inhibitor therapy, and of optimal lipid-lowering, PCI

Table 42.1 Trials of medical therapy versus revascularization: percentage of enrolled women

Trial	% Women
ACIP[32]	14
MASS[33]	18
RITA-2[35]	18
AVERT[34]	16
COURAGE (Clinical Outcomes Utilizing Revascularization and Aggressive Drug Evaluation)	(enrolling)

provided greater anginal relief and improvement in exercise tolerance than did medical therapy. The percentage of women in these trials is displayed in Table 42.1. Nonetheless, there was an excess of procedure-related complications in women.[31–35] Although women in these trials had greater in-hospital mortality, there was similar long-term survival for both sexes. Because of the substantial under-representation of women in these clinical trials, no firm conclusions can be provided for women. Potential data may derive from the ongoing COURAGE (Clinical Outcomes Utilizing Revascularization and Aggressive Drug Evaluation) trial.[36]

Clinical trials of lipid-lowering in women (see also Chapter 4)

The substantial benefit of pharmacologic lipid-lowering in women has been documented in recently reported clinical trials of both primary and secondary prevention. Over 8000 women have been enrolled in statin trials, almost 5000 of them randomized in the Heart Protection Study.[37] Risk reduction is comparable for both sexes.

However, information is lacking for women in trials of pharmacotherapy designed to raise high-density lipoprotein (HDL) cholesterol and lower triglyceride levels, with both these lipid abnormalities potentially posing a greater problem for women than for men. Opportunities exist to define specifically for women the role of niacin, fibrates, and other newly identified categories of drugs advocated to alter these lipid components, including newer PPAR (peroxi-somel proliferator-activated receptor) activators and CETP (cholestryl ester transport protein) inhibitors.

Data are also not available for women on the effects of dietary supplements such as soluble fiber, soy protein, or plant sterol or stanol esters designed to lower levels of low-density lipoprotein (LDL) cholesterol.

Of interest is the Women's Healthy Lifestyle Project,[38] a 5-year randomized controlled trial of diet and exercise designed to explore whether these interventions could prevent both the weight gain and the increase in LDL cholesterol occurring in the menopausal transition. Benefit was evident at 18 months among the 489 participants in weight, body mass index, total cholesterol, LDL cholesterol, systolic blood pressure, and glucose levels. At 18 months, 80% of the intervention women as compared with 45% of the control group were without weight gain.

Additional cardiovascular clinical research studies

In patients without heart failure or ventricular dysfunction at high risk of cardiovascular events, the ACE inhibitor ramipril decreased the composite endpoint of MI, stroke or cardiovascular death by 22%.[39] Beneficial effect was similar in the Heart Outcomes Prevention Evaluation (HOPE) study women (27% of participants) and men.[40]

The Women's Health Study is an ongoing randomized controlled trial of aspirin and vitamin E for the primary prevention of CVD involving 28 263 premenopausal women.[41] In a nested case–control study of the 122 women with cardiovascular events, the highest quartile of high sensitivity C-reactive protein (CRP) and the total cholesterol/HDL ratio independently predicted risk. The question is raised as to whether the addition of high sensitivity CRP to lipid-based screening might better identify women at risk for cardiovascular events.

Hypertension (see also Chapter 31)

There is clinical trial evidence of important effects of age and race on hypertension treatment in women. A summary of 11 randomized clinical trials conducted between 1996 and 1998 provided information derived from 23 000 women.[42] The treatment of hypertension decreased both the relative and absolute risks of cardiovascular morbidity and mortality in women older than 55 years of age and in African American women of all ages. White women aged 30–54 years showed no statistically significant benefit or harm from treatment of hypertension; a potential explanation is the better 'usual care' of these women. In younger women the number needed to treat for benefit was four times greater than in an older population of women.

Heart failure (see also Chapter 29)

The sex-based distribution of patients in heart failure trials is presented in Table 42.2; women constituted about 21% of the study participants. This raises concern in that women constitute more than half of all hospitalized patients with heart failure. Equally of concern is the lack of percentage increase of women participants in heart failure trials from 1985 to the present.[43]

Specifically, in clinical trials of beta-blocker therapy of heart failure, women comprised 23% of participants in the Metoprolol Extended-Release Randomized Intervention Trial in Heart Failure (MERIT HF) trial;[44,45] women were the only subgroup for whom mortality benefit was not demonstrated. Nonetheless, when mortality data were pooled from MERIT-HF, Cardiac Insufficiency Bisoprolol Study (CIBIS-II), and Carvedilol Prospective Randomized Cumulative Survival (COPERNICUS), providing a larger number of deaths for analysis, there was comparable survival benefit for women and men.

An overview of ACE inhibitor therapy for heart failure involved 30 randomized clinical trials.[46] Women did not share with men either the decrease in mortality or the decrease in the combined endpoint of mortality and heart failure hospitalization. The question must be raised as to whether women benefit less from ACE inhibitor therapy or whether under-enrollment of women limited the statistical power to ascertain benefit. A more recent meta-analysis that included 12 763 patients, 2396 of them women, in

Table 42.2 Sex-based distribution of patients in heart failure trials

Trial	Year	No. of patients	% Women
CONSENSUS	1987	253	30
Captopril-Dig	1988	300	17
SOLVD (T)	1990	2569	23
SOLVD (P)	1992	4228	11.5
PROMISE	1991	1088	22
RADIANCE	1993	178	24
US Carvedilol	1996	1094	23
DIG	1997	6800	22
CIVIS II	1999	2647	20
MERIT-HF	1999	3991	23
COPERNICUS	2001	2289	20
Total		25437	21.4

three ACE inhibitor trials showed no significant heterogeneity of benefit by sex.[47] A subsequent survival meta-analysis including 11 674 men and 2898 women showed no overall difference in ACE therapy benefit by sex, but only for women with symptomatic left ventricular systolic dysfunction; asymptomatic women did not demonstrate survival benefit.[48]

The initial report of the DIG (Digitalis Investigation Group) trial defined no survival benefit, but a decrease in heart failure hospitalizations, for the total cohort. Analysis of sex-based differences in the response to digitalis identified that the adverse effect on mortality was confined to women.[49]

Opportunities for further exploration of clinical trial data regarding women with heart failure due to left ventricular systolic dysfunction derive from the Randomized Aldactone Evaluation Study (RALES), with a 27% representation of women.[50] To be defined is whether sex differences are present in benefit of aldosterone blockade with spironolactone, as outcomes were not specified for the subgroup of women. Selective aldosterone blockade with eplerenone in patients with heart failure following MI,[51] with 29% of participants women, showed comparable reduction in morbidity and mortality in both sexes.

Examination is warranted of the ventricular systolic dysfunction secondary to anthracycline chemotherapy for breast cancer, a disease and therapy involving predominantly women. These individuals have been excluded from most randomized controlled trials of heart failure therapies owing to both trial design and their limited potential for survival. The question must be raised as to whether the appropriate heart failure therapies are comparable to those for other etiologies of left ventricular systolic dysfunction.[52]

Potential benefits for women may derive from exploring heart failure with intact left ventricular systolic function, i.e. diastolic dysfunction, a problem that predominates in older women, for most of whom hypertension is etiologic. Symptoms of such heart failure impair the quality of life of these women and exacerbations entail an excess of hospitalizations and medical care costs. The optimal pharmacotherapy remains uncertain and delineation of efficacious therapy is likely to improve clinical outcomes of heart failure for women.

Finally, peripartum cardiomyopathy deserves specific examination. Is the therapy comparable to that of other causes of left ventricular systolic dysfunction? Should therapy be continued after systolic function normalizes, based on documentation of impaired contractile reserve in this setting? A national registry for peripartum cardiomyopathy has been proposed, but has not yet been implemented.[52]

The American Heart Association (AHA) evidence-based guidelines for prevention of CVD in women

In 2004 the American Heart Association, with 11 co-participating organizations and 22 other endorsing agencies published evidence-based guidelines for the prevention of cardiovascular disease in women.[53] Reflecting the under-representation of women in clinical trials of cardiovascular prevention, an additional citation to the usual strength of recommendations was included, a generalizability index of the evidence to women. A generalizability index (GI) = 1 means that it is very likely that the results can be generalized to women; GI = 2 indicates that it is somewhat likely that the results can be generalized to women. A designation of 3 indicates that it is unlikely that the results generalize to women and a GI of 0 means that the authors were unable to project whether the results can be generalized to women.

Summary – opportunities to improve women's cardiovascular health

A revised methodology for clinical research is needed. Well designed and implemented cardiovascular clinical research studies must be conducted, both for problems specific to women (single-sex trials) and to insure adequate representation of women in trials of cardiovascular problems common to both sexes. Scientifically rigorous analysis and reporting of sex-specific comparisons are requisite to address the unique cardiovascular health needs of women.

This equity in the research arena should provide a reliable database to guide both clinical decision-making by health professionals and by women and to formulate public health recommendations applicable to women.

References

1. Wizemann TM, Pardue M-L (eds.). *Exploring the Biological Contributions to Human Health. Does Sex Matter?* Committee on Understanding the Biology of Sex and Gender Differences. Board on Health Sciences Policy, Institute of Medicine. Washington, DC: National Academy Press, 2001.
2. Meinert CL, Gilpin AK, Ünalp A, Dawson C. Gender representation in trials. *Control Clin Trials* 2000; **21**:462–75.
3. US General Accounting Office. Report to Congressional Requesters. *Women's Health: Women Sufficiently Represented in New Drug Testing, but FDA Oversight Needs Improvement.* Washington, DC: US General Accounting Office; July 2001. GAO-01–754.

Available at:
http//www.gao.gov/new.items/d01754.pdf [accessed June 7, 2004].

4. Harris DJ, Douglas PS. Enrollment of women in cardiovascular clinical trials funded by the National Heart, Lung, and Blood Institute. *N Engl J Med* 2000; **343**:475–80.

5. National Institutes of Health, US Department of Health and Human Services. *Monitoring Adherence to the NIH Policy on the Inclusion of Women and Minorities as Subjects in Clinical Research: Comprehensive Report (Fiscal Year 1999 & 2000 Tracking Data): Blue Report.* Bethesda, MD: National Institutes of Health, December 2002. Available at: http://www4.od.nih.gov/orwh/bluerpt.pdf [accessed June 7, 2004].

6. Johnson SM, Karvonen CA, Phelps CL, Nader S, Sanborn BM. Assessment of analysis by gender in the Cochrane Reviews as related to treatment of cardiovascular disease. *J Women's Health* 2003; **12**:449–57.

7. Agency for Healthcare Research and Quality. Results of systematic review of research on diagnosis and treatment of coronary heart disease in women. Evidence Report/Technology Assessment Number 80. US Department of Health and Human Services, Public Health Services. AHRQ Pub. No. 03-E035, May 2003.

8. Agency for Healthcare Research and Quality. Diagnosis and treatment of coronary heart disease in women: systematic reviews of evidence on selected topics. Evidence Report/Technology Assessment No. 81. US Department of Health and Human Services, Public Health Services. AHRQ Pub. No. 03-E037, May 2003.

9. Barrett-Connor E, Grady D. Hormone replacement therapy, heart disease, and other considerations. *Annu Rev Public Health* 1998; **19**:55–72.

10. Writing Group for the PEPI Trial. Effects of estrogen or estrogen/progestin regimens on heart disease risk factors in postmenopausal women. The Postmenopausal Estrogen/Progestin Interventions (PEPI) Trial. *JAMA* 1995; **273**:199–208.

11. Wenger NK. Menopausal hormone therapy. Is there evidence for cardiac protection? In: Shaw LJ, Redberg RF (eds). *Contemporary Cardiology: Coronary Disease in Women: Evidence-Based Diagnosis and Treatment.* Totowa, NJ: Humana Press, 2004: 321–48.

12. US Food and Drug Administration. Center for Drug Evaluation and Research. Estrogen and estrogen with progestin therapies for postmenopausal women. Available at www.fda.gov/cder/druginfopage/estrogens_progestins/default.htm [accessed June 7, 2004].

13. Writing Group for the Women's Health Initiative Investigators. Risks and benefits of estrogen plus progestin in healthy postmenopausal women: principal results from the Women's Health Initiative randomized controlled trial. *JAMA* 2002; **288**:321–33.

14. Shumaker SA, Legault C, Rapp SR, et al., for the WHIMS Investigators. Estrogen plus progestin and the incidence of dementia and mild cognitive impairment in postmenopausal women. The Women's Health Initiative Memory Study: a randomized controlled trial. *JAMA* 2003; **289**:2651–62.

15. Rapp SR, Espeland MA, Shumaker SA, et al., for the WHIMS Investigators. Effect of estrogen plus progestin on global cognitive function in postmenopausal women. The Women's Health Initiative Memory Study: a randomized controlled trial. *JAMA* 2003; **289**:2663–72.

16. The Women's Health Initiative Steering Committee. Effects of conjugated equine estrogen in postmenopausal women with hysterectomy. The Women's Health Initiative Randomized Controlled Trial. *JAMA* 2004; **291**:1701–12.

17. Hulley S, Grady D, Bush T, et al., for the Heart and Estrogen/progestin Replacement Study (HERS) Research Group. Randomized trial of estrogen plus progestin for secondary prevention of coronary heart disease in postmenopausal women. *JAMA* 1998; **280**:605–13.

18. Grady D, Herrington D, Bittner V, et al., for the HERS Research Group. Cardiovascular disease outcomes during 6.8 years of hormone therapy. Heart and Estrogen/Progestin Replacement Study Follow-up (HERS II). *JAMA* 2002; **288**:49–57.

19. Viscoli CM, Brass LM, Kernan WN, Sarrel PM, Suissa S, Horwitz RI. A clinical trial of estrogen-replacement therapy after ischemic stroke. *N Engl J Med* 2001; **345**:1243–9.

20. Clarke SC, Kelleher J, Lloyd-Jones H, Slack M, Schofield PM. A study of hormone replacement therapy in postmenopausal women with ischaemic heart disease: the Papworth HRT Atherosclerosis Study. *Int J Obstet Gynaecol* 2002; **109**:1056–62.

21. Waters DD, Alderman EL, Hsia J, et al. Effects of hormone replacement therapy and antioxidant vitamin supplements on coronary atherosclerosis in postmenopausal women. A randomized controlled trial. *JAMA* 2002; **288**:2432–40.

22. Hodis HN, Mack WJ, Azen SP, et al., for the Women's Estrogen-Progestin Lipid-Lowering Hormone Atherosclerosis Regression Trial Research Group. Hormone therapy and the progression of coronary-artery atherosclerosis in postmenopausal women. *N Engl J Med* 2003; **349**:535–45.

23. The ESPRIT Team. Oestrogen therapy for prevention of reinfarction in postmenopausal women: a randomised placebo controlled trial. *Lancet* 2002; **360**:2001–8.

24. Lee PY, Alexander KP, Hammill BG, Pasquali SK, Peterson ED. Representation of elderly persons and women in published randomized trials of acute coronary syndromes. *JAMA* 2001; **286**:708–13.

25. Maggioni AP, Franzosi MG, Santoro E, White H, Van de Werf F, Tognoni G. The risk of stroke in patients with acute myocardial infarction after thrombolytic and antithrombotic treatment. Gruppo Italiano per lo Studio della Sopravvivenza nell'Infarto Miocardico II (GISSI-2), and The International Study Group. *N Engl J Med* 1992; **327**:1–6.

26. Hochman JS, Tamis JE, Thompson TD, et al., for the Global Use of Strategies to Open Occluded Coronary Arteries in Acute Coronary Syndromes IIb Investigators. Sex, clinical presentation, and outcome in patients with acute coronary syndromes. *N Engl J Med* 1999; **341**:226–32.

27. Lagerqvist B, Säfström K, Ståhle E, Wallentin L, Swahn E, FRISC II Study Group Investigators. Is early invasive treatment of unstable coronary artery disease equally effective for both women and men? FRISC II Study Group Investigators. *J Am Coll Cardiol* 2001; **38**:41–8.

28. Fox KAA, Poole-Wilson PA, Henderson RA, et al., for the Randomized Intervention Trial of unstable Angina (RITA) Investigators. Interventional versus conservative treatment for patients with unstable angina or non-ST-elevation myocardial infarction: the British Heart Foundation RITA 3 randomised trial. *Lancet* 2002; **360**:743–51.

29. Cannon CP, Weintraub WS, Demopoulos LA, et al., for the TACTICS-Thrombolysis in Myocardial Infarction 18 Investigators. Comparison of early invasive and conservative strategies in patients with unstable coronary syndromes treated with the glycoprotein IIb/IIIa inhibitor tirofiban. *N Engl J Med* 2001; **344**:1879–87.

30. Säfström K, Swahn E and the FRISC study group. Early symptom-limited exercise test for risk stratification in post menopausal women with unstable coronary artery disease. *Eur Heart J* 2000; **21**:230–8.

31. Haymart MR, Dickfeld T, Nass C, Blumenthal RS. Percutaneous coronary intervention vs. medical therapy: what are the implications for women? *J Women's Health Gender Based Med* 2002; **11**:347–55.

32. Davies RF, Goldberg AD, Forman S, et al., for the ACIP Investigators. Asymptomatic Cardiac Ischemia Pilot (ACIP) study two-year follow-up. Outcomes of patients randomized to initial strategies of medical therapy versus revascularization. *Circulation* 1997; **95**:2037–43.

33. Hueb WA, Bellotti G, de Oliveira SA, et al. The Medicine, Angioplasty or Surgery Study (MASS): a prospective, randomized trial of medical therapy, balloon angioplasty or bypass surgery for single proximal left anterior descending artery stenoses. *J Am Coll Cardiol* 1995; **26**:1600–5.

34. Pitt B, Waters D, Brown WV, et al., for the Atorvastatin versus Revascularization Treatment Investigators. Aggressive lipid-lowering therapy compared with angioplasty in stable coronary artery disease. *N Engl J Med* 1999; **341**:70–6.

35. RITA-2 trial participants. Coronary angioplasty versus medical therapy for angina: the second Randomised Intervention Treatment of Angina (RITA-2) trial. *Lancet* 1997; **350**:461–8.

36. O'Rourke RA, Boone WE, Weintaub WS, Hardigan P. Clinical implications of the Atorvastatin VErsus Revascularization Treatment (AVERT) study. *Curr Pract Med* 1999; **2**:225–7.

37. Heart Protection Study Collaborative Group. MRC/BHF Heart Protection Study of cholesterol lowering with simvastatin in 20,536 high-risk individuals: a randomized placebo-controlled trial. *Lancet* 2002; **360**:7–22.

38. Simkin-Silverman LR, Wing RR, Boraz MA, Meilahn EN, Kuller LH. Maintenance of cardiovascular risk factor changes among middle-aged women in a lifestyle intervention trial. *Womens Health* 1998; **4**:255–71.

39. The Heart Outcomes Prevention Evaluation Study Investigators. Effects of an angiotensin-converting-enzyme inhibitor, ramipril, on cardiovascular events in high-risk patients. *N Engl J Med* 2000; **342**:145–53.

40. Lonn E, Roccaforte R, Yi Q, et al., on behalf of the HOPE Investigators. Effect of long-term therapy with ramipril in high-risk women. *J Am Coll Cardiol* 2002; **40**:693–702.

41. Ridker PM, Hennekens CH, Buring JE, Rifai N. C-reactive protein and other markers of inflammation in the prediction of cardiovascular disease in women. *N Engl J Med* 2000; **342**:836–43.

42. Quan A, Kerlikowske K, Gueyffier F, Boissel J-P, and the INDANA Investigators. Efficacy of treating hypertension in women. *J Gen Intern Med* 1999; **14**:718–29.

43. Heiat A, Gross CP, Krumholz HM. Representation of the elderly, women, and minorities in heart failure clinical trials. *Arch Intern Med* 2002; **162**:1682–8.

44. MERIT-HF Study Group. Effect of metoprolol CR/XL in chronic heart failure: Metoprolol CR/XL

Randomized Intervention Trial in Congestive Heart Failure (MERIT-HF). *Lancet* 1999; **353**:2001–7.

45. Ghali JK, Pina IL, Gottlieb SS, Deedwania PC, Wikstrand JC, on behalf of the MERIT-HF Study Group. Metoprolol CR/XL in female patients with heart failure. Analysis of the experience in Metoprolol Extended-Release Randomized Intervention Trial in Heart Failure (MERIT-HF). *Circulation* 2002; **105**:1585–91.

46. Garg R, Yusuf S. Overview of randomized trials of angiotensin-converting enzyme inhibitors on mortality and morbidity in patients with heart failure. *JAMA* 1995; **273**:1450–6.

47. Flather MD, Yusuf S, Køber L, et al., for the ACE-Inhibitor Myocardial Infarction Collaborative Group. Long-term ACE-inhibitor therapy in patients with heart failure or left-ventricular dysfunction: a systematic overview of data from individual patients. *Lancet* 2000; **355**:1575–81.

48. Shekelle PG, Rich MW, Morton SC, et al. Efficacy of angiotensin-converting enzyme inhibitors and beta-blockers in the management of left ventricular systolic dysfunction according to race, gender, and diabetic status. A meta-analysis of major clinical trials. *J Am Coll Cardiol* 2003; **41**:1529–38.

49. Rathore SS, Wang Y, Krumholz HM. Sex-based differences in the effect of digoxin for the treatment of heart failure. *N Engl J Med* 2002; **347**:1403–11.

50. Pitt B, Zannad F, Remme WJ, et al., for the Randomized Aldactone Evaluation Study Investigators. The effect of spironolactone on morbidity and mortality in patients with severe heart failure. *N Engl J Med* 1999; **341**:709–17.

51. Pitt B, Remme W, Zannad F, et al., for the Eplerenone Post-Acute Myocardial Infarction Heart Failure Efficacy and Survival Study Investigators. Eplerenone, a selective aldosterone blocker, in patients with left ventricular dysfunction after myocardial infarction. *N Engl J Med* 2003; **348**:1309–21.

52. Wenger NK. Women, heart failure, and heart failure therapies. *Circulation* 2002; **105**:1526–8.

53. Mosca L, Appel LJ, Benjamin EJ, et al. Evidence-based guidelines for cardiovascular disease prevention in women. AHA Guidelines. *Circulation* 2004; **109**:672–92.

43

Education of women about cardiovascular health

Sharonne N. Hayes, Dalene Bott-Kitslaar and Tammy F.L. Adams

The case for effective cardiovascular education for women

Educating women about heart disease presents many unique challenges and opportunities. This chapter will discuss these challenges and highlight proven effective and novel educational interventions. Heart disease is the single leading cause of death and a significant cause of morbidity among American women. Although cardiovascular disease (CVD) incidence and mortality have generally declined over the past four decades, survival gains in women have been less impressive than those in men. Risk factors for coronary heart disease (CHD) and heart failure in women are well documented and effective behavioral and pharmacologic interventions that reduce death and disability are well established.[1] Despite this, there are alarming trends in the lack of identification and treatment of cardiovascular risk factors by both patients and their health-care providers.[2,3] After myocardial infarction (MI) or stroke it is estimated that over 40% of women have at least two poorly controlled risk factors, putting them at high risk for a subsequent cardiac event.[2] Many women do not understand the direct correlation between their behavior or the presence of risk factors and their likelihood of developing CVD.[4] Knowledge gaps regarding the signs and symptoms of acute MI and

chronic CHD have also been identified in women.[4] Despite this, few clinical or public health educational interventions have targeted women, and most commonly utilized cardiovascular health interventions have not been adequately evaluated in women.[5]

Once CVD is manifest, the need for effective patient education to manage the condition and prevent disease progression becomes even more critical. Patient and family education and counseling and behavioral intervention, guided by health professionals, is a process intended to improve the patient's and/or family's level of knowledge, skill and attitude to adopt or reinforce healthy behaviors effectively. Chronic illness requires patients to understand not only how, but also why they need to alter their behavior to achieve optimal outcomes. As a result, patient education is designated as an integral component of a number of CVD-specific guidelines.[6,7]

Effective education and communication with women about their risks of heart disease and secondary prevention measures are critically important and are associated with more accurate diagnoses, effective treatment, improved compliance, and satisfaction with both their medical care and their providers. In addition, evidence is mounting that effective learning not only results in implementation of healthy lifestyle behaviors but also improves clinical outcomes.[8–11] For example, in a placebo-controlled, multicenter prevention trial of women and men at high risk for developing type 2 diabetes, patients randomized to a 16-lesson lifestyle intervention program had a 58% reduction in development of type 2 diabetes. Treatment with the antihyperglycemic medication metformin resulted in only a 31% reduction compared with the placebo group.[8]

Unfortunately, while evidence for the efficacy of preventive and therapeutic lifestyle modification continues to grow, the gap between current recommendations for cardiovascular risk reduction and the typical woman's risk profile is also growing, particularly among nonwhite women. Effective patient education is particularly important in today's health-care environment in which women are discharged from the hospital after minimal stays, leading some women to call their events 'drive by' heart attacks. In addition, women often lack the physical and mental capacity to concentrate on learning during a fast-paced hospital admission. Many patient educators have creatively adapted their programs to maintain follow-up and continuity into the outpatient setting, since it is extremely difficult to fully meet inpatient educational needs. Comprehensive outpatient cardiac rehabilitation programs have been shown to be particularly effective in women. Participants experience significant improvements in quality of life, reduced rehospitalization rates, and lower morbidity and mortality associated with CVD.[12-14] Unfortunately, these programs are significantly underutilized, particularly by women, due to lack of referrals, increased dropout rates and unaddressed barriers to participation. Barriers to participation for older women often include transportation issues and lack of social and financial support, while work and family responsibilities present difficulties for younger women. The population of patients who may potentially benefit from cardiac rehabilitative services has become increasingly diverse, challenging programs to fully meet the educational needs of all participants, including women, with little or no incremental resources.

The education of women about heart disease is a wide-ranging topic. It includes not only what has traditionally occurred in the inpatient and outpatient setting provided by health-care providers, but also community and public health messages about cardiovascular risks and prevention, recognition of signs and symptoms, and taking appropriate action

during a cardiovascular emergency. One-on-one educational interventions are not always available, practical, or affordable. With advances in and wider availability of technology, newer patient education media have been developed including the use of individualized risk assessment tools, interactive web-based education, and individual and population-targeted tailored videos.

Patient education is not only clinically effective but has been shown to be a cost-effective intervention for health-care providers. Bartlett et al. found that, on average, 3–4 dollars were saved for every dollar spent on patient education programs.[15] If the financial benefits were not sufficient to justify the need to develop effective patient education for women, in the United States patient education is a requirement for accreditation by the Joint Commission on Accreditation of Healthcare Organizations (JCAHO). Accreditation is required for reimbursement of medical services by Medicare, Medicaid and many nonfederal insurers, and for federal funding of research and graduate medical education programs. The JCAHO patient-focused standards require that patients receive education and training specific to their needs as appropriate to the care, treatment, and services provided.[16] Education should be based on the patient's learning needs, taking into account cultural and religious beliefs, readiness to learn, and physical and cognitive barriers to learning.[16] Some legal experts have interpreted

---

Box 43.1   JCAHO accreditation requirements for patient education programs

- Formal plan of care, treatment, and services
- Basic health practices and safety
- Safe and effective medication use
- Nutrition interventions, modified diets, oral health
- Safe and effective use of medical equipment or supplies (when provided by the organization)
- Pain assessment, risks and importance and methods of effective pain management
- Habilitation or rehabilitation techniques to help patients reach maximum possible independence

JCAHO, Joint Commission on Accreditation of Healthcare Organizations.

these standards to require that health literacy levels of patients be assessed as part of the educational process.[17] The Joint Commission further recommends education in specific areas 'that (are) appropriate to the patient's condition and assessed needs and the organization's scope of services' (Box 43.1). While these topics are clearly within the purview of cardiovascular education for women, and there is compelling evidence for the benefits and necessity of patient education, many factors can interfere with successful implementation.

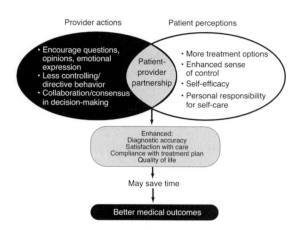

Figure 43.1
Improvement of clinical outcomes via participatory educational experiences.

Gender considerations in cardiovascular education

Various patient populations may require different health messages and modes of delivery of these messages in order to be effective. Women and men have fundamental differences in communication styles and educational preferences in medical settings, such as educator type, educational venue, and group versus individual teaching. For example, when educators lecture or direct recommendations to men, male patients often interrupt the educator or interject their opinions. Women in similar situations tend to sit and listen and are less likely to interrupt or challenge the information. In general, women express more feelings and talk more about relationships with their physicians than men, and they tend to expect certain conversational patterns that encourage interaction. However, many physicians do not provide this encouragement, assuming that patients will speak up if they have an opinion or question. In these situations, some women simply sit, listen, and ask no questions. When providers are faced with a female patient who speaks up or questions them, providers sometimes perceive this behavior as an affront to their authority.

Studies have shown that participatory educational experiences, as opposed to controlling and directive behavior by providers, improve clinical outcomes (Fig. 43.1).[18–21] Women particularly benefit, in terms of better outcomes (diabetes and lipid control, weight loss), from increased 'partnership building' behavior (the provider asks for opinions, concerns) and patient-centered responses (encouragement,

reassurance) by providers and educators.[19] The potential advantage of this partnership building and patient-centered care is that women tend to be more adherent to prescribed recommendations and satisfied with their health care when they are involved in the educational and decision-making process. In addition to women's different educational needs, social, economic, and ethnic differences also demand a more individualized approach if education is to be effective. Learning needs also vary depending upon whether the patient is acutely or chronically ill, or does not perceive herself as ill at all, as is the case of many primary prevention efforts. Receptivity to educational efforts tends to be highest when patients are symptomatic, but very ill women may not be able actively to participate in learning.

Educational theory and practical application

The patient education process is dynamic and needs continual assessment, planning, implementation, and evaluation. The health-care provider's role in educating a patient today is no longer to simply tell her what to do, but rather to first assess and then meet her educational needs. Simply transmitting knowledge, no matter how thoughtfully and competently that information is packaged, is not sufficient to result in behavior change in women with or at risk for heart disease if they do not believe the treatment or behavior change is worthwhile. Cardiovascular education requires establishing a relationship, providing individualized instruction using a variety of interventions, empowering the patient, negotiating, planning steps to action, and goal setting.[22] For a variety of reasons, many physicians shy away from preventive counseling and patient education efforts. They commonly cite time constraints, lack of reimbursement, poor infrastructure and system support, inadequate provider training, and lack of self-efficacy (the belief that one will be successful performing a task) as reasons that they avoid patient education. Although most physicians have received little formal training in counseling behavior changes, these skills can be learned in relatively short, focused sessions. These techniques can be effectively incorporated, in one form or another, in even the busiest practices, particularly if the infrastructure is supportive.[23] The challenge to providers is often the need to deal not only with the most pressing issues (e.g. symptoms, medication side effects) but also to provide education in a cost and time efficient episode of care. Physicians should recognize and seize the educational opportunity that an acute care visit affords. Sick or symptomatic patients are usually far more receptive to preventive advice at these times, and are motivated to make changes to avoid further discomfort or hospitalization.

The conditions for optimal learning are, by nature, multiple. They depend not only on the content of what must be learned and the knowledge patients are able to mobilize, but also on the individual woman's readiness and receptivity to learning and baseline beliefs. Women's attitudes and beliefs about the etiology of their disease, the efficacy of proposed treatment, and their ability to follow recommendations, profoundly affect their willingness to make behavior changes or adhere to pharmacologic therapy. These issues must be addressed before any new information, particularly if it conflicts with her previously held beliefs, can be assimilated. The patient must be able to discern the similarities and differences between already-held beliefs and knowl-

edge and the new information, and then integrate the two and resolve any contradictions. If simple provision of information was all that was necessary to change patient behavior, the vast majority of smokers and obese women would quit smoking, eat less, and exercise more.

Several frameworks are available to explain how adults learn and to enhance health-care providers' skills in educating patients. Adult learning theory[24–26] emphasizes that adults learn in order to solve problems and make decisions. They are most often (and often only) interested in information that they perceive can solve their problems. Adult learning is self-directed and must be defined as relevant by the patient. It draws on previous life experiences, and is influenced by developmental tasks and roles. Learning occurs experimentally, and the application of learning has to occur immediately. An example of this learning theory is the experience of a postoperative coronary artery bypass surgical patient learning proper wound care.

The Stages of Change or Transtheoretical model of learning[27] emphasizes the process of readiness to change and motivation. To be effective, patient education interventions must be appropriate for the patient's current stage of change for that educational topic. Educational interventions appropriate for one stage may not be appropriate for another. For example, cognitive strategies may be used more effectively in the early stages (e.g. education about healthy diet) while behavioral strategies may be more appropriate in the later stages (learning to prepare one meatless meal each week). The behavior change model also helps explain why many patients are aware that they need to make lifestyle changes, but because they are not yet at the action stage, they have not made changes.

The stages of change (precontemplation, contemplation, preparation, action, and maintenance) are not necessarily linear, and regression may occur to earlier stages. Precontemplation occurs when the patient is not yet considering or intending to make a change. She may be unaware of the need to change, may be resistant to change or be overwhelmed. Education interventions at this stage may be aimed at increasing awareness of healthy lifestyles and their benefits. Contemplation occurs when the patient is considering making the change. She may know that she is participating in unhealthy behaviors but has not yet made plans to change. At this stage, the patient may feel that the barriers to change are greater than the benefits. To progress to the next stage women must perceive that the benefits of a behavioral change outweigh the cost (time, inconvenience, etc.). During this stage they often cite time constraints or objection by their family as reasons not to implement healthy lifestyle behaviors. Suggesting that modeling healthy behaviors will improve their family's health, or that investing time in improving their own health will make them better able to care for their families, can be motivating. Educational interventions at this stage may be aimed at promoting the benefits of change and overcoming perceived barriers. During the preparation stage, patients identify the specific steps required to make the desired change, start making small changes, and resolve potential barriers. Educational interventions may be aimed at developing an action plan and encouraging the patient's belief that she can succeed (increasing perceived self-efficacy). When the patient is ready to change, has mechanisms in place to support the lifestyle change, and is actively making changes, she is in the action stage. As she makes changes she can expect periods of relapse into previous behavior. In the maintenance stage the patient has adopted the change as part of her lifestyle, and the changes have become routine. At this point, educational interventions should be aimed at sustaining her efforts, preventing relapse, and developing strategies for regaining control if relapse occurs.

The Health Belief model[28] identifies elements that are important in an individual patient's behavior and health-care decisions and is helpful in understanding successes and failures during attempts at behavior change. Motivation to change is influenced by perceptions of susceptibility to and the severity of illness and whether the perceived benefits of treatment are greater than the barriers and costs. Maslow's hierarchy of needs principle[29] states that behavior is motivated by unmet needs. Lower level needs such as air, water, food, sleep, safety, and security, must be met before higher needs can be satisfied. Clearly, adoption of new behaviors will be more challenging if there is no safe place to walk or insufficient funds to purchase healthy food. Application of this model in patient education recognizes the necessity of meeting lower level needs first.

The social learning model[30] is based on self-efficacy, i.e. past experiences in making changes affect the ability to make changes in the future. The patient's confidence that she will be successful affects her ability to change. For example, previous success at smoking cessation, even with an intervening relapse, is associated with an increased probability of success in a subsequent attempt. In other instances, behavior is learned through observing and modeling another individual's behavior. This is driven by the desire to adopt behaviors for which the outcome is valued and is encouraged by the perception that she already is or would like to be similar to the model. Examples of the social learning model are making a serious attempt at smoking cessation after observing the success of a friend or spouse or viewing an educational video of a woman exhibiting healthy behaviors with whom the patient can identify. Effective patient education uses a combination of these models, often in combination with other sound educational principles, to help women adopt attitudes, behaviors and relationships and to support their physical, mental, emotional, and spiritual health.

The patient education process: women's unique needs and barriers to learning

In clinical settings, the patient education process includes five steps: learning needs assessment, planning, implementation, evaluation, and documentation in the medical record. Much of the initial assessment step can and should occur during the typical history and physical examination, augmented by questionnaires and information gathered by other members of the health-care team. The health-care provider establishes rapport with the patient, asks open-ended questions to elicit concerns and beliefs, maintains eye contact and notes any nonverbal communication. Through this process, the health-care provider identifies the 'need-to-know' versus 'nice-to-know' educational topics and determines the patient's readiness to learn, motivation to change, and preferred learning style. The patient's social and occupational background, perceptions of her condition and proposed treatment, and her priorities and motivation for seeking treatment and behavior change must all be assessed. Previous efforts at behavior change and perceptions of past counseling experiences should also be explored. Patient age, personal preferences, available social support, and a number of other factors will affect the approaches taken during education and behavior change.[31]

A critical component of the learning needs assessment is the identification of potential barriers to learning (Box 43.2). Unlike physical barriers, low educational and literacy levels are often not readily apparent, due to inaccurate assumptions by providers and embarrassment on the part of the patient, but are critical to address in order to meet educational needs. According to the National Work Group on Literacy and Health, in the US one in four adults are functionally illiterate, defined as reading at the third grade level or lower.[17] As a group, they have poorer physical and psychological health than those with better reading skills. Individuals who read at this level are unable to read and understand medication directions, and appointment instructions, or to read a consent form. Women from lower socioeconomic groups are over-represented in this group, composed predominantly of older individuals who have not completed a high school education. Although a disproportionate number of patients with low literacy skills belong to minority groups, the largest absolute numbers are white and born in the US. Addressing the educational needs of this group has great potential to reduce health-care costs. Patients with the lowest literacy level average more outpatient visits per year, and have a 52% greater likelihood of hospitalization than those with adequate literacy skills.[32] Nonwritten educational materials in the form of well-designed computer-based programs, videos, and one-on-one sessions are effective methods to increase knowledge and reduce anxiety in patients with low literacy skills.[17]

It is also important to recognize that provider preconceptions regarding educational needs that are based on a woman's educational level, ethnicity, or social class may actually interfere with optimal care and adherence to recommendations. Low socioeconomic status, widowhood, and lack of social support, along

---

Box 43.2 Common barriers to learning

Patient-related
- Physical – impaired vision or hearing, uncontrolled pain
- Cognitive – low health literacy, impaired mental capabilities
- Education
- Language/communication style
- Insufficient financial resources
- Lack of motivation
- Emotional – depression, anxiety
- Access/transportation – rural, safety or cost concerns
- Role constraints
- Lack of support systems – caregiving, social pressures, work demands
- Health and wellness beliefs
- Lifestyle and cultural practices
- Religious beliefs

Health-care provider- and system-related
- Lack of reimbursement
- Time pressure
- Inadequate training or skills
- Lack of self-efficacy
- Belief that patients do not want education
- Expectations of patient noncompliance
- Lack of confidence in the efficacy of education
- Uncertainty about conflicting recommendations
- Lack of system support

---

with low education level are markers for lower levels of participation in health-care decisions and are independent risk factors for development of CHD and poor outcomes. Therefore, less educated women and those in lower socioeconomic classes are doubly disadvantaged, due to their relatively passive communication styles and physician misperceptions of information needs. Explanations and appropriate educational materials tend to be offered to those who need it least (well-educated individuals) and those who need education the most are least likely to receive it.[33,34]

While socioeconomic disparities, non-English speaking, and belonging to an ethnic minority correlate with increased CVD mortality, morbidity, and risk factors,[5] these high-risk women benefit from a variety of educational interventions. While often considered 'hard to reach', when given appropriate tailored information regarding preventive screening recommendations, these women have screening rates that exceed that of the US average.[35] When no educational material exists to address the needs of the target patient population, efforts should be made to develop appropriate materials to meet these educational and cultural needs.

While cultural and language barriers to learning may be obvious, other less readily apparent barriers may be more important for some women. Psychosocial support, alleviation of psychosocial stress, and diagnosing and treating depression and anxiety can be critical to the success of educational efforts, particularly in women who have heart disease.[36] Women adjust to the diagnosis of CHD more poorly than men, with higher anxiety and depression scores, and more pain and sleep disturbances. These factors are associated with worse outcomes and increased hospitalizations. Gender differences in perceptions of illness and recovery have also been identified. Failure to address these issues and acknowledge women's 'other' priorities, such as her perceived and real responsibilities to her family, can lead to significant frustration on the part of the patient and educator. Negotiation with the patient and family, family education, and additional resources may be necessary to be successful.

Another potential barrier to learning for women is age. The stage of life in which women experience their peak incidence of CVD is delayed as compared with men. This can lead to additional challenges, such as more frequent co-morbid conditions and mobility concerns, when counseling about therapeutic lifestyle modifications. However, it should not be assumed that older patients are resistant to or incapable of lifestyle change. In diabetic patients who received intensive therapeutic lifestyle modification interventions the oldest patients experienced the most dramatic improvements in diabetes control.[37]

Once barriers and learning needs have been assessed, the next step of the patient education process is the development of the educational intervention plan in collaboration with the patient and her family. During this process, mutually agreed upon, realistic goals should be set. Identification of appropriate patient education materials that support the intended messages and determination of who should deliver the education occurs at this stage. This is followed by implementation of the planned educational interven-

tions. Some women may be best served by referral to another health-care provider, community resource or interactive media. Educating patients on behavioral change is time-consuming and time constraints are cited as the most common reason physicians are unable to communicate important information to patients. Collaboration with other providers such as nurses, dietitians, exercise specialists, and nicotine dependence counselors can be valuable resources for education and assessing patient progress. Most of these professionals, unlike physicians, have had formal training in patient education techniques.

After implementation of the educational plan, effectiveness of the intervention is evaluated and the process is documented. Evaluation, whether by follow-up visits, non-face-to-face contact, or by assessment of therapeutic endpoints (lipids, weight loss, blood pressure control), leads to reassessment and development of a follow-up plan for additional educational interventions. Documentation of the educational process in the medical record is important to provide communication between health-care providers, allow reassessment of learning needs at subsequent patient visits, and to satisfy the legal, medical services reimbursement, and accreditation requirements of health-care organizations.[25,26]

Individual education for women in the outpatient setting: practical applications and 'what works'

Health-care providers are no longer viewed as paternalistic figures, dispensing advice regarding treatment in a unilateral fashion. Patient education enables patients to participate knowledgeably in a mutual decision-making process with their health-care providers to help choose treatment options and give informed consent. Patient education also enhances the ability to comply with the plan of care prescribed by the health-care provider. Office visits can be intimidating to many women, and allowing a woman to have an active role in her care removes, or at least decreases, the likelihood of intimidation.[10] Women in particular have become more consumer savvy, playing a more active role in their care. This promotes ownership and empowerment in the decision-making process and sets up a nonthreatening environment by placing provider and patient on level ground. In addition, for cardiovascular education to be effective, it must take place in the broad variety of settings in which women seek care.[38] During their reproductive years, and often well beyond, women receive their health care predominantly through obstetrician-gynecologists, family planning clinics, family practitioners, and other generalists. Developing appropriate educational practices in these diverse clinical settings to provide for cardiovascular risk reduction interventions will ultimately be necessary to reach the majority of women.

Empowering women in the educational process begins with the first provider–patient interaction. Starting the visit by asking patients open-ended questions such as 'Tell me what brings you here?' or 'What can I do for you?' allows the patient to take charge of the visit. It also validates that the provider is truly interested in what the patient has to say. This also quickly clarifies for the provider the woman's perception of the primary focus of the visit. Throughout the patient visit, using good interview techniques such as active listening and motivational interviewing is important. Motivational interviewing is a framework developed by Miller and Rollnick[39] that facilitates a patient's awareness that behavioral change is necessary or desirable. It is based on the premise that the health-care provider's role is to assist patients in identifying at-risk behaviors and helping them move toward healthier behaviors, thereby improving their health. This typically occurs in two stages, first by developing rapport with the patient and second, by facilitating movement through problem-solving and behavior change.[10,39] Through motivational interviewing the provider assists the patient to see that she is empowered and has a sense of control over the educational process and utilizes facilitated problem-solving techniques to help the patient implement change. Providers must be skilled in using open-ended questions, which encourage patients to elaborate, rather than using closed questions, which generally elicit yes or no responses.[39,40] This process of 'assisted' or 'facilitated' education and self-management appears to be even more appealing and effective for women than for men (Box 43.3).

One of the first steps in effecting behavioral change is to guide the patient to a 'self-awareness' of her risk factor or undesirable behavior. Physicians often make inappropriate assumptions regarding their patient's level of awareness about 'obvious' unhealthy behaviors such as smoking or obesity, and do not feel obligated or inclined to offer education or support. They perceive that they may antagonize the patient if they address these issues. To the contrary, such interventions in smokers are actually associated with higher satisfaction levels, even if they express no interest in quitting at the time of the visit.[41] Focusing on one behavioral change that targets one risk factor, as opposed to multiple interventions may offer women a more focused, intense strategy for behavior change, increasing success rates.[5] This can be facilitated by 'self-monitoring' and ultimately, 'self-management'. To facilitate this, patients should be asked to record a specific behavior over a determined period of time. For example, a journal or diary of the timing and quantity of food intake, activity level, and stimuli that

---

Box 43.3 Principles and practice of motivational interviewing

1. *Express empathy* – A patient-centered approach where the interviewer accepts and understands the patient's perspective. This builds rapport and increases patient's self-esteem which promotes change.

2. *Develop discrepancy* – Create and increase patient's awareness of current behaviors and their conflict with long-term goals, beliefs, and values. Assist the patient to recognize the importance and need for change.

3. *Roll with resistance* – Avoid arguing, which is counterproductive. Reframe resistance to create momentum for change. Through reframing, the patient is presented with new information and perspectives and can be directed to develop solutions to facilitate change. Reluctance and ambivalence are normal and to be expected, but resistance that persists should signal the need for a different approach.

4. *Support self-efficacy* – A patient's belief that they can successfully implement change is a key element to achieving their goal. It is enhanced by the provider's assertion and belief in the patient's ability to make desired changes.

Adapted from reference 39.

provoke overeating can set the stage for setting goals for change.[42] Technologically aware women also have the option of using their personal digital assistant or computer to log their exercise or dietary intake of calories, fat, or salt. The convenience and novelty of this approach may be attractive to some women. These quantitative and qualitative recording activities allow patients to identify problem areas themselves and gives the provider accurate and objective information that can be used to make recommendations and set realistic and individualized goals. Goal setting with a patient must be more detailed and specific than simply telling her to 'exercise more'. Focusing on small steps or improvements, such as encouraging a nonthreatening goal of 10-minute daily exercise sessions in a woman who is completely sedentary, can be helpful in promoting success. Using quantitative and concrete tools, such as pedometers, can be motivating and is an excellent method to determine the patient's baseline activity level and set goals for small positive incremental changes[43] and provides an objective method of tracking progress toward her goal. An important component of successful behavioral change is an advance discussion regarding expected setbacks and disappointments and to have a plan in place to deal with them. These temporary lapses are normal and should not discourage continued pursuit of goals.

Evidence supports continued follow-up and monitoring of progress by both patient and health educator.[44,45] Arranging follow-up to assess progress toward goals is not only clinically relevant, but can also provide the motivation necessary for the patient to work toward additional or more advanced goals. Follow-up can be managed face-to-face or non-face-to-face, via telephone or e-mail. With more widespread availability of computers and Internet access by both providers and patients, creative means of communication with patients regarding their progress, and provision of ongoing support through the use of interactive secure websites is gaining in popularity. These options are particularly appealing in situations where frequent office visits are inconvenient or impossible. Non-face-to-face care via telephone has been shown to be an effective adjunct to care in managing heart failure and diabetes and is associated with lower morbidity and rates of hospitalization.[46,47] The benefits of these interventions in women with asymptomatic conditions such as hypertension or hyperlipidemia is less well studied but shows promise.

When patients are not successful in meeting goals, providers should avoid labels, such as 'noncompliant'. The focus should be shifted toward viewing the patient's lack of success as the absence of mutual agreement by the provider and patient (concordance) regarding the desired goals. It is more likely that the patient did not feel empowered to carry out the behavioral change or lacked the necessary tools to do so.

Tailored patient information

Women who understand their disease process and have educational support are more successful in implementing behavior changes than those who do not. Targeting the provided information and interventions to an individual's specific needs is recognized as increasingly important, especially in the current mind-numbing environment of 'information overload'. Modifying the provided educational activities and information considering specific needs, patient age, stage of life, educational level, ethnic and socioeconomic status, and motivational stage can improve both outcomes and patient satisfaction.[48–50] Numerous studies have shown the benefit of providing tailored information to women regarding the importance of preventive care such as breast and cervical cancer screening. Tailored information is more effective than nontailored information, especially in higher-risk patient groups, primarily because it has the ability to provide an individually focused message.[35] Gender studies regarding communication support the value that women place on personalized information.

A major source of health information is the Internet. Women seek information from the Internet independently, often using this information to confirm their suspicions or fears about their illness, to clarify information received from their health-care providers and to assist in medical decision-making. Women frequently arrive at their medical appointments with a copy of the results of a recent Internet search, seeking the expert opinion of their provider.

This can be an excellent opportunity to address not only the patient's specific concerns, but also to encourage her continued attempts at self-education and discuss the issue of the quality and reliability of information available on the Internet. Many patients believe much of what they access online and do not realize that no expertise or qualifications are needed to post outdated, misleading, false, and commercial information. Directing patients to quality information, usually found on sites run by well-known medical institutions, universities, professional organizations, and the government, and providing patients with information to assess the reliability of these sources can greatly enhance both the quality of the information received and the patient-provider relationship (see Appendix).

A number of these sites offer individualized, interactive resources such as cardiovascular risk assessment tools; health trackers to monitor blood glucose, blood pressure, cholesterol and exercise; and treatment decision-making tools. By design, these allow patients to assess information they need. The website of the American Heart Association[51] offers several programs designed for, or individualized for, women. Heart Profilers® is a disease-specific program to individualize and profile several cardiac risk factors and conditions. It provides a review of various treatment options, suggestions for optimizing the patient's interactions with health-care providers, and access to medical journal articles and research studies written in lay terms. Choose To Move® is a 12-week online physical activity program designed specifically for women that encourages regular exercise and healthy eating. Simple Solutions® provides periodic e-mail tips for living a heart-healthy lifestyle, including recipes and an online exercise log.

The Internet also provides opportunities to provide education and behavioral change interventions that minimize face-to-face interaction. This can be used to the patient and provider's advantage for women who prefer this option or have no convenient face-to-face educational alternatives and as an adjunct to conventional teaching methods. Internet-based programs have been shown to be effective for several behavioral interventions including smoking cessation and short-term weight loss. The addition of targeted e-mails to a basic Internet program may be even more effective. One study of obese diabetics (90% women) who received e-mail counseling and Internet education showed them to lose twice the weight as those who received Internet interaction alone. Weight loss in the combined approach group was comparable to weight loss associated with individual face-to-face counseling.[52]

The Comprehensive Health Enhancement Support System (CHESS),[53] an Internet-based education and behavioral program, was developed to assist patients coping with chronic health conditions and to promote positive health behaviors. Password-protected modules have been created for patients with heart disease and a number of other conditions. Each module contains resources specific to the disease or condition. These include health-care provider-facilitated online discussion groups, 'ask an expert' and 'frequently asked question' pages, tools for personal journaling, a health tracker, and decision and planning guides that lead to the development of a personal 'action plan'. Additionally, there are patient stories and videos, links to recommended websites, scientific journals, and lay press articles, a consumer guide, and local and national resource directories. While not specifically designed for women, participation in the cardiac disease module has been shown to result in improvements in exercise duration and understanding of heart disease in both women and men.[54] Research suggests that women utilize CHESS at least as much as men do, and that it is effective over a broad range of age and educational levels. Low-income individuals and minorities are as likely to use the tool as more affluent patients and nonminorities, but tend to use different services. For example, minorities tend to access the information-gathering services and health trackers more and the communication and discussion services (e.g. chat rooms) less.[53]

Technology offers the opportunity to develop unlimited tailored patient education messages. Additionally, computerized tailored patient information, incorporated into a unified electronic medical record, allows the measurement of patient outcomes associated with behavior modification. One such example is the Women's Cardiovascular Risk Assessment Tool used by the Mayo Clinic Women's Heart Clinic. It was developed to provide women with a detailed, personalized report of their cardiovascular and women's health risks. The risk assessment consists of 85 pen-and-paper questions that are scanned into a computer program where a complex set of algorithms and messages generate information specifically tailored to the patient-provided responses. Each woman receives a 10–15 page report outlining her risks of CVD and other selected health problems and specific advice for risk modification.

Tailored 'coaching' by health-care personnel with mailed prompts and a limited number of periodic scheduled telephone calls has also been shown to be effective in improving compliance with dietary and exercise recommendations in both women and men with heart disease.[45] In a multicenter trial, despite the lack of prescription of medication by the coaches, the information provided by them about target risk factor levels and advice to seek physician follow-up, led to a favorable effect on blood pressure, weight loss, dietary fat intake, anxiety levels, symptoms, and perception of general health and mood. There was a 21% reduction in total cholesterol levels in the coached group compared with a 7% reduction in the usual care group.[45]

Patient education videos can also deliver tailored patient education to women by modeling specific behaviors in a gender and culturally sensitive manner. They are effective vehicles to demonstrate desired attitudes and behaviors, increase knowledge, aid in decision-making regarding treatment options, and to reduce pre-procedure anxiety. The knowledge gained from videos has been associated with increased patient involvement in the medical decision-making process, which can be particularly valuable in meeting the needs of non-English-speaking women and low literacy learners.[55] The take-home video format provides consistent educational messages and allows the patient to determine the time and place to view the video. The convenience of this format encourages multiple viewings and sharing of the video with the family.

The role of cardiac rehabilitation (see also Chapter 21)

Prior to the mid-1960s, patients who experienced a MI were essentially 'put to bed' for 6–8 weeks with only cautious recommendations for gradual progression to limited exercise, a practice that undoubtedly contributed to significant excess morbidity and mortality. Early cardiac rehabilitation programs focused primarily on exercise with an emphasis on physical rehabilitation and return to work. The efficacy of exercise training and cardiovascular risk reduction obtained through these early cardiac rehabilitation programs resulted in decreased mortality and improved quality of life for both female and male cardiac patients.[56] Subsequent programs encompassing a more comprehensive, multifaceted and multidisciplinary approach to cardiovascular risk reduction, including psychosocial interventions, have been associated with a further reduction in recurrent coronary event rates as well as slowing of progression of atherosclerosis.[57,58] Cardiovascular rehabilitation programs provide an opportunity for ongoing patient education with measurable outcomes related to behavioral changes for both primary and secondary prevention of cardiovascular risks. Rehabilitation programs utilize various teaching and learning modalities requiring active participation to optimize cardiovascular outcomes. Recommended core components of a comprehensive program include baseline patient assessment, nutritional counseling, risk factor management (lipids, hypertension, weight, diabetes, and smoking), psychosocial management, physical activity counseling, and exercise training.[7,59]

The highest risk patients have been shown to derive the greatest benefits from cardiac rehabilitation in terms of relative risk reduction. Women and the elderly particularly benefit from these interventions[60] but are the least likely to enter or complete a rehabilitation program. Only about 15% of eligible women compared with 25% of men participate in cardiac rehabilitation.[61] The lack of participation by women is not entirely understood, but a number of barriers have been identified. Physicians are less likely to refer women and the elderly to cardiac rehabilitation,[14] perhaps due to the lack of knowledge that rehabilitation programs are equally, if not more, efficacious in women.[60,62] The lack of physician referral is likely a significant factor in women's under-representation in cardiac rehabilitation programs, since one of the major predictors of participation is the strength of the physician's recommendation.[61] The fact that women are typically older and have more co-morbidities than men when they first experience a cardiovascular event also contributes to lower enrollment and follow-through with a rehabilitation program. More women than men with heart disease are widowed, lack social and financial support, and are unable to drive. Younger women may experience difficulty due to family and work responsibilities and the lack of identification with the other, mostly male, participants. Adherence with cardiac rehabilitation programs is also lower in women. Although adherence is associated with improved outcomes, women are more likely than men to drop out of rehabilitation, especially in the first 3–6 months.[63]

One likely factor in women's lower participation and adherence rates is that they have documented different, and often unmet, needs and expectations from their rehabilitation programs. Some women find women-only exercise sessions and small group teaching preferable to mixed-sex exercise sessions and one-on-one teaching. Moore[64] interviewed participants who had completed a cardiac rehabilitation program to assess preferences. Women preferred more emphasis on psychosocial support and stressed that it was important for the staff to be sensitive to their emotional needs and empathize with their life crises. They valued the support and comfort of knowing that they were closely monitored but disliked frequent weight checks. They preferred a variety of exercise options including stationary bicycles and treadmills, but did not want to experience pain or leave feeling exhausted. They also perceived that men received preferential treatment for exercise times.

Cardiovascular rehabilitation programs benefit women and are a vital part of educating and promoting behavioral change to reduce cardiovascular risks. To maximize participation, adherence and benefit, physicians must emphasize to all eligible patients, especially women, the importance of these programs to their overall health and recovery and address individual learning needs. Involvement by family members in these discussions, screening for and treating depression and anxiety, and identifying other barriers to participation is critical.

Community and large-scale education and behavioral interventions

Population-based interventions have been used to raise awareness about heart disease risks, promote healthy behaviors and educate the public about symptoms and appropriate action to take during a cardiovascular emergency.[65–70] These range from large-scale international, national, and community-wide campaigns, to more limited or targeted programs based in work sites, places of worship, or educational institutions. Most community-wide interventions use a combination of mass media campaigns, along with more individualized approaches that may include incentives, self-help groups, screening, feedback, and targeted educational materials. Many of these programs also incorporate environmental (safe routes to school, walking trails) or policy (smoke-free restaurants, healthy school lunches) interventions into their plan to improve outcomes.[71] With few exceptions, these interventions have not specifically or separately targeted women, and due to lack of gender-specific data analysis and reporting, outcome data in women are quite limited.[5,38]

When developing these programs, creative strategies are often required to reach ethnically diverse populations and those with limited resources. Care must be taken to assure that the health interventions are consistent with the shared beliefs, values, and practices of the target population. Nutritional information, for example, should focus on foods and cooking methods already used by that ethnic group. Women's preferred source of health information must also be considered. Low income and minority women get most of their health information from medical sources, television and radio, and personal contacts, while print and Internet sources rank higher among higher socioeconomic and white women.[4,8,72] Other studies have suggested that selecting case managers who are of the same ethnic group as the participant may enhance the effectiveness of behavioral interventions.[8]

Several effective programs have been developed that provide culturally appropriate interventions and educational materials to improve health behaviors in populations of women with common cultural backgrounds and a high or increasing prevalence of risk factors. Women, particularly African Americans and Hispanics, often value and participate in church experiences and may be attracted to health promotion programs in places of worship that encompass the inter-relationship of spiritual, mental, and physical health. Church-based health promotion programs have successfully targeted mid-life women to promote physical activity, weight loss, and other healthy behaviors.[73,74] Many of these initiatives have been associated with high levels of compliance due to the social and faith-based support that accompanies these programs. Other health interventions have been found more effective in women than men. For example, Hispanic women exposed to Spanish language smoking cessation messages during a community-wide intervention were more likely than men to recall and act on the information.[75]

Another example of a successful initiative is 'Heart Disease on the Mend', a multifactorial risk reduction program that utilized a case management approach in a largely non-English-speaking, culturally diverse (Hispanics, Asians, blacks, and whites), predominantly female group of individuals at high risk for CVD. Physicians, nurses, and nutritionists counseled patients on smoking cessation, nutrition, physical activity, weight loss, and stress management. There were significant improvements in lipid profiles, blood pressure, fasting glucose, physical activity, and nutrition scores in the intervention group compared with usual care.[76]

A major challenge to public educational efforts for women has been the historical lack of recognition by women and their physicians that heart disease is a significant health threat to women. Only 13% of women cited heart disease as their greatest health threat in a 2003 American Heart Association-sponsored survey.[4] While this was a significant improvement over the 2000 survey,[77] the majority of women still believed that cancer, specifically breast cancer, was a more significant personal health risk. Interestingly, almost half (46%) of surveyed women correctly identified heart disease as the leading cause of death in women. The fact that an individual woman's assessment of her own cardiovascular risk is in contrast with her awareness of the population risk suggests that women do not 'personalize' their knowledge about heart disease. As a result, they are often less likely to make preventing heart disease a personal priority or recognize early warning signs.

In response to this documented lack of knowledge and awareness, the National Heart, Lung and Blood Institute (NHLBI) and numerous partner organizations developed the 'Heart Truth' campaign.[78] This wide-ranging awareness and educational program is aimed at women aged 40–60 years, when a woman's risk of heart disease starts to rise more steeply. Key messages of the Heart Truth campaign are that heart disease can develop in anyone, not just men and the elderly, and that heart disease is largely preventable. The campaign is a departure from 'business as usual' for the NHLBI, that began with the early and direct involvement of many partners and stakeholders from the earliest planning stages, and the outsourcing of some aspects of project development to a major public relations firm. The end result is an edgy, personal, campaign with images of all types of women with heart disease, most of whom do not 'look the part'. The goal of the campaign is to encourage women to talk to their health-care providers about risk factors and to take action to control them. The centerpiece of the Heart Truth campaign is the 'Red Dress Project'. It was launched with a collection of red dresses donated by 19 leading fashion designers and a signature 'Red Dress' lapel pin during Fashion Week in New York City in 2003. The tag line, 'Heart disease doesn't care what you wear; it's the number one killer of women' is paired with images of appealing women both with and without heart disease. In addition to involvement by the fashion industry, several magazines with a large female readership have increased their cardiovascular health education content. This has had significant impact since the popular press, and particularly magazines, are an important source of health information for women.[4]

The Heart Truth's message has already reached many more younger women than many prior educational efforts. The depth and breadth of this campaign is certainly one of the most ambitious to date, and it will be important to assess the full impact of the Heart Truth and partner organization efforts. Several Heart Truth partners, including the National Coalition for Women with Heart Disease and the American Heart Association, have been active in engaging their membership and the public and developing parallel educational efforts to reach their own constituencies and reinforce the Heart Truth's core messages. The ultimate success of Heart Truth will be dependent upon engaging health-care providers as partners to reinforce the campaign messages and provide appropriate preventive counseling and screening for risk factors.

Science and Leadership Symposium for Women with Heart Disease

Several novel educational programs have been developed to meet specific needs for education of women with heart disease. One such program is the *Science and Leadership Symposium for Women with Heart Disease*, jointly sponsored by the National Coalition for Women with Heart Disease and Mayo Clinic. The goal of this annual program is to educate a select and diverse group of women with heart disease about heart disease, its risks, diagnosis, and treatment. The curriculum also provides participants with the knowledge, confidence, and skills necessary for public speaking and media interviews so as to educate other women in their home communities. This rigorous 4-day course requires advance preparation, active participation, and post-symposium reading and assessments. The participants, many of whom are under age 50 and come from a variety of socioeconomic and ethnic backgrounds, agree to provide at least 4 hours of community service and education per month upon completion of the course. Women with heart disease often describe feeling isolated or ashamed of their condition and many have never met another woman with heart disease. A crucial component of the symposium is the opportunity to meet and interact with other women with the same cardiac condition and develop supportive relationships that are frequently maintained after the course ends. These relationships are facilitated by providing the graduates with ongoing education, individual problem-solving, communication venues, and regular follow-up by both sponsoring organizations. As a result, symposium participants have been extremely effective in raising awareness and developing educational and support programs in their communities.

Summary

Providing effective education for women about CVD and its risks is critical to the success of any effort to reduce their burden of disease and improve clinical outcomes. While proven techniques and programs are available, their effectiveness in women is often unknown and they are typically grossly underutilized. Targeted interventions that involve women as partners in their treatment and that address gender and cultural needs are most likely to succeed at both the individual and community level. Improving access to and utilization of effective interventions to those individuals most likely to benefit from them will continue to be a challenge. More research is needed to determine the best practices to meet the cardiovascular educational needs of women.

References

1. Mosca L, Appel LJ, Benjamin EJ, et al. Expert Panel/Writing Group. Evidence-based guidelines for cardiovascular disease prevention in women. *Circulation* 2004; **109**:672–92.

2. Qureshi AI, Suri MF, Guterman LR, Hopkins LN. Ineffective secondary prevention in survivors of cardiovascular events in the US population: report from the Third National Health and Nutrition Examination Survey. *Arch Intern Med* 2001; **161**:1621–8.

3. Schrott H, Bittner V, Vittinghoff E, Herrington D, Hulley S. Adherence to National Cholesterol Education Program treatment goals in postmenopausal women with heart disease. *JAMA* 1997; **277**:1281–321.

4. Mosca L, Ferris A, Fabunmi R, Robertson RM. Tracking women's awareness of heart disease. An American Heart Association National Study. *Circulation* 2004; **109**:573–9.

5. Krummel DA, Matson Koffman DM, Bronner Y, et al.

Cardiovascular health interventions in women: what works? *J Womens Health Gend Based Med* 2001; **10**:117–36.

6. Konstam M, Dracup K, Baker D. Heart failure: evaluation and care of patients with left-ventricular systolic dysfunction. Clinical Practices Guideline No. 11. Rockville, MD: Agency for Health Care Policy and Research, Public Health Services, US Department of Health and Human Services, 1994.

7. Wenger N, Froelicher E, Smith L. Cardiac rehabilitation. Clinical Practice Guideline No. 17. Rockville, MD: Department of Health and Human Services, Agency for Health Care Policy and Research and the National Heart, Lung, and Blood Institute, 1995.

8. Diabetes Prevention Program (DPP) Research Group. The Diabetes Prevention Program (DPP): description of lifestyle intervention. *Diabetes Care* 2002; **25**:2165–71.

9. Ketola E, Sipila R, Makela M. Effectiveness of individual lifestyle interventions in reducing cardiovascular disease and risk factors. *Ann Intern Med* 2000; **32**:239–51.

10. Burke L, Fair J. Promoting prevention: skill sets and attributes of healthcare providers who deliver behavioral interventions. *J Cardiovasc Nurs* 2003; **18**:256–66.

11. Lorig K, Sobel D, Stewart A, et al. Evidence suggesting that a chronic disease self-management program can improve health status while reducing hospitalization: a randomized trial. *Med Care* 1999; **37**:5–14.

12. Bock BC, Albrecht AE, Traficante RM, et al. Predictors of exercise adherence following participation in a cardiac rehabilitation program. *Int J Behav Med* 1997; **4**:60–75.

13. Wenger NK, Froelicher ES, Smith LK, et al. Cardiac rehabilitation as secondary prevention. Agency for Health Care Policy and Research and National Heart, Lung, and Blood Institute. *Clin Pract Guidel Quick Ref Guide Clin* 1995: 1–23.

14. Ades PA, Waldmann ML, Polk D, Coflesky J. Referral patterns and exercise response in the rehabilitation of female coronary patients aged greater than or equal to 62 years. *Am J Cardiol* 1992; **69**:1422–5.

15. Bartlett E. Cost-benefit analysis of patient education. *Patient Educ Couns* 1996; **26**:87–91.

16. Joint Commission on Accreditation of Healthcare Organizations. *2004 Automated Hospitals.* Oakbrook Terrace: Joint Commission Resources, Inc., 2004.

17. Communicating with patients who have limited literacy skills: report of the National Work Group on Literacy and Health. *J Fam Pract* 1998; **46**:168–76.

18. Street RL, Piziak V, Carpentier W, et al. Provider-patient communication and metabolic control. *Diabetes Care* 1993; **16**:714–21.

19. Kaplan S, Gandek B, Greenfield S, Rogers W, Ware J. Patient and visit characteristics related to physicians' participatory decision-making style. Results from the Medical Outcomes Study. *Med Care* 1995; **33**:1176–87.

20. Legg England S, Evans J. Patients' choices and perceptions after an invitation to participate in treatment decisions. *Soc Sci Med* 1992; **34**:1217–25.

21. Shulman B. Active patient orientation and outcomes in hypertensive treatment: application of a socio-organizational perspective. *Med Care* 1979; **17**:267–80.

22. Houston Miller N, Hill M, Kottke TE, Ockene I. The multilevel compliance challenge: recommendations for a call to action. *Circulation* 1997; **95**:1085–90.

23. Ockene I, Hebert J, Ockene J, Merriam P, Hurley T, Saperia G. Effect of training and a structured office practice on physician delivered nutrition counseling: the Worcester-Area Trial for Counseling in Hyperlipidemia (WATCH). *Am J Prev Med* 1996; **12**:252–8.

24. Knowles M, Holton E, Swanson R. *The Adult Learner: the Definitive Classic in Adult Education and Human Resource Development.* Woburn: Butterworth-Heinemann, 1998.

25. Rankin S, Stallings KD. *Patient Education Principles & Practice.* Philadelphia: Lippincott Williams, 2001.

26. Klug Redman B. *The Practice of Patient Education.* St. Louis: Mosby, 2001.

27. Prochaska J, DiClemente C. Transtheoretical therapy: toward a more integrative model of change. *Psychother Theory Res Pract* 1982; **19**:276–88.

28. Rosenstock I, Strecher V, Becker M. Social learning theory and the Health Belief Model. *Health Educ Q* 1988; **15**:175–83.

29. Maslow A. *Motivation and Personality.* New York: Harper & Row, 1970.

30. Bandura A. *Social Foundations of Thought and Action: A Social Cognitive Theory.* Englewood Cliffs: Prentice-Hall, 1986.

31. Marcus BH, Forsyth LH. Tailoring interventions to promote physically active lifestyles in women. *Womens Health Issues* 1998; **8**:104–11.

32. Baker DW, Parker RM, Williams MV, Clark WS, Nurss J. The relationship of patient reading ability to self-reported health and use of health services. *Am J Public Health* 1997; **87**:1027–30.

33. Street RL. Information-giving in medical consultations: the influence of patient's communicative styles and personal characteristics. *Soc Sci Med* 1991; **32**:541–8.

34. Pendleton D, Bochner S. The communication of medical information in general practice consultations as a function of patient's social class. *Soc Sci Med* 1980; **14**:669–73.

35. Rimer BM, Lyna P, Glassman B, Yarnall K, Lipkus I, Barber L. The impact of tailored interventions on a community health center population. *Patient Educ Couns* 1999; **37**:125–40.

36. Marcuccio E, Loving N, Bennett SK, Hayes SN. A survey of attitudes and experiences of women with heart disease. *Womens Health Issues* 2003; **13**:23–31.

37. Knowler W, Barrett-Connor E, Fowler S, et al. Reduction in the incidence of type 2 diabetes with lifestyle intervention or metform Diabetes Prevention Program Research Group. *N Engl J Med* 2002; **346**:393–403.

38. Whitlock EP, Williams SB. The primary prevention of heart disease in women through health behavior change promotion in primary care. *Women's Health Issues* 2003; **13**:122–41.

39. Miller WR, Rollnick S. *Motivational Interviewing: Preparing People for Change.* New York: Guilford Press, 2002.

40. Shinitzky H, Kub J. The art of motivating behavior change: the use of motivational interviewing to promote health. *Public Health Nurs* 2001; **18**:178–85.

41. Solberg L, Boyle R, Davidson G, Magnan S, Link Carlson C. Patient satisfaction and discussion of smoking cessation during clinical visits. *Mayo Clin Proc* 2001; **76**:138–43.

42. Serdula MK, Khan LK, Dietz WH. Weight loss counseling revisited. *JAMA* 2003; **289**:1747–50.

43. Tudor-Locke C. Taking steps toward increased physical activity: using pedometers to measure and motivate. Series 3. *Res Digest* 2002; **17**:1–8.

44. Hughes S. The use of non face-to-face communication to enhance preventive strategies. *J Cardiovasc Nurs* 2003; **18**:267–73.

45. Vale MJ, Jelinek MV, Best JD, et al. Coaching patients On Achieving Cardiovascular Health (COACH): a multicenter randomized trial in patients with coronary heart disease. *Arch Intern Med* 2003; **163**:2775–83.

46. West J, Miller N, Parker K, et al. A comprehensive management system for heart failure improves clinical outcomes and reduces medical resource utilization. *Am J Cardiol* 1997; **79**:58–63.

47. Piette J, Weinberger M, Kraemer F, McPhee S. Impact of automated calls with nurse follow-up on diabetes treatment outcomes in a Department of Veterans Affairs Health Care System: a randomized controlled trial. *Diabetes Care* 2001; **24**:202–8.

48. Prochaska J, DiClemente C, Velicer W, Rossi J. Standardized, individualized, interactive, and personalized self help program for smoking cessation. *Health Psychol* 1993; **12**:399–405.

49. Bock B, Marcus B, Pinto BM, Forsyth LH. Maintenance of physical activity following an individualized motivationally tailored intervention. *Ann Behav Med* 2001; **23**:79–87.

50. Strecher V, McEvoy-DeVellis B, Becker MH, Rosenstock IM. The role of self-efficacy in achieving health behavior change. *Health Educ Q* 1990; **13**:73–91.

51. American Heart Association. http://www.american-heart.org/presenter.jhtml?identifier=1200000 [accessed Feb 4, 2004].

52. Tate DF, Jackvony EH, Wing RR. Effects of Internet behavioral counseling on weight loss in adults at risk for type 2 diabetes: a randomized trial. *JAMA* 2003; **289**:1833–6.

53. Gustafson D, Hawkins R, Boberg E, et al. CHESS: 10 years of research and development in consumer health informatics for broad populations, including the underserved. *Int J Med Inform* 2002; **65**:169–77.

54. Gustafson D. Pilot study of CHESS heart disease module. CHESS Completed Studies. CHESS Health Education Consortium. http://chess.chsra.wisc.edu/Chess/Research/Completed%20Studies/research_completed_CHESShdpilot.htm [accessed January 31, 2004].

55. Krouse H. Video modeling to educate patients. *J Adv Nurs* 2001; **33**:748–57.

56. Mullen P, Mains D, Velez R. A meta-analysis of controlled trials of cardiac patient education. *Patient Educ Couns* 1992; **19**:143–62.

57. Haskell W, Alderman E, Fair J, et al. Effects of intensive multiple risk factor reduction on coronary atherosclerosis and clinical cardiac events in men and women with coronary artery disease. The Stanford Coronary Risk Intervention Project (SCRIP). *Circulation* 1994; **89**:975–90.

58. Dusseldorp E, van Elderen T, Maes S, Meulman J, Kraaji V. A meta-analysis of psychosocial programs for coronary heart disease patients. *Health Psychol* 1999; **18**:506–19.

59. Balady G, Ades PA, Comoss P, et al. Core components of cardiac rehabilitation/secondary prevention programs: a statement for healthcare professionals from the American Heart Association and the American Association of Cardiovascular and Pulmonary Rehabilitation Writing Group. *Circulation* 2000; **102**:1069–73.

60. Ades PA, Maloney A, Savage P, Carhart RL Jr. Determinants of physical functioning in coronary

patients: response to cardiac rehabilitation. *Arch Intern Med* 1999; **159**:2357–60.

61. Ades PA, Waldmann ML, McCann WJ, Weaver SO. Predictors of cardiac rehabilitation participation in older coronary patients. *Arch Intern Med* 1992; **152**:1033–5.

62. Cannistra LB, Balady GJ, O'Malley CJ, Weiner DA, Ryan TJ. Comparison of the clinical profile and outcome of women and men in cardiac rehabilitation. *Am J Cardiol* 1992; **69**:1274–9.

63. Oldridge N. Patient compliance. In: Pollock N, Schmidt D (eds). *Heart Disease and Rehabilitation.* Champaign: Human Kinetics, 1995: 393–404.

64. Moore S. Women's view of cardiac rehabilitation programs. *J Cardiopulm Rehab* 1996; **16**:123–9.

65. Luepker R, Murray D, Jacobs D, et al. Community education for cardiovascular disease prevention: risk factor changes in the Minnesota Heart Health Program. *Am J Public Health* 1994; **84**:1383–93.

66. Carleton R, Lasater T, Assaf AR, Feldman H, McKinlay S. The Pawtucket Heart Health Program: community changes in cardiovascular risk factors and projected disease risk. *Am J Public Health* 1995; **85**:777–85.

67. Brownson R, Smith C, Pratt M, et al. Preventing cardiovascular disease through community-based risk reduction: the Bootheel Heart Health Project. *Am J Public Health* 1996; **86**:206–13.

68. Commit Research Group. Community intervention trial for smoking cessation (COMMIT): I: Cohort results from a four-year community intervention. *Am J Public Health* 1995; **85**:183–92.

69. Luepker RV, Raczynski JM, Osganian S, et al. Effect of a community intervention on patient delay and emergency medical service use in acute coronary heart disease: the Rapid Early Action for Coronary Treatment (REACT) Trial. *JAMA* 2000; **284**:60–7.

70. Kottke T, Brekke M, Brekke L, et al. The Cardiovision 2020 baseline community report card. *Mayo Clin Proc* 2000; **75**:1153–9.

71. Task Force on Community Services. Recommendations to increase physical activity in communities. *Am J Prev Med* 2002; **22**:67–72.

72. Benjamin-Garner R, Oakes JM, Meischke H, et al. Sociodemographic differences in exposure to health information. *Ethn Dis* 2002; **12**:124–34.

73. Peterson J, Atwood J, Yates B. Key elements for church-based health promotion programs: outcome-based literature review. *Public Health Nurs* 2002; **19**:401–11.

74. Quinn M, McNabb W. Training lay health educators to conduct a church-based weight loss program for African American women. *Diabetes Educ* 2001; **27**:231–8.

75. Marin G, Perez-Stable E. Effectiveness of disseminating culturally appropriate smoking-cessation information: Programa Latino Para Dejar de Fumar. *J Natl Cancer Inst Monogr* 1995; **18**:155–63.

76. Haskell W, Berra K, Clark A, et al. Heart disease on the mend: a multifactor risk reduction program in the medically underserved. Late-Breaking Clinical Trial Abstracts. *Circulation* 2003; **108**:2723 (abstract).

77. Mosca L, Jones W, King K, Ouyang P, Redberg R, Hill M. Awareness, perception, and knowledge of heart disease risk and prevention among women in the United States. American Heart Association Women's Heart Disease and Stroke Campaign Task Force. *Arch Fam Med* 2000; **9**:506–15.

78. The Heart Truth. A National Awareness Campaign for Women About Heart Disease. http://www.nhlbi.nih.gov/health/hearttruth/index.htm [accessed February 6, 2004].

Appendix
Select annotated patient education Internet resources

www.americanheart.org

The American Heart Association website targets both professional and lay audiences with information on clinical guidelines and cardiovascular statistics and extensive content on many cardiovascular conditions. There are several individualized web-based educational programs, a separate women's heart health section and Spanish language material.

www.bhf.org.uk

The website of the British Heart Foundation (BHF). There is information for professional and lay users and a separate section on women with heart disease.

www.cdc.gov

The Centers for Disease Control and Prevention (CDC) website provides updates and recommendations on current public health concerns, including heart disease. The heart disease section provides detailed information and publications on cardiovascular disease and statistics. Appropriate for both professional and lay audiences.

www.healthfinder.gov

healthfinder® was developed by the US Department of Health and Human Services and several other Federal agencies. It is a key resource for government and nonprofit health and human services information with links to carefully selected information and websites from over 1700 health-related organizations.

http://www.hearttruth.gov

The Heart Truth website supports the National Heart, Lung, and Blood Institute's national awareness campaign for women about heart disease. It has multimedia information for women about heart disease prevention and detection and a rich collection of downloadable fact sheets and slide presentations for use by both lay people and medical professionals. Patient stories and educational materials aimed at Latinas African American women and Spanish speakers are available. There is a 'toolkit' for planning and implementing community education events.

www.mayoclinic.com

MayoClinic.com provides useful, up-to-date information and news about heart disease, a variety of women's health topics and a broad range of other diseases and conditions. Mayo Clinic health experts have developed interactive cardiovascular risk management tools, a health tracker, and links to medical information and news.

www.medlineplus.gov

MEDLINEplus provides reliable health information from the National Library of Medicine for both health professionals and consumers. There are also lists of hospitals and physicians, a medical encyclopedia and dictionary, health information in Spanish, prescription and nonprescription drug information, and links to thousands of clinical trials.

www.nhlbi.org

The National Heart, Lung, and Blood Institute (NHLBI) website provides information to patients, the public, health professionals and researchers about diseases of the heart and blood vessels. Downloadable patient education materials in English, Spanish and several other languages, as well as materials for women with low literacy levels, are excellent.

www.4woman.gov

The National Women's Health Information Center is a free website, sponsored by the US Department of Health and Human Services. There is an extensive list of women's health topics in several languages with material designed for both health professionals and lay audiences.

www.womenheart.org

WomenHeart: The National Coalition for Women with Heart Disease is a national organization founded by women with heart disease and is dedicated to reducing death and disability among women living with heart disease. This website is an excellent patient and provider resource, containing current news and information regarding heart disease, community initiatives, support services for women and an extensive list of links.

Index